Essentials of MANAGEMENT OF NURSING SERVICE AND EDUCATION

Essentials of
MANAGEMENT OF NURSING SERVICE AND EDUCATION

Second Edition

Nisha Clement MSc (OBG) PhD (N)
Associate Professor
Department of Obstetrics and Gynecological Nursing
ESIC College of Nursing
Bengaluru, Karnataka, India

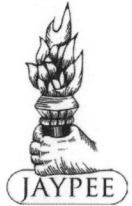

JAYPEE BROTHERS MEDICAL PUBLISHERS
The Health Sciences Publisher
New Delhi | London

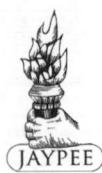 **Jaypee Brothers Medical Publishers (P) Ltd.**

Headquarters
Jaypee Brothers Medical Publishers (P) Ltd
EMCA House
23/23-B, Ansari Road, Daryaganj
New Delhi - 110 002, India
Landline: +91-11-23272143, +91-11-23272703
+91-11-23282021, +91-11-23245672
Email: jaypee@jaypeebrothers.com

Corporate Office
Jaypee Brothers Medical Publishers (P) Ltd
4838/24, Ansari Road, Daryaganj
New Delhi 110 002, India
Phone: +91-11-43574357
Fax: +91-11-43574314
Email: jaypee@jaypeebrothers.com

Overseas Office
J.P. Medical Ltd
83 Victoria Street, London
SW1H 0HW (UK)
Phone: +44 20 3170 8910
Fax: +44 (0)20 3008 6180
Email: info@jpmedpub.com

Website: www.jaypeebrothers.com
Website: www.jaypeedigital.com

© 2022, Jaypee Brothers Medical Publishers

The views and opinions expressed in this book are solely those of the original contributor(s)/author(s) and do not necessarily represent those of editor(s) of the book.

All rights reserved. No part of this publication may be reproduced, stored or transmitted in any form or by any means, electronic, mechanical, photocopying, recording or otherwise, without the prior permission in writing of the publishers.

All brand names and product names used in this book are trade names, service marks, trademarks or registered trademarks of their respective owners. The publisher is not associated with any product or vendor mentioned in this book.

Medical knowledge and practice change constantly. This book is designed to provide accurate, authoritative information about the subject matter in question. However, readers are advised to check the most current information available on procedures included and check information from the manufacturer of each product to be administered, to verify the recommended dose, formula, method and duration of administration, adverse effects and contraindications. It is the responsibility of the practitioner to take all appropriate safety precautions. Neither the publisher nor the author(s)/editor(s) assume any liability for any injury and/or damage to persons or property arising from or related to use of material in this book.

This book is sold on the understanding that the publisher is not engaged in providing professional medical services. If such advice or services are required, the services of a competent medical professional should be sought.

Every effort has been made where necessary to contact holders of copyright to obtain permission to reproduce copyright material. If any have been inadvertently overlooked, the publisher will be pleased to make the necessary arrangements at the first opportunity.

Inquiries for bulk sales may be solicited at: jaypee@jaypeebrothers.com

Essentials of Management of Nursing Service and Education

First Edition: 2016
Second Edition: **2022**
ISBN: 978-93-90595-44-0
Printed at: Sterling Graphics Pvt. Ltd.

Dedicated to

Shri Jitendar P Vij
Group Chairman
M/s Jaypee Brothers Medical Publishers (P) Ltd
New Delhi, India

Preface to the Second Edition

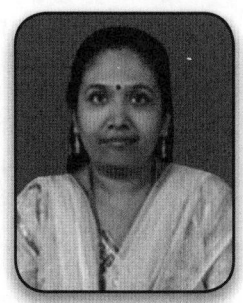

It gives me immense pleasure to draft this second edition *Essentials of Management of Nursing Service and Education*. First of all I would like to thank my Lord Almighty for his blessings that helped me to complete this textbook in time. Strong nurse management helps to encourage nurses to work as units. Strong communication and teamwork are essential for providing quality to patient care and to achieve teamwork. Nurses in management positions should encourage staff members to collaborate and help each other willingly. By learning this subject each nursing student will be able to demonstrate the skills required by the nurse manager to create an effective work environment, understand human resource procedure and processes utilized by nurse leaders and managers. Each nurse will be skilled enough to formulate mission, vision, philosophy and objectives in management process, practise human resource and staff development in management of nursing service in the hospital and community, implement the elements, principles and techniques of material management in hospital service, apply nursing care standards, policies, procedure and practices in hospital management, have better knowledge in concepts, theories and techniques of organizational behavior and human relations, adapt to every ethical, legal responsibility and professional advancements in nursing, demonstrate leadership abilities in professional practice setting and apply leadership and management principles to achieve quality safety outcome. This book has been prepared as per Indian Nursing Council (INC) syllabus. Contents are divided into 25 chapters. Each chapter is written in simple and lucid language, illustrated with simple diagrams, required tables and boxes. It is teacher and student-friendly textbook drafted to the examination point of view, and interestingly exercises are given at the end of each chapter that motivates student to learn furthermore. I am sure that every student who reads this book is sure to get good marks in their examination.

I wish all the best for all the students!

Nisha Clement

Preface to the First Edition

It gives me immense pleasure to introduce this book *Essentials of Management of Nursing Service and Education* to the nursing community. First of all, I would like to thank the Almighty for his wonderful blessings to complete this book. Today's nursing community requires tireless organization and control in order to bring the alignment in provision of quality nursing care. Student nurses should be groomed with leadership and organization capabilities which will help them to gain knowledge in management of clinical/community health nursing services and nursing educational programs. Therefore, in future, they will be able to organize, control, supervise, delegate their responsibilities and operationalize their activities as full-fledged professional nurse. This book will definitely help all nursing fraternity to gain their knowledge in this field. This is suitable for GNM, PB BScN, BScN and MScN, and all nursing teachers can use this as reference material. It is based on the requirement of Indian Nursing Council syllabus, organized in eight sections, simple English is used, illustrated with adequate tables and diagrams, and whole book has 78 chapters. It also has model question papers (five years) that gives better idea to present the content in the examination. Every nursing student who will use the book sincerely will become good leader, manager and excellent nurse educator.

I wish all the best for all readers!

Nisha Clement

Acknowledgments

I am thankful to the Almighty, who strengthens me with his abundant blessings through innumerable means, helping me in all my accomplishments.

I thank my dear parents Mr Babu Jacob and Mrs Kunjumol Babu, for their powerful prayers and blessings that always strengthen my life. I convey my sincere thanks to my beloved sister and brother-in-law Mrs Sheeba Babu and Mr Sathesh. I take this opportunity to thank my little ones, Cibin, Cynthia and Cavin.

I thank my dear husband Dr I Clement, the power force behind me and the man behind the successful release of this book. My heartfelt thanks to Shri Sommana (Former Minister, Government of Karnataka, and Chairman of VSS Group of Institutions, Bengaluru, Karnataka, India) for his constant support and encouragement.

My sincere thanks to my guru BT Basavanthappa (Principal, Rajarajeshwari College of Nursing, Bengaluru) and PV Ramachandran (Chairman, College of Nursing, Sri Ramachandra University, Chennai, Tamil Nadu, India), a great philosopher and an internationally renowned teacher of nursing, who helped me in discovering the world of knowledge.

I am also grateful to Dr Sanjeeva Reddy (Head, Department of Obstetrics and Gynecology, Sri Ramachandra University, Chennai) and Dr OS Ravendran (Professor, Counseling Psychology, Sri Ramachandra University, Chennai).

Special thanks to Dr Jeyaseelan Manickam Devadasan (Dean), Dr Tamilmani (Principal), Professor Mrs Jessie Sudarsanam (Head, Department of Medical Surgical Nursing), and all my teachers and students of Annai JKK Sampoorani Ammal College of Nursing, Namakkal, Tamil Nadu.

My sincere thanks to Shri Jitendar P Vij (Group Chairman), Mr Ankit Vij (Managing Director), Mr MS Mani (Group President), Dr Madhu Choudhary (Publishing Head–Education), Ms Pooja Bhandari (Production Head), Ms Sunita Katla (Executive Assistant to Group Chairman and Publishing Manager), Ms Samina Khan (Executive Assistant to Publishing Head–Education), Mr Rajesh Sharma (Production Coordinator), Ms Seema Dogra (Cover Visualizer), Ms Geeta Rani (Proofreader), Mr Akshay Thakur (Typesetter), Mr Nitin Bhardwaj (Graphic Designer), and staff of Bengaluru Production Unit/Bengaluru Branch of M/s Jaypee Brothers Medical Publishers (P) Ltd, New Delhi.

Contents

Chapter 1: Introduction to Management — 1

- Definitions *1*
- History of Star Wars of Management *2*
- Functional Concept of Management *4*
- Scope of Management *5*
- Nature of Management *6*
- Management as a Science *6*
- Characteristics of Management *7*
- Need of Management *8*
- Differences between Management and Administration *8*
- Levels of Management *9*
- Management Skills *10*
- Managerial Roles *11*

Chapter 2: Principles and Theories of Management — 14

- Management Process *14*
- Elements of Management Process *14*
- Principles of Management *16*
- Scalar Chain *17*
- Theories in Nursing Management *18*
- Scientific Management *18*
- Classic Organization Theories *20*
- Human Relations Theories *21*
- Theories Based on Behavioral Sciences *22*
- Modern Management Theories *24*
- Implications of Management Theories in Nursing *26*

Chapter 3: Functions and Factors of Management — 29

- Elements of Management Process *29*
- Classifications of Management Function *31*
- Functions of Management *31*
- POSDCORB *32*
- Management Needs Resources *32*
- Factors Affecting on Management *32*
- Environmental Factors Affecting Management *33*
- Factors Affecting Financial Management *34*

Chapter 4: Nursing Management and Role of Nurse Manager — 36

- Definition *36*
- Mission Statement of Nursing Management *36*
- Vision of Nursing Management *37*
- Philosophy of Nursing Management *37*
- Goals of Nursing Management *38*
- Nursing Management Roles *39*
- Concept of Nurse Manager *39*
- Qualities of an Effective Manager *39*
- Types of Nurse Managers *40*
- Skills Needed for Nurse Manager *40*
- Functions of Good Nurse Manager *42*
- Characteristics of Successful Manager *42*
- Clinical Responsibilities of Nurse Manager *42*
- General Role of the Manager *44*
- Nurse Manager Job Duties *44*
- Strategical Techniques of Nurse Manager *45*
- Common Problems of Nurse Manager *46*
- Future of Nurse Managers *46*

Chapter 5: Healthcare and Development of Nursing Services in India — 48

- Definitions *48*
- Health System *48*
- History of Healthcare System *49*
- Healthcare Delivery System *50*
- Center Level Healthcare Administration *50*
- The Directorate General of Health Services *52*
- State Level Healthcare Administration *53*
- District Level Healthcare Administration *54*
- Community Level Healthcare Administration *55*
- Healthcare Delivery System in India *56*
- Urban Health Services *56*
- Nursing Services *59*
- Recent Trends and Issues of Nursing Service and Management *60*

Chapter 6: Planning Nursing Services — 63

- Definition *63*
- Meaning of Planning *63*
- Mission Statement of Nursing Service *64*
- Vision Statements *64*
- Nursing Service Philosophy *65*
- Scope of Planning in Nursing Service *65*
- Nursing Service Policies, Procedures and Manuals *65*
- Functional, Operational and Strategic Planning *66*
- Strategic Planning in Nursing *67*
- Operational Planning in Nursing *69*

- Program Planning: Gantt Chart and Milestone Chart 70
- Characteristics of Planning 72
- Importance of Planning 72
- Essentials of Good Planning 73
- Principles of Planning 73
- Steps Involved in Planning 74
- Components of Planning 75
- Factors Affecting Planning 75
- Types/Classifications of Plans 76
- Advantages of Planning 77
- Components of Safety Management Plan 77
- Planning Hospital and Patient Care Unit (Ward) 78
- Planning of Patient Care Unit 79
- Planning for Emergency and Disaster 80
- Triage 84

Chapter 7: Organizing 87

- Definition 87
- Objectives of Organizing 87
- Principles of Organizing 88
- Features of Organizing 88
- Element of Organizing 89
- Functions of Organizing 89
- Importance of Organizing Function 89
- Organizing as a Process—Assignment, Delegation and Coordination 90
- Assignment 90
- Delegation 92
- Coordination 94
- Hospital: Types, Functions and Organization 96
- Organizational Development 99
- Organizational Structure 100
- Organizational Charts 104
- Organizational Effectiveness 105
- Hospital Administration Control and Line of Authority 107
- Concepts of Line of Organization 107
- Line and Staff Organization 108
- Hospital Statistics including Hospital Utilization Indices 109
- Nursing Care Delivery Systems and Trends 111
- Role of Nurse in Maintenance of Effective Organizational Climate 113

Chapter 8: Staffing 117

- Meaning of Staffing 117
- Definition 117
- Objectives of Staffing 118
- Mission and Philosophy of Staffing 118
- Components of Staffing 119
- Factors Affecting Staffing 119
- Functions of Staffing 120
- Staffing Process 120
- Principles of Staffing 121
- Importance of Staffing 122
- Steps Involved in Staffing Process 122
- Patient Classification System 123
- Staff Scheduling 124
- Duty Roster 126
- Staffing Activities in Nursing 128
- Recruitment 130
- Selection 132
- Deployment 133
- Training 133
- Development 135
- Credentialing 137
- Retaining 137
- Promoting 139
- Transfer 141
- Terminating 142
- Superannuation 143
- Norms of Staffing Staff Inspection Unit 145
- Categories of Nursing Personnel Including Job Description of All Levels 146
- Assignment and Nursing Care Responsibilities 154
- Employee Turnover 160
- Employee Absenteeism 161
- Staff Welfare 162
- Employee Discipline 165
- Employee Grievances 169

Chapter 9: In-service Education 172

- Definitions 172
- Purpose, Aims and Objectives 173
- Scope of in-service Education 173
- Need for in-service Program 173
- Importance of in-service Education 174
- Principles of in-service Education 174
- Characteristics of Good in-service Education 174
- Factors Affecting in-service Program 174
- Components of in-service Education 174
- Approaches to in-service Education 175
- Organization of in-service Education 175
- Evaluation Methods Used 178
- Problems Related to in-service Education 179
- Suggestions for Improvement 179
- Nursing in-service Education 179
- Adult Education/Learning 180

Chapter 10: Material Management 186

- Definition 186
- Meaning of Material Management 187
- Purpose of Material Management 187

- Aim of Material Management *187*
- Goals of Material Management *187*
- Scope of Material Management *187*
- Objective of Material Management *188*
- Principles of Purchasing and Material Management *189*
- Material Management Process *189*
- Functions of Materials Management *190*
- Procurement *190*
- Procurement Cycle Steps *191*
- Inventory Management *193*
- Role of Nurse Manager *194*
- Advantages of Material Management *194*
- Role of a Nurse in Material Management *194*
- Inventory Control *195*

Chapter 11: Nursing Audit — 199

- History of Nursing Audit *199*
- Definition *199*
- Meaning of Auditing *200*
- Objectives of Audit *200*
- Objectives of Nursing Audit *200*
- Goals of Nursing Audit *200*
- Characteristics of Audit *200*
- Characteristics of Nursing Audit *200*
- Steps in Audit Process *201*
- Types of Audit *201*
- Methods of Audit *201*
- Principles of Auditing *202*
- Techniques of Auditing/Audit Techniques *202*
- Ethical Principles *203*
- Benefits of Audit *203*
- Nursing Auditor *203*
- Nursing Audit System *204*
- Advantages of Nursing Audit *204*
- Disadvantages of Nursing Audit *204*
- Audit Committee *204*
- Reliability of Audit Evidence *205*
- Procedure for Obtaining Audit Evidence *205*
- Audit Process *206*
- Steps of Audit Cycle *206*
- Nursing as a Total Quality Controls *207*
- Uses of Nursing Audit *208*
- Role and Functions of Nurse Manager for Effective Quality Care *208*

Chapter 12: Directing or Leading — 210

- Definitions *210*
- Meaning of Direction *210*
- Nature of Direction *211*
- Characteristics of Direction *211*
- Principles of Directing *211*
- Elements of Directing *212*
- Functions of Direction *212*
- Importance of Direction *213*
- Techniques of Directing *213*
- Advantages of Direction *214*
- Supervision *214*
- Guidance *218*
- Participatory Management *219*
- Interprofessional Collaboration *222*
- Management by Objectives *224*
- Team Management *228*
- Assignments *230*
- Rotations *232*
- Maintenance of Discipline *233*
- Leadership in Management *235*

Chapter 13: Leadership — 239

- Definition *239*
- Nature of Leadership *239*
- Elements of Leadership *240*
- Characteristics of Leadership *240*
- Principles of Leadership *241*
- Leadership Techniques *241*
- Importance of Leadership *242*
- Leadership Theories *242*
- Qualities of Good Leader *243*
- Difference between Leadership and Management *244*
- Factors Influencing Leadership *244*
- Leadership Styles *245*
- Skills Required in Leadership *248*
- Leadership Competencies *249*
- Situational Leadership Style *249*
- Transformational Leadership Style *251*
- Leadership Development *252*
- Effective Leadership in Nursing *254*
- Qualities of Nurse Leader *254*
- Leadership Styles in Nursing Management *254*
- Mentorship in Nursing *255*
- Preceptorship in Nursing *256*
- Delegation *259*
- Power and Politics *262*
- Politics *263*
- Empowerment *264*
- Mentoring *266*
- Coaching *268*
- Decision-making *269*
- Problem-solving *271*
- Conflict Management *273*
- Negotiation *275*
- Implementing Planned Change *277*

Chapter 14: Controlling — 281

- Definitions *281*
- Features of Controlling Function *281*

- Need of Controlling for Organizations 282
- Elements of an Effective Control System 282
- Process of Controlling 283
- Importance of Controlling 283
- Principles of Controlling 284
- Limitations of Controlling 284
- Traditional Techniques of Control 285
- Sound Control System 286
- Advantages of Controlling 286
- Standards 287
- Policies 290
- Procedures 293
- Protocols 294
- Nursing Performance 295
- Audit 296
- Patient Satisfaction 300
- Nursing Rounds 301
- Documentation—Records and Reports 304

Chapter 15: Total Quality Management 309

- Meaning of Total Quality Management 309
- History of Total Quality Management 309
- Definition 309
- Concept of Total Quality Management 309
- Objectives of Total Quality Management 310
- Principles of Total Quality Management 310
- Phases of Total Quality Management 311
- Elements of Total Quality Management 311
- Components of Total Quality Management 312
- Total Quality Management Tools 313
- Functions of Total Quality Management 314
- Quality Assurance 314
- Quality and Safety 321
- Program Evaluation and Review Technique 324
- Benchmarking 326
- Activity Plan (Gantt Chart) 330
- Critical Path Analysis 331

Chapter 16: Organizational Behavior and Human Relations 334

- Definition 334
- Objectives of Organizational Behavior 335
- Meaning of Organizational Behavior 335
- Nature of Organizational Behavior 335
- Characteristics of Organizational Behavior 336
- Elements of Organizational Behavior 336
- Levels of Organizational Behavior 337
- Principles of Organizational Behavior 337
- Factors Influence Organizational Behavior 337
- Organizational Behavior Model 338
- Approaches to Organizational Behavior 338
- Scope of the Organizational Behavior 339
- Importance of Organizational Behavior 339
- Limitations of Organizational Behavior 339
- Group Dynamics 339
- Review: Interpersonal Relationship 342
- Human Relations 348
- Public Relations in the Context of Nursing 354
- Relations with Professional Associations and Employee Unions 361
- Collective Bargaining 365
- Motivation 372
- Morale Building 377
- Communication in the Workplace 380
- Assertive Communication 384
- Committees—Importance in the Organization, Functioning 385

Chapter 17: Financial Management 390

- Financial Management 390
- Financial Planning 393
- Strategic Financial Management 395
- Budget 396
- Proposal, Projecting Requirement for Staff, Equipment and Supplies for: Hospital and Patient Care Units and Emergency and Disaster Units 404
- Budget Audit 405
- Cost-Benefit Analysis 407

Chapter 18: Nursing Informatics/Information Management 410

- History of Health Informatics 410
- History of Nursing Informatics 411
- Definition 411
- Meaning of Nursing Informatics 411
- Concept of Nursing Informatics 411
- General Purposes Nursing Informatics 412
- Scope of Nursing Informatics 412
- Application of Nursing Informatics 413
- Nursing Informatics Areas 414
- Importance of Nursing Informatics 415
- Nursing Informatics Inpatient Care 415
- Nursing Informatics Model 416
- Competencies of Nursing Informatics 416
- Nursing Career in Informatics 417
- Duties of Nurse in Informatics 418
- Benefits of Computer Automation in Healthcare 418
- Legal Issues in Nursing Informatics 418
- Current Trends and Issues 419
- Patient Records 419
- Nursing Records 421
- Use of Computers in Hospital, College and Community 425

- Use of Computers in Hospital *426*
- Computers in Nursing *427*
- Computers Application in Healthcare *429*
- Telemedicine *429*
- Telenursing *433*
- Electronic Medical Records *436*
- Electronic Health Records *438*

Chapter 19: Personnel Management—Review 442

- Definition *442*
- Meaning of Personal Management *442*
- Objectives of Personnel Management *443*
- Nature of Personnel Management *443*
- Characteristics of Personnel Management *443*
- Elements of Personnel Management *444*
- Scope of Personnel Management *444*
- Role of Personnel Manager *444*
- Functions of Personnel Management *444*
- Roles of a Personnel Manager *448*
- Emotional Intelligence *449*
- Resilience Building *451*
- Stress Management *454*
- Time Management *456*
- Career Planning *458*

Chapter 20: Establishment of Nursing Educational Institutions 462

- Aims of Nursing Education *462*
- Nursing Programs in India *463*
- Coordination with Regulatory and Affiliating Bodies *466*
- Organization of ANM Program *471*
- Organization of GNM Program *474*
- Organization of Basic-Bachelor of Science in Nursing Program *480*
- Clinical Facilities *485*
- Organization of PBBSc(N) Program *486*
- Organization of MSc(N) Program *487*
- Master of Philosophy Program in Nursing *490*
- Doctorate of Philosophy in Nursing (PhD in Nursing) *490*
- Accreditation of Nursing Educational Institutions *491*
- Inspections of Nursing Colleges *493*
- Staffing in College of Nursing *493*

Chapter 21: Planning and Organizing Educational Institutions 499

- Philosophy, Objectives and Mission of The Nursing College *499*
- Curriculum Planning *500*
- Factors Affecting Curriculum Development *502*
- Planning Teaching and Learning Experiences *507*
- Organizing Clinical Facilities for Nursing Students *510*
- Master Rotation Plan *511*
- Clinical Rotation Plan *512*
- Budget Planning for College of Nursing *514*
- Budget Audit *517*
- Records and Reports for Students, Staff, Faculty and Administrative *517*
- Committees and Functioning *520*

Chapter 22: Staffing and Student Selection 526

- Performance Appraisal *526*
- Staff Welfare *537*

Chapter 23: Directing and Controlling 542

- Guidance and Counseling *542*
- Quality Management in Nursing Institutions *549*
- Educational Audit in Nursing Education *550*
- Program Evaluation in Nursing Course *552*
- Evaluation of Performance in Nursing Education *553*
- Maintaining Discipline in Nursing Colleges *554*

Chapter 24: Professional Considerations 557

- Nursing as a Profession *557*
- Ethical Issues in Nursing *563*
- Code of Ethics and Professional Conduct *567*
- Legal Issues in Nursing *571*
- Expanded Role of the Nurse *580*

Chapter 25: Professional Advancement 584

- Continuing Education in Nursing *584*
- Career Opportunities in Nursing *588*
- Professional Organization Membership *604*
- Research Activities in Nursing *608*
- Publications in Nursing *611*

Index *617*

CHAPTER 1

Introduction to Management

LEARNING OBJECTIVES

- History of Star Wars of Management
- Concept of Management
- Scope of Management
- Nature of Management
- Management as a Science
- Characteristics of Management
- Need of Management
- Differences between Management and Administration
- Levels of Management
- Management Skills
- Managerial Roles

■ INTRODUCTION

Management is often included as a factor of production along with, machines, materials and money. According to the management guru Peter, Drucker (1909-2005), the basic task of management includes both marketing and innovation. Practice of modern management originates from the 16th century study of low-efficiency and failures of certain enterprise, conducted by the English statesman Sir Thomas More (1478–1535). Management consists of the interlocking functions of creating corporate policy and organizing, planning, controlling and directing organizations resources in order to achieve the objectives of that policy.

Management can be defined as art and skill of getting things done through others is called management. More elaboration is given by George R Terry. According to **Terry** "Management is the distinct process consisting of planning, organizing, activating, and controlling activities performed to determine and accomplishes the objectives by the use of people and resources."

Figure 1.1 shows concept of management.

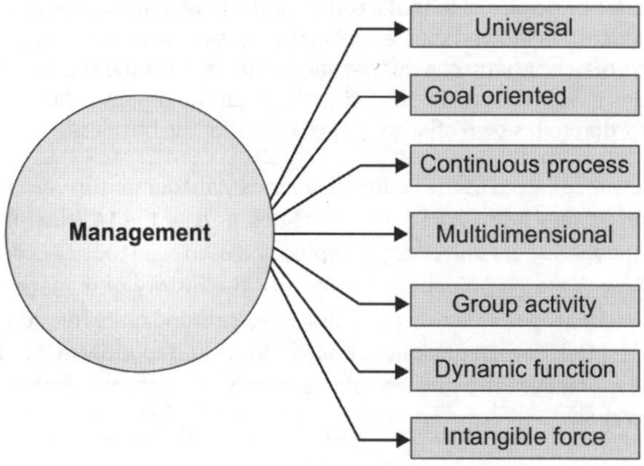

Fig 1.1: Concept of management.

■ DEFINITIONS (BOX 1.1)

- "Management is an art of knowing what is to be done and seeing that it is done in the best possible manner." (Planning and controlling). —*FW Taylor* (Father of Scientific Management)
- "Management is to forecast, to plan, to organize, to command, to coordinate and control activities of others." —*Henry Fayol* (Father of Modern Management)
- "Management is the process by which co-operative group directs actions towards common goals." —*Joseph Massie*
- "Management is that process by which managers create, direct, maintain and operate purposive organization through systematic, coordinated and cooperative human efforts." —*McFarland*
- "Management is the coordination of all resources through the process of planning, organizing, directing and controlling in order to attain stated goals." —*Henry Sisk*

Box 1.1: Definition of management.

- Management is the coordination of all resources through the process of planning, organizing, directing, and controlling in order to attain stated objectives.
- Management is the art of knowing what you want to do and then seeing that it is done in the best and cheapest way.
- Management is concerned with seeing that the job gets done; its tasks all center on planning and guiding the operations that are going on in the enterprise.
- Management is a multipurpose organ that manages a business and manages managers and manages workers and work.
- Management consists in guiding human and physical resources into dynamic, hard-hitting organization unit that attains its objectives to the satisfaction of those served and with a high degree or morale and sense of attainment on the part of those rendering the service.

Chapter 1: Introduction to Management

- "Management is a social and technical process that utilizes resources, influences human action and facilitates changes in order to accomplish an organization's goals."
  —**Tho Harmann, William Scott**
- "Management is a process of working with and through others to achieve organizational objectives in a changing environment, central to this purpose is the effective and efficient use of limited resources."
  —**Rovert Kreitner**
- "Management may be defined as the art of securing maximum results with a minimum of effort so as to secure maximum prosperity and happiness for both employer and employee and give the public the best possible service".
  —**John Mee**
- "Management is distinct process consisting of planning, organizing, actuating, activating and controlling, performed to determine and accomplish the objectives by the use of people and resources."
  —**George**

■ HISTORY OF STAR WARS OF MANAGEMENT

Sl. No.	Contributors	Description
1.	**Frederick W Taylor (1856–1915)**	**Frederick Winslow Taylor (1856–1915)** was an American inventor and engineer that applied his engineering and scientific knowledge to management and developed a theory called scientific management theory. His two most important books on his theory are Shop Management (1903) and The Principles of Scientific Management (1911). Frederick Taylor's scientific management theory can be seen in nearly all modern manufacturing firms and many other types of businesses. His imprint can be found in production planning, production control, process design, quality control, cost accounting, and even ergonomics. If you understand the principles of scientific management, you will be able to understand how manufacturers produce their goods and manage their employees. You will also understand the importance of **quantitative analysis**, or the analysis of data and numbers to improve production effectiveness and efficiency.
2.	**Gantt. Henry L Gantt (1861–1919)**	**Henry Laurence Gantt's** legacy to management is the Gantt Chart. Accepted as a commonplace project management tool today, it was an innovation of world-wide importance in the 1920s. But the Chart was not Gantt's only legacy; he was also a forerunner of the Human Relations School of management and an early spokesman for the social responsibility of business. Gantt is often seen as a disciple of Taylor and a promoter of the scientific school of management. In his early career, the influence of Taylor and Gantt's aptitude for problem-solving resulted in attempts to address the technical problems of scientific management. Such as Taylor, Gantt believed that it was only the application of scientific analysis to every aspect of work which could produce industrial efficiency, and that improvements in management came from eliminating chance and accidents. Gantt made four individual and notable contributions.
3.	**Harrington Emerson (1853–1936)**	**Harrington Emerson** (August 2, 1853–September 2, 1931) was an American efficiency engineer and business theorist who founded the management consultancy firm Emerson Institute in New York City in 1900. He is known for his pioneering contributions to scientific management where he developed a contrasting approach to efficiency. Harrington Emerson (1853–1931) was one of America's pioneers in industrial engineering and management and organizational theory. His major contributions were to install his management methods at many industrial firms and to promote the ideas of scientific management and efficiency to a mass audience. One of the most erudite and cosmopolitan personalities associated with the scientific management movement, Emerson established a modestly successful consulting business as an "efficiency engineer", an author of books on industrial efficiency, and a promoter and popularize of the movement.
4.	**Charles Babbage (1792–1871)**	**Charles Babbage** (1792–1871) is known as the patron saint of operations research and management science. Babbage's scientific inventions included a mechanical calculator (his "difference engine"), a versatile computer (his "analytical engine"), and a punch-card machine. Babbage's most successful book, On the Economy of Machinery and Manufacturers, published in 1832, described the tools and machinery used in English factories. It discussed the economic principles of manufacturing, and analyzed the operations; the skills used and suggested improved practices. He showed that reducing the tasks of manufacturing to their simplest activities increases the numbers of people who can do them and, thus, reduces the average wage which needs to be paid. According to him, a work should be divided into mental and physical efforts and a worker should be paid a bonus in proportion to his own efficiency and success of the business.
5.	**Henry Fayol**	**Henry Fayol**, a French industrialist, is now recognized as the Father of Modern Management. In year **1916**, Fayol wrote a book entitled "Industrial and General Administration". In this book, he gave the **14 Principles of Management**. These 14 principles of management are universally accepted and used even today. According to Henry Fayol, all managers must follow these 14 principles. Students of the history of management thought will be familiar with the name "Henry Fayol". References to his name are found quite frequently in management texts and Ansoff has argued that Fayol "anticipated imaginatively and soundly most of the more recent analyses of modern business practice". The purpose of this brief guide is to introduce you to some of the works by and about Henry Fayol.

Sl. No.	Contributors	Description
6.	Max Webber (1864–1920)	**Max Webber** was the first to observe and write on bureaucracies which developed in Germany during the 19th century. He considered them to be efficient, rational and honest, a big improvement over the haphazard administration that they replaced. The German government was better developed than those in the United States and Britain and was nearly equal to that of France. Max Weber holds a leading position. He was the first to use the term "bureaucracy" as well as the first to analyze it comprehensively. Indeed analysts today speak of a "Weberian bureaucracy," meaning one that fits his ideal type closely. On the other hand, many have found negative features about bureaucracy. It can over conform to its rules and procedures, treating an individual like a number and generating red tape. It can ignore the wishes of elected leaders. It can displace goals, perhaps advancing the interests of the employees rather than the people it is supposed to serve. Weber ignores the issue of democratic control of bureaucracy.
7.	James Mooney (1884-1957)	**James D Mooney (1884-1957)**: Mooney studied mechanical engineering and eventually became a key member of General Motors' top management team. In 1931, he wrote Onward Industry! The book is considered by many scholars to be a significant contribution to administrative management theory. James D Mooney (18 February 1884–21 September 1957) was an engineer and corporate executive at General Motors who played a role in international affairs in the 1930s and early 1940s. His career was disrupted when he was accused of Nazi sympathies in 1940.
8.	Mary Parker Follett (1868-1933)	**Mary Parker Follett (1868-1933)** defined management as: "the art of getting things done through people". Her ideas are contradictory to the idea of scientific management, as she believed that managers and subordinates should fully collaborate. Power is central to her ideas. Power is created and organized by organizations, and according to her it is legitimate and inevitable. Regarding to power Follett used the term "integration," to refer to noncoercive power-sharing based on the use of her concept of "power with" rather than "power over." Her ideas were formulated in three principles: 1. Functions are specific task areas within organizations. The appropriate degree of authority and responsibility should be allocated to them so tasks can be accomplished. 2. Responsibility is expressed in terms of an empirical duty: People should manage their responsibility on the basis of evidence and should integrate this effectively with the functions of others. 3. Authority flows from an entitlement to exercise power, which is based upon legitimate authority.
9.	Lewin Kurt Lewin (1890–1947)	In 1946, social scientist **Kurt Lewin** launches the Research Center for Group Dynamics at the Massachusetts Institute of Technology. His contributions in change theory, action research, and action learning earn him the title of the "father of organization development." **Field Theory:** Influenced by Gestalt psychology, Lewin developed a theory that emphasized the importance of individual personalities, interpersonal conflict and situational variables. Lewin's Field Theory proposed that behavior is the result of the individual and the environment. This theory had a major impact on social psychology, supporting the notion that our individual traits and the environment interact to cause behavior. Lewin is best known for his work in the field of organization behavior and the study of group dynamics. His research discovered that learning is best facilitated when there is a conflict between immediate concrete experience and detached analysis within the individual. His cycle of action, reflection, generalization, and testing is characteristic of experiential learning.
10.	McGregor Douglas McGregor (1932)	He conducted pioneering study in the field of industrial relations. Douglas McGregor remains one of the most influential thinkers in the sphere of human relations. His concepts of Theory X and Theory Y introduced a new philosophy to motivational thinking with. Theory X assumed that workers were inherently lazy and needed to be supervised and motivated. This was the conventional managerial thinking at the time. "Theory Y was based on the principle that people want and need to work, want to be given responsibility, and should be encouraged to take it and commit themselves actively to the objectives of the organizations they work for. It underlay the thinking of the human relations school of management that developed and flourished in the latter part of the 20th century."
11.	Rensis Likert	**Dr Rensis Likert** has studied human behavior within many organizations. After extensive research, Dr Rensis Likert concluded that there are four systems of management. According to Likert, the efficiency of an organization or its departments is influenced by their system of management. His theory of management is based on his work at the University of Michigan's institute for social research. Likert categorized his four management systems as follows; He identified three variables in organizations. 1. The casual variable includes leadership behavior. 2. The intervening variables are perceptions, attitudes and motivations. 3. The end results variables are measures of profits, costs and productivity.

Sl. No.	Contributors	Description
12.	Ludwig von Bertalanffy	**Karl Ludwig von Bertalanffy** (September 19, 1901, Atzgersdorf near Vienna–June 12, 1972, Buffalo, New York) was an Austrian-born biologist known as one of the founders of general system theory (GST). GST is an interdisciplinary practice that describes systems with interacting components, applicable to biology, cybermetrics, and other fields. Bertalanffy proposed that the classical laws of thermodynamics applied to closed systems, but not necessarily to "open systems," such as living things. His mathematical model of an organism's growth over time, published in 1934, is still in use today. Ludwig von Bertalanffy (1901–1972) has been one of the most acute minds of the XX century. Here are miscellanea of passages from his **General System Theory**. The first part of the text focuses on the function of the theory of systems and on the main features of closed and open systems. The second part presents a conception of the human being not as a robot or a moron aiming at reducing tensions by satisfying biological needs, but as an **active personality system** creating his own universe, who revels in accepting challenges, solving problems and expressing his artistic inclinations.
13.	Luther Gulick	**POSDCORB** is an acronym widely used in the field of management and public administration that reflects the classic view of administrative management. Largely drawn from the work of French industrialist Henry Fayol, it first appeared in a 1937 staff paper by Luther Gulick and Lyndall Urwick written for the Brownlow committee. The acronym stands for steps in the administrative process: **P**lanning, **O**rganizing, **S**taffing, **D**irecting, **C**oordinating, **R**eporting and **B**udgeting. In his piece "Notes on the Theory of Organization", a memo prepared while he was a member of the Brownlow Committee, Luther Gulick asks rhetorically "What is the work of the chief executive? What does he do?" POSDCORB is the answer, "designed to call attention to the various functional elements of the work of a chief executive because 'administration' and 'management' have lost all specific content."
14.	Lyndall Urwick	**Edward Brech** (1909–2006) joined Urwick Orr and Partners in 1938 as a management consultant, initially working with Lyndall Urwick to produce the renowned three volumes work The Making of Scientific Management. In Urwick Orr he played a leading role in the introduction of management training and techniques and also wrote copiously on his own account. In 1959, he was seconded to Unilever and in 1965 was appointed as Chief Executive of the Construction Industry Training Board. On his retirement, he returned to research, initially through the pursuit of a PhD, which he was granted at the age of 85. He built on his PhD to produce a monumental series of five volumes collectively titled The Evolution of Modern Management in 2002 and then moved to this biography of his old employer, mentor and co-author, Lyndall Urwick, on which he was working when he died.

FUNCTIONAL CONCEPT OF MANAGEMENT (FIG. 1.2)

Management is a continuous, lively and fast developing science. Management is needed to convert the disorganized resources of men, machines, materials and methods into a useful and effective enterprise. Management is a pipeline, the inputs are fed at the end and they are preceded through management functions and ultimately we get the end results or inputs in the form of goods, services, productivity, information and satisfaction.

Management is a comprehensive word which is used in different sciences in the modern business and industrial world. In the narrow sense, it signifies the technique of taking work from others. In this way, a person who can take work from others is called manager. In the wide sense, the management is an art, as well as science, which is concerned with the different human efforts so as achieve the desired objective.

Concepts of Management

Management = Manage + Men + T (Tactfully) basically, there are 5 concepts of management. They are:

1. **Functional concept:** Management basically is the task of planning, coordinating, motivating and controlling the efforts of other towards the goals and objectives of the organization. According to this concept, management is what a manager does (planning, executing, and controlling)
2. **Human relation concept:** According to this concept, Management is the art o getting things done through and with people in organized groups. It is the art of creating an environment in which people can perform and individuals could cooperate towards attaining of group goals. It is an art of removing blanks to such performance a way of optimizing efficiency in reaching goals.
3. **Leadership and decision making concept:** According to this concept, management is the art and science of preparing, organizing, directing human efforts applied to control the forces and utilize the materials of nature for the benefits to man.

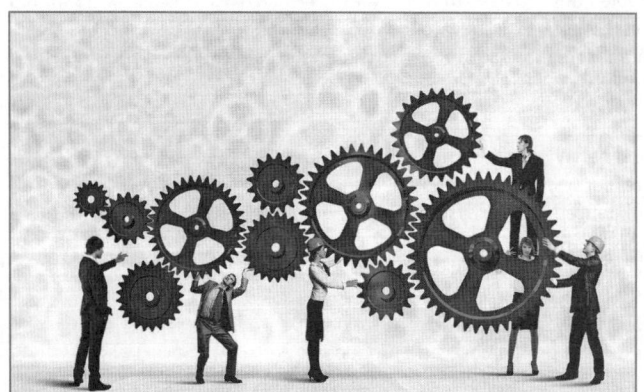

Fig. 1.2: Functional concept of management.

4. **Productive concept:** According to this concept, management may be defined as the art of securing maximum prosperity with a minimum effort so as to secure maximum prosperity and happiness for both employer n employee and provide best services thereby.
5. **Integration concept:** According to this concept, management is the coordination of human and material resources towards the achievement of organizational objectives as well as the organization of the productive functions essential for achieving stated or accepted economic goal.

Haimann's Concept of Management (Fig. 1.3)

These above definition of management, given by different writers and authorities, are found giving different senses. Virtually, the five concepts are found developed by the authorities emphasizing in different aspects. However, it has been realized by many that it will not be fair to define management based upon any one aspect. Management can be taken as process-managerial process or social process either engage in planning, organizing, staffing, directing and controlling or mobilizing the group activities to achieve the corporate goals.

To overcome the limitations of the above concepts, Theo Haimann, the leading management expert has explained three basic concepts of management as under:
1. **Management as a process:** Management is a process. It includes the process of planning, controlling, coordinating, motivating, and staffing. These processes are the series of interrelated sequential functions. Processes refer to accomplish these mentioned activities. Management is the efforts of organizational members to accomplish the organizer's objectives. This concept is very simple because:
   - It is very simple and very easy to understand
   - It indicates functions of management as a process
   - It recognizes management as a universal process
2. **Management as a discipline:** The term management is used as a subject of instructions. It is a specific branch of knowledge which is studied in campuses and schools like economics, sociology, mathematics, political science, etc., the scholars of management have found that the information and management are used in practical life for better functioning. The scope of management is being increased day to day as a discipline
3. **Management as a noun:** The word management itself refers as a noun. There are many kinds of employees in an organization. Some people are involved in managerial function and some are involved in operating functions. The individuals who manage the organization and departments are managers. As a noun, the term management is used as single name of managers, board of directors, managing directors; departmental managers etc., are included in management.

Management as an Activity

According to this approach management consists of those activities, which are performed by managers in attaining the predetermined objectives of the business. This approach may be referred to Henry Fayol, who classified management activities into the following categories:
1. **Technical**—referred to production department.
2. **Commercial**—relates to buying, selling and exchange.
3. **Financial** concerned with maximum utilization of capital.
4. **Security** concurred with protection of property and person.
5. According concerned with maintenance of accounts, presentation and statistics and
6. Management concerned to planning, organizing, commanding, coordinating and controlling.

Management as a Group of Personnel

According to this approach human factor plays an important role in accomplishing business objectives. Management is concerned with those who have been managing the affairs of the business. Managers are assigned duties and are also granted requisite authority to perform their duties efficiently and thus, management is effective direction, coordination and control of individual and group efforts to accomplish business objective. This approach is advocated by management authorities, such as Taylor, Wilson and others. They have defined management as following. As per FW Taylor's approach, "Management is the art of knowing exactly what you want your men to do and then seeing that they do it in the best and cheapest way."

■ SCOPE OF MANAGEMENT (FIG. 1.4)

Management is needed in all types of organized activities. Moreover, management principles are applicable to all types of organizations, including profit-seeking organizations (industrial firms, banks, insurance companies, small business, etc.) and not-for-profit organizations (governmental organizations, healthcare organizations. educations organizations, churches, etc.). Any group of two or more people working to achieve a goal and having resources at its disposal is engaged in management. Obviously, a manager's job is somewhat different in different types of organizations, exists in unique environments, and uses different technology. However, all organizations need the common basic activities:

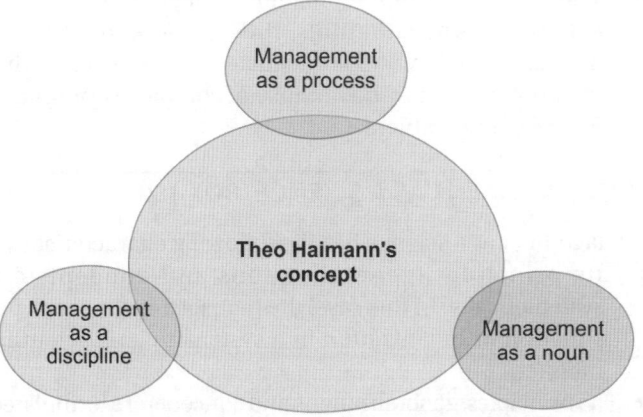

Fig. 1.3: Haimann's concept of management.

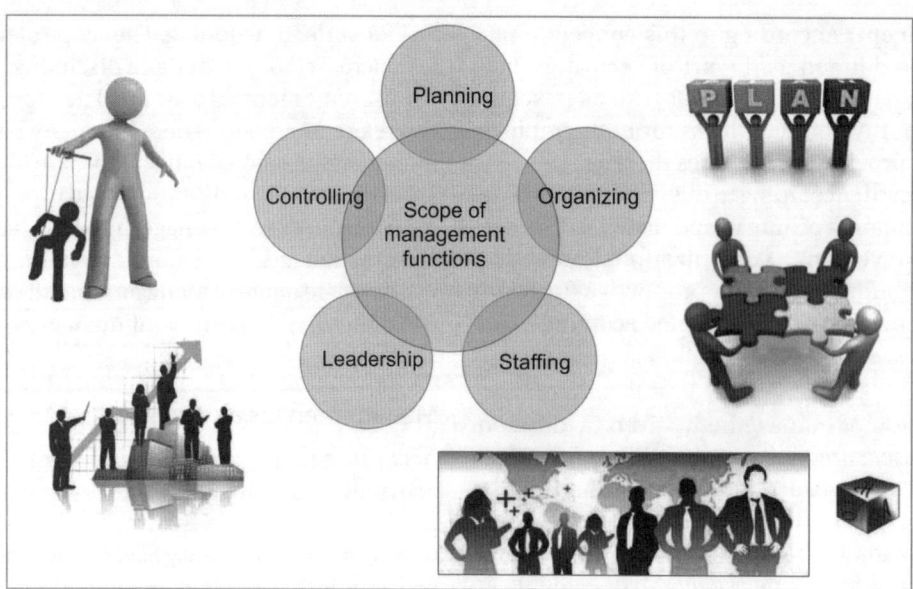

Fig. 1.4: Scope of management.

planning, organizing, leading, and controlling. Management is also universal in that it uses a systematic body of knowledge including economics, sociology, and laws. This knowledge can be applied to all organizations, whether business, or government, or religious, and it is applicable at all levels of management in same organizations.

■ NATURE OF MANAGEMENT (FIG. 1.5)

Management involves characteristics of both art and science. While certain aspects of management make it a science, certain others which involve application of skills make it an art. Every discipline of art is always backed by science which is basic knowledge of that art. Similarly, every discipline of science is complete only when it is used in practice for solving various kinds of problems. Whereas under "science" one normally learns the "why" of a phenomenon, under "art" one learns the "how" of it.

In the words of Robert H Hilkert: "In the area of management, science and art are two sides of the same coin". In the beginning of development of management knowledge, it was considered as an art. There was a jungle of management knowledge. Any one used it to get things done in his own way. But later by codifying and systemizing the management, it became a science as well as being an art.

Nandan choudhary = Management as an Art = Management as an art has the following characteristics:

- Just like other arts it has practical application. The knowledge of management should be learned and practiced by managers, just as medical or legal practitioners practice their respective sciences. In this sense, management is an art.
- The manager gains experience by continuous application of management knowledge. This experience helps them to develop more skills and abilities for translating management knowledge into practice.
- Application of management knowledge calls for innovativeness and creativity.
- The fourth reason to consider management as an art is that in many situations, theoretical knowledge of management may not be adequate or relevant for solving the problem. It may be because of complexity or unique nature of the problem.

■ MANAGEMENT AS A SCIENCE (BOX 1.2)

Management as a science has the following characteristics:
- Its principles, generalizations and concepts are systematically. In this case, the manager can manage the situation or organization in a systematic and scientific manner.
- Its principles, generalizations and concepts are formulated on the basis of observation, research, analysis and

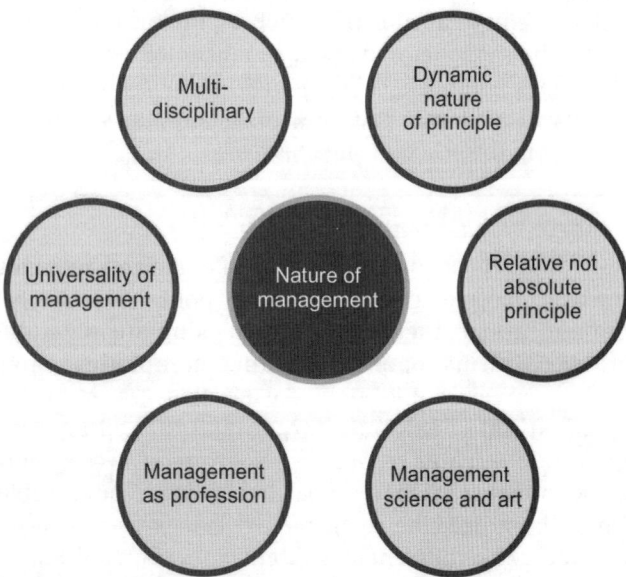

Fig. 1.5: Nature of management.

Box 1.2: Management as an Science.
- Systematic decision—making
- Output may vary, the input being the same
- Principles of management are universally accepted
- Process of management are universally followed

experimentation, as is the case with the principles of other sciences.
- Like other sciences, management principles are also based on relationship of cause and effect. It states that same cause under similar circumstance will produce same effect. Suppose if workers are paid more (cause), the produce more (effect).
- Management principles are codified and systematic, and can be transferred from one to another and can be taught.
- Management principles are universally applicable to all types of organizations. There is no tailor—made answer to a question—Is management a science or art? To ascertain the nature of management with respect of science or art, there is a need to know the exact meaning of the words 'science' or 'art' and subsequently, their application to management.

CHARACTERISTICS OF MANAGEMENT

- **Management as a continuous process:** Management can be considered as a process because it consists of planning, organizing, activating and controlling the resources (personnel and capital) of an organization. So they are used to the best advantage in achieving the objectives of the organization. None of the managerial functions would produce the ultimate results in the absence of all other basic functions. Hence, we can say that management is a continuous process.
- **Management as a discipline:** Since the boundaries of management are not exact as that of any other physical sciences, it may not fit in very well for being addressed as discipline. However, its status as a discipline increases because it continuously discovers many aspects of business enterprises and also passes on the verified knowledge to the practitioners of the managerial process.
- **Management as a career:** As a career or occupation, management is a broad concept- Management itself can be regarded as a career, but it also presents a variety of interesting and challenging careers focused on specialized occupations in the fields, such as marketing, finance and personnel.
- **Management as an applied science:** Even though management is a science so far as it possesses a systematized body of knowledge and uses scientific methods of research, it is not an exact science, such as natural sciences which deal with living phenomena, such as botany and medicine. Hence, management is definitely a social science, such as economics or psychology and has the same institutions which these and other social sciences have.

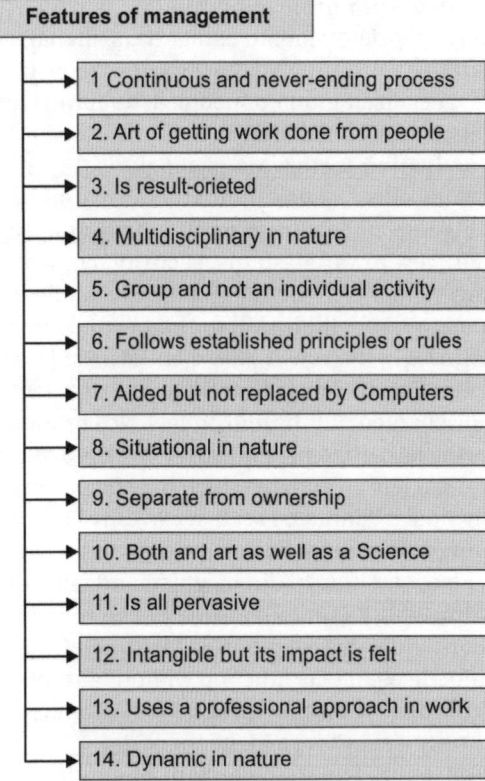

Fig. 1.6: Features of management.

Box 1.3: Need and scope of management.
- Management purpose is to formulate effective **organizational strategies** and **efficiently based** on the missions **objectives and goals**.
- It deals with both **internal and external environment**.
- It concerned with all kind of sources, i.e., **Human, Financial, Material, Machines, Technology and Technical**.
- Management functions include: **Planning, Organizing, Directing, Staffing and Controlling**.
- Managers should possess **varied skills** in order to play a variety of **roles**.
- It applies to managers at **all levels** in an organization.

Figure 1.6 shows features of management. Needs and scope of management is summarize in **Box 1.3**.
- **Universal application:** Management is a universal activity, applied to any form of activity, economic or otherwise.
- **Goal-oriented:** Management has the task of attaining certain objectives. The success or failure of the management depends on how far it is able to attain the desired goals. It is judged by the extent to which it achieves its targets.
- **Guidance:** The main task of the management is guidance in the utilization of material and human resources in the best possible way. Through optimum utilization of resources it has to ensure that the objectives are attained. The essential element of management is that it gets the work done by coordinating the performance of those who actually perform diverse and specific jobs.

- **Divorced from proprietorship:** Management does not signify proprietorship. In earlier days, management and enterprise were lumped into the same factor. It now refers to a specialized group of people who have acquired the ability to carry out a project.
- **An activating factor:** Management is the factor which activates other factors of production. A manager's skill lies in motivating his workers through guidance, training, incentives, rewards, status, security, control, etc. So a mangers' ability lies in the fact that he is able to motivate others to apply their skill to the best advantage of the enterprise in the accomplishment of its objectives.
- **Management is a human activity:** Management functions are discharged only by individuals. No corporate body or an artificial being can perform the work of a management. Although it is an activity which may be performed by an individual it cannot be seen. It can only be felt.
- **Management signifies authority:** Since, the essence of management is to direct, guide and control, it has to have authority. Authority is the power to compel others to work and behave in a particular manner. Management cannot discharge its function without authority. It is the foundation of management. Since management has authority it stands at a higher pedestal.
- **Leadership:** The management has to lead a team of workers. It must be capable of inspiring, motivating and winning their confidence.

NEED OF MANAGEMENT

- **Direction, coordination and control of group efforts:** In business, many persons work together. They need proper direction and guidance for raising their efficiency. In the absence of guidance, people will work as per their desire and the, orderly working of enterprise will not be possible. Management is needed for planning business activities, for guiding employees in the right direction and finally for coordinating their efforts for achieving best/most favorable results.
- **Orderly achievement of business objectives:** Efficient management is needed in order to achieve the objectives of business activity in an orderly and quick manner.
- **Performance of basic managerial functions:** Planning, Organizing, coordinating and controlling are the basic functions of management. Management is needed as these functions are performed through the management process.
- **Effective communication at all levels:** Management is needed for effective communication within and outside the organization.
- **Motivation of employees:** Management is needed for motivating employees and also for coordinating their efforts so as to achieve business objectives quickly.
- **Success and stability of business enterprise:** Efficient management is needed for success, stability and prosperity of a business enterprise.

Figure 1.7 shows importance of management.

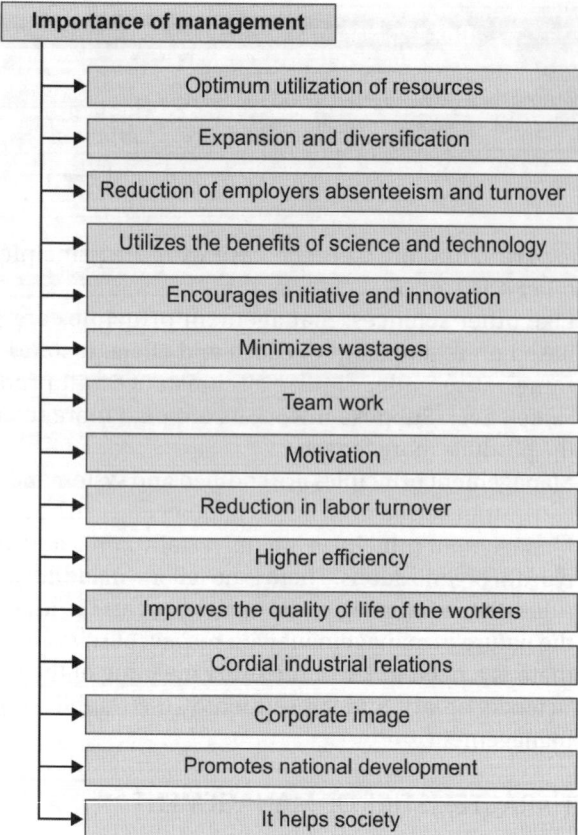

Fig. 1.7: Importance of management.

DIFFERENCES BETWEEN MANAGEMENT AND ADMINISTRATION (TABLE 1.1)

There has been a controversy regarding the interpretation of these two terms. There are different views in this regard: According to first view (William Newman, Peter Drucker, etc.), there is no basic difference between the two terms, and they are interchangeable. If there is any difference, it may perhaps be in their usage in practice. The term administration is used for non-business activities, and management is used for business activities.

According to second view (Kimball, Brech, other British writers, etc.), management is a more comprehensive term which includes administration. Management involves "thinking" and administration involves "doing".

- Management is responsible for planning and organizing, and administration is responsible for directing and controlling. Whereas management refers to a high level of managerial activities, such as goal-setting, policy formulation and strategy making, administration refers to an operative part concerned with lower level management activities such as execution of policies.
- According to third view (Sheldon, Speriegal, Milward, etc.), administration is a more comprehensive term, which includes management. Administration involves "thinking" and management involves "doing".

Table 1.1: Differences between administration and management.

Sl. No.	Basis of difference	Administration	Management
1.	Nature of work	It is concerned about the determination of objectives and major policies of an organization	It puts into action the policies and plans laid down by the administration
2.	Type of function	It is a determinative function	It is an executive function
3.	Scope	It takes major decisions of an enterprise as a whole	It takes decisions within the framework set by the administration
4.	Level of authority	It is a top-level activity	It is a middle level activity
5.	Nature of status	It consists of owners who invest capital in and receive profits from an enterprise	It is a group of managerial personnel who use their specialized knowledge to fulfill the objectives of an enterprise
6.	Nature of usage	It is popular with government, military, educational, and religious organizations	It is used in business enterprises
7.	Decision making	Its decisions are influenced by public opinion, government policies, social, and religious factors	Its decisions are influenced by the values, opinions, and beliefs of the managers
8.	Main functions	Planning and organizing functions are involved in it	Motivating and controlling functions are involved in it
9.	Abilities	It needs administrative rather than technical abilities	It requires technical activities

- Administration is a top level function which concentrates on determination of plans, policies and objectives, whereas management is a lower level function which deals with the execution and direction of policies and operations.
- It does not mean that we need two separate sets of personnel, but each manager performs both the managerial as well as administrative functions.
- At top level more time is spent in administrative activity and as one move down, more time is spent in management activity.

LEVELS OF MANAGEMENT (FIGS. 1.8 AND 1.9)

Top Level of Management

It consists of board of directors, chief executive or managing director. The top management is the ultimate source of authority and it manages goals and policies for an enterprise. It devotes more time on planning and coordinating functions.

Top managers are responsible for the overall direction and operations of an organization. Particularly, they are responsible for setting organizational goals, defining strategies for achieving them, monitoring and implementing the external environment, decisions that affect entire organization. They have such titles as chief executive officer (CEO), president, chairman, division president, and executive vice-president. Managers in these positions are responsible for interacting with representatives of the external environment (e.g., important customers, financial institutions, and governmental figures) and establishing objectives, policies, and strategies.

The main role of the first level manager
- Determines the objectives, policies and plans of the organization.
- Mobilizes (assemble and bring together) available resources.
- Does mostly the work of thinking, planning and deciding.
  Therefore, they are also called as the Administrators and the brain of the organization.
- They spend more time in planning and organizing.
- They prepare long-term plans of the organization which are generally made for 5 to 20 years.
- The top level management has maximum authority and responsibility. They are the top or final authority in the organization.
  They are directly responsible to the shareholders, government and the general public. The success or failure of the organization largely depends on their efficiency and decision making.
- They require more conceptual skills and less technical Skills.

Middle Level of Management

The branch managers and departmental managers constitute middle level. They are responsible to the top management for the functioning of their department. They devote more time to organizational and directional functions. In small organization, there is only one layer of middle level of management, but in big enterprises, there may be senior and junior middle level management. Their role can be emphasized as:

Middle managers are responsible for business units and major departments. Examples of middle managers are department head, division head, and director of the research

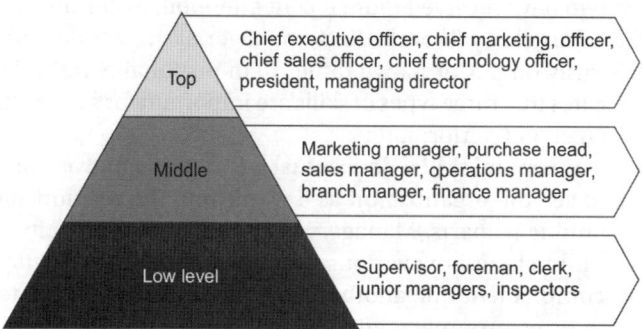

Fig. 1.8: Levels of management.

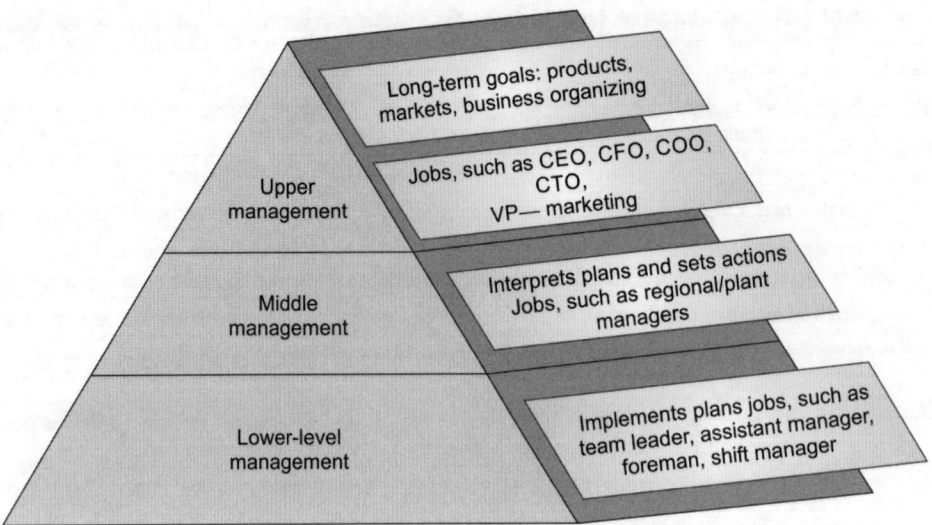

Fig. 1.9: Levels of management and their roles.

lab. The responsibilities of middle managers include translating executive orders into operation, implementing plans, and directly supervising lower-level managers. Middle managers typically have two or more management levels beneath them. They receive overall strategies and policies from top managers and the translate them into specific objective and programs for first-line managers.

The middle level management emphasizes more on following tasks:
- Middle level management gives recommendations (advice) to the top level management.
- It executes (implements) the policies and plans, which are made by the top level management.
- It coordinate the activities of all the departments.
- They also have to communicate with the top level management and the lower level management.
- They spend more time in coordinating and communicating.
- They prepare short-term plans of their departments, which are generally made for 1 to 5 years.
- The middle level management has limited authority and responsibility. They are intermediary between top and lower management. They are directly responsible to the chief executive officer and board of directors.
- Require more managerial and technical skills and less conceptual skills.

Lower Level of Management

Lower level is also known as supervisory/operative level of management. It consists of supervisors, foreman, section officers, superintendent etc. According to RC Davis, "Supervisory management refers to those executives whose work has to be largely with personal oversight and direction of operative employees". In other words, they are concerned with direction and controlling function of management. **First-line managers** are directly responsible for the production of goods and services. Particularly, they are responsible for directing nonsupervisory employees. First-line managers are variously called office manager, section chief, line manager, and supervisor.

- Lower level management directs the workers/employees.
- They develop morale in the workers.
- It maintains a link between workers and the middle level management.
- The lower level management informs the workers about the decisions which are taken by the management. They also inform the management about the performance, difficulties, feelings, demands, etc., of the workers.
- They spend more time in directing and controlling.
- The lower level managers make daily, weekly and monthly plans.
- They have limited authority, but important responsibility of getting the work done from the workers. They regularly report and are directly responsible to the middle level management.
- Along with the experience and basic management skills, they also require more technical and communication skills.

■ MANAGEMENT SKILLS (FIGS. 1.10 AND 1.11)

Regardless of the sort of goals they must meet or their level of authority, managers need to possess conceptual, human, technical, diagnostic, and political skills. The first three skills have long been accepted as important for management; the last two have received more recent attention. According to a classic article by Robert L Katz, managerial success depends primarily on performance rather than personality traits. He indicates that three types of skills are important for successful management performance:

- **Conceptual skills:** Conceptual skill is the cognitive ability to see the organization as a whole and the relationship among its parts. Managers need the mental capacity to understand how various functions of the organization complement one another, how the organization relates to its environment, and how changes in one part of the organization affect the rest of the organization.

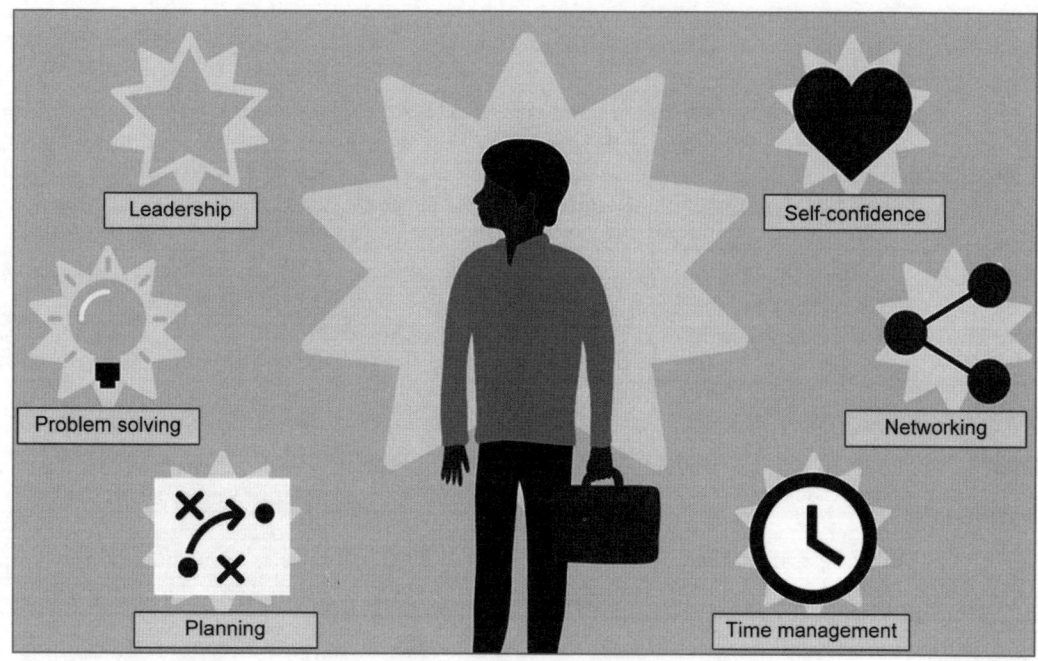

Fig. 1.10: Management skills.

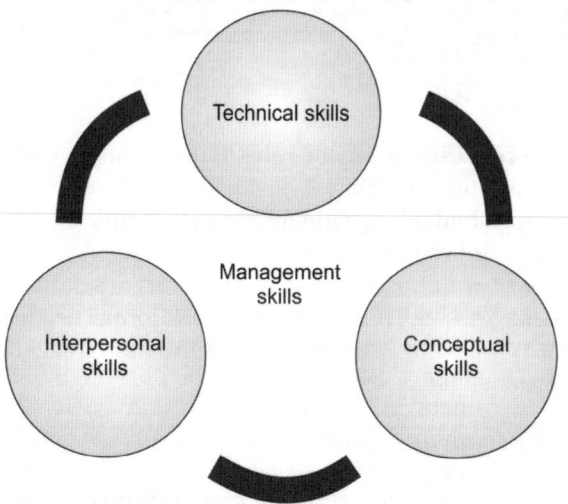

Fig. 1.11: Domains of management skills.

- **Human skills:** The manager needs human skills—the ability to communicate with, understand, and motivate both individuals and groups.
- **Technical skills:** Technical skills are skills necessary to accomplish specialized activities (e.g., engineering, computer programming, and accounting).
- **Diagnostic skills:** Diagnostic skills include the ability to determine, by analysis and examination, the nature of a particular condition. A manager can diagnose a problem in the organization by studying its symptoms. These skills are also useful in favorable situations.
- **Political skills:** Political skill is the ability to acquire the power necessary to reach objectives and to prevent others from taking power. Political skill can be used for the good of the organization and for self-interest.

The extent to which managers need different kinds of skills moves from lower management to upper management. Most low-level managers use technical skills extensively. At higher levels technical skills become less important while the need for conceptual skills grows. However, human skills are very important to all managers

MANAGERIAL ROLES (TABLE 1.2)

Mintzberg's observations and research indicate that diverse manager activities can be organized into ten roles. For an important starting point, all ten rules are vested with formal authority over an organizational unit. From formal authority comes status, which leads to various interpersonal relations, and from these comes access to information, which, in turn, enables the manager to make decisions and strategies. The ten roles are divided into three categories: **interpersonal, informational**, and **decisional**.

Interpersonal Roles

Three of the managers' roles involve basic interpersonal relationships:

1. **The figurehead role:** Every manager must perform some duties of a ceremonial nature (e.g., the president greets the touring dignitaries, the sales manager takes an important customer to lunch). These activities are important to the smooth functioning of an organization.
2. **The leader role:** This role involves leadership directly (e.g., the manager is responsible for hiring a training his own staff). The leader role encompasses relationships with subordinates, including motivation, communication, and influence.
3. **The liaison role**, in which the manager makes contacts inside and outside the organization with a wide range of people: subordinates, clients, business associates, government, trade organization officials, and so on.

Table 1.2: Managerial roles and responsibilities (Henry Mintzberg's Managerial Roles).			
Category	Role	Organizational function	Example activities
Informational	Monitor	Responsible for information relevant to understanding the organization's internal and external environment	Handle correspondence and information, such as industry, societal, and economic news and competitive information
	Disseminator	Responsible for the synthesis, integration, and forwarding of information to other members of the organization	Forward informational e-mails; share information in meetings, conference calls, webcasts, etc.
	Spokesperson	Transmit information to outsiders about organizational policy, plans, outcomes, etc.	Attend management meetings; maintain networks between the organization and stakeholders
Interpersonal	Figurehead	Symbolic leadership duties involving social and legal matters	Attend ceremonies; greet visitors; organize and attend events with clients, customers, bankers, etc.
	Leader	Motivate, inspire, and guide employees' actions; provide opportunities for training; support appropriate staffing	Build trusting relationships with employees; build effective teams; manage conflict
	Liaison	Build and maintain relationships between the organization and outside entities	Work on external boards; create and maintain social networks (real and virtual) with key stakeholders
Decisional	Entrepreneur	Scan the organizational environment for opportunities; foster creativity and innovation	Participate in strategy and review meetings for new projects or continuous improvement
	Disturbance handler	Manage organizational problems and crises	Participate in strategy and review meetings that involve problems and crises; get involved directly with key issues and people
	Resource allocator	Take responsibility for allocation of all types of organizational resources	Create work schedules; make authorization requests; participate in budgeting activities
	Negotiator	Represent the organization during any significant negotiations	Negotiate with vendors and clients; settle disputes about resource allocation

Informational Roles

The processing of information is a key part of the manager's job. Three roles describe the informational aspects of managerial work:
1. **The monitor role:** This role involves seeking current information from many sources. For example, the manager perpetually scans his environment for information, interrogates liaison contacts and subordinates and receives unsolicited information.
2. **The disseminator role:** In their disseminator role, managers pass information to other, both inside and outside the organization.
3. **The spokesperson role:** In their spokesman role, managers send some of their information to people outside the organization about company policies, needs, actions, or plans.

Decisional Roles

The manager plays the major role in his unit's decision-making system. Four roles describe the decisional aspects of managerial work:
1. **The entrepreneur role:** In his entrepreneur role, managers search for improvement his unit to adopt it to changing conditions in the environment.
2. **The disturbance handler role:** This role involves responding to high-pressure disturbances. For example, manager must resolve conflicts among subordinates or between manager's department and other departments.
3. **The resource allocator role:** In their resource allocator role, managers make decisions about how to allocate people, budget, equipment, time and other resources to attain desired outcomes.
4. **The negotiator role:** The negotiations are duties of the manager's job. These activities involve formal negotiations and bargaining to attain outcomes for the manager's unit responsibility.

■ CONCLUSION

Management (or managing) is the administration of an organization, whether it is a business, a not-for-profit organization, or government body. Management includes the activities of setting the strategy of an organization and coordinating the efforts of its employees (or of volunteers) to accomplish its objectives through the application of available resources, such as financial, natural, technological, and human resources. The term "management" may also refer to those people who manage an organization—managers.

■ REVIEW QUESTIONS

Long Essays

1. Define management; explain in brief about history of star wars of management.
2. Enumerate the difference between management and administration.
3. Discuss managerial roles in detail.

Short Essays

1. Haimann's concept of management.
2. Management as a science.
3. Characteristics of management.
4. Levels of management.
5. Management skills.

Short Answers

1. Frederick W Taylor.
2. Henry Fayol.
3. Scope of management.
4. Need of management.
5. Conceptual skills.

BIBLIOGRAPHY

1. George, Claude S. History of Management Thought. Prentice Hall, Englewood Cliffs New Jersey; 1972.
2. Wrege CD, Greenwood RG, Taylor FW. The Father of Scientific Management (Homewood, IL: Business One Irwin. 1991); 253-60.
3. Wren DA, Bedeian AG, Breeze JD. "The foundations of Henry Fayol's administrative theory", Management Decision. 2002; 40 (9): 906-18.
4. Wren DA, Bedeian AG. The evolution of management thought, 6th edition. New York: Wiley; 2009.

CHAPTER 2
Principles and Theories of Management

LEARNING OBJECTIVES

- Management Process
- Elements of Management Process
- Principles of Management
- Theories in Nursing Management
- Scientific Management
- Classic Organization Theories
- Human Relations Theories
- Theories Based on Behavioral Sciences
- Modern Management Theories
- Implications of Management Theories in Nursing

INTRODUCTION

Nursing management is performing leadership functions of governance and decision-making within organizations employing nurses. It includes processes common to all management like planning, organizing, staffing, directing and controlling. It is common for RNs to seek additional education to earn a master of science in nursing or doctor of nursing practice to prepare for leadership roles within nursing. Management positions increasingly require candidates to hold an advanced degree in nursing.

Figure 2.1 shows six M's management.

MANAGEMENT PROCESS (FIG. 2.2)

The management process, such as the nursing process, includes gathering **data**, diagnosing problems, planning, interviewing and evaluating outcomes. But in reality each step of the management process is more complex than the nursing process. The management process consists of working with human and physical resources and organizational and psychological processes within a creative and innovative climate for the realization of organizational goals. Henry Fayol, 1925, first identified the management functions of Planning, Organization, Command, Coordination, and Control. Later, Luther Gulick, 1973, expanded these and introduced seven activities of management: Planning, Organization, Staffing, Directing, Coordinating, Reporting, and Budgeting (POSDCORB).

ELEMENTS OF MANAGEMENT PROCESS (BOX 2.1)

Planning

Planning means to decide in advance what is to be done. It charts a course of actions for the future. It is an intellectual process and it aims to achieve a coordinated and consistent set of operations aimed at desired objectives.

Essentials of Good Planning

- Yields reasonable organizational objectives and develops alternative approaches to meet these objectives.
- Helps to eliminate or reduce the future uncertainty and chance.
- Helps to gain economical operations.
- Lays the foundation for organizing
- Facilitates coordination
- Helps to facilitate control. Dictates those activities to which employers are directed.

Organizing

The management function of organizing can be defined as, elating people and things to each other in such a way that they are all combined and interrelated into a unit capable of

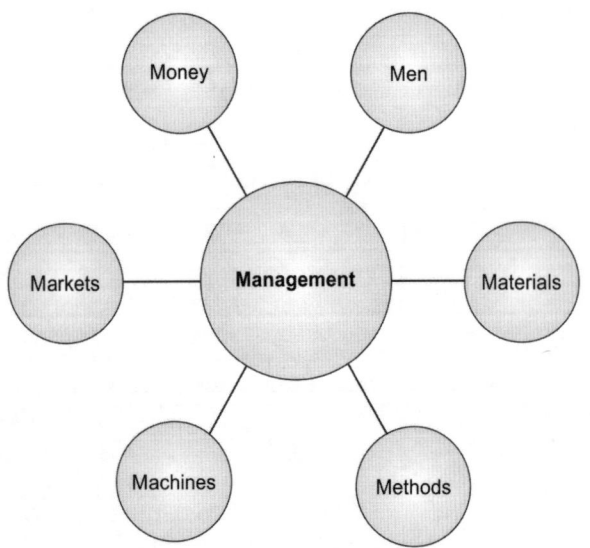

Fig. 2.1: Six M's management.

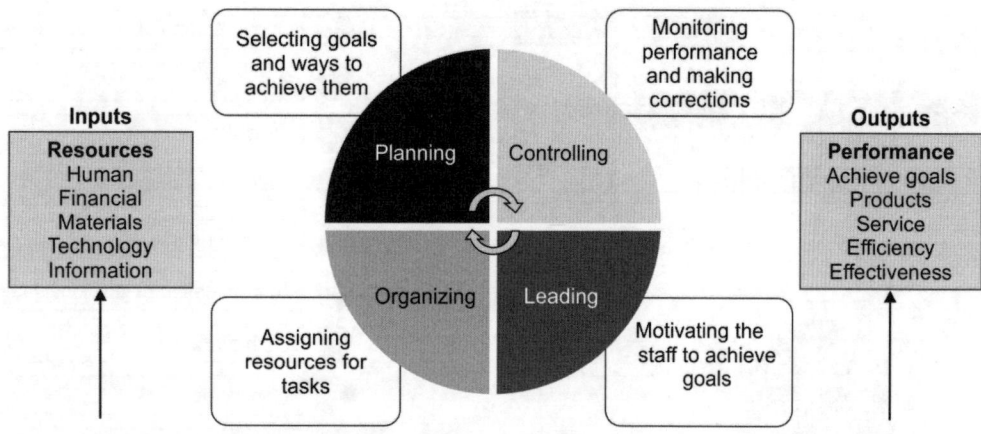

Fig. 2.2: Management process.

> **Box 2.1:** Elements/Components of management process.
>
> - The essential elements/components of management process are four which are actually basic functions of management:
>   - Planning
>   - Organizing
>   - Directing
>   - Controlling
> - We may add some more elements in the management process as follows:
>   - Motivating
>   - Cocoordinating
>   - Staffing
>   - Communicating

Manpower planning involves the following steps: (1) Scrutiny of present personnel strength, (2) Anticipation of manpower needs, (3) Investigation of turnover of personnel.

Directing

Directing means the issuance of orders, assignments and instructions that permit the subordinate to understand what is expected of him and the guidance and overseeing of the subordinate so that he can contribute effectively and efficiently to the attainment of organizational objectives.

Directing includes the following activities: (1) Giving orders, (2) Making supervision, (3) Leading, (4) Motivating, (5) Communicating.

being directed toward the organizational objectives. Work activities required for the organizational performance are separated through:

- Horizontal differentiation (i.e., dividing the organization into operational units for more effective and efficient performance).
- Vertical differentiation (i.e., establishes the hierarchy and the number of levels in the organization)
  - *Responsibility:* Responsibility in an organization is divided among available personnel by grouping the functions that are similar in objectives and content. This should be done in a manner that avoids overlaps and gaps as much as possible. Responsibility may be continuing or it may be terminated by the accomplishment of a single action.
  - *Authority:* When responsibility is given to a person, he must also be given the authority to make commitments, use resources and take the actions **necessary** to carry out his responsibilities.

Staffing

Staffing is the selection, training, motivating and retaining of a personnel in the organization. Before selection we have to make analysis of the **particular** job, which is required in the organization, then comes the **selection** of the personnel. It involves: manpower planning to have the right person in the right place and avoid "square peg in the round hole".

Supervision

Supervision is the activity of the management that is concerned with the training and discipline of the work force. It includes follow up to assure the prompt and proper execution of orders. Supervision is the art of overseeing, watching and directing with authority, the work and behavior of other.

Leading

Leadership is the ability to inspire and influence others to contribute to the attainment of the objectives. Successful leadership is the result of interaction between the leader and his subordinates in a particular **organizational** situation. There are number of styles of leadership that have been identified, such as autocratic, democratic participative leadership. The continuum of leadership styles, ranges from the completely authoritarian situation with no subordinate participation to a maximum degree of democratic leadership, enabling the subordinate to participate in all phases of the decision making process.

Controlling

Controlling can be defined as the regulation of activities in accordance with the requirements of plans. Controlling is an ongoing and continuous process to ensure that activities conform to plan. It include: quality **assurance**, performance appraisal, fiscal accountability, legal and ethical **control** and professional control.

Chapter 2: Principles and Theories of Management

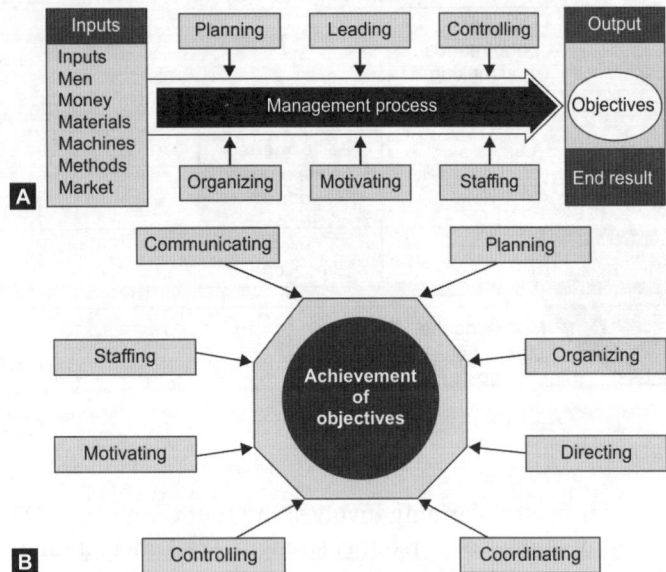

Figs. 2.3A and B: Achievement of objectives by applying management process. (A) Management process; (B) Elements of management process (Functions of management).

Steps of control: The control function, whether it is applied to cash, medical care, employee morale or anything else, involves four steps: (a) established of standards, (b) Measuring performance, (c) Comparing the actual results with the standards. **Figures 2.3A and B** shows achievement of objectives by applying management process.

■ PRINCIPLES OF MANAGEMENT

A principle refers to a fundamental truth. Management principles are the statements of fundamental truth based on logic which provides guidelines for managerial decision making and actions.

The 14 Principles of Management described by Henry Fayol **(Fig. 2.4 and Table 2.1)**.

Division of Labor

- Henry Fayol has stressed on the specialization of jobs.
- All kinds of work must be divided and subdivided and allotted to various persons according to their expertise in a particular area.
- Specialization leads to efficiency and economy in spheres of business.

Party of Authority and Responsibility

- Authority refers to the right of superiors to get exactness from their subordinates whereas responsibility means obligation for the performance of the job assigned.
- If authority is given to a person, he should also be made responsible.
- In a same way, if anyone is made responsible for any job, he should also have concerned authority.
- Authority without responsibility leads to irresponsible behavior whereas responsibility without authority makes the person ineffective.

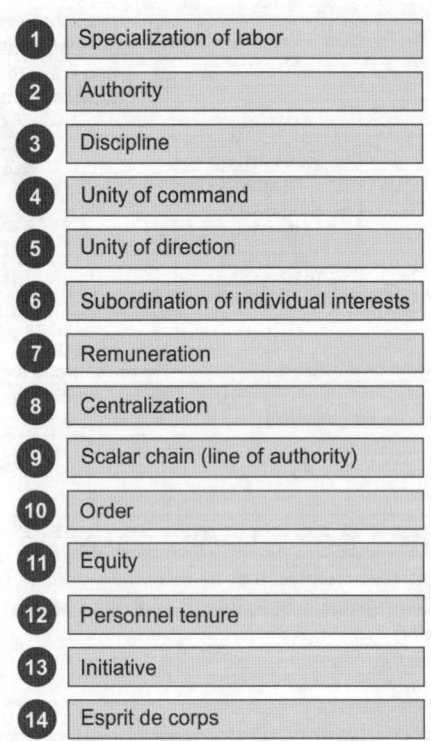

Fig. 2.4: 14 Principles of management described by Henry Fayol.

Table 2.1: Mnemonics of principles of nanagement. Henry Fayol's 14 Principles, Learn it, the easy way!	
DAD U C USSR	O I SEE
D—Division of work	O—Order
A—Authority and responsibility	I—Initiative
D—Discipline	S—Subordination of individual interest to general interest
U—Unity of command	
C—Centralization and decentralization	
U—Unity of direction	E—Equity
S—Scalar chain	E—Esprit de corps
S—Stability of tenure	
R—Remuneration	

Principle of One Boss

- A subordinate should receive orders and be accountable to one and only one boss at a time.
- In other words, a subordinate should not receive instructions from more than one person because:
  - It undermines authority
  - Weakens discipline
  - Divides loyalty
  - Creates confusion
  - Delays and chaos
  - Escaping responsibilities
  - Duplication of work
  - Overlapping of efforts
- Unity of command provides the enterprise a disciplined, stable and orderly existence.

Unity of Direction

- Fayol advocates one head one plan which means that there should be one plan for a group of activities having similar objectives.

- Related activities should be grouped together. There should be one plan of action for them and they should be under the charge of a particular manager.
- In fact, unity of command is not possible without unity of direction.

Equity
- Equity means combination of fairness, kindness and justice.
- It implies that managers should be fair and impartial while dealing with the subordinates.
- They should give similar treatment to people of similar position.
- They should not discriminate with respect to age, caste, sex, religion, relation, etc.
- Equity is essential to create and maintain cordial relations between the managers and subordinate.
- But equity does not mean total absence of harshness.

Order
- This principle is concerned with proper and systematic arrangement of things and people.
- Arrangement of things is called material order and placement of people is called social order.
- **Material order:** There should be safe, appropriate and specific place for every article and every place to be effectively used for specific activity and commodity.
- **Social order:** Selection and appointment of most suitable person on the suitable job.

Discipline
- "Discipline means sincerity, obedience, respect of authority and observance of rules and regulations of the enterprise".
- This principle applies that subordinate should respect their superiors and obey their order.
- Discipline is not only required on path of subordinates, but also on the part of management.
- Discipline can be enforced if:
  - There are good superiors at all levels.
  - There are clear and fair agreements with workers.
  - Sanctions (punishments) are judiciously applied.

Initiative
- It means eagerness to initiate actions without being asked to do so.
- Fayol advised that management should provide opportunity to its employees to suggest ideas, experiences and new method of work.
- It helps in developing an atmosphere of trust and understanding.

Fair Remuneration
- The quantum and method of remuneration to be paid to the workers should be fair, reasonable, satisfactory and rewarding of the efforts.
- As far as possible it should accord satisfaction to both employer and the employees.
- Wages should be determined on the basis of cost of living, work assigned, financial position of the business, wage rate prevailing, etc.
- Fayol also recommended provision of other benefits, such as free education, medical and residential facilities to workers.

Stability of Tenure
- The employees should be appointed after keeping in view principles of recruitment and selection, but once they are appointed their services should be served.
- Time is required for an employee to get used to a new work and succeed to doing it well but if he is removed before that he will not be able to render worthwhile services".

■ SCALAR CHAIN
- The chain of superiors ranging from the ultimate authority to the lowest".
- Every orders, instructions, messages, requests, explanation, etc., has to pass through scalar chain.

Subordination of Individual Interest to General Interest
- As far as possible, reconciliation should be achieved between individual and group interests.
- In order to achieve this attitude, it is essential that:
  - Employees should be honest and sincere.
  - Proper and regular supervision of work.
  - Reconciliation of mutual differences and clashes by mutual agreement. For example, for change of location of plant, for change of profit sharing ratio, etc.

Esprit De Corps (can be achieved through Unity of Command)
- It refers to team spirit, i.e., harmony in the work groups and mutual understanding among the members.
- Esprit De Corps inspires workers to work harder.
- To inculcate Esprit De Corps following steps should be undertaken:
  - There should be proper coordination of work at all levels
  - Subordinates should be encouraged to develop informal relations among themselves.
  - Efforts should be made to create enthusiasm and keenness among subordinates so that they can work to the maximum ability.

Centralization and Decentralization
- Centralization means concentration of authority at the top level. In other words, centralization is a situation in which top management retains most of the decision making authority.
- Decentralization means disposal of decision making authority to all the levels of the organization. In other words, sharing authority downwards is decentralization.

- Anything which increases the role of subordinate is decentralization and anything which decreases it is centralization.
- Fayol suggested that absolute centralization or decentralization is not feasible. An organization should strike to achieve a lot between the two.

Advantages

- Fayol was the first person to actually give a definition of management which is generally familiar today namely 'forecast and plan, to organize, to command, to co-ordinate and to control'.
- Fayol also gave much of the basic terminology and concepts, which would be elaborated upon by future researchers, such as division of labour, scalar chain, unity of command and centralization.

Disadvantages

- Fayol was describing the structure of formal organizations.
- Absence of attention to issues, such as individual versus general interest, remuneration and equity suggest that Fayol saw the employer as paternalistic and by definition working in the employee's interest.
- Fayol does mention the issues relating to the sensitivity of a patient's needs, such as initiative and 'esprit de corps', he saw them as issues in the context of rational organizational structure and not in terms of adapting structures and changing people's behavior to achieve the best fit between the organization and its customers.

THEORIES IN NURSING MANAGEMENT

- The study in the development of management theories can be useful to nursing leaders in creating their own management style.
- No single management theory is sufficient in itself to guide the nursing leaders in every situation **(Table 2.2)**.
- However, selecting from the most applicable theory they may be able to develop their own individual management style and most effective in their situation. Below are some of the most profound management theories developed in different periods. They could be categorized into four main focuses.

Table 2.2: Management theories.	
Theorist	Theory
Taylor	Scientific management
Webber	Bureaucratic organizations
Fayol	Management functions
Gulick	Activities of management
Follett	Participative management
Mayo	Hawthorne effect
McGregor	Theory X and Y
Argyris	Employee participation

- Scientific management **(Table 2.3)**
- Classic organization **(Table 2.4)**
- Human relations **(Table 2.5)**
- Behavioral science **(Table 2.6)**

SCIENTIFIC MANAGEMENT

Scientific principles measurement of the outcome. Among the **Taylor (Fig. 2.5)**:

- Frederick W Taylor (1856–1915) generally recognized as the father of scientific management.
- Through the use of stopwatch studies, he applied the principles of observation, measurement, and scientific comparison to determine the most efficient way to accomplish a task.
- Taylor conducted time-and-motion studies to time workers, analyze their movements, and set work standards.
- He usually found that the same result could be obtained in less time with fewer or shorter motions.
- When the most efficient way to complete a task was determined, workers were trained to follow that method.
- It was management's responsibility to select and train workers rather than allow them to choose their own jobs and methods and train themselves.

Taylor's scientific management reduced wasted efforts, set standards of performance, encouraged specialization, and stressed the selection of qualified workers who could be developed for a particular job.

Frederick W Taylor (1856–1915)

Taylor is recognized as father of scientific management. He conducted time-and-motion studies to time the workers, Analyze their movements and set their standards. He used stop watches. He applied the principles of observation, measurement and scientific comparison to determine the most effective way to accomplish a task.

Achievements of Taylor:

- He trained his workers to follow the time to complete the task given. The most productive workers were hired even when they were paid an incentive or wage.
- Labor costs per unit were reduced as a result.
- Responsibilities of management were separated from the functions of the workers.
- Developed systematic approach to determine the most efficient means of production.
- He considered management function is to plan.
- Working conditions and methods to be standardized to maximize the production.
- It was the management's responsibility to select and train the workers rather than allow them to choose their own jobs and train by themselves.
- He introduced an incentive plan to pay the workers according to the rate of production to minimize workers dissent and reduce resistance to improved methods.
- Increased production and produce higher profits.

Table 2.3: Scientific management theories.

Sl. No.	Theories	Theme	Concepts
1.	Gantt. Henry L Gantt (1861–1919)	Efficiency	1. Refining previous work rather than introducing new concepts 2. Explains relationships between work completed and time needed 3. Bonus remuneration plan to stimulate higher performance 4. Workers are selected scientifically 5. More humanitarian approach by management
2.	Emerson. Emerson (1853–1936)	Conservation and organizations goals and objectives	1. Goals and ideas should be clear and well defined 2. Changes should be evaluated 3. Competent counsel "is essential" 4. Management can strengthen "discipline" 5. Records, including adequate, reliable and immediate information should be available 6. Production scheduling is recommended 7. Standardized schedules to facilitate performance 8. "Efficiency rewards"

Table 2.4: Classical organization.

Sl. No.	Theories	Theme	Concepts
1.	Webber. Max Webber (1864–1920)	Organizations (bases of authority: Iraditional, charisma, legal)	1. The need for legalized, formal authority and consistent rules and regulations for personnel 2. Proposed bureaucracy as an organizational design 3. More rules and regulations and structure to increase efficiency
2.	Mooney. James Mooney (1884–1957)	Directing people and technique of relating functions	1. Coordination and synchronization 2. Functional effects 3. Scalar process 4. Arrange authority into hierarchy

Table 2.5: Human relations.

Sl. No.	Theories	Theme	Concepts
1.	Follett. Mary Parker Follett (1868–1933)	Management: A social process. Asserted participative management	1. Social process aimed at motivating individuals and groups to work toward a common goal 2. Advised that manager should never give orders to an employee 3. Manager should analyze the situation together and both should take orders from the situation

Table 2.6: Behavioral science.

Sl. No.	Theories	Theme	Concepts
1.	Likert. Rensis Likert (1903–1981)	Trust, communication facilitate effectiveness	1. Casual variable of leadership behavior 2. Intervening variable are perceptions, attitudes and motivations. End result variable: measures of profit, costs and productivity 3. Institutions should be structured to facilitate constant interaction among various work groups and stimulate lateral as well as vertical communication

Table 2.7: Comparison between Henry Fayol and FW Taylor.

Basis of difference	Henry Fayol	FW Taylor
Perspective	Top level management	Shop floor level of a factory
Unity of command	Strong proponent	Did not feel important as shown through functional foremanship
Applicability	Universally applicable	Applicable in specialized situations
Basis of formation	Personal experience	Observation and experimentation
Focus	Improving overall administration	Increasing productivity
Personality	Practitioner	Scientist
Expression	Generally theory of administration	Scientific management

The effect of time-motion study of Taylor:
1. Reduced wasted efforts
2. Set standards of performance
3. Encouraged specialization and stressed on the selection of qualified workers who could be developed for a particular job.

Gantt Henry I Gantt (1861–1910)

Gantt was concerned with problems related to efficiency. He contributed to scientific management by refining the previous work of Taylor than introducing new concepts.
1. He studied the amount of work planned or completed on one axis to the time needed or taken to complete a task on the other axis.
2. Gantt also developed a task and bonus remuneration plan whereby workers received a guaranteed day's wages plus a bonus for production above the standard to stimulate higher performance.
3. Gantt recommended to select workers scientifically and provided with detailed instructions for their tasks.
4. He argued for a more humanitarian approach by management, placing emphasis on service rather than profit objectives.
5. He recognized useful non-monetary incentives, such as job security and encouraging staff development.

Emerson (1853–1936)

His emphasis was on conservation and organizational goals and objectives. He defined principles of efficiency related to:
1. Interpersonal relations and to system in management.
2. Goals and ideas should be clear and well-defined as the primary objective is to produce the best product as quickly as possible at minimal expense.
3. Changes should be evaluated-management should not ignore-commonsensel by assuming that big is necessarily better.
4. Competent counsel is essential.

His theory explains about:
1. Management can strengthen discipline or adherence to the rules by justice, or equal enforcement on all records, including adequate, reliable and immediate information about the expenses of equipment and personnel should be available as a basis for decisions.
2. Dispatching or production scheduling is recommended.
3. Standardized schedules, conditions and written instructions should be there to facilitate performance.
4. Efficiency rewards-should be given for successful completion of tasks.
5. Emerson moved further beyond scientific management to classic organizational theory.

Charles Babbage (1792–1871)

Charles Babbage, a scientist mainly interested in mathematics, contributed to the management theory by developing the principles of cost accounting and the nature of relationship between various disciplines. Charles Babbage laid the foundation for much of the work that later come to be known as scientific management. He concentrated on production problems and stressed the importance.
1. Division and assignment of work on the basis of skill and
2. The means of determining the feasibility of replacing manual operations with automatic machinery.

CLASSIC ORGANIZATION THEORIES

1. Classic administration-organization thinking began to receive attention in 1930.
2. It viewed the organization as a whole rather than focusing solely on production, managerial activities and controlling.
3. The concepts of scalar levels, span of control, authority, responsibility, accountability, line-staff relationships, decentralization, and departmentalization became prevalent.

Importance of classic organization theory:
1. The classic administration-organization thinking began to receive attention in 1930.
2. Organization is viewed as whole rather than focusing solely in production.
3. The concepts of scalar levels, span of control, authority, responsibility, accountability, line staff relationships, decentralization, and departmentalization become prevalent.

Henry Fayol (1841–1925)

Fayol was a French industrialist known as father of the management process school concerned with management of production shops. He studied the functions of managers and concluded that management is universal.

Functions of management:
1. Planning policies, programs and procedures.
2. Organization based on hierarchy of authority
3. Directing the business in order to gain optimum return from all workers.
4. Coordination, signifying harmony in activities of the organization and to facilitate its working
5. Control, the errors of the functionaries of organization and ensure that such errors do not occurs.

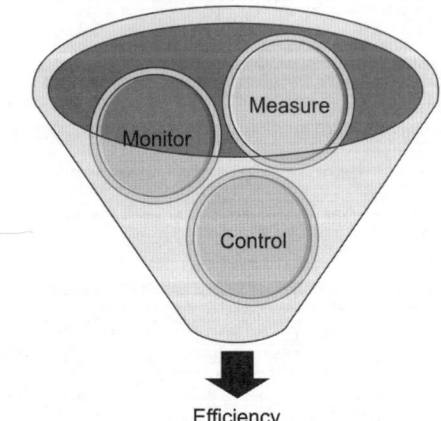

Fig. 2.5: Taylor's scientific management theory.

Table 2.8: Differences between classical and neo-classical approach.

Points of distinction	Classical approach	Neo-classical approach
Organizational focus	Functions and economic demand of workers	Emotion and human qualities of workers
Structure of organization	Impersonal and mechanistic	Social system
Application	Autocratic management and strict rules	Democratic process
Emphasis	Discipline and rationality	Personal security and social demand
Work goal of worker	Maximum remuneration and reward	Attainment of organizational goal
Concept about workers	Economic being	Social being
Content	Scientific management, administration and bureaucratic management	Hawthorne experiment, human relations movement and organizational
Relations in organization	Formal	Informal
Nature of organization	Mechanistic	Organistic

Fayol divided all the work carried out in a business enterprise into the following categories:
- Technical activities (production, manufacture, etc.)
- Commercial activities (buying, selling, personnel, and industrial relations)
- Financial activities (to have optimum use of capitals)
- Security activities (production of property and persons)
- Managerial activities (planning organizing, commanding, directing, coordination control, communication, motivation and leadership)

Principles by which good organization can be recognized. They are as follows:
- The number of organization units should be the minimum needed to cover the major enterprise functions.
- All related functions should be combined within one unit.
- The number of levels of authority should be kept to a minimum.
- There should be room for initiative with the limit of his assigned authority.
- Functions should be assigned so as to minimize cross relations between organizational units.
- No more employees should report to a superior than he can effectively direct and coordinate.

Max Webber Theory (1864–1920)

He is German psychologist. He earned the title of father of organizational theory. His emphasis was on rules instead of individuals and on competencies over favoritism. His conceptualization was on bureaucracy, structure of authority that would facilitate the accomplishment of organizational objectives:

The three bases for authority:
1. **Traditional authority**, which is accepted because it seems things have always been that way, such as the rule of a king in a monarchy.
2. **Charisma**, having a strong influential personality.
3. **Rational legal authority** which is considered rational in formal organizations because the person has demonstrated the knowledge, skills and ability to fulfill the position.

Figure 2.6 shows classical theory of authority.

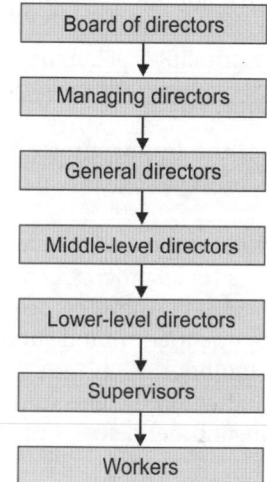

Fig. 2.6: Classical theory of authority.

James Mooney Theory (1884–1957)

Moony believed that management to be the technique of directing people and organization the technique of relating functions. Organization is management's responsibility.

Four universal principles:
1. Coordination and synchronization of activities for the accomplishment of goal.
2. Functional affects the performance of one's job description.
3. Scalar process organizes level of commands.
4. Arrange authority in to a higher Archie.

Consequently people get their right to command from their position in the organization.

■ HUMAN RELATIONS THEORIES

- The human relations movement began in the 1940s with attention focused on the effect individuals have on the success or failure of an organization.
- The chief concerns of the human relations movement are individuals, group process, interpersonal relations, leadership, and communication.
- Instead of concentrating on the organization's structure, managers encourage workers Instead of concentrating

> **Box 2.2:** Principles of human relations theory.
>
> - Human relations theory is characterized by a shift in emphasis from task to worker
> - Go beyond physical contributions to include creative, cognitive, and emotional aspects of workers
> - Based on a more dyadic (two-way) conceptualization of communication.
> - Social relationships are at the heart of organizational behavior-effectiveness is contingent on the social well-being of workers
> - Workers communicate opinions, complaints, suggestions, and feelings to increase satisfaction and production
> - Origins (Hawthorne Studies and work of Chester Barnard)
> - Human Relations School of Management—Elton Mayo (Harvard

on the organization's structure, managers encourage workers to develop their potential and help them meet their needs for recognition, accomplishment, and sense of belonging.

Box 2.2 summarize principles of human relation theory.

Follett Theory (1868–1933)

- Follett stressed the importance of coordinating the psychological and sociological aspects of management in 1920s.
- She perceived the organization's a social system and management as a social process.
- Indicated that legitimate power is produced by a circular behavior where by superiors and subordinates mutually influence one another.
- The law of the situation dictates that a person does not take orders from another person but from the situation.

Lewin Kurt Lewin (1890–1947)

- Lewin focused on the study of group dynamics.
- Lewin maintained that groups have personalities of their own: composites of the members' personalities.
- He showed that group forces can overcome individual interests.
- Lewin advocated democratic supervision.
- His research indicated that democratic groups in which participants solve their own problems and have the opportunity to consult with the leader are most effective.
- Autocratic leadership, on the other hand, tends to promote hostility and aggression or apathy and to decrease initiative.

THEORIES BASED ON BEHAVIORAL SCIENCES

- Behavioral science emphasized the use of scientific procedures to study the psychological, sociological, and anthropological aspects of human behavior in organizations.
- Behavioral scientists indicated the importance of maintaining a positive attitude toward people, training managers, fitting supervisory action to the situation, meeting employees' needs, promoting employees' sense of achievement, and obtaining commitment through participation in planning and decision making.

Emphasis is on:
- Use of scientific procedures to study the psychological
- Sociological
- Anthropological aspects of human behavior in organization.

Behavioral science indicated:
- The importance of maintaining a positive attitude toward people
- Training managers
- Fitting supervisory actions to the situation

McGregor Douglas

McGregor (1932) developed the managerial implications of Maslow's theory.

- He noted that one's style of management is dependent on one's philosophy of humans and categorized those assumptions as Theory X and Theory Y (**Fig. 2.7**).
- In Theory X, the manager's emphasis is on the goal of the organization. The theory assumes that people dislike work and will avoid it; consequently, workers must be directed, controlled, coerced, and threatened so that organizational goals can be met.

According to Theory X:
- Most people want to be directed and to avoid responsibility because they have little ambition.
- They desire security.
- Managers who accept the assumptions of Theory X will do the thinking and planning with little input from staff associates.
- They will delegate little, supervise closely, and motivate workers through fear and threats, failing to make use of their potentials.

In Theory Y, the emphasis is on the goal of the individual:
It is the manager's assumption that people do not inherently dislike work and that work can be a source of satisfaction. Theory Y managers assume:

- That workers have the self-direction and self-control necessary for meeting their objectives and will respond to rewards for the accomplishment of those goals.
- They believe that under favorable conditions, people seek responsibility and display imagination, ingenuity, and creativity.
- They will delegate, give general rather than close supervision, support job enlargement, and use positive incentives such as praise and recognition.

Figure 2.8 shows comparison between Theory X and Theory Y.

Rensis Likert's Theory

Dr Rensis Likert has studied human behavior within many organizations. After extensive research, Dr Rensis Likert concluded that there are four systems of management. According to Likert, the efficiency of an organization or its departments is influenced by their system of management. His theory of management is based on his work at the University of Michigan's institute for social research. Likert categorized

Chapter 2: Principles and Theories of Management

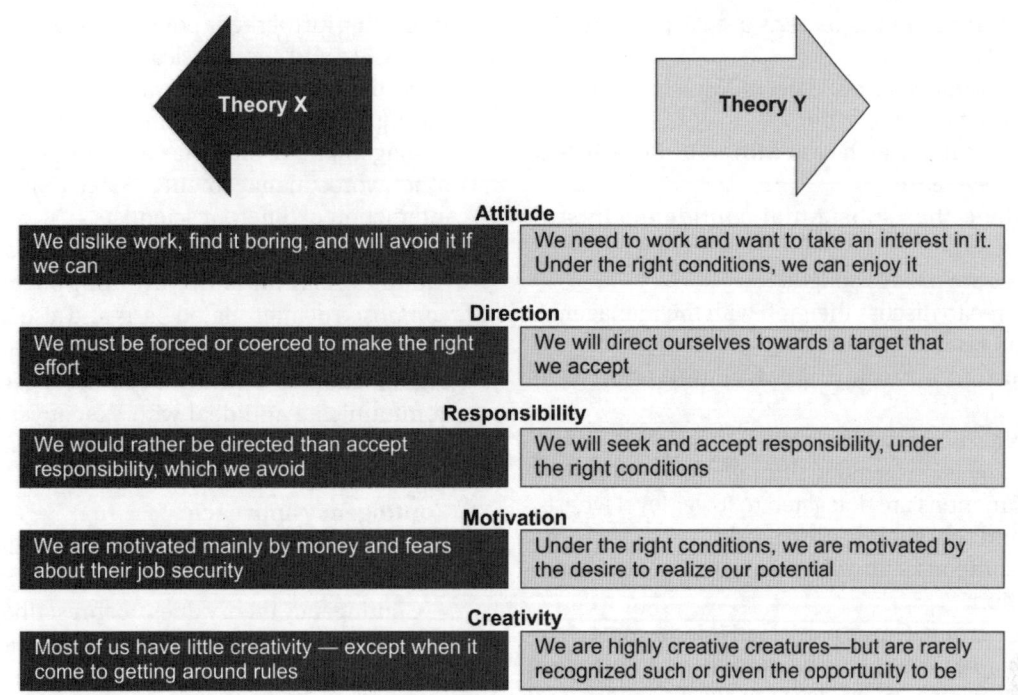

Fig. 2.7: Theory X and Theory Y.

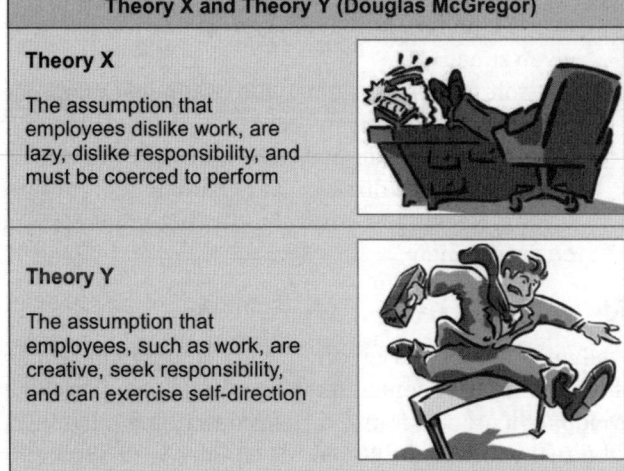

Fig. 2.8: Comparison between Theory X and Theory Y.

Exploitative-authoritative
The leader impose decision on subordinates and uses fear to achieve employee motivation

Benevolent-authoritative
The leader uses rewards to encourage productivity, but management is responsible for all decisions and there is no teamwork

Consultative
The leader listens to subordinates and incorporates some employee ideas, but most subordinates do not feel responsible for the organization's goals

Participative
The leader engages subordinates, solves problems with teamwork, and everyone feels responsible for achieving the organization's goals

Fig. 2.9: The four systems of management—Rensis Likert.

his four management systems as follows; He identified three variables in organizations.

1. The casual variable includes leadership behavior.
2. The intervening variables are perceptions, attitudes and motivations.
3. The end results variables are measures of profits, costs and productivity.

Factors measured by Likert scale: The scale measures several factors related to leadership behavior process:
- Motivation
- Managerial
- Communication
- Decision making process
- Goal setting
- Staff development

Four types of management system according to Likert effects on the management systems **(Fig. 2.9)**:

1. **Exploitive-authoritative:**
   - He associates the first system with the least effective in performance.
   - Managers show less confidence in staff associates and ignore their ideas.
   - Consequently staff associates do not feel free to discuss their jobs with their managers
2. **Benevolent-authoritative:**
   - Staff associates ideas are sometimes sought, but they do not feel free to discuss their jobs with the manager.

- Top and middle management are responsible for setting goals.
- There is minimal communication. Mostly downward and received with suspicion.
- Decisions are made at the top with some delegation.

3. **Consultative system:**
   - The manager has substantial confidence in staff associates.
   - Their ideas are usually sought.
   - They fell free to discuss their job with the manager.
   - Goal setting is fairly general.
   - It has limited accuracy and accepted with some caution.
   - Broad policy is set at the top level.
   - There are decisions making throughout organization.
   - Control functions are delegated to lower level where.
   - Reward and self-guidance are used.
   - There is some resistance from informal groups in the organization.

4. **Participative group:** Group participative is the most effective performance. Managers have complete confidence in their staff associates. Their ideas are always sought, and they feel completely free to discuss their jobs with the manager. Goals are set at all levels. There is a great deal communication—upward, downward, and later that is accurate and received with open mind.

MODERN MANAGEMENT THEORIES

The modern era is characterized by trends in the management through viz:
1. Microanalysis of human behavior, motivation, group dynamics leadership leading to many theories of organization.
2. The macro search for fusion of the many systems in business organization—economic social technical political and quantitative methods in decision-making. Modern management theories era can be further classified as the three streams viz:
   - Quantitative approach
   - System approach
   - Contingency approach

Indicating further refinement, extension and synthesis of all the classical and neo-classical approaches to management.

1. **Quantitative approach:** Management science refers to the application of quantitative methods to management. Management science has an interdisciplinary basis in other words management science is a combination and interaction of different scientists.
2. **System approach:** According to system approach the organization is the unified, purposeful systems composed of interrelated parts and also interrelated with its environment. Each unit must mesh/interact with the organization as a whole, each manager most interact/communicate and deal with executives of other unites and the organization itself must also interact with other organizations and society as whole.
3. **Contingency approach:**
   - The contingency approach can be described as the behavioral approach.
   - Contingency theory does not prescribe the application of certain management principles to any situation.
   - Contingency theory is recognition of the extreme importance of individual manager performance in any given situation.
   - It rests on the extent of manager power and control over a situation and the degree of uncertainty in any given situation.
   - The role of management in the contingency approach is to develop an appropriate management solution for any given organizational environment.
   - It is principally directed at the management practitioner seeking to control a distinct organizational environment.

Ludwig von Bertalanffy

Bertalanffy, biology is credited with coining the general system theory. His contention were that it was possible to develop a theoretical framework for describing relationship in the real world and different disciplines with similarities could be developed into a general systems model (**Fig. 2.10**). The similarities were:
- Study of organization

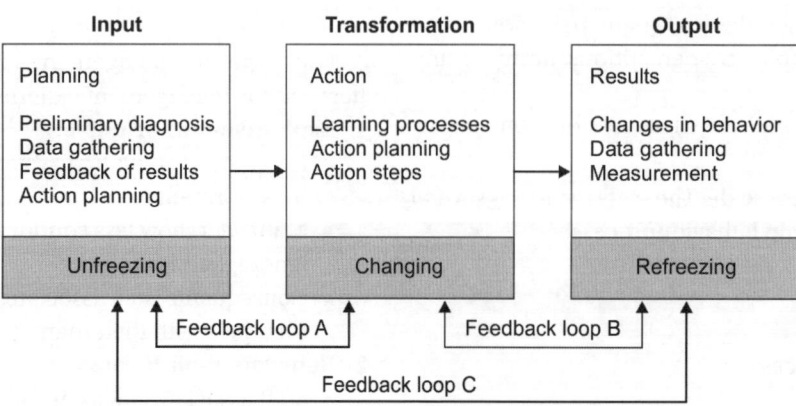

Fig. 2.10: Ludwig von bertalanffy system theory.

- State of equilibrium
- Openness of all systems and their influence on the environment and environment influence on the system.

Luther Gulick

He was influenced by Taylor and Fayol. He used Fayal's five elements of administration viz. Planning, Organizing, Command, Coordination and Control as a framework for his neutral principles. He condensed the duties of administration into a famous acronym: POSDCORB. Each letter in the acronym stands for one of the seven activities of the administrator as given below **(Box 2.3 and Fig. 2.11)**:

1. **Planning (P):** Working out the things that need to be done and the methods for doing them to accomplish the purpose set for the enterprise.
2. **Organizing (O):** Establishment of the formal structure of authority through which work subdivisions are arranged, designed and coordinated for the defined objective.
3. **Staffing (S):** The whole personnel function of bringing in and training the staff, and maintaining favorable conditions of work.
4. **Directing (D):** Continuous task of making decisions and embodying them in specific and general orders and instructions, and serving as the leader of the enterprise.
5. **Coordinating (CO):** all important duties of inter-relating the various parts of the work.
6. **Reporting (R):** Keeping the executive informed as to what is going on, which includes keeping himself and his subordinates informed through records, research and inspection.
7. **Budgeting (B):** All that goes with budgeting in the form of fiscal planning, accounting and control.

> **Box 2.3:** Luther Gulick POSDCORB (1892–1993).
> - His seven-activities acronym, POSDCORB, is a familiar word throughout management practice.
> - Planning, Organizing, Staffing, Directing, Coordinating, Reporting and Budgeting.
> - Concept of Span of control, which addressed the factors limiting the number of people a manager could supervise.
> - Homogeneity of work centered that an organization should not combine dissimilar activities in single agency.
> - In a time where the prevalent theme was the separation of politics and administration, Gulick advocated that it was impossible to separate the two.

Luther Gulick was very much influenced by Fayal's 14 basic elements of administration in expressing his principles of administration as follows:
1. Davison of work or specialization
2. Bases of departmental organization
3. Coordination though hierarchy
4. Deliberate coordination
5. Decentralization
6. Unity of command
7. Staff and line
8. Delegation
9. Span of control

Lyndall Urwick

Lyndall Urwick also one of the classical theorist, attached more important to the structure of organization than the role of the people in the organization. Lyndall Urwick concentrated his efforts on the discovery of principles and identified eight principles of administration applicable to all organization as given below:

1. The principle of objective—that all organizations should be an expression of a purpose.
2. The principle of correspondence—that authority and responsibility must be co-equal.
3. The principle of responsibility—that the responsibility of higher authorities of the work of subordinates is absolute.
4. The scalar principle—that a paramedical type of structure is build up in an.
5. The principle of span control
6. The principle of specialization—limiting ones works to single function.
7. The principle of coordination
8. The principle of definition—clear prescribed of every duty.

Figure 2.12 shows principles of critical thinking.

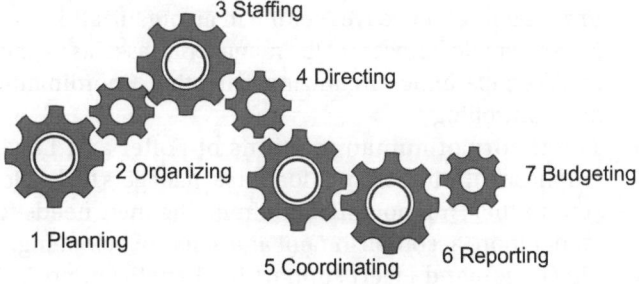

Fig. 2.11: POSDCORB cycle.

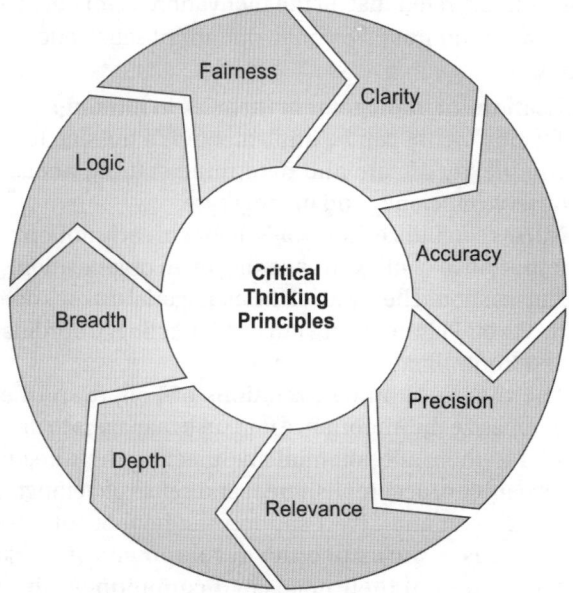

Fig. 2.12: Principles of critical thinking.

Critical Theory versus Critical Thinking

Steffy and Grimes note that a strict natural science approach to social science is native, since subjective or qualitative analysis is important to quantitative research. This holds true for management and, consequently for nursing management. The authors suggest a critical theory approach to organizational science rather than a phenomenological or hermeneutic approach. Phenomenological approach uses second order constructs—interpretations of interpretation. The nurse manager would interpret the meaning of nursing of nursing management experience or observations and arrive at a nursing management theory from aggregate of meanings.

Douglas McGregor (1906–1964)

1. McGregor is the other major theorist associated with the Human Relations School of management.
2. McGregor believes there are two basic kinds of managers. One type of manager, Theory X, has a negative view of employees assuming they are lazy, untrustworthy and incapable of assuming responsibility while the other type of manager
3. Theory Y, assumes employees are trustworthy and capable of assuming responsibility having high levels of motivation.

Herzberg's Two Factor Theory

This theory was developed in 1959. It is based on realization that work motivation and job-satisfaction are two dimensions that influence the productivity of an employee. Herzberg's finding that good working conditions, adequate salary, good physical facilities, good human relation, quality of supervision might contribute to job satisfaction, of employees, which are hygiene factors. Whereas factors, such as recognition of work done, status, opportunities for growth, challenging task, play an important role in creating work motivation for employees, which are the motivation factors. Later, many authors interpreted that all the motivation factors described by Herzberg do not give equal amount of satisfaction to all employees.

Implications of management theories in nursing:
- Taylor's theory can be implemented in nursing to study complexity of care and determine staffing needs and observe efficiency and nursing care.
- Nurses can utilize Emerson's theory of early notion of the importance of objectives setting in an organization.
- Nurses should be aware of the managerial tasks as defined by Fayol: Planning, Organizing, Directing, Coordinating and Controlling.
- The theory of human relations of Follett and Lewin emphasize the importance for nurse managers to develop staff to their full potential and meeting their needs for recognition, accomplishment and sense of belonging.
- Mc Gregon and Likert support the benefits of positive attitudes towards people, development of workers, satisfaction of their needs and commitment through participation.

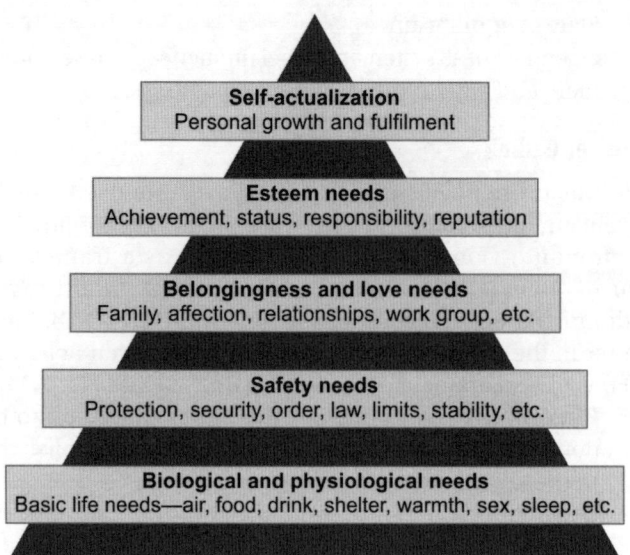

Fig. 2.13: Maslow's needs theory of human needs.

Maslow's Needs Theory (Fig. 2.13)

Maslow's hierarchy of needs is a theory about what sorts of things motivate us as human beings and what sorts of needs we have. Maslow presents a hierarchy of needs in which each level of need must be fulfilled before the individual can think about achieving goals at the next level. Maslow's hierarchy is particularly important for educators.

According to Maslow, the levels of the hierarchy are:

1. **Physiological needs:** These are things we need for physical survival like food, water, and shelter.
2. **Safety needs:** This is our need to feel that we are secure and that our world is stable.
3. **Love and belonging needs:** These are our needs to feel that we belong and are accepted. We need to love and be loved.
4. **Esteem needs:** We need to feel that other people respect us.
5. **Self-actualization needs:** This is our need to reach our full potential as people.

IMPLICATIONS OF MANAGEMENT THEORIES IN NURSING

- Taylor and Gilbreth theories can be replicated in nursing to study complexity of care and determine staffing needs and observe efficiency and nursing care.
- Nurses can utilize Emerson's early notion of the importance of objectives setting in an organization.
- Nurses should be aware of the managerial tasks' as defined by Fayol: Planning, Organizing, Directing, Coordinating, and controlling
- The theory of human relations of Follet and Lewin emphasize the importance for nurse managers to develop staff to their full potential and meeting their needs for recognition, accomplishment and sense of belonging.
- Mc Gregon and Likert support the benefits of positive attitudes towards people, development of workers,

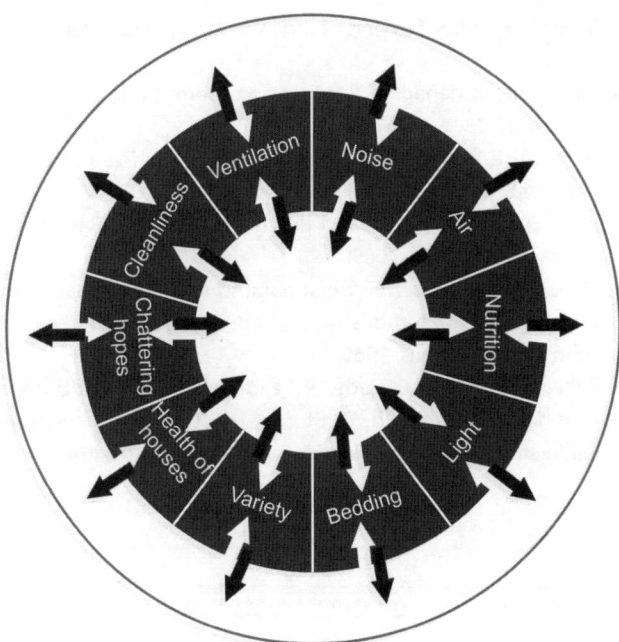

Fig. 2.14: Conceptual framework of Florence Nightingale's environmental theory.

satisfaction of their needs, and commitment through participation.
- Overall, study of the development of management, potential nurse leaders can define the management role, develop leadership style, learn managerial technique and give an insight to how to work with others to accomplish goals.

Figure 2.14 shows conceptual framework of Florence Nightingale's environmental theory.

Application of Maslow's theory in nursing practice:
- **Physiologic needs oxygen:** Evaluate oxygen needs by assessing skin color, vital signs, anxiety levels, responses to activity, and mental responsiveness.
- **Physiologic needs intake and elimination:** Intake and elimination of fluids: measure intake and output, testing the resiliency of the skin, checking the condition of the skin and mucous membranes, and weighing the patient helps assess water balance.
- **Physiologic needs food:** Assessing nutritional status with a variety of indicators, including weight, muscle mass, strength, and laboratory values.
- **Physiologic needs temperature:** Assess as a vital sign
- **Physiologic needs sexuality:** Person's age, sociocultural background, self-esteem, and level of health.
- **Physiologic needs physical:** Physical: intact and functioning neuromuscular and skeletal systems. Rest and sleep age, environment, exercise, stress and drug use.
- **Safety and security needs physical:** Involve both physical and emotional.
  Being protected from potential and actual harm. Physical: Proper hand washing and sterile techniques to prevent infection, use electrical equipment properly, administering medications knowledgeable, teaching parents about dangerous chemicals.
- **Safety and security needs emotional:** Involve both physical and emotional.
- **Being protected from potential and actual harm. Emotional:** Encouraging spiritual practices, allowing as much independent decision making and control as possible, and carefully explaining new and unfamiliar procedures and treatments.
- **Love and belonging needs:** Nurses should always consider this when developing a plan of care. Include family and friends in the care of the patient, establish a nurse-patient relationship based on mutual understanding and trust (demonstrate caring, encouraging communication, and respecting privacy), referring patients t specific support groups.
- **Self-esteem needs:** Changes of a job, death of spouse, body image affect self-esteem. The person's perception of the change rather that the actual change is what affects that individual's self-esteem. Respecting patients values and beliefs, encouraging patients to set attainable goals, and facilitating support form family or significant others.
- **Self-actualization needs:** Acceptance of self and others as they are, focus of interest on problems outside oneself, ability to be objective, feeling of happiness and affection for others, respect for all people, ability to discriminate between good and evil, uses creativity for solving problems and pursuing interest.

CONCLUSION

A managerial principle is a broad and general guideline for decision-making and behavior. For example while deciding about promotion of an employee one manager may consider seniority, whereas the other may follow the principle of merit. One may distinguish principles of management from those of pure science. Management principles are not as rigid as principles of pure science. They deal with human behavior and, thus, are to be applied creatively given the demands of the situation. Human behavior is never static and so also technology, which affects business. Hence all the principles have to keep pace with these changes.

REVIEW QUESTIONS

Long Essays
1. Define management; explain the 14 Principles of Management described by Henry Fayol.
2. Describe classical organization theories.
3. Discuss Maslow's needs theory; explain the application of Maslow's theory in nursing practice.

Short Essays
1. Elements of management process.
2. Scientific management theories.
3. Human relations theories.
4. Theories based on behavioral sciences.
5. Herzberg's two factor theory.
6. Implications of management theories in nursing.

Short Answers

1. Management process.
2. Unity of direction.
3. Scalar chain.
4. Esprit De Corps.
5. Centralization and Decentralization.
6. POSDCORB.
7. Self-actualization.

BIBLIOGRAPHY

1. Bertalanffy L von. 'Problems of General Systems Theory: A New Approach to the Unity of Science'. Hum Biol. 1951;23 (4):302-12.
2. Mayo E. 'The human problems of an industrial civilization' New York: Macmillan; 1933.
3. Miller EJ, Rice A. K 'Systems of Organisation', Tavistock Publications; 1967.
4. Mintzberg H. Managing. San Francisco, Berrett-Kohler Publishers. 2009; p. 26-28.
5. Northouse PG. Leadership: theory and practice. 4th edition. Thousand Oaks, CA: Sage Publications; 2007.
6. Price D. The Principles and Practice of Change, Basingstoke: Palgrave Macmillan; 2009.
7. Schein EH, Bennis WG. 'Personal and Organizational change through Group Methods: The laboratory approach'. New York: John Wiley and Sons; 1965.
8. Zaccaro SJ, Kemp C, Bader P. Leader traits and attributes. In: Antonakis J, Cianciolo AT, Sternberg RJ (Eds). The nature of leadership. Thousand Oaks, CA: Sage; 2004. pp.101-124.

CHAPTER 3

Functions and Factors of Management

Learning Objectives

- Elements of Management Process
- Classifications of Management Function
- Functions of Management
- POSDCORB
- Management Needs Resources
- Factors Affecting on Management
- Environmental Factors Affecting Management
- Factors Affecting Financial Management

INTRODUCTION

Management has been described as a social process involving responsibility for economical and effective planning and regulation of operation of an enterprise in the fulfillment of given purposes. It is a dynamic process consisting of various elements and activities. These activities are different from operative functions, such as marketing, finance, purchase, etc. Rather these activities are common to each and every manager irrespective of his level or status. Effective management and leadership involve creative problem solving, motivating employees and making sure the organization accomplishes objectives and goals. There are five functions of management and leadership: planning, organizing, staffing, coordinating and controlling (**Fig. 3.1**). These functions separate the management process from other business functions, such as marketing, accounting and finance.

ELEMENTS OF MANAGEMENT PROCESS

Planning

- Planning is the primary function of management. It involves determination of a course of action to achieve desired results/objectives.
- Planning is the starting point of management process and all other functions of management are related to and dependent on planning function.
- Planning is the key to success, stability and prosperity in business. It acts as a tool for solving the problems of a business unit.
- Planning plays a pivotal role in business management It helps to visualize the future problems and keeps management ready with possible solutions.

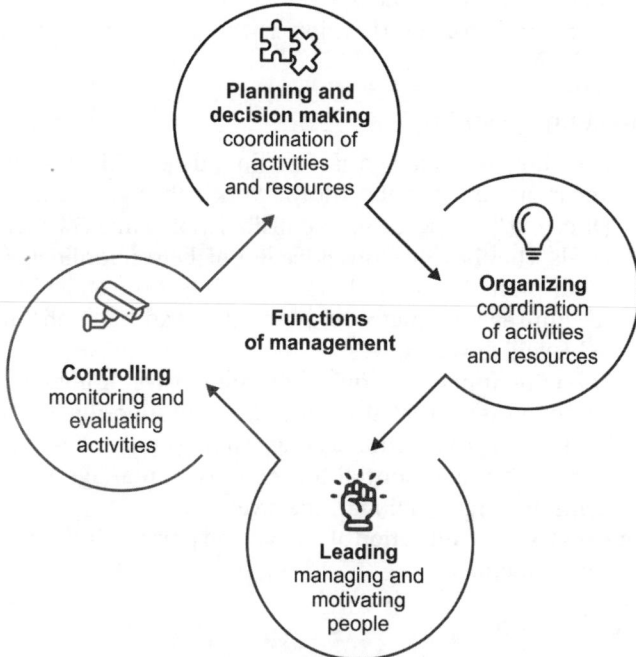

Fig. 3.1: Functions of management.

Organizing

- Organizing is next to planning. It means to bring the resources (men, materials, machines, etc.) together and use them properly for achieving the objectives. Organization is a process as well as it is a structure.
- Organizing means arranging ways and means for the execution of a business plan.
- It provides suitable administrative structure and facilitates execution of proposed plan.

- Organizing involves different aspects, such as departmentation, span of control delegation of authority, establishment of superior-subordinate relationship and provision of mechanism for coordination of various business activities.

Staffing

- Staffing refers to manpower required for the execution of a business plan.
- Staffing, as managerial function, involves recruitment, selection, appraisal, remuneration and development of managerial personnel.
- The need of staffing arises in the initial period and also from time to time for replacement and also along with the expansion and diversification of business activities.
- Every business unit needs efficient, stable and cooperative staff for the management of business activities.
- Manpower is the most important asset of a business unit. In many organizations, manpower planning and development activities are entrusted to personnel manager or HRD manager.
- 'Right man for the right job' is the basic principle in staffing.

Directing (Leading)

- Directing as a managerial function, deals with guiding and instructing people to do the work in the right manner.
- Directing/leading is the responsibility of managers at all levels. They have to work as leaders of their subordinates.
- Clear plans and sound organization set the stage but it requires a manager to direct and lead his men for achieving the objectives.
- Directing function is quite comprehensive. It involves Directing as well as raising the morale of subordinates.
- It also involves communicating, leading and motivating. Leadership is essential on the part of managers for achieving organizational objectives.

Figure 3.2 shows utilization of human and physical resources by management.

Coordinating

- Effective coordination and also integration of activities of different departments are essential for orderly working of an Organization. This suggests the importance of coordinating as management function.
- A manager must coordinate the work for which he is accountable. Coordination is rightly treated as the essence of management.

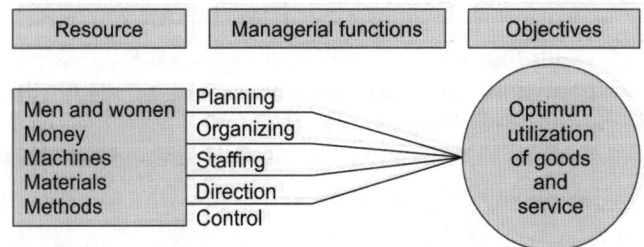

Fig. 3.2: Utilization of human and physical resources by management.

- It may be treated as an independent function or as a part of organisms function. Coordination is essential at all levels of management.
- It gives one clear-cut direction to the activities of individuals and departments.
- It also avoids misdirection and wastages and brings unity of action in the organization.
- Coordination will not come automatically or on its own special efforts are necessary on the part of managers for achieving such coordination.

Controlling

Controlling is an important function of management. It is necessary in the case of individuals and departments so as to avoid wrong actions and activities. Controlling involves three broad aspects:

1. Establishing standards of performance,
2. Measuring work in progress and interpreting results achieved, and
3. Taking corrective actions, if required.

Business plans do not give positive results automatically. Managers have to exercise effective control in order to bring success to a business plan. Control is closely linked with other managerial functions. It is rightly treated as the soul of management process. It is true that without planning there will be nothing to control. It is equally true that without control planning will be only an academic exercise. Controlling is a continuous activity of a supervisory nature.

Motivating

- Motivating is one managerial function in which a manager motivates his men to give their best to the organization.
- It means to encourage people to take more interest and initiative in the work assigned.
- Organizations prosper when the employees are motivated through special efforts including provision of facilities and incentives.
- Motivation is actually inspiring and encouraging people to work more and contribute more to achieve organizational objectives. It is a psychological process of great significance.

Communicating

- Communication (written or oral) is necessary for the exchange of facts, opinions, ideas and information between individual's and departments.
- In an organization, communication is useful for giving information, guidance and instructions.
- Managers should be good communicators. They have to use major portion of their time on communication in order to direct, motivate and coordinate activities of their subordinates.
- People think and act collectively through communication. According to Louis Allen, "Communication involves a systematic and continuing process of telling, listening and understanding".

CLASSIFICATIONS OF MANAGEMENT FUNCTION (FIG. 3.3)

Different experts have classified functions of management. According to George and Jerry, "There are four fundamental functions of management, i.e., planning, organizing, actuating and controlling". According to Henry Fayol, "To manage is to forecast and plan, to organize, to command, and to control". Whereas Luther Gulick has given a keyword 'POSDCORB' where P stands for Planning, O for Organizing, S for Staffing, D for Directing, Co for Coordination, R for Reporting and B for Budgeting. But the most widely accepted are functions of management given by KOONTZ and O'DONNEL, i.e., Planning, Organizing, Staffing, Directing and Controlling. For theoretical purposes, it may be convenient to separate the function of management but practically these functions are overlapping in nature, i.e., they are highly inseparable. Each function blends into the other and each affects the performance of others.

FUNCTIONS OF MANAGEMENT

The basic management functions that make up the management process are described in the following sections (Fig. 3.4):

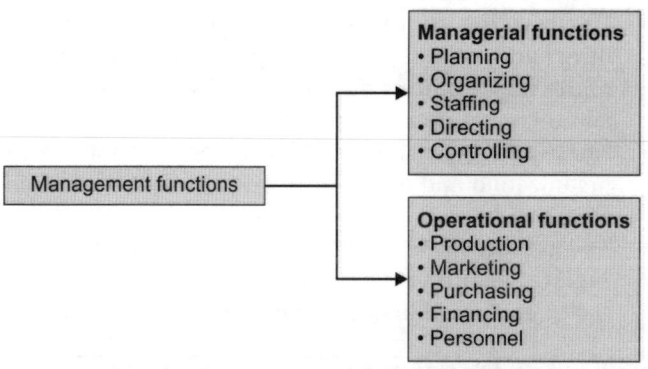

Fig. 3.3: Classifications of management functions.

Planning
- The planning function of management controls all the planning that allows the organization to run smoothly.
- Planning involves defining a goal and determining the most effective course of action needed to reach that goal.
- Typically, planning involves flexibility, as the planner must coordinate with all levels of management and leadership in the organization.
- Planning also involves knowledge of the company's resources and the future objectives of the business.

Organizing
- The organizing function of leadership controls the overall structure of the company.
- The organizational structure is the foundation of a company; without this structure, the day-to-day operation of the business becomes difficult and unsuccessful.
- Organizing involves designating tasks and responsibilities to employees with the specific skill sets needed to complete the tasks.
- Organizing also involves developing the organizational structure and chain of command within the company.

Staffing
- The staffing function of management controls all recruitment and personnel needs of the organization.
- The main purpose of staffing is to hire the right people for the right jobs to achieve the objectives of the organization.
- Staffing involves more than just recruitment; staffing also encompasses training and development, performance appraisals, promotions and transfers.
- Without the staffing function, the business would fail because the business would not be properly staffed to meet its goals.

Coordinating
- The coordinating function of leadership controls all the organizing, planning and staffing activities of the

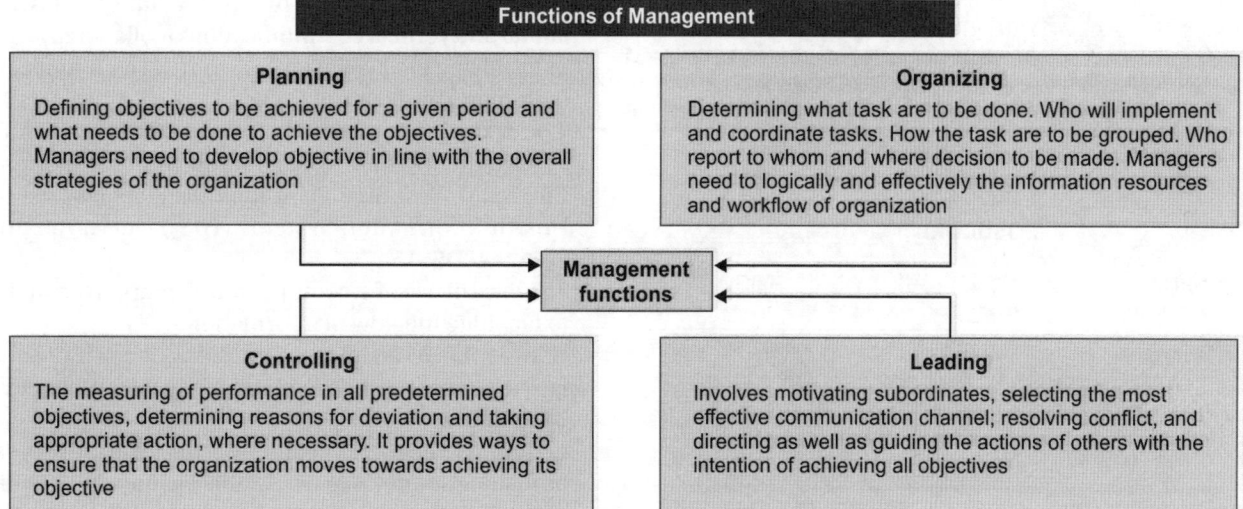

Fig. 3.4: Types of management functions.

company and ensures all activities function together for the good of the organization.
- Coordinating typically takes place in meetings and other planning sessions with the department heads of the company to ensure all departments are on the same page in terms of objectives and goals.
- Coordinating involves communication, supervision and direction by management.

Controlling

- The controlling function of management is useful for ensuring all other functions of the organization are in place and are operating successfully.
- Controlling involves establishing performance standards and monitoring the output of employees to ensure each employee's performance meets those standards.
- The controlling process often leads to the identification of situations and problems that need to be addressed by creating new performance standards.
- The level of performance affects the success of all aspects of the organization.

■ POSDCORB

In 1937, L Urwick and Luther Gulick delineate seven "major activities and responsibilities of any chief executive". By then, the term POSDCORB is employed to delineate the 7 operates of managers: This essentially refers to the various steps or stages involved in a typical administrative process. POSDCORB stands for **(Fig. 3.5)**:

1. **Planning:** This essentially refers to establishing a broad sketch of the work to be completed and the procedures incorporated to implement them.
2. **Organizing:** Organizing involves formally classifying, defining and synchronizing the various sub-processes or subdivisions of the work to be done.
3. **Staffing:** This involves recruiting and selecting the right candidates for the job and facilitating their orientation and training while maintaining a favorable work environment.
4. **Directing:** This entails decision making and delegating structured instructions and orders to execute them.
5. **Coordinating:** This basically refers to orchestrating and interlinking the various components of the work.
6. **Reporting:** Reporting involves regularly updating the superior about the progress or the work related activities. The information dissemination can be through records or inspection.
7. **Budgeting:** Budgeting involves all the activities that under Auditing, Accounting, Fiscal Planning and Control.

■ MANAGEMENT NEEDS RESOURCES

- **The director of nursing resource management:** This individual directs the management of the staffing and payroll functions, nursing supervisors, and the nurse manager of the organization.
- **The staffing and payroll office:** This office is responsible for providing support to the inpatient nursing units and the emergency department for scheduling, staffing and payroll. Its responsibilities include daily staffing, maintaining scheduling changes.
- **The nursing supervisors:** The nursing supervisors direct and evaluate nursing care and related activities of the nursing units on the off-shifts and serve as the administrative resource person within the hospital.
- **Nurse manager:** This individual manages the staff of the organization and the 24-hour operations of the holding areas.
- **The nursing staff:** is comprised of the following positions: registered nurse certified nursing assistants, unit secretaries, and nursing service aides.

■ FACTORS AFFECTING ON MANAGEMENT

- The degree to which management's decision making style affects information flow by making full use of two-way lateral and vertical communications (collaborative styles) or by relying mostly on one-way vertical communications (command and control styles).
- The types of technology used in the performance management system to generate and process information: Enterprise Resource Planning (ERP), specialized tools, Health Information Systems (HIS), Decision Support Systems (DSS).
- The level of use of e-commerce and Internet technologies to facilitate the flow of information.
- **Competition:** Healthcare setting that do not jump quickly into a promising service market may be outmaneuvered by their competitors.
- **Economy:** The overall economy or health of the company's industry also may negatively affect a manager's ability to plan. When sudden downturns occur, planning must be stopped, adjusted or taken in a new direction.

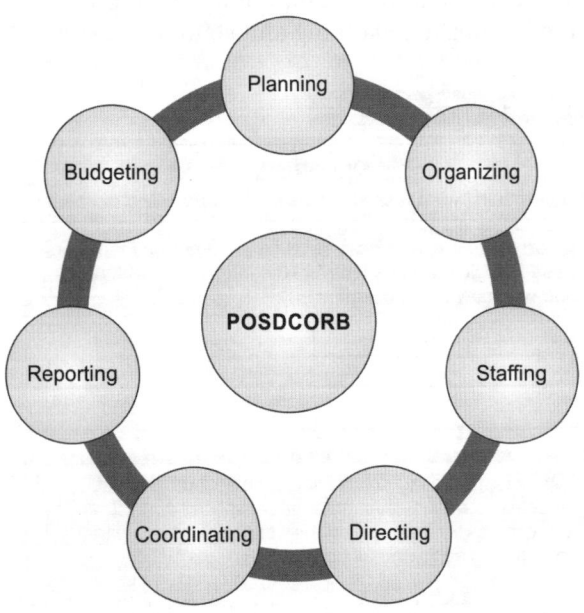

Fig. 3.5: Managerial functions by POSDCORB.

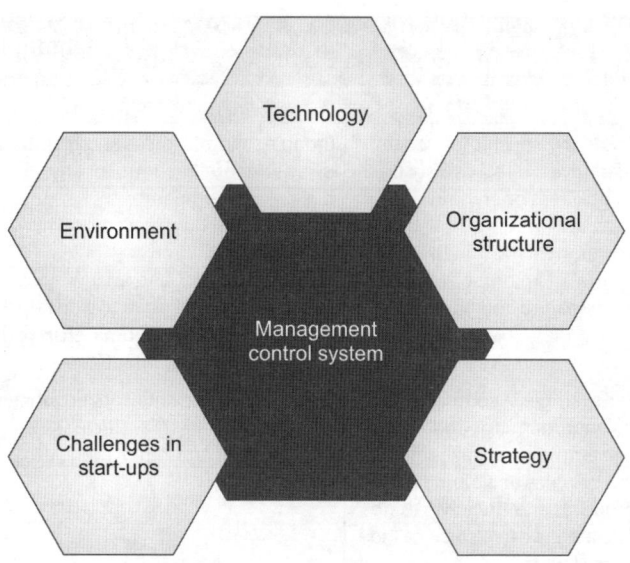

Fig. 3.6: Management control system.

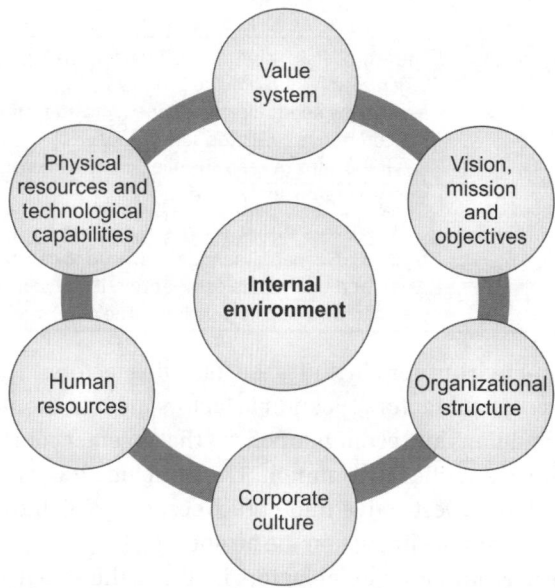

Fig. 3.7: Internal environmental factors affecting management.

Managers must be flexible to changing outside economic conditions even when they are in the midst of planning a project of special interest to them.
- **Managers:** Managers themselves also affect their own planning function. If they are not good planners in general or do not have the experience, education or background in planning required to be successful, they are more likely to plan poorly
- **Information:** When planning occurs, it is vital to have accurate information from consumers, the market, the economy, competitors and other sources.

Figure 3.6 shows management control system.

ENVIRONMENTAL FACTORS AFFECTING MANAGEMENT

Managers who do not have accurate and timely information are more likely to plan poorly and inadequately. The different environmental factors that affect the business can be broadly categorized as internal and has its own external factors.

Internal Factors

Internal factors are those factors which exist within the premises of an organization and directly affect the different operations carried out in a business. These internal factors are **(Fig. 3.7)**:
- **Value system:** It implies the culture and norms of the business. In other words, it means the regulatory framework of a business and every member of the organization has to act within the limits of this framework.
- **Mission and objectives:** Different priorities, policies and philosophies of a business is guided by the mission and objectives of a business.
- **Financial factors:** Financial factors, such as financial policies, financial position and capital structure also affect a business performance and its strategies.
- **Internal relationship:** Factors, such as the amount of support the top management enjoys from its shareholders, employees and the board of directors also affects the smooth functioning of a business.

External Factors

The external factors include all those factors which exists outside the firm and are often regarded as uncontrollable. These external forces can further be categorized as micro-environment and macro-environment.

Micro-environment includes the following factors:
- **Suppliers:** Suppliers are those people who are responsible for supplying necessary inputs to the organization and ensure the smooth flow of production.
- **Competitors:** Competitors can be called the close rivals and in order to survive the competition one has to keep a close look in the market and formulate its policies and strategies as such to face the competition.
- **Marketing intermediaries:** Marketing intermediaries aid the company in promoting, selling and distribution of the goods and services to its final users.

Therefore, marketing intermediaries are vital link between the business and the consumers.

Following are some of the micro-environment factors:

Employees	Employees exert great influence on the organization. It is imperative to find the right people for each job. Organizations need to motivate employees positively and retain specialized talent.
Owners and the management	Investors are major influencers on a company's revenue and operations. It is important that the owners are satisfied with the company. It is the manager's job to balance the aims of the company and the owners.
Consumers	Competition and consumerism has rendered multiple alternatives for the same product in different brands. Organizations recognize that it is in their own interest to keep consumers happy.

Contd...

Contd...

Suppliers	The suppliers or contractors manage the inputs of organizations and provide products or services that a company needs directly or need it to add value to the company's own products or services. It is important to keep suppliers happy to ensure a smooth input supply system.
Competition	Competitors affect profits by trying to divert business. A capable manager will need to constantly study and analyze its competition if the company wants to maintain its position in the market.

Macro-environment includes the following factors:
- **Economic factors:** Economic factors include economic conditions and economic policies that together constitute the economic environment. These include growth rate, inflation, restrictive trade practices, etc. Which have a considerable impact on the business?
- **Social factors:** Social factors includes the society as a whole alongside its preferences and priorities, such as the buying and consumption pattern, beliefs of people their purchasing power, educational background, etc.
- **Political factors:** The political factors are related to the management of public affairs and their impact on the business. It is important to have a political stability to maintain stability in the trade.
- **Technological factors:** A latest technology helps in improving the marketability of the product plus makes it more consumers friendly. Therefore, it is important for a business to keep a pace with the changing technologies in order to survive in the long run.

Following are some of the macro-environment factors:

Political-legal environment	The country's unique political and legal landscape within which organizations function The effects of this are quite visible, e.g., the effect of changing taxes or raising interest rates
Technology	Companies have to carefully evaluate the technological developments that it wishes to embrace as it is a cost intensive factor and provide millions in return to one company and take millions from another
Socio-cultural environment	The means of communication, the country's infrastructure, its education system, the purchasing power of the citizens, family values, work ethics and preferences, etc.

Table 3.1 summarize comparison between microeconomic and macroeconomics factors and **Table 3.2** discuss internal and external factors influencing management decisions.

FACTORS AFFECTING FINANCIAL MANAGEMENT

The routine in financial management activities may be cumbersome for some corporate leaders, but these work streams help companies run efficient businesses. Functions, such as record keeping, financial reporting and fundraising help a firm ease its route to financial success. Factors affecting financial management include government regulations, the state of the economy, securities exchanges and borrowing costs.

Table 3.1: Comparison between microeconomic factors and macroeconomic factors.

Microeconomic factors	Macroeconomic factors
Company-specific influences that have a direct impact on its business operations and success. Components within the control of an organization can be managed and altered.	Broad economic forces and global events are out of control of any business or company. Forces indirectly affect company objectives Volatile and risky, and a savvy manager must be agile to sidestep a cascading macroeconomic crisis to keep the company intact
For example, a company's revenue, earnings and margin. The employees, stakeholders, the production volume of the products and the advertising campaigns can also be called micro factors	For example, the country's economic output, inflation, its political environment, unemployment, etc.

Table 3.2: Internal and external factors influencing financial management decisions.

Internal factors	External factors
• Size of the firm • Nature of business • The legal forms of business organizations • Situation of business cycle • Assets structure • Regulatory and adequacy of income • Economic life of business • Terms of credit • Management philosophy	• Government regulations • Tax system • Economic condition of the country • Political condition of the country • Condition of money market • Condition of capital market

Financial Regulations

- Company principals establish a working rapport with regulators to create a compliant, effective business environment.
- Senior executives understand that adverse legislation can cripple productivity, a prelude to financial losses later on down the road.
- Consequently, top leadership sets up corporate compliance departments to monitor regulatory developments and indicate how they may affect financial activities.
- Occupational Safety and Health Administration rules concerning workplace safety could increase personnel charges in corporate income statements.
- Aside from compliance managers, internal auditors help companies find ways to handle the binomial question of generating profits while complying with the law.

Corporate Solvency

- Solvency is a broad term referring to a borrower's ability to repay a loan and steps the creditor takes to maintain a strong balance sheet.
- Investors pay attention to solvency metrics to determine whether a firm is a good bet or an unfortunate wager.

- Corporate-solvency discussions are hardly a sideshow for financial management professionals.
- They contribute their intellectual knowledge to these talks, helping corporate leadership find ways to operate without piling on too much debt.
- Financial managers also work in tandem with fixed-asset accountants to increase corporate assets, such as equipment, land and machinery

Securities Markets

- Securities markets and businesses enjoy a mutually beneficial relationship.
- Healthy conditions in financial exchanges positively affect corporate financial strategies.
- Well-run, profitable firms move market trends favorably; as investors view corporate profits as a sign the economy is on an upward trajectory.
- Financial exchanges, such as the Tokyo Stock Exchange, Chicago Mercantile Exchange and New York Stock Exchange, enable publicly traded companies to implement their financial strategies, most notably by raising cash and purchasing long-term investments.

Business Lending

- Business lending, or corporate credit, is a vibrant factor in the financial management equation.
- It gives organizations the opportunity to operate in the short term and think confidently about long-term expansion tactics.
- All organizations, including charities, borrow to rein in the occasional cash shortfall resulting from delays in customer payments or donor remittances.
- Finding the right mix of debt and equity is part of a company's formula for success.
- Failure to adequately think about what debt level is appropriate for the firm may cause corporate income to drop.
- Corporate credit refers to financial instruments, such as loans, overdrafts arrangements, credit lines and bonds.

■ CONCLUSION

Management is a set of principles relating to the functions of planning, organizing, directing, and controlling, and the applications of these principles in harnessing physical, financial, human, and informational resources efficiently and effectively to achieve organizational goals. There are numerous factors that affect an organization or the management. Managers can monitor these factors/environments through boundary spanning a process of gathering information about developments that could impact the future of the organization. The four basic functions of management are planning, organizing, leading and controlling. These functions work together in the creation, execution and realization of organizational goals. The four functions of management can be considered a process where each function builds on the previous function. To be successful, management needs to follow the four functions of management in the proper order.

■ REVIEW QUESTIONS

Long Essays

1. Define management process; explain the elements of management process.
2. Describe classifications of management function.

Short Essays

1. POSDCORB.
2. Factors affecting on management.
3. Environmental factors affecting management.
4. Factors affecting financial management.

Short Answers

1. Organizing.
2. Directing (Leading).
3. Macro-environment.
4. Micro-environment.

■ BIBLIOGRAPHY

1. Altaher AM. Knowledge Management Process Implementation 2011. International Journal of Digital Society (IJDS). 2010; 1(4): 265-71
2. Baggett MM, Baggett FB. Move from management to high-level leadership. Nursing Management. 2005; 36(7): 12.
3. Barker AM. Transformational Nursing Leadership: A Vision for the Future. New York: National League for Nursing Press; 1992.
4. Grossman S, Valiga TM. The New Leadership Challenge: Creating the Future of Nursing. Philadelphia: FA Davis; 2000.
5. Hersey P, Campbell R. Leadership: A Behavioral Science Approach. Calif.: Leadership Studies Publishing; 2004.
6. Tappen RM. Nursing Leadership and Management: Concepts and Practice. Philadelphia: FA Davis;2001.
7. Trofino J. Transformational leadership in health care. Nursing Management. 1995; 26(8): 42-7.

CHAPTER 4

Nursing Management and Role of Nurse Manager

Learning Objectives

- Mission Statement of Nursing Management
- Vision of Nursing Management
- Philosophy of Nursing Management
- Goals of Nursing Management
- Nursing Management Roles
- Concept of Nurse Manager
- Qualities of an Effective Manager
- Types of Nurse Managers
- Skills Needed for Nurse Manager
- Functions of Good Nurse Manager
- Characteristics of Successful Manager
- Clinical Responsibilities of Nurse Manager
- General Role of the Manager
- Nurse Manager Job Duties
- Strategically Techniques of Nurse Manager
- Common Problems of Nurse Manager
- Future of Nurse Managers

INTRODUCTION

Nursing management is performing leadership functions of governance and decision-making within organizations employing nurses. It includes processes common to all management, such as planning, organizing, staffing, directing and controlling. It is common for RNs to seek additional education to earn a Master of Science in Nursing or Doctor of Nursing practice to prepare for leadership roles within nursing. Management positions increasingly require candidates to hold an advanced degree in nursing.

Nurse managers have complex, responsible positions in healthcare organizations. Ineffective managers may do harm to their employees, their patients, and to the organization, and effective managers can help their staff members grow and develop as healthcare professionals while providing the highest quality care to their patients (**Fig. 4.1**).

DEFINITION

- Nursing management consists of the performance of the leadership functions of governance and decision-making within organizations employing nurses. It includes processes common to all management, such as planning, organizing, staffing, directing and controlling.
- Management is the process and agency which directs and guides the operations of an organization in realizing established aims.
- A nurse administrator/manager defined as leaders who not only guide the nurses in their department, but also help to adopt new ideas and practices for the betterment of the facility or organization.

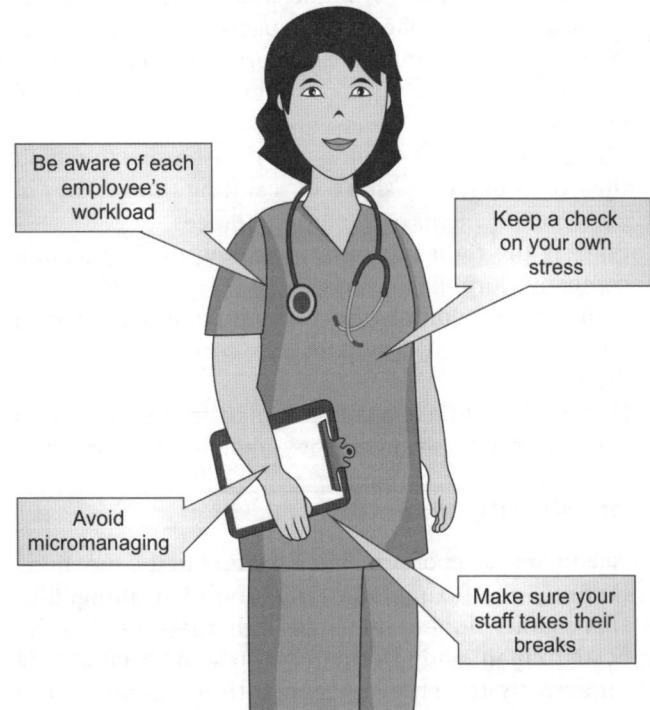

Fig. 4.1: Nurse manager's supervisory role.

MISSION STATEMENT OF NURSING MANAGEMENT

Mission

- A mission statement is a broad general goal of an organization that describes its purpose in the community.
- The mission statement of a small community hospital may indicate that its purpose is to serve the healthcare

needs of the immediate community and provide care for commonly occurring illnesses.
- A large university hospital may have a mission statement that encompasses research, teaching and care for complex problems.
- These two organizations will establish different priorities for spending, choose different technologies as essential to their missions, and structure their staff in different ways.
- These mission statements provide the overall umbrella under which all functions of the organization take place.
- In addition to or even in place of a mission statement a general statement of philosophy may be used. When both are present, they should agree. The philosophy is typically longer and more detailed.

Dimensions of Mission Statements

According to Bart, the strongest organizational impact occurs when mission statements contain 7 essential dimensions:
1. Key values and beliefs
2. Distinctive competence
3. Desired competitive position
4. Competitive strategy
5. Compelling goal/vision
6. Specific customers served and products or services offered
7. Concern for satisfying multiple stakeholders

The mission statement of an; organization describes the purpose for which that organization exists.
- Mission statements provide information and inspiration that clearly and explicitly outline the way ahead for the organization. They provide vision.
- Individuals want productive and meaningful lives. Therefore, the purpose of the organization and of each of its units should be defined a teamwork approach should be properly trained: and all individuals within the organization should be treated with respect.
- Organizational purpose moves and guides the organization toward a perceived goal.
- Many writers indicate that the purpose or mission statement should be created from mission statement should be properly trained and all individual s within the organization should be treated with respect.
- Organizational purpose moves and guides the organization toward a perceived goal.
- The mission or purpose statement incorporates the culture of the organization, including strong leadership, rules and regulations, achievement of goals, and the notion that people are more important than work.
- Employees who participate in developing the vision statement believe in their own abilities and are more committed to the organization.
- The vision statement is shared companywide so that employees live the vision.
- The mental exercise of creating one is more meaningful than the contents of the statement itself. Vision, values, mission or purpose statements are meaningful only to the creators. **Box 4.1** summarizes definition of nursing management and nurse manager and **Table 4.1** discusses differences between management and leadership.

Box 4.1: Definition of nursing management and nurse manager.
- **Nursing management:** It is the body of knowledge related to performing the functions of planning organizing, staffing directing and controlling (evaluating) the activities of a nursing in departmental subunits.
- **Nurse manager:** Person who is responsible for translating the administration's vision into operating plans and acting in the middle and first-line levels of hierarchy.

Table 4.1: Differences between management and leadership.

Management	Leadership
Concentrates on project admin, including reporting and plans	Looks for the essence of information from the reports
Accepts current constraints	Challenges current constraints
Works within the existing organizational structure	Identifies problems with the existing structure and identifies alternatives
Relies on control	Inspires trust
Uses authority of the role to issue instructions	Uses persuasion and motivation to create the environment to follow instructions
Concerned with resources	Concerned with reasons
Concentrates on timeframe, budget, and resources	Concentrates on reasons for project and benefits

VISION OF NURSING MANAGEMENT

- Employees who participate in developing the vision statement believe in their own abilities and are more committed to the organization than employees who do not participate.
- The vision statement is shared companywide so that employees may live the vision. It is updated to keep with technology and trends. A vision statement is sometimes.
- The mental exercise of creating one is more meaningful than are the contents of the statement itself.
- Vision values, mission, or purpose statements are meaningful only to the creators.
- Translated for the community, these statements place value on the way nurses care for people.
- It follows that ethnic populations are considered in developing vision and values statements for nursing entities. Nursing education teaches the meaning of values such as tolerance and compromise.
- Examples of values are informality, creativity, honesty, quality, courtesy, and caring.

PHILOSOPHY OF NURSING MANAGEMENT

A philosophy of nursing is a statement that outlines a nurse's values, ethics, and beliefs, as well as their motivation for being part of the profession. It covers a nurse's perspective regarding their education, practice, and patient care ethics.
- **Cost effectiveness:** In management or administration of any enterprises for organization, the quality, quantity, timing and cost of the necessary to reach the objective of

the enterprises are interrelated factor which must be given constant attention.

- **Execution and control of work plan:** One of the greatest possible contributors to wastage of our precious recourses, whether at the local or national level, is the failure of those at any level of administration, and at all stages in the management of the activity, to base all decision on verifiable facts.
- **Delegation of responsibility and authority:** The delegation of responsibility and authority is an important aspect of successful administration, to place the responsibility for decision at the lowest possible organizational level in order to attain decision as speedily as possible.
- **Human relation and good morale:** Since, the function of administration is to attain an established objective through the management of people, administration if deeply concerned with human relation. Good morale of the staff is essential to the success of any organization.
- **Effective communication:** Effective communication are essential for all aspect of effective administration. Staff must be adequately and correctly informed about plan, methods, schedules, problems events and progress.
- **Flexibility:** Administrators must be completely flexible to meet the changing needs of the situation.

Organizational Philosophy and Philosophy of Nursing Service Administration

- Organizational Philosophy is its explicit and implied view of itself and what it is. Generally, it is expressed in mission statements.
- The philosophy is directly linked to and rooted in the organizations cultural beliefs and values.
- Philosophy depicts the desired nature of the relationships between health service organizations and its customers, employees and external constituents.
- It is a set of beliefs that determines how organizational purposes are achieved and that serves as the foundation for agency objectives, policies and procedures.
- Nurses have the right to know the beliefs about nursing care, nursing practice and nursing management held by the collective group, which they are a part of the nursing department.
- A statement of philosophy is a valuable management tool. Nurses should be given a copy before they join the staff so that they can judge whether their personal philosophy is sufficiently in agreement with the organizational philosophy to enable them to become a contributing member of the department.
- Philosophy statements are relatively enduring documents because stated beliefs are usually expressions of firm commitment to the best that can be achieved and are derived from the broad goals of the agency.
- A useful philosophy has a timeless quality because basic premises change only under unusual conditions.
- Nevertheless, philosophy statements need to be reviewed periodically. If a review by all members of the department reveals that the statement still reflects the guiding beliefs of the collective group, there is no need to revise the document.
- If scrutiny indicates that the statement is not consistent with current agency goals or philosophy or is not effective in directing the actions of the department, then the statement should be rewritten to assure that it meets the criteria of compatibility, attainability, intelligibility, acceptability, measurability and accountability.
- When developing or reevaluating a philosophy, the manager should consider theory, education, practice, research, and nursing's role in the total organization.

GOALS OF NURSING MANAGEMENT

Goals

- Goals are the broad statements of overall intent of an organization or individual. They are usually stated in general terms.
- The purpose of writing goals is to identify where you are going and to enable you to evaluate when you have arrived there.
- A meaningful stated goal is one that succeeds in communicating the intent of those generating the goal.
- It should be stated in such a way that it will be understood clearly by others.
- As a nurse in a healthcare institution, you need to be aware of the existence of several levels of goals: the institutional level, the nursing department level and the nursing unit level.
- The goal levels all need to relate to the health needs of the community, because these are the focus of healthcare.

Institutional Goals

- Based on the community's health needs, the institution forms goals and objectives.
- An institution that focuses thinking on goals for the future and activities that will move the organization toward these goals is referred to as a proactive institution.
- The managers of such institutions spend a great deal of time, money and energy on identifying possible future events and on preparing the institution to deal with them.
- Institutions that do not have specific or future oriented goals are reactive institutions.
- They spend their time reacting to events, that is, "putting out fires" rather than "preventing them."
- A reactive facility would wait until such emergencies occurred and then would handle them as a crisis rather than as an anticipated event.

Nursing Department Goals

- The goals of the institution definitely affect those of nursing service, which must support and complement institutional goals.
- In an institution with an overall goal of developing a mental health program, a nursing department goal may include developing nurses in psychiatry.

- The astute manager of a nursing department must also be proactive about the national issues facing nursing, community needs for nursing, and the needs within the institution itself.
- This manager would formulate goals to help the nursing department meet the challenges of care in the future, because the ultimate nursing department goal is quality client care.

Nursing Unit Goals

- It is important that each employee understand the institutional and nursing department goals, because the group or unit goals develop from them.
- Each nurse should be able to contribute to the formation of unit goals in terms of philosophy of care, quality of care, and development of nursing expertise.
- Helping to formulate the goals for your unit is important, because these goals can also represent your individual goals.
- Unit goals develop from the group as a whole and often include individual goals in the process.
- Development and implementation of goals must be meaningful to the group if they are to be successful.
- The member of the group must feel that they are the originators of the unit goals and objectives.

NURSING MANAGEMENT ROLES

- **Matron:** A matron is the senior nurse who serves as "the head of the general staff of the hospital" and is obeyed by his/her subordinate nurses. Traditionally, matrons wear a dark-blue dress, usually darker than her subordinates, also known as sisters, in addition to a white-starched hat. As such, matrons usually "provide strong leadership and act as a link between Board-level nurses and clinical practice."
- **Director of nursing:** A director of nursing (DON) is a registered nurse who supervises the care of all the patients at a healthcare facility. The director of nursing is the senior nursing management position in an organization and often holds executive titles like Chief Nursing Officer (CNO), Chief Nurse Executive, or Vice-President of Nursing
- **Service directors:** Many large healthcare organizations also have **service** directors. These directors have oversight of a particular service within the facility or system (surgical services, women's services, emergency services, critical care services, etc.).
- **Nurse manager:** The nurse manager is the nurse with management responsibilities of a nursing unit. They typically report to a service director. They have primary responsibilities for staffing, budgeting, and day-to-day operations of the unit.
- **Charge nurse:** The charge nurse is the nurse, usually assigned for a shift, who is responsible for the immediate functioning of the unit. The charge nurse is responsible for making sure nursing care is delivered safely and that all the patients on the unit are receiving adequate care. They are typically the frontline management in most nursing units. Some charge nurses are permanent members of the nursing management team and are called shift supervisors.

CONCEPT OF NURSE MANAGER

- A nurse manager coordinates and manages a nursing staff. She ensures the staff under her runs effectively.
- The nurse manager is efficient around the clock, following all administrative and clinical procedures and polices according to a set of medical guidelines.
- In a manner of superb professionalism, the nurse manger maintains an effective work environment supportive to all nurses and staff. For a nurse manager to be successful in today's healthcare environment, mastery of basic business skills is essential.
- No longer are nurse managers expected to be clinical experts but, instead, must be equipped and skillful in "running their business."
- Mintzberg (1989) divided a manager's activities into three categories: interpersonal, decisional, and informational.
- A nurse manager directs, supervises, and leads the nursing staff of a hospital or medical facility.
- The nurse manager's role is fast-paced, multidimensional, requires organization and critical thinking, and is vital to patient care as they oversee the nurses that provide direct care.

QUALITIES OF AN EFFECTIVE MANAGER (FIG. 4.2)

The effective nurse manager possesses a combination of qualities: leadership, clinical expertise, and business sense. None of these alone is enough; it is the combination that prepares an individual for the complex task of managing a unit or team of healthcare providers. Consider each of these briefly:

- **Leadership:** All of the people skills of the leader are essential to the effective manager. They are skills needed to function as a manager.
- **Clinical expertise:** It is very difficult to help others develop their skills and evaluate how well they have done so without possessing clinical expertise oneself. It is probably not necessary (or even possible) to know everything all other professionals on the team know, but it is important to be able to assess the effectiveness of their work in terms of patient outcomes.
- **Business sense:** Nurse managers also need to be concerned with the "bottom line," with the cost of providing the care that is given, especially in comparison with the benefit received from that care and the funding available to pay for it, whether from insurance, Medicare, Medicaid, or out of the patient's own pocket. This is a complex task that requires knowledge of budgeting, staffing, and measurement of patient outcomes.

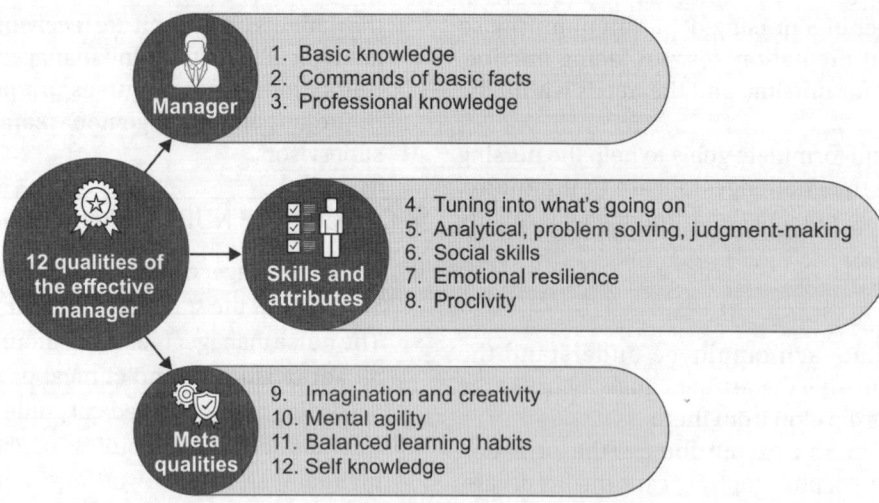

Fig. 4.2: Qualities of effective manager.

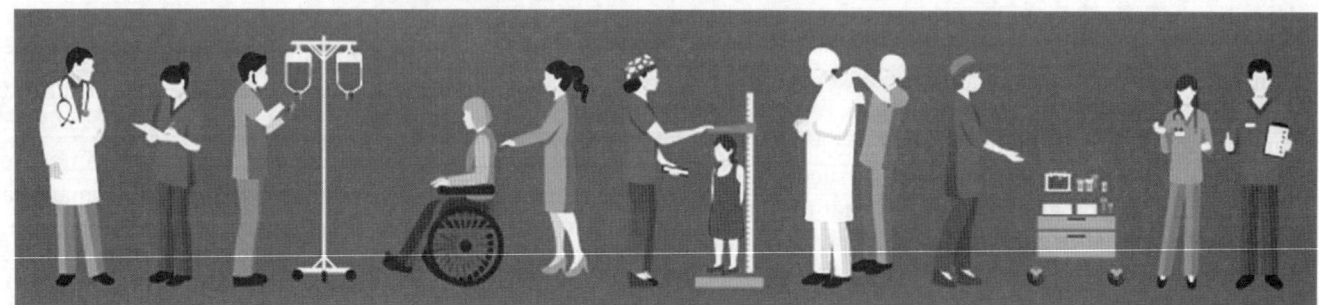

Fig. 4.3: Role of nurse manager in different settings.

TYPES OF NURSE MANAGERS

- **Clinical nurse managers:** As a professional in a hospital, clinic, nursing home, acute care center, or other institution, you would have a broad scope of responsibilities and be regarded as a valuable member of a large, coordinated team. Depending on your specialty and training, you may be heading the nursing staffs in ICU, ER, pediatrics, or other departments.
- **Nursing case managers:** Following a training course of about one year, you may become certified as a Nursing Case Manager. This role has you working closely with individual patients, coordinating treatment, tracking outcomes, and performing research. Some case managers work with insurance companies as well, advocating for the patient while designing a feasible treatment plan.
- **Geriatric care nurse manager:** As opposed to a case managers, a geriatric care manager specializes in senior adults and their care. This role would have you assessing the patient's home, consulting with family and physicians, creating a care plan, and supervising the appointment of home health aides and other support personnel.

Figure 4.3 shows role of nurse manager in different settings.

SKILLS NEEDED FOR NURSE MANAGER

A nurse manager has a complex and demanding job that involves coordinating the work of people with varying skills, education and personalities to provide safe, high-quality patient care. Nurse managers must assume responsibility for staff performance, financial management, resource utilization and patient outcomes, as well as ensuring that care is delivered according to standards of practice and organizational policy. A good nurse manager should provide leadership, ensure the unit or department runs smoothly and be a professional role model for her staff **(Fig. 4.4)**.

Clinical Expertise

- Clinical skills are an important quality in the nurse manager. The staff on a unit looks to the nurse manager for clinical expertise and advice when they have a problem.
- The nurse manager should be able to demonstrate how to change a dressing or start an intravenous line, or be able to make recommendations for managing a particular situation.
- The nurse manager must be committed to ongoing education through reading, formal education and regular clinical practice to ensure she retains her clinical expertise.

Communication Skills

- Communication is a key skill for a nurse manager. The staff on a nursing unit may include nurse aides with minimal education as well as nursing professionals educated at the baccalaureate level or above.
- Nurse managers also interact with doctors, social workers, patients, families, other hospital workers, such

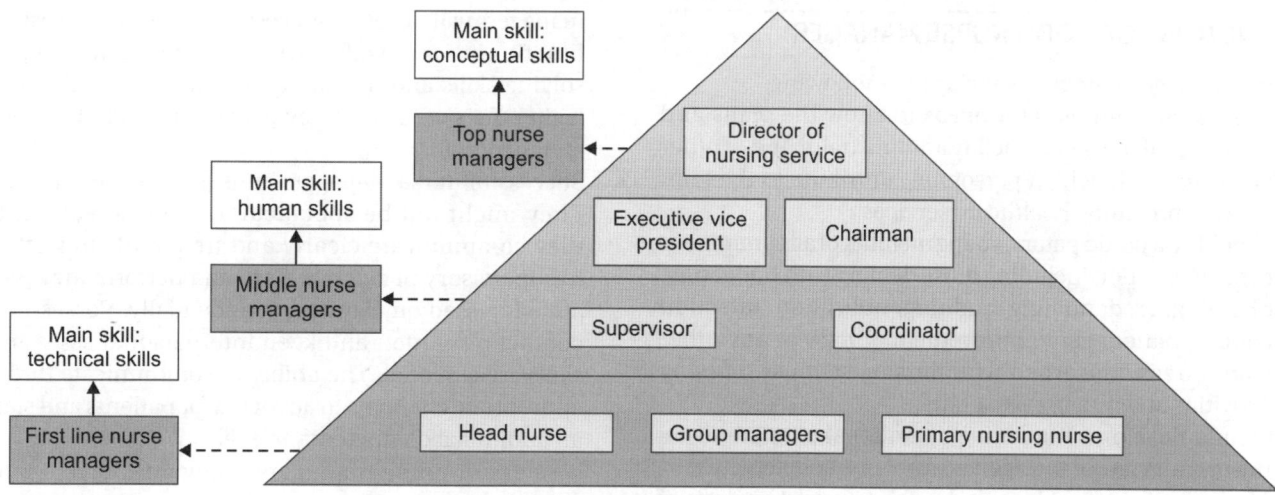

Fig. 4.4: Nurse manager's role in patient care.

as respiratory therapists or lab technicians and senior hospital administration staff.
- Some of the people who work in or seek care from a hospital may have limited English skills.
- In each case, the nurse manager must be able to establish rapport, ensure communication is clear and listen carefully for potential problems or miscommunication.

Flexibility
- A nurse manager must be flexible. Priorities can change quickly in a healthcare setting as patients develop problems.
- Most inpatient hospital units experience daily or even hourly changes in census as patients are admitted or discharged.
- Medical technology also changes regularly, or the lack of a particular item may necessitate a change in supplies or equipment.
- The nurse manager must be able to adjust staffing or care decisions in response to changing needs while also being decisive when necessary.

Managing People
- People management skills are vital for nurse managers. Much of a nurse manager's work is done through others, so a nurse manager must be able to educate and supervise without micromanaging.
- A nurse manager uses conflict resolution and negotiating skills to promote collaboration between staff, physicians and hospital leaders.
- Nurse managers must be able to coach and mentor staff at all levels and to work with the varied strengths and weaknesses of the nursing staff on the unit.

Other Skills
Other important skills for nurse managers are focus on quality and patient safety, attention to patient satisfaction and a good grasp of customer service. The senior leaders look for a nurse manager with financial acumen, strong physician relationships, collegiality and networking ability and the appropriate use of power. Nurse managers should also be creative, innovative and able to multitask, prioritize and self-direct.

- **Advocacy:** In some cases, nurse leaders might have to advocate for staff to ensure a safe and reasonable practice environment. In other cases, they might have to advocate for patient safety and access to quality healthcare. Nurse managers should not be afraid of using their voice and position.
- **Participation:** With so many administrative demands, it is important that nurse managers balance business with patient care. Nurse managers must have superior clinical skills to ensure patient safety and wellbeing.
- **Mentoring:** Successful nurse leaders do not micromanage their staff. They encourage, empower, mentor, and find strengths. They boost creativity and mindfulness.
- **Maturity:** Nurse managers do not immediately take sides in squabbles or assess blame before knowing all the facts. They do not let simmering emotions boil over. Instead, they meet conflict and work through it.
- **Professionalism:** Nurse managers follow their moral compass to ensure all aspects of the profession are met with honesty and integrity. They address people with respect and do not bully.
- **Supportive:** They do not set the bar for expectations unreasonably high. Instead, they use supportive encouragement to challenge employees to success. They coach and mentor.

Box 4.2 summarizes skills of good manager.

Box 4.2: Skills of good manager.

- Superior communication skills
- Leading with transparency and honesty
- Supporting your employees with clear direction and removing their roadblocks for them
- Embracing technology
- Motivating with positive feedback and recognition
- An expert in the field
- Mediating with productivity and calmness
- Promoting cross-level and cross-functional collaboration
- Creating a productive and lively work environment
- Trusting your employees

FUNCTIONS OF GOOD NURSE MANAGER

A nurse manager's functions include the following:
- The nurse administrator needs to know the plans and programs of the health facility administrator and of other departments in which personnel contribute to the joint effort of providing healthcare services.
- Should be a participatory, voting member of all committees of the institution including those dealing with budgeting, planning, credentialing, auditing, utilization, infection control, patient care improvement, library or any other committees concerned with nursing services, nursing activities and nursing personnel.
- Should develop a marketing operational plan based on the overall view of the agency problems and activities.
- Marketing plan should include gathering and analysis of data related to product or service
- Operational plan consist of pinpointing possible strengths, weaknesses, problems and opportunities.
- Before launching a venture, a control plan is made to measure performance of implementation of venture within a time frame.
- Selected and trained personnel will be assigned to compare expected results with actual results for making corrections in all elements of plan and its implementation in future. **Box 4.3** discusses dual role of nurse manager.

CHARACTERISTICS OF SUCCESSFUL MANAGER (FIG. 4.5)

Although most successful managers demonstrate skills that are difficult to measure, examining the common characteristics illuminates the broader base of skills that might be considered.
- Successful nurse managers make their decisions based on what is best for the patient. They are visible on the unit and talk to patients and families regarding their care. The manager advocates for the patient and family by creating an environment conducive to providing quality care.
- Successful nurse managers demonstrate that they value the role of the staff nurse in providing care. The manager does not necessarily need to be an expert in a clinical specialty, but does need to "pitch in" during times of high stress and acuity. When confronted with an obviously stressed staff nurse, the empathetic manager asks the question, "What can I do to help?" On the other hand, managers will never be successful if they are consistently functioning as a staff nurse. Listening and problem-solving skills and the ability to comprehend the issues facing the staff are the key competencies to look for in an individual.
- Successful nurse managers are superb communicators. They might not be spectacular public speakers, but they communicate clearly and frequently to staff and to supervisory personnel. Care and performance issues are addressed quickly and confidentially. Possession of conflict resolution and keen interpersonal assessment skills are essential. The ability to communicate through appropriate channels to advocate for patients and staff is an additional competency to seek.
- Successful nurse managers enjoy and have a talent for mentoring staff nurses. They recognize leadership potential and create opportunities for development of leadership abilities. A high value is placed on education at all levels and a successful manager usually has someone who can step into the role when they are gone.
- Successful nurse managers have the ability to see the broad view of an organization. They recognize the role their area of responsibility plays in the healthcare setting, but they work as a member of a larger team. Experience working in a multidisciplinary group or setting is excellent preparation for the role.

These are a few of the characteristics of successful nurse managers and, granted, these skills are not as easily measured as the number of years of previous nurse manager experience. Yet we all know individuals who are promoted from within because they have exhibited these positive characteristics in another position.

CLINICAL RESPONSIBILITIES OF NURSE MANAGER (FIG. 4.6)

Nurse managers oversee a specific unit in a hospital, such as intensive care or the emergency room. They are responsible for both the clinical and administrative aspects, including supervising nurses and addressing the concerns of patients and their families. Nurse managers not only require specialized nursing expertise, but they also need strong people and communication skills and the ability to take charge.
- **Supervising nurses:** The nurse manager makes all assignments for the nurses she supervises, taking into account their strengths and weaknesses, their experience levels, the types of cases and number of patients requiring care. Using this information, she will assign nurses to specific cases or tasks, and set schedules for all nurses in the unit. She also ensures all nurses fulfill their duties and meet the hospital's expectations. If a nurse does not provide adequate care, is rude to a patient or does not fulfill her assigned tasks, the nurse manager may take disciplinary action and give her directions for improvement.
- **Coaching:** Nurse managers often play a mentoring role, especially to new or young nurses. They frequently

---

Box 4.3: Dual role of nurse manager.

Nurse managers wear two hats: They deliver clinical care and serve as administrative leaders.
- **Represent and support their nursing staff (staff)**
  - Mentor and coach nursing staff
  - Listen to concerns and provide counsel
  - Represent their unit and staff within the hospital
- **Oversee unit-based operations (administration)**
  - Financial
  - Human resources
  - Customer-/patient-focused care delivery
  - Regulation and unit-based protocol

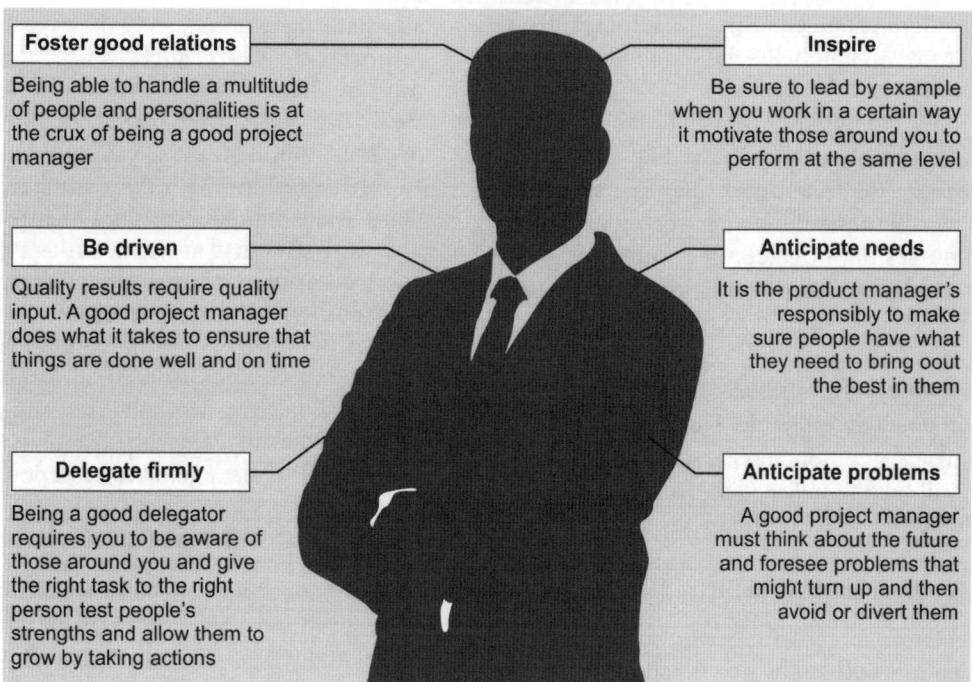

Fig. 4.5: Characteristic of successful manager.

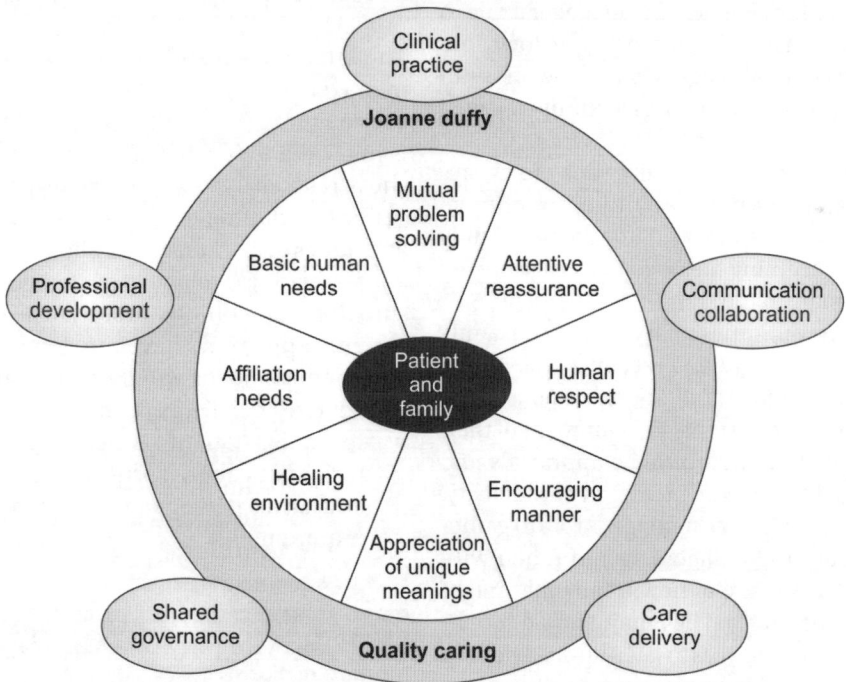

Fig. 4.6: Clinical responsibility of a nurse manager.

supervise these less experienced nurses closely, praising them for a job well done and offering suggestions and advice for improving the quality of care they deliver and their interactions with patients and hospital staff. They also guide veteran nurses, and must be available if one of their nurses needs feedback regarding her job performance or insight into a difficult case. If questions arise regarding a patient's treatment, it is usually the nurse manager who makes the final decision or consults the patient's doctor for a second opinion.

- **Leadership and conflict management:** Effective nurse managers set clear expectations for the nurses in their unit, explaining exactly what is expected of them and outlining guidelines for how they behave toward each other and toward patients and family members. However, even in teams who normally work well together, conflicts occasionally arise. It is the nurse manager's responsibility to defuse the conflict before it harms the team or hinders patient care. She may call in the conflicted parties for a meeting, encouraging them

to discuss their dispute and creating a plan for resolving the conflict in a way that benefits the individual nurses, the team and patients.
- **Patient relations:** When patients or their families have issues about the quality of their care, they often take their concerns to the nurse manager. They may simply be confused or have questions about their treatment plan, or they may feel nurses have treated them rudely or given them sub-par care. Even if a patient or family member is irate, the nurse manager must take time to listen to his concerns and answer his questions. She must also let him know she takes his concerns seriously and wants to ensure he receives the best care possible. During her meeting with the patient or family member, she should also outline the steps she will take to investigate his complaint and remedy the situation.

GENERAL ROLE OF THE MANAGER

- **Creating the vision:** Successful organizations are led by visionary leaders with a clear understanding of the organization's mission statement. This helps everyone focus on the organization's main purpose.
- **Implementing the vision:** It is also the manager's role to implement the mission statement by breaking it down into specific, achievable goals. Managers help the workers to recognize how the work they do relates to the overall goal of the organization.
- **Facilitating change:** Dynamic organizations are always changing, and managers help facilitate the change through their role as change agents. They do this by fully understanding and accepting the need to change and by conveying this rationale to the staff.
- **Mentoring:** Managers who are visionary leaders constantly mentor their staff. It is their role to recognize talent and groom employees for positions of additional responsibility. They contribute to the professional development of their employees by conducting performance appraisals and encouraging personal growth and increased productivity.
- **Gathering information:** It is the manager's role to gather all relevant information. Managers stay in touch with their superiors and are aware of new trends that might be implemented in the future. They maintain an "open-door" policy with their employees to keep up-to-date with issues that might be causing resentment or discontent among them.
- **Evaluating information:** Evaluate information when it is received, to determine who should receive the information and how it will be communicated. Managers use their judgment to decide what is relevant to pass on to their supervisors and what to share with their workers.
- **Communicating:** Managers must communicate information at the most suitable time, using the most appropriate method of communication whether it be face-to-face at a meeting, via electronic technology or in print.
- **Decision-making:** Managers are constantly involved in decision-making, whether it's for smaller issues, such as what time workers will take their breaks or for more important matters, such as firing an employee for a transgression.
- **Building relationships:** A vital management role revolves around the interpersonal relationships with their subordinates and with their superiors. Managers who develop a climate of trust find it easier to do their job. It is easier for them to get their workers to follow directions and it is easier to take direction from their supervisors.
- **Controlling climate:** Managers are responsible for facilitating healthy interpersonal relationships among staff members. Employees are more productive when the relationships in the workplace are supportive and collaborative instead of filled with poisonous back-stabbing. It is the role of the manager to foster a positive climate

NURSE MANAGER JOB DUTIES

The nurse manager is responsible for having an efficient staff working under her through timely and useful professional development courses for nurses and other supporting staff. Under the direction of the nurse manager, staff receives such programs to grow as professionals and a working community. She researches opportunities that help her staff work more proficiently while serving the population to the fullest extent. The interviewing and hiring process also goes to the nurse manager, and working with an approved budget for staff, she can make knowledgeable decisions as to how much staff is needed and in what areas. Along with the hiring process, she is responsible for performance reviews and disciplinary actions, including terminations. She delegates assignments and duties to her nurse staff. She is responsible for monitoring and evaluating availability of medical equipment and making sure it is functioning properly. Through the nurse manger, patients and family have the guarantee that their personal and medical needs will be taken care of properly. **Box 4.4** summarizes behaviors of an effective manager.
- Identifies patient service requirements by establishing personal rapport with potential and actual patients and other persons in a position to understand service requirements.

Box 4.4: Behaviors of an effective manager.

- **Informational**
  - Representing employees
  - Representing the organization
  - Public relations monitoring
- **Interpersonal**
  - Networking
  - Conflict negotiation and resolution
  - Employee development and coaching
  - Rewards and punishment
- **Decisional**
  - Employee evaluation
  - Resource allocation
  - Hiring and firing employees
  - Planning
  - Job analysis and redesign

- Maintains nursing guidelines by writing and updating policies and procedures.
- Maintains nursing operations by initiating, coordinating, and enforcing program, operational, and personnel policies and procedures.
- Assures quality of care by developing and interpreting hospital and nursing division's philosophies and standards of care; enforcing adherence to state board of nursing and state nurse practice act requirements and to other governing agency regulations; measuring health outcomes against standards; making or recommending adjustments.
- Maintains nursing staff by recruiting, selecting, orienting, and training nurses and auxiliary staff.
- Completes patient care requirements by scheduling and assigning nursing and staff; following up on work results.
- Maintains nursing staff job results by coaching, counseling, and disciplining employees; planning, monitoring, and appraising job results.
- Establishes a compassionate environment by providing emotional, psychological, and spiritual support to patients, friends, and families.
- Promotes patient's independence by establishing patient care goals; teaching and counseling patient, friends, and family and reinforcing their understanding of disease, medications, and self-care skills.
- Provides information to patients and healthcare team by answering questions and requests.
- Resolves patient needs by utilizing multidisciplinary team strategies.
- Maintains safe and clean working environment by designing and implementing procedures, rules, and regulations; calling for assistance from other healthcare professionals.
- Protects patients and employees by developing and interpreting infection-control policies and protocols; enforcing medication administration, storage procedures, and controlled substance regulations.
- Maintains patient confidence and protects operations by monitoring confidential information processing.
- Maintains documentation of patient care services by auditing patient and department records.
- Achieves financial objectives by preparing an annual budget; scheduling expenditures; analyzing variances; initiating corrective actions.
- Ensures operation of medical and administrative equipment by verifying emergency equipment availability; completing preventive maintenance requirements; following manufacturer's instructions; troubleshooting malfunctions; calling for repairs; maintaining equipment inventories; evaluating new equipment and techniques.
- Maintains nursing supplies inventory by studying usage reports; identifying trends; anticipating needed supplies; approving requisitions and cost allocations.
- Maintains professional and technical knowledge by attending educational workshops; reviewing professional publications; establishing personal networks; participating in professional societies.
- Maintains a cooperative relationship among healthcare teams by communicating information; responding to requests; building rapport; participating in team problem-solving methods.
- Contributes to team effort by accomplishing related results as needed

STRATEGICAL TECHNIQUES OF NURSE MANAGER

As a manager in the medical field, she must be able present and implement strategies and career minded goals to her staff. She must be able to manipulate databases and other computerized information systems that aid in patient care. Interpersonal skills are required as well so the nurse manager can speak with all staff, patient and family members with respect and dignity. It is important for the nurse manager to be the leading example in safety protocol, ensuring her staff follows these procedures as well. She must have an excellent command of the English language, both oral and written, as well as an extensive knowledge of medical terminology, including diseases, medications and treatment. The following three categories identify several of the business skills that are essential for nurse managers:

Financial Management

- Become knowledgeable with basic financial terminology and definitions. Develop a plan to educate yourself and your direct reports.
- Become proficient in reading and understanding organizational budget reports.
- Be able to develop a basic unit budget. As a nurse manager, it is important to be able to develop a basic unit budget and recognize the different line items and categories that are included in the budget.
- Learn how to monitor and analyze budget variances and be able to develop strategies to address the variances.
- Establish strong working relationships with the finance personnel at your organization. Invite the chief financial officer, controller, or staff accountant to nurse management meetings when appropriate.
- Participate in the selection of programs that influence nursing such as productivity programs, inventory management, and documentation systems.
- If consultants are hired to work with the organization, ensure that nursing has input into the process and outcomes.

Human Resources

- Identify and develop recruitment and retention programs. Successful recruitment and retention strategies are vital to the long-term success of the organization, so nurse managers should take the lead in identifying successful strategies.
- Monitor employee satisfaction on your unit through both informal and formal processes. By being available, open, and visible to your staff, you are able to gauge the satisfaction of the employees on the unit. You should be knowledgeable in the formal survey process that the

organization uses and be able to analyze the data and develop strategies for improvement.
- Similar to your relationship with the finance department, you should also develop a strong working relationship with the human resources department.
- Learn how to effectively handle conflict, negotiation, and delegation.
- Keep current on policies and procedures relating to running your business, including employment issues, salaries, benefits, policies addressing attendance, corrective action, performance evaluations, and legal and regulatory issues such as licensure and accreditation surveys. As a nurse manager, you should fully understand the policies and procedures and be able to effectively discuss with the staff when questions or issues arise.

Strategic Management

- Familiarize with the components of a business plan. As a nurse manager should have the skills to write a simple business plan and be able to conduct a SWOT (strengths, weaknesses, opportunities, threats) analysis.
- Since emergency preparedness has become such an important part of the strategic planning process for all organizations, the nurse manager should participate in the emergency preparedness process, and be knowledgeable about the incident command structure, regulatory and accreditation standards that address emergency preparedness, and specific organizational policies and procedures.
- Participate in the strategic planning process for the organization. The nurse manager should provide input into this process and share in the plan's responsibility for implementation.
- Become proficient in writing organizational and personal goals and objectives.

■ COMMON PROBLEMS OF NURSE MANAGER

Nurse managers juggle increasingly demanding work schedules. They are expected to relate well to patients, junior staff and their own managers. The nurse manager is also the key person other members of the multidisciplinary team will approach when a problem occurs. The job is not made easier by the new expectations placed on the nurse manager. As well as being an expert in nursing, the new nurse manager must be computer and financially literate

Staff Retention

- Many nurses leave their current employment and move onto other jobs. The nurse manager must try to ensure that most staff enjoys the job enough to stay.
- This is not always easy to balance with the need for all staff to work extremely hard under sometimes fraught circumstances.
- Though it may seem unfair, the nurse manager will be held at least partly accountable for high numbers of staff leaving, or high rates of absenteeism.

Balancing Act

- A nurse will be trained to strive for the best possible outcomes for his patients.
- He will naturally want to ensure that they have the best care, are not left waiting for buzzers to be answered, and not rushed. However, the nurse manager often finds that some of these things do happen, and it is difficult to do anything about it.
- This is because of financial constraints and staff shortages, two factors which are often linked.

Giving Feedback

- The nurse manager has to deal with other nursing staff, even when this involves some negative feedback. This is often a very difficult task.
- The nurse manager is only human, she probably wants to be liked, but occasions arise when this has to be secondary to the need to give constructive criticism.
- A good manager can do this in a way that leaves the self-esteem of the other person, and the relationship, intact.

Solutions

- The nurse manager needs coping strategies to deal with some of these problems. He needs an understanding manager or mentor of his own to give support.
- He needs to recognize the crucial need to delegate, and to also the need to have outlets outside of work.
- The nurse manager also needs the support of others within the care setting. This is sometimes given by peer group forums where common problems can be discussed in a non-judgmental manner.

■ FUTURE OF NURSE MANAGERS

- As the current nursing workforce ages and retires, the anticipated shortage of nurses will create opportunities for newly minted nurse managers.
- Researchers have found that nurse managers are vital to overall nurse retention because they influence the quality of work and the stability of a work environment.
- "Strong leadership qualities in the nursing unit manager have been associated with greater job satisfaction, reduced turnover intention among nursing staff, and improved patient outcomes.
- Nurse leaders need to be supported in an effort to retain nurses given ongoing workforce issues and to ensure high-quality patient care," researchers said in the 2014 "Leadership skills for nursing unit managers to decrease intention to leave" study.
- Researchers found there must be cohesive relationships among staff members and better communications with staff for nurse managers to do a better job in the future.
- Continual changes in healthcare and a focus on costs are among the many things that make the role of nurse manager challenges.

"Growing future nurse leaders is a long-term quest that requires both planning and action," authors of the "Growing

Nurse Leaders: Their Perspectives on Nursing Leadership and Today's Practice Environment" study found. "Our emerging leaders will ultimately replace our current leaders and continue the very important work being done to improve nursing practice environments, and most importantly, patient outcomes. Yet succession planning is challenging today in a healthcare environment that is fast-paced and constantly changing."

■ CONCLUSION

Each nursing unit is a component of a larger organization that depends on qualified nurses to manage the business and to understand the "big" picture. Nurse managers are the change agents and leaders in improving the work environment where nurses practice, so it is essential that they have the required skills. Nurse manager promotes and restores patients' health by developing day-to-day management and long-term planning of the patient care area; directing and developing staff; collaborating with physicians and multidisciplinary professional staffs; providing physical and psychological support for patients, friends, and families.

■ REVIEW QUESTIONS

Long Essays

1. Explain mission and vision statement of nursing management.
2. Discuss the functions of good nurse manager.
3. Describe the duties and responsibilities of nurse manager.

Short Essays

1. Philosophy of nursing management.
2. Goals of nursing management.
3. Nursing management roles.
4. Qualities of nurse manager.
5. Types of nurse managers.
6. Skills needed for nurse manager.
7. Functions of good nurse manager.
8. Characteristics of successful manager.
9. Clinical responsibilities of nurse manager.
10. General role of the manager.
11. Strategically techniques of nurse manager.
12. Common problems of nurse manager.
13. Future of nurse managers.

Short Answers

1. Leadership.
2. Clinical expertise.
3. Clinical nurse managers.
4. Communication skills.
5. Mentoring.
6. Professionalism.
7. Decision-making.
8. Strategic management.

■ BIBLIOGRAPHY

1. Baggett MM, Baggett FB. Move from management to high-level leadership. Nursing Management. 2005;36(7):12.
2. Grossman S, Valiga TM. The New Leadership Challenge: Creating the Future of Nursing. Philadelphia: FA Davis; 2000.
3. Hart LB, Waisman CS. The Leadership Training Activity Book. New York: AMACOM; 2005.
4. Hersey P, Campbell R. Leadership: A Behavioral Science Approach. Calif.: Leadership Studies Publishing; 2004.
5. Hunter JC. The World's Most Powerful Leadership Principle. New York: Crown Business; 2004.
6. Kovner CT, Brewer CS, Fairchild S, et al. Newly licensed RNs' characteristics, work attitudes, and intentions to work. American Journal of Nursing. 2007;107(9):58-70.
7. Lombardi DN. Handbook for the New Health Care Manager. San Francisco: Jossey-Bass/AHA Press; 2001.

CHAPTER 5

Healthcare and Development of Nursing Services in India

LEARNING OBJECTIVES

- Health System
- History of Healthcare System
- Healthcare Delivery System
- Center Level Healthcare Administration
- The Directorate General of Health Services
- State Level Healthcare Administration
- District Level Healthcare Administration
- Community Level Healthcare Administration
- Healthcare Delivery System in India
- Urban Health Services
- Nursing Services
- Recent Trends and Issues of Nursing Service and Management

INTRODUCTION

Health has been at the center of human concern since ancient times. Civilizations developed and perished due to wars, conflicts and raging diseases, which left none untouched, save those whose health was taken care of by an organized system. Ancient civilizations that developed in Indus valley, Greece, Rome and Mesopotamia had fairly advanced health systems for their times and the medical practitioners enjoyed a high status in the society due to their practice.

Two renowned medical systems developed in India in ancient times; Ayurveda and Siddha, which were quite similar in concept and practice. Indian systems sought knowledge by which life could be prolonged and some of the popular medical treatises of those times were the Charaka Samhita and the Sushruta Samhita.

DEFINITIONS

- **Health:** Health is defined as, "a dynamic state of complete care physical, mental and social well-being and not merely an absence of disease or infirmity." (WHO)
- **Healthcare:** Healthcare is defined as, "multitude of services rendered to individuals, families or communities by the agents of the health services or professions for the purpose of promoting, preventing, maintaining, monitoring or restoring health."
- **System:** A set of interrelated and independent parts designed to achieve a set of goals.
- **Healthcare system:**
  - Healthcare delivery system is a system in which the services related to healthcare delivered to the target population.
  - Healthcare delivery system is an integral part of the government, responsible to central authority and interrelated in its activities with a general conduct to governmental affairs.

HEALTH SYSTEM

- Health system covers a whole extent of health activities, health programs, institutions providing medical care, such as hospitals, clinics and primary healthcare centers and the policies enunciated by governments to provide optimal healthcare for its citizens.
- In general, health system defines as "Complex of facilities, organizations, and trained personnel engaged in providing health care within a geographical area."
- Health system as described by WHO is the "sum total of all the organizations, institutions and resources whose primary purpose is to improve health."
- Health systems should be accessible, efficient, affordable and of a good quality. **Box 5.1** shows current trends and issues in healthcare.

Health systems usually include the following:
- Development of health policies, plan for their implementation and development of a system of regulation of health services.

Box 5.1: Current trends and issues in healthcare.

- Nursing shortage
- Patient satisfaction
- Managed care
- Transcultural nursing
- National patient safety initiatives
- Evidence-based practice
- Information age
- Genetics
- Globalization of health
- Aging population
- Legal and ethical issues
- Terrorism/bioterrorism/disaster nursing

- Define and develop the institutional framework to deliver the health services within the purview of this system.
- Allocate and mobilize financial and human resources for its functioning.
- Plan, manage and deliver the health services.

Aim of Health Systems

Ultimately aim of health systems is to improve, maintain and restore the health status of the community at a cost that an individual and the community can afford to spend without substantial change in their financial status.

Goals of Healthcare System

A health system has to provide for much more than routine delivery of services. It has to protect the health of its community, treat them with dignity and ensure that it responds fairly to the expectations of the population. The WHO has thus identified three overall goals for the health systems to be:
1. Effective in contributing to better health throughout the entire population.
2. Responsive to people's expectations, including safeguarding patient's dignity, confidentiality and autonomy and being sensitive to the specific needs and vulnerabilities of all population groups.
3. Fair in how individuals contribute to funding the system so that everyone has access to the services available and is protected against potentially impoverishing levels of spending.

Functions of Health System

Healthcare systems fulfill three main functions:
1. Healthcare delivery,
2. Fair treatment to all, and
3. Meeting non-health expectations of the population

Determinants of Health System

- Economic
  - Affordability
  - Availability
- Political
  - Priorities
  - Appropriateness
  - Accessibility
  - Equity
- Cultural
  - Acceptability
  - Utilization
- Participation

Objectives of healthcare system is discussed in **Box 5.2**.

Box 5.2: Objectives of healthcare system.
- To improve health status of population and clinical outcomes of care
- To improve social justice equity in the health status of the population
- To reduce the total economic burden of healthcare
- To raise and pool the resources accessible to deliver healthcare services

Forces Influence the Health System

- New emerging diseases
- Changing disease profile
- Technical and diagnostic advances
- Longevity of life
- Expectations of people
- Subsidies and cross-subsidies
- Increasing non-plan expenditure
- Competing priorities
- Improving awareness among people
- Rising cost of healthcare delivery

HISTORY OF HEALTHCARE SYSTEM

Early History

- India is one of the ancient civilizations of the Indus valley. The excavations in the Indus valley especially Harappa and Mohenjodaro showed planned cities with drainage, house and public baths built of baked bricks suggesting the practice of environmental sanitation in 3000 BC.
- The art of Healthcare in India can be traced back nearly 3500 years, when India was invaded by Aryans, Ayurveda and siddha systems of medicine came into existence.
- The hospital system was developed during the rule of Emperor Ashoka (third century), schools of learning in the healing arts were created.
- Many valuable herbs and medicinal combinations were created. Even today many of these continue to be used.
- The Emperor Ashoka was the first leader in world history to attempt to give healthcare to all of his citizens, thus, it was the India of antiquity which was the first state to give its citizens national healthcare. There were hospitals not only for people, but also for animals.
- During the eleventh century, the Arabic system known as "Unani" was introduced in India by the Arabs and Persians.

Pre-Independence Era

- The British had established their rule in India in 1757. A Royal Commission was appointed to investigate the causes of the extremely unsatisfactory condition of health in the British army stationed in India.
- The commission pointed out the need for the protection of water supplies, construction of drains and prevention of epidemics in civil population for safeguarding the health of the British army.
- An epidemic of plague in 1896 awakened the government to the urgent need of improving public health.
- The All India Institute of Hygiene and Public Health, was established in Calcutta with aid from the Rockefeller foundation.
- The Health Survey and Development Committee (Bhore Committee) was appointed by the Government of India to survey the existing position in regard to health conditions and health organization in the country and to make recommendations for the future development.

- In 1946, the Bhore committee recommended a short-term and long-term program for the attainment of reasonable health services based on concept of modern health practice.

Post-Independence Era

- India became independent in 1947 with new concept of establishing a welfare state.
- The burden of improving the health of people and widening the scope of health measures fell upon the center and states. Government appointed various committees for health analysis in the country.
- The Alma Ata deceleration of 1978 launched concept of "Health for All 2000 AD" and introduced the concept of primary healthcare.
- It was totally state's responsibility to provide primary healthcare to the people and led to the formulation of the first National Health Policy.
- In 1983, 1st National Health Policy was introduced. The major goals of the policy was to provide universal, comprehensive primary health services and articulated the need to encourage private initiative in healthcare service delivery.
- 1980-90 the period of Neoliberal economic and health sector reform that were aimed at increasing the importance of the private sector and desire to utilize private sector resources for addressing public health goals.
- Liberalization of insurance sector to provide health financing system.
- In the year of 2000, the national population policy (NPP) was announced to address the unmet need of contraception, healthcare infrastructure, and health personnel, and to provide integrated delivery for basis reproductive and child care services.
- Near 20 years after the first health policy, the 2nd National Health Policy was introduced in 2002.
- The NPH was set a new policy framework to achieve public health goals by the increasing access to the decentralized public health system by establishing new infrastructure indifferent area and upgrading the infrastructure of existing institutions.
- Recently in 2005, The Government of India has launched the National Rural Health Mission with the goal of improving the availability of and access to quality healthcare by people, especially for rural areas.
- NRHM provides great strength to the rural healthcare delivery system.
- Most recently in 2007, telemedicine and the medical tourism were introduced in the healthcare system of India.

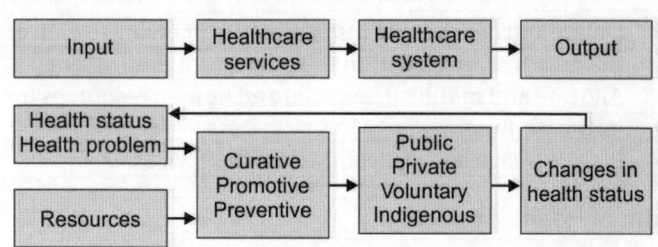

Fig. 5.1: Healthcare delivery system in India.

1. The "inputs" are the health status or health problems of the community; they represent the health needs and health demands of the community. Since, sources are always limited to meet the many health needs, priorities have to be set.
2. The "healthcare services" are designed to meet the health needs of the community through the use of available knowledge and resources. The services provided should be comprehensive and community-based.
3. The "healthcare system" is intended to deliver the healthcare services; it constitutes the management sector and involves organizational matters.
4. The final outcome or output is the changed health status or improved health status of the community which is expressed in terms of lives saved, deaths averted, diseases prevented, etc.

Organization and administration of health system in India: Health administration is the science of the organizing and coordinating government agencies whose purpose is to improve the physical, mental and social well-being of the people of the country. It is a part of the public administration.

1. India is a Union of 28 States and 7 Union territories. Under the Constitution of India, the States are largely independent in matters relating to the delivery of healthcare to the people.
2. Each State has developed own system of healthcare delivery, independent of the Central Government.
3. The Central responsibility of an organization of policy making, planning, guiding, assisting, evaluating, and coordinating the work of the State Health Ministries, so that health services cover every part of the country, In order to achieve the goal to "Health for All – 2020". Health administration governed in India at 4 levels:
   1. National level (Central level)
   2. State level
   3. District level
   4. Community level

HEALTHCARE DELIVERY SYSTEM (FIG. 5.1)

The challenge that exists today in many countries is to reach the whole population with adequate healthcare services and to ensure their utilization. For that, the numerous models have been developed for the delivery of healthcare services. One of the simplest model is:

CENTER LEVEL HEALTHCARE ADMINISTRATION

The official "organs" of the health system at the National Level consist of:
- The Ministry of Health and Family Welfare
- The Directorate General of Health Services; and
- The Central Council of Health and Family Welfare

Union Ministry of Health and Family Welfare

Organization (Fig. 5.2)

The Union Ministry of Health and Family Welfare is headed by a Cabinet Minister, a Minister of State and a Deputy Health Minister. The Union Ministry has three departments:
1. Departments of health
2. Departments of family welfare
3. Departments of Indian Systems of Medicine and Homoeopathy (ISM&H)

Functions of the Union Health Ministry: The functions of the Union Health Ministry are set out in the seventh schedule of Article 246 of the Constitution of India under:
- The Union list and
- The Concurrent list

Union list: The functions given in the Union list are:
- International health relations and administration of port quarantine
- Administration of central institutes, such as the All India Institute of Hygiene and Public Health, Kolkata; National Institute for the Control of Communicable Diseases, Delhi, etc.
- Promotion of research through research centers and other bodies
- Regulation and development of medical, pharmaceutical, dental and nursing professions
- Establishment and maintenance of drug standards
- Census, and collection and publication of other statistical data
- Immigration and emigration
- Regulation of labor in the working of mines and oil fields
- Coordination with States and with other ministries for promotion of health.

Concurrent list: The functions listed under the concurrent list are the responsibility of both the Union and State governments.

The concurrent list includes:
- Prevention of communicable diseases
- Prevention of adulteration of foodstuffs
- Control of drugs and poisons
- Vital statistics
- Labor welfare
- Ports other than major
- Economic and social planning, and
- Population control and family planning

Functions of Department of Medical and Public Health:
- Health Policy preparation
- National Health Programs conduction
- Drug Control
- PFA enforcement

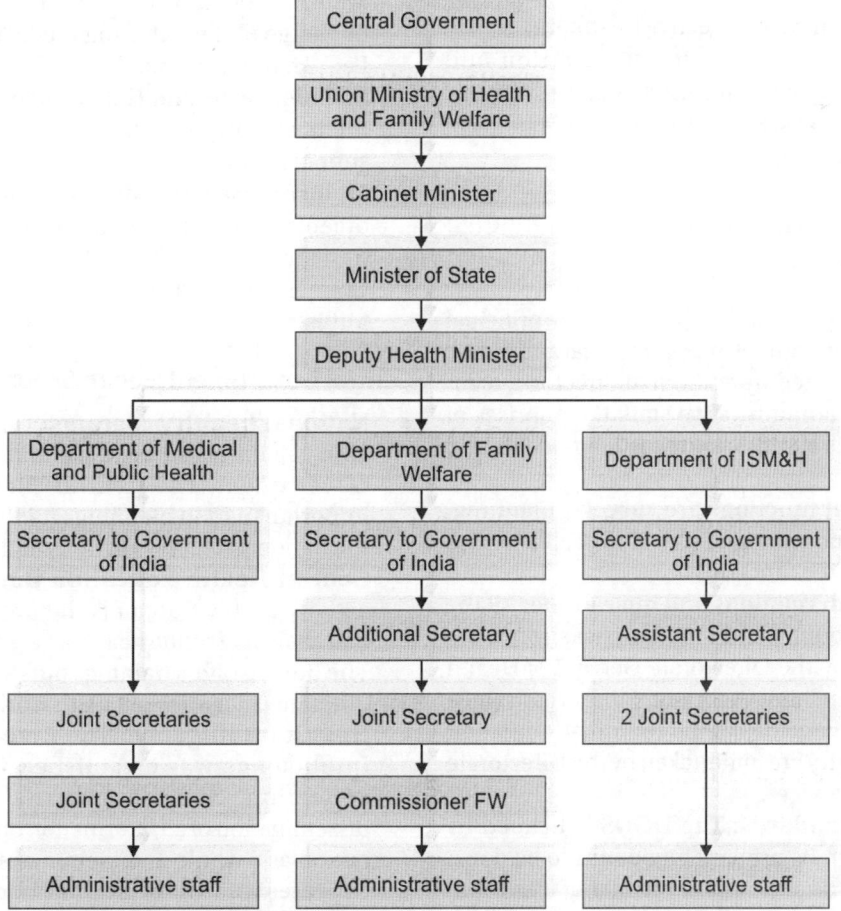

Fig. 5.2: Organization of Union Ministry of Health and Family Welfare.
(ISM&H: Indian System of Medicine and Homeopathy; FW: family welfare)

- Diseases control
- Communicable/noncommunicable
- Supplies and disposal maintenance
- CME and trainings
- Medical education and research
- Vital statistics and health intelligence
- International support

Functions of Department of Family Welfare:
- Policy preparation and planning
- Information collection and evaluation
- Contraceptive-research/supply
- Seeking international support for Family Welfare
- EPI/UIP/CSSM/RCH/ARI/ORT—trainings and area development
- Maternal and child health services
- Information, education and communication (IEC)
- Rural health services
- Paraprofessional training
- NGO support
- Development of subcenter

Functions of Department of IMS &H: The functions of the Department of IMS&H are:
- Upgrade the educational standards in the Indian Systems of Medicines and Homoeopathy colleges in the country;
- Strengthen existing research institutions and ensure a time-bound research program on identified diseases for which these systems have an effective treatment;
- Draw up schemes for promotion, cultivation and regeneration of medicinal plants used in these systems;
- Evolve Pharmacopoeial standards for Indian Systems of Medicine and Homoeopathy drugs.

THE DIRECTORATE GENERAL OF HEALTH SERVICES

Organization (Fig. 5.3)

Directorate General of Health Services (DGHS) is the principal adviser for the Union Government in both medical and public health matters. He is assisted by additional director, a team of deputies and a large administrative staff. It comprises of three units—medical care and hospital, public health and general health.

Functions: The general functions are surveys, planning, coordination, programming and appraisal of all health matters in the country. The specific functions are:
- **International health relations and quarantine:** All the major ports in the country and international airports are directly controlled by the Directorate General of Health Services. All matters relating to the obtaining of assistance from international agencies and the coordination of their activities in the country are undertaken by the Directorate General of Health Services.
- **Control of drug standards:** The DGHS is headed by the Drugs Controller. Its primary function is to lie down and enforce standards and control the manufacture and distribution of drugs through both Central and State Government Officers.

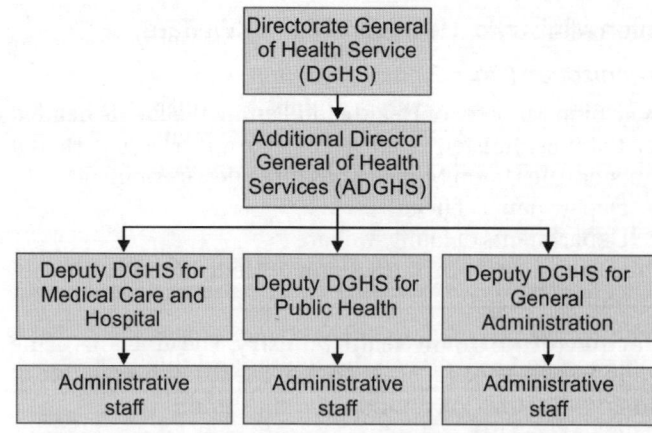

Fig. 5.3: Organization of Directorate General of Health Service.

- **Medical store depots:** The Union Government runs medical store depots. These depots supply the civil medical requirements of the Central Government and of the various State Governments. These depots also handle supplies from foreign agencies. The Medical Stores Organization endeavors to ensure the highest quality, cheaper bargain and prompt supplies.
- **Postgraduate training:** The DGHS is responsible for the administration of national institutes, which also provide postgraduate training to different categories of health personnel.
- **Medical education:** The Central Directorate is directly in charge of the following medical colleges in India: the Lady Harding, the Maulana Azad and the medical colleges at Puducherry, and Goa. Besides these, there are many medical colleges in the country which are guided and supported by the Center.
- **Medical research:** Medical Research in the country is organized largely through the Indian Council of Medical Research, founded in 1911 in New Delhi. The funds of the Council are wholly derived from the budget of the Union Ministry of Health.

Central Government Health Scheme

- **National health programs:** Health programs of this kind can hardly succeed without the help of the Central Government. The Central Directorate plays a very important part in planning, guiding and coordinating all the national health programs in the country.
- **Central Health Education Bureau:** An outstanding activity of this Bureau is the preparation of education material for creating health awareness among the people. The Bureau offers training courses in health education to different categories of health workers.
- **Health intelligence:** The Central Bureau of Health Intelligence was established in 1961 to centralize collection, compilation, analysis, evaluation and dissemination of all information on health statistics for the nation as a whole. It disseminates epidemic intelligence to States and international bodies. The Bureau has an Epidemiological Unit, a Health Economics Unit, a National Morbidity Survey Unit and a Manpower Cell.

- **National medical library:** The Central Medical Library of the Directorate General Health Services was declared the National Medical Library in 1966. The aim is to help in the advancement of medical, health and related sciences by collection, dissemination and exchange of information.

Central Council of Health

The Central Council of Health was set up by a Presidential Order on 9 August, 1952 under Article 263 of the Constitution of India for continuous consultation, mutual understanding and cooperation between the Center and the States in the implementation of all the programs and measures pertaining to the health of the nation.

Organization: The Union Health Minister is the Chairman and the State Health Ministers are the members.

Functions: The functions of the Central Council of Health are:
- To consider and recommend broad outlines of policy in regard to matters concerning health in all its aspects such as the provision of remedial and preventive care, environmental hygiene, nutrition, health education and the promotion of facilities for training and research.
- To make proposals for legislation in fields of activity relating to medical and public health matters and to lay down the pattern of development for the country as a whole.
- To make recommendations to the Central Government regarding distribution of available grants-in-aid for health purposes to the States and to review periodically the work accomplished in different areas through the utilization of these grants-in-aid.
- To establish any organization or organizations invested with appropriate functions for promoting and maintaining cooperation between the Central and State Health administrations.

STATE LEVEL HEALTHCARE ADMINISTRATION

- Organizational structure at the state level is on the similar pattern as that as that as the central level (**Fig. 5.4**). Health being a state subject, the state government has autonomy in dealing with health matters.
- At present there are 28 States in India, with each state having its own health administration.

State Ministry of Health and Family Welfare

- The State Ministry of Health is headed by a Minister of Health and Family Welfare and a Deputy Minister of Health and Family Welfare. These are political appointments and they are elected members of legislative assembly.
- They have political responsibilities, responsibilities towards their constituencies as per their political agenda, and responsibilities for administration and management of Health and Family Welfare services in their state.

Health Secretariat

- The State Health and Family Welfare Minister is assisted for all administrative aspects of healthcare by the Health Secretariat, that is the official organ of his Ministry.
- The Health Secretariat is headed by the secretary who is assisted by Additional, Deputy and Assistant Secretaries and other hierarchy of administrative staff.

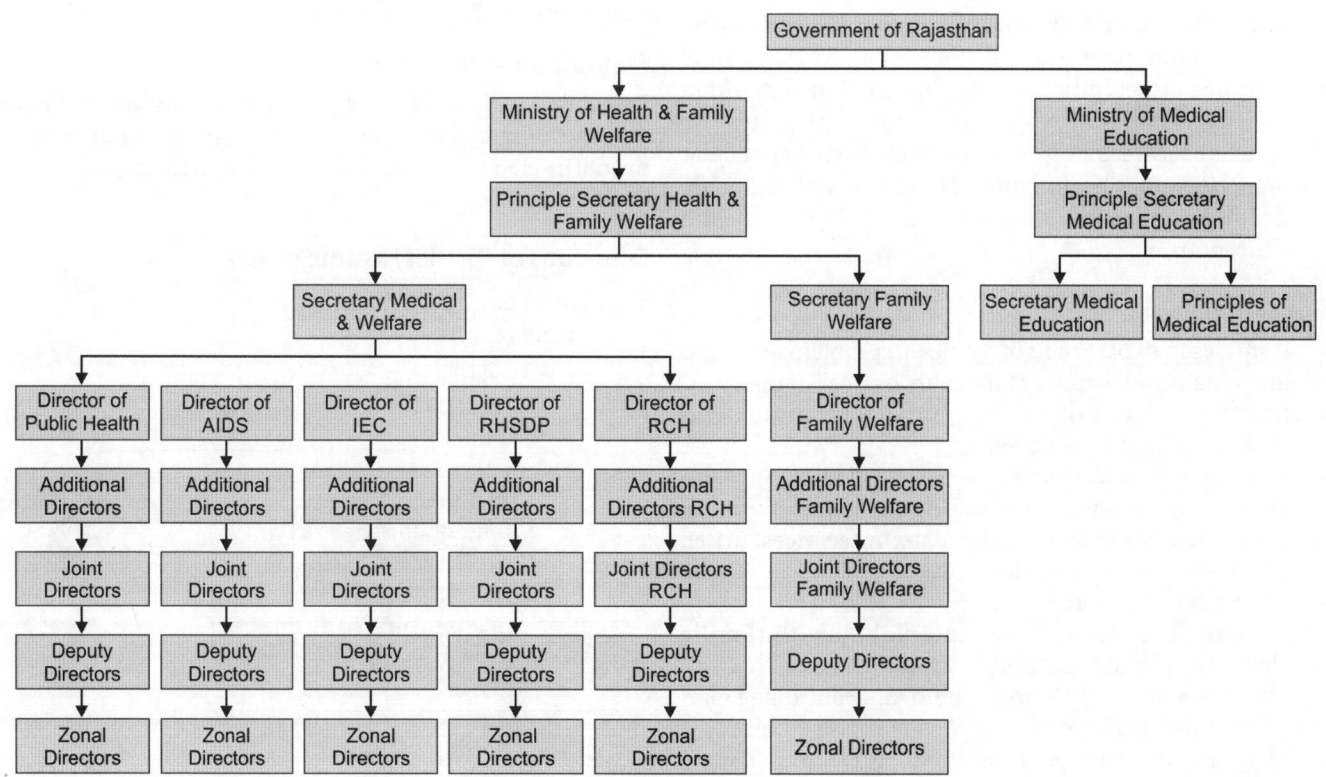

Fig. 5.4: Organizational setup at state level.

Functions: The major functions which are performed by the secretariat include helping minister in:
- Formulation, review and modification of broad policy outlines.
- Execution of policies programs, etc.
- Coordination with Government of India and other State Governments.
- Control for smooth and efficient functioning of administrative machinery.

State Health Directorate

- The State Health Directorate is the technical wing of state Ministry of Health and Family Welfare.
- Before independence, the Medical and Public Health Services at the State level like at the Center were also administered by two separate departments headed by surgeon General and Inspector General of civil hospitals and Director of Public Health Services respectively.
- After independence these two departments' medical health and public health were integrated into State Directorate of Health Services as recommended by Dr. Bhore committee report in 1946.
- State Health Directorate is headed by Director of health services. In some States, he is designated as Director of Health and Family Welfare.
- He is the chief technical advisor to the stale Government on all matters of Medical, Public Health and Family welfare.
- He is assisted by a number of Deputy and Assistant Directors to plan and provide healthcare services to meet healthcare needs of the State as per Government health policy.
- The Deputy and Assistant Directors of Health may be of two types-regional and functional. The Regional Directors inspect all the branches of public health within their jurisdiction, irrespective of their specialty. The Functional Directors are usually specialists in a particular branch of public health, such as mother and child health, family planning, nutrition, tuberculosis, leprosy, health education, etc.

Functions

- It studies in department of the health problem and need of the state and planning for health services in the state.
- Implementation of national health programs and evaluating their achievements.
- Promoting providing and supervising all types of health services in the state, such as primary health services; school health services; family planning services; MCH; occupational health services, etc.
- Collection of vital statistics.
- Encouraging reproductive and child health (family welfare maternal health, etc.)
- Improvement of nutrition program and controlling food adulteration and also sanitation in milk and edibles.
- Medical and nursing education, training of nurses, female health workers and other health workers.
- Controlling rural and urban health services through district medical officer.
- Providing feedback to the state health ministry regarding health.
- Following the directives of union ministry of health/state health ministry.

DISTRICT LEVEL HEALTHCARE ADMINISTRATION

District—an administrative unit defined geographical boundary and population. Within each district again, there are six types of administrative areas—Subdivisions, Tehsils (Talukas), Community Development Blocks, Municipalities and Corporations (urban area), Panchayats (Villages):
- District is peripheral most planning unit
- It is a self-contained segment of National Health System
- Middle level management organization
- The principal unit of administration in India is the district under a Collector.
- It is a link between the State/regional structure on one side and the peripheral level structures such as PHC/subcentre on the other side.

Organization

Chief Medical and Health Officer

Chief Medical and Health Officer (CM and HO) is a Director of Health and Family Welfare service at the district in rural area and are overall in-charge of the health and family welfare programs in the rural area. CM&HO is assisted by Deputy CMO, RHC Officer and programme Officers. Deputy CMO and RHC officer are assisted by Block CMOs. **Figure 5.5** shows organizational setup at district level.

Principle Medical Officer

Principle Medical Officer (PMO) is a Director of Health and Family Welfare service at the district in urban area and is overall in-charge of the health and family welfare programmes in urban area.

Functions of District Health System

- Liaison between field units and headquarter
  - Field reports

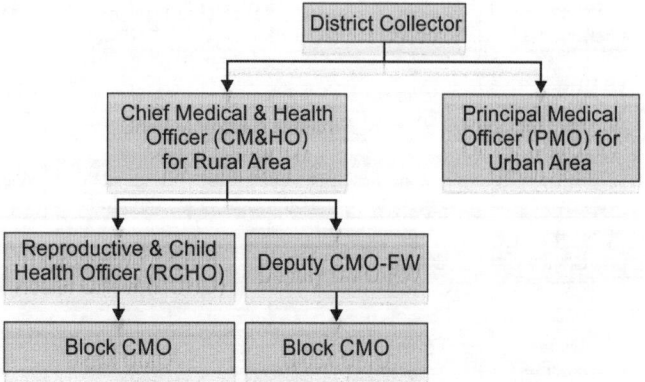

Fig. 5.5: Organizational setup at district level.

- Inspections
- Meetings
■ Implementation of policy and programs
■ District level planning and action plans
■ Rationale use of finance and resources
■ Communication management: Plans/schedules/progress/problems
■ Control and monitoring

COMMUNITY LEVEL HEALTHCARE ADMINISTRATION

Community Health Center

Community health Center (CHC) has been established for every 80,000 to 120,000 population and this center provides the basic specialty services in general medicine, Pediatric, surgery, obstetrics and gynecology.

Functions of CHC

- Care of routine and emergency cases in medicine
- Care of routine and emergency cases in surgery
- 24 hour delivery services, including normal and assisted deliveries.
- Essential and emergency obstetric care
- FP services including laparoscopic services
- Newborn care
- Routine and emergency care of sick children
- Other management including nasal packing, tracheotomy, foreign body removal, etc.

Organization

Center	Population norms	
	Plain area	hilly/tribal/difficult area
CHC	1,20,000	80,000
PHC	30,000	20,000
Subcenter	5000	3000

- All the national health programs (NHP) should be delivered through the CHC.
- Other:
  - Blood storage facility
  - Essential laboratory services
  - Referral services

Figure 5.6 shows rural healthcare system in India.

Staffing Pattern at CHC

Existing clinical manpower
- General Surgeon — 1
- Physician — 1
- Obstetrician/Gynecologist — 1
- Pediatrician — 1

Existing Support Manpower

- Nurse-midwife — 7+2
- Dresser — 1
- Pharmacist/Compounder — 1
- Lab technician — 1

Community Health Center (CHC)
A 30 bedded hospital/referral unit for 4 PHCs with four medical specialists Surgeon, Physician, Gynecologist and Pediatrician supported by 21 paramedical and other staff

↓

Primary Health Center (PHC)
A referral unit for 6 subcenter 4–6 bedded manned with a medical officer in charge and 14 subordinate paramedical staff

↓

Subcenter (SC)
Most peripheral contact point between primary healthcare system & community manned with one MPW (F) ANM & one MPW (M)

Fig. 5.6: Rural healthcare system in India.

- Radiographer — 1
- Ophthalmic assistant — 1
- Ward boy/nursing orderly — 2
- Sweepers — 2
- Chowkidar — 1
- OPD attendant — 1
- Data Entry Operator — 5
- OT attendant — 1
- Registration Clerk — 1

Primary Health Center Level

At present, there is one primary health center covering about 30,000 (20,000 in hilly, desert and difficult terrains) or more population. Many rural dispensaries have been upgraded to create these PHCs. The bed strength of primary health center is 6. (but can be raised up to 10)

Functions of PHC

- Medical care
- MCH including family planning
- Safe water supply and basic sanitation
- Prevention and control of locally endemic diseases.
- Collection and reporting of vital statistics
- Education about health
- National health programs as relevant
- Referral services
- Training of health guides, health workers local dais and health assistants.
- Basic laboratory services

Staffing Pattern of PHC

- Medical Officer — 1
- Pharmacist — 1
- Nurse Midwife — 1
- Health Worker (female)/ANM — 1
- Block Extension Educator — 1
- Health Assistant (Male) — 1
- Health Assistant (Female) — 1
- UDC (Upper Division clerk) — 1
- LDC (Lower Division clerk) — 1
- Lab Technician — 1

- Driver   1
- Class IV   4
- Total   15

Subcenter Level

The subcenter is the peripheral outpost of exiting healthcare delivery system in rural areas. It provides interface with community at the grass root level providing all the primary health services. One subcenter for every 5000, population in general and one for every 3000 population in hilly, tribal and backward areas. Each subcenter is manned by one male and one female multipurpose health worker.

Functions of Subcenter

1. Mother and child healthcare
2. Family planning and immunization
3. It is proposed to extend the facilities at all subcenters for IUD insertion, and simple laboratory investigation, such as routine examination of urine for albumin and sugar.
4. The work at subcenters is supervised by male and female health assistants.
5. According to the revised norm, one female HA will supervise the work of 6 female health workers.

Staffing Pattern of Subcenter

- Health Worker (Female)/ANM   1
- Health Worker (Male)   1
- Voluntary Worker   1
- Total   3

HEALTHCARE DELIVERY SYSTEM IN INDIA

Healthcare services in general are rendered by the government through a network of health centres from the grassroots areas to the block level in the rural areas and through hospitals, dispensaries, maternal, child health and family welfare centers in the urban areas. The hospitals in the sub-divisional, Talukas level, district level, etc., provide referral services to the infrastructure in the rural area. There are also voluntary and private agencies which are functioning to deal with the health problems of people **(Fig. 5.7)**.

Public or Government Sector

Public sector is government sponsored system. It is funded by the public funds which are generated through general taxes. The services are rendered to the people at large in rural and urban areas by three tier system developed at the block level, district and state level.

Rural Health Service

- The health services in the rural areas are rendered through a network of infrastructure developed from within the village and in continuum up to block level.
- The major emphasis is on promotive and preventive healthcare services and comprises primary healthcare.
- At the village level, elementary services are rendered by trained village health guides, birth attendants (local dias) and anganwari workers.
- They belong to the village they serve and are non-governmental functionaries.
- They are included in the healthcare delivery system to promote and encourage community participation and to have a link between the community and the health functionaries.
- The village health guide provide simple treatment for common minor ailments, first aid during accidents and emergency, care to mother and children including family planning, health education, etc.
- The trained birth attendants work under the supervision and guidance of female health worker and provide personal and skillful care during prenatal period, give health education on child care, immunization, nutrition, and family planning.
- Anganwari workers work in anganwaries and carry on the responsibility of health check-ups, supplementary nutrition, immunization, non-formal education of children enrolled in anganwari. They coordinate with the ANMs in their areas for some of the functions, e.g., immunization and health check-up of children. Each one serves a population of 1000 in the village.
- The continuum of health centers which provide primary healthcare services include subcenters, primary health centres and community health centres.
- The subcenter serve a population of 5000 in plain area and 3000 in hilly, tribal and backward areas.
- The limited primary healthcare services which are provided from subcenters include; maternal and child health, family planning, prevention and control of communicable diseases, treatment of minor ailments, record of vital events, emergency care, maintenance of record and reports, supervision and training of dais and village health guides.

The services are rendered by ANMs, i.e., health workers (F) and health worker (M) under the supervision and guidance of health supervisor (F and M) respectively.

URBAN HEALTH SERVICES

- The services in the urban areas are rendered through district hospitals and medical college hospitals.
- There are also hospitals and institutes of higher education and research which are under Central Government and provide general as well as referral services.
- In addition to these hospital services, there are maternal and child health, family welfare centers, family planning clinics, dispensaries, maternity homes, community hospitals run by local government to provide specific primary level services to defined population. **Figure 5.8** shows urban health care delivery model.

Health Insurance System

In India health insurance system is restricted to factory/industrial workers and their families and central government employees and their families. They are covered by two different very well organized health insurance schemes. These are:

Chapter 5: Healthcare and Development of Nursing Services in India

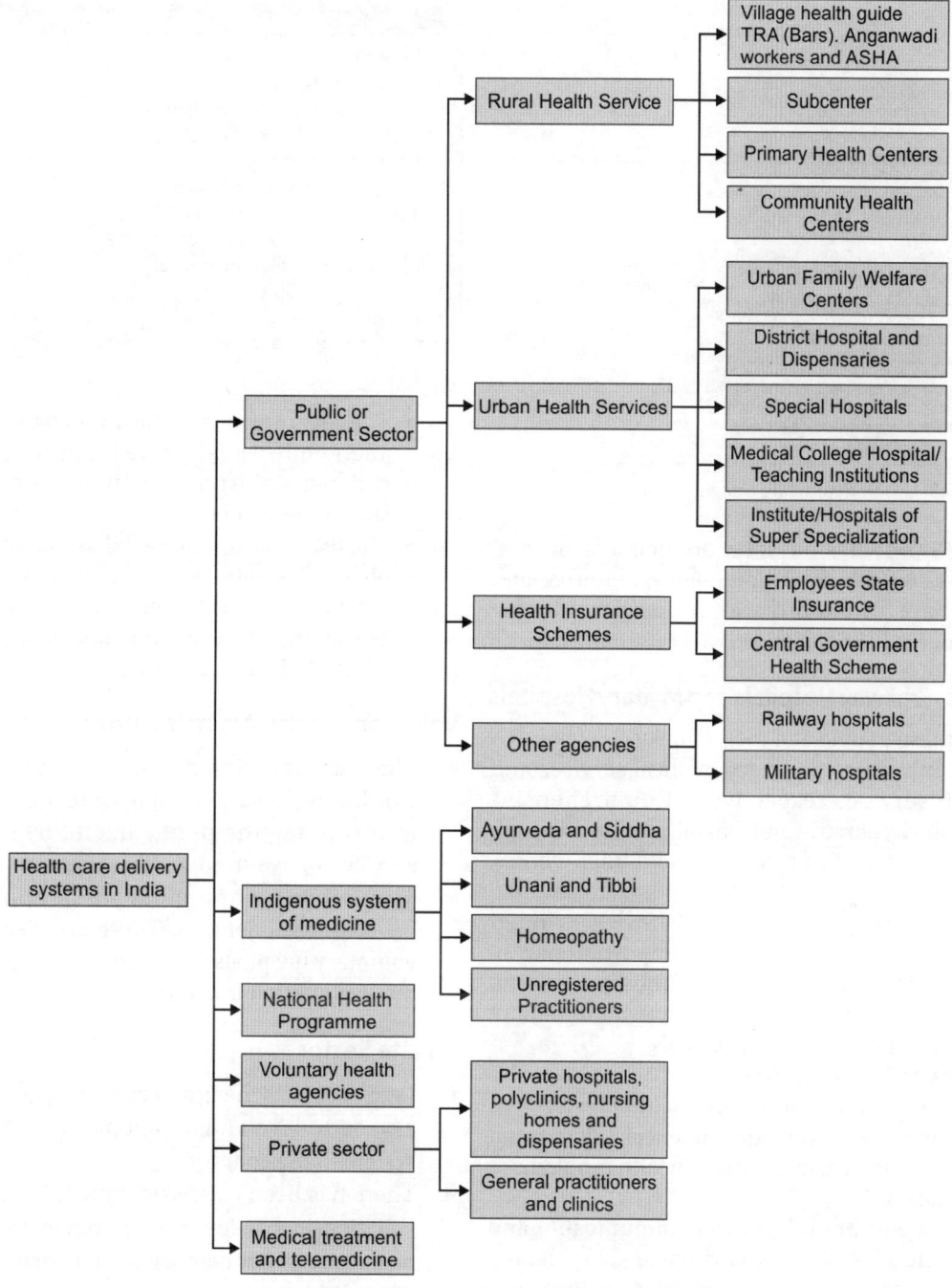

Fig. 5.7: Healthcare delivery model.

1. **Employees State Insurance:** The ESI scheme was started under the parliament Act in 1948 to provide medical benefits in kind and cash during sickness, employment injury, maternity, etc., the scheme is based on the contributions from the employer, employees and the government.
2. **Central Government Health Scheme:**
   - This scheme is for the Central Government Employers. To start with it was introduced in Delhi in 1954 to provide comprehensive healthcare to central government employees.
   - Gradually, it was extended to other cities not only to central government employees and their family members but also other autonomous organizations employees, members of parliament, retired central government servants, and widow receiving family pensions, Governors and retired judges.
   - The scheme is on the cooperative efforts and contribution basis from the employees and employer for their mutual benefits.
   - The services are given through a network of dispensaries, governmental hospitals, and identified private specialized hospitals in various systems of medicine.

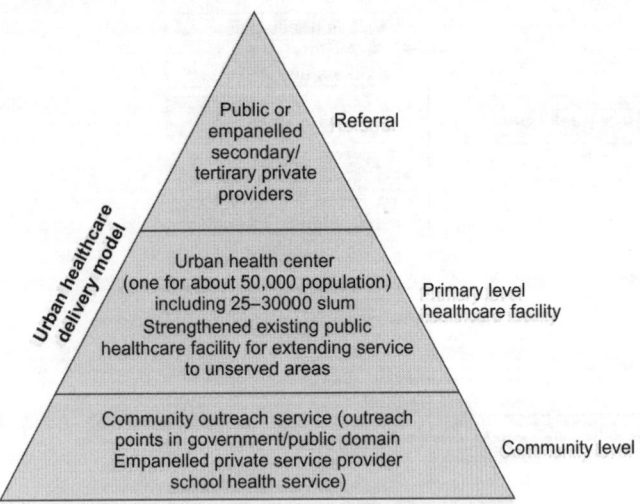

Fig. 5.8: Urban healthcare delivery model.

- The CGHS provides outdoor, domiciliary, indoor, specialists consultations, emergency, maternal and child welfare and family welfare services. It also supplies optical and dental aids at reasonable rates.

Other Agencies—railway Hospitals and Military Hospitals

The services to these people and their families are rendered by specially organized armed forces medical services and railways health services respectively. Comprehensive preventive, promotive, curative and rehabilitative services are rendered through especially organized health units, clinics, hospitals, etc.

- **Indigenous system of medicine [AYUSH]:** The indigenous systems of medicine form an important part of public system of healthcare delivery in both rural and urban areas. Services are rendered through out-patient departments, dispensaries and hospitals.
- **National Health Program (Box 5.3)**
  - In addition to various levels of healthcare services through public system, the government of India has put in lot of efforts to deal with various health problems at the national level.
  - These problems are related to communicable and noncommunicable diseases, environmental sanitation problem, nutritional problems, population problems, etc.

Box 5.3: National Health Programs.

To improve the health status of people, to control communicable diseases, improvement of environment sanitation, control of population, etc., the Central Government launched the National Health Programmes.
- **Programmes for Communicable Diseases**
  - National Vector Borne Diseases Control Programme (NVBDCP)
  - Revised National Tuberculosis Control Programme
  - National Leprosy Eradication Programme
  - National AIDS Control Programme
  - Universal Immunization Programme
  - National Guinea worm Eradication Programme
  - Yaws Control Programme
  - Integrated Disease Surveillance Programme

Box 5.4: Voluntary health agencies in India.
- Indian Red Cross Society
- Hind Kusht Nivaran Sangh
- Indian Council for Child Welfare
- Tuberculosis Association of India
- Bharat Sevak Samaj
- Central Social Welfare Board
- The Kasturba Memorial Fund
- Family Planning Association of India
- All India Women's Conference
- Professional Bodies
- International Agencies

- The government of India through its ministry of health and family welfare have launched ongoing various national health programs in successive five year plans since independence.
- The technical and material assistance have also been obtained by various international and bilateral agencies in planning and implementation of these programs.
- These organizations include WHO, UNICEF, World Bank, UNFPA, DANIDA, etc.

Voluntary Health Agencies (Box 5.4)

- There are varieties of nongovernmental organizations which are voluntary in nature and contribute tremendously in furthering the public health by providing health services, or health education, by advancing research, etc.
- The NGOs complement and supplement role of government agencies. There are also "not for profit" voluntary hospitals which generate funds to sustain and provide charitable services, e.g., Holy Family Hospital.

Private Sector

- Like voluntary health sector, the private health sector also occupies an important place in healthcare delivery system in the country.
- There has been extensive growth in the private owned facilities since independence, but more so during the last decade, there has been significant increase in the number of medical practitioners.
- They range from herbal and witch doctors to modern unqualified or quasi-qualified "quacks" to qualified practitioners of different system of medicine, many of whom also indulge in quackery.
- The different system of medicine includes Allopathy or Modern Medicine, Homeopathy, Ayurveda, Unani and Siddha. Apart from these, there is other, such as Yoga, Naturopathy and Chiropractice.
- There are large numbers of practitioners who have not qualified in any of the recognized systems.
- It is this diversity and complexity which is in part responsible for lack of regulation and quality control in private practice.

- Further, those who are qualified in modern medicine tend to locate themselves in urban areas and all others are equally locating themselves in urban areas and all others are equally located in urban and rural areas. There are three times more allopathic in urban than in rural areas.
- There has been increase in the number of private hospitals including those owed by the voluntary agencies.
- The private consultants are attached to these hospitals. They participate in the services organized by the hospital as well as they have their own private OPD/clinics and cases in hospital.
- The fee which is charged for the services varies depending upon the level, standard, popularity, etc., of the hospital; consultant; locality, etc., there is no uniform pattern and there is no control over this.
- The system is beyond the reach of even an average middle class family. It is not an organized system of providing healthcare services. Efforts are being put into maintain the standards through legislation related to Nursing Homes and Hospitals and Consumer Protection Act.
- The various diagnostic facilities are on the increase to assist in making diagnosis, but these are very expensive and often exploited liberally. The government is putting in efforts to involve Medical Council of India and Indian Medical Association to regulate the system, etc.

Medical Truism and Telemedicine

- Medical tourism is one of the major external drivers of growth of the Indian healthcare sector.
- This is a developing concept whereby people from world over visit India for their medical and relaxation needs.
- Most common treatments are heart surgery, joint replacement, orthopedic surgery, gastroenterology, ophthalmology, transplants, urology, cosmetic surgery and dental care.
- Hospitals groups, such as The Global Hospitals Group, MIOT Hospitals, Fortis Healthcare and Apollo hospitals, Max Hospitals, Dharamshila Cancer Hospital and Research Centre have increased their presence in international market for medical tourism.
- In the current rapidly changing healthcare scenario, the magnitude of the problem associated with healthcare delivery is enormous and extremely dynamic. However, present day technology has the solution for this problem.
- User-friendly equipment with compatibility to integrate technologies, such as telemedicine makes the solution simpler.
- Telemedicine system is growing rapidly in India, nearing 700 million rural populations of India will benefit enormously from digital data transmission related to healthcare.
- Both public and private entities are aggressively pursuing the use of telemedicine to hasten diagnostics and treatment of a variety of diseases.
- Private hospitals, such as Apollo Hospital Group, Escorts Heart Institute and Fortis Healthcare are providing these services in India.

Challenges in Health System
- Manpower—number and norms
- Rural/Urban differential
- Geographical divide across states
- S-E groups—accessibility/reach
- Gaps between policy and action
- Health sector expenditure
- Newer infections

Role of Nurse in Healthcare Delivery System
- Care—provide
- Planner
- Sensitive observer
- Educator manager
- Organizer
- Evaluator
- Controller
- Administrator

NURSING SERVICES

Nursing service is the part of the total health organization which aims at satisfying the nursing needs of the patients/community. In nursing services, the nurse works with the members of allied disciples, such as dietetics, medical social service, pharmacy, etc., in supplying a comprehensive program of patient care in the hospital.

Definition of nursing services: WHO expert committee on nursing defines the nursing services as the part of the total health organization which aims to satisfy major objective of the nursing services is to provide prevention of disease and promotion of health.

Organization of Nursing Services

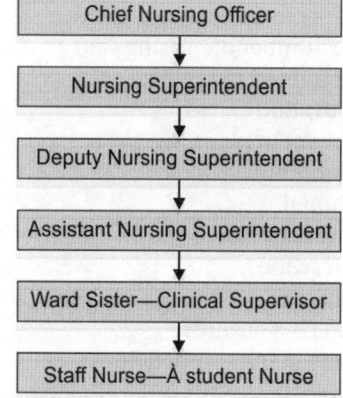

Objective of Nursing in Ward
- Maximum comfort and happiness by way of pleasant surroundings.
- Qualitative/comprehensive care to the patient
- Care based on the patient's needs.
- Accurate assessment of illness.
- Adequate material resources at all times.
- Health education to the patient and attendants
- Managerial skills as and when required
- Privacy at all levels

Effective Nursing

An effective nursing is always based on nursing process which is an organized and systematic approach to nursing care, that prioritizes patient assessment and management.

Entire nursing process consists of four phases:
- **Assessment:** Not only initial but integral ongoing component of the whole nursing process.
- **Planning and implementation:** In this, the nurse formulates and implements the care.
- **Evaluation:** Decides whether the action taken has met the identified needs or not. This is the final step of care. Also, review of the whole care plan. Without this no quality care or comprehensive care is possible to provide.

Factors to be considered in planning hospital nursing services:
- Number and type of patient
- Number of beds and type of ward
- The services required.
- Procedures/techniques necessary for care
- Number and type of personal needed to perform care effectively
- Physical facilities
- Provisional of equipment and supplies

SIU norms

- 1 Nursing sister for 3:6 staff nurses
- 1 ANS for 4:5 nursing sisters
- 1 DNS for 7:5 ANS
- 1 Nursing superintendent for 250-500 beds
- 1 CNO for 500 or more beds

Problems and challenges faced by the nursing administrator:
- Lack of adequate training
- Problem of personnel management
- Inadequate number of nursing staff
- Shortage of trained manpower
- Lack of motivation
- No involvement in planning
- No career mobility
- Poor role model
- Non-nursing activities
- No research scope
- No proper authority
- Professional risk/hazards
- No autonomy in nursing activities

Constrains and barriers in nursing services administration:
- Planning of nursing manpower
- Management and development
- Staff development
- Development/awards
- Nursing legislation
- Trained nurse managers
- Diversification in nursing profession
- Leadership inadequacy
- Lack of strength, weakness, opportunity and threat
- Lack of awareness to meet social, economic and technical changes in the Society and Consumer Protection Act.
- Lack of communication
- Nursing care audit

Day to day problem in nursing services:
- Shortage of nurses
- Lack of motivation
- Negative attitude
- Lack of training
- Lack of team approach
- Inactive participation of programs
- Lack of IPR
- Less involvement in patients care by the nursing supervisors.
- Lack of supervision

Foreseen for better nursing service administration in the next millennium:
- Accountability
- Autonomy of professional activities
- Awareness of CPA
- Independent nursing practices
- Renewal of licenses based on education and examination
- Specialty nursing
- Nursing care audit
- Qualitative nursing care
- Separate nursing budget
- Diploma in nursing management
- Nursing research

RECENT TRENDS AND ISSUES OF NURSING SERVICE AND MANAGEMENT

Nursing Trends refers to direction towards which the different nursing event have moved or are moving as well as the opinion in and around nursing that are found in and about nursing profession.

There are different changes in profession

Social Change:
- Nursing profession severs to meet the need to the society particularly the need related to health and well being.
- The changes in society will influence to bring about changes in nursing profession.
  - At present, efforts are made by government of India to deliver the healthcare to the community especially in rural area.
  - Overall improvement in the education of people with ever growing awareness about health and health need.
- Now women are more educated and take up jobs out of home to sever and earn.
- Advancement of technology, e.g., automatization, industrialization, urbanization.
- After independence, government began to make serious efforts to meet health need of nation by implementing recommendation of Bhore committee.

Changes in other profession:
- Medical profession is fast-changing profession and the era of specialization and super specialization has come.
- Modern healthcare facility, such as ICU, ICCU, renal unit, organ transplant unit, etc.

- Biomedical science have for advanced resulting in newer diagnostic equipment such as scanner, new drugs, monitoring system in field of healthcare all over the world.

Changes in nursing profession itself in the country:
- Trends to take up education leading to bachelor degree in nursing, master degree as well as doctoral degree.
- Trends related to tuition fee, e.g., paid stipends, free hiring, accommodation, food and uniform, but service is expected from the nurse.
- Trends related to changes in working condition for nurses.

Change taking place in other countries in nursing world:
- Fast growing trends to post basic degree programmes.
- INC promotes sharing of ideas and common interest between members of national organization.
- Exchange of professional literature, such as international review, professional journals, articles, etc.

Current trends and issues in nursing:
- **Reduction in distance through seedy communication:** Mobile, video conference has made it possible for the nurses to reach patient, doctor and other profession whenever need arise. Along with verbal and nonverbal communication skill, nurses also need to gain competencies in using information and technology.
- **Computerization for patient care management:** Easy reference on direction for patient care, record keeping, reporting, compilation of information, stock monitoring, auditing are some of the function which have taken over. Ability to use computers for patient care management has become essential qualification for nurses.
- **Quality assurance in nursing care:** Public know their right.
- **Decentralized approach to care management:** This make each and every nurse responsible and accountable for the care of assigned patient.
- **Continuing nursing education:** It has become essential to keep up with the changing needs of patient care. Nurses have to continuously update themselves with new and innovative approaches in patient care management.
- **Evidence based practice:** For this, nurses should have scientific bend of mind and dynamic approach to patient care.
- **Nurse patient ratio:** Adherence to nurse patient ratio is necessary for providing quality care.
- **Conduct of nursing research:** Having knowledge is essential for the nursing profession. This is possible only through research and dissemination of research finding.
- **Nursing audits:** Audit is required to keep the activities on the right track. It builds knowledge for the profession.
- **Higher education for senior position in nursing:** Nursing leader can guide and monitor the nursing team effectively.
- **Independent nurse practitioners:**

Issues in nursing:
- Renewal of nursing registration
- Diploma v/s Degree in nursing for registration to practice nursing
- Specialization in clinical area
- Nursing care standards

Issues in nursing education:
- Nursing training school multiplied.
- Lack of independent building for school and college.
- Lack of independent principal for school and college.
- Inadequate hostel facility for student
- Shortage of qualified teacher in nursing
- Inadequate library facilities
- Less supply of AV aids
- Less promotional opportunities for teachers of both school and college.
- Very less or no stipend for nursing student.

CONCLUSION

Health systems and polices have a critical role in determining the manner in which health services are delivered, utilized and affect health outcomes. 'Health' being a state subject, despite the issuance of the guidelines by the central government, the final prerogative on implementation of the initiatives on newborn care lies with the states. Nursing profession is considered a caring profession to begin with; it was an art and a vocation. Now, it is considered a scientific profession nursing care is defined as the care of the patient with regard to nursing needs, with the ever increasing dimension of medical sciences quantitatively and qualitatively nursing care is becoming more and more complex with its management services.

REVIEW QUESTIONS

Long Essays
1. Define healthcare, aims, goals and functions of healthcare system.
2. History of healthcare system: explain the pre-independence Era and post-independence Era.
3. Describe State level healthcare administration.
4. Explain Healthcare delivery system in India.
5. Recent trends and issues of nursing service and management.

Short Essays
1. Forces influence the health system.
2. Organization and administration of health system in India.
3. Union Ministry of Health and Family Welfare.
4. Functions of department of medical and public health.
5. Directorate General of Health Services.
6. Central Government Health Scheme.
7. Health Secretariat.
8. District Level Healthcare Administration.
9. Chief Medical and Health Officer (CM and HO).
10. Community level Healthcare Administration.
11. Urban Health Services.

Short Answers
1. Functions of the Union Health Ministry.
2. Functions of Department of IMS&H.
3. Central Health Education Bureau.
4. National Health Programs.
5. Central Council of Health.
6. State Health Directorate.

7. Functions of District Health System.
8. Community Health Centre.
9. Staffing Pattern at CHC.
10. Functions of subcenter.
11. Employees State Insurance.
12. Indigenous system of medicine.
13. National Health Program.
14. Voluntary health agencies.
15. Challenges in health system.
16. Definition of nursing services.
17. SIU norms.

BIBLIOGRAPHY

1. Blais K, Hayes J. Professional Nursing Practice Concepts and Practices, 7th edition. NJ: Pearson; 2016.
2. Diwakar G. Healthcare delivery system in India. The Heinz school review. 2006;3(2):34-36.
3. Emanuel EJ, Emanuel LL. What is accountability in healthcare? Ann Intern Med. 1996;124:229-39.
4. George S. Healthcare delivery system; www.social science research network. 2005; (5):19-21.
5. Kishore J.' National Health Programs of India' published by Century Publications edition. 2010; pp. 63-9.
6. Madura G. India launches National Rural Health Mission. British Medical Journal. 2005;4(3):33-5.
7. Park K. 'Textbook of preventive and social medicine' published by Banarsidas. Bhanot edition. 2009; p765-75.
8. Rao M, Rao KD, Shiva Kumar AK, Chatterjee M, Sundararaman T. Human resources for health in India. The Lancet. 2011; 377: 587-98.
9. Reddy KS, Patel V, Jha P, Paul VK, Kumar AK, Dandona L, et al. Towards achievement of universal healthcare in India by 2020: A call to action. Lancet. 2011;377:760-8.
10. Roy S. Primary healthcare in India. Health Popul Perspect Issues. 1985;8:135-67.
11. TNAI; Textbook of manual of community health,(3):141-3.

CHAPTER 6

Planning Nursing Services

LEARNING OBJECTIVES

- Meaning of Planning
- Mission Statement of Nursing Service
- Vision Statements
- Nursing Service Philosophy
- Scope of Planning in Nursing Service
- Nursing Service Policies, Procedures and Manuals
- Functional, Operational and Strategic Planning
- Strategic Planning in Nursing
- Operational Planning in Nursing
- Program Planning: Gantt Chart and Milestone Chart
- Characteristics of Planning
- Importance of Planning
- Essentials of Good Planning
- Principles of Planning
- Steps Involved in Planning
- Components of Planning
- Factors Affecting Planning
- Types/Classifications of Plans
- Advantages of Planning
- Components of Safety Management Plan
- Planning Hospital and Patient Care Unit (Ward)
- Planning of Patient Care Unit
- Planning for Emergency and Disaster
- Triage

INTRODUCTION

Planning as a basic function of management is a principal duty of all managers. It is a systematic process and requires knowledgeable activity based on sound managerial theory. Being the first element of management defined by Fayol, planning is making a plan of action to provide for the foreseeable future. This plan of action must have unity, continuity, flexibility, and precision.

Planning is a continuous process, beginning with the setting of goals and objectives and then laying out a plan of action for accomplishing them, putting them into play, reviewing the process and the outcomes, providing feedback to personnel, and modifying plans as needed. As planning is put into action, the management functions of organizing, leading, and evaluating are implemented, making all management functions interdependent.

Figure 6.1 shows levels of management.

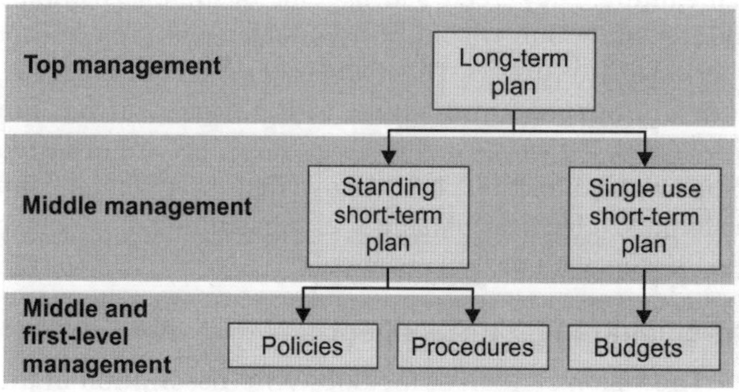

DEFINITION

Different authors have given different definitions of planning from time to time. The main definitions of planning are as follows:

- According to Alford and Beatt, "Planning is the thinking process, the organized foresight, the vision based on fact and experience that is required for intelligent action."
- According to Theo Haimann, "Planning is deciding in advance what is to be done. When a manager plans, he projects a course of action for further attempting to achieve a consistent coordinate structure of operations aimed at the desired results. According to Billy E Goetz, "Planning is fundamentally choosing and a planning problem arises when an alternative course of action is discovered."
- According to Koontz and O' Donnell, "Planning is an intellectual process, conscious determination of course of action, the basing of decision on purpose, facts and considered estimates."
- According to Allen, "A plan is a trap laid to capture the future."

MEANING OF PLANNING

- Planning is a deliberative, systematic phase of the nursing process that involves decision making and problem solving.

Fig. 6.1: Levels of management.

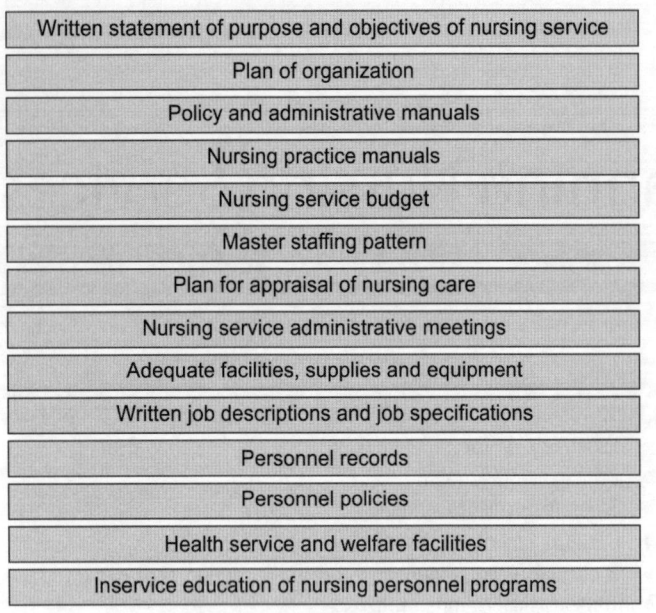

Fig. 6.2: Essential characteristics of a nursing service.

- In planning, the nurse refers to the client's assessment data and diagnostic statements for direction and formulating client goals and designing the nursing strategies required to prevent, reduce or eliminate the client's health problems planning means to decide in advance what is to be done.
- It charts a course of actions for the future. It is an intellectual process and it aims to achieve a coordinated and consistent set of operations aimed at desired objectives.
- Planning is the fundamental management function, which involves deciding beforehand, what is to be done, when is it to be done, how it is to be done and who is going to do it.
- It is an intellectual process which lays down an organization's objectives and develops various courses of action, by which the organization can achieve those objectives. It chalks out exactly, how to attain a specific goal.
- Planning bridges the gap from where we are to where we want to go. It includes the selection of objectives, policies, procedures and programs from among alternatives. A plan is a predetermined course of action to achieve a specified goal.
- It is an intellectual process characterized by thinking before doing. It is an attempt on the part of manager to anticipate the future in order to achieve better performance. Planning is the primary function of management.

Figure 6.2 shows essential characteristics of a nursing service.

■ MISSION STATEMENT OF NURSING SERVICE

A Mission Statement defines the organization's purpose and primary objectives. Its prime function is internal-to define the key measure or measures of the organization's success-and its prime audience is the leadership team and stockholders. Mission statements are the starting points of an organization's strategic planning and goal setting process. They focus attention and assure that internal and external stakeholders understand what the organization is attempting to accomplish.

Mission and purpose: Mission and purpose are used interchangeably, though at theoretical level, there is a difference between two. Mission has external orientation and relates the organization to the society in which it operates. A mission statement helps the organization to link its activities to the needs of the society and legitimize its existence. Purpose is also externally focused but it relates to that segment of the society to which it serves; it defines the business which the institution will undertake.

- At is most basic, the mission statement describes the overall purpose of the organization.
- If the organization elects to develop a vision statement before developing the mission statement, ask "Why does the image, the vision exist—what is it's purpose?" This purpose is often the same as the mission.
- Developing a mission statement can be quick culture-specific, i.e., participants may use methods ranging from highly analytical and rational to highly creative and divergent, e.g., focused discussions, divergent experiences around daydreams, sharing stories, etc. Therefore, visit with the participants how they might like to arrive at description of their organizational mission.
- When wording the mission statement, consider the organization's products, services, markets, values, and concern for public image, and maybe priorities of activities for survival.
- Consider any changes that may be needed in wording of the mission statement because of any new suggested strategies during a recent strategic planning process.
- Ensure that wording of the mission is to the extent that management and employees can infer some order of priorities in how products and services are delivered.
- When refining the mission, a useful exercise is to add or delete a word from the mission to realize the change in scope of the mission statement and assess how concise is its wording.
- Does the mission statement include sufficient description that the statement clearly separates the mission of the organization from other organizations?

■ VISION STATEMENTS

Vision statements reflect the ideal image of the organization in the future. They create a focal point for strategic planning and are time bound, with most vision statements projected for a period of 5 to 10 years. The vision statement communicates both the purpose and values of the organization. For employees, it gives direction about how they are expected to behave and inspires them to give their best. Shared with customers, it shapes customers' understanding of why they should work with the organization.

Developing a Vision Statement

- The vision statement includes vivid description of the organization as it effectively carries out its operations.

- Developing a vision statement can be quick culture-specific, i.e., participants may use methods ranging from highly analytical and rational to highly creative and divergent, e.g., focused discussions, divergent experiences around daydreams, sharing stories, etc. Therefore, visit with the participants how they might like to arrive at description of their organizational vision.
- Developing the vision can be the most enjoyable part of planning, but the part where time easily gets away from you.
- Note that originally, the vision was a compelling description of the state and function of the organization once it had implemented the strategic plan, i.e., a very attractive image toward which the organization was attracted and guided by the strategic plan. Recently, the vision has become more of a motivational tool, too often including highly idealistic phrasing and activities which the organization cannot realistically aspire.

NURSING SERVICE PHILOSOPHY

The nursing service philosophy is a statement of beliefs that flows from and is congruent with the institution's philosophy. The belief system of the nursing philosophy should reflect the nursing division member's ideas and ideals for nursing and should be endorsed by others. Nursing is a healthcare service mandated by society; the practice of nursing stems from the beliefs and ideals of the nursing service department. In the first area, nursing theory, the task for the nurse manager is to decide whether and how to incorporate theory different methods may be considered.

1. One method is to use an eclectic approach, selecting ideas and constructs from various nursing theories and incorporating these into the philosophy.
2. A second method is to use one theory throughout the philosophy.
3. A third approach is to adopt a theory, then attach the entire document describing the theory to the philosophy and refer to the theory at appropriate places in the philosophy.
4. A second set of values related to nursing/nursing practice center around practice, education and research.
5. Values specific to education are essential content for most departments of nursing. The beliefs may focus on the need for continuing education off staff members.
6. The third value related to the concept of nursing practice is research and this includes the department's commitment to applying research findings or supporting others in their research efforts.
7. The beliefs held about the areas of impact of administration will influence the formation of philosophy.
8. The last content area related to nursing/nursing practice is nursing's role in overall organization.

SCOPE OF PLANNING IN NURSING SERVICE

- **Top management (Nursing directors, chief nurses, directors of nursing and their assistants):** Set the overall goals and policies of the organization. Scope of responsibility is the overall management of the organization.
- **Middle management (Nursing supervisors):** Direct the activities that actually implement the broad operating policies, such as staffing and delivery of services to the units headed by the senior or head nurses. Formulation of policies, rules and regulations, methods and procedures for personnel for intermediate level planning for ongoing activities and projects are done in coordination with top management and those in the lower level.
- **Lower or first level management (Head nurses or senior nurses including charge nurses or team leaders):** Do the daily schedules, or weekly plans for the administration of direct patient care in their respective units.

Factors to be considered in planning hospital nursing services:
- Number and type of patient
- Number of beds and type of ward
- The services required
- Procedures/techniques necessary for care
- Number and type of personal needed to perform care effectively.
- Physical facilities
- Provisional of equipment and supplies

NURSING SERVICE POLICIES, PROCEDURES AND MANUALS

Nursing procedure manuals are an important resource for practice, but ensuring that the correct procedure can be located when needed is an ongoing challenge. This poster presents an approach used to automatically index nursing procedures with standardized nursing terminology.

Box 6.1 summarizes policies related to nursing service and **Box 6.2** shows policies manual for nursing department.

In recognition of providing the highest possible quality and safety of patient care, as well as the importance of maintaining the mutually shared goal of patient care with hospital administration and nursing staff, a nursing staffing committee has been established.

1. The nursing staffing committee, made of one-half (1/2) (or 3) direct care nursing staff and one-half (1/2) (or 3) hospital administration, will meet quarterly at a minimum to review staffing effectiveness and any related issues.

Box 6.1: Policies related to nursing service.
- Employment—recruitment rules, qualification
- Job description
- Working hours
- Workload, working facilities
- Policies for breakage and losses
- Special allowances—special duty/hard duty allowance, medical allowance
- Promotional opportunities
- Career development
- Accommodation
- Transport
- Special incentives
- Occupational hazard

> **Box 6.2:** Policies manual for nursing service department.
>
> It includes:
> - Description of the structure, function and organization of the nursing department
> - Identification of current departmental administrative and clinical nursing practice, policies and procedures that are applicable to nursing department
> - Duty hours and its rotation
> - Reporting on and off duty
> - Type of uniforms
> - Staff education
> - Identification of current hospital and medical staff policies and procedures related specifically to nursing

> **Box 6.3:** Essential elements.
>
> - A written statement of the purpose and objectives
> - A plan of organization
> - Policy and administrative manuals
> - Nursing practice manuals
> - Nursing service budget
> - A master staff planning
> - Plans of appraisal of nursing
> - Nursing service administrative meetings
> - Advisory committees

Results of this review will be shared through quarterly hospital board reports and annual human resource reporting.

2. A written report of the committee's findings to the Director of Legislative Counsel Bureau:
   2.1. The written report will include establishment of the committee, activities and progress of the staffing committee, and a determination of the efficacy of the staffing committee.
3. The hospital staffing plan will be reviewed and revised as needed. The staffing plan will set forth:
   3.1. The number, skill mix and classification of licensed nurses required in each unit of the hospital. The experience of the clinical and nonclinical support staff with which the nurses collaborate, supervise or otherwise delegate assignments will be taken into account.
   3.2. A description of the types of patients who are treated in each unit, including, without limitation the type of care required by the patients; A description of the activities in each unit, including, without limitation, discharges, transfers and admissions.
   3.4. A description of the size and geography of each unit
   3.5. A description of any specialized equipment and technology for each unit
   3.6. Any foreseeable changes in the size or function of each unit
   3.7. Sufficient flexibility to allow for adjustments based upon changes in a unit of the hospital. Essential element is discussed in **Box 6.3**.
4. The nursing staffing committee will consider the following in monthly meetings:
   4.1. Methods of improving patient care as it related to staffing
   4.2. Review and discuss assignments and workloads
   4.3. Review and discuss issues related to patient acuity and staffing factors
   4.4. Review and discuss issues related to per diem employees and agency staffing
   4.5. Review and discuss issues related to floating, including orientation requirements
   4.6. Review and discuss issues related to nursing recruitment and retention;
   4.7. Review and discuss methods for reducing overtime.
5. The nursing staffing committee will assess staffing effectiveness by analyzing a minimum of two (2) clinical indicators and two (2) human resource indicators. Actions related to staffing will be taken as needed upon completion of this review. With any staffing disputes, the staffing committee will handle and resolve them by a two-thirds (2/3) majority.

FUNCTIONAL, OPERATIONAL AND STRATEGIC PLANNING

Planning occurs at three levels: strategic, functional and operational.

Strategic Planning

- Strategic planning is the managerial decision process that matches the firm's resources (such as financial assets and workforce) and capabilities (the things, it is able to do well because of expertise and experience) to its market opportunities for long-term growth.
- In strategic plan, top management (CEO, managing director, chairman or other top executives) define the firm's purpose and specify what the firm hopes to achieve over the next five or so years.
- For example, set an objective of increasing total revenues by 20% in the next five years.
- For large firms, such as Walt Disney that have a number of self-contained divisions or strategic business units (such as theme park, movie, TV, cruise line), strategic planning occurs both at overall corporate level and at the individual business unit level.

Functional Planning

In nursing, planning helps to ensure that clients or patients will receive the nursing services they want and need and that these services are delivered by satisfied nursing workers. Planning should be based on objectives that should be framed in terms of making a product or providing a service for the community.

- The next level planning is functional planning (or tactical planning). This level gets its name because it is accomplished in by the various functional areas of the firm, such as marketing, finance, human resources.
- Function director usually do this. The functional planning marketing department conducts is referred to as marketing planning. Elements of planning is shown in **Box 6.4**.

Chapter 6: Planning Nursing Services

Box 6.4: Elements of planning.

- All objectives should be SMART
  - S = Specific (concerned with specific area or activity)
  - M = Measurable (the outcomes can be measured to demonstrate that the objective has been achieved)
  - A = Attainable (the outcome is possible to achieve)
  - R = Realistic (achievable with available resources)
  - T = Time-framed (achievable within the time)
- We need to constantly review our objectives by measuring the outcomes, so that we can change the way that we are working, if necessary.

- The person in charge of such planning is Director of Marketing, or Chief Marketing Officer (CMO).
- Example of objective: to gain 40% of particular market by introducing three distribution outlets during the coming year.
- This objective would be part of functional area plan. Functional planning typically includes both a broad five-year plan to support the firm's strategic plan and detailed annual plan for the coming year.

Operational Planning

- Still further down the planning ladder are the first-line managers. In the marketing department, first-line managers include people, such as sales managers, marketing communications managers and marketing research managers.
- These managers are responsible for planning at a third level called operational planning.
- This level of planning focuses on the day-to-day execution of the functional plans and includes detailed annual, semi-annual or quarterly plans.
- Operational plans might show exactly how many units of a product a salesperson needs to sell per month or how many TV commercials the firm will place on certain channels during a season.
- At the operational planning level, for example, a company communications manager may develop plans to promote the new products to potential customers, while the sales manager may develop quarterly plan for the company's sales force. Both of these activities are forms of operational planning.

Table 6.1 shows differences between strategic, functional and operational planning.

STRATEGIC PLANNING IN NURSING

Drucker defines strategic planning as "a continuous, systematic process of making risk-taking decisions today with the greatest possible knowledge of their effects on the future; organizing efforts necessary to carry out these decisions and evaluating results of these decisions against expected outcome through reliable feedback mechanisms." Nursing administrators can increase effectiveness through strategic planning, which can promote professional nursing practice and the long-range goals of the organization and the division of nursing **(Figs. 6.3 ad 6.4)**.

Table 6.1: Differences between strategic, functional and operational planning.

Strategic planning	Functional planning	Operational planning
Planning done by top-level corporate management	Planning done by top functional-level management, such as marketing director	Planning done by supervisory managers
• Define the mission • Evaluate the internal and external environment • Set organizational or business unit objectives • Establish the business portfolio (if applicable) • Develop growth strategies	• Perform situation analysis • Set marketing objectives • Develop marketing strategies • Implement marketing strategies • Monitor and control marketing strategies	• Develop action plans to implement marketing plan • Use marketing metrics to monitor how the plan is working

Meaning of Strategic Planning

- Strategic planning in nursing is concerned with what nursing should be doing. Its purpose is to improve allocation of scarce resources, including time and money, and to manage the agency for performance.
- Strategic planning provides strategic forecasting from one year up to more than twenty years.
- It should involve top nurse managers and representatives of all levels of nursing management and practice.
- It will include analysis of such factors as projected technological advances, the internal and external environments, the nursing and healthcare market and industry, the economics of nursing and health care, availability of human and material resources, and judgments of top management.
- In today's world, the strategic planning process is used to acquire and develop new healthcare services and product lines, including new nursing services and products.
- Strategic planning is also used to remove outdated services and products. Both activities present moral and ethical dilemmas for the managers and practitioners of nursing.
- Strategic planning can foster better goals, better corporate values, and better communication about corporate direction.
- It can lead to changes in operating management and organization. Strategic planning can produce better management strategy and analysis and can forecast and mute external threats.

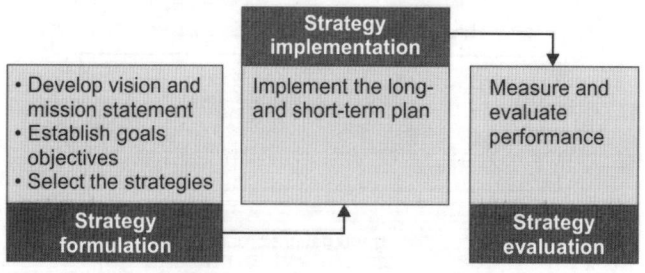

Fig. 6.3: Strategic planning phases.

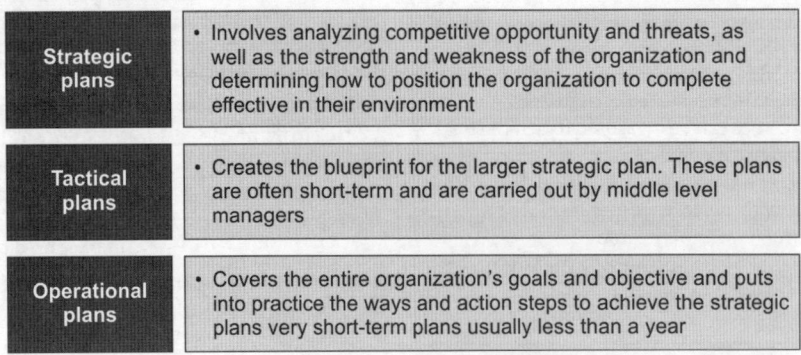

Fig. 6.4: Strategic planning.

Process for crafting a strategic plan:
Odiorne recommends the following process for crafting a strategic plan:
- Identify the major problems of your organization, determining where you are headed and where you want to be. This is "gap analysis," a technique to examine markets, products, customers, employees, finances, technology, and community relations. Cabinets or task forces from each area may be helpful in doing gap analysis and identifying major problems.
- Examine outside influences that relate to the key problems of your organization. Focus on the few major issues.
- **List the critical issues:** Those that affect the entire organization, have long-term impact, and are based on irrefutable evidence rather than media hype.
- Rank the critical issues according to their importance to your organization and plan accordingly: "must do" and "to do" and "important but not urgent." Then divide them into "success producers" and "failure preventers."
- Decide the critical issues to all organization managers.
- Include time in the budget.

Strategic plans should be developed from the bottom up, the front line where business occurs. The written plan should be shared with everyone, should not be slavishly followed, as it will be constantly affected by change, and should be modified every year. **Figure 6.5** shows functional nursing care delivery model.

Strategic planning can be used to improve nursing management:
- To provide accountability and monitoring of performance; to tie merit to performance.
- To set up more formal planning programs and require divisional and unit planning.

> **Box 6.5:** Concept of strategic planning.
>
> - Strategic planning is also "a process of defining the values, purpose, vision, mission, goals and objectives of an organization. Through the planning process, a jurisdiction or agency identifies the outcomes it wants to achieve through its programs and the specific means by which it intends to achieve these outcomes."
> - Strategic planning can be:
>   – A process for setting future directions
>   – A means to reduce risk
>   – A vehicle for training managers and direct supports
>   – A process for making strategic decisions
>   – A way to develop consensus among managers and direct supports
>   – A means to develop a written long-range plan.
>   – A sound strategic plan will:
>   - Serve as a framework for decisions or for securing support/approval
>   - Provide a basis for more detailed planning

- To integrate strategic plans with operational and financial plans.
- To improve knowledge of and training in strategic planning.
- To increase top management involvement and commitment.
- To improve focus on competition, market segments, and external factors.
- To improve communication from top administration and nursing management.
- To allow better execution of plans.
- To be more realistic, and less rationalizing and vacillating.
- To improve the development of nursing management strategies.
- To improve the development and communication of nursing management goals.
- To put less emphasis on raw numbers.
- To anticipate the future and plan for it.
- To develop the annual budget.
- To focus on quality outputs that will improve nurse performance and productivity, decrease losses, and increase return on equity.

Box 6.5 shows concepts of strategic planning.

Phases of Strategic Planning Process

Phase 1: The Mission and the Creed:
- Develop statements that define the work, the aims, and the character of the division of nursing.

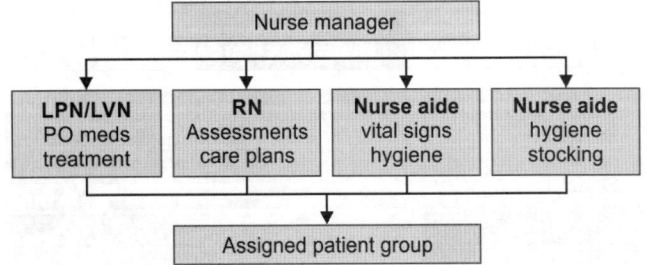

Fig. 6.5: Functional nursing care delivery model.

- These include idea statements of shared values and beliefs. They are called mission (or purpose) and creed (or philosophy) statements and relate to personnel, patients, community, and all other potential customers.

Phase 2: Data Collection and Analysis:
- Collect and analyze data about the healthcare industry and nursing. Such data should include internal forces that define the work and affect employees, clients, stockholders, and creditors; technological advances; threats; opportunities to improve growth and productivity; external forces, such as competition, communities, government and political issues, and legal requirements; marketing and public relations or image; trends in the physical and social work environments; and communication.
- Use simple and complex forecasting techniques, including trend lines, group consensus, nominal group process, and a qualitative decision matrix that uses probabilities based on conditions of certainty, risk, and uncertainty.

Phase 3: Assess Strengths and Weaknesses:
- Define those factors from the data analysis that influence the management of the division of nursing.
- List them as strengths or opportunities that will facilitate effectiveness and achievement of goals and objectives or as weaknesses or threats that will impede achieving goals and objectives.
- Define the current position and strength of the unit.

Phase 4: Goals and Objectives:
- Write realistic and general statements of goals.
- Break the goals down into concrete written statements of objectives the division of nursing intends to accomplish in the next three to five years.

Phase 5: Strategies:
- Identify untoward conditions that could develop in achieving each objective. Note administrative actions to avoid or manage them.
- Use this information to modify goals and objectives, making contingency plans for alternative actions.
- Define the organization needed for doing and implementing strategic plans. It should be interactive if cross-functional activities are involved in a matrix organization.

Phase 6: Timetable:
- Develop a timetable for accomplishing each objective.
- Identify by geographic units as well. This phase will produce or become part of the plans.

Phase 7: Operational and Functional Plans:
- Provide guidelines or general instructions that lead the functional and operational nurse managers to develop action plans to implement the goals and objectives.
- These will include detailed actions, policies, practices, communication and feedback, controlling and evaluation plans, budgets, timetables, and persons to be held accountable.

Phase 8: Implementation: Put the plans to work.

Phase 9: Evaluation:
1. Provide for formative evaluation reports before, during, and after the operational plan is implemented.
2. Provide for summative evaluation that is quantified.
3. Report actual versus expected results.
4. Frequently evaluate the strategic mission and plan. Provide continuous feedback that can be used to modify and update the plan.
5. Use people who implement the plan to evaluate it.

OPERATIONAL PLANNING IN NURSING (FIG. 6.6)

Operational management is the organization and directing of the delivery of nursing care. It includes such planning as creating a budget, creating an effective organizational structure that encompasses a quality monitoring process, and directing nurse leaders, an administrative staff, and new programs.

- Operational plans are everyday working management plans developed from both long-range objectives and the strategic planning process and short range or tactical plans.
- In development of operational objectives, new strategic objectives can emerge or old ones can be modified or discarded.
- Strategic and tactical plans are made into operational plans and carried out at all levels of nursing management, not just at the patient-care level.
- Operational managers develop goals, objectives, strategies, and targets to set the strategic plan in motion.
- They match each unit goal or objective to a strategic goal or objective. Their objectives can be much more detailed and specific than the strategic objectives.
- Numerous operational objectives can support one strategic objective.
- All aspects of an operational plan are based on goals and their achievement.
- The individual leadership style determines whether goal setting will be of the top-down or bottom-up variety.
- Bottom-up goal setting is participatory, using guidelines from the operational manager.
- Participatory goal setting is believed to increase workers' commitment and achievement.
- Increased participation leads to greater group cohesiveness, which in turn fosters increased morale, increased motivation, and increased achievement and productivity.
- Individuals, including professional nurses, can ensure greater relative success in achievement of goals by building in some slack in terms of projected resources and time.
- Nurses who reject goals of participating staff should explain their reasons for rejection. Participation in goal setting does not alone ensure success
- The goal is to plan, assess progress toward goals and objectives at all levels, and provide feedback to all levels of management.
- Efficiency is also a goal; all levels of management should guard against unnecessary time spent in meetings. As organizing changes are occurring, controlling activities are in operation and activities are being evaluated.

Chapter 6: Planning Nursing Services

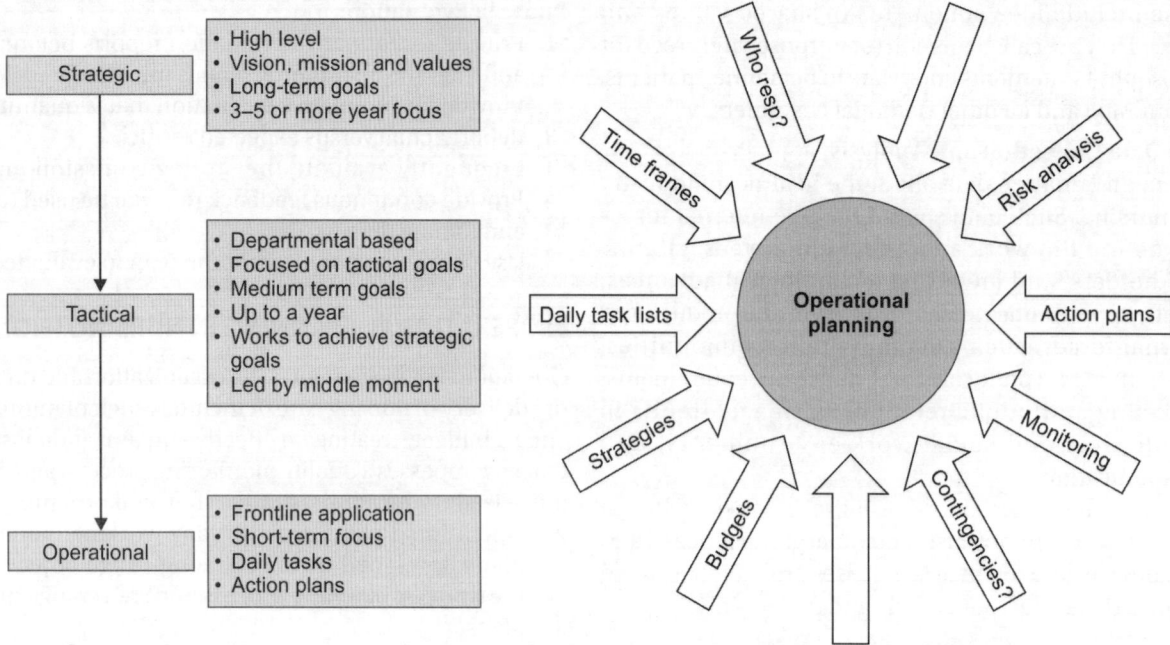

Fig. 6.6: Operational planning.

Nature of Planning

They are as follows:
- **Planning is a mental activity:** Planning is not a simple process. It is an intellectual exercise and involves thinking and forethought on the part of the manager.
- **Planning is goal-oriented:** Every plan specifies the goals to be attained in the future and the steps necessary to reach them. A manager cannot do any planning, unless the goals are known.
- **Planning is forward looking:** Planning is in keeping with the adage, "look before you leap". Thus planning means looking ahead. It is futuristic in nature since it is performed to accomplish some objectives in future.
- **Planning pervades all managerial activity:** Planning is the basic function of managers at all levels, although the nature and scope of planning will vary at each level.
- **Planning is the primary function:** Planning logically precedes the execution of all other managerial functions, since managerial activities in organizing; staffing, directing and controlling are designed to support the attainment of organizational goals. Thus, management is a circular process beginning with planning and returning to planning for revision and adjustment.
- **Planning is based on facts:** Planning is a conscious determination and projection of a course of action for the future. **Box 6.6** shows strategic versus operational planning.

> **Box 6.6:** Strategic versus operational planning.
> - **Strategic planning:** The process of developing a mission and long-range objectives and determining in advance how they will be accomplished.
> - **Operational planning:** The process of setting short-range objectives and determining in advance how they will be accomplished.
> - **Strategy:** A plan for pursuing the mission and achieving objectives.

Purposes of Planning

The following are some reasons for planning:
- Planning increases the chances of success by focusing on results, not on activities.
- It forces analytic thinking and evaluation of alternatives, therefore improving decisions.
- It establishes a framework for decision making that is consistent with top management objectives.
- It orients people to action instead of reaction.
- It includes day-to-day and future-focused managing.
- It helps to avoid crisis management and provides decision-making flexibility.
- It provides a basis for managing organizational and individual performance.
- It increases employee involvement and improves communication.
- It is cost-effective.

PROGRAM PLANNING: GANTT CHART AND MILESTONE CHART

Program planning is the process by which a program is conceived and brought to fruition. Program planning involves multiple steps including the identification of a problem, selection of desired outcomes, and assessment of available resources, implementation, and evaluation of the program. Program planning is sometimes called program design or program design planning.
- A program is created when an organization identifies a need and creates a plan for addressing that need.
- In order to be successful, a program must have specific goals and a process for meeting those goals.
- Program planning is the means by which this objective is achieved. Various models, such as the logic model or evidence-based model, may be used to create a program plan.

- When planning, an organization will consider the problem that has been identified, potential solutions and desired outcomes, and the resources available to implement the program.
- Support and participation by stakeholders, or other interested parties, and ongoing program evaluations are key elements of solid program planning.

Gantt Chart (Fig. 6.7)

A Gantt chart is a visual presentation used in project management to show overview of timeline for project activities and their inter-dependence. Each project task or activity is represented with a bar chart clearly displaying start and end date. Thus the length of the bar shows the duration required for a task to complete. This way multiple tasks when displayed as bar charts, shows work breakdown structure on a timeline. Essentially Gantt chart shows when an activity starts, completes, how long it will take to complete an activities and also overall project, which is a project schedule.

Definition: A Gantt chart is a useful graphical tool which shows activities or tasks performed against time. It is also known as visual presentation of a project where the activities are broken down and displayed on a chart which makes it is easy to understand and interpret.

Brief History

- Gantt chart is a legacy left behind by Henry Laurence Gantt in 1910. Henry Gantt was a mechanical engineer, management consultant and industry expert.
- He introduced Gantt chart to visualize schedule and actual progress of projects.
- Its first major implementation or usage was well known–World War One (WW1) when US army used Gantt charts to manage arms production and logistic projects.
- Henry Gantt experimented with Gantt chart and presented variations of it.
- The Gantt chart we see and use today (along with task dependencies) was introduced by Wallace Clark.
- Interestingly Wallace Clark used to work in Henry Gantt's company and was considered as Henry Gantt's disciple.

Importance of Gantt Chart

There have been few tools or techniques used to identify and manage project activities before Gantt chart came into existence, such as:

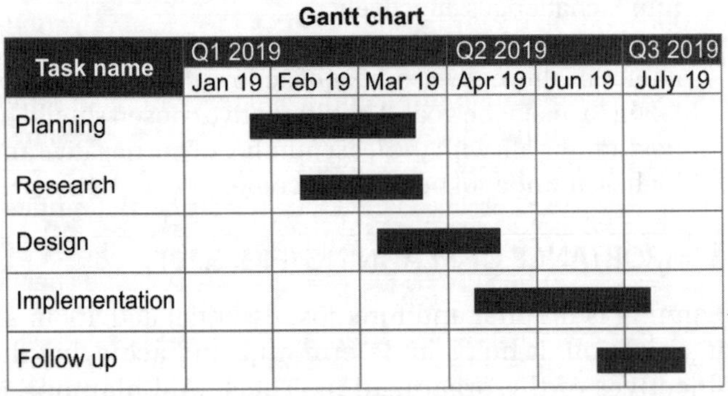

- Message board
- Post-it boards
- To do lists/Task lists

However, these tools and techniques could not give a better picture about a project schedule. And this is where Gantt chart stands out:

- It shows breakdown structure.
- It shows dependencies.
- It shows expected timeline.
- It shows current progress.
- It shows schedule baseline.
- It shows resources assigned.
- It shows task priority.
- It shows critical path.
- It shows smallest as well as longest task.

Advantages of Gantt Chart

There are distinct advantages of a Gantt chart, primarily from project managers', project stakeholders' perspective. It is easy for stakeholder's to understand the timeline, it brings clarity to everyone: when a project is going to start and expected to complete, team can manage its time accordingly, it also establishes accountability among stakeholders, it enables team to better coordinate project activities thereby enabling team to improving overall efficiency.

- It is easy to understand.
- It gives clarity of dates.
- It enables time management.
- It brings efficiency.
- It ensures accountability in terms of timeline.
- It expects coordination among stakeholders in order to deliver things as per Gantt timeline.

Steps to Create a Gantt Chart

- In order to create Gantt chart, first project manager needs to identify high level tasks, and then break those down into smaller actionable subtasks.
- Further he can identify efforts and duration required for those smaller set of tasks, link, sequence project tasks. And now it is a time to plot bar chart against each of the task.
- Fortunately we do not have to use pen and paper to draw Gantt chart; neither have we to use MS Excel spreadsheet for the same.
- Project management tools, such as ZilicusPM make it easier for project manager to create Gantt chart online easily.
- Interactive Gantt chart makes it even quick and simpler. You can also find real life examples how Gantt chart is used by various businesses.

Disadvantages of Gantt Chart

However Gantt chart has its own limitations. Let's look at those briefly.

- Tedious if one needs to keep it updating regularly
- Can become unmanageable for detailed project plan
- Unclear amount of work expected
- Not easy to view everything on a single paper

Gantt chart

Task name	Q1 2019			Q2 2019		Q3 2019
	Jan 19	Feb 19	Mar 19	Apr 19	Jun 19	July 19
Planning		■■■				
Research			■■■			
Design				■■■		
Implementation					■■■■	
Follow up						■■

Fig. 6.7: Gantt chart.

Milestone Chart

Milestones are key elements or points in time that can be identified in the progress of a program or project. A Milestone chart provides a sequential list of the various tasks to be accomplished in the program or project (tasks, in turn, can be broken down into specific activities if this level of detailed is warranted) and an increased awareness of the interdependencies between tasks. The list of tasks and milestones are displayed adjacent to a time scale.

Advantages of Milestone Chart

Milestone chart is a modification over the original Gantt chart. Small notes on milestone charts are:
- Controlling can be easily done and inter relationships between other similar activities can be easily established.
- These points are those that can be easily identified over the main bar.
- Milestones are key events of a main activity represented by a bar.
- These specific points in time that mark the completion of certain portions of the main activity.
- If the activity is broken or sub divided into a number of subactivities, each one of which can be easily recognized during the progress of the project.
- The beginning and end of these subdivided activities or tasks are termed as milestones.

Figure 6.8 shows standard symbols.

CHARACTERISTICS OF PLANNING (FIG. 6.9)

- **Managerial function:** Planning is a first and foremost managerial function provides the base for other functions of the management, i.e., organizing, staffing, directing and

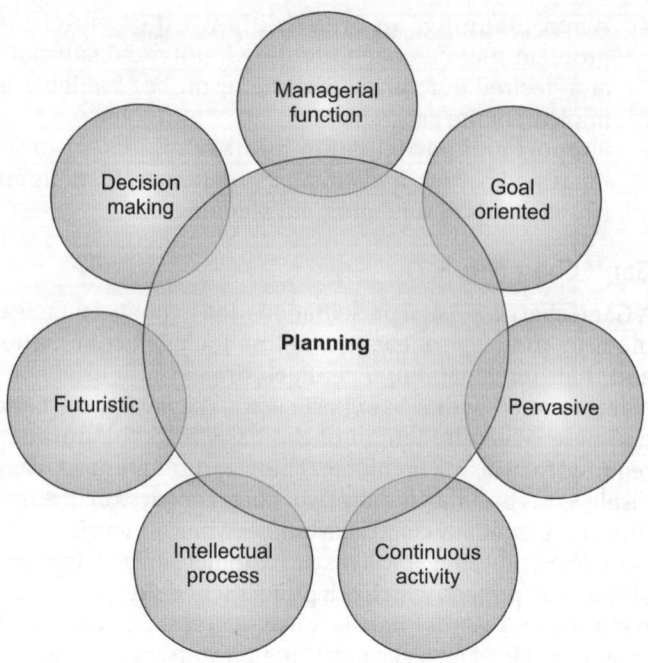

Fig. 6.9: Characteristics of planning.

controlling, as they are performed within the periphery of the plans made.

- **Goal oriented:** It focuses on defining the goals of the organization, identifying alternative courses of action and deciding the appropriate action plan, which is to be undertaken for reaching the goals.
- **Pervasive:** It is pervasive in the sense that it is present in all the segments and is required at all the levels of the organization. Although the scope of planning varies at different levels and departments.
- **Continuous process:** Plans are made for a specific term, say for a month, quarter, and year and so on. Once that period is over, new plans are drawn, considering the organization's present and future requirements and conditions. Therefore, it is an ongoing process, as the plans are framed, executed and followed by another plan.
- **Intellectual process:** It is a mental exercise at it involves the application of mind, to think, forecast, imagine intelligently and innovate, etc.
- **Futuristic:** In the process of planning, we take a sneak peek of the future. It encompasses looking into the future, to analyse and predict it so that the organization can face future challenges effectively.
- **Decision making:** Decisions are made regarding the choice of alternative courses of action that can be undertaken to reach the goal. The alternative chosen should be best among all, with the least number of the negative and highest number of positive outcomes.

IMPORTANCE OF PLANNING (FIG. 6.10)

Planning is the first and foremost essential activity in all organization. It helps in determining and achieving the objectives of the organization. The sound planning is important condition for effective management.

Standard symbols have been adapted for air force milestone schedule the most common symbols used and their meanings are shown below:

Basic symbol	Meaning
⇧	Schedule completion
⬆	Actual completion
◇	Previous scheduled completion-still in future
◆	Previous scheduled completion-date passed

Representative uses		Meaning
◇	⇧	Anticipated slip-rescheduled completion
◆	⇧	Actual slip-rescheduled completion
◆	⬆	Actual slip-actual completion
	⬆	Actual completion ahead of schedule
⬆	⇧	Time span action
⇧	⇨	Continuous action

Fig. 6.8: Standard symbols.

Chapter 6: Planning Nursing Services

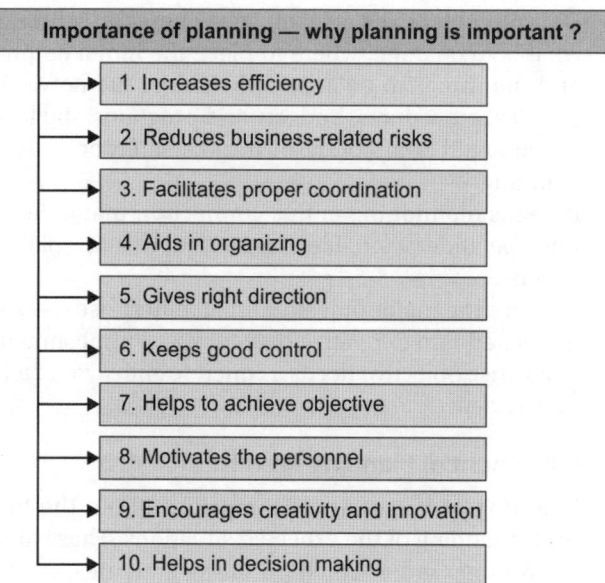

Fig. 6.10: Importance of planning.

It helps the organization in the following ways:
- **Making objectives clear:** It makes objectives clean, clear, and specific, it also serves as guide for deciding what action should be taken in present and future conditions.
- **Planning provides direction:** Planning helps the organization to keep on the right path. It provides definite direction to manager to decide what to do and when to do it.
- **It reduces risk and uncertainty:** It helps organization to predict future events and prepare to take necessary actions against unexpected events. It is helpful in assessing and meeting future challenges. As per view of Peter F Drucker, "Planning enables a manager to affect rather than accept the future".
- **Planning is economical:** As per views of Koontz and O' Donnell," Planning substitutes jointly directed effort against uncoordinated, piecemeal activity, an even flow of work for an uneven flow, and deliberate decisions for snap judgments". The effective plans coordinate organizational work and economical.
- **Planning provides the basis for control:** Planning provides the standard against which the actual performance can be measured and evaluated. There is nothing to control without planning and without proper control. Plans serve as yardsticks for measuring performance.
- **Planning facilitates decision making:** Planned targets serve as the criteria for the evaluation of different alternatives so that the best one may be chosen with the help of planning hasty decisions and random actions can be avoided.
- **Planning improve efficiency of operations:** It is rational activity that leads to efficient and economical operations, planned action is always better than unplanned. Planning makes the task of managing more efficient and effective manner. It helps to minimize the cost of operations and improves the competitive strength of an organization.
- **Planning improves morale:** If the role of employee is cleared and well defines goals, then the employee feels highly motivated and contributes his full potential towards accomplishment of objectives. Planning improves the behavioral climate in the organization and reduces the friction between departments.
- **Effective coordination:** According to Koontz and O' Donnell "Plans are selected courses along with the management desires to coordinate group action." The effective coordination integrates the physical and human resources between departments.
- **Planning encourages innovation and creativity:** Planning compels the managers to be creative and innovative all the time. It forces managers to find out new and improved ways of doing things in order to remain competitive and avoid the threats in the environment.

ESSENTIALS OF GOOD PLANNING

- Yields reasonable organizational objectives and develops alternative approaches to meet these objectives.
- Helps to eliminate or reduce the future uncertainty and chance.
- Helps to gain economical operations.
- Lays the foundation for organizing.
- Facilitates coordination.
- Helps to facilitate control.
- Dictates those activities to which employers are directed.

PRINCIPLES OF PLANNING (FIG. 6.11)

- Planning must focus on purposes. It should always be based on a clearly defined objective.
- Planning is a continuous and iterative process which includes series of steps, so continuity and flexibility should be maintained in planning cycle.
- Planning should be simple and there should be provision for proper analysis and classification of actions.

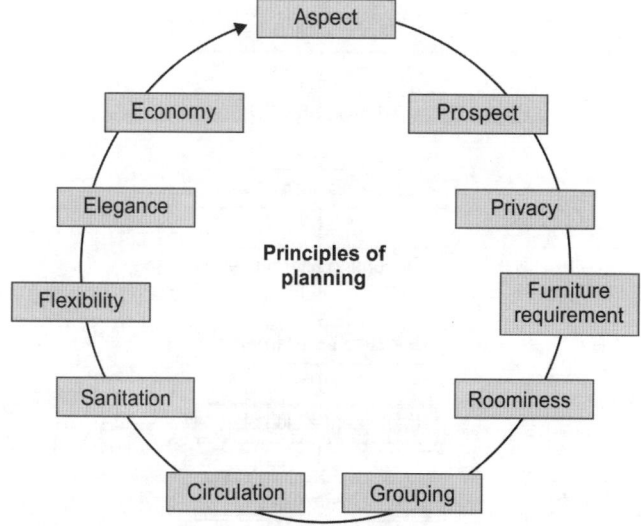

Fig. 6.11: Principles of planning.

- In planning, there should be a good harmony with organization and environment-political as well as economical, etc.
- Planning is hierarchical in nature and must have an organizational identification.
- Planning should be pervasive activity covering the entire organization with all its departments, sectors, and different levels of administration, and it should be balanced.
- Planning must be precise in its objective scope and nature. It should be realistic in its scope and pinpoint the expected results.
- In planning, the provision should be made to use all available resources.
- Planning should always be documented so that the entire concerned are fully committed to the implementation of the program.

STEPS INVOLVED IN PLANNING (FIG. 6.12)

Planning is a process which embraces a number of steps to be taken. Planning is an intellectual exercise and a conscious determination of courses of action. Therefore, it requires courses of action. The planning process is valid for one organization and for one plan, may not be valid for other organizations or for all types of plans, because various factors that go into planning process may differ from organization to organization or from plan to plan. For example, planning process for a large organization may not be the same for a small organization. However, the major steps involved in the planning process of a major organization or enterprise are as follows:

Establishing Objectives

- The first and primary step in planning process is the establishment of planning objectives or goals.
- Definite objectives, in fact, speak categorically about what is to be done, where to place the initial emphasis and the things to be accomplished by the network of policies, procedures, budgets and programs, the lack of which would invariably result in either faulty or ineffective planning.
- It needs mentioning in this connection that objectives must be understandable and rational to make planning effective.
- Because the major objective, in all enterprise, needs be translated into derivative objective, accomplishment of enterprise objective needs a concrete endeavor of all the departments.

Establishment of Planning Premises

- Planning premises are assumptions about the future understanding of the expected situations. These are the conditions under which planning activities are to be undertaken. These premises may be internal or external.
- Internal premises are internal variables that affect the planning. These include organizational polices, various resources and the ability of the organization to withstand the environmental pressure.
- External premises include all factors in task environment like political, social technological, competitors' plans and actions, government policies, market conditions.
- Both internal factors should be considered in formulating plans. At the top level, mainly external premises are considered. As one moves downward, internal premises gain importance.

Determining Alternative Courses

- The next logical step in planning is to determine and evaluate alternative courses of action.
- It may be mentioned that there can hardly be any occasion when there are no alternatives. And it is most likely that alternatives properly assessed may prove worthy and meaningful.
- As a matter of fact, it is imperative that alternative courses of action must be developed before deciding upon the exact plan. **Figure 6.13** shows planning elements.

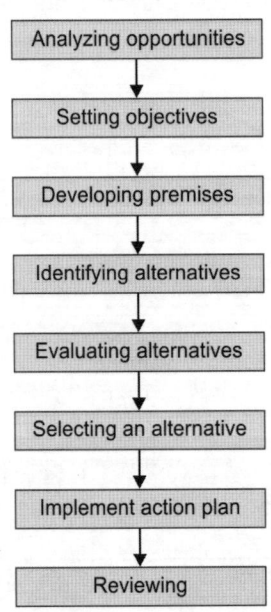

Fig. 6.12: Steps involved in planning.

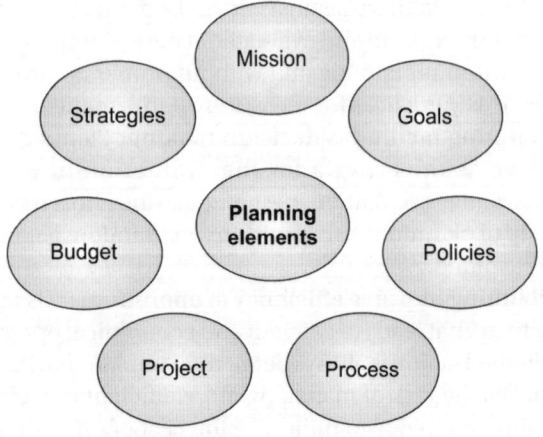

Fig. 6.13: Planning elements.

Evaluation of Alternatives

- Having sought out the available alternatives along with their strong and weak points, planners are required to evaluate the alternatives giving due weight-age to various factors involved, for one alternative may appear to be most profitable involving heavy cash outlay whereas the other less profitable, but involve least risk.
- Likewise, another course of action may be found contributing significantly to the company's long-range objectives although immediate expectations are likely to go unfulfilled.
- Evidently, evaluation of alternative is a must to arrive at a decision.
- Otherwise, it would be difficult to choose the best course of action in the perspective of company needs and resources as well as objectives laid down.

Selecting a Course of Action

- The fifth step in planning is selecting a course of action from among alternatives.
- In fact, it is the point of decision-making-deciding upon the plan to be adopted for accomplishing the enterprise objectives.

Formulating Derivative Plans

- To make any planning process complete the final step is to formulate derivative plans to give effect to and support the basic plan.
- For example, if Indian Airlines decide to run Jumbo Jets between Delhi an Patna, obliviously, a number of derivative plans have to be framed to support the decision, e.g., a staffing plan, operating plans for fuelling, maintenance, stores purchase, etc.
- In other words, plans do not accomplish themselves. They require to be broken down into supporting plans.
- Each manager and department of the organization is to contribute to the accomplishment of the master plan on the basis of the derivative plans.

Establishing Sequence of Activities

- Timing a sequence of activities are determined after formulating basic and derivative plans, so that plans may be put into action.
- Timing is an essential consideration in planning. It gives practical shape and concrete form to the programs.
- The starting and finishing times are fixed for each piece of work, so as to indicate when the within what time that work is to be commenced and completed.
- Bad timing of programs results in their failure. To maintain a symmetry of performance and a smooth flow of work, the sequence of operation shaped be arranged carefully by giving priorities to some work in preference to others.
- Under sequence it should be decided as to who will do what and at what time.

Feedback or Follow-up Action

- Formulating plans and chalking out of programs are not sufficient, unless follow-up action is provided to see that plans so prepared and programs chalked out are being carried out in accordance with the plan and to see whether these are not kept in cold storage.
- It is also required to see whether the plan is working well in the present situation. If conditions have changed, the plan current plan has become outdated or inoperative it should be replaced by another plan.
- A regular follow-up is necessary and desirable from effective implementation and accomplishment of tasks assigned.
- The plan should be communicated to all persons concerned in the organization.
- Its objectives and course of action must be clearly defined leaving no ambiguity in the minds of those who are responsible for its execution.
- Planning is effective only when the persons involved work in a team spirit and all are committed to the objectives, policies, programs, strategies envisaged in the plan.

COMPONENTS OF PLANNING

- **Objectives:** Objectives are basic plans which determine goals or end results of the projected action of an enterprise. By setting goals, objectives provide the foundation upon which structure of plan can be built.
- **Policies:** Policies are written statements or oral understanding. In some, they are general terms for governing actions in repetitive situations. Realization of objectives is made easy with the help of policies, as policies provide standing solutions to problem.
- **Procedures:** Procedures indicate the specific manner in which a certain activity is to be performed. They are more definite and specific guides to action, but only for fulfillment of objectives.
- **Program:** Program welds together different plans for implementing them into completely and orderly course of action. Programs are necessary for both repetitive (routine planning) and non-repetitive (creative planning) course of action.
- **Budget:** Budgets are plans continuing statements of expected results in numerical terms; i.e., rupees, man-hours, product units and so forth.

FACTORS AFFECTING PLANNING

Planning is a key component of managers' job functions. They design and devise ways to improve their companies and departments. However, factors inside and outside the company can affect managerial planning for better or worse. Fail-proof planning does not exist, but taking steps to mitigate any negative effects of planning can help ensure project success. Planning enables managers to adjust the environment in which their companies operate instead of only reacting to changes.

Competition

- Companies that do not jump quickly into a promising product or service market may be outmaneuvered by their competitors.
- Planning may take a backseat to entering the profitable, emerging market for a new product or service when a company wants to beat its competitors.
- In some cases, the higher costs of completing the project before competitors that comes from a lack of thorough planning do not have negative effects on the business.
- The higher profits that come from beating competitors to customers more than compensates for them. However, a hurried entrance into a new market can cost the company money in the long run and not make full use of managers' planning abilities.

Economy

- The overall economy or health of the company's industry also may negatively affect a manager's ability to plan. When sudden downturns occur, planning must be stopped, adjusted or taken in a new direction.
- If the economy improves significantly, managers may scrap former plans and begin new ones.
- Managers must be flexible to changing outside economic conditions even when they are in the midst of planning a project of special interest to them.

Managers

- Managers themselves also affect their own planning function. If they are not good planners in general or do not have the experience, education or background in planning required being successful, they are more likely to plan poorly.
- They may not fully commit to the planning process, as it can be complicated and time-consuming.
- They also may sacrifice their visions of the long-term for solving short-term problems.
- Managers may rely too much on their planning departments to construct and organize the vision for a project.
- The responsibility to plan still rests with them. Managers also may focus too much on the variables they can control instead of the variables that they cannot, such as the economy.

Information

- When planning occurs, it is vital to have accurate information from consumers, the market, the economy, competitors and other sources.
- Managers who do not have accurate and timely information are more likely to plan poorly and inadequately.

■ TYPES/CLASSIFICATIONS OF PLANS (FIG. 6.14)

Plans can be classified based on importance, period of planning, level, formality, and approach.

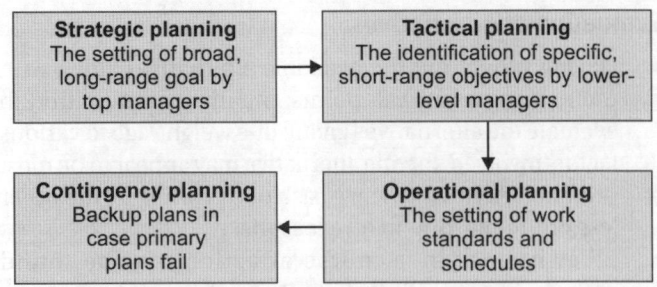

Fig. 6.14: Classification of plan.

Based on Importance

- Plans can be strategic, tactical, or operational. Strategic plans are important, future-oriented plans that form the hub of fulfilling the vision.
- Usually, they concern the entire organization. Tactical plans are required to implement strategic plans.
- Examples, are redesigning the shop floor layout or closing a few non-performing outlets of a retail chain.
- Operational plans are related to day-to-day functioning, such as production, delivery, or purchase operation.
- Take for instance, the plan of Precision Connectors to deliver connectors to the two-wheeler manufacturer, which is an illustration of operational plans.

Based on Time

- Plans can be short, medium, or long-term. Short-term usually refers to plans of one year or less; medium term, to two to five years; and long-term, to five to 10 or even 20 years. It depends on the nature of the project.
- Some projects, such as building the Metro in Mumbai or Bangalore may have a short-term plan that covers 50 km of Metro in five years; a medium-term plan that covers 200 km in 10–12 years, and a long-term plan that covers 300 or 400 km of rail that in 20 to 30 years.

Based on Level

- A plan can be called corporate level, business level, or functional level plan.
- The Tatas entering the airlines business is an example of corporate-level plan and Precision Connectors becoming an OEM is an example of a business-level plan.
- Functional-level plans are made by departments, for example, a plan on how the marketing department will achieve its goals.

Based on Formality

A plan can be formal or informal. It is formal when planning is done as per the defined steps and documented, and informal when the documentation is not very rigorous.

Based on Approach

- A plan can be called proactive when it is meant to meet an anticipated situation. For instance, a compensation plan based on a three-year salary negotiation is a proactive plan to ensure industrial peace.

- If the same compensation plan came up as a result of a flash strike, it would be a reactive plan.
- The former leads to growth and the latter helps to regain balance and to ensure survival.

ADVANTAGES OF PLANNING

An organization without planning is like a sailboat minus its rudder. Without planning, organization, are subject to the winds of organizational change. Planning is one of the most important and crucial functions of management. According to Koontz and O'Donnell, "Without planning business becomes random in nature and decisions become meaningless and adhoc choices." According to Geroge R Terry, "Planning is the foundation of most successful actions of any enterprise." Planning becomes necessary due to the following reasons:

- **Reduction of uncertainty:** Future is always full of uncertainties. A business organization has to function in these uncertainties. It can operate successfully if it is able to predict the uncertainties. Some of the uncertainties can be predicted by undertaking systematic. Some of the uncertainties can be predicted by undertaking systematic forecasting. Thus, planning helps in foreseeing uncertainties which may be caused by changes in technology, fashion and taste of people, government rules and regulations, etc.
- **Better utilization of resources:** An important advantage of planning is that it makes effective and proper utilization of enterprise resources. It identifies all such available resources and makes optimum use of these resources.
- **Increases organizational effectiveness:** Planning ensures organizational effectiveness. Effectiveness ensures that the organization is in a position to achieve its objective due to increased efficiency of the organization.
- **Reduces the cost of performance:** Planning assists in reducing the cost of performance. It includes the selection of only one course of action amongst the different courses of action that would yield the best results at minimum cost. It removes hesitancy, avoids crises and chaos, eliminates false steps and protects against improper deviations.
- **Concentration on objectives:** It is a basic characteristic of planning that it is related to the organizational objectives. All the operations are planned to achieve the organizational objectives. Planning facilitates the achievement of objectives by focusing attention on them. It requires the clear definition of objectives so that most appropriate alternative courses of action are chosen.
- **Helps in coordination:** Good plans unify the inter-departmental activity and clearly lay down the area of freedom in the development of various sub-plans. Various departments work in accordance with the overall plans of the organization. Thus, there is harmony in the organization, and duplication of efforts and conflict of jurisdiction are avoided.
- **Makes control effective:** Planning and control are inseparable in the sense that unplanned action cannot be controlled because control involves keeping activities on the predetermined course by rectifying deviations from plans. Planning helps control by furnishing standards of performance.
- **Encouragement to innovation:** Planning helps innovative and creative thinking among the managers because many new ideas come to the mind of a manager when he is planning. It creates a forward-looking attitude among the managers.
- **Increase in competitive strength:** Effective planning gives a competitive edge to the enterprise over other enterprises that do not have planning or have ineffective planning. This is because planning may involve expansion of capacity, changes in work methods, changes in quality, anticipation of tastes and fashions of people and technological changes, etc.
- **Delegation is facilitated:** A good plan always facilitates delegation of authority in a better way to subordinates.

Table 6.2: Advantages and disadvantages of planning.

Advantages	Disadvantages
Forces organizations to look ahead	Can be time consuming and expensive
Improved fit with the environment	May be difficult in rapidly changing markets
Better use of resources	Can become a straightjacket
Provides a direction/vision	Some unplanned for opportunities may be missed
Helps monitor progress	Can become bureaucratic
Ensures goal congruence	Is less relevant in a crisis

Table 6.2 summarizes advantages and disadvantages of planning.

COMPONENTS OF SAFETY MANAGEMENT PLAN

- **Management policy statement:** This document shall be signed by the top executive of the company acknowledging management's responsibility and commitment to a safety plan and their intention to comply with all applicable local, state, and federal safety requirements and appropriate industry standards. Management shall commit resources, responsibility, and accountability to all levels of management and to each employee for the safety program.
- **Responsibility** for safety shall be defined in writing for executive and middle level operating management, supervisors, safety coordinator, and employees.
- **Inspections** shall be made of all areas of the work place at least quarterly by a supervisor at the site. A written report (check list or narrative) is to be completed for each inspection and retained for a period of one year. The report will be designed to cover the identification of recognized unsafe conditions, unsafe acts, and any other items inherent in a particular job. The form will include a space to indicate any corrective action taken. The responsibility for the correction of defects is to be designated by management.

- **An accident investigation** of any job-related injury that requires a visit to a clinic or physician shall be initiated by the injured employee's supervisor as soon as possible on the shift the accident occurs. The accident investigation report will include information required to determine the basic causes of the accident by asking the questions who, what, where, when, and how. Corrective action to be taken and/or recommended to prevent a recurrence of a similar accident will be implemented. Complex accidents may require technical assistance to ensure an accurate investigation; however, the injured employee's supervisor should be included on the investigation team.

  The accident investigation report shall include information on the injured person, his or her job, what happened, basic causes, corrective actions required, the time frame to make corrections, and who will be responsible for seeing that corrections are implemented.

- **Safety meetings** shall be held by a supervisor with all of his/her employees at least quarterly. A record will be kept showing the topics discussed, date of meeting, and the names of the persons attending.

  Safety meeting topics will be designed to instruct the employees on how to perform their jobs productively, efficiently, and safely. Hazard recognition and hazard control procedures; selection, use, and care of personal protective equipment; job procedures review; and good housekeeping are examples of the information employees should receive at a safety meeting.

  A review of the recent work area inspection results, the workers' compliance with safety procedures, and the accident investigations that occurred since the last safety meeting should be covered in the safety meeting.

- **Safety rules:** Management shall develop specific safety rules that apply to the operations being performed. The rules should be short, concise, simple, enforceable, and stated in a positive manner. The safety rules are to be followed and adhered to by all management personnel and all employees. The rules shall be written with a copy provided to each employee and documented.

- **Training:** Management shall implement a training program that will provide for orientation and training of each new employee, existing employees on a new job, or when new equipment, processes, or job procedures are initiated. The training provided will consist of, but not be limited to, the correct work procedures to follow, correct use of personal protective equipment required, and where to get assistance when needed. This training should be accomplished by the employee's supervisor but may be done by a training specialist or an outside consultant, such as a vendor or safety consultant. Training shall be provided to all persons in operating supervisory positions in conducting safety meetings, conducting safety inspections, accident investigation, job planning, employee training methods, job analysis, and leadership skills.

- **Record keeping:** In addition to OSHA logs, which are retained for five years (a federal requirement), each firm shall maintain other safety records for a period of one year from the end of the year for which the records are maintained (a state requirement). These will include inspection reports, accident investigation reports, minutes of safety meetings and training records.

- **First aid:** Management shall adopt and implement a first aid program which will provide for a trained first aid person at each job site on each shift. A first aid kit with proper supplies for the job exposures will be maintained and restocked as needed. Emergency phone numbers for medical services and key company personnel must also be maintained.

- **Emergency preparedness program:** Management shall develop a written emergency preparedness plan to ensure to the extent possible the safety of all employees, visitors, contractors, and vendors in the facility at the time of emergency situations, such as but not limited to natural disasters, fire, explosions, chemical spills and/or releases, bomb threats, and medical emergencies. Emergency shutdown and startup procedures will be developed in industries having equipment that requires several steps to properly shutdown and secure. Employees shall be trained in these procedures to reduce the incidences of additional injuries, property damage, and possible release of hazardous materials to the environment. Emergency plans shall comply with all governmental regulations and state and local emergency response committee requirements.

PLANNING HOSPITAL AND PATIENT CARE UNIT (WARD)

Essential hospital service required for the community can be met most economically only with adequate thought given to planning, design, construction and operation of health care facilities. A design expert says, 'we have got to design 'smart' hospitals that respond to present needs while anticipating future changes'.

Hospital Planning

- Planning is the forecasting and organizing the activities required to achieve the desired goals.
- All successful hospitals, without exception are built on a triad of good planning, good design and construction and good administration.
- To be successful, a hospital requires a great deal of preliminary study and planning.
- It must be designed to serve people.
- It must be staffed with competent and adequate number of efficient doctors, nurses, and other professionals.
- A strong management essential for the daily functioning of a facility; must be included in the plans of a new hospital.
- Hospital building differs from other building types in the complex functional relationship that exist between the various parts of the hospital.

- Apart from providing right environment for patients and care providers, it should also be sensitive to the needs of visitors.
- It is thus imperative to examine the emerging issues, analyze the challenges, appreciate the emerging trends and study the various strategic options available for planning, designing and construction of a hospital.

Principles of Planning Hospital Units

- **Protection:** Protection from unwanted and unnecessary disturbances in order to help speedy recovery
- **Separation:** Separation of dissimilar activities
- **Control:** Control over the untoward incidents
- **Circulation:** Proper integration of departments

Objectives of Planning Hospital Units (Box 6.7)

- **Provide quality care:** Quality medical services and enhancing patient satisfaction
- **Provide maximum comfort:** Comfort in terms of safety, security, convenience and privacy—avoiding slippery floors, direct sunlight, etc.
- **Enhance staff satisfaction:** Staff motivation and safe working environment
- **Patient relatives and visitors convenience:** Comfortable stay, safe environments, etc.
- Maintenance and cost of services

Factors in Hospital Planning

- Community interest over individual interest.
- Preventive services over curative services
- Services catering to the weaker sections of the community
- Rural over urban
- Regionalized planning

Hospitals must meet two basic fundamental needs

- Must meet the needs of the patients it is going to serve adequately
- It must be in size and proportion which the owner or promoters will be able to build and operate.

Guiding Principles for Hospital Planning

- High quality patient care
- Effective community orientation
- Economic viability
- Sound structural plan

Box 6.7: Objectives of planning hospital units.

- **Provide quality care:** Quality medical services and enhancing patient satisfaction
- **Provide maximum comfort:**
  - Comfort in terms of safety, security, convenience and privacy
  - Avoiding slippery floors, direct sunlight, etc.
- **Enhance staff satisfaction:** Staff motivation and safe working environment
- **Patient relatives and visitors convenience:** Comfortable stay, safe environments, etc.
- Maintenance and cost of services

PLANNING OF PATIENT CARE UNIT

Hospital is an institution or the organization for the treatment, care, and cure of the sick and wounded, for the study of disease, and for the training of physicians (teaching hospitals), nurses, and allied health care personnel. The hospital is divided into blocks and each block is divided into wards/units A ward is that area of the hospital where all amenities—physical, social and especially medical care—are made available to facilitate patient's treatment and make the patients feel at home till they are discharged. In other words, a ward is a temporary home for the patients admitted there.

Nursing Unit

A nursing unit is an area in a hospital or other healthcare delivery setting where patients with similar needs are grouped to facilitate the delivery of care by health care professionals trained in that specialty

- typically a nurse manager/Head nurse/Assistant nurse supervisor is in-charge of the unit
- As planning is put into action, the management functions of organizing, leading, and evaluating are implemented, making all unit management functions interdependent

Patient care unit means a unit or department that is included within a general acute care hospitals license that provides direct patient care including but not limited to nursing units, diagnostic imaging, emergency department, or rehabilitation and behavioral health. "Patient handling" means lifting, transferring, repositioning or mobilizing of part or all of a patient's body.

Planning must focus on purposes:

- It should always be based on clearly defined objectives.
- Continuity and flexibility should be maintained in planning cycle.
- Planning should be simple and there should be provision for proper analysis and classification of actions.
- In planning there should be good harmony with organization and environment.
- Planning is hierarchical in nature and must have an organizational identification.
- Planning should cover the entire setup, all connected departments, and different levels of administration, and it should be balanced.
- It should be realistic in its scope and pinpoints the expected results.
- Provision should be made to use available resources.
- Planning should always be documented.

Cleaning a Patient Unit

Scope of responsibility: Nursing service personnel are responsible for the bed, bedside cabinet, chair, overbed table (when used), lamp, and curtain or cubicle partition. In addition, when custodial housekeeping services are not available, the medical specialist is also responsible for the floor and windowsills within the patient unit area and the adjoining bathroom.

Types of Cleaning

The two types of unit cleaning are termed concurrent and terminal.

1. Concurrent unit cleaning is the cleaning of a unit daily or in accordance with local standing operating procedure (SOP). A similar procedure is required on a regularly scheduled basis for a long-term patient to ensure that any accumulation of dust and germs is eliminated.
2. Terminal unit cleaning is the cleaning of a unit, when the patient is discharged, transferred, or dies. This type of cleaning includes more activity than the daily (concurrent) cleaning of the area.
   a. **Equipment:** The equipment required to clean a patient unit follows:
      - Wheeled utility cart
      - Wheeled laundry camper
      - Cleaning cloths
      - Wastebasket with paper bag or plastic liner
      - Basin of prescribed detergent-germicide solution.
   b. **Terminal cleaning procedure**
      1. Assemble the equipment in the utility room and take it to the patient unit.
      2. Clear the bedside cabinet (and overbed table if used). Check for any personal articles left by the patient and turn them in to the ward master. Place all utensils and any reusable treatment equipment on the cart. Discard waste in the wastebasket. Place any unused linen in the unit in the laundry hamper.
3. Strip the bed. Remove the pillow, placing the pillow on the chair and the pillowcase in the hamper.
   - Lower the Gatch bed. Loosen the bedding all around, walking around the bed and lifting the mattress edge to release the linen without snagging it on the bedsprings.
   - Check to see that no articles are concealed in the linen folds. Roll each piece toward the foot of the bed.
   - Check the pocket of discarded pajamas and bathrobe.
   - Place all linen in the hamper. Fold woolen blankets, if used, and place them on the cart for special laundry.
4. Clean the bed. Wash the top of the plastic mattress cover and inspect it for any tears. Rinse the cloth frequently and use it damp but not dripping wet. a. Replace any damaged cover. Turn the clean surfaces of the mattress together, toward the head of the bed.
   - Wash the bottom half of the bed frame and all crevices. Lower the Gatch bed at the knee.
   - By grasping the clean fold of the mattress, lift and swing its clean side crosswise on the clean half of the spring and wash the exposed surface.
   - Place the pillow on the unwashed upper half of the spring. Wash the top surface of the pillow.
   - Place the pillow clean side down on the clean mattress surface and wash the other side.
   - Wash the upper spring, raising the head portion of the bed, to complete bed cleansing.
- Wash the cabinet, inside and out. Complete the unit cleaning by washing the chair, bed lamp (cord unplugged), signal cord, and overbed table.
- If you are responsible for the floor, sweep and mop it and wash the windowsills. Wash your hands when the cleaning is completed and remake the bed for a new occupant.
- Discard the waste. If cleaning cloths are to be reused, place them in the laundry hamper.
- Wash the collected utensils and place them in the utensil boiler (sanitizer) for a 30-minute boiling period. Wash the utility cart and return it to the storage place.
- Wash hands
- Remove the clean utensils from the utensil boiler. Dry and return them to the storage shelf.

Nursing Care

This may be considered under three main groups:

I. **Concerned with the comfort and well being of every patient:**
   - The kind of reception patient receives
   - Insistence on careful cleaning and daily dusting and checking of empty units for condition and completeness of equipment.
   - Before admission deciding where to place patient.
   - Set the standard for the quality of care given.
   - Helping her staff to improve their nursing ability, for seeking and utilizing their contributions in planning and evaluating the care of the patient.
   - Look into general comforts of the patient and his/her relatives.

II. **Those which are concerned with the carrying-out of medical treatment:**
   - Review of equipment to determine completeness, availability for use, cleanliness, safety, and convenience in placement
   - Staff orientation to operation, purpose, and aftercare of them
   - Quantities of supplies on hand
   - Supervision to assure specific and intended use of equipments
   - Convenient and easy access of them
   - Provision for ordering on an emergency basis

III. **Those which are concerned with education:** The head nurse in a hospital where student nurse receives their education has responsibilities in addition to the other administrative duties.
   - Orientation program for new nursing staff, student nurse and domestic staff—Participation in ward teaching
   - In-service education of nursing personnel
   - Assignment of duties
   - Keeping her knowledge up-to-date
   - Supervision
   - Ensuring good quality nursing care

PLANNING FOR EMERGENCY AND DISASTER

Emergency and disaster planning involves a coordinated, cooperative process of preparing to match urgent needs

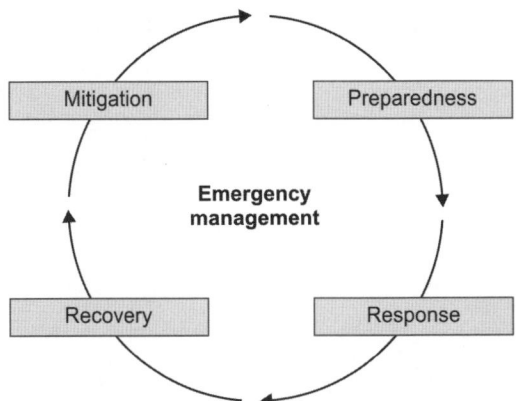

Fig. 6.15: Emergency management.

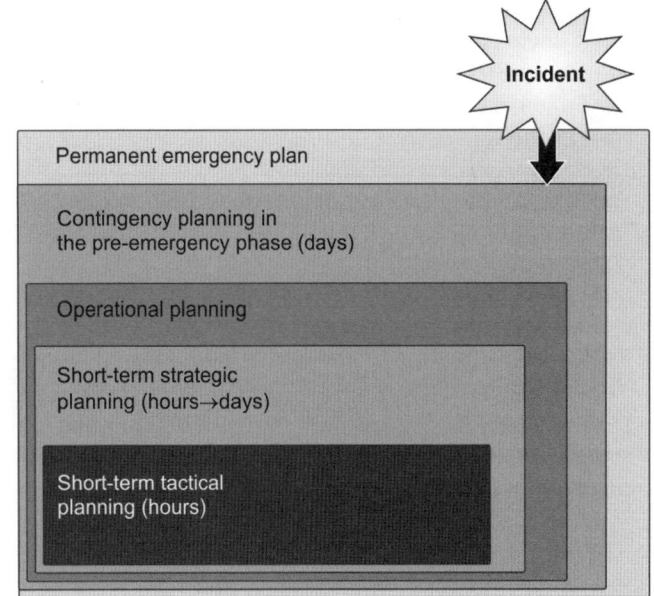

Fig. 6.16: Emergency response planning.

with available resources. The phases are research, writing, dissemination, testing, and updating. Hence, an emergency plan needs to be a living document that is periodically adapted to changing circumstances and that provides a guide to the protocols, procedures, and division of responsibilities in emergency response **(Fig. 6.15)**.

- Emergency planning is an exploratory process that provides generic procedures for managing unforeseen impacts and should use carefully constructed scenarios to anticipate the needs that will be generated by foreseeable hazards when they strike.
- Plans need to be developed for specific sectors, such as education, health, industry, and commerce.
- They also need to exist in a nested hierarchy that extends from the local emergency response (the most fundamental level), through the regional tiers of government, to the national and international levels.
- Failure to plan can be construed as negligence because it would involve failing to anticipate needs that cannot be responded to adequately by improvisation during an emergency.
- Plans are needed, not only for responding to the impacts of disaster, but also to maintain business continuity while managing the crisis, and to guide recovery and reconstruction effectively.
- Dealing with disaster is a social process that requires public support for planning initiatives and participation by a wide variety of responders, technical experts and citizens.
- It needs to be sustainable in the light of challenges posed by nonrenewable resource utilization, climate change, population growth, and imbalances of wealth. Although, at its most basic level, emergency planning is little more than codified common sense, the increasing complexity of modern disasters has required substantial professionalization of the field.

Emergency Response: Planning and Organization (Fig. 6.16)

- **Location:** There are two essential location requirements:
  1. It must be on ground floor and easily accessible to both ambulatory and ambulance patients, and there should be minimal separation between it and radiology department.
  2. Secondly, the emergency department should have ready access to the acute patient care areas, e.g., operation theater, ICU, blood bank, etc.

  Emergency department must be designed; usually 1000 sq ft is required for daily patient load of 100 patients.
- **Stretcher, trolley, wheelchair store:** A store for stretcher, trolley and wheelchairs should be located adjacent to the entrance.
- **Ambulance attendants, police, mass media room:** An equipped room of about 10 m^2 near the entrance hall with attached toilet serves the needs of above personnel.
- **Work area:** It should be spacious with enough room for personnel and patients.
- **Waiting area for emergency department patients:** The main function of this is to be the passageway to patient examination and treatment area.
- **Waiting area for relatives:** Patient relatives should not be allowed in the work areas of emergency department. Waiting room with recreational facilities may be provided.
- **Visitor's toilet:** It should be provide near the main waiting space.
- **Nurse's station and administrative office:** This should be next to the entrance and manned on 24 hour basis. It should be provided with multiple telephones, bulletin board with duty roster of doctors on call and directive pertaining to the emergency department should be displayed. Nurses work room should be well stocked with drugs, IV fluids.
- **Examination and treatment area:** This area should always be in readiness to receive patients at all times, and should consist of a large room and number of separate smaller rooms for examination and treatment. It should be well illuminated space with oxygen supply, resuscitation

equipment, suction, portable X-ray, electrocardiographs, and Boyle's apparatus.

- **Equipment:**
  - Stretchers
  - On-the wall oxygen unit
  - On-the wall suction unit
  - BP apparatus, otoscope, stethoscope, opthalmoscope; etc.
  - Spot lights
  - Utility table
  - Airways and resuscitation bags
- **Resuscitation room:** The patient is to be stabilized in this room before shifting to treatment or recovery room, or to ICU or nursing unit. It should be well equipped with resuscitation equipment, ECG machine and X-ray viewing screening with facility for performing minor operative procedures.
- **Operation room:** A self sufficient operation room to serve patients who need minor surgery and no admission or who are critically ill, etc., in emergency department.
- **Fracture room:** A separate fracture room equipped similar to OT and additional facilities for reduction of closed fractures under local anesthesia can be planned with hospitals with turnover of emergency patients in excess of 15,000 per annum.
- **Plaster room:** It is needed for treatment of fractures and application plasters.
- **Care of burns:** A separate room with 20 m² area should be reserved for immediate care of burn patients. An observation ward of about 6–8 beds for patients to be kept under observation overnight or 24 hours.
- **Isolation room:** For obstetric patients, pediatric patients.
- **Other rooms:** These should be planned based on the local needs:
  - Room for dead bodies
  - Pantry 7 m²
  - Storage space
  - Utility and soiled linen room 7 m²
  - Cleaners room-house keepers room 4 m²
  - Change room duty rooms 9 m²
  - Conference room and reference library 8 m²

Figure 6.17 shows phases of disaster management.

Emergency Response: Staffing Pattern

- **Senior physician**/Surgeon/Orthopedic surgeon who should be in-charge.
- **Casualty officers:** In medium size hospital, one casualty medical officer is required to work round the clock. In large size hospital with heavy work load in casualty more than one officer may be posted. Alternately only one doctor is posted. It should be possible to mobilize help if the need arises. Doctors posted in casualty need to have experience as resident medical officer for at least one year.

  They should also have some orientation training for (a) emergency services, (b) procedures required for critically ill, (c) communication skill and public relations, (d) legal procedures.

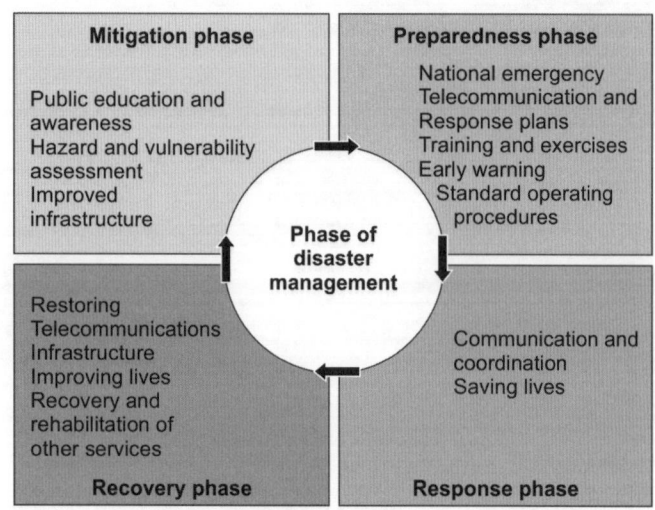

Fig. 6.17: Phases of disaster management.

- **Specialist doctors** may be called as and when necessary.
- **Nursing staff:** (a) sister in charge who will be in overall charge of entire emergency care area, (b) Staff nurses:
  - One staff nurse round the clock in casualty examination room.
  - Depending on number of beds in the observation ward and turnover rate one or two staff nurses round the clock.
  - One staff nurse round the clock in operation theatre.

  It is desirable to mobilize staff nurses from the area having no work to the area having more work. She should not be confined to the geographical area. Her work will be activity based.
- **Labor staff:**
  - For cleaning the place
  - For shifting patient's
  - Carry messages on call book
  - Carry pathology samples
  - Get pathology reports
    a. This is especially true in light of the increasing role in emergency response of information and communications technology.
    b. Disaster planners and coordinators are resource managers, and in the future, they will need to cope with complex and sophisticated transfers of human and material resources.
    c. In a globalizing world that is subject to accelerating physical, social, and economic change, the challenge of managing emergencies well depends on effective planning and foresight, and the ability to connect disparate elements of the emergency response into coherent strategies.

Table 6.3 shows functional differences between different sizes of event of planning.

Planning Process

- Planning emergency actions is a process; it is not a one-time event. While the plan may detail specific objectives

Chapter 6: Planning Nursing Services

Table 6.3: Functional differences between different sizes of event.

	Incidents	Major incidents	Disasters	Catastrophes
Size of impact	Very localized	Fully or partially localized	Widespread and severe	Extremely large in the physical and social sphere
Size of response	Local resources used	Mainly local resources used, with some mutual assistance from nearby areas	Intergovernmental, multi-agency, multi-jurisdictional response needed	Major national and international resources and coordination are required
Plans and procedures activated	Standard operating procedures used	Standard operating procedures used; emergency plans may be activated	Disaster or emergency plans activated	Disaster or emergency plans activated, but huge challenges may overwhelm them
Impact on response resources needed for response	Local resources will probably be sufficient	Local resources and some outside resources needed	Extensive damage to resources in disaster area; major inter-regional transfers of resources	Local and regional emergency response systems paralyzed and in need of much outside help
Involvement of public in response	Public generally not involved in response	Public largely not involved in response	Public extensively involved in response	Public overwhelmingly involved in response
Challenges to post-event recovery	No significant challenges to recovery	Few challenges to recovery processes	Major challenges to recovery from disaster	Massive challenges and significant long-term effects

and preparedness actions, these will need to be corrected and refined during an actual emergency.

- Planning may be ineffective if all affected parties are not included in the process.
- Those that are charged with implementing preparedness or emergency activities are more likely to comply if they feel that their views are incorporated into the planning process.
- Experience shows that plans created by an external person or by an isolated individual or agency are usually not valued and used. Therefore, a team approach is desirable.
- A team approach allows for diverse perspectives to be shared during the planning stage.
- It also helps ensure that the team has access to precise and complete information.

Communication and Coordination of Plans

- In the process of formulating and updating specific aims and objectives, national societies should communicate with and coordinate their plans with those of government agencies and nongovernmental organizations involved in disaster response.
- This will improve planning, reduce duplication of efforts, make plans more realistic and increase the overall effectiveness of disaster response.
- Through direct coordination, agencies can clearly divide responsibility for different operations and plan their actions accordingly.
- Similarly, representatives of various agencies working in one area (e.g., health, shelter and food distribution) may organize planning subgroups.
- Joint development and updating of preparedness plans can serve as the basis for coordination among agencies.
- Besides the Red Crescent/Red Cross Societies, other agencies that may be involved with disaster response operations include:
  - Ministries and committees for emergencies and civil defense

> **Box 6.8:** General principles of emergency medical care.
> - Triage
> - **Primary survey using Asset-based Community Development (ABCD) approach:** Airway, breathing, circulation and disability
> - **Secondary survey using EFGHI approach:**
> - Exposure to environment
> - Full set of vital signs
> - Give comfort measures
> - History collection
> - Inspect the posterior surface

- Fire brigades
- Health departments, ministries or agencies
- Militia divisions
- International agencies (in major disasters)
- Local authorities and affected populations

Within the national society itself, it is critical that the headquarters office and its branch societies at the district (or state) and the local community level clarify their respective roles and responsibilities in disaster preparedness and response and establish the necessary communication and coordination mechanisms among the different levels.

Box 6.8 summarizes general principles of emergency medical care.

Emergency Admission

If the ambulance is sent to receive the patient in emergency. The ambulance driver on the staff with the patient in ambulance communicates with the staff in casualty about the patient arrival and condition of the patient if possible.

- Patient is taken in casualty as soon as he/she comes in the hospital.
- A casualty doctor checks the patient's vital and initiate the emergency treatment as per the evidence based medicine protocols.
- At the same time, the relatives are sent for counseling to billing in charge the consultant is called and the patient

is transferred to ward/ICU/OT according to his condition for further management.

In case of MLC admission: A medicolegal case is a case of injury/illness where the attending doctor, after eliciting history and examining the patient, thinks that some investigation by law enforcement agencies is essential.

Cases that are to be treated as medicolegal:
- All cases of injuries and burns
- All vehicular, factory or other unnatural accident cases specially when there is a likelihood of patient's death or grievous hurt.
- Cases of suspected or evident sexual assault.
- Cases of suspected or evident criminal abortion.
- Cases of unconsciousness where its cause is not natural or not clear.
- All cases of suspected or evident poisoning or intoxication.
- Cases referred from court or otherwise for age estimation.
- Cases brought dead with improper history creating suspicion of an offence.
- Cases of suspected self-infliction of injuries or attempted suicide
- Any other case not falling under the above categories but has legal implications.

TRIAGE (FIG. 6.18)

Triage refers to the evaluation and categorization of the sick or wounded when there are insufficient resources for medical care of everyone at once. Triage is used in a number of situations in hospital, including:
- In mass casualty situations, triage is used to decide who is most urgently in need of transportation to ICU (generally, those who have a chance of survival, but who would die without immediate treatment), whose injuries are less severe and to determine which patients should be seen and treated immediately.
- Triage may be used to prioritize the use of space or equipment, such as operating rooms, in a crowded medical facility.

Rationale: To save the lives of the people and avoid medical complications of the patients received in a disaster or mass casualty situation.

Various Personnel Responsible
- Casualty medical officer
- RMO in-charge
- Triage nurse
- Nurse on call

Procedure
- In a disaster or mass casualty situation, immediately after receiving the patients, the first step is to check the vital signs of the patients, i.e., heart rate, respiration and blood pressure in order to identify seriously ill persons who must receive immediate care.
- The victims are grouped into four categories, depending on the urgency of their needs; it involves a color-coding scheme using red, yellow, green, white, and black tags:
  - **Red tags:** (immediate) are used to label those who cannot survive without immediate treatment but who have a chance of survival.
  - **Yellow tags:** (observation) for those who require observation (and possible later re-triage). Their condition is stable for the moment and, they are not in immediate danger of death. These victims will still need hospital care and would be treated immediately under normal circumstances.
  - **Green tags:** (wait) are reserved for the "walking wounded" who will need medical care at some point, after more critical injuries have been treated.
  - **White tags:** (dismiss) are given to those with minor injuries for whom a doctor's care is not required.
  - **Black tags:** (expectant) are used for the deceased and for those whose injuries are so extensive that they will not be able to survive given the care that is available.
- The triage nurse will coordinate with the various departments for the availability of equipment, facilities and resources.
- The triage nurse will supervise the transportation of the patients, their safety.
- The CMO billing will counsel the patient's relatives so that there is no panicky situation

Figure 6.19 shows triage categories. **Figure 6.20** shows triage assessment criteria. **Box 6.9** summarizes characteristics of triage nurse.

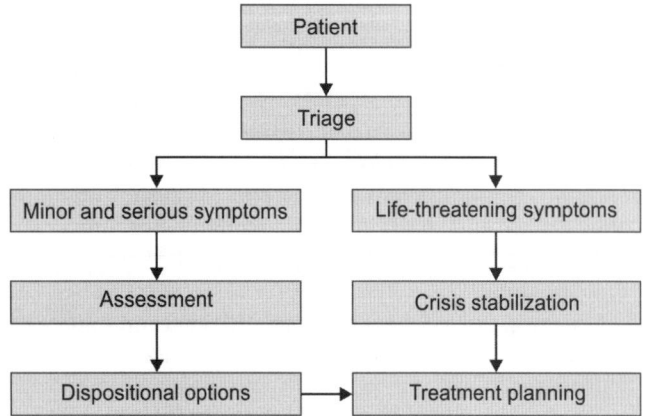

Fig. 6.18: Triage management.

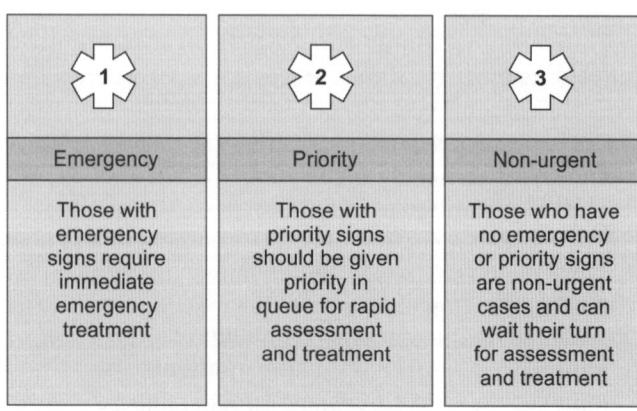

Fig. 6.19: Triage categories.

	1 resuscitation	2 urgent (15 min)	3 less urgent (60 min)	4 not urgent (180 min)
A	Obstructed airway stridor	Threatened airway		
B	SpO_2 <80 RR >35 or <8	SpO_2: 80–89 RR: 31–35	SpO_2: 90–94 RR: 26–30	$SpO_2 \geq 95$ RR: 80–25
C	HR > 130 Bp_{sys} < 80	HR: 121 – 130 HR <40 BT_{sys}: 80–89	HR: 111–120 HR: 40–49	HR: 50–110
D	GCS ≤8	GCS: 9–13	GCS = 14	GCS = 15
E		Tp >40 Tp <32	Tp: 38.1–40.0 Tp: 32–34	Tp: 34.1–38.0

Fig. 6.20: Triage assessment criteria.

> **Box 6.9:** Characteristics of triage nurse.
> - Extensive knowledge to emergency medical treatment
> - Adequate training and competent skills, language, terminology
> - Ability to use the critical thinker process
> - Good decision maker

Triage Nursing

Triage consists of rapidly classifying the injured on the bases of severity of their injuries and the likelihood of their survival with prompt medical intervention.

- **Golden hour:** A seriously injured patient has one hour in which they need to receive advanced trauma life support. This is referred to as the golden hour.
- **Immediate or high priority:** Higher priority is granted to victims who's immediate or long-term prognosis can be dramatically affected by simple intensive care. Immediate patients are at risk for early death. They usually fall into one of two categories. They are in shock from severe blood loss or they have severe head injury. These patients should be transported as soon as possible.
- **Delayed or medium priority:**
  - Delayed patients may have injuries that span a wide range
  - They may have severe internal injuries, but are still compensating

  Delayed patients have:
  - Respirations under 30/minutes
  - Capillary refill under 2 seconds
  - Can do—follow simple commands
- **Minor or minimal or ambulatory patients:** Patients with minor lacerations, contusions, sprains, superficial burns are identified as—minor/minimal
- **Expectant or least priority:**
  - Morbid patients who require a great deal of attention with questionable benefit have the lowest priority.
  - Patients with whom there are signs of impending death or massive injuries with poor likelihood of survival are labeled as expectant.

CONCLUSION

Planning is also a management process, concerned with defining goals for a company's future direction and determining the missions and resources to achieve those targets. To meet objectives, managers may develop plans, such as a business plan or a marketing plan. The purpose may be achievement of certain goals or targets. Planning revolves largely around identifying the resources available for a given project and utilizing optimally to achieve best scenario outcomes.

REVIEW QUESTIONS

Long Essays
1. Define planning; explain mission and vision in planning.
2. Describe functional, operational and strategic planning.
3. Explain program planning by using Gantt chart.
4. Discuss in detail about planning in nursing care unit.
5. Enumerate planning for emergency and disaster.
6. Define triage; explain the triage procedures.

Short Essays
1. Nursing service philosophy.
2. Scope of planning in nursing service.
3. Operational planning in nursing.
4. Steps to create a Gantt chart.
5. Characteristics of planning.
6. Principles of planning.

7. Steps involved in planning.
8. Components of planning.
9. Factors affecting planning.
10. Types/classifications of plans.
11. Components of safety management plan.
12. Phases of disaster management.

Short Answers

1. Policies related to nursing service.
2. Strategic planning in nursing.
3. Strategic planning phases.
4. Importance of Gantt chart.
5. Milestone chart.
6. Importance of planning.
7. Essentials of good planning.
8. Objectives of planning hospital units.
9. Emergency response planning.

BIBLIOGRAPHY

1. Douglass LM. The effective nurse-leader and manager. 5th edition. Mosby: St. Louis; 1996.
2. Ellis JR, Hartley CL. Managing and coordinating nursing care. 3rd edition. Lippincott: Philadelphia; 1995.
3. Marquis BL, Huston CJ. Leadership and Management Functions in Nursing- Theory and application. 5th edition. Philadelphia: Lippincott Williams and Wilkins; 2006.
4. Marquis BL, Hutson CJ. Leadership roles and management functions in nursing– Theory and application. 5th edition. Philadelphia: Lippincott Williams and Wilkins; 2006.
5. Ward MJ, Price SA. Issues in nursing administration. St. Louis: Mosby; 1991.
6. Wehrich H, Koontz H. Management: A global perspective. 11th edition. New Delhi: Tata McGraw-Hill Publishing company Ltd; 2005.

CHAPTER 7

Organizing

LEARNING OBJECTIVES

- Organizing as a Process—Assignment, Delegation and Coordination
- Hospital—Types, Functions and Organization
- Organizational Development
- Organizational Structure
- Organizational Charts
- Organizational Effectiveness
- Hospital Administration, Control and Line of Authority
- Hospital Statistics Including Hospital Utilization Indices
- Nursing Care Delivery Systems and Trends
- Role of Nurse in Maintenance of Effective Organizational Climate

■ INTRODUCTION

The word "organizing" refers to a process of a managerial function. Studying organization structure helps one to clarify the principle features of the organization's anatomy and study the similarities as well as the distinctions among different organizations. The term "Organization" may be dealt in two contexts. Organizing is the function of management which follows planning. It is a function in which the synchronization and combination of human, physical and financial resources takes place. All the three resources are important to get results. Therefore, organizational function helps in achievement of results which in fact is important for the functioning of a concern (**Fig. 7.1**) and Purpose of organizing is summarizes in **Box 7.1**.

■ DEFINITION

- According to Chester Barnard, "Organizing is a function by which the concern is able to define the role positions, the jobs related and the coordination between authority and responsibility. Hence, a manager always has to organize in order to get results.
- "Organizing is the process of defining and grouping the activities of the enterprise and establishing authority relationships among them" —***Theo Haimman***
- "To organize a business is to provide it with everything useful to its functioning: raw materials, machines and tools, capital and personnel". —***Henry Fayol***
- "In its broadest sense organizing refers to relationship between various factors present in a giving endeavor or enterprise". —***William Spriegel***
- "Organizing is the establishing of effective authority relationships among selected work, persons and work places in order for a group to work together efficiently". —***GR Terry***

> **Box 7.1:** Purposes of organizing.
> - Divides work to be done into specific jobs and departments.
> - Assigns tasks and responsibilities associated with individual jobs.
> - Coordinates diverse organizational tasks.
> - Clusters jobs into units.
> - Establishes relationships among individuals, groups, and departments.
> - Establishes formal lines of authority.
> - Allocates and deploys organizational resources.

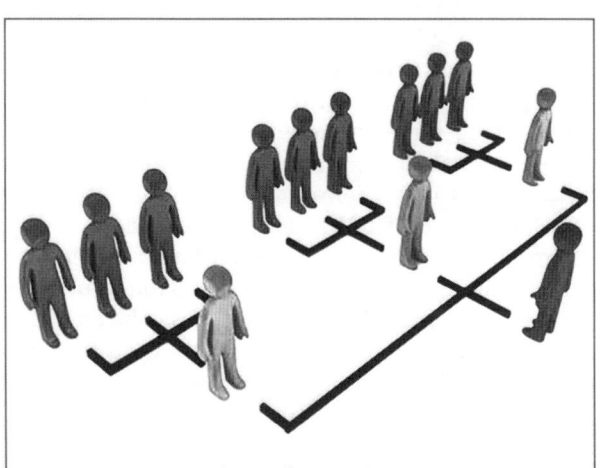

Fig. 7.1: Organizing.

■ OBJECTIVES OF ORGANIZING

- **Helps to achieve organizational goal:** Organization is employed to achieve the overall objectives of business firms. Organization focuses attention of individual's objectives towards overall objectives.
- **Optimum use of resources:** To make optimum use of resources, such as men, material, money, machine and method, it is necessary to design an organization properly.

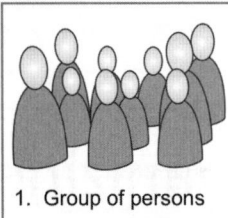
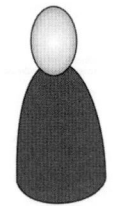
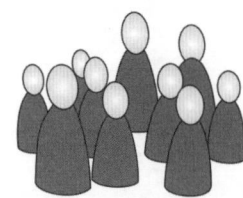

1. Group of persons
2. Common objectives
3. Division of work
4. Cooperative efforts
5. Communication
6. Central authority
7. Rules and regulations
8. Dynamic element

Fig. 7.2: Nature of organizing.

Box 7.2: Principles of organizing.
The success of any organization depends on its principles. Basic principles should be observed.
1. **Unity of objective:** If the aim is one to all employees and managers, success will follow.
2. **Efficiency:** Doing maximum work at minimum cost is efficiency.
3. **Span of management:** Managers have long time to direct a number of executives.
4. **Division of work:** Proper departmentalization (each department has it's own function and job)
5. **Functional definition:** When duties of every one is defined

Work should be divided equally and qualified people should be given the right jobs to reduce the wastage of resources in an organization.

- **To perform managerial function:** Planning, organizing, staffing, directing and controlling cannot be implemented without proper organization.
- **Facilitates growth and diversification:** A good organization structure is essential for expanding business activities. Organization structure determines the input resources needed for expansion of a business activity; similarly organization is essential for product diversification, such as establishing a new product line. it also stimulates creativity in managers by organizing.
- **Humane treatment of employees:** Organization has to operate for the betterment of employees and must not encourage monotony of work due to higher degree of specialization. Now, organization has adapted the modern concept of systems approach based on human relations and it discards the traditional productivity and specialization approach. **Figure 7.2** shows nature of organizing.

PRINCIPLES OF ORGANIZING (BOX 7.2)

- Principle of Consideration of Unity of Objectives
- Principle of Specialization
- Principle of Coordination
- Principles of Scaler Chain
- Principle of Commensurate Authority and Responsibility
- Principle of Ultimate Responsibility
- Principle of Efficiency
- Principle of Delegation
- Principle of Unity of Command
- Principle of Span of Control
- Principle of Balance
- Principle of Communication
- Principle of Personal Ability
- Principle of Exception
- Principle of Flexibility
- Principle of Departmentation
- Principle of Division of Work
- Principle of Definiteness
- Principle of Discipline
- Principle of Simplicity
- Principle of Separation of Line and Staff Function
  Line function should be separated from the staff functions
- Principle of Continuity of Operations
- Principle of Leadership
- Principle of Definition
- Principle of Work Assignment
- Principle of Employee Participation

FEATURES OF ORGANIZING

The features of organizing are stated as here under:

- **Division of work:** The total work should be divided into many parts for effective performance of the work. Each part of work is to be performed by one person or a group of persons.
- **Achieving organizational objective:** There is a need of coordination among the employees in the organization. The division of work is done keeping in view the overall objectives of the organization. The organizing process is framed in such a way so as to achieve organizational objectives smoothly.
- **Authority-responsibility structure:** The position of each of the executives is defined with regard to the extent of authority and responsibility vested in him to discharge his duties. Organizing arranges for the delegation of authority and responsibility. It tries to bring harmony, authority, and responsibility.
- **Grouping of activities:** Activities are needed to be grouped on certain well-defined basis, such as function, product, customer, process, territory, etc. This grouping process is called departmentation. It helps in achieving the benefits of specialization and administrative control.
- **Scalar (step-by-step) principle:** Authority is delegated from the upper level to the lower level and the responsibility flows from the lower level to the upper level of organizational hierarchy. Provision is to be made for the accountability of the assigned duties. Each employee of an organization must know where his accountability lies. **Figure 7.3** shows organizing process.
- **Installing sound communication system:** The success of management depends upon effective system of communication. It helps the management by providing

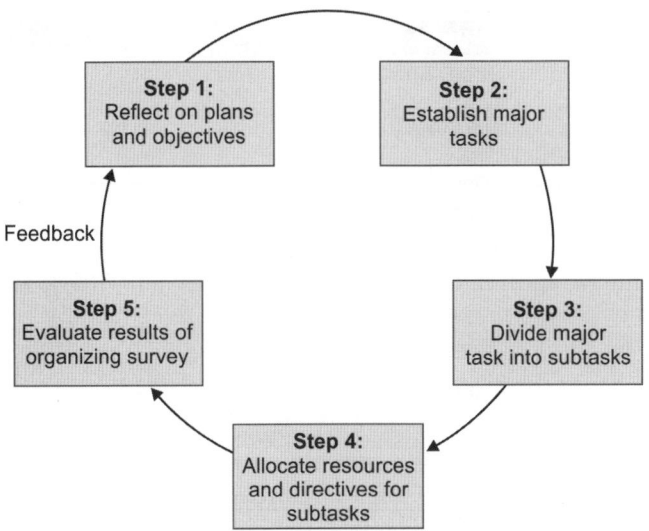

Fig. 7.3: Organizing process.

information about the duties, responsibilities, authority, positions, and jobs. Coordination can be maintained among various related departments by making exchange of information on a regular basis.
- **Flexibility:** The organizing process should be flexible so that any change can be incorporated as and when required. It ensures the ability to adapt and adjust the activities in response to the change taking place in the external environment. The programs, policies, and strategies can be changed as and when required if the provision for flexibility is made in the organizing process.
- **Coordination:** Coordination ensures the unity of action in the realization of a common objective. It is an arrangement of group effort to achieve organizational goals. Coordination of different personnel and departments are needed for ensuring higher efficiency and effectiveness.

ELEMENT OF ORGANIZING

The basic elements of organizing are as follows:
- **Division of work:** It means dividing the work into specific tasks with deadlines to their completion. Once the work is divided, the tasks are distributed to different functional areas of the organization as production, marketing, finance and personnel.
- **Grouping of activities:** The tasks are grouped into different departments on the basis of similarity of their features. This is called departmentation.
  The common forms of departmentation are as follows:
  - Functional departmentation (Grouping activities by functions performed)
  - Product departmentation (Grouping activities by product line)
  - Customer departmentation (Grouping activities on the basis of common customers or types of customers)
  - Geographic departmentation (Grouping activities on the basis of territory)
  - Process departmentation (Grouping activities on the basis of product or service or customer flow)
- **Distribution of authority:** Once the departments are created, members are given authority to perform the tasks assigned. Authority specifies the discretion of employee over his work. In a formally designed organization structure, employees' behavior is bound by rules, regulations and policies but in a comparatively less formal organization structure, they have a great deal of freedom in deciding how they perform their work.
- **Coordination:** When people perform tasks assigned to them at different levels in different departments, it has to be ensured that the tasks are related to each other and aim at unified goals. This requires coordination amongst the tasks of all the organizational members. Coordination is the act of organizing, making different people or things work together for a goal or effort to fulfill desired goals in the organizations.

FUNCTIONS OF ORGANIZING

A manager performs organizing function with the help of following steps:
- **Identification of activities:** All the activities which have to be performed in a concern have to be identified first. For example, preparation of accounts, making sales, record keeping, quality control, inventory control, etc. All these activities have to be grouped and classified into units.
- **Departmentally organizing the activities:** In this step, the manager tries to combine and group similar and related activities into units or departments. This organization of dividing the whole concern into independent units and departments is called departmentation.
- **Classifying the authority:** Once the departments are made, the manager likes to classify the powers and its extent to the managers. This activity of giving a rank in order to the managerial positions is called hierarchy. The top management is into formulation of policies, the middle level management into departmental supervision and lower level management into supervision of foremen.
- **Coordination between authority and responsibility:** Relationships are established among various groups to enable smooth interaction toward the achievement of the organizational goal. Each individual is made aware of his authority and he/she knows whom they have to take orders from and to whom they are accountable and to whom they have to report. A clear organizational structure is drawn and all the employees are made aware of it.

IMPORTANCE OF ORGANIZING FUNCTION (BOX 7.3)

- **Specialization:** Organizational structure is a network of relationships in which the work is divided into units and departments. This division of work is helping in bringing specialization in various activities of concern.
- **Well defined jobs:** Organizational structure helps in putting right men on right job which can be done by selecting people for various departments according to their qualifications, skill and experience. This is helping

Chapter 7: Organizing

> **Box 7.3:** Organizing function.
> - A management process
> - Identifying and establishing jobs, positions, and chain of command
> - Facilitate communication
> - Identifying skills employees
> - Arraying physical, financial, and human resources for efficient use
> - Provides for information flow
> - Goal is to make business run smoothly

> **Box 7.4:** Methods of patient assignment.
> - Case method nursing or total patient care
> - Functional nursing
> - Team nursing or modular nursing
> - Primary nursing
> - Case management or managed care
> - Progressive patient care

in defining the jobs properly which clarifies the role of every person.

- **Clarifies authority:** Organizational structure helps in clarifying the role positions to every manager (status quo). This can be done by clarifying the powers to every manager and the way he has to exercise those powers should be clarified so that misuse of powers does not take place. Well defined jobs and responsibilities attached helps in bringing efficiency into managers working. This helps in increasing productivity.
- **Coordination:** Organization is a means of creating co-ordination among different departments of the enterprise. It creates clear cut relationships among positions and ensure mutual cooperation among individuals. Harmony of work is brought by higher level managers exercising their authority over interconnected activities of lower level manager.
- **Effective administration:** The organization structure is helpful in defining the jobs positions. The roles to be performed by different managers are clarified. Specialization is achieved through division of work. This all leads to efficient and effective administration.
- **Growth and diversification:** A company's growth is totally dependent on how efficiently and smoothly a concern works. Efficiency can be brought about by clarifying the role positions to the managers, coordination between authority and responsibility and concentrating on specialization.
- **Sense of security:** Organizational structure clarifies the job positions. The roles assigned to every manager are clear. Coordination is possible. Therefore, clarity of powers helps automatically in increasing mental satisfaction and thereby a sense of security in a concern. This is very important for job-satisfaction.
- **Scope for new changes:** Where the roles and activities to be performed are clear and every person gets independence in his working, this provides enough space to a manager to develop his talents and flourish his knowledge. A manager gets ready for taking independent decisions which can be a road or path to adoption of new techniques of production. This scope for bringing new changes into the running of an enterprise is possible only through a set of organizational structure.

ORGANIZING AS A PROCESS—ASSIGNMENT, DELEGATION AND COORDINATION

Organizing essentially consists of establishing a division of labor. The managers divide the work among individuals and group of individuals. And then they coordinate the activities of such individuals and groups to extract the best outcome. Organizing also involves delegating responsibility to the employees along with the authority to successfully accomplish these tasks and responsibilities. One major aspect of organizing is delegating the correct amounts of responsibilities and authority.

ASSIGNMENT

The nurse manager makes all assignments for the nurses she supervises, taking into account their strengths and weaknesses, their experience levels, the types of cases and number of patients requiring care. Using this information, she will assign nurses to specific cases or tasks, and set schedules for all nurses in the unit. She also ensures all nurses fulfill their duties and meet the hospital's expectations. **Box 7.4** summarizes methods of patient assignment.

Definition

- Assignment refers to "a written delegation of duties to care for a group of patients by trained personnel assigned to the unit."
- Patient assignment, a specialty capitation method in which patients choose a provider in each specialty represented. Capitation payments are then distributed accordingly to the providers selected.
- A patient assessment according to Basford and Slevin (1995) is a carefully thought out approach to gathering information and analysis of the data' in simple terms, i.e., building a picture of the patient. This is especially so in this assessment as building a picture of the patient is essential in order to determine care.

Process of Organizing Patient Care

The head nurse or the nurse in charge should carry out their duties and responsibilities through applying the following steps:

- **Planning:** It is a process of developing a course of action for meeting the needs of patient. In planning, the head nurse decides what should be done, when, how, where, by whom and to whom.
- **Assigning:** Assignment of patient and nursing activities are written in the assignment sheet by the head nurse/nurse in charge, based on the principles of assignment.
- **Leading:** Includes issuing instructions, motivation, and coordination of activities, by making rounds, checking performance and conducting conferences.
- **Evaluating:** By reviewing nursing performance and patient progress to be compared by the assignment and nursing care plan.

> **Box 7.5:** Role of nurse managers.
>
> - Managing, supervising and assisting the nursing staff, as well as providing administrative support and patient care.
> - Assigning nurses and support staff to patients.
> - Develop and implement training courses and organize seminars to help educate and train new nurses and staff.
> - Document the performance of nurses, perform evaluations and counsel nurses on unsatisfactory performance.
> - Creating schedules, maintaining adequate supplies and informing staff of changes to protocol.

- **Reporting:** The head nurse prepares a nursing unit report "e.g., shift report" which includes patient's needs, special observations, census, bed number, all critically-ill and postoperative patients, and patient's needs special preparation on. **Box 7.5** shows role of nurse managers.

Method of Patient Care Delivery

Case Method

It is the oldest patient care delivery method. In this method, one professional nurse assumes total responsibility of providing complete care for one or more patients (1–6) while she is on duty. This method is used frequently in intensive care units and in teaching nursing students. **Figure 7.4** shows purpose of functional method.

Advantages

- High degree of autonomy
- Lines of responsibility and accountability are clear
- Patient receives holistic, unfragmented care

Disadvantages

- Each RN may have a different approach to care
- Not cost-effective
- Lack of RN availability

Functional Method

This method focuses on getting the greatest amount of tasks in the least time. In this method, the nursing care is divided into tasks and each staff member is assigning to perform one or two tasks for all patients in the unit according to the level of skill required for performance as follows:

Advantages

- Care is provided economically and efficiently
- Minimum number of RNs required, so it is efficient when there is a shortage in the staff or there is limited number of professional nurses.
- Tasks are completed quickly.
- Useful in emergency situations.

Disadvantages

- Care may be fragmented.
- Patient may be confused with many care providers.
- Caregivers feel unchallenged.
- Lack of communication among the different persons who care for the patient.
- Neglecting the humanity of the patient and the individual needs of the patient will be lost in an effort to get the work done. **Figure 7.5** shows functional nursing care delivery model.

Team Nursing

Team nursing was developed because of social and technological changes in world war-II drew many nurses away from hospitals, learning haps, services, procedures and equipment became more expensive and complicated, requiring specialization at every turn. It is an attempt to meet increased demands of nursing services and better use of knowledge and skills of professional nurses (**Box 7.6**).

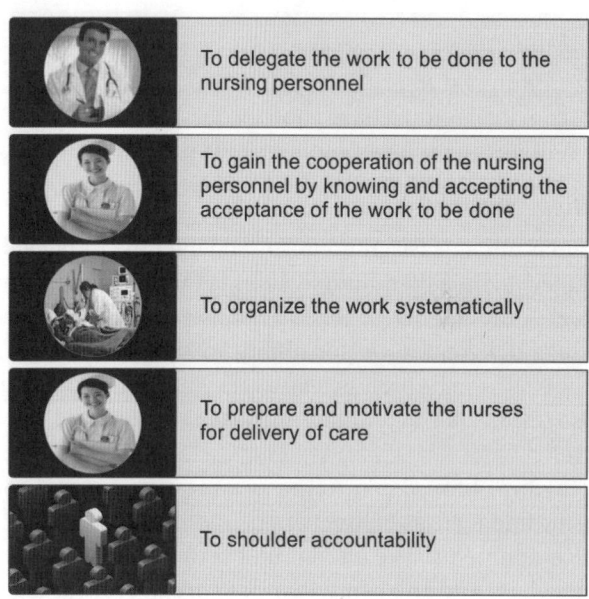

Fig. 7.4: Purpose of functional method.

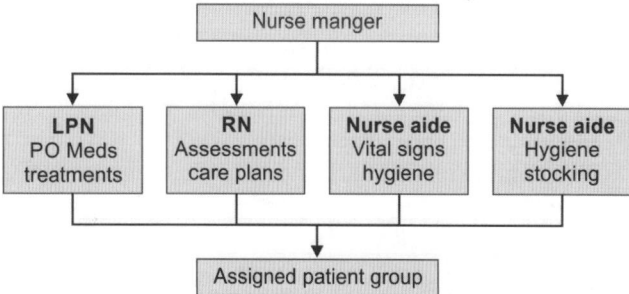

Fig. 7.5: Functional nursing care delivery model.

> **Box 7.6:** Team nursing.
>
> - Team nursing is based on philosophy in which groups of professional and nonprofessional personnel work together to identify, plan, implement and evaluate comprehensive client-centered care.
> - In team nursing an RN leads a team composed of other RNs, LPNs or LVNs and nurse assistants or technicians.
> - The team members provide direct patient care to group of patients, under the direction of the RN team leader in coordinated effort.
> - The charge nurse delegates authority to a team leader who must be a professional nurse. This nurse leads the team usually of 4 to 6 members in the care of between 15 and 25 patients.
> - The team leader assigns tasks, schedules care, and instructs team members in details of care.

Definition: Team nursing is based on philosophy in which groups of professional and non-professional personnel work together to identify, plan, implement and evaluate comprehensive client-centered care. The key concept is a group that works together toward a common goal, providing qualitative comprehensive nursing care (Kron 1978).

Advantages
- High-quality, comprehensive care with a high proportion of ancillary staff.
- Team members participate in decision making and contribute their own expertise.

Disadvantages
- Continuity suffers if daily team assignments vary.
- Team leader must have good leadership skills.
- Insufficient time for planning and communication.

Modular Nursing

Modular nursing assignment is used when the nursing staff includes technical and nurse aides, as well as professional nurses. Although two or three persons are assigned to each module, the greatest responsibility for the care of assigned patients falls on the professional nurse. The professional nurse is also responsible for guiding and teaching non-professional nurse.

Definition: Modular nursing is a modification of team nursing and focuses on the patient's geographic location for staff assignments. The patient unit is divided into modules or districts, and the same team of caregivers is assigned consistently to the same geographic location.

Advantages
- Continuity of care is improved when staff members are consistently assigned to the same module
- The RN as team leader is able to be more involved in planning and coordinating care.
- Geographic closeness and more efficient communication save staff time.

Disadvantages
- Costs may be increased to stock each module with the necessary patient care supplies (medication cart, linens and dressings).
- Long corridors, common in many hospitals, are not conducive to modular nursing.

Primary Nursing Method

This method is the best in an agency with an all-professional nurse staff. It is a comprehensive, continuous and coordinated nursing process for meeting the total needs of each patient (**Box 7.7**).

Advantages
- High-quality, holistic patient care
- Establish rapport with patient
- RN feels challenged and rewarded

> **Box 7.7:** Primary nursing care.
> - It was developed in the 1960s with the aim of placing RNs at the bedside and improving the professional relationships among staff members.
> - It supports a philosophy regarding nurse and patient relationship.
> - This method is based on the concept of 'my patient-my nurse" In this nursing care delivery system, each registered nurse is assigned to the care of group of patient for which she plans complete 24 hours care and writes the nursing care plan.
> - He/she is responsible for coordinating and implementing all the necessary nursing care that must be given to the patient during the shift.

Disadvantages
- Primary nurse must be able to practice with a high degree of responsibility and autonomy
- RN must accept 24-hour responsibility
- More RNs needed; not cost-effective

Case Management

Case management is a process of monitoring an individual patient's healthcare by the case manager, for the purpose of maximizing positive outcomes and containing costs (**Fig. 7.6**).

Advantages
- **For the patient:**
  - Establishing and achieving a set of "expected" or standardized patient care outcomes for each patient.
  - Facilitating early patient discharge or discharge within an appropriate length of stay.
  - Using the fewest possible appropriate healthcare resources to meet expected patient care outcomes.
  - Facilitating the continuity of patient care through collaborative practice of diverse health professionals.
- **For the nurse:**
  - Enhancing nurse's professional development and job satisfaction.
  - Facilitating the transfer of knowledge of expert clinical staff of novice staff.

■ DELEGATION

This is a concept concerned with the division of labor and organizational effectiveness. When the organizational grows, irrespective of size, the activities cannot be managed by one boss. Particularly in medium and large-sized business houses many levels of management prevail. The leaders or managers of these levels should have authority responsibility and accountability to carry out the tasks assigned to them. "Delegation" refers to this. **Figure 7.7** shows delegation in nursing.

Purpose of Delegation (Fig. 7.8)

The following are five purposes of delegating
1. Assigning routine tasks
2. Problem solving
3. Changes in the nurse manager's own job emphasis
4. Capability building
5. Assigning tasks for which the nurse manager does not have time.

Chapter 7: Organizing

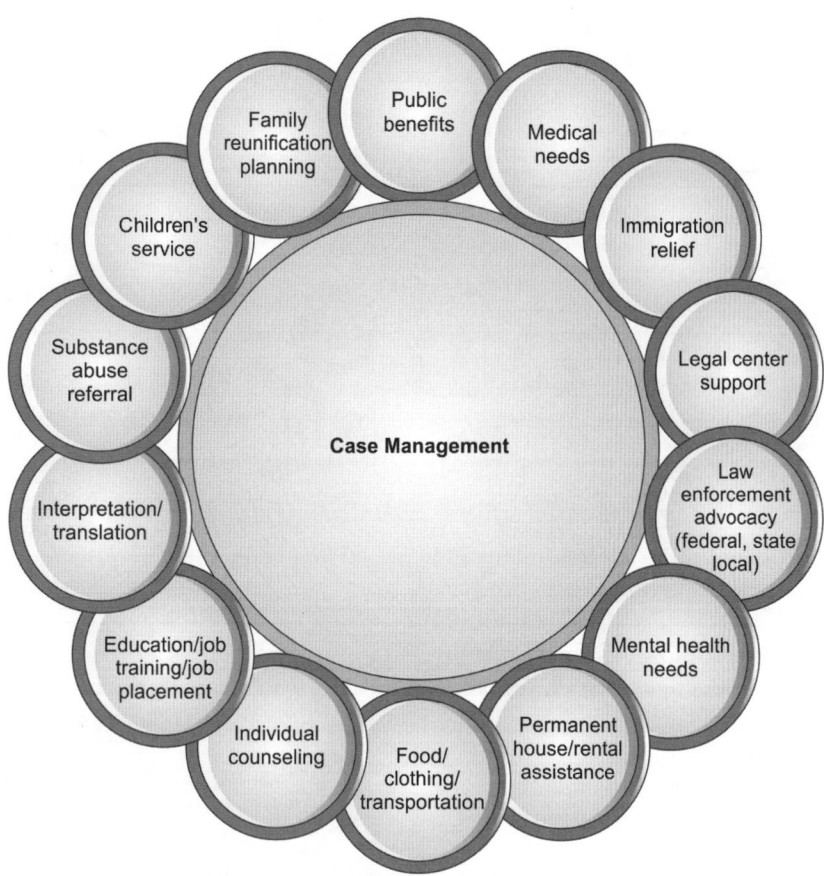

Fig. 7.6: Case management.

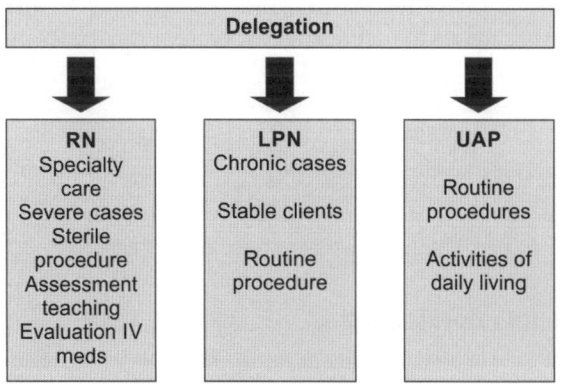

Fig. 7.7: Delegation in nursing.

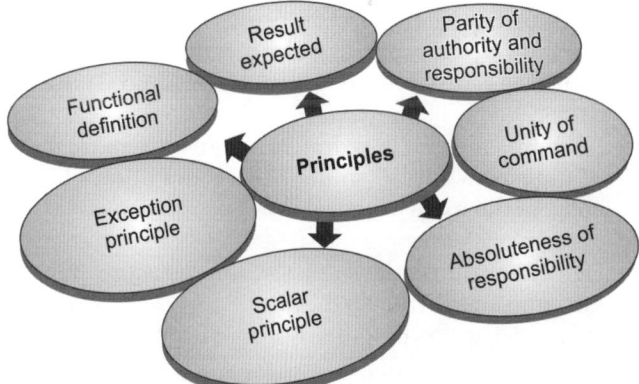

Fig. 7.8: Principles of delegation.

Principles of Delegation

- Select the right person to whom the job is to be delegated.
- Delegate both interesting and uninteresting tasks.
- Provide subordinates with enough time to learn.
- Delegate gradually
- Delegate in advance
- Consult before delegating
- Avoid gaps and overlaps

Four Steps in Delegation

1. The determination of results expected.
2. The assignment of tasks
3. The delegation of authority for accomplishing the tasks.
4. The responsibility and accountability

Types of Delegation (Fig. 7.9)

There are formal and informal delegations:
1. **Formal delegation:** The formal delegation is found in the exercise of authority defined by organizations role.
2. **Fimak delegation:** Fimak delegation is "down ward delegation" and is effective to the extent of the acceptance and respect for formal authority.
3. **Informal delegation:** Informal delegation occurs because people want to do something not they are told to do. It is something that is not formally required to be

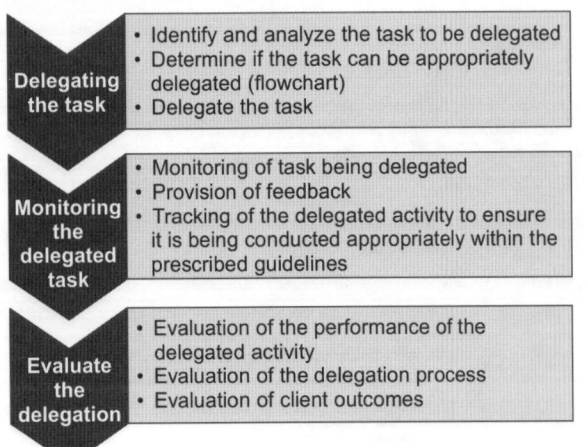

Fig. 7.9: Types of delegation.

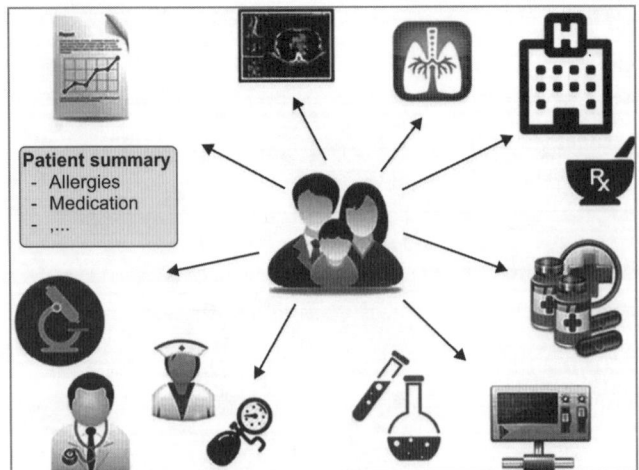

Fig. 7.10: Delegation of patient assignment.

done. When there is problem in the exercise of formal authority, informal delegation is accepted.

4. **Bottom-up delegation:** In 1st hour organizations informal group leaders, without formal authority assume authority to restrict supply and workers accept such informal delegations.
5. **Lateral delegation:** In modern organization, few positions are independent and team work exists in members of a group entrusting the authority, responsibility to others in the group at their level.

Advantages of Delegation

- Delegation serves as a vehicle of coordination. The various levels of the organization are used more appropriately.
- A sound system of delegation tends to develop an increased sense of responsibility and enhanced potential work capacity of individual employees.
- It reduces the executive burden—it relieves the superior of time-consuming, minor duties and allows him to concentrate more effectively on major responsibilities of his own position.
- Delegation minimizes delay when decisions have no longer to be referred up the line.
- Proper delegation of authority is conductive to an effective control over operation.
- As delegation provides the means of multiplying the limited personal capacity of the superior it is instrumental for encouraging and diversification of business.

Delegation of patient assignment is shown in **Figure 7.10** and **Figure 7.11** shows role of nurse in patient care.

COORDINATION

Coordination expresses the principles of organization in toto; nothing less. Coordination is the orderly arrangement of group effort to provide unity of action in the pursuit of common purpose. It is the beginning and end of all organized efforts. A manager is mainly a coordinator.

Definition: Coordination is a continuous process by which managers achieve the integrated common goals. It is therefore, the responsibility of manager to establish better coordination.

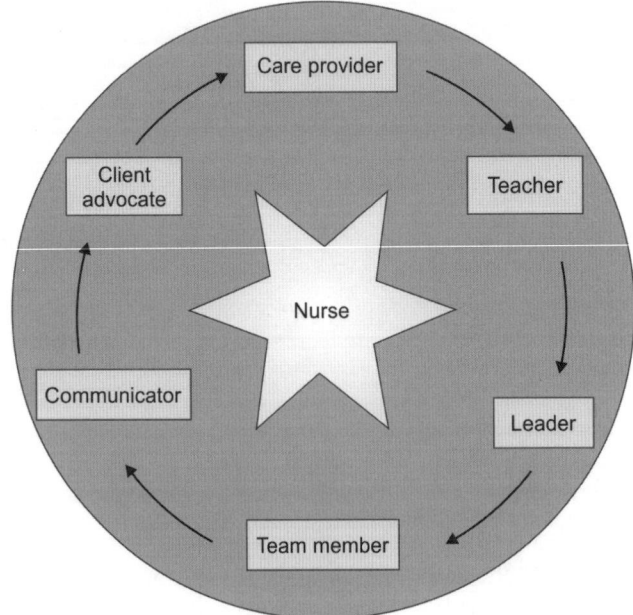

Fig. 7.11: Role of nurse in patient care.

Need for Coordination

We all are aware of the fact that there are several departments in an organization, such as finance, purchase, production, sales, human resource, marketing, research and development etc., and the work of all the departments are interlinked, and interdependent. Further, there are three levels in organizational hierarchy, wherein:

1. **Top-level:** Comprises of the Board of Directors, Chief Executives, Managing Directors, etc.
2. **Middle-level:** Comprises of departmental heads and managers.
3. **Lowest-level:** Comprises of supervisors, first-line managers and foreman.

Principles of coordination are:

- Early start
- Personnel contract
- Continuity
- Reciprocal relationship

- Dynamism
- Simplified organization
- Self-coordination
- Clear-cut objectives
- Clear definition of authority and responsibility
- Effective communication
- Effective supervision

Features of Coordination

The important features of coordination are:
- It is essential for group efforts and not for individual efforts.
- It is a continuous and dynamic process.
- Coordination emphasizes the unity of efforts
- Helps in the integration of functions
- It is the responsibility of every manager in the organization.

Types of Coordination

Coordination can be of the following types:
1. **Internal and external coordination:** Coordination between the activities of departments and people working within the organization is known as internal coordination. Coordination between activities of the organization with units outside the organization (Government, customers, suppliers, competitors, etc.) is known as external coordination.
2. **Vertical and horizontal coordination:** Both these types of coordination are the forms of internal coordination. Vertical coordination is achieved amongst activities of people working at different levels. It coordinates the activities of top managers with those of middle and lower level managers.

   Horizontal coordination is achieved amongst activities of different departments working at the same level. It is "the linking of activities across departments at similar levels. It links the activities of four primary departments-production, finance, personnel and sales". **Figure 7.12** shows coordination in patient care.

Essential Elements of Coordination

- **Balancing:** Efforts, jobs and activities of all departments must be balanced. In other words, the entire work must be divided and assigned to each department evenly.

- **Timing:** Timing involves scheduling of operations in a suitable order. Time schedules for beginning and completing the jobs must be fixed well in advance and efforts should be taken to complete them as per the schedule.
- **Integration:** Integration refer to the unification of all unrelated and diverse activities in such a manner as to accomplish the job efficiently.

Importance of Coordination (Fig. 7.13)

The importance of coordination is discussed below:
- **Growth of organization:** As time passes, organization grows in size, resulting in an increased volume of work. There will be numerous employees to handle the work, which are hired for different departments.
- **Locational differences:** Big corporations are located at different locations, even in different countries, which do not allow people to meet and communicate frequently.
- **Diversification of business:** When a company decides to diversify its business, by entering into new markets with a new product, the company starts new divisions or ventures, to undertake the activities.
- **Specialization:** In specialization, tasks are assigned to the employees as per their expertise or specialization in the specific field. Coordination helps in bringing together all the talented and experienced employees together, to maintain a harmonious relationship between various groups.
- **Synergy:** It is a universal fact that the combined effort of two people is always greater than those working separately.

Benefits of Coordination

The smooth functioning of the enterprise depends on effective coordination. Chester I Barnard even went to the extent of saying that Thus, coordination is considered as the essence of manager-ship because of the following benefits it offer:
1. Coordination ensures unity of direction through arranging spontaneous collaboration on the part of different departments.
2. It promotes the efficiency of the enterprise and employees.

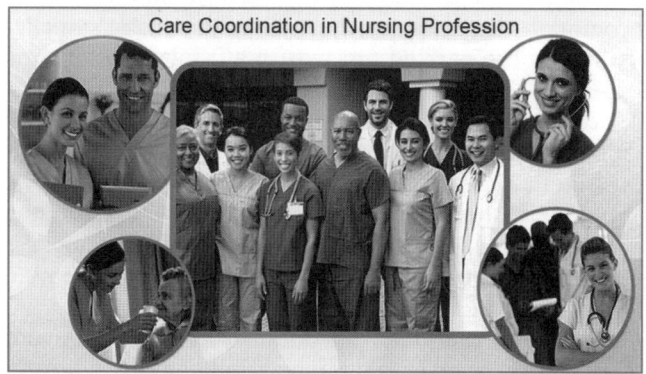

Fig. 7.12: Coordination in patient care.

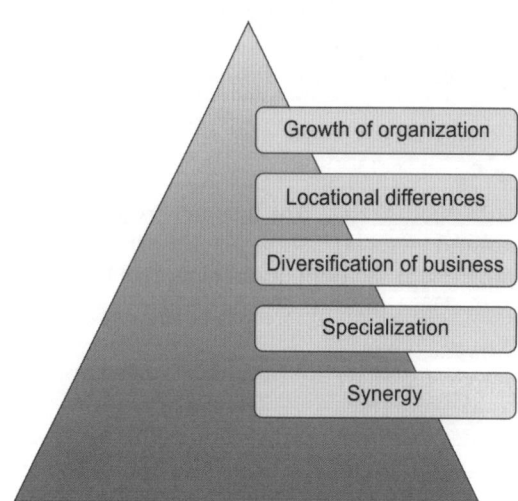

Fig. 7.13: Importance of coordination.

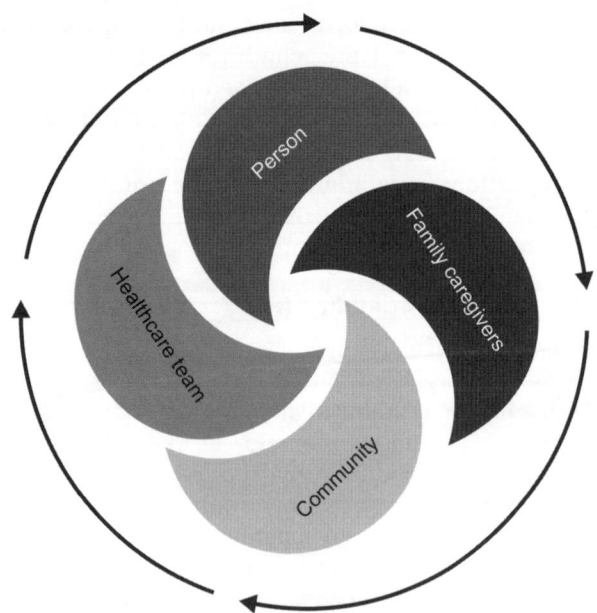

Fig. 7.14: Coordination in health care.

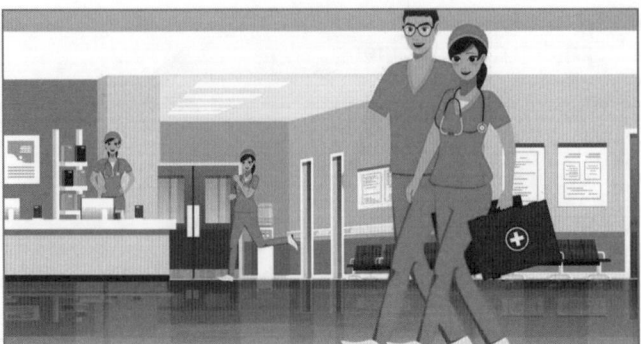

Fig. 7.15: Structure of hospital.

3. It increases employee morale and provides job satisfaction and avoids conflicts between employees.
4. It is a creative force, i.e., it creates something new out of the group which is always greater than isolated or individual efforts.
5. It develops team spirit and ensures a favorable environment for work.
6. It avoids interruptions on operations due to omission or wrong allocation of duties.
7. It eliminates inconsistencies in the objectives and policies.
Figure 7.14 shows coordination in health care.

HOSPITAL: TYPES, FUNCTIONS AND ORGANIZATION

The English word 'hospital' originates from the Latin word "HOSPILE" and also some viewed that it comes from the French word 'hospitale' as do the words 'hostel' and 'hotel'. The three words hospital, hostel, hotel, all are derived from same source, are used in different sense, but basically the meaning of the word will be same. For example, in hotel, hotel authorities take care of the clients, who wish to stay there and client will receive the hospitality according to their ability.

Definition

1. **According to WHO:** "The hospital is an integral part of a social and medical organizations, the function of which is to provide for the population complete healthcare, both 'curative' and 'preventive' and whose outpatient services reach out to the family and it's environment; the hospital is also a center for the training of health workers and biosocial research.
2. **According to Steadman's medical dictionary:** Hospital is an institution for the care, cure and treatment of the sick and wounded, for the study of diseases and for the training of doctors and nurses.

Objectives of the Hospital

As stated in the definition and philosophy of the hospital, its main objective is to:
1. Provide optimum health services to all people irrespective of race, color, caste, and creed and regardless of socio-economical status.
2. Provide care, cure, and preventive service to all people irrespective of race, color, caste, creed and economic and social status.
3. Protect the human rights of clients while taking care in its jurisdiction/in all areas of its services.
4. Provide training for professionals, i.e., doctors, nurses, pharmacists, dentists and others technical personnel who are involving in healthcare services.
5. Provide in-service/continuing education in all discipline professional/technical personnel involving healthcare. For updating their knowledge, skills, etc.
6. Participate/conduct research (and investigations in basic and applied biomedical, social and technological sciences) that will benefit patient care, improve the community health status, the management of hospital services and the education of individual who perform the required service.
7. Define its leadership role in the community and possibly the region depending upon its size, type and facilities in relation to regional area planning of hospital. **Figure 7.15** show structure of hospital.

Scope of Hospital

As stated in the objectives of the hospital, an optimum healthcare service have the basis of scientific method, and should be applied in a personalized manner with full recognition and attention to personal dimensions in client needs and are carried out within a framework of social responsibility. It should be available and accessible to everyone who needs it through his own community. The optimum health services consist of following elements.

- **Team approach:** The care of the needy person will be taken by the team of professional members (Doctors, Nurses, etc.) arid paraprofessionals, technicians under the leadership of medically qualified persons with integration and coordination.
- **Contents of service:** A spectrum of services that includes diagnosis, specific treatment, rehabilitation, education and prevention.

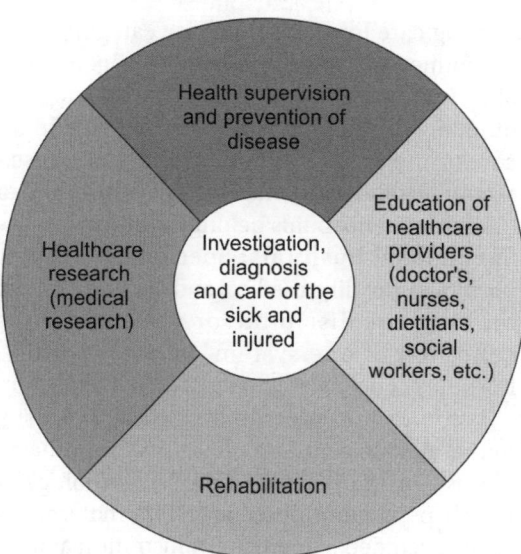

Fig. 7.16: Diagnosis and care of sick.

- **Coordination Clients' care** will cover the coordinate efforts of all agencies, which have the required facilities at all levels.
- **Continuity of care:** Continuity of client care will be available and rendered by the particular agency with specific services whenever needed.
- **Integration organization** of the hospital care of both ambulatory and non-ambulatory patients into a continuum with common integrated services.
- **Evaluation and research:** Periodic evaluation programs and provision of conducting research included in the optimum health services for adequacy in meeting needs of the patients and the community. **Figure 7.16** shows diagnosis and care of sick.

Functions of the Hospital

- **Patient care of the sick** and injured and restoration of the health of a diseased person without any discrimination.
- **Diagnosis and treatment of disease:** There are diagnosis and treatment services to in-patients. Within this broad function, there are many subdivisions of medical, surgical, obstetrical, gynec, pediatric, psychiatric and other forms of care and rehabilitation. Involved in the entire inpatient services are, various modalities, including nursing, dietics, pharmaceutical skills, laboratory and X-ray services and varying refinement of diagnosis and therapy.
- **Out-patient services:** There are services to out-patients with an equally wide range of specialties and technical modalities.
- **Medical education and training:** Hospital provides professional and technical education for many classes of health personnel. They must work in hospital to receive proper training of their choice, i.e., medical, nursing, pharmacy, dental, lab technicians, X-ray technicians, etc.
- **Medical and nursing research:** Since accumulation of different types of patients, the hospital provides the basis for scientific investigation into causes, diagnosis, treatment and nursing management of diseases, and hospital administration, ward/unit administration in hospitals.
- **Prevention of disease and promotion of health:** Hospital provides services to surrounding populations that may be preventive care and promoting their health. There are many ways that hospitals, as centers for technical skills, can offer services to people before they are sick or can protect patients from the hazards of disease beyond that for which they have come to the hospital.

Classifications of Hospitals (Box 7.8)

Hospitals have been classified in many ways. Each hospital is distinct in its characteristic as it differs in structure, functions, performance and the community it serves. However, we can classify the hospitals into different types depending upon different criteria. The most commonly accepted criteria for classification of the modern hospital are according to:

I. **Classification according to length of stay of patient:** A patient stays for a short-term in a hospital for treatment of disease that is acute in nature, such as pneumonia, peptic ulcer, gastroenteritis, etc. A patient may stay for a long-term in a hospital for treatment of diseases that are chronic in nature, such as tuberculosis, leprosy, cancer, psychosis. The hospital according to long-term and short-term also known as chronic-care hospital and acute care hospitals respectively. **Figure 7.17** shows types of acute care.

II. **Classification according to clinical bases:** These are hospitals licensed as general hospital; treat all kinds of diseases, but major focus on treating speed disease or conditions, such as heart disease, or cancer, or ophthalmic or maternity, etc.

III. **Classification according to ownership control:** On the basis of ownership or control, hospitals can be divided into four categories:
  1. **Public hospitals:** Public hospitals are those run by the central or state governments or local bodies on

---

Box 7.8: Classifications of hospital.

Basing on bed capacity (Size)
a. Small hospital (Up to 100 beds)
b. Medium hospital (More than 100 to less than 300 beds)
c. Large hospital (More than 300 beds)

Basing on type of care:
a. Primary care
b. Secondary care
c. Tertiary care

By teaching affiliation:
a. Teaching hospital
b. Non-teaching hospital

Basing on system of medicine:
a. Allopathic hospital
b. Ayurvedic hospital
c. Homeopathic hospital
d. Unani hospital
e. Hospitals of other system of medicine

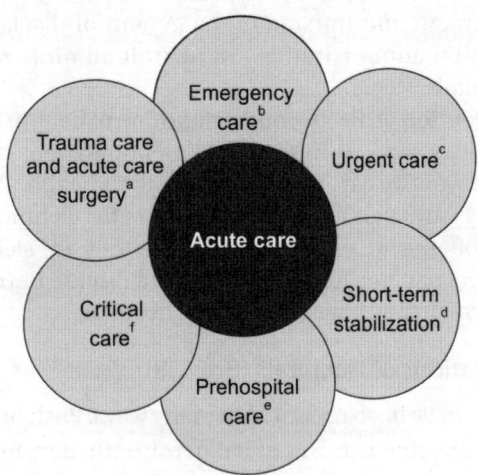

Fig. 7.17: Types of acute care.

noncommercial lines. These may be general hospital or specialized hospitals or both.

2. **Voluntary hospitals:** Voluntary hospitals are those which are established and incorporated under the Societies Registration Act 1860; or Public Trust Act 1882 or any other appropriate act of central or state governments. They are run with public or private funds on a non-commercial basis.
3. **Private nursing hospitals/Nursing homes:** Private nursing hospitals/nursing homes are generally owned by an individual doctor or a group of doctors. They run the hospital or nursing home on a commercial basis. They accept patient suffering from infirmity, advanced age, illness, injury, chronic, disability, etc. But, do not admit patient suffering from communicable disease, alcoholism, drug addiction or mental illness. Usually, they prefer patient from wealthy families.
4. **Corporate hospitals:** Corporate hospitals are, which are public limited companies formed under the companies Act. They are normally run on commercial lines. They can be either general or specialized or both (e.g., Hinduja hospital, Mallya hospital, Apollo Group of Hospitals).

IV. **Classification according to the objectives:** According to the objectives, hospitals can be classified into four categories.
  1. **Teaching-cum-research hospital:** Teaching/cum/research hospital is a hospital to which a college is attached for medical/Nursing/dental/pharmacy education. The main objective of these hospitals is teaching based on research and the provision of healthcare is secondary, e.g., AIIMS, New Delhi, PGIMER, Chandigarh, JIPMER, Puducherry, KR Hospital, Mysuru, Victoria hospital, Bengaluru belong to this type.
  2. **General hospitals:** General hospitals are those which provide treatment for common diseases and conditions. All establishments permanently staffed by at least two or more doctors, who can offer inpatient accommodation and provide active medical and nursing care for more than one category of medical discipline, such as general medicine, general surgery, obstetrics and gynecology, pediatrics, etc. The main objective of these hospitals is to provide medical care to the people. While teaching and research is secondary and incidental, e.g., all district and taluk or PHC or rural hospitals belong to this type.
  3. **Specialized hospitals:** Specialized hospitals are hospitals providing medical and nursing care primarily for only one discipline or a specific disease or condition of one system. In other words, these hospitals concentrate on a particular aspect or organ of the body and provide medical and nursing care in that field, e.g., tuberculosis, ENT, ophthalmology, leprosy, orthopedics, pediatrics, cardiology, mental health/psychiatric, oncology, STDs, maternal, etc. The specialized department, administration attached to a general hospital will not be considered as specialized hospital.
      – **Isolation hospitals:** Isolation hospital is a hospital in which the persons are suffering from infections/communicable diseases requiring isolation of the patients, e.g., Epidemic Diseases Hospital, Bengaluru.

V. **Classification according to size:** On the basis of health committee report, it is recommended that the following pattern of development of hospitals to be adopted according to size, i.e., bed strength.
  1. Teaching hospital 500 (bed to be increased according to the number of students).
  2. District hospital 200 (may be raised up to 300 beds depending upon population).
  3. Taluk hospital 50 (may be raised depending upon population to be served).
  4. Primary health centers 6 (may be increased up to 10 depending upon needs).

VI. **Classification according to management:**
  1. Union Government/Government of India all hospitals administered by the Government of India, e.g., hospital run by the railways, military/defense, or public sector undertakings of the Central Government.
  2. State Governments all hospitals administered by the state/union territory. Government authorities and public sector undertaking operated by the state/union territories, including the police, prison, irrigation department, etc.
  3. Local bodies all hospitals administered by local bodies, i.e., municipal corporation, municipality, zila parishad, panchayat, e.g., corporation maternity homes.
  4. Autonomous bodies, all hospitals established under special act of parliament or state legislation and founded by the central/state government/union territory, e.g., AIIMS, New Delhi, PGIMER, Chandigarh, NIMHANS, Bengaluru, KMIO, Bengaluru.
  5. Private all private hospitals owned by an individual or by a private organization, e.g., MAHE, Manipal, Manipal Hospital, Bengaluru, Hinduja hospital, Mumbai.

6. Voluntary agencies, all hospitals operated by a voluntary body/a trust/charitable society registered or recognized by the appropriate authority under central/state government laws. This includes hospitals run by missionary bodies and cooperatives.

VII. **Classification according to system:** According to the system of medicine, we can classify the hospital as follows:
1. Allopathic hospitals
2. Ayurvedic hospitals
3. Homeopathic hospitals
4. Unani hospitals
5. Hospitals of other systems of medicine

ORGANIZATIONAL DEVELOPMENT

Organization development (OD) as a practice involves an ongoing, systematic process of implementing effective organizational change. OD is both a field of applied science focused on understanding and managing organizational change and a field of scientific study and inquiry. It is interdisciplinary in nature and draws on sociology, psychology, particularly industrial and organizational psychology, and theories of motivation, learning, and personality **(Figs. 7.18 and 7.19)**.

Definition

Organizational development is a critical and science-based process that helps organizations builds their capacity to change and achieve greater effectiveness by developing, improving, and reinforcing strategies, structures, and processes.

Objectives of OD

1. To increase the level of interpersonal trust among employees
2. To increase employees' level of satisfaction and commitment

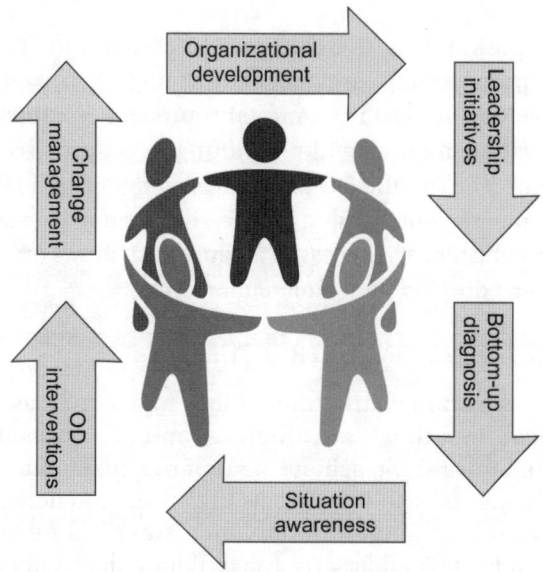

Fig. 7.18: Organization development.

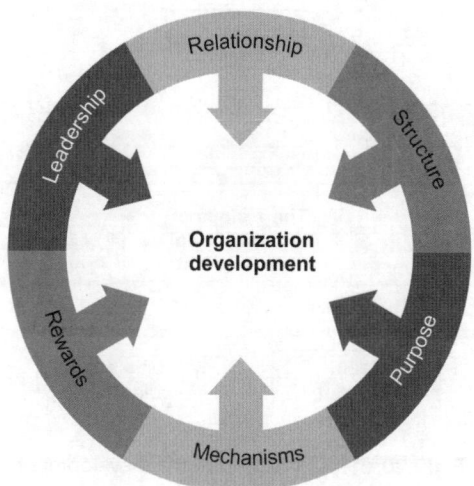

Fig. 7.19: Organization development strategies.

3. To confront problems instead of neglecting them
4. To effectively manage conflict
5. To increase cooperation and collaboration among employees
6. To increase organizational problem-solving
7. To put in place processes that will help improve the ongoing operation of an organization on a continuous basis

Goal of Organizational Development

1. The ultimate goal of organizational development is to increase the organization's competitiveness in order to create a business that wins in the marketplace.
2. This can be done through increasing profits, margins, market share, morale, cultural values, or other sources of competitive advantage.

Organization Development Interventions

There are many possible intervention strategies from which to choose. Several assumptions about the nature and functioning of organizations are made in the choice of a particular strategy. Beckhard lists six, such assumptions:

1. The basic building blocks of an organization are groups (teams). Therefore, the basic units of change are groups, not individuals.
2. An always relevant change goal is the reduction of inappropriate competition between parts of the organization and the development of a more collaborative condition.
3. Decision making in a healthy organization is located where the information sources are, rather than in a particular role or level of hierarchy.
4. Organizations, subunits of organizations, and individuals continuously manage their affairs against goals. Controls are interim measurements, not the basis of managerial strategy.
5. One goal of a healthy organization is to develop generally open communication, mutual trust, and confidence between and across levels.

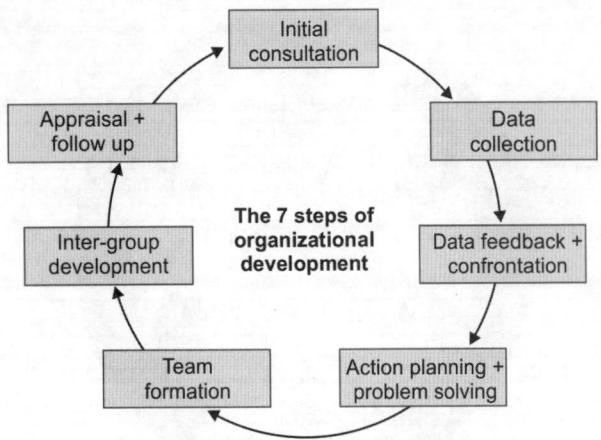

Fig. 7.20: Steps of organizational development.

6. People support what they help create. People affected by a change must be allowed active participation and a sense of ownership in the planning and conduct of the change. **Figure 7.20** shows steps of organizational development.

Characteristics of Organizational Development

- Organizational development is an educational strategy for bringing a planned change.
- It is related to real problems of the organization.
- Laboratory training methods based on experienced behavior are primarily used to bring change.
- OD uses change agent (or consultant) to guide and affect the change. The role of change agent is to guide groups towards more effective group processes rather than telling them what to do.
- There is a close working relationship between change agents and the people who are being changed.
- OD seeks to build problem-solving capacity by improving group dynamics and problem confrontation.
- OD reaches into all aspects of the organization culture in order to make it more humanly responsive.
- OD is a long-term approach (of 3 to 5 years period) and is meant to elevate the organization to a higher level of functioning by improving the performance and satisfaction of organization members.
- OD is broad-based and describes a variety of change programs. It is concerned not only with changes in organizational design but also with changes in organizational philosophies, skills of individuals and groups.
- OD is a dynamic process. It recognizes that the goals of the organization change and hence the methods of attaining them should also change.
- OD utilizes systems thinking. It is based on open, adaptive systems concept. The organization is treated as an interrelated whole and no part of the organization can be changed without affecting other parts.
- OD is research based. Change agents conduct surveys, collect data, evaluate and then decisions are taken.
- OD uses group processes rather than individual process. It makes efforts to improve group performance.
- OD is situational and contingency oriented.

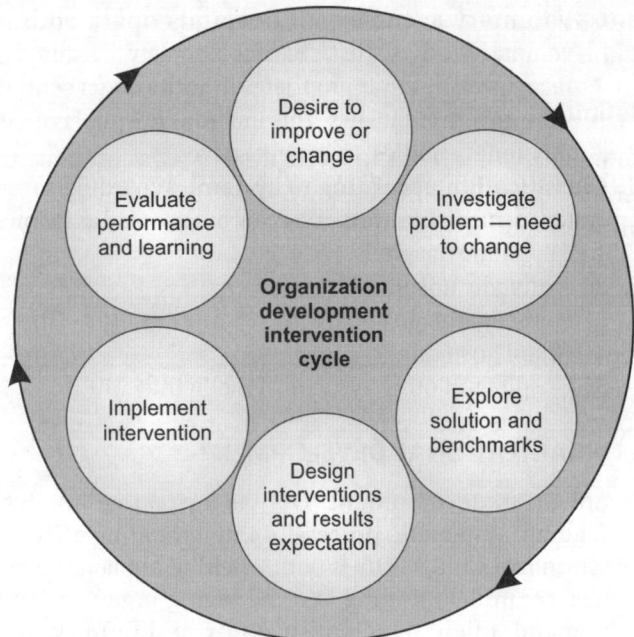

Fig. 7.21: Organizational development intervention cycle.

- Organization development and management development are complementary rather than conflicting.

Steps in organizational development (OD): Lawrence and Lorsch have provided the following steps in organizational development:

- **Problem identification-diagnosis:** OD program starts with the identification of the problem in the organization. Correct diagnosis of the problem will provide its causes and determine the future action needed.
- **Planning strategy for change:** OD consultant attempts to transform diagnosis of the problem into a proper action plan involving the overall goals for change, determination of basic approach for attaining these goals and the sequence of detailed scheme for implementing the approach.
- **Implementing the change:** OD consultants play an important role in implementing change.
- **Evaluation:** OD is a long-term process. So, there is a great need for careful monitoring to get process feedback whether the OD program is going on well after its implementation or not. This will help in making suitable modifications, if necessary. **Figure 7.21** shows organizational development intervention cycle.

ORGANIZATIONAL STRUCTURE

An organizational structure defines how activities, such as task allocation, coordination, and supervision are directed toward the achievement of organizational aims. Organizational structure affects organizational action and provides the foundation on which standard operating procedures and routines rest. It determines which individuals get to participate in which decision-making processes, and thus to what extent their views shape the organization's actions.

Definition

An organizational structure is a system that outlines how certain activities are directed in order to achieve the goals of an organization. These activities can include rules, roles, and responsibilities. The organizational structure also determines how information flows between levels within the company.

Types of Organizational Structures

Four types of common organizational structures are implemented in the real world.

Functional Structure (Fig. 7.22)

- The first and most common is a functional structure. This is also referred to as a bureaucratic organizational structure and breaks up a company based on the specialization of its workforce.
- Most small-to-medium-sized businesses implement a functional structure.
- Dividing the firm into departments consisting of marketing, sales, and operations is the act of using a bureaucratic organizational structure.

Divisional or Multidivisional Structure

- The second type is common among large companies with many business units.
- Called the divisional or multidivisional structure, a company that uses this method structures its leadership team based on the products, projects, or subsidiaries they operate.
- A good example of this structure is Johnson and Johnson. With thousands of products and lines of business, the company structures itself so each business unit operates as its own company with its own president.

Flatarchy Structure

- Flatarchy, a newer structure, is the third type and is used among many startups. As the name alludes, it flattens the hierarchy and chain of command and gives its employees a lot of autonomy.
- Companies that use this type of structure have a high speed of implementation.

Matrix Structure

- The fourth and final organizational structure is a matrix structure. It is also the most confusing and the least used.
- These structure matrixes employees across different superiors, divisions, or departments.
- An employee working for a matrixed company, for example, may have duties in both sales and customer service.

I. Formal Organization

A formal organization is one in which position, responsibility, authority and accountability at each level is clearly defined. In such an organization, authority is delegated from higher to lower levels, and the whole stricture is designed to accomplish the objectives of the organization. A formal organization is bound by rules, systems, procedures and methods as laid down by the top management from time to time **(Fig. 7.23)**.

Components of organization: According to George R Terry, there are four basic components of a formal organization.
1. The work-which is divisionalized
2. Persons-who are assigned to and perform the divisionalized jobs
3. The environment-under which the work is done; and
4. The relationships-among persons or work units.

A formal organization is systematically planned and is based on the principle of the delegation of authority and the principle of responsibility. It makes use of organization charts and attempts to maintain a balance among the various types of work to be done, each being given the importance that its true value deserves.

The advantages of formal organization include:
- Avoidance of role conflict
- Avoidance of overlapping of authority and responsibility
- Advantages of specialization

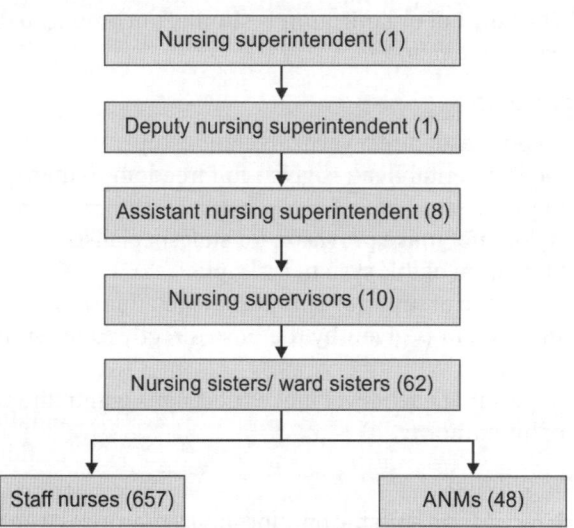

Fig. 7.22: Functional structure.

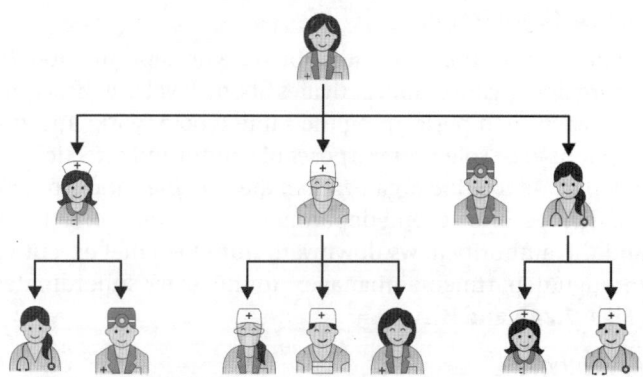

Fig. 7.23: Formal organization.

- Defining and standardizing systems, rules, policies and procedures of an enterprise, etc.

Limitations
- It does not recognize informal relationships.
- It creates problem of communication.
- It emphasizes structure rather than people.

II. Informal Organization

An informal organization always exists together with a formal organization in every enterprise. In an organization, people evolve informal groups among themselves which are bound together by common social, technological work or other interests. Such groups make up an informal organization. It is an accepted fact that wherever people work together, social relationships and groupings are bound to arise on account of their frequent contact with one another which give rise to informal organizations. Such organizations are not needed by formal organizations, and therefore, they find no place in organization charts or manuals. They establish their own unwritten rules, which are usually followed by individuals in the formal organization; but they form an integral part of formal organizations.

Advantages

The advantages of informal organizations are:
- It provides a useful channel of communication.
- It covers the deficiencies of the formal organization.
- It influences the formal organization to work carefully and
- It brings mutuality among group members who derive job satisfaction by an exchange of ideas and views, etc.

Limitations
- It may tend to act on the basis of mob psychology.
- It may be a source of rumors of wastage of time.
- It may tend to oppose change.

The informal organization is a reality in every enterprise, and every manager should accept this fact. He should utilize it as a part of the total organization, as an effective channel of communication; as a forum for the exchange of idea; and as an instrument for obtaining support from the informal group. As a matter of fact, informal organizations are complementary to formal organizations and are in no way less important.

III. Line Organization

A line organization may either be pure or departmental. In a pure line organization, activities at one level are the same, with each man performing the same type o work; and the divisions exist solely for purposes of control and direction. In a departmental line organization, the activities and workers are divided into several departments on a functional basis and the authority flows downward from the chief executive through departmental managers to the lower subordinates **(Figs. 7.24A and B)**.

Advantages

The advantages of a line organization are:

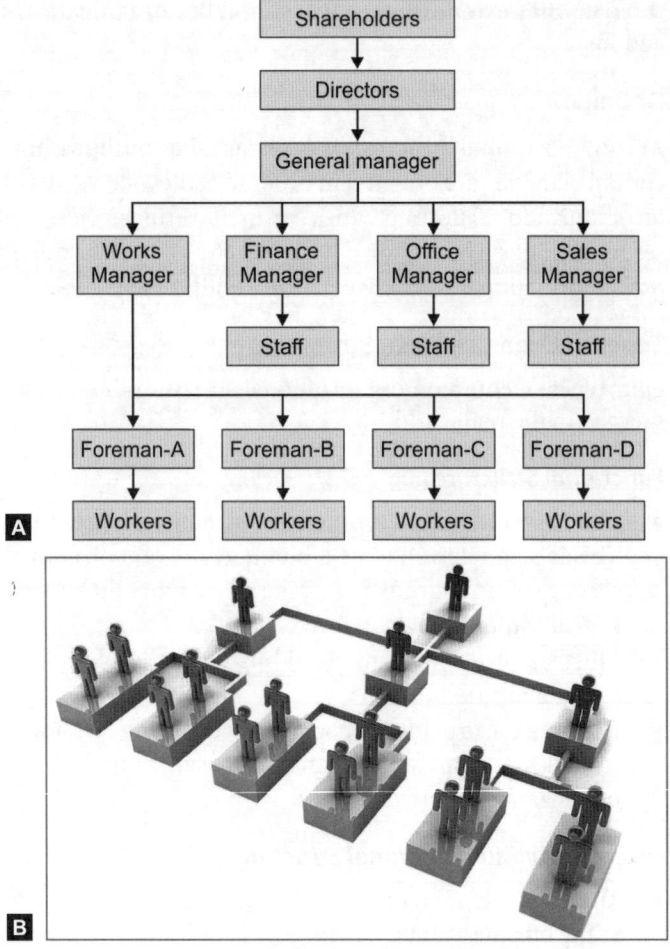

Figs. 7.24A and B: Line of organizations.

- It follows the principle of the chain of command and single accountability.
- Authority and responsibility are clearly stated and identified.
- Effective control can be exercised over supervisors.
- Discipline is no problem.
- It ensures flexibility and quick action.
- This form of organization is simple, uncomplicated and easily understood.

Characteristics
- It consists of direct vertical relationships.
- Departmental head is given full freedom to manage his department.
- It does not make provision for staff specialists.
- Operation of this system is simple.
- Existence of superior-subordinate relationship.
- Instruction is given by the boss directly to his subordinates.
- Superior at each level makes decisions within the scope of his authority.

Disadvantages
- It is rigid and suitable only for small enterprises where the number of employees is small.

- The entire organization becomes dependent on a few line supervisors or executives. Their absence may be fatal to the organization.
- The services of functional specialists are not utilized. Specialization is difficult to practice.
- It is sometimes characterized by an absence of team work, working together towards a common end.
- In such an organization, managerial planning, research and development activities may be neglected because of greater reliance on line authority.

IV. Functional Organization

Functional organization is an organizational structure which combines all aspects of one activity or several related activities which are called "Functions", such as production, finance, marketing, HRD, etc. It is structured according to products dealt or service rendered in the organization. It is the most logical and basic form of departmentation. Functional organization leads to specialize in business skills. It also makes it easier to mobilize specialized skills to needy areas of the business **(Fig. 7.25)**.

Advantages

- **Specialization:** It ensures maximum use of the principle of specialization at every work point.
- **Efficiency:** Since, the workers have to perform a limited number of functions, their efficiency would be very high.
- **Mass production:** Due to specialization and standardization, large-scale production can be undertaken without much inconvenience.
- **Cooperation:** As there is no scope for one-man control in the organization, there is the possibility of promoting cooperation.
- **Relief to the executives:** Since instructions from specialists flow directly to the lower levels, the line executives are free from worries about the technical problems faced by the workers.
- **Flexibility:** Any change in the organization can be introduced without disturbing the whole organization and hence there is an element of flexibility in this type of organization.

Disadvantages

- **Conflict amongst foremen:** Under this type, foreman of equal rank will be many in number and this may lead to conflict among them.
- **Discipline:** Since workers have to work under different bosses, it is difficult to maintain discipline among them.
- **Lack of coordination:** There are several functional experts in the organization and this may create the problem of coordination.
- **Speed of action:** As control is divided among the various specialists, the speed of action is very much hampered.
- **Lack of fixed responsibility:** If there is any unsatisfactory progress, it is difficult for the top management to fix responsibility.
- **Expensive:** As a large number of specialists to be appointed under this system, it is very expensive and small firms cannot afford it.

V. Matrix Structure

The matrix structure groups employees by both function and product simultaneously. A matrix organization frequently uses teams of employees to accomplish work, in order to take advantage of the strengths, as well as make up for the weaknesses, of functional and decentralized forms. An example would be a company that produces two products, "product a" and "product b". Using the matrix structure, this company would organize functions within the company as follows: "product a" sales department, "product a" customer service department, "product a" accounting, "product b" sales department, "product b" customer service department, "product b" accounting department **(Fig. 7.26)**.

Weak/functional matrix:

- A project manager with only limited authority is assigned to oversee the cross-functional aspects of the project.
- The functional managers maintain control over their resources and project areas.

Balanced/functional matrix:

- A project manager is assigned to oversee the project. Power is shared equally between the project manager and the functional managers.

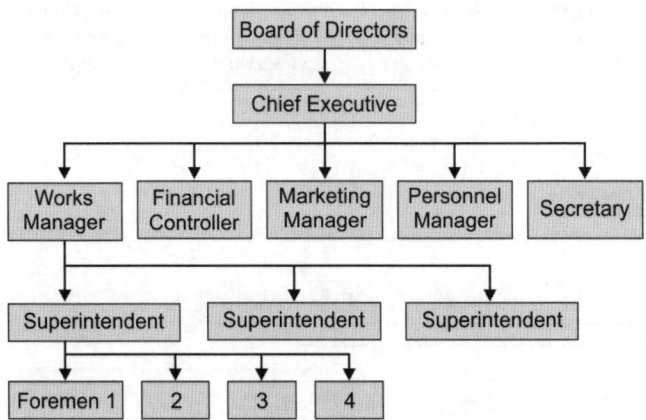

Fig. 7.25: Functional organization.

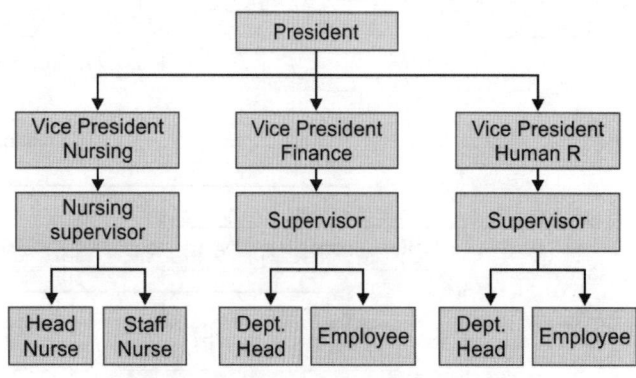

Fig. 7.26: Matrix organizational structure.

- It brings the best aspects of functional and projectized organizations. However, this is the most difficult system to maintain as the sharing of power is a delicate proposition.

Strong/project matrix: A project manager is primarily responsible for the project. Functional managers provide technical expertise and assign resources as needed.

ORGANIZATIONAL CHARTS

An organizational chart is the visual representation of this vertical structure. It is therefore very important for an organization to take utmost care while creating the organizational structure. The structure should clearly determine the reporting relationships and the flow of authority as this will support good communication-resulting in efficient and effective work process flow.

The definition of an organization chart or "org chart" is a diagram that displays a reporting or relationship hierarchy. The most frequent application of an org chart is to show the structure of a business, government, or other organization.

Definition: An organization chart is a graphic portrayal of the various positions in the organization and the formal relationships among them. It serves as a blue print. **Figure 7.27** shows organization chart in nursing and **Figure 7.28** shows flat organizational design.

Types of Organization Charts

There are many. But all the organization charts are classified into two broad categories.

1. **Vertical charts:** This is called top to down chart, lowest position is shown at the bottom. It is most widely used.
2. **Horizontal charts:** This is called left to right chart, highest position is placed at extreme right and the lowest is at the extreme left.

Advantages or Uses of Organization Chart

- It shows clearly the various positions and how they relate to one another.
- It shows at a glance the lines of authority and responsibility.
- It provides a basis of planning organizational change.
- It provides guidance to outsiders to whom they should contact.
- It serves as a valuable guide to the new personnel.
- It helps to point out inconsistencies and deficiencies.
- It provides a framework for classification and evaluation of personnel.
- It provides clues to the lines of promotion.
- It also facilitates communication.

Principles of Organization Charts

- Should have a clear title.
- Should clearly show the lines of authority.
- Positions of equal ranks must be shown at the same level.
- Solid lines must be used to indicate the line of authority.
- Staff relationships by dotted lines.
- Complete chart should be on a single sheet.
- Colors may be used to indicate different departments.

Limitations

- Fails to recognize informal relationships.
- Does not represent flexibility.

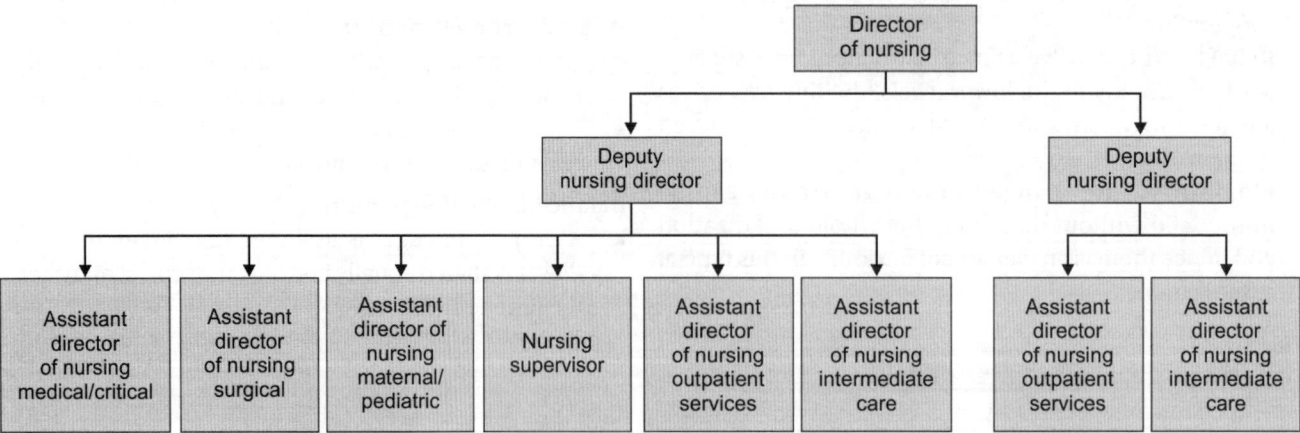

Fig. 7.27: Organization chart in nursing.

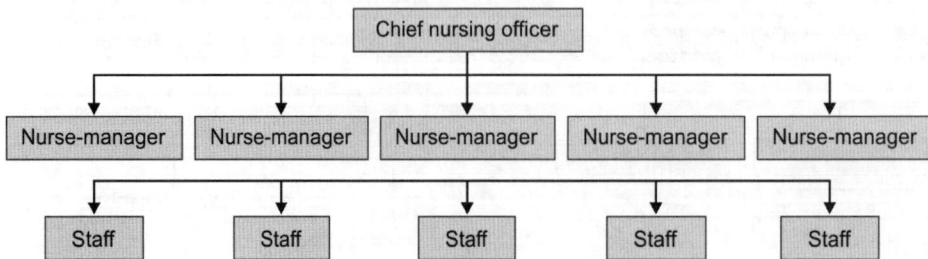

Fig. 7.28: Flat organizational design.

- It introduces bureaucratic rigidity in the formal relationships.
- Shows the relationships which is supposed to exist rather than what actually exist.
- Fail to show how much authority and responsibility an individual can exercise due to over simplification.
- Poorly designed charts cause confusion and misunderstanding.
- They may create superiority and inferiority feelings and lead to conflicts in the organization.

Uses of Organization Chart

Organizational charts are useful in a number of ways. Here are a few of the ways the company or group can benefit from an org chart.
- Show work responsibilities and reporting relationships.
- Allow leadership to more effectively manage growth or change.
- Allow employees to better understand how their work fits into the organization's overall scheme.
- Improve lines of communication.
- Create a visual employee directory.
- Present other types of information, such as business entity structures and data hierarchies.

ORGANIZATIONAL EFFECTIVENESS

Organizational effectiveness can be defined as the efficiency with which an association is able to meet its objectives. This means an organization that produces a desired effect or an organization that is productive without waste **(Fig. 7.29)**.
- Organizational effectiveness can be defined as the efficiency with which an association is able to meet its objectives. This means an organization that produces a desired effect or an organization that is productive without waste.
- Organizational effectiveness is about each individual doing everything they know how to do and doing it well; in other words, organizational efficiency is the capacity of an organization to produce the desired results with a minimum expenditure of energy, time, money, and human and material resources.
- The desired effect will depend on the goals of the organization, which could be, for example, making a profit by producing and selling a product.
- An organization, if it operates efficiently, will produce a product without waste.
- If the organization has both organizational effectiveness and efficiency, it will achieve its goal of making a profit by producing and selling a product without waste.
- In economics and the business world, this may be referred to as maximizing profits.

Definition

Organizational effectiveness is defined as a concept to measure the efficiency of an organization in meeting its objectives with the help of given resources without putting undue strain on its employees. It is about how the company can produce the target quota of products, how efficient its process is, and how much waste is produced.

Systems of Organizational Effectiveness (Fig. 7.30)

The Six Systems are broader in scope than functional departments and must be understood independently and interdependently as part of an integrated whole. These Six Systems set up the conditions and components necessary to create a healthy, high-performing organization.

1. **Leadership:** To achieve high performance or sustain results, leaders must define and refine key processes and execute them with daily discipline. They must translate vision and values into strategy and objectives, processes and practices, actions and accountabilities, execution and performance.
2. **Communication:** Everything happens in or because of a conversation, and every exchange is a potential moment of truth—a point of failure or critical link in the success

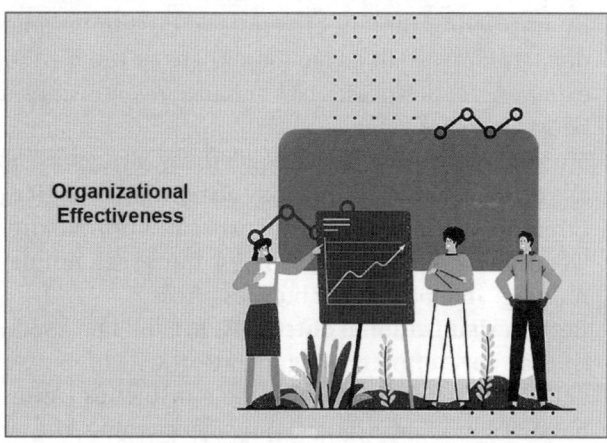

Fig. 7.29: Organizational effectiveness.

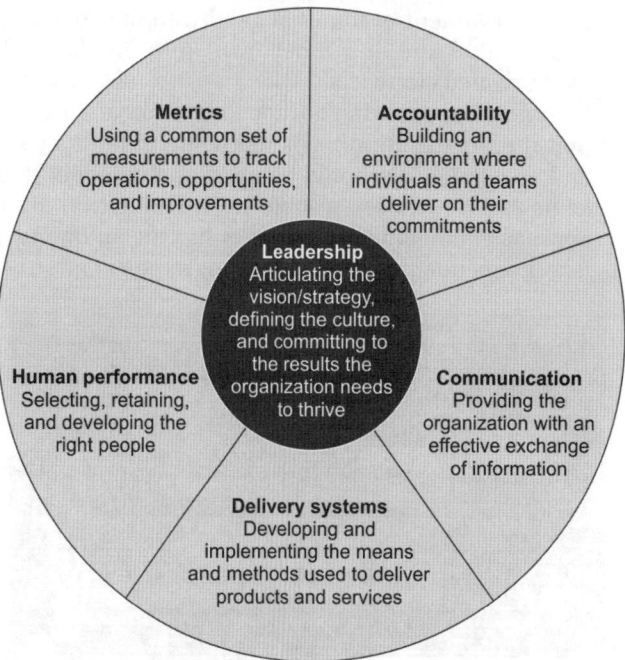

Fig. 7.30: Systems of organizational effectiveness.

chain. Strategic communication ensures that the impact of the message is consistent with your intentions, and results in understanding.
3. **Accountability:** Leaders translate vision and strategic direction into goals and objectives, actions and accountabilities. Performance accountability systems clarify what is expected of people and align consequences or rewards with actual performance.
4. **Delivery:** The best organizations develop simple processes that are internally efficient, locally responsive, and globally adaptable. Complexity is removed from the customer experience to enable them to engage you in ways that are both elegant and satisfying. Establishing and optimizing operational performance is an ongoing journey.
5. **Performance:** The human performance system is designed to attract, develop, and retain the most talented people. The idea is to hire the best people and help them develop their skills, talents, and knowledge over time.
6. **Measurement:** A system of metrics, reviews, and course corrections keeps the business on track. Organizations need concrete measures that facilitate quality control, consistent behaviors, and predictable productivity and results.

Approaches to Organizational Efficiencies (Fig. 7.31)

- **Goal approach:** The goal approach refers to optimal profit by offering the best service that will lead to high productivity. The limitation of the goal approach is that it is a bit difficult to identify the real goal and not the ideal goal
- **System-resource approach:** The system resource approach puts its onus on the interdependency of processes that align the organization with its environment. It takes the form of input-output transactions and includes human, economic and physical resources. The limitation of this approach is that acquisition of resources from the environment becomes aligned with the goal of the organization and thus it becomes quite similar to the goal-oriented approach.
- **Functional approach:** The functional approach assumes that the organization has already identified its goals, and now the focus should be upon attainment of these goals and how to serve society. The limitation of this approach is that the organization has the autonomy to take independent action for attaining its goals and so why

will it accept serving society as its ultimate goal. Effective organizations demonstrate strength in five key areas are shown in **Figure 7.32**.

Factors Affecting Organizational Effectiveness

- **Casual variables:** These are independent variables that can be altered by the organization and its management, for instance, its policies, skills and behavior and leadership and business strategies. The casual variables can determine the course of development within an organization.
- **Intervening variables:** These are motivation, performance goals, attitude, loyalty and perception of the employees and their capacity for efficient decision-making, communication, and interaction. The intervening variables show the health of an organization.
- **End-result variables:** These are loss, costs, earnings, and productivity. The end-result variables reflect the achievements of an organization.

Importance of Organizational Effectiveness

Ultimately, factors, such as the above have significant impacts on many business functions.

Benefits of Organizational Effectiveness

The benefits of effectiveness in an organization can include improved:

- **Employee engagement and performance:** Employee productivity is directly tied to the outcomes and performance of individual business units. This, in turn, affects the organization's performance.
- **Better management:** Improved management can mean better manager training, increased communication between managers and frontline employees, updated managerial policies and procedures, among other things.
- **Decreased costs:** Efficiency in any business unit can decrease costs. Those savings can come from any area that is causing waste–outdated processes, obsolete technology, ineffective workflows, and so forth.
- **Improved customer engagement and value:** A main goal of any business is to maximize customer value. By improving the effectiveness of customer-related departments, such as customer care or the customer experience—businesses can enhance relationships and boost customer value.
- **More efficient use of technology:** Today, all organizations use digital technology. But they do not always use it well. Effective digital adoption efforts can improve digital workflows, data insights, business processes, employee training, and many other business areas.
- **Better organizational outcomes:** It should be apparent that a more effective organization will be better at achieving its goals and strategic priorities. And the better it can achieve its goals and meet its aims, the more profitable it will be.

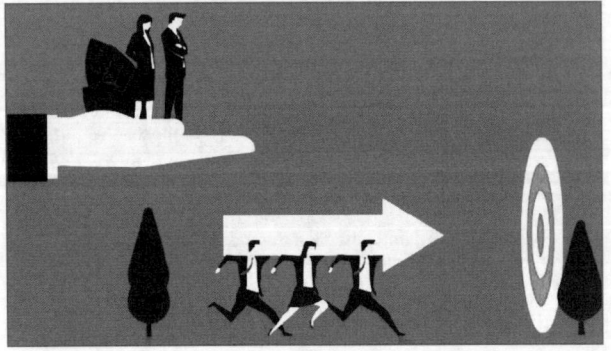

Fig. 7.31: Approaches to organizational efficiencies.

Chapter 7: Organizing

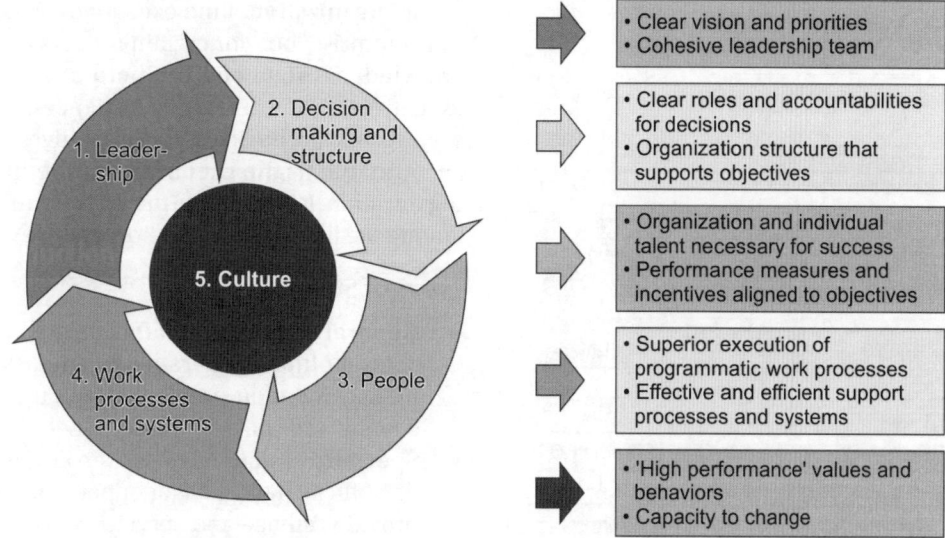

Fig. 7.32: Exhibit 1: Effective organizations demonstrate strength in five key areas.

HOSPITAL ADMINISTRATION CONTROL AND LINE OF AUTHORITY

Hospital administration is the management of the hospital as a business. The administration is made up of medical and health services managers—sometimes called healthcare executives and healthcare administrators—and their assistants. Hospital administrators are responsible for organizing and overseeing the health services and daily activities of a hospital or healthcare facility. They manage staff and budgets, communicate between departments and ensure adequate patient care amongst other duties (**Box 7.9**).

Responsibilities of a Hospital CEO

Some of the responsibilities for a hospital CEOs may include:
- Creating a positive and productive work culture through leadership
- Setting the standards for excellence in operations
- Hiring and ensuring qualified staff
- Maintaining high quality in the delivery of patient care
- Implement clinical policies and procedures
- Administer compliance with hospital policies (State and Federal rules and regulations)
- Developing relationships with the medical community, referring physicians, and the media
- Ensure fiscal performance

Box 7.9: Line of authority.

- It is a hierarchical form of authority.
- Manager to direct the work of an employee.
- It is the employer-employee authority relationship that extends from top to bottom.
- Line manager directs the work of employees and makes certain decisions without consulting anyone.
- It is small level enterprise.
- Top management has complete control.
- An example of a line manager is a marketing executive.

Hospital Administrator Responsibilities

- Serve as a liaison among governing boards, medical staff and department managers.
- Organize, control and coordinate services as per the hospital board regulations.
- Perform all duties within HIPAA regulations.
- Oversee the development and implementation of programs and policies for patient services, quality assurance, public relations and department activities.
- Evaluate personnel and prepare daily reports.
- Assist with recruitment, consenting, screening and enrolment of personnel.
- Practice financial acumen in managing budgets.
- Authorize admissions/treatment as per agreed protocols.
- Ensure that stock levels are adequate and orders are made on time.
- Communicate medical results to patients under clinical supervision.
- Sterilize instruments in accordance with OSHA requirements.
- Complete timely and accurate documentation of patient visits.

CONCEPTS OF LINE OF ORGANIZATION

A line of organization may either be pure or departmental. In a pure line organization, activities at one level are the same, with each man performing the same type o work; and the divisions exist solely for purposes of control and direction. In a departmental line organization, the activities and workers are divided into several departments on a functional basis and the authority flows downward from the chief executive through departmental managers to the lower subordinates (**Fig. 7.33**).

Advantages

- It follows the principle of the chain of command and single accountability.

Chapter 7: Organizing

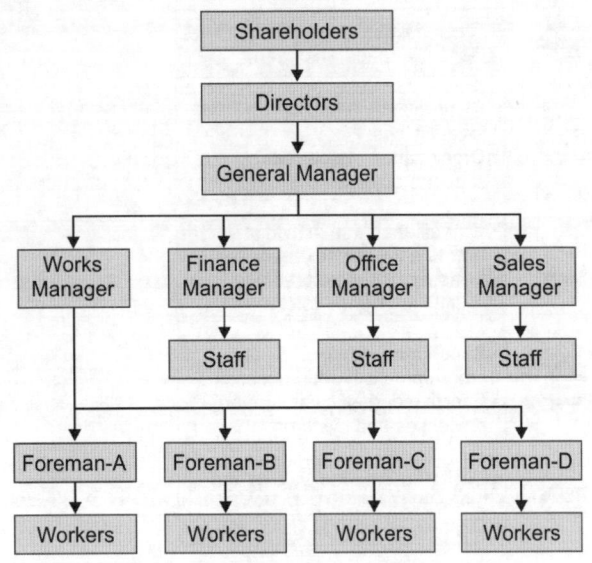

Fig. 7.33: Concepts of organization.

- Authority and responsibility are clearly stated and identified.
- Effective control can be exercised over supervisors.
- Discipline is no problem.
- It ensures flexibility and quick action.
- This form of organization is simple, uncomplicated and easily understood.

Characteristics

- It consists of direct vertical relationships.
- Departmental head is given full freedom to manage his department.
- It does not make provision for staff specialists.
- Operation of this system is simple.
- Existence of superior-subordinate relationship.
- Instruction is given by the boss directly to his subordinates.
- Superior at each level makes decisions within the scope of his authority.

Disadvantages

- It is rigid and suitable only for small enterprises where the number of employees is small.
- The entire organization becomes dependent on a few line supervisors or executives. Their absence may be fatal to the organization.
- The services of functional specialists are not utilized. Specialization is difficult to practice.
- It is sometimes characterized by an absence of team work, working together towards a common end.
- In such an organization, managerial planning, research and development activities may be neglected because of greater reliance on line authority.

LINE AND STAFF ORGANIZATION

In a line and staff organization, the line executives or supervisors assume the power of command and direction in the enterprise, while staff managers merely serve in an advisory capacity and do not play a directive or executive role in the organization. Line executive's acts independently in the enterprise; but, for certain matters requiring specialized knowledge, they need the help of staff executives. Line executives under certain circumstances, act on their own and even against the advice of staff executives, for they are directly accountable to the executives at the higher levels in the organization. It is desirable to have a harmonious relationship among the line and staff authorities.

Types of Staff

- **General staff:** Such staff is located at the head office/central office/corporate office to assist and advise top management on problems faced by the organization in general and shared by different departments.
- **Specialized staff:** It refers to an arrangement where each line official has a advisor or personal assistant. Such staff provides advice and service to the line executives with whom they are attached.

Advantages of Line and Staff Organization

- It enables an enterprise to secure the full benefits of the specialized knowledge of its staff.
- It permits line personnel to concentrate on the basic activities of the business because the necessary advice and services are provided by the staff. It thus improves efficiency and performance.
- The principles of the unit of command and unit of direction are followed, for line executives exercise full authority over their staff.
- It facilitates executive training and management development. **Figure 7.34** shows staff line hierarchy.

Disadvantages

The disadvantages of a line and staff organization are:

- It often creates confusion between line and staff executives.

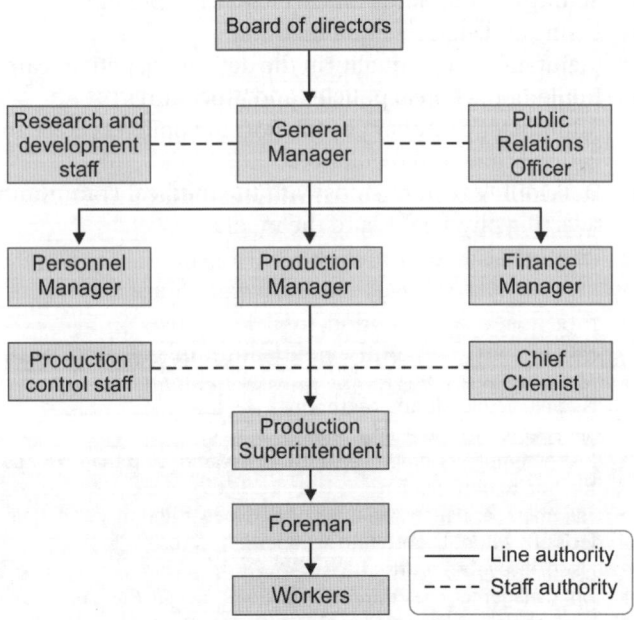

Fig. 7.34: Staff line hierarchy.

- If staff undermines line authority, or if line ignores staff's advice, a conflict may arise and the job of the chief executive may become complicated. A lot of his time may be wasted in the resolution of line and staff conflicts.
- Staff authority, because it is not responsible to a higher authority, may act recklessly.
- Line authority may, by not implementing the advice of the staff, make the Staff absolutely ineffective.
- The line department may not admit, and probably may not realize that, without staff help; it would do a poor job.
- The expensive staff personnel may become a burden on the cost of the production if its services are not properly utilized.

HOSPITAL STATISTICS INCLUDING HOSPITAL UTILIZATION INDICES

Importance of hospital statistics to ensure the generation of accurate hospital statistical report. Hospital statistical reports shall be made available at all times. Serves as a management tool in the effective management and operation of the hospital.

Definition

Hospital statistics defined as information obtained from hospital indoor and outdoor facilities regarding quality of care, utilization of services, quantity of services delivered, workload and other hospital related administrative and logistic details.

Uses of Hospital Statistics

- Measure of evaluation of quality of care
- Helps in planning
- Allocation of resources in different areas
- Identify deficiencies at various levels; i.e., input, process and outcome
- Evaluate effectiveness and efficiency of the administration

Types of Hospital Statistics (Box 7.10)

1. **Reports related to hospital beds daily census:** Daily average attendance, bed occupancy rate, bed turn over, interval bed turn over, rate total patient days care, vacancy rate hospital beds, sanctioned beds, functional bed, bed supply rate
2. **Reports related to admission/discharge/death admission:** Daily admission, total admission over a period discharge: Daily discharge, total discharge over a period, average length of stay deaths, daily number of deaths, total deaths over a period, total deaths over 48 hours, total deaths under 48 hours, net death rate, gross death rate, postoperative death rate, anesthetic death rate.
3. **Work load statistics:** Total number of outputs new cases/Repeat cases, total number of operations, total number of X-rays average OPD patients per day total cesarean sections per day, average number of food served per day.
4. **Hospital care evaluation statistics:** HAI rate postoperative complication rate, autopsy rate, percentage of agreement between final and pathological diagnosis, gross result of treatment; i.e., patients recovered, improved or not relieved.

Box 7.10: Types of hospital statistics.

Reports related to hospital beds
- Daily census
- Daily average attendance
- Bed occupancy rate
- Bed turn over interval
- Bed turn over rate
- Total patient days care
- Vacancy rate
- Hospital beds
- Sanctioned beds
- Functional bed
- Bed supply rate

---

5. **Indices related to population at risk:** Admission rate, hospitalization rate per person, bed-population index
6. **Other type of classifications:**
   a. Patient movement statistics: Admission, discharge, deaths
   b. Morbidity statistics: Patients under various diagnoses
   c. Administrative statistics: Manpower, material, money-finance
   d. Hospital service statistics: No. of operations, utilization indicators

Hospital Utilization Statistics

- **Admission:** The formal acceptance by a hospital or other inpatient healthcare facility of a patient who is to be provided with room, and continuous nursing service in an area of the hospital or facility where patients generally reside at least overnight. Admission rate number of admission per 1000 population in a year.
- **Discharge:** Discharge from the hospital is the point at which the patient leaves the hospital and either returns home or is transferred to another facility, such as one for rehabilitation or to a nursing home. Discharge involves the medical instructions that the patient will need to fully recover. Uses of hospital statistics is shown in **Box 7.11**.

Hospital Beds

- WHO defines a hospital bed as a bed that is regularly maintained and staffed for the accommodation and full-time care of a succession of inpatients and is situated in wards or a part of the hospital where continuous medical care for inpatients is provided.
- Total number of beds excludes bed compliments of the hospital for normal, healthy newborn babies in maternity ward; but includes incubators used for premature babies.

Box 7.11: Uses of hospital statistics.

- Measure of evaluation of quality of care
- Helps in planning
- Allocation of resources in different areas
- Identify deficiencies at various levels; i.e., input, process and outcome
- Evaluate effectiveness and efficiency of the administration

- **Sanctioned bed:** It is the official bed capacity of the hospital. CMH, Dhaka: 1100 beds (Soon to upgrade to 1500 beds) functional bed. This is the actual functional status of beds in a hospital.

Bed-days or Patient-days

- A bed-day is a day during which a person is confined to a bed and in which the patient stays overnight in a hospital.
- It is the unit of measure denoting the services rendered to one in-patient day in the hospital.
- One full day is counted when admission before mid-day and discharge after mid-day. Patient-day should not include data for healthy newborn infants.
- Bed supply rate (Bed to population ratio) BSR = (No. of beds available ÷ No. of population served) × 1000 Bangladesh: 0.6 beds/1000 population WHO Standard: 5 beds/1000 population vacancy rate = 100% – Occupancy rate

Bed turnover rate, average number of patients cared for a bed during a given period. BTR = (No. of discharges including deaths for a given period of time ÷ **Average bed count for that period of time**) × 100 Indicates:

- An important measure of hospital utilization indices. Gives the net effect of changes in occupancy rate and average length of stay (ALS).
- Example: In a particular hospital, there were 2358 discharges in the year 2009. Number of beds in that hospital in 2009 was 300. Hospital bed turnover rate = 2358/300 = 7.86. **Box 7.12** summarizes other type of classification of hospital statistics.

Average Bed Occupancy

- Average number of days during which the bed is occupied by a patient in the course of a given period of time.
- Average daily census (ADC) average number of patients in the hospital at a given time per day.
- This is the ratio of the total number of in-patient days (Excluding newborn) to total number of days in the same period. ADC= Total patient days ÷ Number of calendar days in a period.
- For example, the total number of inpatient service days provided for the 1st week of May is 1729. Average daily census is 1729/7 = 247.

Average Length of Stay (ALOS)

- Length of stay is a term which is used to calculate a patient's day of admission in the hospital till the day of discharge, i.e., the number of days a patient stayed in a hospital for treatment.

Box 7.12: Other type of classification.
- **Patient movement statistics:** Admission, discharge, deaths
- **Morbidity statistics:** Patients under various diagnosis
- **Administrative statistics:** Manpower, material, money-finance
- **Hospital service statistics:** No. of operations, utilization indicators

---

- Formula for calculating average length of stay: (Total inpatient days of care/Total discharges) = Average length of stay (In days)—the average length of stay in hospitals (ALOS) is often used as an indicator of efficiency.
- All other things being equal, a shorter stay will reduce the cost per discharge.
- Total length of stay = 6 + 11 + 5 + 8 = 30 days average length of stay = Total length of stay/Total number of discharges = 30/4 = 7.5 days given, number of patients = 4.

Number of Patients' Day (Service Days)

- In a year, number of beds × 365 × 100 bed occupancy rate (BOR) BOR is the average occupancy of hospital beds in percentage.
- It is the ratio between beds used and beds provided. The beds occupancy rate is calculated based on the midnight bed census at each hospital. [For example, the BOR for Monday is based on the bed census taken at 0000 hours Tuesday].
  - 80–85% BOR is ideal for good quality of patient care.
  - 15–20% beds are vacant for emergency, maternity, isolation, intensive care (Dead Space Beds).
  - 100% occupancy means over-utilization.
  - Occupancy less than 80% is uneconomical
- Example: In the month of June 4000 inpatients days were served in a hospital with 150 beds. Given, total number of inpatient days = 4000. Available beds = 150. June has 30 days. So, number of days in the period = 30 BOR = Total number of inpatient days for a given period × 100/ Available beds × Number of days in the period = 4000 × 100/150 × 30 = 400000/4500 = 88.889%

Bed Turn Over Interval (TOI) Turnover Interval (TOI)

- Average length of time (in days) that elapses between the discharge of one inpatient and the admission of the next inpatient to the same bed.
- It is the average period in days that a bed remains empty.

Calculation of Turnover Interval (TOI) (Fig. 7. 35)

- TOI = (Available staffed bed days – Occupied bed days)/ Inpatient discharges.
- Inpatient discharges include deaths, transfers out to other specialties/significant facilities and transfers out to other hospitals.
- **Interpretation:**
  - Negative TOI indicates scarcity of beds and over-utilization.
  - Long positive TOI s indicative of under-utilization because of defective admission procedures or poor quality medical care.
  - Short positive TOI is indicative of optimum utilization.
  - TOI is 'zero' when bed occupancy rate is 100%.

Gross Death Rate

- Ratio of total deaths to total discharges including deaths. In general hospital, it should not exceed 3%. Gross death rate = (Total death in a period ÷ Total discharge) × 100

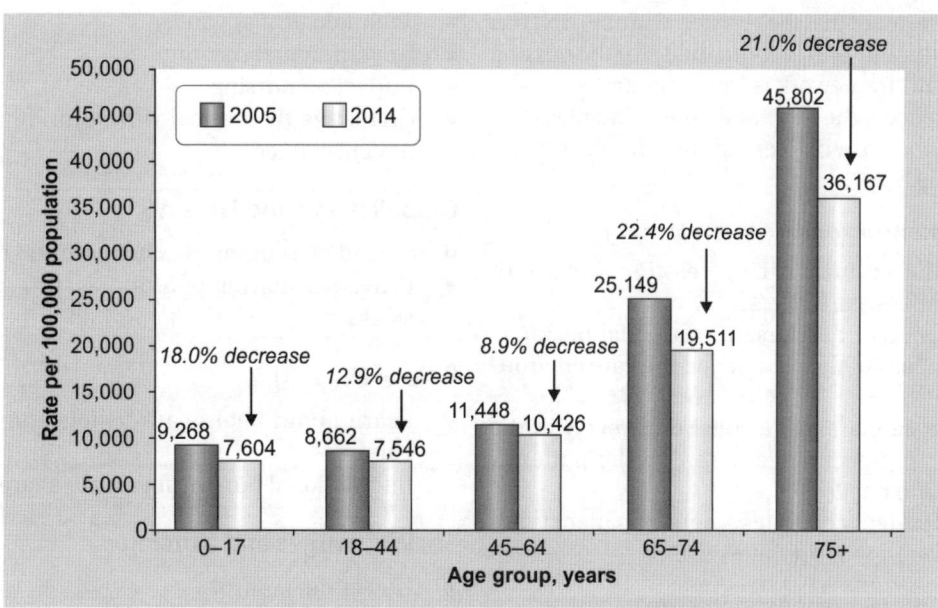

Fig. 7.35: Calculation of turnover interval (TOI).

- Formula: r = (n/t) × 100 Where, r = (Hospital) gross death rate n = Number of deaths of inpatients in a period t = Number of discharges (Including deaths) in the same period.

Net Death Rate

- A death rate, also known as the institutional death rate that does not include deaths, which occur within 48 hours of admission (24 hours of admission in some countries).
- Anesthetic death rate = (No. of deaths due to anesthesia ÷ No of patients anesthetized during that period) × 5000
- It should be less than 1 in 5000 postoperative death rate = (Deaths within 10 days of surgery ÷ Total operations during that period) × 100 usual value is 1–2% (Depending on nature of surgery)
- Autopsy rate = (Number of pathological autopsies performed ÷ Number of deaths during that period) × 100 Patients who are dead on arrival (DOA) at the hospital and fetal deaths are excluded from both the numerator and the denominator.
- Autopsy rate more than 15–20% indicates enquiry type of medical staff, progressive in outlook.
- Cesarean section rate = (Total CS performed ÷ Total live-births during that period) × 100 – Normal value is 3–4%.

NURSING CARE DELIVERY SYSTEMS AND TRENDS

A nursing care delivery system defines the way we use our nursing values to care for our patients, families, colleagues, and selves. The care delivery system is actually a subsystem of the professional practice model that describes our approach to delivering patient care by:

- Detailing assignments, responsibilities and authority to accomplish patient care;
- Determining who is going to perform what tasks, who is responsible, and who makes decisions; and
- Matching number and type of caregivers to patient care needs.

Relationship Based Care (Fig. 7.36)

Nurses adopted Relationship Based Care (RBC) as our nursing care delivery system. In RBC, the patient and family are always the central focus with an emphasis on the development of collaborative relationships needed to provide excellent patient care. There are three crucial relationships in RBC:

1. Relationship with patients and their families. Care givers demonstrate unwavering respect for the patient and family and actively engage them in all aspects of care.
2. Relationship with colleagues. Care givers are committed to a common purpose and respect each colleague's unique contribution to the team.
3. Relationship with self. Care givers balance the demands of their role with their personal and professional health and well-being.

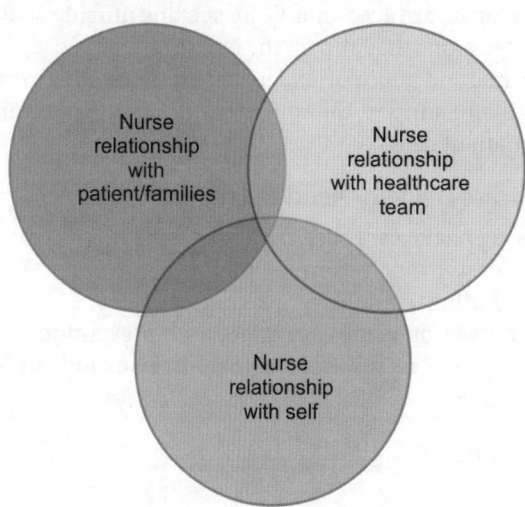

Fig. 7.36: Relationship based care in nursing.

RBC is built on the tenet that the registered nurse (RN) has the authority, responsibility and accountability for the nursing process. How the RBC framework is implemented varies by setting but always reflects the PPM and core principles. The building blocks of the care delivery system in all settings include the following:

Nurse-Patient Relationship and Decision Making

- RNs develop therapeutic caring relationships with patients and families/care givers.
- The scope/duration of the nurse-patient relationship is defined by the needs of the patient and the care environment.
- Decisions about care are made collaboratively with the patient or their representative based on the patient's values, beliefs, and needs.
- Nurses serve as patient advocates when the patient is not able or available to speak for themselves.

Work Allocation and/or Patient Assignments

- RNs are involved in the planning and implementation of staffing plans that meet the needs of the patient/family.
- Patient/nursing care assignments are based on the care environment, the needs of the patient and family, and staff competency.
- While supporting continuity of care, work allocations and/or assignments may vary based on changing needs.

Communication between Healthcare Team Members

- RNs actively participate in established processes for planning and evaluating interdisciplinary care.
- RNs communicate directly with other members of the healthcare team, taking an active role in coordinating the patient's care.
- Formal and informal leaders serve as a resource to nursing staff and support the role of the RN in the coordination of patient care.

Management of the Unit or Environment of Care

- Nursing staff are accountable for recognizing issues in the environment of care and actively working to resolve them.
- Managers are accountable for seeking nursing staff input in decisions that impact the environment of care.
- Formal and informal leaders serve as a resource to nursing staff and support the role of the RN in the coordination of patient care.

Healthcare Delivery Need to Change

- Rising healthcare cost
- Increasing elderly population
- Expanding technology
- Emphasis on acute care rather than prevention
- Insurance reimbursement that rewarded increased spending

Cause and Effect

Cause

- Consumer demands
- Technological advances
- Governmental scrutiny
- Impact on nursing
- Challenge theoretical viewpoint, practice models, and patient services

Globalization and Nursing

- Spread of a common culture around the world
- Universal sharing of attitudes, products, industry, and stocks

Role of Nursing

- Learn about healthcare beliefs and practices of other cultures
- International nursing forums to share nursing practice

Social Changes and Nursing

- Consumer control
- Desire to make own choices
- Conventional vs alternative therapies
- Question health information
- Research independently
- Demand more preventive care
- Judge value of healthcare service orientation
- Aging
- Majority population
- Multiple healthcare needs
- New technology
- Telemedicine

Current Trends affecting the Vision of Nursing

- Dominant role in healthcare delivery systems
- Geriatrics a prominent specialty
- Leadership role in determining/implementing policy
- Provide holistic care (integration of multiple facets)
- Technology enhanced quality care
- Quality care based upon outcome criteria
- Emphasis on case-management
- Increased nursing involvement in making policy and governmental decisions affecting healthcare
- Education more user-friendly
- Expanding cultural knowledge and practice

Healthcare Settings and Services

- **Acute care hospitals:** Acute care hospitals are the most commonly known healthcare facility. Acute care implies that a client in the hospital has a serious condition that needs to be closely monitored by healthcare professionals, particularly nurses. Acute care facilities admit clients for short periods of time, usually only a matter of a few days. Clients are often very sick and need a great deal of nursing care.
- **Intensive care units:** Intensive care units (ICUs) that care for the critically ill are found in acute care facilities. ICUs may specialize in medical, surgical, respiratory, coronary, burn, neonatal, and pediatric care areas. ICUs provide

Table 7.1: Types and settings of services.	
Types of healthcare services	Delivery settings
Preventive care	• Public health programs • Community programs • Personal lifestyles
Primary care	• Physician office/clinic • Self-care • Alternative medicine
Specialized care	Specialist clinics
Chronic care	• Primary care settings • Specialist provider clinics • Home health • Long-term care facilities • Self-care • Alternative medicine

care for clients by specially trained nurses. Many ICUs use high-tech equipment and health status monitors.

- **Subacute care facilities**: Many hospitals have areas that are classified as subacute care or step-down units. A person may move to a subacute unit when the level of acuity of care has decreased. However, the client is not considered ready for discharge. A client may be transferred from an ICU to a step-down unit before being discharged from the hospital.
- **Specialized hospitals are facilities that** admit only one type of client. Examples include government veteran hospitals, psychiatric, or pediatric hospitals. Specialized hospitals may also have units for medical, surgical, or intensive care. Other types of specialized hospitals include facilities for the developmentally or mentally disabled. Some facilities care for specific conditions, such as head and spinal cord injuries or substance abuse.
- **Although its primary function is** to provide healthcare, the hospital performs other functions. For example, your clinical facility has the added role of education, and many large hospitals, particularly those affiliated with a university, also play an important role in research.
- **With acute care facilities sending** individuals home earlier to recover from surgery or illness, the need for home healthcare has increased. In some cases, nursing care is available 24 hours a day in the home. However, in most cases, the family and other lay caregivers need to take responsibility for some care. Nurses are vital in teaching individuals how to perform care in the home. **Table 7.1** summarizes types of healthcare services and delivery settings.

Trends in Healthcare Delivery

- **Robots:** Robots have joined the healthcare team in many hospitals, where they deliver medications, meals, linens, lab specimens, equipment and supplies. They reduce costs, decrease delivery times, improve employee satisfaction, and allow nurses and other clinical staff to focus their time and attention on direct patient care.
- **Telemedicine:** Health systems and clinics will turn toward telemedicine to increase rural patients' access to health services, whether primary or specialty care. Some emergency medical services are adding teleconferencing systems to stretchers, enabling emergency department physicians to assess the patient while en route to the hospital.
- **Addressing simple illnesses:** Web-based, virtual doctors visits are gaining in popularity, enabling patients to "see" a doctor 24 hours a day without leaving their home or office for treatment of simple illnesses, such as a sore throat or urinary tract infection, and allowing the limited supply of physicians to care for a growing number of patients.
- **Empowering patients:** Technology also can provide patients with more affordable and convenient care, such as clinical decision support programs. Hwang said software that sorts through symptoms and offers treatment options could decrease cost and increase satisfaction.

ROLE OF NURSE IN MAINTENANCE OF EFFECTIVE ORGANIZATIONAL CLIMATE

Organizational climate is the shared perception of employees who work and live in the organization. It is the sum of individual perceptions regarding the organizational procedures, policies and practices. It represents the psychological environment of the organization consisting of individual opinions framed upon micro events that happen to them as well as to others around, over a period of time **(Figs. 7.37 to 7.39)**.

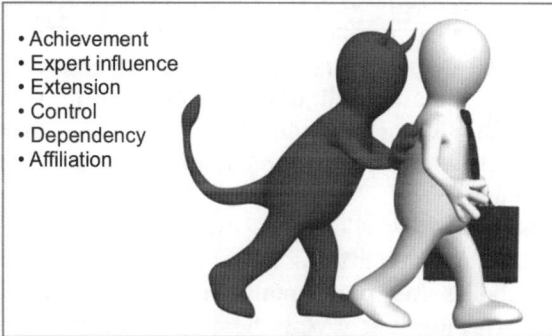

Fig. 7.37: Organizational climate motives.

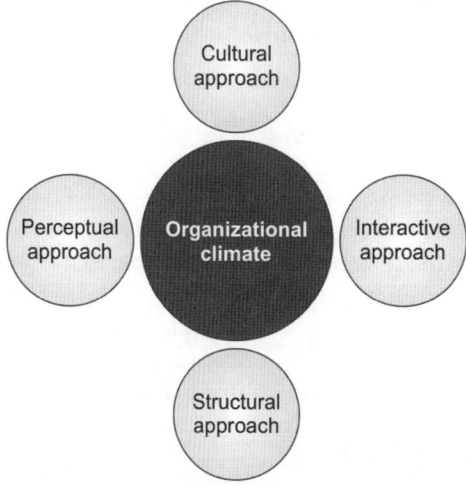

Fig. 7.38: Organization climate approaches.

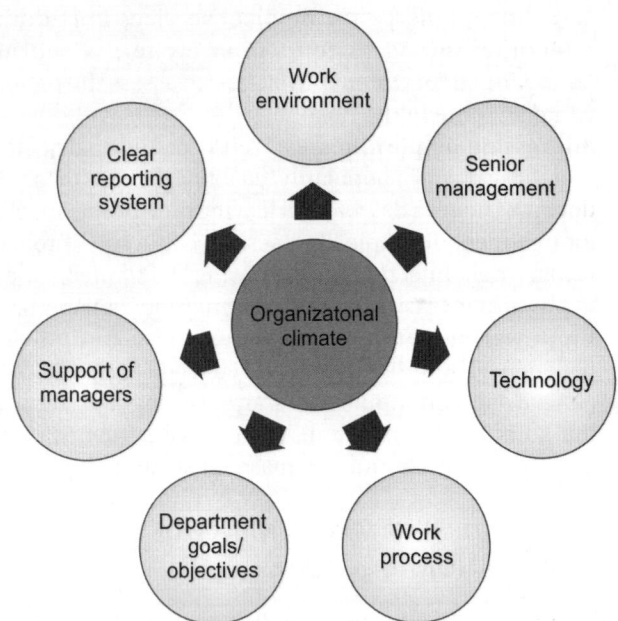

Fig. 7.39: Organization climate areas.

- It is the set of measurable properties of the work environment, perceived directly or indirectly by the members, influencing their work and satisfaction
- The organizational climate facilitates the firm to identify to the deficiencies in connection with different organizational factors, such as organizational structure, employee compensation system, communication level, physical atmosphere, organizational culture, etc.
- It is the apparent trait of a firm and its sub-systems as replicated in the mode in which an organization deals with its associates, team members and organizational problems.
- It is comparatively enduring excellence of the in-house atmosphere that is experienced by its employees which influences their performance and can be described in terms of the values of a specific set of behaviors in the firm.
- Organizational climate is comprised of a mixture of norms, values, expectations, policies and procedures that influence work motivation, commitment and ultimately individual or work unit performance.

Measuring Climate

Measurement of climate seeks to identify the components of both bad and good climate, both in absolute terms and perceptual terms. While there are commercial instruments that measure climate, there are powerful arguments for having one tailor-made to the organization, and that change as the organization changes.

Generally, the areas of interact to measure are:
- External environment-organizational interface with it
- Organizational leadership/mission
- Organizational structure/systems
- Organization and you
- Management practices
- Working-co-workers/teams/supervisor
- Self-at work-the role, development, opportunities, motivation, commitment, stress
- Self-outside work-how work affects the life (good/bad)-vice-versa.

Climate is worthwhile to understand and measure because there are organizational and human benefits a 'good' climate, and powerful disadvantages of many kinds of bad climate.

'Good' Climate has been linked to desirable outcomes, such as:
- Job satisfaction
- Confidence in management
- Affective commitment
- Intention to quit
- Emotional exhaustion
- Faith in organizational
- Performance

Desirable good behaviors, such as:
- Risk-taking (strategic)
- Departure from the status quo
- Open communication
- Trust
- Operational freedom, and
- Employee development

'Bad' Climate has been linked to:
- Turnover
- Stress
- Sickness
- Poor performance
- Error rate
- Wastage
- Accidents

Desirable bad behaviors, such as:
- Sabotage
- Absenteeism
- Go-slow
- Bullying

The dimensions of organizational climate is:
- **Challenge:** The emotional involvement of the members of the organization in its operations and goals. A high—challenge climate is seen when the people are experiencing joy and meaningfulness in their job, and, therefore, they invest much energy. Low challenge means feelings of alienation and indifference; the common sentiment and attitude is apathy and lack of interest for the job and the organization.
- **Freedom:** The independence in behavior exerted by the people in the organization. In a climate with much of this kind of freedom people make contacts and give and receive information; discuss problems and alternatives; plan and take initiatives of different kinds; and make decisions.
- **Idea support:** The ways new ideas are treated. In a supportive climate, ideas and suggestions are received in an attentive and supportive way by bosses and workmates. People listen to each other and encourage initiatives. Possibilities for trying out new ideas are

created. The atmosphere is constructive and positive. When idea support is low, the reflexive "no" prevails. Every suggestion is immediately refuted by a counter-argument. Fault finding and obstacle rising are the usual styles of responding to ideas.
- **Trust/Openness:** The emotional safety in relationships. When there is a strong level of trust, everyone in the organization dares to put forward ideas and opinions. Initiatives can be taken without fear of reprisal and ridicule in case of failure. Communication is open and straightforward.
- **Dynamism/Liveliness:** The eventfulness of life in the organization. In the highly dynamic situation, new things are happening all the time and alterations between ways of thinking about and handling issues often occur. There is a kind of psychological turbulence which is described by people in those organizations as "full speed", "go", breakneck", "maelstrom", and the like.
- **Playfulness/Humor:** The spontaneity and ease that is displayed. A relaxed atmosphere with jokes and laughter characterizes the organization which is high in this dimension. The opposite climate is characterized by gravity and seriousness. The atmosphere is stiff, gloomy, and cumbrous. Jokes and laughter are regarded as improper.
- **Debates:** The occurrence of encounters and clashes between view points, ideas, and differing experiences and knowledge. In the debating organization many voices are heard and people are keen on putting forward their ideas.
- **Conflicts:** The presence of personal and emotional tensions (in contrast to conflicts between ideas) in the organization. When the level of conflict is high, groups and single individuals dislikes each other and the climate can be characterized by "warfare", plots and traps are usual elements in the life of the organization. There is gossip and slander. In the opposite case, people behave in a more mature manner; they have psychological insight and control of impulses.
- **Risk taking:** The tolerance of uncertainty in the organization. In the high risk-taking case, decisions and actions are prompt and rapid, arising opportunities are taken and concrete experimentation is preferred to detailed investigation and analysis. In a risk-avoiding climate, there is a cautious, hesitant mentality. People try to be on the "safe side", they decide "to sleep on the matter", they set up committees and they cover themselves in many ways before making a decision.
- **Idea time:** The amount of time people can use (and do use) for elaborating new ideas. In the high idea-time situation, a possibility exists to discuss and test impulses and fresh suggestions that are not planned or included in the task assignment; and people tend to use these possibilities. In the reverse case, every minute is booked and specified. The time pressure makes thinking outside the instructions and planned routines impossible.

Role of nurse in maintenance of effective organizational climate: Nurses in the organization have to be well conversant with rites, rituals, policies, etc. This can only bring sense of belongings among employees and further help in the growth of organization. Organization climate is of great significance for utilization of human relations and resources at all levels.

- Organizational climate has a major influence on motivation, productivity, commitment, empowerment and job satisfaction.
- It is also a major motivating factor responsible for satisfaction and dissatisfaction of nurses and affects the quantum of their turnover.
- A positive work climate encourages and sustains staff motivation. Managers can often turn their work groups around by applying leadership and management practices that promote on-the-job clarity, support, and challenge.

Patience
- Nurses must be patient and help people overcome anxiety and the importance of patience should be realized by everyone as it makes people better generally—building empathy towards others is crucial in the medical profession.
- Patience helps us accept other people as the way they are, thus anger and stress are two things that are enough to ruin a person's health.

Organization
- A nurse's to do list can change rapidly, therefore, organizational skills are crucial and an organized nurse will function better in everyday activities.
- An organized nurse can manage their time effectively and know how to allocate hours in a day to prepare for, conduct and follow up on events and activities.
- Highly organized nurses can easily access and analyze procedures designed to handle various problems when they arise.
- Nurses with excellent organizational skills are more productive and make better overall impressions and as a result receive promotion.

Technical Savvy
- Technology continues to expand and the healthcare is certainly no exception.
- Today's hospital workforce consists of four unique generations: Traditionalists, baby boomers, generation X, and generation Y but as computer.
- Updates occur and new technology emerges the baby boomer and generation X nurses continue to call on the expertise of the youngest generation.
- Technology is coming to the bedside at a rapid pace - Health technology can do a lot to improve patient care and having technical skills leads to better and more efficient communication, thus a nurse interacting with a patient can retrieve needed information and act on it quickly.

Adaptability
- A nurse must be adaptable to change because things now change at a far greater speed and pace than ever

before with rapid changes in technology, diversity and society, hospitals need nurses who are open to new ideas and flexible enough to work through challenging issues, such as dealing with challenging priorities and workloads.

- Adaptability is something a nurse must bring with them to the job. By learning how to be more adaptable a nurse will become better equipped to respond when faced with a crisis.
- Every medical environment wants a nurse who fits within the existing work environment and is able to anticipate, respond to and manage change on a day-to-day basis.

REVIEW QUESTIONS

Long Essays

1. Define organizing; explain the purpose, objectives and principles of organizing.
2. Define assignment and explain method of patient care delivery.
3. Define delegation; explain the purposes, principles and advantages of delegation.
4. Define hospital; discuss the objectives, scope and functions of the hospital.
5. Define organizational development; explain the objectives, goals and characteristics of organizational development.
6. Discuss in detail about nursing care delivery systems and trends.

Short Essays

1. Enumerate the features of organizing.
2. Functions of organizing.
3. Enumerate the advantages and disadvantages of functional method.
4. Primary nursing method—advantages and disadvantages.
5. Discuss the types of delegation.
6. Features and types of coordination.
7. Classifications of hospital.
8. Types of organizational structures.
9. Informal organization.
10. Organizational charts.
11. Organizational effectiveness.
12. Hospital administration control and line of authority.
13. Describe the role of nurse in maintenance of effective organizational climate.
14. Trends in healthcare delivery.

Short Answers

1. Division of work.
2. Element of organizing.
3. Organizing function.
4. Methods of patient assignment.
5. Process of organizing patient care.
6. Case method.
7. Purpose of functional method.
8. Modular nursing.
9. Case management.
10. Team nursing.
11. Importance of coordination.
12. Flatarchy structure.
13. Principles of organization charts.
14. Line of organization.
15. Factors affecting organizational effectiveness.
16. Telemedicine.

BIBLIOGRAPHY

1. Charles G, James LR. "The cross-level effects of culture and climate in human service teams". Journal of Organizational Behavior. 2002;23(6):767-94.
2. Etzioni, Amitia. Modern Organizations. Englewood Cliffs, NJ: Prentice-Hall; 1964.
3. Herman RD, Renz DO. Advancing Nonprofit Organizational Effectiveness Research and Theory: Nine Theses. Nonprofit Management and Leadership. 2008; 18 (4):399-415.
4. Hunter ST, Bedell KE, Mumford MD. Climate for creativity: A quantitative review. Creativity Research Journal. 2007;19(1):69-70.
5. Richard, et al. Measuring Organizational Performance: Towards Methodological Best Practice. Journal of Management; 2009.

CHAPTER 8

Staffing

LEARNING OBJECTIVES

- Definition, Objectives, Components and Functions of Staffing and Scheduling
- Staffing—Philosophy, Staffing Activities
- Recruiting, Selecting, Deployment
- Training, Development, Credentialing, Retaining, Promoting, Transfer, Terminating, Superannuation
- Staffing Units—Projecting Staffing Requirements/Calculation of Requirements of Staff Resources Nurse Patient Ratio, Nurse Population Ratio as per SIU Norms/IPH Norms, and Patient Classification System
- Categories of Nursing Personnel Including Job Description of All Levels
- Assignment and Nursing Care Responsibilities
- Turnover and Absenteeism
- Staff Welfare
- Discipline and Grievances

INTRODUCTION

Staffing is that part of the process of management which is concerned with acquiring, developing, employing, appraising, remunerating and retaining people so that right type of people are available at right positions and at right time in the organization. In the simplest terms, staffing is 'putting people to jobs'. After an organization's structural design is in place, it needs people with the right skills, knowledge, and abilities to fill in that structure **(Fig. 8.1)**.

People are an organization's most important resource, because people either create or undermine an organization's reputation for quality in both products and service. In addition, an organization must respond to change effectively in order to remain competitive. The right staff can carry an organization through a period of change and ensure its future success. Because of the importance of hiring and maintaining a committed and competent staff, effective human resource management is crucial to the success of all organizations.

MEANING OF STAFFING

Staff management is the function of managing all employees in the organization, including the development of staff skills through training and other forms of staff development as well as the identification, development and implementation of training needs and programs available for staff. Employees include permanent, temporary, and part-time employees, people working under scholarships, traineeships, apprenticeships and similar relationships. Human resource management (HRM), or staffing, is the management function devoted to acquiring, training, appraising, and compensating employees.

- Staffing involves choosing competent and suitable personnel for different positions in the organization.
- Staffing may be defined as the management function of employing and developing human resources for carrying out various managerial and nonmanagerial activities of the organization.
- Staffing basically involves matching jobs and individuals.
- Staffing involves making people suitable to jobs, while organizing is concerned with creation of jobs. **Box 8.1** summarizes nature of staffing.

DEFINITION

- "Staffing is the function by which managers build an organization through the recruitment, selection, and development of individuals as capable **employees**".
  —*McFarland*
- According to AK Singh, "Staffing is the process of providing jobs to deserving people, through the function

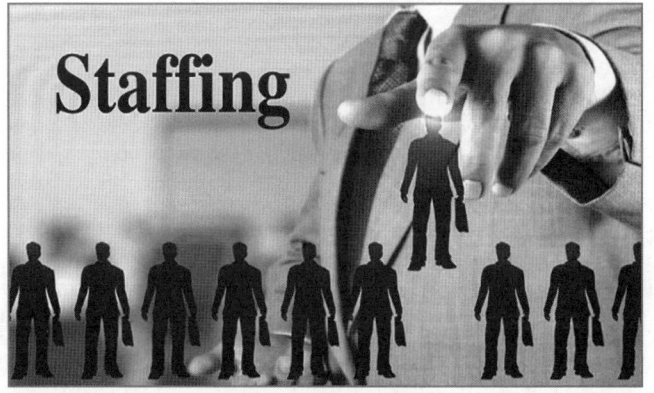

Fig. 8.1: Staffing process.

Box 8.1: Nature of staffing.

- It is a significant function of management.
- It is an important part of management process.
- It is continuous activity function of management.
- It is concerned with human resources of an organization.
- It is separate from physical factors, because it is complicated and sensitive function.
- It deals with the maximum utilization of human resources, such as direction, coordination and control.

of recruitment, selection and training with-a-view to getting benefits from them, for the achievement of pre-set goals of organization".

- According to Theo Heimann, "Staffing is concerned with the placement, growth and development of all those members of the organization whose function is to get the things done through the efforts of other individuals."

OBJECTIVES OF STAFFING (FIG. 8.2)

- Provide an all professional nurse staff in critical care units, operating rooms, labor and emergency room
- Provide sufficient staff to permit a 1:1 nurse-patient ratio for each shift in every critical care unit
- Staff the general medical, surgical, obstetrics and gynecology, pediatric and psychiatric units to achieve a 2:1 professional-practical nurse ratio.
- Provide sufficient nursing staff in general, medical, surgical, obstetrics and gynecology, pediatric and psychiatric units to permit a 1:5 nurse patient ratio on a day and afternoon shifts and 1:10 nurse–patient ratio on night shift.
- Involve the heads of the nursing staffs and all nursing personnel in designing the department's overall staffing program.
- Design a staffing plan that specifies how many nursing personnel in each classification will be assigned to each nursing unit for each shift and how vacation and holiday time will be requested and scheduled.
- Hold each head nurse responsible for translating the department's master staffing plan to sequential eight weeks time schedules for personnel assigned to her/his unit.
- Post time schedules for all personnel at least eight weeks in advance.
- Empower the head nurse to adjust work schedules for unit nursing personnel to remedy any staff excess or deficiency caused by census fluctuation or employee absence.
- Inform each nursing employee that requests for specific vacation or holiday time will be honored within the limits imposed by patient care and labor contract requirements.
- Reward employees for long-term service by granting individuals special time requests on the basis of seniority.

MISSION AND PHILOSOPHY OF STAFFING

Staff is selected very carefully, not only for their qualifications and experience, but also for their love of children. We understand that continuity of care for the children is paramount and for that reason we are totally committed to promoting staff loyalty. There is nothing worse for a child's development at nursery then to experience constantly changing faces due to staff turnover.

Mission

- To ensure maximum utilization of human resources.
- To discover and obtain competent personal for various job.
- Adequate staffing ensures continuous survival and growth of enterprise.
- To improve job satisfaction, morale of employees through objective assessment.
- To meet the crisis at the time of emergency.
- To deliver good quality of care and attain job satisfaction and patient satisfaction.

Philosophy of Staffing (Box 8.2)

- The nurse administrator believes that it is possible to match (nurse) staff's or employees knowledge and skill to the patient care, therefore, it save way to attain the job satisfaction with quality of care.

Box 8.2: Philosophy of staffing in nursing.

- Nurse administrators believe that it is possible to match employee's knowledge and skills to patient care needs in a manner that optimizes job satisfaction and care quality.
- Nurse administrators believe that the technical and humanistic care needs of clinically-ill patients are so complex that all aspects of that should be provided by professional nurses.
- Nurse administrators believe that the health teaching and rehabilitation needs of chronically-ill patients should be provided by professional and technical nurses.
- Nurse administrators believe that patient assessment, work quantification and job analysis should he used to determine the number of personnel in each category to assigned to care for patients of each type (e.g., coronary care respiratory failure, etc.)
- Nurse administrators believe that a master staffing plan and policies to implement the plan in all units should be developed centrally by the nursing heads and staff of the hospital.
- Nurse administrators believe that staffing plan should be administered at the unit level by the head nurse, so that selected plan details, such as shift-start time, number of staff assigned on holidays, and number of employees assigned to each shift can be modified to accommodate the unit workload and workflow.

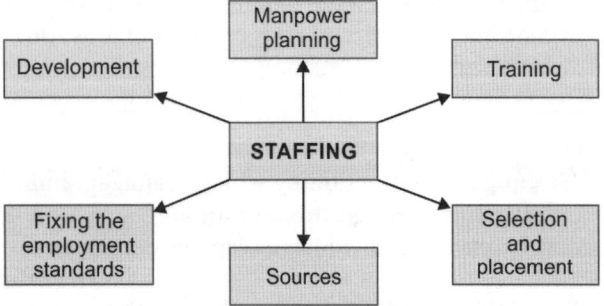

Fig. 8.2: Objectives of staffing.

- Nurse administrator believes that only professionally trained nurse can provide a high quality of patient care.
- Nurse administrator believes that only professionally skillful nurse can handle critically-ill patients by providing technical and humanistic care.
- Nurse administrator believes that a professional nurse can treat chronically-ill patient, provide health education, and provide rehabilitative care which is more complex.
- Nurse administrator believes that by determining patient needs and doing patient assignment only job quantification and job analysis can be done.
- Nurse administrator believes that all sorts of nursing related plans, e.g., master rotation plan, duty roster should be done only by nursing heads.
- Nurse administrator believes that staffing plan to be delegated to each unit level head nurse so that each ward activities, details of each shift are planned well.

COMPONENTS OF STAFFING (FIG. 8.3)

- **Job analysis:** It involves the collection of job-related information to prepare job description and job specification. Job description includes detail information about what a person has to do while being in specific job. Job specification indicates the qualification, training work experience and other personnel requirement to perform a particular job.
- **Human resource planning:** It involves an estimation of demand and supply of manpower to fulfill current and future HR requirement of the organization.
- **Recruitment and selection:** Recruitment is the process of making a pool of qualified candidates. It starts with the invitation of application and ends with the development of a list of qualified candidates. Selection involves the process of reviewing application blanks, organizing interviews and test and informing candidates.
- **Training and development:** Training and development is required to develop the skill and ability to motivate employees to work. Depending on the training needs, of the employees on the job (inside the organization) and off the job (outside the organization) training in organized.
- **Performance appraisal:** It is a process of evaluation employees' performance related strength and weaknesses. Performance is measured against criteria set previously. The result of evaluation is used for determining training needs, making promotion decision and providing reward based on the employees' performance.
- **Compensation and benefits:** Compensation is for rewarding people through pay, incentives and benefits for the work done. Compensation and benefits are great source of motivating employees, so the packages must be adequate, equitable and acceptable to the employees.
- Health and safety
- Employee relation

FACTORS AFFECTING STAFFING (TABLE 8.1)

Staffing is one of the most important functions of management. In fact, it is the process of filling vacant position by appointing the right personnel at the right job, at the right time. Hence, everything will occur in the right manner. It is universal truth that human resource is one of the greatest parts of every organization, because in any organization all other resources, such as money, material, machine, etc., can be utilized efficiently and effectively by the positive efforts of the human resource. Thus, it is too important that each and every personnel in organization should be appointed at the right job, according to their ability, talent, aptitude and specializations.

Internal Factors Affecting Staffing

- **Promotion policy:** Staffing is affected by the promotion policy of the organization. If the organization has a good promotion policy with prospects to career growth and development, only then efficient people will be attracted to the organization. Internal promotions are better for lower and middle-level jobs. This is because it increases the morale and motivation of the staff. However, for top level jobs, the 'RIGHT' person must be selected. The right person may be from within the organization, or he/she may be selected from outside.

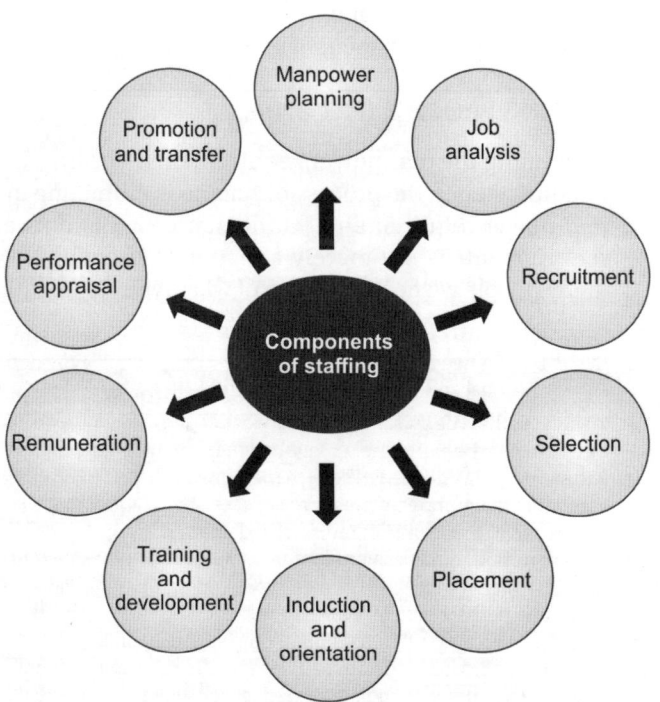

Fig. 8.3: Components of staffing.

Table 8.1: Factors affecting staffing.	
Internal environment	External environment
Promotion policy	Labor laws
Future growth plans of organization	Pressure from sociopolitical group
Technology used	Competition
Support from top management	Educational standards
Image of the organization	Other external factors

- **Future growth plans:** Staffing is also affected by the future growth plans of the organization. If the organization wants to grow and expand then it will need many talented people. In order to grow and expand, the organization must select experts and give them continuous training and development.
- **Technology used:** Staffing is also affected by the technology used by the organization. If the organization uses modern technologies then it must have continuous training programs to update the technical knowledge of their staff.
- **Support from top management:** Staffing is also affected by the support from top management. If the top management gives full support to it then the organization can have scientific selection procedures, scientific promotion and transfer policies, continuous training programs, career development programs, etc.
- **Image of organization:** Staffing is also affected by the image of the organization in the job market. If it has a good image then staffing will attract the best employees and managers. An organization earns a good image only if it maintains good staffing policies and practices. This includes job security, training and development, promotion, good working environment, work culture, etc.

External Factors Affecting Staffing

- **Labor laws:** Labor laws of the government also affect the staffing policy of the organization. For example, the organization has to support 'Social equality and upliftment' policies of the government by giving job reservations to candidates coming from depressed classes, such as scheduled castes (SC), scheduled tribes (ST), other backward classes (OBC), etc., and even to those who are physically handicapped (PH). It is mandatory for an organization not to recruit children in their workforce and stop child labor. The provisions of 'Minimum Wages Act' guide an organization to fix minimum salaries of employees and stop their economic exploitation.
- **Pressure from sociopolitical groups:** Staffing is also affected by activities of sociopolitical groups and parties. These groups and parties put pressure on the organization to grant jobs only to local people. The concept of '*Sons of Soil*' is becoming popular in India.
- **Competition:** In India, there is a huge demand for highly qualified and experienced staff. This has resulted in competition between different organizations to attract and hire efficient staff. Organizations often change their staffing policies, offer attractive salaries and other job benefits in order to add the best minds in their workforce.
- **Educational standards:** Staffing is also affected by the educational standards of an area. If the educational standard of a place is very high then the organization will only select qualified and experienced staff for all job positions. For example, some IT companies in India only prefer skilled candidates with computer or IT Engineering degree for the post of software developer.
- **Other external factors:** Staffing is also affected by other external factors, such as trade unions, social attitude towards work, etc.

■ FUNCTIONS OF STAFFING (BOX 8.3)

The managerial function of staffing involves manning the organization structure through proper and effective selection, appraisal and development of the personnel's to fill the roles assigned to the employers/workforce.

- **Staffing is an important managerial function:** Staffing function is the most important managerial act along with planning, organizing, directing and controlling. The operations of these four functions depend upon the manpower which is available through staffing function.
- **Staffing is a pervasive activity:** As staffing function is carried out by all managers and in all types of concerns where business activities are carried out.
- **Staffing is a continuous activity:** This is because staffing function continues throughout the life of an organization due to the transfers and promotions that take place.
- **The basis of staffing function is efficient management of personnel's:** Human resources can be efficiently managed by a system or proper procedure, that is, recruitment, selection, placement, training and development, providing remuneration, etc.
- **Staffing helps in placing right men at the right job:** It can be done effectively through proper recruitment procedures and then finally selecting the most suitable candidate as per the job requirements.
- **Staffing is performed by all managers:** Depending upon the nature of business, size of the company, qualifications and skills of managers, etc. In small companies, the top management generally performs this function. In medium and small scale enterprise, it is performed especially by the personnel department of that concern.

■ STAFFING PROCESS (FIG. 8.4)

- **Estimating the manpower requirements:** The first and foremost step in the process of staffing is estimating the manpower requirements. Understanding manpower requirements is not merely a matter of knowing how many people we need, but also of what type. Estimation

---

Box 8.3: Functions in staffing.

- Identifying the type and amount of service needed by agency client.
- Determining the personnel categories that have the knowledge and skill to perform needed service measures.
- Predicting the number of personnel in each job category that will be needed to meet anticipated service demands.
- Obtaining, budgeted positions for the number in each job category needed to service for the expected types and number of clients.
- Recruiting personnel to fill available positions.
- Selecting and appointing personnel from suitable applicants.
- Combining personnel into desired configurations by unit and shift.
- Orienting personnel to fulfill assigned responsibilities.
- Assigning responsibilities for client services to available personnel.

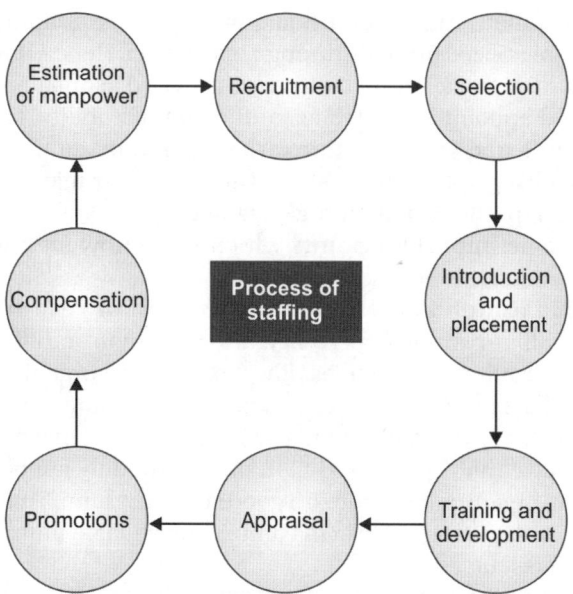

Fig. 8.4: Processing steps in staffing.

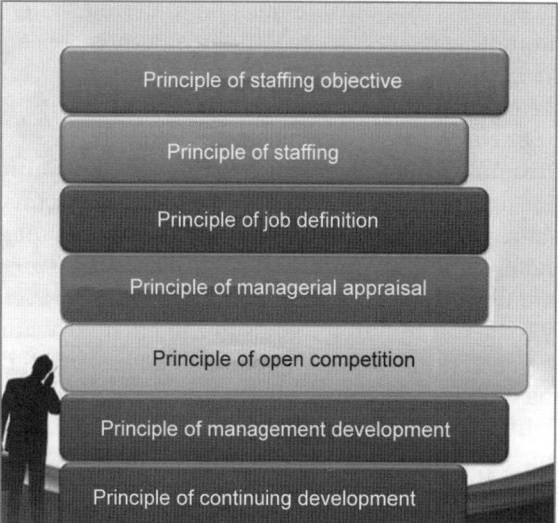

Fig. 8.5: Major staffing principles.

of manpower requirements involves workload analysis and workforce analysis.

- **Recruitment:** Recruitment may be defined as the process of searching for prospective employees and stimulating them to apply for jobs in the organization.
- **Selection:** Selection is the process of choosing from among the pool of the prospective job candidates that is developed at the stage of recruitment.
- **Placement and orientation:** Placement refers to the employee occupying the position or post for which the person has been selected. Orientation is introducing the selected employee to other employees and familiarizing him with the rules and policies of the organization.
- **Training and development:** Training and development of employees is very important in order to improve their skills and to give them an opportunity for their career advancement.
- **Performance appraisal:** It refers to rating or evaluating the current performance of employees according to certain predetermined standards. Transfers and promotions of the staff are based on performance appraisal.
- **Promotion and career planning:** It is necessary for every organization to keep promotion and career plans of an employee into consideration so as to ensure job satisfaction.
- **Compensation:** Organizations pay wages and salaries to their employees for whom they need to establish wages and salary plans. There are various ways to prepare different pay plans depending upon the worth of the jobs.

PRINCIPLES OF STAFFING (FIG. 8.5)

Staffing process of management assists in obtaining the right talent and also nurturing it. Staffing principles which are universally accepted are not present. Nonetheless, identifying valuable principles for effectively grasping and performing staffing function was done by Heinz Weihrich and Harold Koontz, which were here under.

- **Principle of the purpose of staffing:** Qualified personnel who are able and keen to carry on organizational roles is the main purpose of managerial staffing. It is proved that lack of the said qualities leads to failure.
- **Principle of staffing:** High managerial quality depends on clarity of defining organizational roles and human needs, good methods of managerial assessment and the training given to employees. Organizations without recognized job descriptions, efficient appraisals or any methods for training and development have to depend on outside resources to fill the managerial positions. Alternatively, organizations using individual's potentials effectively in the enterprise are doing so by utilizing the systems methodology of staffing and human resource management.
- **Principle of job definition:** Precise identification of the managerial results is needed to define the magnitude of their positions. Organizational roles of people have different features, such as pay, status, power, direction and the likelihood of achievement that makes managers to function well.
- **Principles of managerial appraisal:** Identification of the managerial activities and clarity of various objectives are needed for precise managerial appraisal against these criteria. The principle implies that the performance of managers is determined by the measurement of verifiable goals against the standards of managerial performance. Managerial appraisal takes into account the main managerial jobs, such as planning, organizing, staffing, directing and controlling.
- **Principle of open competition:** Encouragement of open competition amongst candidates for management positions depends entirely on the full commitment of an enterprise on quality management. Many firms have chosen managers with insufficient abilities because of breach of these principles. Good candidates who can

be chosen from outside must be preferred rather than promoting candidates within the enterprise because of social pressures. Simultaneously, by using this principle, the enterprise is obliged to correctly evaluate its people by providing them with chances for growth.

- **Principle of management training and development:** For achieving effective development programs and activities, it is important to integrate more managerial training and development with the management methods and objectives. According to the systems approach, the managerial functions, goals of the enterprise and the managers' professional requirements are correlated with the training and growth efforts.
- **Principle of training objectives:** The training objectives must be stated correctly in order to achieve them. To aid the effectiveness of training efforts, it is necessary for analyzing training needs as the foundation for giving direction to development. This principle focuses on the importance of training for the needs of the enterprise and individual development.
- **Principles of ongoing development:** Managers must practice self-development as an ongoing process for fulfilling the commitment of an enterprise towards managerial excellence. This principle states that managers must continuously learn in the present day competitive environment. Managerial knowledge and approaches must be continuously updated and re-examined and their skills must be enhanced in order to get positive results in an enterprise.

IMPORTANCE OF STAFFING (FIG. 8.6)

Staffing is one of the most essential functions for every organization. In fact, in the absence of a good staffing system no organization can exist for a long duration. Because in every organization all the resources like, money, material, machine, etc., are utilized properly through man power. Hence, it is too important that all the personnel (employees) in organization should appoint at the job according to their ability, talent, aptitude and specializations which can only be possible through a good staffing system. Thus, it is clear that staffing is too important for every organization.

Some important points which show how staffing is important for every organization:

- **Maximum and efficient utilization of resources:** Staffing plays an important role in maximum and efficient utilization of resources. Because in every organization all the resources, such as money, material and machine, etc., are utilized efficiently through specialized man power and specialized man power can only appoint in an organization through a good staffing system. Thus, we can say that it helps in maximum and efficient utilization of resources.
- **Reduces cost of production:** Staffing also plays an important role in reducing cost of production. Because it helps in appointing right person at the right job, at the right, time so that no wastage and mistakes can be made by efficient personnel during the production of products. Hence, it is clear that it assists in reducing cost of production.
- **For job satisfaction:** Staffing is an important source for employee's job satisfaction. Because by means of this system jobs are allocated among the personnel are according to their ability, talent, aptitude and specializations which give employees more satisfaction regarding their jobs. As a result of that they give their hundred percent efforts behind their jobs.
- **For meeting present and future needs of employees:** Staffing is very important for fulfilling present as well as future needs of employees. Because it gives a clear picture to organization that in coming year how much positions will be vacant and new positions will be established. So that organization can fulfil those vacant and new positions by appointing the deserved candidates. Thus, it is clear that staffing fulfils present and future needs of employees in organization.
- **For maintaining coordination among the employees:** Staffing plays a prominent role in establishing unity and coordination among the employees. Because it assigns their jobs according to their ability, talent, aptitude and specializations which makes them involved in their tasks and ensure healthy and cooperative relationship among the employees.

STEPS INVOLVED IN STAFFING PROCESS (FIG. 8.7 AND BOX 8.4)

- **Manpower requirements:** The very first step in staffing is to plan the manpower inventory required by a concern in order to match them with the job requirements and demands. Therefore, it involves forecasting and determining the future manpower needs of the concern.

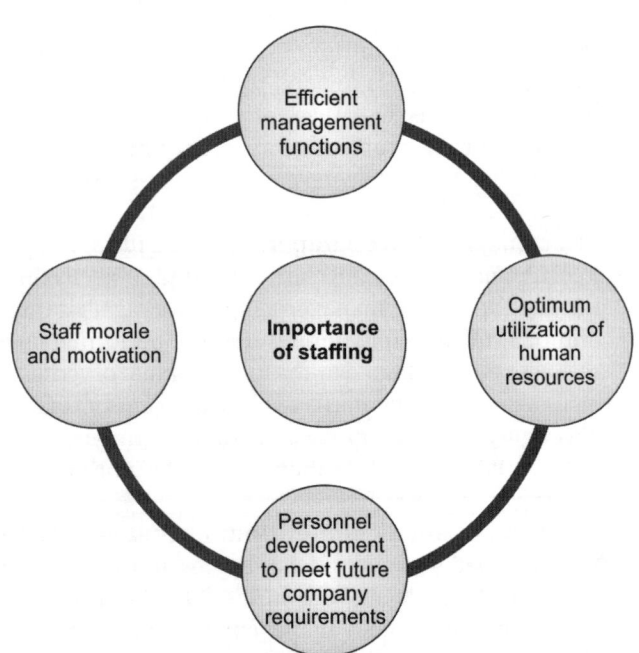

Fig. 8.6: Importance of staffing.

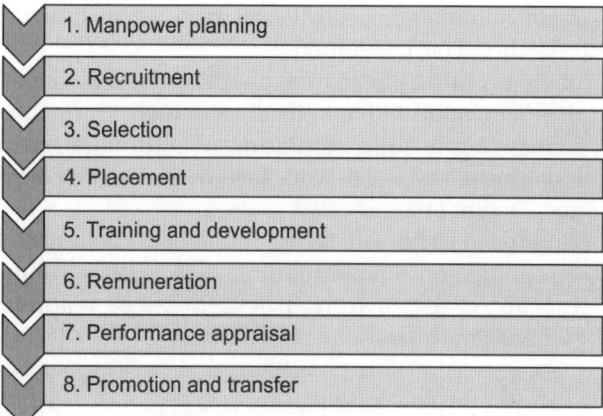

Fig. 8.7: Staffing process.

> **Box 8.4:** Staffing process—steps involved in staffing.
> - **Manpower requirements:** The very first step in staffing is to plan the manpower inventory required by a concern in order to match them with the job requirements and demands.
> - **Recruitment:** Once the requirements are notified, the concern invites and solicits applications according to the invitations made to the desirable candidates.
> - **Selection:** This is the screening step of staffing in which the solicited applications are screened out and suitable candidates are appointed as per the requirements.
> - **Orientation and placement:** Once screening takes place, the appointed candidates are made familiar to the work units and work environment through the orientation programs, placement takes place by putting right man on the right job.
> - **Training and development:** Training is a part of incentives given to the workers in order to develop and grow them within the concern. Training is generally given according to the nature of activities and scope of expansion in it. Along with it the workers are developed by providing them extra benefits of indepth knowledge of their functional areas. Development also includes giving them key and important jobs as a test or examination in order to analyze their performances.
> - **Remuneration:** It is a kind of compensation provided monetarily to the employees for their work performances. This is given according to the nature of job-skilled or unskilled, physical or mental, etc. Remuneration forms an important monetary incentive for the employees.
> - **Performance evaluation:** In order to keep a track or record of the behavior, attitudes as well as opinions of the workers towards their jobs. For this regular assessment is done to evaluate and supervise different work units in a concern. It is basically concerning to know the development cycle and growth patterns of the employees in a concern.
> - **Promotion and transfer:** Promotion is said to be a non-monetary incentive in which the worker is shifted from a higher job demanding bigger responsibilities as well as shifting the workers and transferring them to different work units and branches of the same organization.

- **Recruitment:** Once the requirements are notified, the concern invites and solicits applications according to the invitations made to the desirable candidates.
- **Selection:** This is the screening step of staffing in which the solicited applications are screened out and suitable candidates are appointed as per the requirements.
- **Orientation and placement:** Once screening takes place, the appointed candidates are made familiar to the work units and work environment through the orientation programmes. Placement takes place by putting right man on the right job.
- **Training and development:** Training is a part of incentives given to the workers in order to develop and grow them within the concern. Training is generally given according to the nature of activities and scope of expansion in it. Along with it, the workers are developed by providing them extra benefits of in-depth knowledge of their functional areas. Development also includes giving them key and important jobs as a test or examination in order to analyze their performances.
- **Remuneration:** It is a kind of compensation provided monetarily to the employees for their work performances. This is given according to the nature of job-skilled or unskilled, physical or mental, etc. Remuneration forms an important monetary incentive for the employees.
- **Performance evaluation:** In order to keep a track or record of the behavior, attitudes as well as opinions of the workers towards their jobs. For this regular assessment is done to evaluate and supervise different work units in a concern. It is basically concerning to know the development cycle and growth patterns of the employees in a concern.
- **Promotion and transfer:** Promotion is said to be a non-monetary incentive in which the worker is shifted from a higher job demanding bigger responsibilities as well as shifting the workers and transferring them to different work units and branches of the same organization.

Steps of Staffing in the Hospital

1. Determine the number and types of personnel needed to fulfil the philosophy, meet fiscal planning responsibilities, and carryout the chosen patient care management organization.
2. Recruit, interview, select, and assign personnel based on established job description performance standards.
3. Use organizational resources for induction and orientation.
4. Ascertain that each employee is adequately socialized to organizational values and unit norms.
5. Use creative and flexible scheduling based on patient care needs to increase productivity and retention.
6. Develop a program of staff education that will assist employees meeting the goals of the organization.

PATIENT CLASSIFICATION SYSTEM

The patient classification system (PCS), also known as patient acuity system, is a tool used for managing and planning the allocation of nursing staff in accordance with the nursing care needs. Thus, PCS is used to assist nurse leaders determine workload requirements and staffing needs. There are different kinds of PCS available, but the three most commonly used are:

1. **Descriptive:** This is a purely subjective system wherein the nurse selects which category the patient is best suited.

> **Box 8.5:** Categories of patient classification systems.
> - Category 1: Self-care requiring from 1 to 2 hours per day
> - Category 2: Minimal care requiring from 3 to 4 hours
> - Category 3: Intermediate care requiring from 5 to 6 hours
> - Category 4: Modified intensive care requiring from 7 to 8 hours
> - Category 5: Requiring from 10 to 14 hours

2. **Checklist:** Another subjective system, wherein the patient is assigned to a numerical value based on the level of activity in specific categories. The numerical value is added up to give the nurse an overall rating.
3. **Time standards:** This is another method where the nurse assigns a time value based on the various activities needed to be completed for the patient. This time value is sum up and converted to an acuity level.

Among these three, the most commonly used is the descriptive kind of Patient Classification System. These are subdivided into four classifications, namely **(Box 8.5)**:

1. **Self-care/minimal care:** The first classification of patients who are recovering and normally requires only diagnostic studies, minimal therapy, less frequent observations, and daily care for minor conditions and are awaiting elective surgery.
2. **Moderate care:** The patient in this category is moderately ill or under the recovery stage from a serious illness or operation. They require nursing supervision or assistance that is related to ambulating and caring for their own hygiene.
3. **Maximum care:** Patient needs close attention and complete care all through the shift. The nurses initiate, supervise and perform most of the patient's activities.
4. **Intensive care:** The last category or classification, wherein the patients are acutely ill and high level of nurse dependency is required. Intensive therapy and/or intensive nursing care are needed because of the unstable condition of the patient. Frequent evaluation, observation, monitoring and adjustment of therapy are also required. Patients in these levels include those in critical conditions or in life and death situations.

But whatever PCS is used, this will be applied to forecast staffing needs within each department. Nurses should be informed of the patient care ratios that are relevant to each department and should understand how to predict the staffing needs.

STAFF SCHEDULING

Staffing and scheduling are human resource allocations that select and assign employees to tasks within an organization, and specify when and for how long those tasks should be performed. In this context, an individual employee is a member of the staff and that staff member is assigned a specific schedule of work hours. By properly managing staffing and scheduling an employer can help to increase employee satisfaction and reduce safety risks **(Fig. 8.8 and Box 8.6)**.

Definition

- Staffing and scheduling are human resource allocations that select and assign employees to tasks within an organization, and specify when and for how long those tasks should be performed.
- Staffing is human resources planning to fill positions in an organization with qualified personnel.
- Scheduling is implementation of staffing pattern by assigning personnel to work specific hours and days in a specific unit or area.
- Staffing mix is the skill level of individuals delivering the required care. In nursing it includes registered nurses (RNs), licensed practical nurses (LPNs), nursing assistants and unlicensed assistive personnel.

Concept of Staff Scheduling

The objective of the nurse-scheduling problem is to determine the rotating shifts of the nursing staff over a schedule period (weekly or monthly). A nurse schedule includes the work shifts and days-off of the nursing staff, ensuring that all the combinations of shifts and days-off meet the manpower requirements of each shift (including total number of staff members, daily minimum number of staff members, and number of senior staff members required), and at the same time the number of basic days-off of each staff member should be fulfilled.

- In general, there are a lot of types of work shifts and days-off in shift schedules.
- The most common ones include the 2-shift rotation (i.e., 12-hour day shift and 12-hour night shift) and the 3-shift rotation (i.e., 8-hour day shift, 8-hour evening shift, and 8-hour night shift).
- Regular days-off allow the nursing staff to rest, and each staff member is entitled to the same number of days-off.
- Due to diverse personal lifestyles and different degrees of physical tolerance for continuous working days, the nursing staff usually have different preferences for work shifts and days-off.

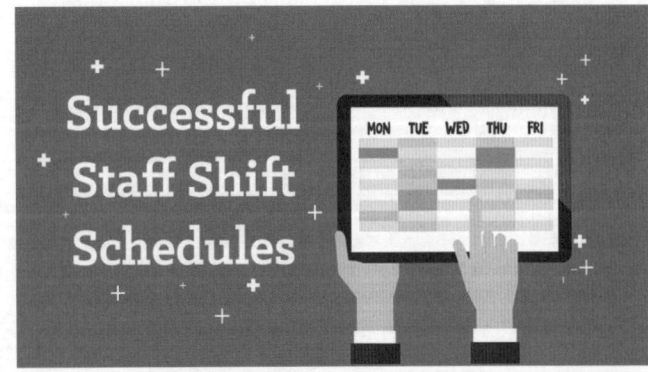

Fig. 8.8: Preparing staff shift schedules.

> **Box 8.6:** What is staff scheduling?
> - Staff scheduling problems are concerned with scheduling a workforce so as to meet demand which varies with the time of day and with the day of week.
> - The major challenge is providing a reasonable labor cost and customer satisfaction while meeting this varying demand.

Major Dimensions of Nursing Intensity

- Severity of client illness (the medical condition and how ill the person is abnormality and instability of physiological condition)
- Client dependency (need for assistance with ADLs activities of daily living)
- Complexity of nursing care
- Time (the hours of direct and indirect care received by a client)

Types of Staffing Schedules (Box 8.7)

Centralized Scheduling

The schedule done by the upper manager for all nurses in all departments manually or by computer.

Advantages

- Fairness to employees through consistent, objective, and impartial application of policies and opportunities for cost containment through better use of resources.
- Relieves nurse managers from time-consuming duties, freeing them for other activities.

Computer can be used for centralized scheduling. The advantage of this include cost-effectiveness through the reduction of clerical staff and better use of professional nurses by decreasing the time spent in non-patient care activities; unbiased, consistent scheduling; equitable application of agency policy; developed in advance so employees know what their schedule are and can plan their personal live accordingly.

Disadvantages

Lack of individualized treatment of employees is a chief complaint.

Decentralized Scheduling

When managers are given authority and assume responsibility, they can staff their own units through decentralized scheduling.

Advantages

- Personnel feel that they get more personalized attention with decentralized scheduling.
- Staffing is easier and less complicated when done for a small area instead of for the whole agency.
- Managers can work together to solve chronic staffing problems.

Box 8.7: Staff scheduling system.

- Provides automated 4–6 weeks schedule applying organizational policies
- Provides electronic tracking of staff trends
- Enforces organizational policies example no day shift after night shift
- Provides the tools to offer fair distribution of overtime and rotation of shifts
- Provides seamless tools to enhance staff satisfaction upon requesting time off, swap or floating

---

Box 8.8: Different types of shift.

- **Straight shift:** Staff work a specified number of hours continuously
- **Split shift:** Staff normally work a specified number of hours-then have a few hours off duty and return to work
- **Rotating shift:** Three shifts of 8 hours rotate—6–2, 2–10, 10–6
- **Alternating shift:** Staff work either a specified number of early and late shifts each week or one week early and one week late.

Disadvantages

- Some staff members may receive individualized treatment at the expense of others.
- Work schedules can be used as a punish reward system.
- Because it is consuming time, takes managers away from other duties or forces them to do the scheduling while off duty.
- It may use resources less efficiently and consequently make cost containment more difficult. **Box 8.8** summarizes different types of shift.

Self-scheduling

Self-scheduling is a system that is coordinated by staff nurses. Staff may negotiate before and after work and during break and lunchtime. They may also write notes to each other and Waite for responses.

Advantages

- Help create a climate where professional nursing can be practiced.
- Saves the manager considerable scheduling time and changes the role of the manager from supervisor to coach.
- Increases staff member's ability to negotiate with each others.
- Increased perception of autonomy, increased job satisfaction, increased cooperative atmosphere, improved team spirit, improved morale, decreased absenteeism, reduced turnover.

Alternating or Rotating Work Shifts

- Some nurses may work all three shifts within 7 days.
- Create stress for staff nurses.
- Body rhythms need time to adjust to the discrepancy between the person's activity cycle and the new demands of the environment. The ability of the body functions to adjust varies considerably among individuals. It may take 2–3 days to 2 weeks for a person to adjust to a different sleep-wake cycle.
- It effects the health of nurses and the quality of their work. Anorexia, digestive disturbances, disruption in bowel habits, fatigue, and error proneness.

Permanent Shift

Advantages

- Permanent shift relieve nurses from stress and health-related problems associated with alternating and rotating shifts.
- Provide social, educational, and psychological advantages.
- Staff can participate in social activities.

- They can continue their education by planning courses around their work schedules.
- Child care arrangement can be stable.
- Fewer health problems and less tardiness, absenteeism, and turnover.

Disadvantages

- Managers may have difficulty in evaluating the evening and night shifts.
- The staff of permanent shift not develops an appreciation for the workload or problems of other shifts.

Block, Cyclical, Scheduling

Block or cyclical, scheduling uses the same schedule repeatedly. The schedule repeats itself every 6 weeks.

Advantages

- Personnel know their schedules in advance and consequently can plan their social live.
- Absenteeism will be less.
- Establish stable work groups and decrease floating, thus promoting team spirit and continuity of care.

Variable Staffing

Method in which the number and mix of staff are determined by patient needs.

- Eight hour shift in a five day workweek 5-day, 40-hours workweek
- The shift usually 7 AM to 3:30 PM, 3 PM to 11:30 PM, and 11 PM to 7:30 AM and a half hour overlap time between shifts to provide for continuity of care.

Ten hour shift in four day workweek: The main problem was fatigue. The long weekends and off were attractions. There is time to finish work, peak workloads can be covered, and there is decreased overtime and decreased costs.

Twelve-hour shift in seven day workweek:

- The better use of personnel lowers staffing requirements; this consequently lowers the cost per patient day.
- Fewer communication gaps and better continuity of care. Improved nurse-patient relations, job satisfaction and morale.
- Working relations are improved. Team development is possible. No blames for problems.
- Total time off is increased, with an increased usefulness for other duties. Travel time is reduced. Overtime pay has been of some concern.

■ DUTY ROSTER (BOX 8.9)

In nursing management of any unit, time planning for the workers is a prerequisite for successful nursing operations because patterning of work and non-working hours directly affect the employee's productivity, work satisfaction and job tenure. So, scheduling id defined as a pattern of on-off duty hours for employees in a particular unit. Many different approaches to nurse staffing and scheduling are being tried in an effort to satisfy needs of the employees and meet workload demands for patient care. These include

> **Box 8.9:** Duty roster.
> - Duty roster of nursing staff for accident and emergency for the month of June 2009 is attached in the next slide.
> - If you can observer carefully, at any given point of time the average nurses available in this department is three.
> - Due to adjustments in duty so as to complete 208 hours of service per month there would be some additional allocation seen.
> - However, the intended nursing staff allocation to this department is three.

game theory, modified work weeks (10 to 12 hours shift), team rotation, premium day, weekend nurse staffing. Such approaches should support the underlying purpose, mission, philosophy and objectives of the organization and the division of nursing and should be well defined in a staffing philosophy, statements and policies.

Objectives or Purpose of Duty Roster

- To ensure adequate patient care while over staffing is avoided.
- To achieve desirable distribution of days off.
- To ensure fair treatment of nursing staff.
- To let individual know in advance what their schedules are.
- To achieve good unit management.
- To determine when the help is required from relief nurse.

Principles of Planning Duty Roster (Fig. 8.9)

- **Coverage:** Nursing coverage must be provided 24 hours a day, seven days a week with the right number and mix of the staff.
- **Continuity:** Continuity of quality and quality care.
- **Flexibility:** The ability of the scheduling system to handle change and consider individual preferences as much as possible.
- **Stability:** The extent to which nurses know in advance their future days off and on duty and in consistent with stable staffing policies.

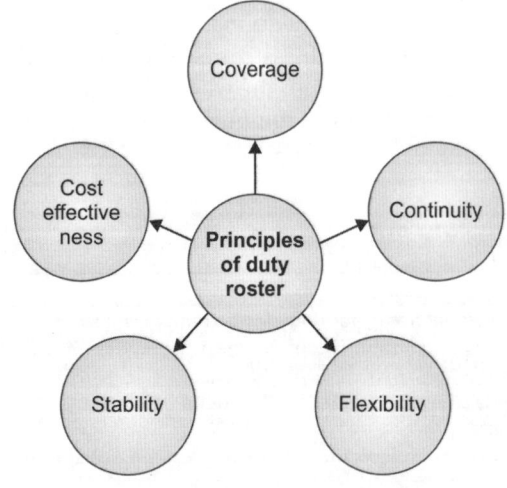

Fig. 8.9: Principles of duty rosters.

> **Box 8.10:** Before planning the duty roster.
> - Consider the amount of cover required.
> - Consider the types of shifts.
> - Make sure that all duties are covered.
> - Sufficient cover of all grades of staff-each shift.
> - Fair allocation of weekend work.
> - Take into account break periods.

- **Cost effectiveness:** The ability to assign the needed staff without over staff and ensuring maximum utilization of nurse's time and skills.
- **Modified work week:** This using 10 and 12 hour shifts and other methods are common place. A nurse administrator should be sure work schedules are fulfilling the staffing philosophy and policies, particularly with regard to efficiency. Also, such schedules should not be imposed on the nursing staff but should show a mutual benefits to employer, employees and the client served.

Planning Duty Roster (Box 8.10)

When writing the rota the following rules should apply:

- An identified nurse in-charge will be rostered and highlighted on each shift
- There will be an appropriate agreed skill mix on each shift which should be spread evenly throughout the 7 day working week.
- Staff numbers on shifts will be consistent in line with set establishments.
- Roster requests will be agreed and prioritized by the ward manager, provided that roster rules in regard to cover, skill mix and annual leave can be met.
- Requests will be granted in a fair and equitable way. Electronic rostering will facilitate an equitable allocation of requests to individual staff.
- Only in exceptional circumstances will staff who are employed on set hours or term time contracts, request alternative shifts or days off. This will require negotiation with another member of staff to cover their set shift.
- Flexibility will be promoted within the ward team
- Any duty rota changes must be legible, trackable and agreed with the ward manager or designated deputy.
- The annual leave allocation will not exceed or drop below the agreed weekly quota for each individual area (*see* section Annual Leave)
- Careful consideration by the ward manager and matron, should be given to the appropriateness of rostering two members of staff who are in personal relationship, onto the same shifts. This should be discussed fully with the staff in question.

The following details should be displayed on each duty roster:

- Trust logo
- Ward/Department/Unit name
- First name and surname of each member of staff
- Clinical grade of each member of staff
- Professional qualification of each member of staff to include NVQ qualification for HCSW's
- WTE and hours to be worked over the roster period for each member of staff
- Actual hours rostered for the roster period for each member of staff
- Tally of actual numbers of RN's on each shift.
- Tally of actual numbers of HCSW's on each shift
- Ongoing tally of hours worked, i.e., show positive or negative balance of hours worked by staff
- Vacancies expressed for each grade
- Signature of ward manager
- Signature of matron
- Show a key of the abbreviations and times of shifts worked in that ward area
- Clearly show meal break allowances for each shift

Ward Managers Shift Patterns

To facilitate effective leadership, availability and achieve optimum visibility, the ward manager should work a:

- Minimum of 4 day shifts each week, ideally 5 day shifts
- Maximum one late shift per week
- Maximum 9.5 hour shifts, ideally 7.5 hour shifts
- Maximum 2 weekend shifts each 4 week period
- Not work regular night shifts unless there is an exceptional clinical need or unresolved staffing problem.
- Band 7s who work in departments where they do not fulfill the ward manager role will be expected to work the shifts required by the department.

Out of Hours Senior Nurse Cover

Out of hours senior nursing cover to maintain professional leadership and the management of staffing trust wide, 7.30–8 PM. This rota will be hosted on the G drive maintained by the lead nurse for workforce. The shifts on the rota will be allocated to ensure equitable cover for all weekends, bank holidays and evenings.

- Agreed shifts—late 15.00–20.00,
- Weekend and bank holidays 07.30–14.00 and 13.45–19.45

Guide to Compiling Duty Roster (Part A)

- Use roster sheet as provided by health agencies.
- Do not cut sheets—always use full size and fill one sheet before going on to new sheet.
- Compile roster for one full calendar month in advance.
- Fill in headings-name of department-month dates and days of week.
- Rule lines in red to divide into complete weeks, e.g., from Saturday of the previous week to Friday of the following week.
- Write full name and designation of each staff member in left hand column.
- Ensure that the names of all staff including those on leave and new members are recorded accurately.

Level	Nurse #	Name	Week 1 S S M T W T F	Week 2 S S M T W T F	Week 3 S S M T W T F	Week 4 S S M T W T F	Day	Night	Total	% of Days	% of Nights
Staff Nurse 1	1	GM	N N N _ _ N N	_ _ N N _ _ _	_ _ D _ D D _	_ D D D _ _ _	8	7	15	53%	47%
	2	EH	D D _ _ D D D	_ D D D _ _ _	_ _ _ _ N N _	N N _ _ N N N	8	7	15	53%	47%
	3	MB	_ _ D D D _ _	_ D D D _ N N N	N _ _ _ N N N	_ N N _ _ _ _	6	9	15	40%	60%
	4	M.R	_ _ _ N N _ _	N N _ _ D D D N	_ D D D _ _ _	D D D _ _ D D	10	5	15	67%	33%
	6	DM	N N _ _ N N N	_ _ N N _ _ _	_ _ D D D _ _	D D _ N N N _	5	10	15	33%	67%
Staff Nurse 2	1	VA	_ _ N N N _ _	D D D _ _ _ D	D N N _ N N N	_ _ N N _ _ _	5	10	15	33%	67%
	2	EB	_ D D D _ N N	_ _ N N N _ _	N N _ _ _ N N	_ _ N N N _ _	3	12	15	20%	80%
	4	MD	_ D D _ _ D D	_ D D _ _ D D N N	N N N _ _ N N	_ _ _ _ _ _ _	8	7	15	53%	47%
	5	NT	N N _ _ _ N N	_ N N _ _ D D D	_ _ D D D _ _	D D D _ _ _ _	9	6	15	60%	40%
	6	RS	_ N N N _ _ _	N N _ _ N N N _	_ N N _ _ D D D	_ _ _ _ D D _	5	10	15	33%	67%
	7	CC	N N _ _ _ N N	_ D D D _ _ _	D D D _ _ N N _	_ N N N _ _ _	6	9	15	40%	40%
	8	RC	_ N N _ _ _ N N	N N N _ _ _ _	_ D D D _ _ D D	_ D D D _ _ _	8	7	15	53%	47%
NA	1	MN	D D D _ _ D D	_ _ D D _ _ _	D D D _ _ _ D D	_ _ _ D D _ _	15	0	15	100%	0%
		TDS	2 4 4 2 2 3 3	3 3 5 2 4 4 4	3 4 4 4 5 4 4	3 4 3 4 2 3 4 4					
		TNS	4 4 4 4 4 4 4	4 4 3 3 4 4 4	3 3 3 3 3 3 3	3 3 3 4 4 3 3					

(TDS: total day staff; TNS: total night staff; MDS: min day staff; MNS: min night staff; D: day shift; n: night shift; SN1: staff nurse 1; SN2: staff nurse 2; Na: nurse aid)

Fig. 8.10: Manual schedule for psychiatry unit.

- When staff leaves the department through transfer or resignation, draw two lines in red through remaining days of the month, indicating the new department, or resignation, or end of contract.
- Enter leave by ruling a line between the agreed dates. For example, 30 days AL + 45 days ML — 15.12.2007
- Use accepted symbols only

Guide to Compiling Duty Roster (Part B)

- Before starting, check request book for any special requests.
- All shifts M (morning), A (afternoon), N (night) should be written in blue felt pen.
- DO (day off), PH (public health holiday) should be written in top right corner, e.g., PH6, etc.
- Asterisk (*) the name of the staff nurse in charge for each shift.
- Count numbers on each shift according to grade, total and record on roster.
- Duty roster should be submitted to nursing officer NS for checking and approval one week before they are due to come into force.
- Staff who resigns at any time during the year are only entitled to the number of PHs occurring up to the date of resignation.
- Copy of the completed roster checked and signed by the ward in charge and nursing officer is to be submitted to nursing administration not later than 26th/27th day of each month. **Figure 8.10** shows manual schedule for psychiatry unit.

STAFFING ACTIVITIES IN NURSING

Staffing function is related to the employment of nursing personnel of all types. It includes various types of activities to get the right type of nurses on the right job. It is concerned with the filling of various type of positions or jobs in the nursing organization with suitable nursing personnel.

Definition

- **WHO expert committee** on nursing defines the nursing services as the part of the total health organization which aims to satisfy major objective of the nursing services is to provide prevention of disease and promotion of health.
- **Nursing services:** Nursing service is the part of the total health organization which aims at satisfying the nursing needs of the patients/community. In nursing services, the nurse works with the members of allied disciples, such as dietetics, medical social service, pharmacy, etc., in supplying a comprehensive program of patient care in the hospital.

Essentials of Nursing Service

The outcome of our journey is the achievement of the eight essentials of a Magnet Designated facility; fundamentals to create an environment that:

1. Embraces patient care as the priority
2. Promotes interdisciplinary collaboration
3. Encourages professional development
4. Supports evidence-based autonomous practice
5. Provides adequate staffing
6. Recruits and retains qualified and competent staff
7. Shares control for professional practice
8. Provides excellent leadership and management

Through our nursing vision, values, and philosophy it is our passion to promote excellence in nursing practice and support the health system's mission to improve the health of the communities we serve with quality and compassion by providing extraordinary nursing care.

Together with professional care, warmth, friendliness and the sharing of joys and sorrows help to make each hospital and hospice a place where hearts can be lightened, work enjoyed, happiness shared and health restored. The care provided by the nurse and other staff and the ethos of the hospital are formed and shaped by the traditions, principles. The values on which their clinical care is based include a profound respect for human life and for each individual person irrespective of color, race, creed, gender, and sexual orientation, physical or mental disabilities.

Classification of Nursing Practice Personnel

The department consists of two main classifications:
1. **Professional nursing personnel:** They are director, assistants, supervisors, first-line managers (RN) and staff nurses.
2. **Nonprofessional nursing personnel:** They are practical nurses (assistant nurses), nurse aides, orderlies and clerks. **Box 8.11** summarizes staffing activities.

Functions of the Nursing Service Department

- To plan, provide and evaluate nursing care for patient and families.
- To define and implement the philosophy, objectives and standards for nursing care of the patients.
- To provide and implement a departmental plan of administrative authority which delineates responsibilities and duties of each category of nursing personnel.
- To coordinate the functions of the department with the functions of all other departments.

Box 8.11: Staffing activities.
- Recruitment
- Recruitment planning
- Recruitment challenges
- Recruitment sources
- Electronic recruiting
- Recruitment yield pyramid
- Legal issue
- Selection
- Selection process
- Interview components techniques
- Types of interviews
- Interviewing and legal considerations
- Assessment centers

- To estimate the requirements of the department.
- To interpret hospital and nursing practice objectives to the patients and community.
- To participate in the formulation of personnel policies, to implement established policies and evaluate their effectiveness.
- To develop an effective system of nursing records and reports.
- To estimate needs for facilities, supplies and equipment.
- To participate in financial planning.
- To participate in studies and research projects for the improvement of patient care and hospital services.
- To provide and implement continuing education program for all nursing personnel.
- To participate in and or facilitate all educational programs of students in the health care field.

Specific Functions of Nursing Unit

- Provide and maintain the highest quality patient care with the lowest possible cost.
- Furnish the most desirable environment (safe, comfortable and pleasant) for patients and health service personnel, i.e., medical and nursing staff as well as the other hospital personnel.
- Consider needs of patients families and significant others.
- Provide adequate space to facilitate the carrying out of all the activities needed, i.e., using different types of equipment with minimum waste of personnel time, i.e., wide doors and corridors, wheel chair with IV stand, patient movement in their beds with attached apparatus- improves quality care.
- Promote job satisfaction of the health personnel.

Factors Influencing Nursing Service

These factors include:
- The type of service to be provided, i.e., medical, surgical, obstetrics, gynecology, pediatrics, psychiatric, etc. The acuteness of the service.
- The experience of the nurses who are to give the patient care.
- The number of non-nurses who involve in patient care, their quality and stability of service.
- The amount of quality of teaching given in-service preparation.
- The physical facilities available.
- The amount, type, location of equipment and supplies.
- The number of working hours of nurses and the flexibility in hours.
- The morale of the workers.
- The method of assignment.

For organizing functions to be productive and facilitate meeting the organizations needs, the leader must know the organization and its members well. The roles and functions of the leader/manager in organizing groups for patient care are:

Leadership Roles Associated with Organizing Patient Care

- Periodically evaluates the effectiveness of the organizational structure for the delivery of patient care.

- Determines if adequate resources and support exist before making any changes in the organization of patient care.
- Examines the human element in work redesign and supports personnel during adjustment to change.
- Inspires the work group toward a team effort.
- Inspires subordinates to achieve higher levels of education, clinical expertise, competency, and experience in differentiated practice.
- Ensures that chosen nursing care delivery models advance the practice of professional nursing.

Management Functions Associated with Organizing Patient Care

- Examines the unit philosophy to ensure that it supports any change in the patient care delivery system.
- Selects a patient care delivery system that is most appropriate to the needs of the patients being served.
- Uses scientific research and current literature to analyze proposed changes in nursing care delivery models.
- Uses a patient care delivery system that maximizes human and physical resources as well as time.
- Ensures that nonprofessional staff are appropriately trained and supervised in the provision of care.
- Organizes work activities to attain organizational goals.
- Groups activities in a manner that facilitates communication and coordination within and between departments.
- Organizes work so that it is cost-effective as possible.
- Makes changes in work design to facilitate meeting organizational goals.
- Clearly delineates criteria to be used for differentiated practice roles.

Nursing service management is one of the prerequisite for good nursing care.

Management of work, management of personnel and maintenance of records and reports are important in ward management.

Common Nursing Service Activities

Hygiene, nutrition, medications, fluid management, skin and wound care, respiratory care, circulatory care, elimination, mobility, special diagnostic and treatment procedures, health teaching and daily activities of living. After care descriptors have been selected, the levels of care, intensity is defined for each descriptor. The level is differentiated by the amount of nursing time and frequency of each care measure.

- **The factor system** is referred to as objective because specifying particular indicators or factors associated with patient care helps to ensure objectivity by the rater.
- **Prototype evaluation system:** This is considered subjective and uses broad descriptive categories to describe the patient and needs. Characteristics are listed for a typical patient in each of the categories.
  - **Type-I:** Patients with acute, episodic disease or disability who will return to their pre-illness level to functioning and for whom the goal is to relieve existing health problem.
  - **Type-II:** Patients with chronic disease with acute episode of illness, but has potential to return to pre-episodic level of functioning where the chronic health problem can be managed by self or the family.
  - **Type-III:** Patients with chronic disease where return to pre-illness level of functioning, but potential to increase level of functioning with care goal is rehabilitation to a maximum level of functioning with agency support.
  - **Type-IV:** Patients with chronic disease who cannot be maintained at home without ongoing agency support.
  - **Type-V:** Patient with end stage of illness. However, the most effective patient classification system is one that is specifically tailored to the clinical situation where it will be used. **Figure 8.11** shows common Nursing Service approaches.

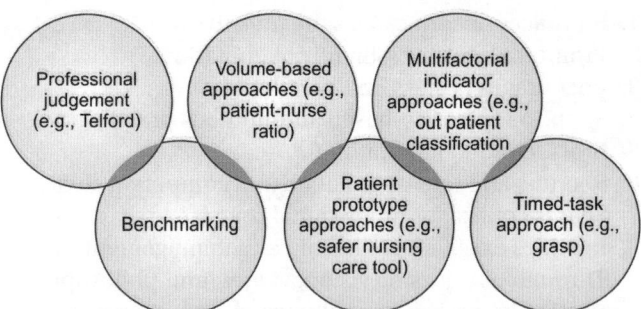

Fig. 8.11: Common nursing service approaches.

Role and Responsibilities

There are six main roles and functions of the nurse manager listed by American Organization of Nurse Executives (AONE):

1. The nurse manager is accountable for excellence in the clinical practice of nursing and the delivery of patient care on a selected unit or area within the health care institutions.
2. The nurse manager is accountable for managing human, fiscal and other resources needed to a manage clinical nursing practice and patient care.
3. The nurse manager is accountable for facilitating development of licensed and unlicensed nursing and healthcare personnel.
4. The nurse manager is accountable for ensuring institutional compliance with professional, regulatory, and government standards of care.
5. The nurse manager is accountable for planning as it relates to the units or areas, department, and organization as a whole.
6. The nurse manager is accountable for facilitating cooperative and collaborative relationship among disciplines/departments to ensure effective delivery of quality care.

RECRUITMENT

Recruitment refers to the discovery and developments of the sources of require personnel so that sufficient number of candidates will always be available for employment in the organization. It involves identifying an attracting job candidate who has the required abilities, attitudes and motivation so as to meet the manpower requirements of the enterprise.

Definition: Recruitment has been defined as "the process of searching of prospective employees and stimulating them to apply for jobs in the organizations".

Methods of Recruitment

- **Transfer:** A transfer refers to the shifting of an employee from one job to another without a drastic change in the responsibilities and status of the employee.
- **Promotion:** It involves shifting an employee to a higher position carrying higher responsibilities, higher status and more pay.
- **Advertisements:** Advertising in newspaper or trade and professional journals is a very popular source of recruitment.
- **Employment agencies:** The government of India has set up a network of employment exchanges throughout the country. These exchanges maintain detailed records of job seeker and refer appropriate candidates to the employers.
- **Educational institutions:** Colleges and institutes of management and technology have become a popular source of recruitment for technical professional and managerial jobs.
- **Recommendations:** Applicants introduced by present employees, for their friends and relatives may prove to be a good source of recruitment.
- **Casual callers:** Many well reputed business organizations draw a steady stream of unsolicited applicants in their offices. Such job seekers can be a valuable source of manpower.
- **Direct recruitment:** Under this source of recruitment a notice is placed on the notice board of the enterprise specifying the details of the jobs available.
- **Labor contracts:** Labors contract maintain close contracts with laborers and they can provide the required number of workers at short notice. **Figure 8.12** shows recruitment and selection.

Factors Affecting Recruitment

Internal Factors include the following
- Budget constraints
- Expected or trend of employee separations
- Production levels
- Sales increases or decreases
- Global expansion plans

External Factors might include the following
- Changes in technology
- Changes in laws
- Unemployment rates
- Shifts in population
- Shifts in urban, suburban, and rural areas
- Competition

Importance of Recruitment

Recruitment is one of the most fundamental activities of the HR team. If the recruitment process is efficient, then:
- The organization gets happier and more productive employees
- Attrition rate reduces
- It builds a good workplace environment with good employee relationships.
- It results in overall growth of the organization.

Purpose and importance of recruitment in an organization:
- It determines the current and future job requirement.
- It increases the pool of job at the minimal cost.
- It helps in increasing the success rate of selecting the right candidates.
- It helps in reducing the probability of short term employments.
- It meets the organization's social and legal obligations with regards to the work force.
- It helps in identifying the job applicants and selecting the appropriate resources.
- It helps in increasing organizational effectives for a short and long term.
- It helps in evaluating the effectiveness of the various recruitment techniques.
- It attracts and encourages the applicants to apply for the vacancies in an organization.

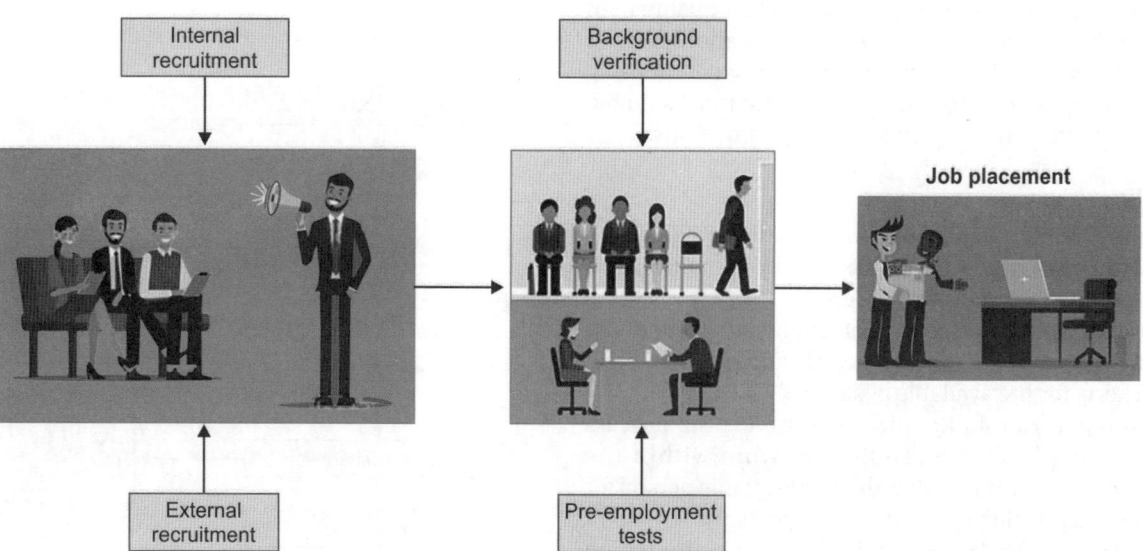

Fig. 8.12: Recruitment and selection.

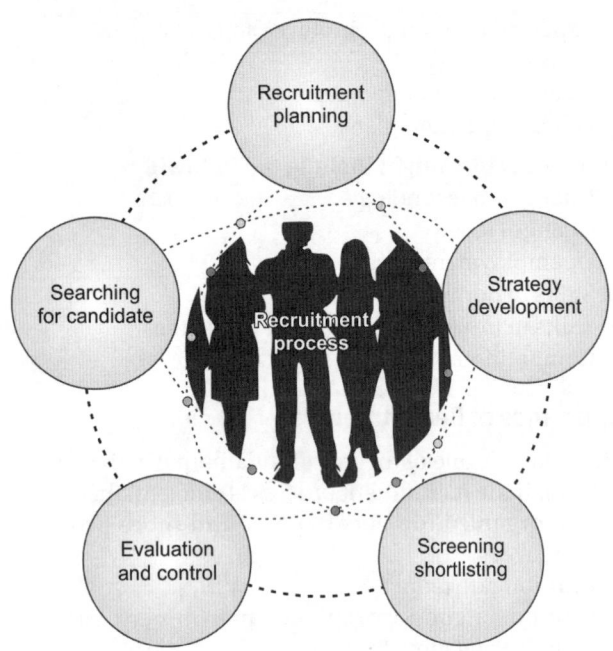

Fig. 8.13: Recruitment process.

- It determines the present futures requirements of the organization and plan according.
- It links the potential employees with the employers.
- It helps in increasing the success ratio of the selection process of prospective candidates.
- It helps in creating a talent pool of prospective candidates, which enables in selecting the right candidates for the right job as per the organizational needs. **Figure 8.13** shows recruitment process.

SELECTION

After recruitment, selection procedure has to be implemented. Selection process relates to the securing of relevant information about an applicant. This information can be obtained in different ways. Selection is actually matching people with the job. It is only the quality human force that matters much in the organizations. It is essential; therefore, to select quality men for placing them in right positions render quality services. Selection of men is a critical activity. It is a process of choosing from among the candidates from outside, the most suitable persons for the current position or for future positions.

Definition

- David and Robbins said, "Selection process is a managerial decision-making process as to predict which job applicants will be successful if hired."
- According to RM Hodgetts, "Selection is the process in which an enterprise chooses the applicants who best meet the criteria for the available positions."
- According to Harold Koontz, "Selection is the process of choosing from the candidates, from within the organization or from outside, the most suitable person for the current position or for the future positions."
- Dale Yoder said, "Selection is the process by which candidates for employment are divided into classes those who will be offered employment and those who will not."

Steps of Selection Procedures

1. Initial screening
2. Completion of the application form
3. Employment tests
4. Job interview
5. Conditional job offer
6. Background investigation
7. Medical examination
8. Permanent job offer

Figure 8.14 shows steps in selection process.

Importance of the Selection Process

- Proper selection and placement of employees lead to growth and development of the company. The company can similarly, only be as good as the capabilities of its employees.
- The hiring of talented and skilled employees results in the swift achievement of company goals.
- Industrial accidents will drastically reduce in numbers when the right technical staff is employed for the right jobs.
- When people get jobs, they are good at, it creates a sense of satisfaction with them and thus their work efficiency and quality improves.
- People who are satisfied with their jobs often tend to have high morale and motivation to perform better.

The major differences between recruitment and selection:

Recruitment	Selection
Recruitment is defined as the process of identifying and making the potential candidates to apply for the jobs.	Selection is defined as the process of choosing the right candidates for the vacant positions.
Recruitment is called as a positive process with its approach of attracting as many candidates as possible for the vacant jobs	Selection is called as a negative process with its elimination or rejection of as many candidates as possible for identifying the right candidate for the position.

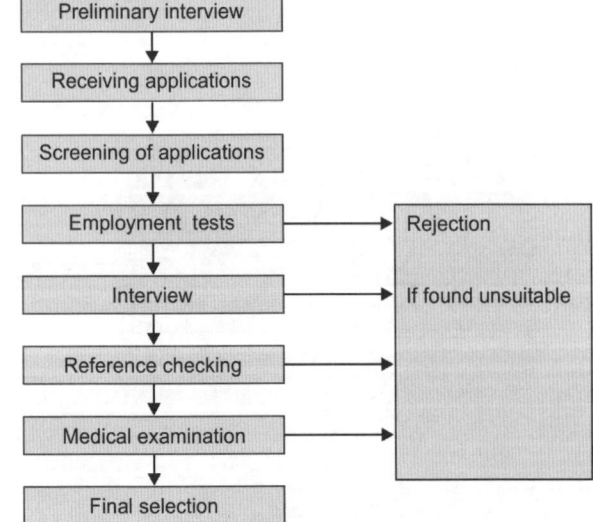

Fig. 8.14: Steps in selection process.

Advantages of Selection

A good selection process offers the following advantages:
- It is cost-effective and reduces a lot of time and effort.
- It helps avoid any biasing while recruiting the right candidate.
- It helps eliminate the candidates who are lacking in knowledge, ability, and proficiency.
- It provides a guideline to evaluate the candidates further through strict verification and reference-checking.
- It helps in comparing the different candidates in terms of their capabilities, knowledge, skills, experience, work attitude, etc.

■ DEPLOYMENT

Deployment is defined as the movement of staff from ones' current assignment to another to meet operational needs. He mentions such programs as including the training and development, reward system, performance evaluation programs and employee assistance programs and the employee deployment programs.
- Deploy means arrange, manage or give position to their employees.
- **Deployment in nursing:** Staff nurses having qualification of BSc or MSc nursing being deployed as teaching faculty in schools and colleges, i.e., redesignation form staff nurse to tutor/lecturer.

Objectives

- Delivering change faster and at optimum cost and minimized risk
- Successful and on schedule deployment of release package.
- New or changed services are capable of delivering the agreed service requirements.
- There is knowledge transfer to enable the customers and users to optimize their use of service to support their business activities.
- Minimal unpredicted impact on the production services, operation and support organization.
- Customers, users and service management staff are satisfied with service transition practices and outputs.

Deployment Management Process (Fig. 8.15)

- **Release management support:** It provides guidelines and support for the deployment of releases.
- **Release planning:** The objective of this process is to assign authorized changes to release packages. It also defines the scope of releases.
- **Release build:** This process deals with building releases and ensures all components are ready to enter the testing phase.
- **Release deployment:** The objective of this process is to deploy new release in the live environment and also arrange training for end users and operating staff.

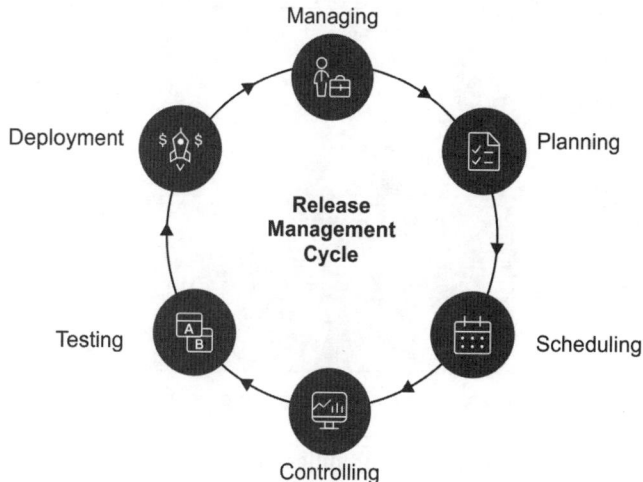

Fig. 8.15: Release/deployment management cycle.

- **Early life support:** The purpose of this process is to resolve operational issues during initial period after release deployment.
- **Release closure:** This process deals with closing a release after verifying if activity logs and CMS contents are up to date.

■ TRAINING

Management training is training activity that focuses on improving an individual's skills as a leader and manager. There may be an emphasis on soft skills, such as communication and empathy, which enable better team work and more progressive relationships with the people they manage.

Definition

- "Training is the act of increasing the knowledge and skills of an employee for doing a particular job."
  —*Edwin B Flippo*
- "Training is a process by which the attitudes, skills and abilities of employees to perform specific jobs are increased."
  —*Micheal J Jucious*
- "Training is the organized procedure by which people learn knowledge and/or skill for a definite purpose."
  —*EFL Breach*

Objectives

The objectives of training are as given here:
- To provide the knowledge about the working system, process and principles, etc.
- To provide the objective, plans and programs of the enterprise to employees
- To give the knowledge about new and innovative techniques of work performance
- To provide the norms, provisions, regulations and approaches concerning of the concern
- To raise the level of moral, enthusiasm, work spirit and work culture among employees

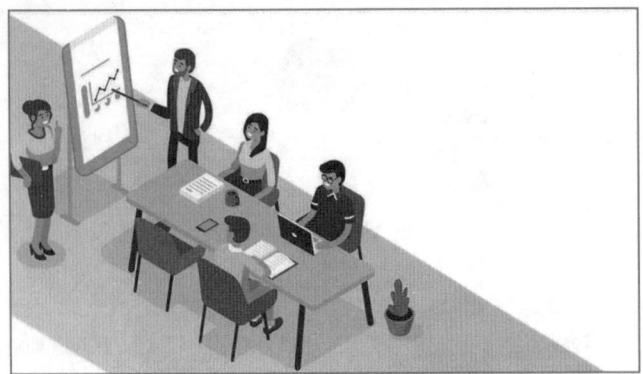

Fig. 8.16: How to design a winning employee training process.

- To enhance the potentialities for career development of employees
- To develop a suitable procedure of recruitment, selection and induction program
- To encourage new and innovative skills, efficiencies, capabilities, methods and techniques in operational scenario. **Figure 8.16** shows how to design a winning employee training process.

Types of Training

Generally given training in:
- Organization and control of production, maintenance and materials handling at the departmental levels.
- Planning, allocation and control of work and personnel.
- Planning their own work and allocation of time to their various responsibilities.
- Effect of industrial legislation at the departmental level.
- Cost factors and costs control
- Accident prevention
- Training of subordinates
- Communication, effective instructing, report-writing
- Handling and settling human/labor problems
- Leadership for effective working of the undertaking

Characteristics

The various important characteristics of training are:
- Training must be help to create an attitudinal change by creating awareness of the overall process.
- Training helps to perform the role of different sections of employees, the managerial responsibility and the importance of communication and participation
- It must enhance skills in organizational and managerial areas
- It must make orient new entrants in the organization to the discipline and culture requirement of the organization
- Proper orientation and training should be given to the new entrants.
- An effective training program should process the following characteristics.
- Training programs should be chalked out after identifying needs or goals.
- It should have relevance to the job requirements.
- An effective training program should be flexible.
- It should make due allowance for the differences among the individuals in regard to ability, aptitude, learning capacity, emotional make-up, etc.
- A good training performance should prepare the trainee mentally before they are imparted any job knowledge or skills.
- Training programs should be conducted by well qualified and experienced trainers.
- An effective training program should have the support from top management.
- Top management can gently influence the quality of training in the organization by the policies it adopts and the extent to which it supports training programs.
- An effective training program should be supported by critical appraisal of the outcome of the training efforts.

Need for Training (Fig. 8.17)

The need for training of employees arises due to the following factors:
- **Higher productivity:** It is essential to increase productivity and reduce cost of production for meeting competition in the market. Effective training can help increase productivity of workers by imparting the required skills.
- **Quality improvement:** The customers have become quality conscious and their requirement keep on changing. To satisfy the customers, quality of products must be continuously improved through training of workers.
- **Reduction of learning time:** Systematic training through trained instructors is essential to reduce the training period. If the workers learn through trial and error, they will take a longer time and even may not be able to learn right methods of doing work.
- **Industrial safety:** Trained workers can handle the machines safely. They also know the use of various safety devices in the factory. Thus, they are less prone to industrial accidents.
- **Reduction of turnover and absenteeism:** Training creates a feeling of confidence in the minds of the workers. It gives them a security at the workplace. As a result, labor turnover and absenteeism rates are reduced.

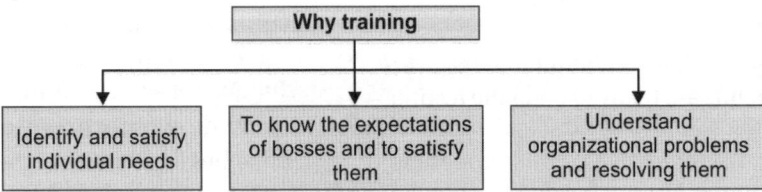

Fig. 8.17: Need and importance of training.

- **Technology update:** Technology is changing at a fast pace. The workers must learn new techniques to make use of advance technology. Thus, training should be treated as a continuous process to update the employees in the new methods and procedures.
- **Effective management:** Training can be used as an effective tool of planning and control. It develops skills among workers and prepares them for handling present and future jobs. It helps in reducing the costs of supervision, wastages and industrial accidents. It also helps increase productivity and quality which are the cherished goals of any modern organization. **Figure 8.18** shows steps in training process and **Figure 8.19** shows formal training program.

DEVELOPMENT (FIGS. 8.20 AND 8.21)

Employee development is defined as a process where the employee with the support of his/her employer undergoes various training programs to enhance his/her skills and acquire new knowledge and skills.

- Human resource development is the training and development of a company's workforce.
- Human resource development may be conducted formally, through training and education, or informally, through mentorship and coaching.
- Human resource development is important for cultivating an engaged and motivated workforce and leads to superior business results.

Definition

- "A conscious and systematic process to control the development of managerial resources in the organization for the achievement of goals and strategies."
- "It is a program of training and planned personal development purporting to prepare and aid managers in their present and future jobs." —*Yoder*

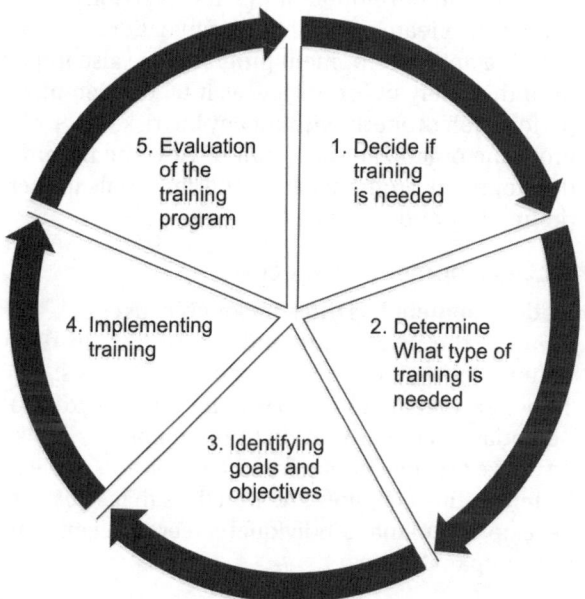

Fig. 8.18: Steps in training process.

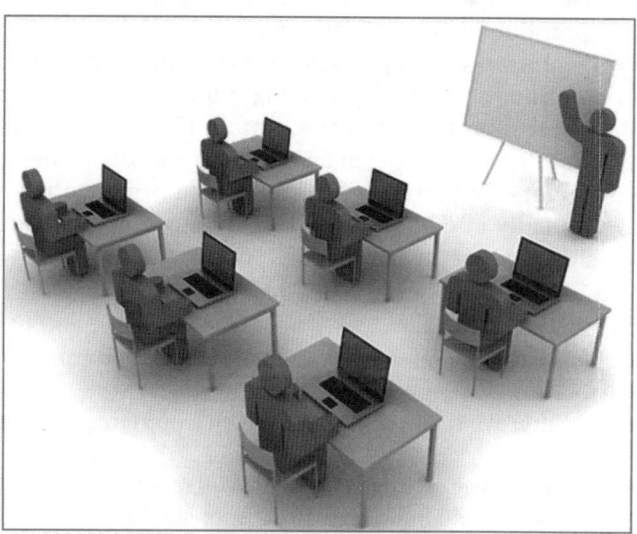

Fig. 8.19: Formal training program.

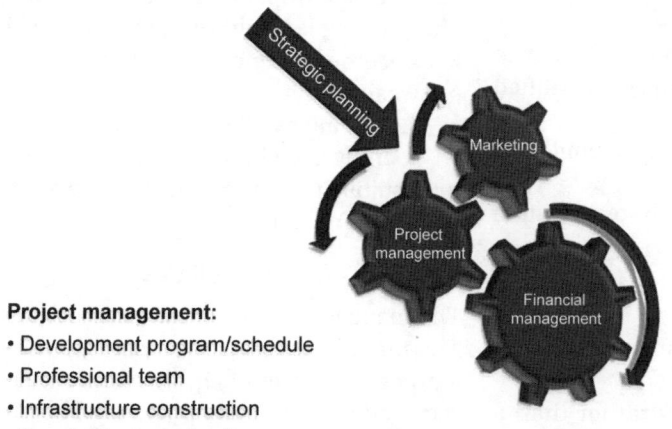

Marketing:
- Market determination
- Marketing strategy
- Sales
- Transfer of product

Project management:
- Development program/schedule
- Professional team
- Infrastructure construction
- Top structure construction

Financial management:
- Feasibility
- Budget
- Cash flow
- Funding

Fig. 8.20: Development management.

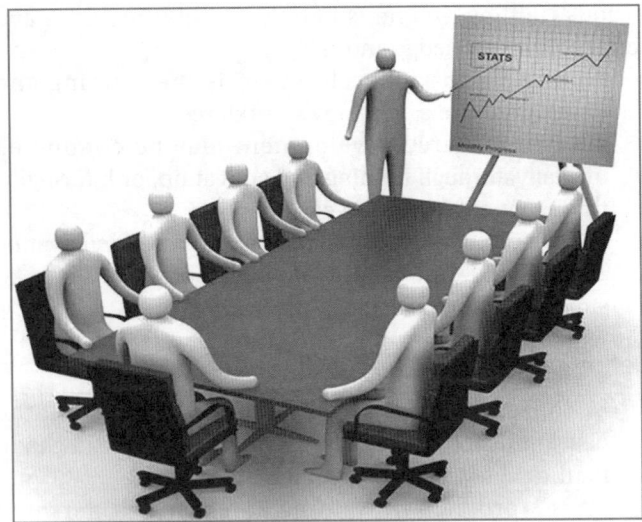

Fig. 8.21: Training and development in organization.

Objectives

- **Individual objectives:** Help employees in achieving their personal goals, which in turn, enhances the individual contribution to an organization.
- **Organizational objectives:** Assist the organization with its primary objective by bringing individual effectiveness.
- **Functional objectives:** Maintain the department's contribution at a level suitable to the organization's needs.
- **Societal objectives:** Ensure that an organization is ethically and socially responsible to the needs and challenges of the society.

Purposes

- To sustain better performance of managers throughout their careers.
- To improve the existing performance of managers at all levels.
- To encourage existing managers to increase their capacity to assume and handle greater responsibility.
- To enable the organization to have the availability of required number of managers with the required skills to meet the present and anticipated (future) needs of the organization.
- To replace elderly executives who have risen from the ranks by highly competent and academically qualified professionals.
- To provide opportunities to the executives to fulfil their career aspirations.
- To ensure that the managerial resources of the organization are utilized optimally.

Characteristics of Development

The characteristics of management development are as follows:
- It is an organized process of learning rather than a haphazard or trial and error approach.
- It is a long-term process as managerial skills cannot be developed overnight.
- It is an ongoing exercise rather than a "one-shot" affair. It continues throughout an executive's entire professional career because there is no end to learning.
- Management development aims at preparing managers for better performance and helping them to realize their full potential.
- Executive development is guided self-development. An executive can provide opportunities for development of its present and potential managers.

Importance of Training and Development

- In Human Resource Management (HRM) training and development is important aspect when company wants optimum utilization of their manpower.
- Training and development is a key for the succession planning of the organization as it helps in improvement of skills, such as team management and leadership.
- Training and development activities are vital to motivate the employee and to increase their productivity.
- Training and development in HRM is significant aspect to develop a team spirit in the organization.
- Training and development programs are also important from the safety point of view as it teaches employee to perform job properly without any life risk.
- From the organizational point of view the training and development programs are important tools to increase profitability and enhance corporate image.

Career Development—Objectives

Career development has three major objectives:
1. To meet the immediate and future human resource requirements of the company on a timely basis.
2. To better update the company and the individual about potential career path within the company.
3. To utilize existing human resource programs to the fullest by integrating activities and practices that select, assign, develop, and manage individual careers in alignment with the company's plan.

Career Development Process

Career planning entails an individual and organizational requirements and options that can be matched in a variety of ways. Thus, career planning is the process through which employees:
- Become aware of their interests, values, strengths and weakness.
- Collect information about job options within the company.
- Identify and choose career goals.
- Establish action plans to achieve those specific career goals and objectives.

Manager's Responsibilities

The manager should act as a catalyst and sounding board. The manager should show an employee how to go about a process and then help the employee understand what is required of him in the position. The immediate manager facilitates guidance and encouragement. The manager typically verifies the employee's readiness for job mobility. Moreover, managers are often the primary source of information about position openings, training courses, and other development options.

CREDENTIALING (BOX 8.12)

Credentialing is the process of establishing the qualifications of licensed medical professionals and assessing their background and legitimacy. Many healthcare institutions and provider networks conduct their own credentialing, generally through a credentialing specialist or electronic service, with review by a credentialing committee. It may include granting and reviewing specific clinical privileges, and allied health staff membership.

Definition

- Credentialing is the process of establishing the qualifications of licensed medical professionals and assessing their background and legitimacy.
- Credentialing is the process of obtaining, verifying, and assessing the qualifications of a practitioner to provide care or services in or for a healthcare organization. Credentials are documented evidence of licensure, education, training, experience, or other qualifications.

Credentialing: Credentialing refers to ways in which professional competence is ensured and maintained. Three processes are used for credentialing in nursing. They are accreditation, licensure and certification.

Licensure: Licensure is a specialized form of credentialing based on laws passed by a state legislature. A license is a legal document that permits a person to offer to the public skills and knowledge in a particular jurisdiction, where such practice would otherwise be unlawful without a license

Purpose of credentialing: Credentialing is the process of obtaining, verifying, and assessing the qualifications of a practitioner to provide care or services in or for a health care organization. Credentials are documented evidence of licensure, education, training, experience, or other qualifications.

Examples of credentials include academic diplomas, academic degrees, certifications, security clearances, identification documents, badges, passwords, user names, keys, powers of attorney, and so on.

Credential Management Services

The credential management services (CMS) in the Federal ICAM architecture include Sponsorship, Registration, Issuance, Maintenance, and Revocation.

- **Sponsorship:** Formally establish that a person or entity requires a credential. Keywords: Sponsor, Authorizing Official, Affiliation, Request
- **Registration:** Collect the information needed from a person or entity to issue them a credential. Keyword: Enrollment
- **Issuance:** Assign a credential to a person or entity. Keywords: Activation, Token
- **Maintenance:** Maintain a credential throughout its lifecycle. Keywords: Renewal, Reset, Suspension, Reissuance
- **Revocation:** Withdraw a credential from a person or entity, or deactivate an authenticator. Keywords: Termination.

Credentialing in Nursing

Credentialing allows nurses to gain formal recognition of their level of expertise and skill in their clinical practice, their leadership, their education and their research in a way that is recognizable to colleagues, employers, patients and the public.

- Credentialing is the process of assessing the background and legitimacy of nurses to practice at an advanced level through assessing their qualifications, experience and competence.
- Credentialing allows nurses to gain formal recognition of their level of expertise and skill in their clinical practice, their leadership, their education and their research in a way that is recognizable to colleagues, employers, patients and the public. **Figure 8.22** shows types of credentialing.

RETAINING

Employee retention involves taking measures to encourage employees to remain in the organization for the maximum period of time. Organization is facing a lot of problems in employees retaining these days. Employees stay and leave organizations foe some reasons. The reason may be personal or professional. These reasons should be understood by the employer and should be taken care of. The organizations are becoming aware of these reasons and adopting many strategies for employee retention.

Definition

According to the Business Dictionary, employee retention refers to "an effort by a business to maintain a working environment which supports current staff in remaining with the company."

Box 8.12: Nursing credentialing.

- **Licensure:**
  - Restrictive: Governmental requirement for practice
  - Protects practice and title
  - To protect public from incompetent practitioners
  - Usually includes examination/assessment
- **Certification:**
  - Voluntary: Non-governmental; not required for practice
  - Recognizes individual's advanced knowledge and skill
  - To inform public that-certified individuals have certain degree of knowledge and skill
  - Usually includes examination/assessment

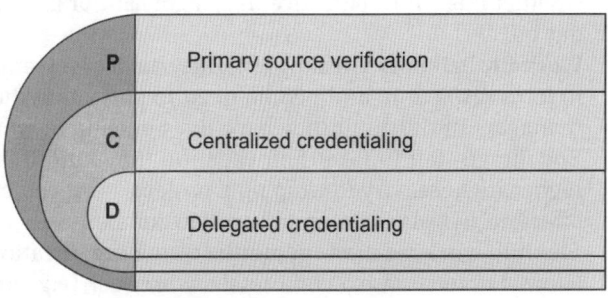

Fig. 8.22: Types of credentialing.

Meaning

Employee retention refers to the ability of an organization to retain its employees. Employee retention can be represented by a simple statistic (for example, a retention rate of 80% usually indicates that an organization kept 80% of its employees in a given period). Employee retention refers to the ability of an organization to retain its employees. However, many consider employee retention as relating to the efforts by which employers attempt to retain the employees in their workforce.

Methods of Improve Employee Retention

- **On boarding and orientation:** Every new hire should be set up for success from the very start. The on boarding process should teach new staff members not only about the job, but also the company culture and how they can contribute and thrive.
- **Mentorship programs:** Pairing a new employee with a mentor is a great component to add to the continuing on boarding process. Mentors can offer guidance and be a sounding board for newcomers, welcoming them into the company.
- **Employee compensation:** It Is absolutely essential in this competitive labor market for companies to offer attractive compensation packages. That includes salaries, of course, but also bonuses, paid time off, health benefits and retirement plans.
- **Perks:** Whether it Is paid time off for volunteering, occasional catered lunches or free snacks and coffee every day, perks can make your workplace stand out and boost employee morale.
- **Wellness offerings:** Keeping employees fit, mentally, physically and financially, is just good business.
- **Communication and feedback:** Keeping open lines of communication are a formal way of describing a practice that's essential for employee retention.
- **Annual performance reviews:** Even if you have met with employees throughout the year to check on their job satisfaction, never skip a regular big-picture conversation.
- **Training and development:** Make it a priority to invest in your workers' professional development and seek opportunities for them to grow. Some companies pay fees and travel for employees to attend conferences or industry events each year, provide tuition reimbursement, or pay for continuing education training.
- **Recognition and rewards systems:** Every person wants to feel appreciated for the work they do. Make it a habit to thank your direct reports when they go the extra mile, whether it is with a sincere email, a gift card or an extra day off.
- **Work-life balance:** A healthy work-life balance is essential to job satisfaction, and people need to know that their managers understand they have lives outside of work. Encourage staff to take their vacation time, and if late nights are necessary to wrap up a project, see if you can offer late arrivals or an extra day off to compensate.
- **Flexible working arrangements:** Some organizations allow staff to choose a compressed workweek (e.g., four 10-hour days) or flextime, where employees are on the clock, say, from 6 AM to 4 PM or 10 AM to 7 PM. The ability to telecommute-and avoid sitting in traffic-one or two days a week can be a significant stress reliever and retention booster.
- **Dealing with change:** Every workplace has to deal with change, and staff will look to leadership for reassurance. If your organization is going through a merger, a layoff or another big shift, keeping your staff as informed as you can will help you manage the rumor mill.
- **Fostering teamwork:** When people work together, make sure everyone, not just your team's stars, has a chance to contribute ideas and solutions. Further foster culture of collaboration by accommodating individuals' working styles and giving them the latitude to make smart decisions.
- **Acknowledge milestones large and small:** Whether the team just finished a huge project under budget or an employee celebrated a 10-year work anniversary, seize the chance to celebrate together with a shared meal or group excursion. **Figure 8.23** shows employee retention techniques and **Figure 8.24** shows factors affecting employee retention. **Figure 8.25** shows employee retention strategies.

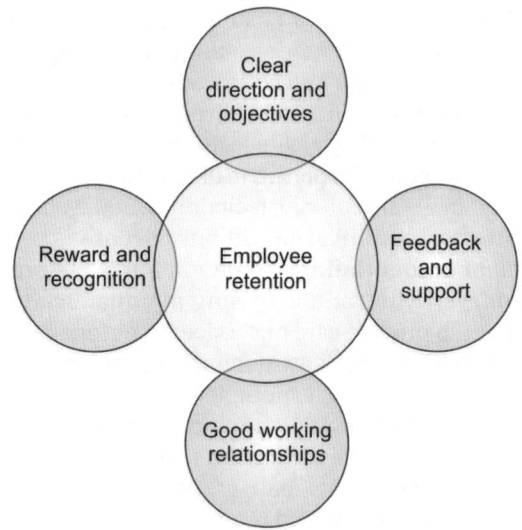

Fig. 8.23: Employee retention techniques.

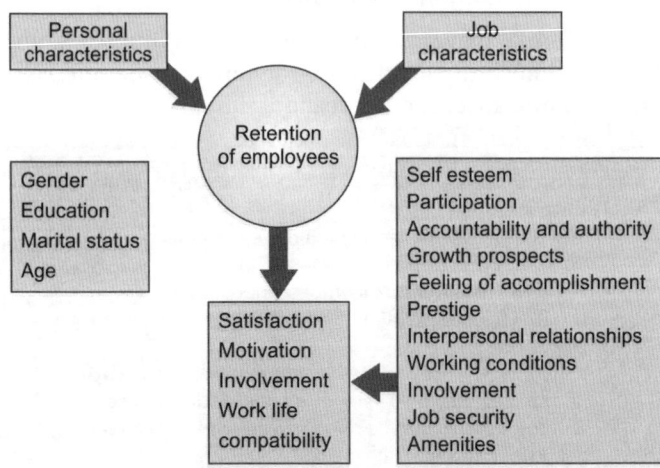

Fig. 8.24: Factors affecting employee retention.

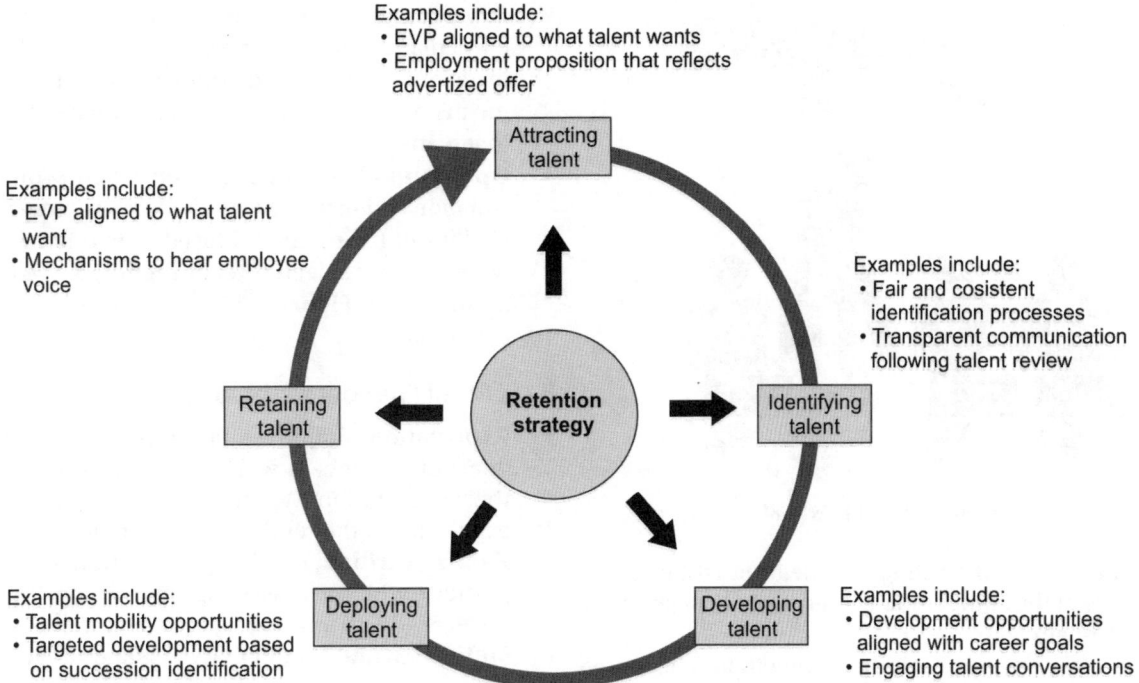

Fig. 8.25: Employee retention strategies.

Advantages

- Avoids and or reduces hiring costs.
- Retaining employees reduces training costs.
- It builds a team of skilled and experienced employees.
- Retaining experienced staff creates a positive impact on customer services.
- Retention activity fosters loyalty towards the organization amongst employees.
- Encourages friendly environment and fosters bonding amongst employees.
- It facilitates smooth workflow of internal processes.
- It increases the quantity of work delivered.
- It enhances the quality of the work produced.
- It increases revenue for the organization.

Disadvantages

- It promotes groupism amongst old employees which creates an insecure environment for new employees.
- Improper mixing of staff affects productivity and ensures poor quality of work.
- Excessive liberty to staff just to maintain work flow affects quantity and quality both.
- Flexible work timings rarely justify the work delivered.
- Retaining non-delivering staff kills the productivity and creativity of knowledgeable employees.
- Retaining spoon-fed and complaining employees add to the cost of the organization.

■ PROMOTING

"Promotion" is a term which covers a change and calls for greater responsibilities and usually involves higher pay and better terms and conditions of service and, therefore, a higher status or rank. Promotion is an upward movement or advancement of an employee in the organization to another job which commands better pay, prestige or status and higher challenges, responsibilities, opportunities, better working environment and hours of work facilities.

Meaning

Employee promotion means the ascension of an employee to higher ranks. It involves an increase in salary, rank, responsibilities, status, and benefits. This aspect of the job is what drives employees the most.

Definition

- According to Scott and Clothier—"A promotion is the transfer of an employee to a job which pays more money or one that carries some preferred status."
- According to Paul Pigors and Charles A Myers, Promotion is advancement of an employee to a better job—better in terms of greater responsibility, more prestige or status, greater skills and especially increased rate of pay or salary.

Objectives

There are number of objectives for which organizations promote their employees:

- For the optimum utilization of the employees' skill, knowledge at the appropriate level in the organizational hierarchy resulting in organizational effectiveness and employee satisfaction.
- For the development of competitive spirit and inculcate the enthusiasm in the employees to acquire the skill, knowledge, etc., needed for the higher level jobs.
- To develop competent internal source of employees ready to take up jobs at higher levels in the changing environment.

Chapter 8: Staffing

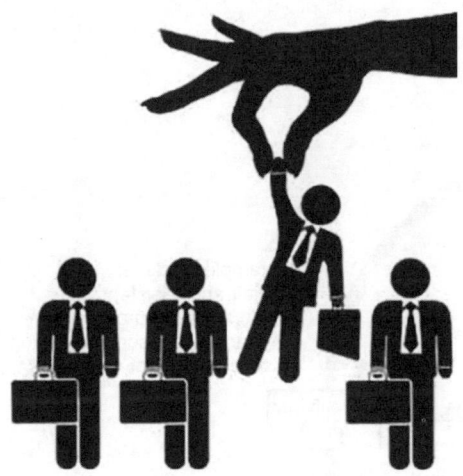

Fig. 8.26: Staff selecting method.

- For the promotion of a feeling of content with the existing conditions of the company and a sense of belongingness to the company.
- To promote employee's self-development and be ready for the promotion as and when their turn of promotion occurs.
- To promote interest in training, development programs and in team development areas.
- To get rid of the problems created by the leaders of workers' unions by promoting them in the officers' levels where they are less effective in creating problems.

Types of Employee Promotion

- **Horizontal promotion:** This kind of promotion rewards an employee with an increase in pay, but little to no change in responsibilities. It is also regarded as an up-gradation of an employee. In the educational sector, an example of this is the move from lecturer to senior lecturer.
- **Vertical promotion:** This refers to an upward movement of employees with a change in skills and experience. It brings a change in salary, responsibility, status, benefits, etc. In the marketing industry, this can be the promotion of a marketing supervisor to the marketing manager.

    Due to its nature, it can also change the nature of the job as well. This can be a shift from functional head to the chief executive, both being very different jobs.

- **Dry promotion:** A promotion that employees are not particularly fond of. This promotion refers to an increase in responsibilities and status without the benefits. It means no increase in pay or any financial benefits for that matter.
- **Open and closed promotion:** Open promotion is a situation where in every individual of an organization is eligible for the position. Closed promotion is a situation wherein only selected team members are eligible for a promotion. **Figure 8.27** shows criteria for employee promotion.

Benefits of Employee Promotion

- **Expectation:** Employee Promotion is one of the main goals of employees working hard. Thus, it turns into their expectation. When employers do not fulfill these expectations, they end up losing employees.
- **Reduce attrition:** Employee promotion often includes a pay raise which acts as a huge motivation. This in return further reduces attrition.
- **Motivation and productivity:** As stated above, employee promotion is a big tool for career advancement and employee retention. It is because when employees get a chance to grow they stick with a company. This motivation ultimately correlates to higher productivity.
- **Cost-efficient:** Internal employee promotion involves less cost than hiring new ones.
- **Career growth:** Employee promotion facilitates the very important career path and growth of an individual.
- **Need to manage:** Employee promotion often brings new responsibilities that initiate a sense of management. This sense of management is a key factor in employee satisfaction as it helps them grow.
- **Rewards and recognition:** Employee promotion is a crucial element of an organization's rewards and recognition program. This reduces retention, employee engagement, and motivation. **Figure 8.28** shows managing promotions and transfer.

Benefits of Promotion

- Recognizes and promotes employee performance, ambition, and morale
- Boosts motivation and increases employee loyalty
- Encourages retention
- Develops competitive spirit in the workplace
- Grooms future leaders
- Reduces employee resistance and discontent

Box 8.13 summarizes promotion policy

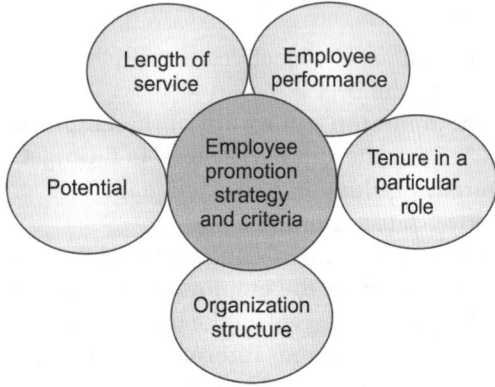

Fig. 8.27: Criteria for employee promotion.

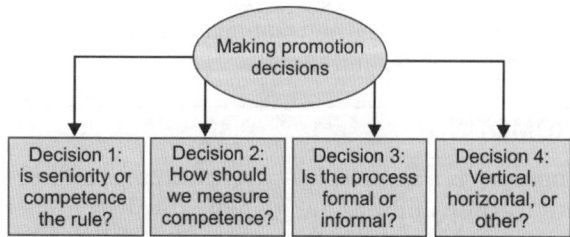

Fig. 8.28: Managing promotions and transfer.

> **Box 8.13:** Sound promotion policy.
> - Uniform
> - Consistent—applied uniformly to all employees
> - Fair and impartial
> - Systematic line of promotion channel
> - Equal opportunities
> - Clear-cut norms for judging the merit, etc.
> - Appropriate authority should make the final decision
> - Favoritism should be avoided
> - Must contain promotional counseling, encouragement, guidance and follow-up
> - Definite basis for promotion

■ TRANSFER

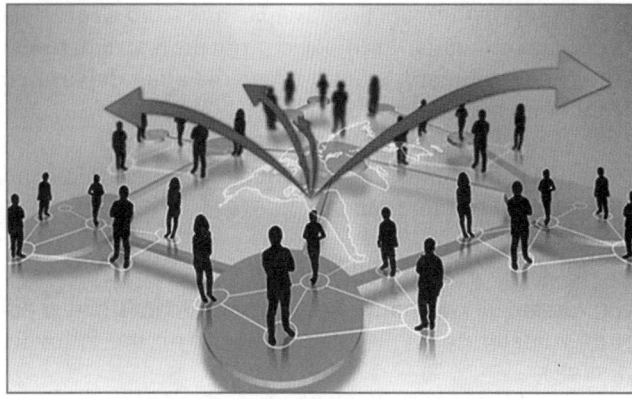

Fig. 8.30: Employee transfer method.

Employee transfer is the most important part of an organization which allows the company to shift, the employee from one department to the other. This process is usually a horizontal movement in an organization where there is no change in the employee's responsibilities.

Definition

- According to Edwin Flippo, a transfer "is a change in job where the new job is substantially equal to the old in terms of pay, status and responsibilities".
- Dale Yoder, "A transfer involves the shifting of an employee from any job to another without special reference to change responsibility or compensation".

Meaning

Transfer means a change in job assignment. It refers to a horizontal or lateral movement of an employee from one job to another in the same organization without much change in his status or pay package. Transfer causes a shift of individual from one job to another without there being any marked change in his responsibilities, skills and other benefits.

Types (Fig. 8.29)

The transfers are mainly comprised of four major categories, which are production, replacement, remedial and versatility transfer.

- The transfers which take place in the production type are the ones which transfer the employees, with their consent, to another department because the organization is lacking requirement of manpower in it.
- Replacement type of transfers are the ones in which a new member is added to a department to reduce the stress on the existing employee.

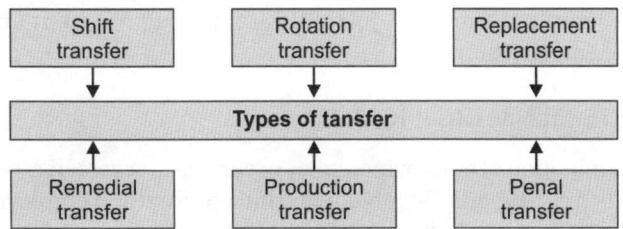

Fig. 8.29: Types of transfer.

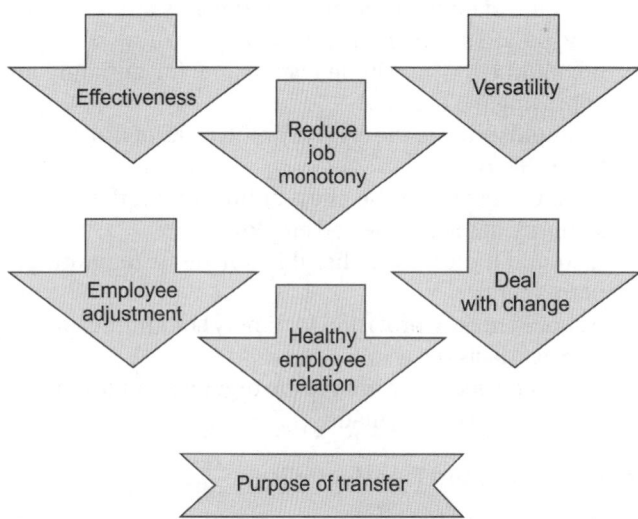

Fig. 8.31: Purposes of transfer.

- Remedial transfer, as the name suggests, happens when there was a mistake during the hiring process, and hence, making sure that the employee goes to the department where they are comfortable.
- Versatility transfer is the most interesting and by far the most useful for the company, which transfers the employees throughout the departments for knowledge transfer. This is very much possible with the HRM tool because the interests and the progress of the employees can be easily tracked. **Figure 8.30** shows employee transfer method and **Figure 8.3**1 shows purposes of transfer.

Objectives

The following are some of the objectives of transfer of employees in a company:
- To meet the exigencies of the company's business.
- To meet the request of an employee.
- To correct incompatibilities of employee relations.
- To suit the age and health of an employee.
- To provide creative opportunities to deserving employees.
- To train the employee for later advancement and promotion. This involves actually job rotation.
- To deal with fluctuations in work requirements or exigencies at work, such as situations when there is

slackness in the work in one department and an overload of work in another, an employee from the first department may be temporarily transferred to the other department as found necessary.
- To correct erroneous placement.
- To place the employee in another department where he/she would be more suitable.

Principles of Transfer Policy

Every organization should have a clear, unambiguous and sound transfer policy. It must be based on the following principles:
- It should clearly indicate the types and circumstances under which a transfer will be made.
- It should state the frequency of transfers and minimum time period between the transfers.
- It should tell who will be responsible for initiating and approving the transfers.
- It should indicate the criteria or the basis of transfer and follow it strictly.
- It should point out the effect of transfer on the pay and seniority of the transferred employee.
- It should indicate whether this transfer is temporary or permanent.
- It should make a provision for timely communicating the transfer decision.
- It should specify the area of the organization over which the transfers can be made.

Essentials of Good Transfer Policy

- **Written form:** It should be in writing and be made known to all the employees of the organization.
- **Clarity:** The policy should clearly state the types of transfers and the circumstances under which transfers will be made.
- **Rate of pay:** The policy should also specify the rate of pay which is to be given to the transferee.
- **Intimation:** The policy ensures that fact of transfer would be intimated to the person concerned well in advance.
- **Retention of seniority:** It should be mentioned whether an employee will retain the seniority at his credit permanently or for a temporary period or lose it altogether.
- **Not frequent:** The policy ensures that transfers should not be made frequently and not for the sake of transfer only.
- **Bases:** The policy should also mention the basis for or grounds of transfers.
- **Indication of the authority:** The policy should indicate the authority in some officer who will be responsible for initiating and implementing transfers.
- **Area:** This policy should specify the units or areas, over which transfer would take place, i.e., whether transfers can be made only within a sub-unit or also between departments, divisions and plants.
- **Requirement of training:** It should be prescribed in the policy whether the training or retraining is required on the new job.

Problems Associated with Transfer

Despite these benefits, some problems are associated with transfer.
They are:
- Adjustment problems to the employee to the new job, place, environment, superiors and colleagues,
- Transfers from one place to another cause much inconvenience and cost to the employee and his family members relating to housing, education of children, etc.,
- Transfer from one place to another result in loss of mandays,
- Company initiated transfers result in reduction in employee contribution, and
- Discriminatory transfers affect employee morale, job satisfaction, commitment and contribution.

Advantages

Main advantages of transfer are highlighted as under:
- **Increases motivation:** It increases motivation and productivity through avoidance of monotony.
- **Relations improvement:** It improves supervisor-employee relations.
- **Ensures future promotions:** It develops the employees for future promotions.
- **Increases productivity:** It increases the productivity and effectiveness of the organization overall.
- **Improvement:** It improves the skills of the existing employees.
- **Provides job satisfaction:** It provides greater job satisfaction to the existing employees.
- **Stabilization:** It helps to stabilize fluctuating work requirements.
- **Remedial:** It remedies faulty placements.

Disadvantages

Transfer process is criticized on the following grounds:
- **Adjustment problems:** Adjustment problems to the employee to the new job, place, environment, superior and colleagues.
- **Inconvenient:** Transfers from one place to another is caused much of inconvenience and cost to the employee and his family members relating to housing, education to children, etc.
- **Loss of time:** Transfer from one place to another result in loss of many days.
- **Reduces contribution of employees:** Company initiated transfers result in reduction in employee contribution.
- **An adverse effect:** Discriminatory transfers affect employee morale, job satisfaction, commitment and contribution.

■ TERMINATING (FIG. 8.32)

Termination of employment may occur due to several reasons which can broadly be categorized into external and employee related factors. Employee related factors usually encompass lack of performance, breach of the employment terms,

Chapter 8: Staffing

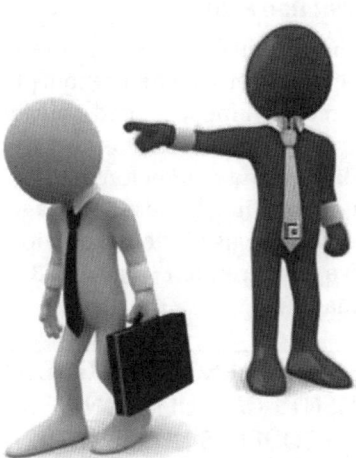

Fig. 8.32: Employee termination.

misconduct, inefficiency, or simply loss of confidence by the employer in the employee.
- A termination from employment is the ending of an employee's job.
- Termination of employment can be voluntary, in which it is the employee's decision, or involuntary, when it is the employer's decision.
- If someone is wrongfully terminated from employment, they may be able to bring their case to court.

Definition
Termination of employment refers to the end of an employee's work with a company. An employee may be terminated from a job of their own free will or following a decision made by the employer.

Someone who has been terminated from employment is no longer employed and their job is ended.

Most common types of termination letters:
- Termination letter due to layoffs/downsizing.
- Termination letter for cause (misconduct/performance/attendance, etc.)
- Termination of business contract.

Reasons (Box 8.14)
In general, there are half-dozen categories of acceptable reasons for termination:
- Incompetence, including lack of productivity or poor quality of work
- Insubordination and related issues, such as dishonesty or breaking company rules
- Attendance issues, such as frequent absences or chronic tardiness
- Theft or other criminal behavior including revealing trade secrets
- Sexual harassment and other discriminatory behavior in the workplace
- Physical violence or threats against other employees

Types (Box 8.15)
There are two types of job terminations:

Box 8.14: Cause of termination.
- Poor job performance
- Lack of fit with organization
- Inability to perform job responsibilities
- Conflict with managers and other employees
- Misconduct
- Many instances of employment separation
- For poor performance, including lack of punctuality, absenteeism, or failure to desired results
- For resisting change
- For negativism
- For insubordination
- For not conforming to company values
- For questionable character or ethical lapses
- For criminal acts

Box 8.15: Types of termination.
1. Retirement
2. Resignation
3. Breach of contract
4. Frustration of contract
5. Ending of a fixed term contract
6. Non-confirmation of a probationer
7. Retrenchment
8. Dismissal (misconduct and pool performance)
9. Constructive dismissal

---

1. **Voluntary:** A voluntary termination of employment is a decision made by the employee. Voluntary termination includes resignation or retirement.
2. **Involuntary:** Employment termination is involuntary when an employee is terminated by the employer

After Termination
Once an employee has been terminated, they may be able to collect certain kinds of payments:
- **Unemployment:** The ability to receive unemployment and other benefits after being dismissed may depend on the reasons provided for your dismissal, as well as your state.
- **Severance pay:** Some companies may offer severance pay, particularly if the dismissal is due to company-related changes, such as restructuring or downsizing.
- **Dismissal compensation:** Many companies outline dismissal compensation benefits in their employee handbook. Some offer weekly compensation for varying weeks with a cap or ceiling on the benefit. Others may offer a lump sum payment. However, there is no obligation for payment until you are covered by a contract or employment agreement that provides for it.
- **Healthcare:** The employee may be eligible to continue group health benefits for a period of time after a job loss.

■ SUPERANNUATION (BOX 8.16)

Superannuation is an organizational pension program created by a company for the benefit of its employees. It is also referred to as a company pension plan. Funds deposited

> **Box 8.16:** Superannuation.
> - **Superannuation** refer to a pension granted upon retirement
> - In general, a **pension** is an arrangement to provide people with an income when they are no longer earning a regular income from employment
> - Retirement plans may be set up by employers, insurance companies, the government or other institutions, such as employer associations or trade unions.

in a superannuation account will grow, typically without any tax implications, until retirement or withdrawal.

- Superannuation is more commonly referred to as a company pension plan.
- Superannuation's are usually defined-benefit or defined-contribution plans.
- A retiree with superannuation is typically less concerned about outliving their retirement funds.

Definition

- Superannuation is an organizational pension program created by a company for the benefit of its employees. It is also referred to as a company pension plan. Funds deposited in a superannuation account will grow, typically without any tax implications, until retirement or withdrawal.
- Superannuation benefit is a retirement benefit offered by an employer to its working class. Superannuation is an organizational pension program created by a company for the benefit of its employees. It is also referred to as a company pension plan.

Purpose of the Bill

The purpose of the Superannuation (Objective) Bill 2016 (the Bill) is to establish the primary objective of the superannuation system, and to provide that subsidiary objectives can be prescribed by regulation. The Bill will also require the preparation of a 'statement of compatibility' for future Bills or regulations relating to changes in superannuation.

Types of Superannuation Benefit

Superannuation benefit is classified into the following in India based on the investment and benefit it offers:

Defined benefit plans:
- As the name itself suggests, in this kind of superannuation, the benefit derived is already fixed irrespective of contribution to the plan.
- The predetermined benefit is based on various factors, such as a number of years of service in the organization, salary, age at which employee starts reaping the benefit.
- This is comparatively complex and risk of generating such benefit lies on employer.
- Upon retirement, an eligible employee receives a fixed amount which is determined by the pre-existing formula, at regular intervals.

Defined Contribution Plans

- This superannuation benefit is opposite to defined benefit plan. While in case of a defined benefit plan, the benefit is fixed and predetermined, defined contribution plan has a fixed contribution and benefit is directly correlated with the contribution and market forces.
- This type of benefit is better to manage and the risk is with the employee as he does not know how much he will receive at retirement. **Figure 8.3**3 shows types of superannuation.

STAFFING UNITS—PROJECTING STAFFING REQUIREMENTS/CALCULATION OF REQUIREMENTS OF STAFF RESOURCES NURSE PATIENT RATIO, NURSE POPULATION RATIO AS PER SIU NORMS/IPH NORMS, AND PATIENT CLASSIFICATION SYSTEM

The nurse-to-patient ratio is one of the determining factors of the patient outcome. The higher workload and lower nurse-to-patient ratio increases the risk of medication errors, iatrogenic complications, hospital morbidity, prolonged hospital stay and compromised patient safety.

- The nurse-to-patient ratio for intensive care units recommended by SIU is 1:1; while NABH recommended 1:1 for ventilated patients and 1:2 for non-ventilated patients.
- These recommendations are in line with international norms. However, the ratio recommended by INC was significantly lower, i.e., only 1:3 or 1:1.
- Most of the research studies conducted in critical care units of the selected tertiary care hospitals in India also highlighted the required nurse-patient ratio of less than 1:1 in different ICUs.
- Nurse staffing norms in India are not updated since a long and they are far behind from international norms and estimated ratios in some of the research studies conducted in India. However, recommendations given by NABH are most recent and realist, practical and feasible to use in India
- A single norm for all the wards and hospitals cannot be used for a fair estimation of nursing human resource needs. While estimating nurse-to-patient ratio estimation different factors, such as unit workload, patients' dependency, skill mix, available proportion of nurses' productive and non-productive activities, and variations in time and nursing care activities during the shift should be considered

General wards: 1:6; Super specialty wards: 1:4; high

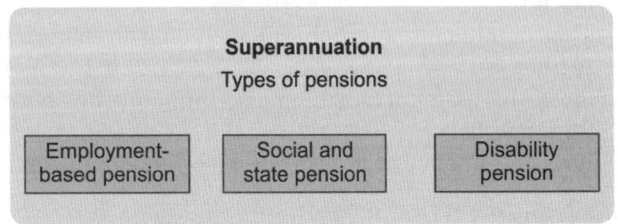

Fig. 8.33: Types of superannuation.

dependency units: 1:3; ICUs and postoperative recovery rooms: 1:1 (ventilator beds) and 1:2 (non-ventilator beds); emergency and trauma: 1:1 (ventilator beds) and 1:2 (non-ventilator beds); labor room: 02 nurse per labor table; antenatal/postnatal ward: 1:4; pediatric ward: 1:5; neonatal ICU 1:1; acute respiratory/burns unit: 1:2; palliative care unit: 1:4; major OT: 02 nurses for each table; minor OT: 1:1; Chemotherapy/Daycare Unit: 1:3; OPD procedure rooms: 1:1 and OPDs: 1:50 patients; infection control nurse: 01 for every 100 beds; and 10–15 nurses for the work of diabetes nurse educator, wound care nurse, stoma nurse, dialysis nurse, organ transplant coordinator nurse, Peripherally inserted central venous catheter (PICC) line care nurse and nurse research assistants. Further, there must be 45% additional nurses for the leave reserve and in-charge nurses must have the flexibility to distribute nurses as per workload in each shift. Further extensive studies are needed to provide staffing standards for nurses, based on the available workload of tertiary care hospitals. **Box 8.17** summarizes objectives of staffing in nursing.

NORMS OF STAFFING STAFF INSPECTION UNIT (BOX 8.18)

Norms

- Norms are standards that guide, control, and regulate individuals and communities. For planning nursing manpower we have to follow some norms.
- The nursing norms are recommended by various committees, such as; the Nursing Man Power Committee, the High-power Committee, Dr Bajaj Committee, and the Staff Inspection Committee, TNAI and INC.
- The norms has been recommended taking into account the workload projected in the wards and the other areas of the hospital.
- All the above committees and the staff inspection unit recommended the norms for optimum nurse-patient ratio, such as **1:3** for non-teaching hospital and 1:5 for the teaching hospital.

Box 8.17: Objectives of staffing in nursing.
- Provide an all professional nurse staff in critical care units, operating rooms, labor and emergency room
- Provide sufficient staff to permit a 1:1 nurse-patient ratio for each shift in every critical care unit
- Staff the general medical, surgical, obstetrics and gynecology, pediatric and psychiatric units to achieve a 2:1 professional-practical nurse ratio.
- Provide sufficient nursing staff in general, medical, surgical, obstetrics and gynecology, pediatric and psychiatric units to permit a 1:5 nurse-patient ratio on a day and afternoon shifts and 1:10 nurse-patient ratio on night shift.
- Involve the heads of the nursing staffs and all nursing personnel in designing the department's overall staffing program.
- Design a staffing plan that specifies how many nursing personnel in each classification will be assigned to each nursing unit for each shift and how vacation and holiday time will be requested and scheduled.

Box 8.18: Staff inspection unit (SIU) norms.
- The Staff Inspection Unit (SIU) is the unit which has recommended the nursing norms in the year 1991-92. As per this SIU norm the present nurse-patient ratio is based and practiced in all central government hospitals.
- **Recommendations of SIU:**
  - The norm has been recommended taking into account the workload projected in the wards and the other areas of the hospital.
  - The posts of nursing sisters and staff nurses have been clubbed together for calculating the staff entitlement for performing nursing care work which the staff nurse will continue to perform even after she is promoted to the existing scale of nursing sister.

- The Staff Inspection Unit (SIU) is the unit which has recommended the nursing norms in the year 1991-92. As per this SIU norm the present nurse-patient ratio is based and practiced in all central government hospitals.

Recommendations of SIU:
- The norms for providing staff nurses and nursing sisters in Government hospital is given in annexure to this report. The norm has been recommended taking into account the workload projected in the wards and the other areas of the hospital.
- The posts of nursing sisters and staff nurses have been clubbed together for calculating the staff entitlement for performing nursing care work which the staff nurse will continue to perform even after she is promoted to the existing scale of nursing sister.
- Out of the entitlement worked out on the basis of the norms, 30% posts may be sanctioned as nursing sister. This would further improve the existing ratio of 1 nursing sister to 3.6. Staff nurses fixed by the government in settlement with the Delhi nurse union in May 1990.
- The assistant nursing superintendent are recommended in the ratio of 1 ANS to every 4.5 nursing sisters. The ANS will perform the duty presently performed by nursing sisters and perform duty in shift also.
- The posts of Deputy Nursing Superintendent may continue at the level of 1 DNS per every 7.5 ANS
- There will be a post of Nursing Superintendent for every hospital having 250 or beds.
- There will be a post of 1 Chief Nursing Officer for every hospital having 500 or more beds.
- It is recommended that 45% posts added for the area of 365 days working including 10% leave reserve (maternity leave, earned leave, and days off as nurses are entitled for 8 days off per month and 3 National Holidays per year when doing 3 shift duties).

Most of the hospital today is following the SIU norms. In this the post of the Nursing Sisters and the Staff Nurses has been clubbed together and the work of the ward sister is remained same as staff nurse even after promotion. The Assistant Nursing Superintendent and the Deputy Nursing Superintendent have to do the duty of one category below of their rank.

In addition to the 10% reserve as per the extent rules, 45% posts may be added where services are provided for 365 days in a year/24 hours.

The norms are based on hospital beds.
- Chief Nursing Officer: 1 per 500 beds
- Nursing Superintendent: 1 per 400 beds or above
- DNS: 1 per 300 beds and 1 additional for every 200 beds
- ANS: 1 for 100–150 beds or 3–4 wards
- Ward sister: 1 for 25–30 beds or one ward. 30% leave reserve
- Staff nurse: 1 for 3 beds in teaching hospital in general ward and 1 for 5 beds in non-teaching hospital +30% leave reserve
- Extra nursing staff to be provided for departmental research function.
- For OPD and emergency: 1 staff nurse for 100 patients (1: 100) + 30% leave reserve
- For intensive care unit: (ICU)- 1:1 or (1:3 for each shift) +30% leave reserve.
- It is suggested that for 250 bedded hospitals there should be One Infection Control Nurse (ICN).

For specialized departments, such as operation theater, labor room, etc. 1:25 +30% leave reserve. Norms are not based on Nursing Hours or Patient's Needs here.

CATEGORIES OF NURSING PERSONNEL INCLUDING JOB DESCRIPTION OF ALL LEVELS (FIG. 8.34)

A job description is the statement of the basic purpose of the job, the significant tasks to be carried out, the extent of authority vested in the post, and the upward downward and horizontal relationships necessary for the performance of the job.
- Nursing personnel are among the largest no of healthcare professionals working in the various fields of healthcare they work from the lowest level of care to the highest level.
- They work in the varied settings namely—hospital/clinical areas, community area, educational settings, and holistic setting.

The nurses working in the clinical settings:
- The topmost nursing officers are nursing directors Synonymous (Nursing Superintendent/principal Matron/ Matron in chief).
- Giving general supervision, delegation, coordinating interdepartmental functions, collaboration with the hospital administration and the staff nurses.

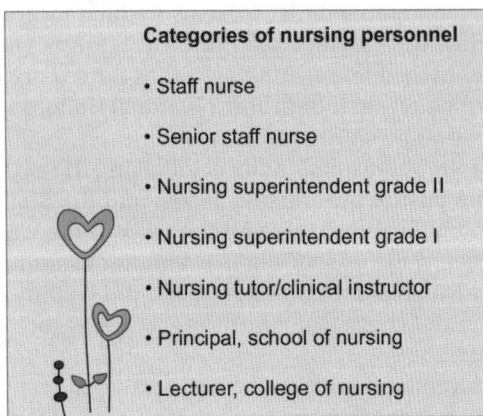

Fig. 8.34: Categories of nursing personnel.

Nursing Director
Roles and responsibilities:
- Formation of the aims and the objectives policies of the new nursing services
- Staffing based on the nursing requirement according to the accepted standards of the medical standards
- Planning and directing the nursing care
- Coordinating the interdepartmental activities
- Maintaining the supplies and the equipment
- Budgeting
- Keeping records and reports

Chief Nursing Officer
- Chief officer for all the staff nurses in hospital. She does planning, coordination, supervision, controlling, reporting to higher medical officer and delegating the work schedules to other nurses.
- Follows and adapts PCS, which helps to recruit, assign and allocate the required staff at the right place and time.
- Explains the job description, supervision and delegating responsibilities to each staff nurse.
- Report to CEO, conducts round in the hospital regularly to check out functioning, cleanliness of the hospital.
- Takes attendance, plan and implement the duty roster for the staff nurses.
- Recruits the staff needed, coordinates work with the entire department.
- Conducts in-service education, encourages continuing education.
- Conducts nursing audit, does anecdotal reporting to evaluate nursing care.
- Make all staff observes and follows code of ethics and regulation of the hospitals.
- Has authority to terminate any nurse if she misbehaves or violates hospital regulations.
- Encourages and participates in all round development of nurses, especially in nursing research activities.

Nursing Sister Grade I/Assistant Nursing Superintendent

The Nursing Sister Grade I is responsible to the Assistant Nursing Superintendent or the total care of patients in the wards and supervision of the Nursing Sister Grade II, student nurses and domestic staff. She would also be assisted by Nursing Sister Grade II, Clinical and Domestic staff. The main aim of the sister Grade I should be to foster team spirit in her area of works as a team leader. **Table 8.2** shows the nurse-patient ratio as per the SIU norms.

Nursing Care of Patients
- Assess the total needs of patients and prepare plan of nursing care.
- Admission and discharge of patients.
- Demonstrate and carry out efficient nursing care, taking care of personal comfort and toilet of patients, administration of drugs and treatment, observation and recording of vital parameters.
- Supervise patient's diet.

Table 8.2: The nurse-patient ratio as per the SIU norms.

1. **General ward**	1:6
2. **Special ward** (pediatrics, burns, neurosurgery, cardiothoracic, neuromedicine, nursing home, spinal injury, emergency wards attached to causality)	1:4
3. **Nursery**	1:2
4. **ICU**	1:1 (Nothing mentioned about the shifts)
5. **Labor room**	1:1 per table
6. **OT**	Major—1:2 per table Minor—1:1 per table

7. **Casualty:**
  a. Casualty main attendance up to 100 patients per day thereafter
  b. For every additional attendance of 35 patients
  c. Gyne/obstetric attendance
  d. Thereafter every additional attendance of 15 patients
	3 staff nurses for 24 hours, 1:1 per shift
	1:35
	3 staff nurses for 24 hours, 1:1/shift
	1:15

8. **Injection room OPD**	Attendance up to 100 patients per day 1 staff nurse • 120–220 patients: 2 staff nurses • 221–320 patients: 3 staff nurses • 321–420 patients: 4 staff nurses
9. **OPD** Name of the department • Blood bank • Pediatric • Immunization • Eye • ENT • Preanesthetic • Cardio lab • Bronchoscopy lab • Vaccination antirabies • Family planning • Medical • Dental • Central sample collection center • Orthopedic • Gyne • X-ray • Skin • VD center • Chemotherapy • Neurology • Microbiology • Psychiatry • Burns	 1 2 2 1 1 1 1 1 1 2 1 1 1 1 2 2 3 2 2 2 1 2 1 2

- Attending rounds with Medical/Nursing personnel.
- Assist medical staff in examination of patients and treatment.
- Participate and help with clinical investigations/procedures.
- Demonstrate and carry out preoperative and post-operative care of patients.
- Maintenance of patient's records.
- Care of patient's personal effects in accordance with hospital rules.
- Giving and receiving reports
- Follow prescribed rules in case of accident or death of a patient.
- Give information and health education to patients and their attendants.
- Intimation to nursing supervisors of any emergency or unusual occurrence in the ward.

Ward Management

- Handing over and takeover charge of patients at the end of the shift.
- Assignment of work to nursing sister Grade II and domestic staff.
- Coordinate and facilitate work of other staff, e.g., physical therapist, social worker, dietitian, voluntary worker, etc.
- Maintaining good interpersonal relationship among all categories of staff and with patients and their relatives.
- Maintain cleanliness of ward, its annexes and environments.
- Proper upkeep and repairs of linen and ward equipment.

- Make indents for drugs, surgical supplies, stores and issue.
- Keep custody of dangerous drugs and record of their administration.
- Daily check of emergency drugs and life savings equipments.
- Maintenance of stock registers inventories.
- Investigate complaints, if any.

Teaching and Supervision

- Orientation of new staff and student nurses.
- Participate in service education of nursing personnel and attend staff meetings.
- Impart planned and incidental teaching.
- Supervise sister Grade II and student nurses.
- Supervise domestic staff.
- Consult and cooperate with nursing tutor in arranging clinical teaching.
- Perform any other duty as may be specified from time to time.

Nursing Superintendent: Grade II

Educational qualifications:

- General education: As prescribed for staff nurse
- Professional education: As prescribed for staff nurse
- Registration: As prescribed for staff nurse, registered with Karnataka Nursing Council.
- Experience: Should have experience as senior staff nurse.
- **Standard norms:** Since, it is the second level nursing supervisory role, it needs at least the Nursing Superintendent Grade II for three senior staff nurses (1:3).
- **Job summary:** She/he is responsible for developing and supervising nursing services of a department or a floor consisting of two or more wards or units managed by the senior staff nurses. These units may be inpatient wards, out-patient department clinics, operation theaters, obstetric units, central supply department, etc., she/he is responsible to the nursing Superintendent Grade I.

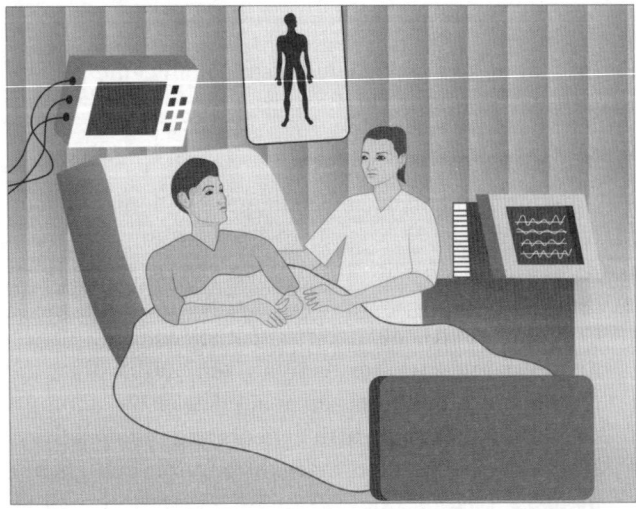

Fig. 8.35: Patient management.

Patient Care and Ward/Unit Management (Figs. 8.35 and 8.36)

- Organizes and plans nursing care activities of the department of floor according to the hospital policies and service needs.
- Plans staffing pattern and the other necessary requirements of her/his department.
- Complies and submits nursing statistics to the concerned authorities.
- Conducts and attends to the departmental and interdepartmental meetings/conferences from time to time.
- Makes regular rounds of her/his department.
- Ensures to the safety and general dealings of the department.
- Looks into general comforts of the patient and his/her relatives.
- Receives report from the Night Supervisor of her/his departments.
- Evaluates nature and quantum of care required in each unit/ward.
- Makes rotation plan for the nursing staff and domestic staff under her/his jurisdiction.
- Plans ward management with the each ward/unit.
- Reinforces the principles of good ward management in ward.
- Helps ward/unit supervisors to procure their ward/unit.
- Supervises the proper use and care of the equipment and supplies in the department.
- Acts as the public relation officer of the unit and deals with the problems faced by the ward supervisor if any, especially with Group "D" employees, patient at tenders.
- Keeps the nursing superintendent Grade I and office informed of the needs of the nursing units/wards under her/his charge and of any special problem/problems.
- Officiates in the absence of Nursing Superintendent Grade I.

Educational Function

- Arranges classes and clinical teaching of nursing students in the department, related to the specialty experience.
- Implements the ward teaching program and clinical experience of the students with the help of doctors and nurses.
- Does counseling and guidance of staff and students.
- Arranges and conducts staff development programs of her/his department.
- Assists in planning for and participation in the training of auxiliary personnel.

General

- Escorts Nursing Superintendent Grade I, Medical Superintendent, and special visitors for hospital rounds.
- Arranges and participates no professional and social function of staff and students.

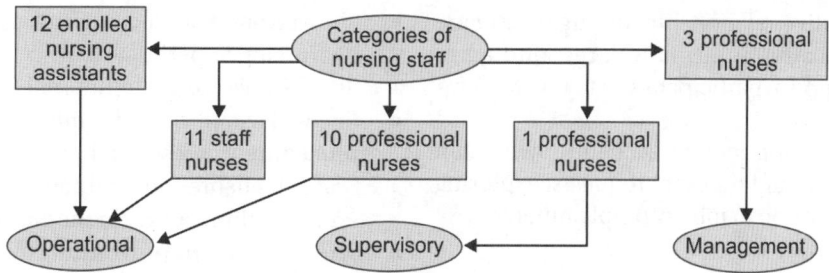

Fig. 8.36: Ward management/Staff management system.

- Acts as a Liaison Officer between the nursing department and higher hospital authorities.
- Carries out any other duties delegated by the Nursing Superintendent Grade I.

Nursing Supervisor

A nurse supervisor manages all of the registered nurses on their team. They may also interact with patients, but they are mainly in charge of making sure the entire operation is running smoothly and everything is up to code. If something goes wrong, the nurse supervisor is responsible for taking action. It is up to them to make sure their team is properly trained and that everything is running correctly. A nurse supervisor's duties include scheduling hours and assigning nurses to particular patients. They must also evaluate their team to ensure they are giving the best care possible to their patients. Supervisors may be involved in hiring nursing staff.
Nurse supervisor job purpose: Promotes and restores patients' health by developing day-to-day management and long-term planning of the patient care area; directing and developing staff; collaborating with physicians and multidisciplinary professional staffs; providing physical and psychological support for patients, friends, and families.

Nurse Supervisor Job Duties

- Accomplishes nursing human resource objectives by selecting, orienting, training, assigning, scheduling, coaching, counseling, and disciplining employees; communicating job expectations; planning, monitoring, appraising job contributions; recommending compensation actions; adhering to policies and procedures.
- Meets nursing operational standards by contributing information to strategic plans and reviews; implementing production, productivity, quality, and customer-service standards; resolving problems; identifying system improvements.
- Meets nursing financial standards by providing annual budget information; monitoring expenditures; identifying variances; implementing corrective actions.
- Identifies patient service requirements by establishing personal rapport with potential and actual patients and other persons in a position to understand service requirements.
- Maintains nursing guidelines by writing and updating policies and procedures.
- Assures quality of care by developing and interpreting hospital and nursing division's philosophies and standards of care; enforcing adherence to state board of nursing and state nurse practice act requirements and to other governing agency regulations; measuring health outcomes against standards; making or recommending adjustments.
- Completes patient care requirements by scheduling and assigning nursing and staff; following up on work results.
- Establishes a compassionate environment by providing emotional, psychological, and spiritual support to patients, friends, and families.
- Promotes patient's independence by establishing patient care goals; teaching and counseling patient, friends, and family and reinforcing their understanding of disease, medications, and self-care skills.
- Provides information to patients and healthcare team by answering questions and requests.
- Resolves patient needs by utilizing multidisciplinary team strategies.
- Maintains safe and clean working environment by designing and implementing procedures, rules, and regulations; calling for assistance from other health care professionals.
- Protects patients and employees by developing and interpreting infection-control policies and protocols; enforcing medication administration, storage procedures, and controlled substance regulations.
- Maintains patient confidence and protects operations by monitoring confidential information processing.
- Maintains documentation of patient care services by auditing patient and department records.
- Ensures operation of medical and administrative equipment by verifying emergency equipment availability; completing preventive maintenance requirements; following manufacturer's instructions; troubleshooting malfunctions; calling for repairs; maintaining equipment inventories; evaluating new equipment and techniques.
- Maintains nursing supplies inventory by studying usage reports; identifying trends; anticipating needed supplies; approving requisitions and cost allocations.
- Maintains professional and technical knowledge by attending educational workshops; reviewing professional publications; establishing personal networks; participating in professional societies.

- Maintains a cooperative relationship among healthcare teams by communicating information; responding to requests; building rapport; participating in team problem-solving methods.
- Accomplishes organization goals by accepting ownership for accomplishing new and different requests; exploring opportunities to add value to job accomplishments.

Head Nurse

The ward sister is the first level supervisor and team leader of the unit. She is directly accountable to the Nursing Superintendent through Deputy Nursing Superintendent for ward management and patient care.

Duties and responsibility in relation to patient care: She will be responsible—

- To organize and make plan of all nursing activities of her unit for patient care according to hospital policy and rules.
- To establish and reinforce the prepared standard protocol for patient care.
- To take the report of her unit from the on duty staff nurse and will read and sign the report book.
- To make bed to bed round of the department with staff and students.
- To supervise direct patient care of the unit and provide direct care to seriously-ill patients as and when situation arises.
- To assign staff nurses, student nurses for nursing care, specially for acute-ill, dangerously-ill patient and postoperative cases.
- To coordinate with other department for patient care and for smooth running of the unit.
- To supervise dietary arrangement, serving of diet and feeding of the helpless patient.
- To supervise, guide and direct the staff Nurses and students to carry out treatment of the patients as prescribed by the physician/surgeon of the unit.
- To check all the records of the patient related to diagnosis, condition and treatment and ensure proper maintenance of records.

Duties and responsibilities related to ward management and supervision

- She will take active part to maintain cleanliness of the ward with the help of Assistant Superintendent and Ward Master.
- She will ensure safety and comfort of the patient of the unit.
- She will make duty roster of the staff nurses, student nurses and work assignment.
- She will check the attendance of all nurses posted in her unit and report to the office of Nursing Superintendent.
- She will indent and procure the ward supplies, equipment and drugs.
- She will check the inventory regularly and keep the stock register up to date.
- She will maintain the records of non-serviceable articles and make arrangement for condemnation.
- She will maintain stock register and it will be countersigned by Nursing Superintendent.
- She will face the audit (Internal and external) periodically.
- She will establish and reinforce the standard of nursing procedure as prescribed.
- She will ensure the maintenance of waste management and infection control of the ward.
- She will ensure prevention of wastage and misuse of supplies and drugs.
- She will act as a liaison officer between ward and administration.
- She will maintain good public relation in her unit.
- She will maintain ward statistics and submit to concern authority regularly.
- She will deal with adverse situation and report to the concerned authority.
- She will report any theft or loss to the higher authority through Nursing Superintendent.
- She will report any medicolegal cases in the ward to the concern authority.
- She will write and submit performance report of the staff and send to the office of the Nursing Superintendent.
- She will make arrangement for keeping the patients belongings in safe custody as per laid down policy of the hospital.
- She will maintain daily patient's census of the unit and report about the critically-ill patients to the Nursing Superintendent.
- She will perform any other duty allotted to her by the Nursing Superintendent/Deputy Nursing Superintendent in the interest of the public and when necessary.
- She will perform morning, evening and night duty in the interest of the hospital.

Duties and responsibilities in relation to nursing education: She will be responsible—

- To organize and oversee the orientation program of staff and student.
- To encourage and participate in staff development program in her unit.
- To implement the practical part of the Nursing Educational Programme.
- To guide the student for formulation of nursing care pan, nursing care studies for the patient.
- To evaluate the students performance in the ward and report accordingly.
- To assist and supervise the student for incidental teaching, health education program (formal and informal) for the patients and their relatives.
- To help in Medical and Nursing Research.

Ward In charge Nurse

Roles:

- Report to the head nurse for any issue.
- Plan control and supervise the activity of the subordinates and also ensure that the staff are allocated at required areas and provide good care to the patients.

- Ensure ward cleanliness, safety and security for all the patients in the ward.
- Oversee the patients' conditions regularly and to care for the concerns of doctors who take care of the patients.
- Conduct ward rounds with staff nurse and plan her daily activities accordingly.
- Coordinate the shift schedule, day/night off in the coordination with the head nurse.
- Meet the healthcare needs of all patients in the ward.

Responsibilities
- Record patients' medical records and monitor vital signs.
- Supervising nursing staff and monitoring their needs.
- Coordinating daily administrative duties, including schedules, nursing assignments and patient care.
- Overseeing patient admissions, transfers and discharges.
- Mentoring and training new staff and providing support and guidance to all staff members.
- Monitoring medical charts and providing compassionate care and assistance to patients and families.
- Liaising with doctors and administrators and communicating any protocol changes to staff.
- Ensuring compliance with all health and safety regulations.
- Recording and maintaining accurate reports.
- Identifying issues or emergencies and responding in a calm and efficient manner.

Senior Nursing Officer

Job Role:
- To utilize professional skill and knowledge to assess, plan, implement and evaluate the clinical care of patients without supervision and incorporating the standards and philosophy of the unit.
- To demonstrate effective communication skills with all professionals involved in the patient pathways, with an open, polite and professional attitude.
- To manage all resources effectively and efficiently.
- To be a professional role model and mentor for all multi-professional teams
- Will provide, demonstrate and maintain a high standard of professional nursing care.
- Demonstrate the ability to work within a team, to supervise, nurture, counsel and develop the knowledge and skills of junior staff.
- To initiate/facilitate developments with the Senior Sister/Matron to include all aspects of unit, division, trust policies and procedures.
- To be responsible in the absence of the senior sister for managing the unit.
- Works within Nursing and Midwifery Councils code of conduct at all times.
- Adhere to confidentiality at all times especially with sensitive data and deal with sensitive situations.
- Respect all patients, careers and staff and contribute to a clean, safe and friendly environment.
- Participate in the provision of the Critical Care Outreach Service recognizing and advising in the management of the acutely ill/deteriorating patient on general wards and emergency department.
- Regularly follow up patients on the general ward after a period of critical illness in ICU.

Direct Patient Care
- Provide a source of specialist knowledge for junior nurses and doctors throughout the trust.
- Assesses, plans, implements and evaluate the clinical care of patients without supervision and incorporates the standards and philosophy of the unit.
- Takes an accurate and comprehensive nursing history of individual patients, setting realistic short and long-term goals to aid recovery with the cooperation of the patients.
- Is able to apply knowledge to prevent potential problem due to treatment, justifying intervention with recent relevant research.
- Work with medical staff to understand their patient's specific requirements and also their organizational requirements.
- Works closely with the Multidisciplinary Team providing them with professional and clinical nursing expertise.
- Is able to give patients a balanced view of risks and benefits of symptom management methods.
- Is able to confidently initiate alternatives if planned interventions are not satisfactory.
- Assist in the transfer of critically ill patients to other departments within the Trust and other Hospitals.
- Ensure all staff are taught the use and care of special equipment and instructed in the use of new equipment.
- Utilize special medical equipment to treat patients with organ failure, maintaining patient safety and ensuring machines are adequately decontaminated after use and properly assembled prior to use.

Communication
- Is able to demonstrate pro-active communication strategies to meet the needs of patients, relatives and colleges.
- Be approachable and able to perform as a role model/mentor for junior staff.
- Liaise with nursing and non-nursing colleagues and offer advice, guidance and counsel as appropriate.
- Anticipates patient's reaction and plans appropriate style in view of patient problems and lifestyle.
- Respects confidentiality at all times especially with sensitive personal data.
- Assist the Senior Sister to investigate any complaints.
- Maintains accurate and legible nursing records as stipulated by the NMC.
- Uses knowledge and underpinning skills to interpret measurements and clinical observation reporting to medical staff with the urgency the individual situation requires and follows through to a satisfactory conclusion.
- Maintains good and effective liaison links with other wards and departments throughout the hospital.

Education and Development

- To demonstrate continuous personal development of professional knowledge and skills, taking ownership for revalidation
- Demonstrate a professional approach to leadership and management of staff. Achieved or planned Leadership Course
- Is able to identify the learning needs of patient/relatives and modify approach accordingly to their response.
- Provides clinical support and advice to junior members of staff.
- Ensure there exists an environment which is conducive to learning and professional development.
- Actively participates in teaching programs/sessions for patients, relatives, nursing colleagues and other healthcare professionals.
- Facilitates and mentors student nurses and junior colleagues. Achieved or planned Mentorship Course.
- Participates in staff selection and recruitment and encourages staff retention.
- Participates in staff development and induction programs.
- Participates in staff appraisal and review. Monitors performance of own team, linking in with senior sister.
- Monitor standards of behavior/performance amongst staff taking remedial action where necessary.
- Is able to reflect on own experience and identify own learning needs, actively seeking to meet those needs through their appraisal.
- Participates in clinical reflection/Critical incident/Clinical supervision to facilitate reflective practice and so improve standards of care and own professional accountability and responsibility.
- Attends ward, directorate and trust meetings as appropriate and use them as a forum for the exchange of views and ideas to promote nursing development and improves standards of care, i.e., safety thermometer, clinical governance, clinical leadership meeting.

Resource Management

- Organizes own time and supervises that of junior staff.
- Monitor nursing staff's attendance for duty, professional appearance and behavior and report all absences and marked repeated deviations to the senior sister.
- When in charge of a shift monitors performance of staff on duty supervising and supporting where necessary. Update E-rostering where appropriate
- Ensures sufficient staffing level/skill mix according to patient's dependency and clinical need, liaising with Matron where appropriate
- Liaising with Nurse Bank office as appropriate within financial constraints.
- Develop an adequate understanding of budgetary management for the clinical area.
- Challenges existing practice, leading new initiatives for more effective use of resources.
- Maintains own knowledge and adherence to trust policies and procedures.

Junior Staff Nurse

Educational qualifications:

- General pre-university course/10+2 or equivalent exam.
- Professional: 3 years General Nursing/9 months/6 months Midwifery/Psychiatric Nursing Diploma/Certificate, recognized by Indian Nursing Council or Revised General Nursing and midwifery/Psychiatric Nursing Diploma/Certificate Recognized by Indian Nursing Council. Or Basic BSc Nursing from a Recognized University according to Indian Nursing Council norms.
- Registration: Registered with the Karnataka State Nursing Council/Indian Nursing Council (INC)/Respective State Nursing Councils Standard Norms and Inc (Nurse-Patient Ratio)

General wards: (a) 1:3 (Hospital attached with school or college of nursing) (b) 1:5 (Hospital not attached with school or college of nursing).

Job summary: Staff nurse is a first level professional nurse who provides direct patient care to one patient or group of patients assigned to her/him during duty shift and assist in management of wards/units/special departments. She/he is directly responsible to Senior Staff Nurse or ward in charge nurse/Nursing Superintendent Grade II.

Duties and Responsibilities

Direct Patient Care

- Carry out the procedures of admission and discharge of the patient
- Makes beds of serious patients and helps or guides students or Group "D" employees to make beds, by supplying linen.
- Maintains personal hygiene and comforts of the patient.
- Attends to the nutritional needs of the patient and feeds the helpless patients.
- Maintains clean and safe environment for the patient.
- Implements and maintains ward policies and routines.
- Coordinates patient care with other team members.
- Take rounds with the doctors when called to list new orders and see that they are carried out.
- Performs various technical tasks related to nursing care:
  - Administration of medication, i.e., tablets, injections, infusions and transfusion on prescription or according to standing instructions.
  - Assisting doctors in various medical and surgical diagnostic procedures by preparing patients and getting ready with required things.
  - Performing simple diagnostic procedures, viz, urinalysis hemoglobin percent, etc.
  - Collecting and sending of specimens for laboratory diagnostic procedures.
  - Recording of vital signs, i.e., temperature, pulse, respiration and blood pressure.
  - Performing gastric lavage, giving enema, etc.
  - Prepares patients for operations and see that he/she is sent to operation theater with all necessary papers and medications.

- Takes care of eyes, ears, back, bowel, bladder, perineum, and breast, etc., whenever needed.
- Observers all patients conditions and take suitable action accordingly and/or reports changes to ward in charge and/or the doctor.
- Give expert bedside nursing to all patients.
- Attends last officers in case of a patient dying during shifts and arrange to preserve dead body in mortuary, or hand over the body with respect to concerned family members/relatives/authorities.

Ward/Unit Management

- Helps the ward in charge to carry out her/his work or act as ward in charge during their absence.
- Maintains general cleanliness of the ward and the sanitary annexure.
- Supervises the duties of Group "D" employees and guides them and reports accordingly.
- Writes the diet register and supervises the distribution of diet and report, if any necessary.
- Maintains scheduled poisonous drug registers.
- Supervises nursing care and other tasks carried out by the students.
- Maintains duly room trays, sterilizes instruments and see that procedural trays are in readiness.
- Take over from duty nurse of the previous, new and serious patients, instruments, supplies, drugs, etc., and handover the same accordingly.
- Maintains all the records pertaining to ward/unit.
  - Maintains case papers, investigation reports, etc.
  - Maintains vital signs charts, intake-output charts and other special charts, if necessary.
  - Takes special care of medicolegal case papers and records
  - Writes day and night orders and maintains ward statistics.

Operation Theater Management

- Maintains aseptic environment of the operation theater.
- Autoclaving of articles, instruments, gloves, linen, etc., required for various types of surgery.
- Receives patients from the ward intact for surgery.
- Prepares anesthetic trolley and trolley for surgery, according to type and procedures.
- Assist the surgeon and anesthetist in every step, skillfully while performing various types of surgery.
- Indenting and procuring surgical instruments, drugs, gloves, suturing materials and O_2, N_2, CO_2, etc., required for operation theater.
- Maintains records and reports pertaining to the operation theater.
- Maintains safety of the Boyle's apparatus, oxygen cylinder, nitrogen cylinder, anesthetic drugs, and autoclave, etc., in the operation theater.

Management of Labor Room

- Preparation of expectant mother for aseptic safe delivery.
- Conducts normal deliveries and reports.
- Attends and assists the doctors in all obstetrical emergencies.
- Attends and assists in difficult and abnormal deliveries.
- Takes care of the newborn and premature babies.
- Maintains records and reports pertaining to labor room.
- Indent and procure necessary drugs, supplies linen, etc., to labor room.

Management of Postoperative/ICU/Burns Units

- Indent and procurement of all the necessary equipments, drugs, O_2 cylinders, which are required for the units.
- Operates ECG, EEG, cardiac resuscitation, etc., or other sophisticated high-tech machines whenever needed or assist the doctors in operating such machines.

Psychiatric Unit

- Assists the doctors in admission and discharge of patients.
- Prepares patient for ECT and other procedures, and therapies.
- Assists in management of aggressive, suicidal as grief as other symptoms of the patient.
- Maintains records and reports of the units.

Educational Function

- Helps in orientation of new staff and students.
- Teaches and guides the domestic staff (Group D) for handling bedpans, urinals, etc.
- Carries out health teaching for individual or group of patients.
- Extends cooperation and participates in clinical teaching.
- Provides and demonstrates methods and procedure whenever needed.
- Participates in in-service education programs.
- Plans and implements formal and informal health education programme and teaching program.
- Assists and extends cooperation in medical and nursing research program.

Graduate Nurse/Student Nurse

- The nurse directly provides patient care.
- Learns the policies of the hospital and ward, and works according to the standards of care.
- Provides health education and direct skilled work
- She works under the supervision of the senior nurse and holds authority over the Nursing Assistants and the Aids.

Nurses Working in the Community Areas

- The nurses working in the community level are also a large part of the healthcare delivery system.
- They work at various levels and provide care to various levels.
- They can be broadly classified as—female health worker and community health nurse.

Community Health Nurse

There are various community health nurse levels in various states of India. Generally, they can be classified as:
- **DPHNO:** District Public Health Nursing Officer
- **BPHN:** Block Public Health Nurse
- **PHN:** Public Health Nurse/Lady Health Visitor
- **ANM:** Axillary Nurse Midwife/Female Health Workers

Axillary Nurse Midwife (ANM)/Female Health Workers

Roles and responsibilities:
- Registers and cares for the prenatal and postnatal mothers at home.
- Registers and follows up all the eligible couples
- Provides nutritional advice and immunization to mother and children.
- Carries out family planning services and including the distribution of the contraceptives
- Provides treatment to minor ailments
- Notifies communicable diseases
- Maintains the records and registers all the services provided and vital events like birth and death.
- Participates in the various disease control programs.
- Conducts surveys of all subcenter areas and maintains records about every family.
- Coordinates activities with the block level
- Functions in the field of administration and supervision, education training personnel, health services and research.

Community Health Nurse (Fig. 8.37)
- Qualified community health nurse is one who has undergone general training, and basic education in the community health nursing.

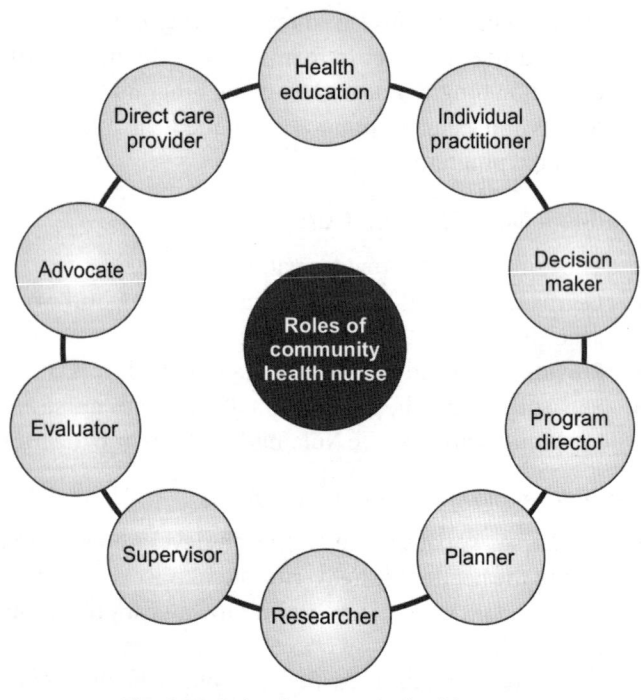

Fig. 8.37: Role of community health nurse.

- She must have BSc Nursing with a registration to work as a community health nurse.

ASSIGNMENT AND NURSING CARE RESPONSIBILITIES

Planning of patient assignment is not a mere matter of dividing up the patients among the available members of the staff, but it is assigning an individual patient or group of patients to nurses according to the patient's nursing care needs and nurses ability to give care to those assigned patients.

Objectives of Patient Assignment
- To promote the patient with the best possible nursing care.
- To plan assignments which are interesting and stimulating to professional growth?
- To provide a broad education and experience for each student nurse.
- To achieve good ward management.

Principles of Patient Assignment (Box 8.19)
- Equal case load depending on staff ability and hours.
- Patient assignment should be made according to the needs of each patient and of the nurse's ability to give him the care.
- In hospital where student nurses are being educated, assignment must necessarily revolve round the requirements for the student's education.
- For nurses to grow in professional competence, assignments must be varied and challenging to their ability.
- Activities are better performed when each one is made responsible for a single person.
- If there are not enough nurses on duty to carry the nursing load. It is preferable to overload the graduate staff nurses than the students or nonprofessional works.
- Assignments of patients and duties should not be changed frequently than is absolutely essential.
- The care required by all patients in the group assignments to one nurse must be considered when making assignments.
- Assignments planning are closely related to time planning. If patients are to receive good care in the late afternoon and early evening, usually as many nurses are required during these periods as during the morning hours.
- The best use will be made of nurse's time, if the patients assigned to one nurse are geographically close together.

Patient Care Delivery System

One important function of the professional nurse at the first-line management position of nursing service department is organizing the activities of the staff into a workable pattern to meet patient needs. She/he should establish effective relationships between the activities to be performed, the workers to perform them.

Definition of assignment: Assignment refers to "a written delegation of duties to care for a group of patients by trained personnel assigned to the unit."

> **Box 8.19:** Principles of patient assignment.
> - Made by head nurse for each individual nurse
> - Planned weekly and revised daily to ensure continuity of care
> - Must be balanced among nursing staff
> - Never assign same task to more than one nurse
>
> **Based on:**
> - Nursing needs of each patient
> - Skill, experience, capabilities of each staff
> - Job description

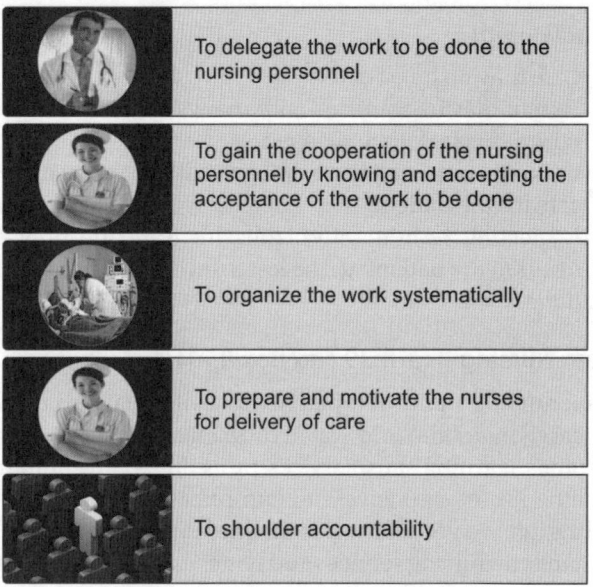

Fig. 8.38: Purpose of patient assignment.

Purposes of assignment (Fig. 8.38):
- To delegate the work to be done to the nursing personnel.
- To gain the cooperation of the nursing personnel by knowing and accepting the acceptance of the work to be done.

Principles of personnel assignment:
- Made by the head nurse or nurse in charge for each individual nurse.
- Based on:
  - Nursing needs of each patient and approximate time required to care for him.
  - The capabilities, skill level, previous experience and the interest of the staff members.
  - Job description
- Planned weekly, and revised daily if necessary to assure continuity of care.
- Take into account all the direct, indirect and unit activities
- Consider the geographical location of the unit and the assigned duties to save nurse's time and effort.
- Must be balanced among nursing staff.
- Never to assign the same task to more than one nurse.

Process of organizing patient care: The head nurse or the nurse in charge should carry out their duties and responsibilities through applying the following steps:
1. **Planning:** It is a process of developing a course of action for meeting the needs of patient. In planning, the head nurse decides what should be done, when, how, where, by whom and to whom.
2. **Assigning:** Assignment of patient and nursing activities are written in the assignment sheet by the head nurse/nurse in charge, based on the principles of assignment.
3. **Leading:** Includes issuing instructions, motivation, and coordination of activities, by making rounds, checking performance and conducting conferences.
4. **Evaluating:** By reviewing nursing performance and patient progress to be compared by the assignment and nursing care plan.
5. **Reporting:** The head nurse prepares a nursing unit report "e.g., shift report" which includes patient's needs, special observations, census, bed number, all critically ill and postoperative patients, patients needs special preparation on.

Methods of patient care delivery: (methods of assignment):
The traditional methods
- Case method
- Functional method
- Team method
- Modular nursing
- Primary nursing method

The advanced method: Case management

Case Method

It is the oldest mode of organizing patient care. In this method, nurses assume total responsibility for meeting all the needs of assigned patients during their time on duty. It involves the assignment of one or more clients to a nurse for a specific period of time, such as shift. Complete care, including treatments, medication administration and nursing care planning, is the assigned nurse's responsibility.

Merits

- The nurse can see better and attend to the total needs of clients due to the time and proximity of interactors. Co-ordination of all aspects of care is the main responsibility of the nurse; which includes physical, emotional, medical regimen, teaching and all other aspects related to it.
- Continuity of care can be facilitated with care.
- Client/nurse interaction/rapport can be developed by virtue of intensity of time and proximity of those involved.
- Client may feel more secure, knowing that one person is thoroughly familiar with the needs and the course of treatment of his/her disease.
- Educational needs of the clients can be closely monitored.
- Family and friends become better known by nurse and get more involved in the care of the client.
- Work load for the unit can be equally divided among the available staff.
- Nurse's accountability for their function is built-in. **Table 8.3** shows nursing care delivery models.

Demerits

- Many clients do not require the inherent care of intensity in this type of service.

Chapter 8: Staffing

Table 8.3: Nursing care delivery models.

Direct patient care functions	Indirect patient care functions
Assessment	
Monitoring	Clinical practice
Prioritizing goals	Education/research
Care coordination	Leadership
Therapeutic interventions	Operations
Evaluation	Personnel management
Communication	Quality improvement
Patient education	System coordination

Box 8.20: Functional nursing.

This system emerged in 1930's in USA
- **Meaning:**
  – Individual care givers are assigned to specific tasks rather than being assigned to certain patients or clients. It is based on a division of labor similar to an assembly line.
  – This model is also referred to as task method. Functional nursing evolved during the depression when RNs went from being private practitioners to becoming employees for the job security.
- **Origin:** Once world war II was broke out resulted in severe shortage of nurses in US. Many nurses entered the military to care for the soldiers. To accommodate this shortage, hospitals increased their usage of auxiliary personnel.

- This method must be modified if nonprofessional health workers are to be used effectively.
- Nurses are not enough to comply the demand of this model; cost-effectiveness must be considered.
- It is difficult for nurses to use this method to become involved in long-term planning and evaluation of care.
- The greatest disadvantage to case nursing occurs, when the nurse is inadequately trained or prepared to provide total care to the patient.

Functional Method (Box 8.20)

Emerged during 1950s, due to shortage of nurses. This method focuses on getting the greatest amount of tasks in the least time. In this method, the nursing care is divided into tasks and each staff member is assigning to perform one or two tasks for all patients in the unit according to the level of skill required for performance as follows:
- **Registered professional nurses:** Responsible for administering medication to all unit patients, another for changing dressings and administering ordered treatments (such as postural drainage or warm compresses) for all patients.
- **Technical nurses:** Responsible for taking vital signs and recording intake and output for all patients in the unit, while another might is giving baths to all bedridden patients.
- **Nurse aides:** Responsible for making beds for all ambulatory patients and assisting mobility-impaired patients to move in bed or walk in the hall.
- **Unit clerk:** Responsible for answering telephone, delivering messages, recording admissions and discharges, etc.

Advantages
- Care is provided economically and efficiently
- Minimum number of RNs required, so it is efficient when there is a shortage in the staff or there is limited number of professional nurses
- Tasks are completed quickly
- Useful in emergency situations.

Disadvantages
- Care may be fragmented
- Patient may be confused with many care providers
- Caregivers feel unchallenged
- Lack of communication among the different persons who care for the patient.
- Neglecting the humanity of the patient and the individual needs of the patient will be lost in an effort to get the work done.

Team Nursing (Fig. 8.39 and Box 8.21)

Team nursing was developed because of social and technological changes in World War-II drew many nurses away from hospitals, learning haps, services, procedures and equipment became more expensive and complicated, requiring specialization at every turn. It is an attempt to meet increased demands of nursing services and better use of knowledge and skills of professional nurses.

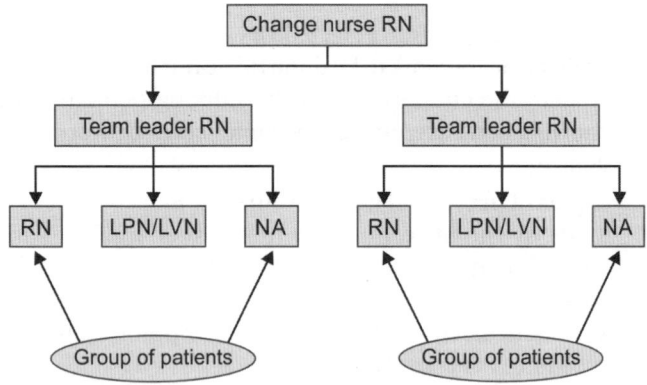

Fig. 8.39: Team nursing.

Box 8.21: Team nursing.

- Team nursing is the delivery of nursing care by a designated group of staff members including both professional nurses and non-professional staff.
- This method of nursing care was introduced in early 1950's.
- Several elements are considered necessary:
  – Team leader is the delegated authority to make assignments for team members and guide the work of the team. The leader of the team should be a registered nurse, not a practical nurse
  – The leader is expected to use a democratic or participative style in interactions with team members.
  – The team is responsible for the total care given to an assigned group of patients or clients.

Definitions

- Team nursing is based on philosophy in which groups of professional and non-professional personnel work together to identify, plan, implement and evaluate comprehensive client-centered care. The key concept is a group that works together toward a common goal, providing qualitative comprehensive nursing care. —*Kron 1978*
- Team nursing was designed to accommodate several categories of personnel in meeting the comprehensive nursing needs of a group of clients. —*Donavan 1975*

Concept of team nursing: The concept of team nursing was introduced in the early 1950s. It is a method of nursing assignment that binds professional, technical and nurse aides into small teams. This method allows for efficient utilization of technical and/or nurse's aide through the direct supervision, guidance, and teaching of professional nurses.

Objectives: The objective of team nursing is to give the best possible quality of patient care by utilizing the abilities of every member of the staff to the fullest extent and by providing close supervision both of patient care and of the individual who give it.

Process of implementing the team method: One registered nurse in the team is appointed by the head nurse to serve as a team leader. The team members commonly consist of at least one professional nurse, one technical nurse, nursing students and nursing aides. All team members may receive reports about their patients' care needs from the team leader or team member on previous shift.

The team leader usually assigns:
- **Professional nurse** to care for the most seriously-ill patients, to ensure informed observation and skilled interventions. Often, the team leader assigns the **technical nurse** to bath, feed, and move and change dressings for patients.
- **Aides** are assigned to make beds, assist ambulatory patients with bathing and grooming, testing urine and performing simple nursing care procedures.
- **Team leader** usually administers medications and monitors parenteral fluid therapy for all patients assigned to the team. Without team planning and communication through the team conferences, team nursing may become in reality just a variation of the functional method.

Functions of team nursing: The two important points of functioning are:
1. The head nurse must know at all times the condition of the patients and the plan for their care and must be assured that assignments and workmanship contribute to quality nursing.
2. The team leader must have freedom to use their initiative and the opportunity to nurse, supervise, and teach unencumbered by the responsibility for administrative detail.

Functions of registered nurse:
- In the team nursing RN functions as a team leader and coordinates the small group (no more than four or five) of ancillary personnel to provide care to a small group of patients.
- As coordinator of the team, the RN must know the condition and needs of all patients assigned to the team and plan for the individualized care for each patient.
- The team leader is also responsible for encouraging a cooperative environment and maintaining clear communication among all team members.
- The team leader's duties include planning care, assigning duties, directing and assisting team members, giving direct patient care, teaching and coordinating patient activities.
- The team leader assigns each member specific responsibilities dependent on the role.
- The members of the team report directly to the team leader, who then reports to the charge nurse or unit manager.
- Communication is enhanced through the use of written patient assignments, the development of nursing care plans, and the use of regularly scheduled team conferences to discuss the patient status and formulate revisions to the plan of care.
- However, for team nursing to succeed, the team leader must have strong clinical skills, good communication skills, delegation ability, decision-making ability, and the ability to create a cooperative working environment.

Advantages

- High-quality, comprehensive care with a high proportion of ancillary staff.
- Team members participate in decision making and contribute their own expertise.

Disadvantages

- Continuity suffers if daily team assignments vary
- Team leader must have good leadership skills
- Insufficient time for planning and communication

Modular Nursing (Box 8.22)

Modular nursing assignment is used when the nursing staff includes technical and nurse aides, as well as professional nurses. Although two or three persons are assigned to each module, the greatest responsibility for the care of assigned patients falls on the professional nurse. The professional nurse is also responsible for guiding and teaching non-professional nurse.

Definition

Modular nursing is a modification of team nursing and focuses on the patient's geographic location for staff assignments (Magargal 1980).
- The patient unit is divided into modules or districts, and the same team of caregivers is assigned consistently to the same geographic location.
- Each location, or module, has an RN assigned as the team leader, and the other team members may include LVN/LPN or UAP. —*Yoder Wise 2003*
- Just as in the team nursing, the team leader in the modular nursing is accountable for all patient care and is

Chapter 8: Staffing

> **Box 8.22: Modular nursing.**
> - It is a modification of team nursing In modular nursing, staff are geographically assigned to patients for whom they coordinate and provide comprehensive care. It focuses on geographic location of patient rooms and assignment of staff members.
> - It was developed by Magargal in 1987.
> - **Delivery model:**
>   - The total unit is divided into modules or districts and the same team of staff is assigned consistently to the module. Modular nursing is enhanced when nursing units are physically designed and built with this nursing delivery system in mind, but it can also be used in nursing units that are not so designed. Each module has a modular or team leader RN, who assigns the patient to module staff.
>   - Each module ideally consists of at least one RN, one LPN/LVN and one nursing assistant. A charge nurse will coordinate the work of all the modules in a unit. She expects the module leaders to be accountable for patient care but assist in problem solving when necessary. Staff nurses work independently or together, depending on the size of a modular districts. Modules may have same or different number of patients.

responsible for providing leadership for team members and creating a cooperative work environment.

- The concept of modular nursing calls for a smaller group of staff providing care for a smaller group of patients.
- The goal is to increase the involvement of the RN in planning and coordinating care.
- Communication is more efficient among a smaller group of team members. —*Marquis and Huston, 2003*
- The success of the modular nursing depends greatly on the leadership abilities of the team leader.

Advantages: (Yoder Wise 2003)

- Continuity of care is improved when staff members are consistently assigned to the same module
- The RN as team leader is able to be more involved in planning and coordinating care.
- Geographic closeness and more efficient communication save staff time.

Disadvantages: (Yoder Wise 2003)

- Costs may be increased to stock each module with the necessary patient care supplies (medication cart, linens and dressings).
- Long corridors, common in many hospitals, are not conducive to modular nursing.

Note:

- Modular nursing is similar to team nursing because professional and non-professional employees cooperate in caring for patients under the leadership of a professional nurse.
- Module nursing is similar to primary nursing because each pair or trio of nursing personnel are responsible for the care of the patients in their caseload from admission to discharge, following discharge and during subsequent admissions to the agency.
- As with primary nursing, the worker pair or trio arrange or another pair or trio to care for their assigned patients on alternate shifts and days off.

Progressive Patient Care

Progressive client care is a method in which client care areas or units provide various levels of care, e.g., (1) intensive care unit for the critically ill, (2) post-intensive care unit, (3) regular care units, (4) convalescent unit, and (5) self-care unit. Here the clients are evaluated with respect to all level (intensity) of care needed. As they progress towards increased self-care (as they become less ethically-ill or in need of intensive care or monitoring) they are marked to units/wards staffed to best provide the type of care needed. The merits and demerits of progressive patient care are as follows:

Merits

- Efficient use is made of personnel and equipment.
- Clients are in the best place to receive the care they require.
- Use of nursing skills and expertise are maximized due to different staffing patterns of each unit.
- Clients are moved towards self-care, independence is fostered where indicated.
- Efficient use and placement of equipment is possible.
- Personnel have greater probability to function towards their fullest capacity.

Demerits

- There may be discomfort to clients who are moved often.
- Continuity care is difficult, even though possible.
- Long-term nurse/client relationships are difficult to arrange.
- Great emphasis is placed on comprehensive, written care plan.
- There is often times difficulty in meeting administrative need of the organization, staffing evaluation and accreditation. **Figure 8.40** shows elements of progressive patient care (PPC).

Primary Nursing Method

This method is the best in an agency with an all-professional nurse staff. It is a comprehensive, continuous and coordinated nursing process for meeting the total needs of each patient **(Fig. 8.41)**.

Basic Concepts in Primary Nursing

- **Patient assessment** by a primary nurse, who plans the care to be given by secondary or associate nurse when the primary nurse is off duty. The 24 hours responsibility for care is put into practice through the primary nurse's written directive on a preplanned communication assignment.
- **Complete communication** of care given in the nursing staff daily reporting method.
- **Discharge planning** including teaching, family involvement and appropriate references.

Process for Implementing Primary Nursing Method

- **The head nurse:**
  - Assigns primary nurse to patients by matching the skills of the nurse to the needs of the patients.

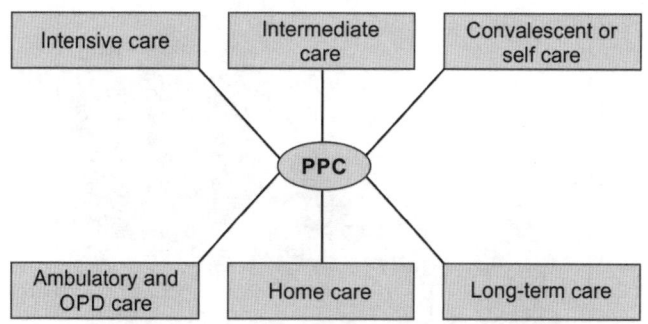

Fig. 8.40: Elements of progressive patient care (PPC).

- Ensures proper scheduling for all shifts so that if primary nurse is off the unit an associate nurse is available for care.
- Guides, counsels and evaluates care given.
- May also assign herself to patients either as a primary nurse or associate nurse.
- **Professional staff nurse:**
  - **Primary nurse:** Functions of primary nurse include performing the following:
    – Conducting an admission (initial) assessment
    – Developing, planning, implementing, and revising the nursing care plan
    – Directing care in her absence
    – Collaborating with physicians and families
    – Making referrals
    – Teaching health concepts
    – Making discharge plans
  - **Associate nurse:** Associate nurse may be professional or technical nurse. She carries out the nursing care planned by the primary nurse when she is not on duty.

Technical nurse: Carry out the nursing tasks assigned by the primary or associate nurses in giving the care.

Nurse aides: Their activities are focusing away from direct contact with the patient and can be utilized as messengers and transporters.

Ward clerk: Responsible for the non-nursing functions of administrative duties.

Advantages

- High-quality, holistic patient care
- Establish rapport with patient
- RN feels challenged and rewarded.

Disadvantages

- Primary nurse must be able to practice with a high degree of responsibility and autonomy
- RN must accept 24-hour responsibility
- More RNs needed; not cost-effective

Case Management

Case management is a process of monitoring an individual patient's health care by the case manager, for the purpose of maximizing positive outcomes and containing costs. The case manager has graduate-level preparation or is at an advanced level of nursing practice. The case manager role requires not only advanced nursing skills but also advanced managerial and communication skills.

The case manager is an individual "professional nurse" assigned responsibility for this process.

Case Manager's Approaches

- **Case managers employed by the hospitals** follow a patient from the time admission is planned through the time of discharge. This case manager might plan the admitting process to ensure that all preadmission work-ups are completed and that the patient is being admitted at the appropriate time to facilitate follow-up through on problems.
- **Case managers in private practice** may focus on a particular group of client. For example, the geriatric case manager focuses on managing care for the older client. The private case manager is paid by the client or family usually based on the hours of service provided. The case manager may help the family to identify all the options for care and treatment, ask questions to obtain greater understanding of the overall problem, and work with the family in the decision-making process.

Case management tools: The case manager uses two tools, Case Manager Plan (CMP), and Critical Path Diagnosis (CPD) to, design, map, track, monitor, and adjust the patient's course through the care-treatment process.

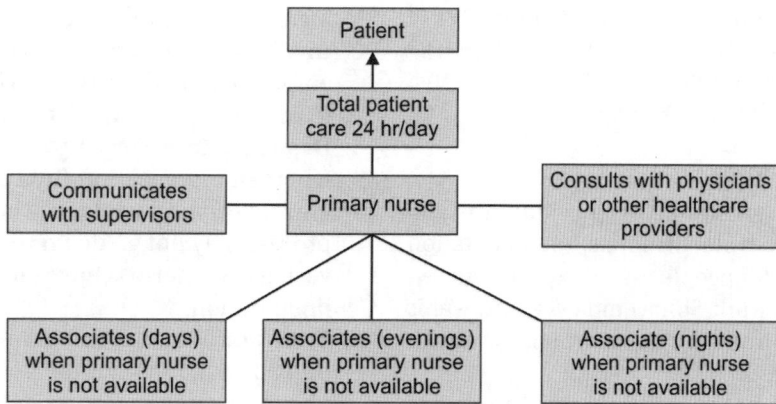

Fig. 8.41: Primary nursing method.

- **Case manager plan (CMP):** It is a multicolumn plan with accompanying time line that includes medical and nursing diagnosis, desired care outcomes, intermediate daily goals to supports each outcome, and the daily activities required of nurse, physicians, and other care givers to achieve intermediate goal.
- **Critical path diagnosis (CPD):** It is an abbreviated, one-page version of the required physician and nurse action listed in the CMP, together with the exact data on which all key events must occur to achieve the desired outcome by the target date.

The case manager evaluates the patient's progress toward care and treatment goal daily by comparing signs, symptoms, and assessment data against information in the CMP and CDP then tracking variances from the expected course of progress.

Advantages

- **For the patient:**
  - Establishing and achieving a set of "expected" or standardized patient care outcomes for each patient.
  - Facilitating early patient discharge or discharge within an appropriate length of stay.
  - Using the fewest possible appropriate healthcare resources to meet expected patient care outcomes.
  - Facilitating the continuity of patient care through collaborative practice of diverse health professionals.
- **For the nurse:**
  - Enhancing nurse's professional development and job satisfaction.
  - Facilitating the transfer of knowledge of expert clinical staff of novice staff.

EMPLOYEE TURNOVER (FIG. 8.42)

Turnover is the number or percentage of an employer's workforce that must be replaced due to the voluntary and involuntary separation of employees from employment. Voluntary turnover includes leaving employment to retire, illness, returning to school and better career opportunities, while involuntary turnover includes layoffs and terminations for poor performance or disciplinary problems.

Definition

A common definition of employee turnover is the loss of talent in the workforce over time. This includes any employee departure, including resignations, layoffs, terminations, retirements, location transfers, or even deaths.

Causes of Employee Turnover

High employee turnover is taxing. It costs precious time and money and can result in a loss of staff morale. Your reputation could also be tarnished, with people assuming your organization is a terrible place to work. Some employee turnover is inevitable. For example, retirement, relocation and leaving for schooling cannot be avoided.

- **Lack of growth and progression:** Opportunity for growth and development is very important for retaining

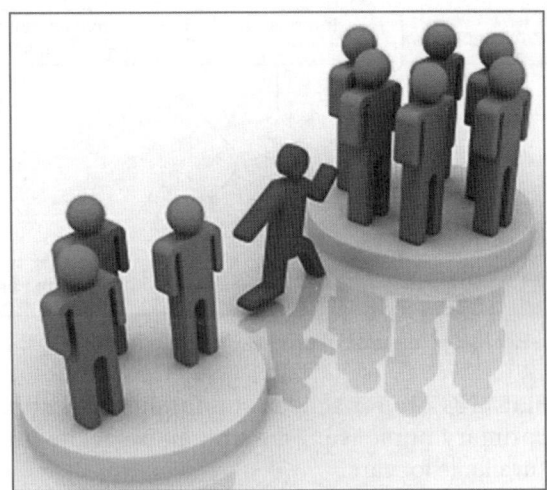

Fig. 8.42: Employee turnover.

good employees. If an employee feels trapped in a dead-end position, they are likely to look towards different companies for the chance to improve their status and income.
- **Being overworked:** It might seem natural that, in periods of economic pressure, employer asks the staff to take on extra responsibilities.
- **Lack of feedback and recognition:** Feedback is the first step to ensuring your employees succeed, so avoiding this process can be detrimental to their success.
- **Little opportunity for decision-making:** Micromanaging stamps out the opportunity for innovation, which is not what you want. Stifled, over managed employees are likely to grow frustrated with the lack of freedom, which contributes to high turnover.
- **Poor employee selection:** Finding the perfect employee is difficult, but forcing a match with an employee that is clearly not right for the company culture or values will never end well.

Types

Employee turnover is primarily of 4 types:
1. **Voluntary turnover:** This type of turnover is when an employee decides to voluntarily leave the organization. It is the employee's choice to disassociate from the organization, without pressure from any external forces.
2. **Involuntary turnover:** This type of turnover is when an employee is fired, or asked to leave the organization due to various factors (which cannot always be pinpointed).
3. **Desirable turnover:** Turnover is considered desirable when an organization fires or loses underperforming employees and replaces them with new hires. This process may not go down well with a lot of employees, yet it is essential to keep the momentum going within the organization.
4. **Undesirable turnover:** Undesirable turnover is when an organization loses it is top performing employees. Some employees leave a deeper impact than others, those are the employees that are difficult to replace.

Effects of Labor Turnover

There must be some labor turnover due to personal and unavoidable causes. It has been observed by employers that a normal labor turnover, which is between 3% and 5%, need not cause much anxiety. But a high labor turnover is always detrimental to the organization. The effect of excessive labor turnover is low labor productivity and increased cost of production.

- Frequent changes in the labor force give rise to interruption in the continuous flow of production with result that overall production is reduced.
- New workers take time to become efficient. Hence, lower efficiency of new workers increases the cost of production.
- Selection and training costs of new workers recruited to replace the workers who have left increase the cost of production.
- New workers being unfamiliar with the work give more scrap, rejects and defective work which increase the cost of production.
- New workers being inexperienced workers cause more depreciation of tools and machinery. Due to faulty handling of new workers, breakdown of tools and machinery may also occur very often and hamper production.
- New workers being inexperienced workers are more prone to accidents. Consequently, all costs associated with accidents, such as loss on account of output lost, compensation for the injured workers, damage of materials and equipment due to accidents, etc., increase the cost of production. **Box 8.23** summarizes example of labor turnover.

Reduction of Labor Turnover

As already pointed out, normal labor turnover is advantageous because it allows injection of fresh blood into the firm. But excessive labor turnover is not desirable because it shows that labor force is not contended. Therefore, every effort should be made to remove the avoidable causes which give rise to excessive labor turnover. Following steps may be taken to reduce the labor turnover:

- A suitable personnel policy should be framed for employing the right man for the right job and giving a fair and equal treatment to all workers.
- Good working conditions which may be conducive to health and efficiency should be provided.
- Fair rates of pay and allowances and other monetary benefits should be introduced.
- Maximum non-monetary benefits (i.e., fringe benefits) should be introduced.
- Distinction should be made between efficient and inefficient workers by introducing incentive plans whereby efficient workers may be rewarded more as compared to inefficient workers.
- An employee suggestion box scheme should be introduced whereby workers who suggest improvements in the method of production should be suitably rewarded.
- Men-management relationships should be improved by encouraging labor participation in management.

EMPLOYEE ABSENTEEISM

Absenteeism is a pattern or habit of an employee missing work, often for no good reason.

Definition

Employee absenteeism is defined as the frequent absence of an employee from his/her work. This type of absence is often categorized as a habitual absence which excludes authorized leaves or paid time off.

Reasons for Employee Absenteeism (Fig. 8.43)

- **Low employee engagement:** Employee engagement is a vital part of the 21st-century work culture. In the shorter term, it is the practice followed by corporations to bring employees closer to their workplace.
- **Time theft:** Absenteeism does not always mean being absent for a whole day or two at the workplace. Employees taking unnecessary long breaks, coming late and leaving too early also imply absenteeism.
- **Lack of a flexible work schedule:** Flexible working has become a necessity rather than a privilege for professionals across businesses. Employees have their own social and personal commitments which they need to abide by for enjoying a sound work-life balance.
- **Workplace burnout:** Burnout is one of the major reasons for ill-performance displayed by the employees. This mostly occurs when employees are subjected to rigorous and unscheduled working conditions.

Box 8.23: Labor turnover example.

Early Risers Ltd is a manufacturer of breakfast cereals. Last year, it employed an average of 80 staff. During last year, the business recruited 12 staff to replace 15 who left.

$$\text{Labor turnover} = \frac{\text{Number of employees leaving (15)}}{\text{Average number employed (80)}} \times 100$$
$$= 18.75\%$$

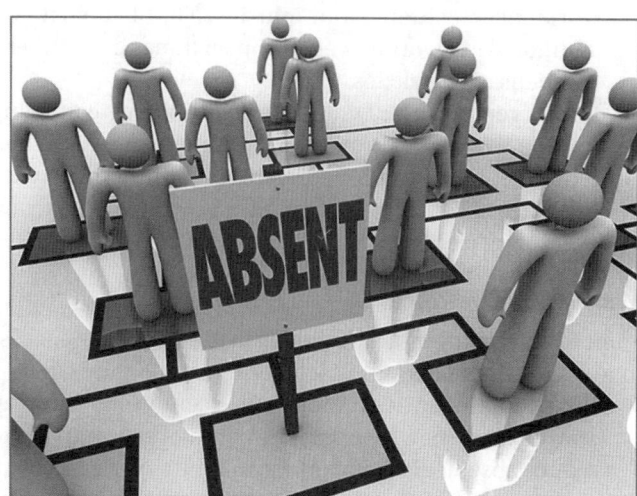

Fig. 8.43: Reasons for employee absenteeism.

- **Substance abuse:** Often employees succumb to unethical means of rejuvenation. Here, one of the most common examples would be alcoholism.
- **Misuse of seniority:** When employees have been a part of the organization for a long time they get accustomed to its operations. Being senior employees they often do not feel the need to inform their counterparts about their absence.
- **Workplace harassment:** Workplace harassment is a very major issue faced by workplaces around the globe. Harassment can be either in verbal or physical form. Such issues have a negative impact on employees' emotional state and their mental health. This also causes a decline in the employees' interest in their work leading to absenteeism.
- **Mental health issues:** All the reasons mentioned above ultimately lead to mental health issues. Having a sound mental health is one of the most important factors that help employees to showcase unbiased performance at work.

Costs/Effects of Absenteeism

It is important to understand what absenteeism costs you in real terms. Missed work days can affect a company in a number of ways. For example:

- **Lost work and wages:** The money comes from wages paid for no work, as well as additional wages for temporary employees or overtime.
- There are **administrative costs** associated with managing employee absenteeism, and over the course of a year, they can add up.
- **Lost productivity:** When employees are disgruntled and missing work, your overall productivity can take a hit. If left unaddressed, reduced productivity can cut into the profits.
- **Quality control:** When employees miss work and others have to pick up the slack, it is inevitable that the people who are putting in extra work will end up making mistakes.
- **Safety issues:** If you have to bring in temp workers or ask others to fill in for an absent employee, their lack of training and experience can lead to an increase in workplace accidents and injuries. That can cost you additional lost work as well as impact things like workers' compensation policies.
- **Employee morale:** One slacking employee can bring down a whole department or a whole company. When employees feel that one person is getting away with excessive absenteeism, it can have a negative impact on everything else in the workplace.

Measures to Overcome

Some ideas employers are beginning to use with some success in reducing (if not curing) absenteeism among their staff:

- **Providing incentives:** Providing incentives to show up at work is one newly popular way employers are trying to reduce absenteeism. Incentives may be as varied as extra vacation days, free gift cards, preferred parking spaces and more.
- **Providing mandatory paid sick leave days:** Offering paid sick leave is a good way to tell which employees are really sick when they are absent. It can also reduce genuine absences when a sick co-worker comes to work and contagious germs are passed around the office.
- **Workplace wellness programs:** There is some research that shows employers who assist employees with maintaining better health and fitness can also cut absenteeism in their workforce. Not only can wellness education teach employees how to stay healthier, but it can also communicate that an employer values their staff enough to invest in their wellbeing.
- **Vacation-friendly corporate culture:** In today's often uncertain economic times, employees can feel reluctant to take a vacation and still feel sure their job will be there on the other side. But this can lead to absenteeism when workers burn out on the job. Encouraging employees to take their vacation days can lower absenteeism rates and also make employees feel more valued.
- **Track attendance:** While this can backfire if used in an overly punitive way, it can also help employers with earlier identification of potential chronically late or absent workers. This provides a chance to fix the issue(s) causing the absenteeism before it becomes even more costly.

STAFF WELFARE

The institution should serve various facilities for the staff members to enable them to function effectively at their work. The institution expects from its staff a commitment to serve, in the spirit of god, the patients and others who come in search of the services. Some of the provisions provided are unique to the institution and we believe will faster a fellowship and friendship amongst the staff to develop a team spirit which is critical for successful medical services.

Purposes of Staff Welfare

- It motivates the staff to work effectively.
- It improves interest to serve to the particular institution.
- It facilitates the staff member to participate with full involvement.
- It improves the team work in the institution.
- It helps to meet the psychological, social and educational need of the employee.
- It helps to meet the psychological, social and educational and of the employee.

Faculty Improvement Techniques

- Encourage and Stimulate faculty
- Take positive attitude towards problems of teachers
- Provide resources and facilities for the implementation of instructions.
- Give recognition to abilities.
- Create a climate which stimulates creative participation by faculty members.
- While making changes in the curriculum, invite suggestions from the faculty.
- Given opportunity to plan, experiment and explore,

- Assist in developing teaching techniques
- Maintain good relation with faculty members.

Staff Welfare Activities (Fig. 8.44)

- The conditions under which the teaching staff have an effect on the implementation of the program besides contributing towards the stability of the staff.
- Frustrations, conflicts, resignations and frequent requesting for transfer can often be reduced when there are clearly defined policies related to hours of work, teaching load, welfare of the staff and other matters.
- The policies should be written down known to everyone. The following are some of the benefits for employee welfare activities; social security measures provided by the institution for the welfare of the employees.
  - Employees provident fund
  - Gratuity benefit
  - Maternity benefit
  - Risk allowances
  - Compensations for work injuries
  - Family pension schemes
  - Employee state insurance

Types of faculty welfare include:

- Opportunity for leave on the basis of leave rules by the institution policies. These leave rules incorporate existing annual leave, maternity leave, sabbatical leave, study leave, leave on loss of pay, official leave.
- Gratuity-cum-retirement benefit scheme
- Hospital concessions
- Staff special superannuation benefit scheme for long-term service.
- Provident fund
- Death benefit schemes
- Providing opportunity to develop cognitive skills by staff development programs, in-service program and continuing education programs. **Figure 8.45** shows staff benefit activities.

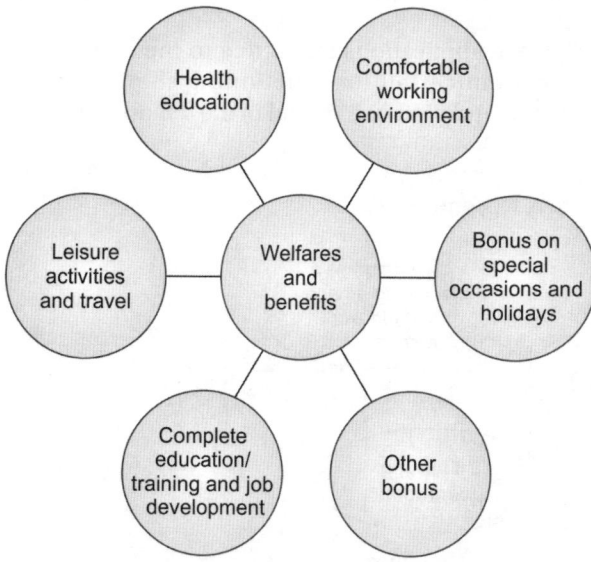

Fig. 8.44: Staff welfare services.

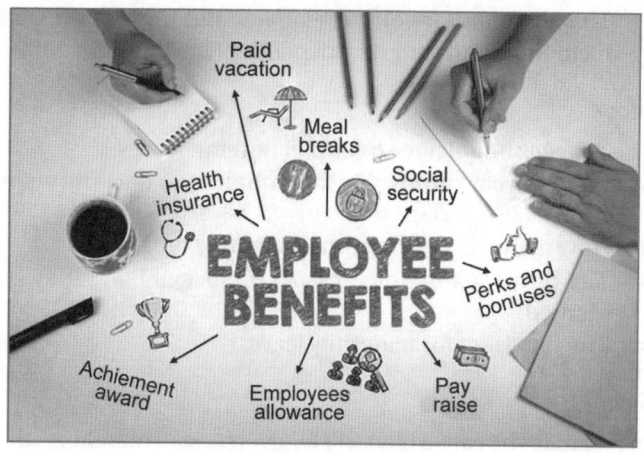

Fig. 8.45: Staff benefit activities.

Formulation of Policies

- Condition under which the teaching staff work, has an effect in the implementation on the program besides contributing towards the stability of the staff trust rations, conflicts, resignations and frequent requests for transfer, can often be reduced when there are clearly defined policies relating to hour of work, teaching load, welfare of staff and other matters.
- Such policies are particularly effective when the staff have been involved in formulating them, when they are known to everyone.
- The following are some of the matters in which it would be helpful to have stated policies and some of the factors to be considered in formulating them are.

Hours of Work

The policy should give direction on:
- The maximum number of working hours per week.
- The number of days off per month, to which the staff is entitled.
- The procedure to be followed regarding public holidays.

Teaching Load

- The policy regarding the maximum teaching load to be carried by each tutor should allow time for preparation for classes and laboratory sessions, student guidance and counseling, evaluation of student assignments, committee work, record keeping and all other functions expected of a tutor.
- A teaching load of 14–16 hours per week will permit attention to these functions.
- In cases where this in not possible, 20 hours of formal teaching per week should not be exceeded.

Residence

- There should be policy regarding the residence of staff quarters facilities.
- Residence for some staff is essential if student's curricular and extracurricular activities are implemented satisfactorily.

- The accommodation for married and unmarried staff including family quarters depends on institution's policy.

Leave

The college should have clear policy about leaves.
- Time of year during which annual leave may normally be taken.
- How many leaves may be taken at one time.
- The purpose for which casual or special leave may be granted.
- The provision for maternity leave.

Sickness

In regard to the care which will be given to staff members who are sick the college policy should state clearly about sick leave, medical expenses, reimbursement facility, etc.

Attendance at Conference and Study Care

The college should state policies regarding the selection and deputation of the staff for further education, including attendance at formal courses, refresher courses, work shop and conferences.

Promotion and Transfer

- Promotion is the transfer of an employee to a job that pays more money or one that enjoys some preferred status.
- A promotion is the advancement of an employee to a better job better in terms of greater responsibilities, more prestige or status, greater skill, and especially increased pay or salary.
- There should be a promotion policy in a college of nursing to motivate the teacher for higher productivity.
- The cadre of promotion must be clearly established and communicated to the employees.
- The promotion policy must consider the merit, potential for advancement and seniority of the employees. It should not be merely on the basis of year of experience.
- Transfer involves the shifting of an employee from one job to another without special reference to changing responsibilities or compensation, placing employees to position more appropriate to their interest or abilities or filling vacancies in a department.

In-service Education

- Service education is an organized educational program which is offered to trained staff during their period of employment and related to improvement of their performance.
- It should contain the element of orientation, training of special skills and continuing education.

Continuing Education

One of the basic aspects of continuing education for teachers is that it covers all those organized and informal means whereby teachers of all ages are encouraged to learn from one another and from society around them continuing education is very essential for the faculty because there has been an explosion of knowledge in medical science and other allied areas. Also the growth of science and technology has mostly contributed to the development of new knowledge in the field of teaching. The scope of continuing education for nursing teachers is very broad and comprehensive. It refers to the education a teacher receives after she has entered into the teaching profession.

Leave Facilities

Leave facilities incorporate existing annual leave, casual leave, compensatory holidays, sick leave, maternity leave sabbatical leave, study leave, leave on loss of pay, official level.

General Rules of Taking Leave

- Leave shall be granted in accordance with the leave rules of institution.
- Leave cannot be claimed by any employee as right.
- The administrative officer concerned shall be the competent authority to sanction by the administrative officer concerned depending up on the necessities.
- Ordinarily no employee shall absent himself or herself from work unless leave is sanctioned. Employees remaining absent unauthorisedly shall be subjected to disciplinary action.
- Normally, leave application shall be made in prescribed forms.
- All leave applications forwarded to the administrative officer concerted for sanctioning shall contain the recommendation of the head of the department.

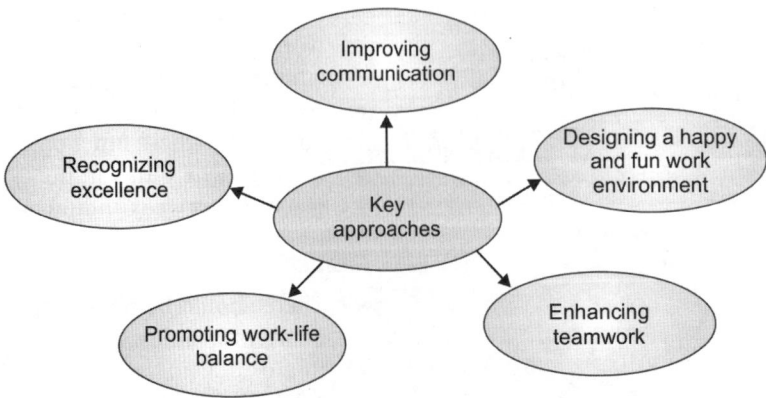

Fig. 8.46: The pride approaches.

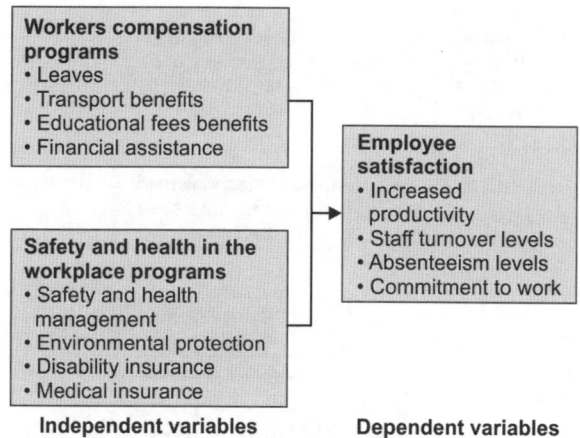

Fig. 8.47: Employee satisfaction.

- The administrative officer concerned shall arrange to intimate the unveiled leave to the credit of the employees of each department.

Annual Leave

- The quantum of annual leave shall be on the following scale.
- Council appointees-35 days, non-council appointees-25 days
- Annual leave for unconfirmed employees shall be calculated on prorate basis on the number of days spent on duty by on employee in the leave year. For arriving at the number of days spent on duty, the days availed on annual leave, casual leave, and sick leave, maternity leave will be taken into account.
- Annual leave cannot follow casual leave. However, casual leave up to a maximum of five days can be added on to the annul leave by prior permission of administrative officer concerned.
- Annual leave shall not be granted in more than three installments in a leave year.

Casual Leave

- Casual leave may be granted to a employees for a total of 10 days in each year subject to the necessities and exigencies of work.
- Casual leave may be either prefixed or suffixed to Sundays or holidays. Casual leave may be availed for half a day.
- Unexpected casual leave up to 2 day may be carried over to the following year to be used within the first six months.

Compensatory and Institutional Holidays

- If any member of staff is on any leave other than official leave on a declared holiday of the institution, no compensatory leave shall be given to him/her. However, if the day off given to a staff member falls on a declared.
- If Christmas, New Year's Day, Republic Day, Good Friday and Independence Day, which are National and Institutional holidays, falls on a Sunday, compensatory leave will be given which may be taken within 6 months.

Sick Leave

- Sick leave with full pay for a total of 15 days may be granted in a leave year.
- In addition to 15 days sick leave full pay as above, sick leave with half pay for a further period up to 18 days may be granted in a leave year. However, this cannot be converted to 9 days sick leave with full pay.
- Sick leave normally be granted only on production of a sick leave recommendation slip issued by the medical officer, staff student health service.
- Sick leave shall be sanctioned according to the number of days indicated in the sick leave slip issued by the staff student health service.

Maternity Leave

Women employees in the institution shall be granted maternity leave for 8 weeks with full pay. Part of the maternity leave may be availed just prior to delivery.

Incentives

- Incentives are provided by some organization in order to attract and retain good employees. Incentives may be monetary and non-monetary.
- The monetary incentives may be the form of payment of bonuses, merit increments, housing facilities, medical care, loans, provision of transportation, education of children, etc.
- The non-monetary incentives are also used to motivate the employees for higher education.
- They are in the form of status and recognition, job security, responsibility; participation is decision making, training facilities, promotion, discipline, team spirit, etc., negative incentives are in the form of fine, demotion, suspension, etc.

EMPLOYEE DISCIPLINE (FIG. 8.48)

Discipline is the backbone of healthy industrial relations. The promotion and maintenance of employee discipline is essential for smooth functioning of an organization. Employee morale and industrial peace are definitely linked with a proper maintenance of discipline. Disciplinary action can also help the employee to become more effective. The actions of one person can affect others in the group.

Meaning

Discipline means a prescribed conduct or pattern of behavior. Employee discipline at workplace can be defined as adherence to the company policies, rules, regulations and processes laid down by the management. With discipline comes self-restraint and responsibility. Discipline is important to business success and each employer wants to maintain discipline at workplace.

Definition

As rightly said by Jim Rohn, "Discipline is the bridge between goals and accomplishment".

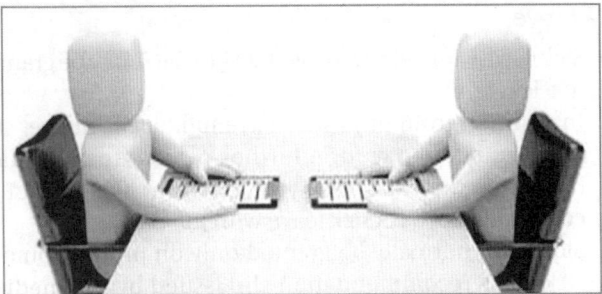

Fig. 8.48: Employee conduct and discipline.

Nature of Discipline

According to Megginson; discipline involves the following three things:
1. **Self-discipline** implies that a person brings the discipline in himself with a determination to achieve the goals that he has set for himself in life.
2. **Orderly behavior** refers to discipline as a condition that must exist for orderly behaviors in the organization.
3. **Punishment** is used to prevent indiscipline. When a worker goes astray in his conduct, he has to be punished for the same and the recurrences of it must be prevented.

Characteristics

- **Immediate:** Just as when you touch a red hot stove, the burn is immediate, similarly the penalty for violation should be immediate/immediate disciplinary action must be taken for violation of rules.
- **Consistent:** Just as a red hot stove burns everyone in same manner; likewise, there should be high consistency in a sound disciplinary system.
- **Impersonal:** Just as a person is burned because he touches the red hot stove and not because of any personal feelings, likewise, impersonality should be maintained by refraining from personal or subjective feelings.
- **Prior warning and notice:** Just as an individual has a warning when he moves closer to the stove that he would be burned on touching it, likewise, a sound disciplinary system should give advance warning to the employees as to the implications of not conforming to the standards of behavior/code of conduct in an organization. **Figure 8.49** shows the discipline process.

Common Issues Related to Employee Discipline (Fig. 8.50)

Nondisciplinary behavior by employees can disturb the decorum of the entire workplace. It can damage the reputation of the organization and adversely affect its profitability and growth. Examine if the following examples related to employee discipline are relevant to the business environment of your organization?

Compliance Issues

- Providing wrong information or hiding factual personal data during recruitment
- Noncompliance with the terms of employment contract, for example, an employee takes up additional job while still working in your organization.

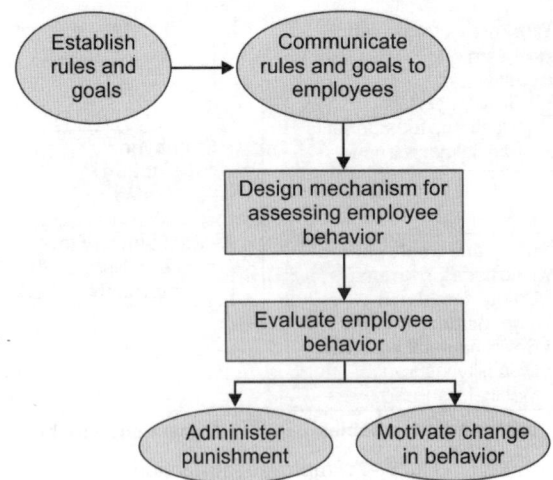

Fig. 8.49: The discipline process.

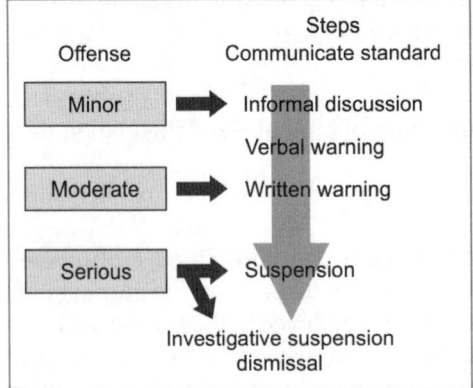

Fig. 8.50: Common issues related to employee discipline.

- Violation of company policies, rules and regulations
- Nonadherence to workplace safety instructions
- Indulgence in theft and fraud in the company
- Absconding without resignation
- False medical, travel and expense claims

Behavioral Issues

- Exhibiting misconduct towards manager, leadership and coworkers
- Reporting late to work or team meetings
- Frequent leave without intimation and approvals
- Indulging in political activities and antisocial activities
- Not completing work assignments on time or repeatedly not meeting goals
- Refusal to attend training programs
- Not marking attendance
- Wasting time on social media and other websites that are not related to work
- Bullying other colleagues
- Sexual harassment

Important Objectives

- To obtain a willing acceptance of the rules and regulations or procedures of an organization so that organizational goals may be attained.

- To develop among the employee a spirit of tolerance and a desire to make adjustments.
- To give direction or responsibility.
- To increase the working efficiency or morale of the employees so that their productivity is stepped up and the cost of production brought down and the quality of production improved.
- To create an atmosphere of respect for the human personality or human relations.

Principles for Maintenance of Discipline

Disciplinary measures have serious repercussions on employees; they should therefore, be based on certain principles, so that they may be fair just and acceptable to employees or their unions.

- As far as is possible, all the rules should be formed in cooperation or collaboration with the representatives of employees.
- All the rules should be appraised at frequent or regular intervals to ensure that they are and continue to be, appropriate, sensible and useful.
- Rules should be uniformly enforced if they are to be effective. They must be applied without exception.
- Penalties for any violation of any rule should be clearly stated in advance.
- Extreme caution should be exercised to ensure that infringements are not encouraged.
- If violations of a particular rule are fairly frequent; the circumstances surrounding them should be carefully investigated and studied in order to discover the cause or causes of such violation.
- Define or precise provisions for appeal or review of all disciplinary actions should be expressly mentioned in the employee's handbook.

Significance of Discipline

Significance of discipline can be explained as under:

From the point of view of an individual:
- Discipline provides self-safety to an individual.
- It enhances an individual's progress.
- An individual needs it for his own satisfaction.

From the point of view of a work group:
- Discipline ensures better teamwork and cohesive.
- A disciplined atmosphere is the key to the progress of the group.
- Discipline ensures higher productivity.
- Discipline enhances morale and motivation of employees.

From the point of view of an organization:
- Discipline ensures higher productivity and quality.
- Discipline helps an organization in attaining maximum profit.
- It is essential better all-round benefits.
- It helps in keeping a check on wastage and costs.
- It helps in developing a sense of belonging.

Factors influences: To be fair and equitable the following factors need to be analyzed:

- **Seriousness of the problem:** The manager must assess how serious is the indiscipline. For example, sexual harassment is more serious than late coming.
- **Duration of the problem:** It must be known for how long the problem continues or how often this happens. First time offence may be less serious than subsequent offences of longer duration.
- **Nature of the problem:** The pattern of the problem calls for more attention. It must be known whether it is a part of emerging problem or a continual problem. Continual problem is a serious one.
- **External influence:** Sometimes, a disciplinary problem may arise which is external to the employee. For example, an employee may fail to appear for an important meeting or performance appraisal due to some accident.
- **Degree of familiarity:** The organization with formal written rules governing the employee conduct is more justified in strictly enforcing disciplinary action taken than the organization where the rules of conduct are informal or vague.
- **Disciplinary practices:** There must be well laid out procedure in assessing disciplinary problems. Equitable treatment must take into consideration the previous actions taken against the employees for similar type of disciplinary violations.
- **Management support:** When the affected employee takes the issue to higher authorities, the manager must be having adequate reasons/data to defend his actions.

Consequences of disciplinary problems: Disciplinary action should have the following consequences:

- **Burns immediately:** If disciplinary action is to be taken, it must occur immediately so the individual will understand the reason for it. With the passage of time, people have the tendency to convince themselves that they are not at fault.
- **Provides warning:** It is very important to provide advance warning that punishment will follow unacceptable behavior. As you move closer to hot stove, you are warned by its heat that you will be burned if you touch it.
- **Gives consistent punishment:** Disciplinary action should also be consistent in that everyone who performs the same act will be punished accordingly. As with a hot stove, each person who touches it is burned the same way.
- **Burns impersonally:** Disciplinary action should be impersonal. There are no favorites when this approach is followed. **Figure 8.51** shows employee disciplinary measures.

Punishment: Minor and Major Punishment

Minor Punishment

- **Oral reprimand:** When a superior officer verbally warns the employee committing the offence, he expresses that he does not approve of his behavior. For example, employee sleeping during working hours or found smoking in the workplace.
- **Written reprimand:** Manager writes up the warnings and mails it to the employee concerned. The employee

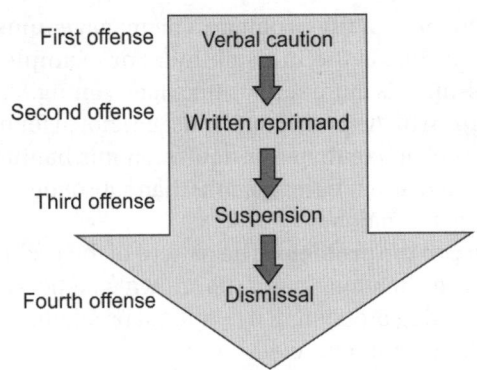

Fig. 8.51: Employee disciplinary measures.

is called for explanation. A copy of his reply is sent to HR department.

- **Punitive suspension:** It is awarded for minor offenses. It may extend for a few days. Employee gets subsistence allowance during the suspension period.
- **Loss of privilege:** Some of the privileges, such as assigning interesting work, shift preferences, leave, flexi hours, choice of machine, etc., may be withdrawn for a given period.
- **Fine:** A deduction may be made from the pay for certain offences, such as damage to the goods, machines and property of the company or for loss of money he has to account for.
- **Transfer:** An employee may be transferred to a far off place or to a different department for the offence committed. It is usually awarded by companies or institutions operating with a network of branches. Government institutions practice this type of punishment.

Major Punishment

- **Pay cut:** Cutting employee's pay for offences relating to damage or loss of property. The loss is recovered from the pay of the employee.
- **Demotion:** When the employee proves himself to be unfit for the present job he is holding, he is downgraded to a lower job carrying lower pay and responsibilities. It has a serious implication on the employee's morale and motivation.
- **Suspension pending enquiry:** It is awarded for serious offence. His regular wages are withheld during the period. The punitive suspension may extend for a longer period say several months till the enquiry is completed. Employee gets subsistence allowance during the suspension period.
- **Discharge:** It is awarded for the gravest offence involving integrity, moral turpitude, etc. There is a stigma attached to the dismissal and he may find it difficult to get employment elsewhere.

Policy Formulation

- It is essential to have a properly laid down and unambiguous company policy that defines the code of conduct expected from employees in various contexts (attendance, leave, employee interactions, customer interactions, sexual harassment, dress code, submission of expenses, etc.).
- The policy should be regularly updated, reviewed and shared with all employees in an easily accessible employee handbook format.
- The consequences of violating the policy must be clearly articulated.
- We recommend that the policy document be shared in your employee portal and employees should be expected to read and accept the document during on-boarding and at least once each year.

Disciplinary Committee

- A disciplinary committee should be formed where employees can report issues pertaining to discipline.
- This committee should take care of discipline management and document all disciplinary actions taken against the defaulters.
- The objective of disciplinary actions should be a transformation in the employee behavior. The disciplinary action therefore should be corrective, rather than destructive and should be carried out with rationality and without any bias.
- Follow the technique of progressive discipline. This type of disciplinary approach follows progression of disciplinary actions **(Box 8.24)**. Start from verbal counseling to

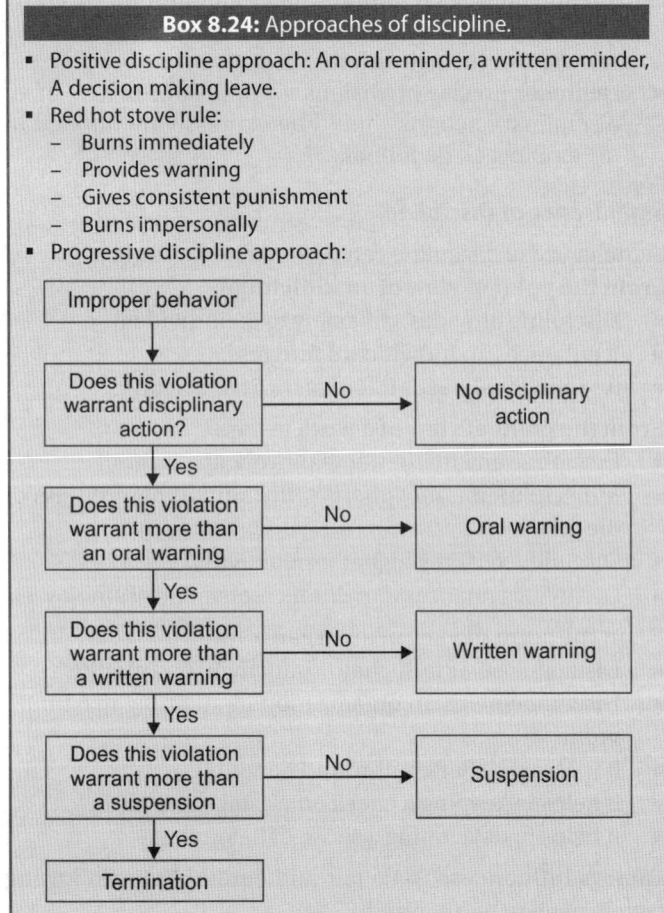

written warning to monetary deductions. And if needed, you can opt for suspension of the concerned employee. Termination of employee services should be a last resort.
- Process of redressal of complaints should be fair, confidential and transparent. Create an online helpdesk to address employee complaints and grievances. Employees should not feel victimized while reporting any disciplinary issue against any co-worker or a senior.

Background Screening

- At the time of recruitment and selection, the recruiters and hiring managers should conduct extensive background checks of candidates before making an offer.
- This can prevent a wrong hire that later results in a disciplinary issue.

Fairness

- Be fair while drafting employment policy.
- While every organization strives to be profitable, the goal should also include long-term sustainability, growth, goodwill and positive employee-employer relationships.
- Rules should not be crafted just for the sake of making rules.

■ EMPLOYEE GRIEVANCES (FIG. 8.52 AND BOX 8.25)

A grievance is any dissatisfaction or feeling of injustice having connection with one's employment situation which is brought to the attention of management. Speaking broadly, a grievance is any dissatisfaction that adversely affects organizational relations and productivity. To understand what a grievance is, it is necessary to distinguish between dissatisfaction, complaint, and grievance.

Features of Grievance

- A grievance refers to any form of discontent or dissatisfaction with any aspect of the organization.
- The dissatisfaction must arise out of employment and not due to personal or family problems.
- The discontent can arise out of real or imaginary reasons. When employees feel that injustice has been done to them, they have a grievance. The reason for such a feeling

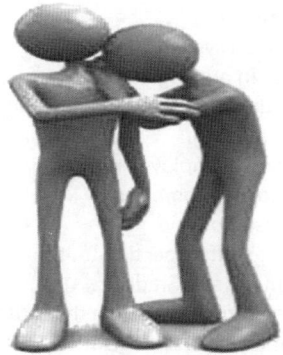

Fig. 8.52: Employee grievance and redressal.

> **Box 8.25:** Employee grievance.
>
> **Grievance** means any type of dissatisfaction or discontentments arising out of factors related to an employee's job which he thinks arc unfair, which may include, complaints concerning wages, hours of work, working conditions, performance evaluations, job assignments, or the interpretation or application of a rule, regulation or policy.
>
> **In an organization, a grievance may arise due to several factors, such as:**
> - Violation of management's responsibility, such as poor working conditions
> - Violation of company's rules and regulations
> - Violation of labor laws
> - Violation of natural rules of justice, such as unfair treatment in promotion, etc.
>
> **Sources of grievance may be categorized under three heads:**
> 1. Management policies
> 2. Working conditions
> 3. Personal factors

may be valid or invalid, legitimate or irrational, justifiable or ridiculous.
- The discontent may be voiced or unvoiced, but it must find expression in some form. However, discontent per se is not a grievance. Initially, the employee may complain orally or in writing.
- Broadly speaking, thus, a grievance is traceable to be perceived as non-fulfillment of one's expectations from the organization.

Causes of Grievances

Grievances may occur due to a number of reasons:
- **Economic:** Employees may demand for individual wage adjustments. They may feel that they are paid less when compared to others. For example, late bonus, payments, adjustments to overtime pay, perceived inequalities in treatment, claims for equal pay, and appeals against performance-related pay awards.
- **Work environment:** It may be undesirable or unsatisfactory conditions of work. For example, light, space, heat, or poor physical conditions of workplace, defective tools and equipment, poor quality of material, unfair rules, and lack of recognition.
- **Supervision:** It may be objections to the general methods of supervision related to the attitudes of the supervisor towards the employee, such as perceived notions of bias, favoritism, nepotism, caste affiliations and regional feelings.
- **Organizational change:** Any change in the organizational policies can result in grievances. For example, the implementation of revised company policies or new working practices.
- **Employee relations:** Employees are unable to adjust with their colleagues, suffer from feelings of neglect and victimization and become an object of ridicule and humiliation, or other inter-employee disputes.
- **Miscellaneous:** These may be issues relating to certain violations in respect of promotions, safety methods,

transfer, disciplinary rules, fines, granting leaves, medical facilities, etc.

Effects of Grievance

Grievances, if not identified and redressed, may adversely affect workers, managers, and the organization.

The effects are the following:

On the production:
- Low quality of production
- Low productivity
- Increase in the wastage of material, spoilage/leakage of machinery
- Increase in the cost of production per unit

On the employees:
- Increase in the rate of absenteeism and turnover
- Reduction in the level of commitment, sincerity and punctuality
- Increase in the incidence of accidents
- Reduction in the level of employee morale.

On the managers:
- Strained superior-subordinate relations.
- Increase in the degree of supervision and control.
- Increase in indiscipline cases
- Increase in unrest and thereby machinery to maintain industrial peace

Need for a formal procedure to handle grievances (Fig. 8.53):
- A grievance handling system serves as an outlet for employee frustrations, discontents, and gripes like a pressure release value on a steam boiler.
- Employees do not have to keep their frustrations bottled up until eventually discontent causes explosion.
- The existence of an effective grievance procedure reduces the need of arbitrary action by supervisors because supervisors know that the employees are able to protect such behavior and make protests to be heard by higher management.
- The very fact that employees have a right to be heard and are actually heard helps to improve morale.
- In view of all these, every organization should have a clear-cut procedure for grievance handling.

CONCLUSION

Staffing is the process of hiring eligible candidates in the organization or company for specific positions. In management, the meaning of staffing is an operation of recruiting the employees by evaluating their skills, knowledge and then offering them specific job roles accordingly. The staffing process is a systematic attempt to implement die human resource plan by recruiting, evaluating and selecting qualified candidates for the job-positions in the organization. Thus, such as planning and organization, staffing is also an important function of management.

REVIEW QUESTIONS

Long Essays

1. Define staffing, explain the objectives, mission and philosophy of staffing.
2. Describe the steps involved in staffing process.
3. Define staff scheduling, explain the dimension and types of staff scheduling.
4. Define duty roster, describe the objectives and principles.
5. Define recruitment, explain the methods and factors involves in recruitment.
6. Explain categories of nursing personnel working in nursing services and enumerate their job description.
7. Define staff welfare, enumerate the purposes and types.

Short Essays

1. Components of staffing.
2. Factors affecting staffing.
3. Functions of staffing.
4. Staffing process.
5. Importance of staffing.
6. Patient classification system.
7. Staffing activities in nursing.
8. Define training, discuss about objectives and types of training.
9. Credentialing in nursing.
10. Methods to improve employee retention.
11. Benefits of employee promotion.
12. Principles of transfer policy.
13. Norms of staffing-staff inspection unit.
14. Nursing Superintendent: Grade II
15. Define employee turnover, explain the causes and types.
16. Reasons for employee absenteeism
17. Employee discipline.
18. Employee grievances.

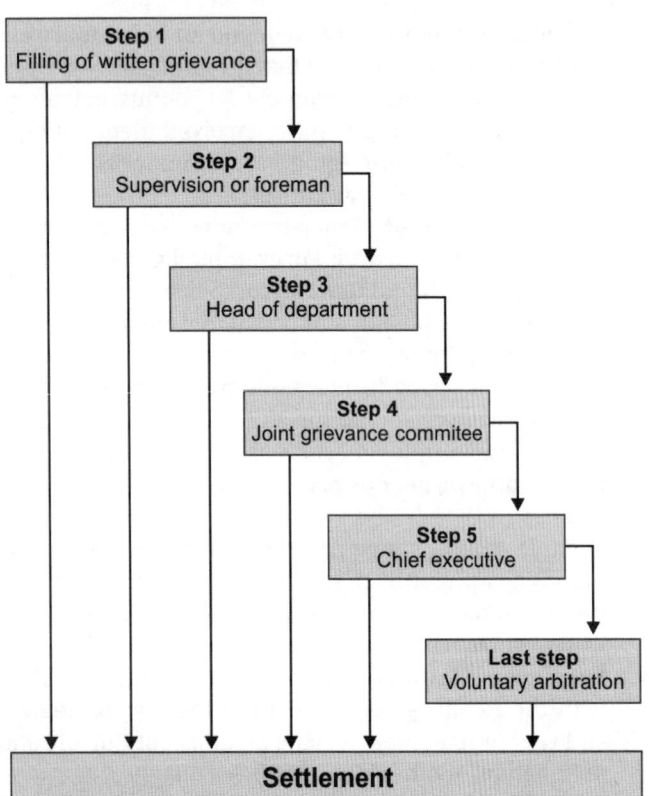

Fig. 8.53: Procedure to handle grievances.

Short Answers

1. Principles of staffing.
2. Manpower requirements.
3. Checklist.
4. Functions of the nursing service department.
5. Factors influencing nursing service.
6. Importance of the selection process.
7. Deployment management process.
8. Importance of training and development.
9. Career development process.
10. Define promotion.
11. Vertical promotion.
12. Types of transfer.
13. Cause of termination.
14. Types of superannuation benefit.
15. Objectives of staffing in nursing.
16. Principles of patient assignment.
17. Patient care delivery system.
18. Progressive patient care.
19. Faculty improvement techniques.
20. Continuing education.
21. Principles for maintenance of discipline.
22. Disciplinary committee.

BIBLIOGRAPHY

1. Aiken L. Hospital nurse staffing and patient mortality, nurse burnout, and job dissatisfaction. JAMA. 2002; 288:1987-93.
2. Anthony MK, Theresa S, Glick J, Duffy M, Paschall F. Leadership and nurse retention, the pivotal role of nurse managers. J Nurs Adm. 2005;35(3):146-55.
3. Basavanthappa BT. Nursing Management and administration. 6th edition. Jaypee Brothers Medical Publishers; New Delhi, 2010. pp. 78-84, 145.
4. Berkow S, Jaggi J, Fogelson R. Fourteen unit attributes to guide staffing. J Nurs Adm. 2007;37(3):150-5.
5. Blegen MA, Goode CJ, Reed L. Nurse staffing and patient outcomes. Nurs res. 1998; 47(1):43-50.
6. Cimiotti JP, Aiken LH, Sloane DM, et al. Nurse staffing, burnout, and health care–associated infection. Am J Infect Control. 2012; 40(6): 486-90.
7. Clark PA, Leddy K, Drain M, et al. "State nursing shortages and patient satisfaction: more RN—better patient experiences," Journal of Nursing Care Quality, 2007; 22(2): 119-27.
8. Clement I. Management of nursing services and education. 1st edition. Elsevier; New Delhi. 2011: pp-47-53,143-47.
9. Duffield C, Diers D, O'Brien-Pallas L, et al. Nursing staffing, nursing workload, the work environment and patient outcomes. Appl Nurs Res. 2011;(4)24:244-55.
10. Finkler SA, Kovner CT. Financial management for nurse managers and executives, 2nd edition. Philadelphia, PA: Saunders; 2000.
11. Gullatte MM. Nurse management: Principles and practice. Pittsburgh, PA: Oncology Nursing Society; 2005.
12. Henderson E. Budgeting: Part one. Nursing Management. 2003;10(1): 33-7.
13. Henderson E. Budgeting: Part two. Nursing Management. 2003;10(2): 32-6.
14. Koontz H, Weihrich H. Management a global perspective. 1st edition. New Delhi: Tata Mc. Graw Hill publishers; 2001.
15. Lehmann-Spitzer R. Nursing management desk reference concepts, skills and strategies. Philadelphia: Saunders; 1994.
16. Lucita M. Nursing: practice and public health administration, 2nd edition. Elsevier: New Delhi; 2013. pp. 57-63.
17. Maenhout B, Vanhoucke M. "An integrated nurse staffing and scheduling analysis for longer-term nursing staff allocation problems," Omega. 2013;41(2):485-99.
18. Marjorie B. Nurse executives' perspectives on succession planning. JONA. 2006, 36(6):304-12.
19. Marrelli TM. The nurse manager's survival guides (3rd edition). St. Louis, MO: Mosby; 2004.
20. Schmidt DY. Financial and operational skills for the nurse manager. Nursing Administration Quarterly.1999;23(4)16-28.
21. Topaloglu S, Selim H. "Nurse scheduling using fuzzy modeling approach," Fuzzy Sets and Systems. 2010; 161(11):1543-63.
22. Vati J. Principles and practice of the nursing management and administration, 1st edition. Jaypee Brothers Medical Publishers; New Delhi; 2013. pp. 218-27.

CHAPTER 9

In-service Education

LEARNING OBJECTIVES

- Nature and Scope of In-service Education Program
- Principles of Adult Learning-review
- Planning and Organizing In-service Educational Program
- Methods, Techniques and Evaluation
- Preparation of Report

INTRODUCTION

In-service education is a type of education that is provided to the employees while they are on the job so as to improve their working capacity and efficiency. The concept of in-service education is in budding form in India, whereas in Western countries, it has grown fully and has become an essential requirement of professional growth of a nurse.

In-service education is defined as learning experiences provided in the working setting for the purpose of assisting staff in performing their assigned functions in that particular agency. It is a planned educational experiences provided in the job setting and closely identified with service in order to help the person to perform more effectively as a person and as a worker. It is a planned instructional or training program provided by an employing agency in the employment setting and designed to increase competence ill a specific area **(Fig. 9.1)**.

DEFINITIONS

- In-service education is defined as learning experiences provided in the working setting for the purpose of assisting staff in performing their assigned functions in that particular agency.

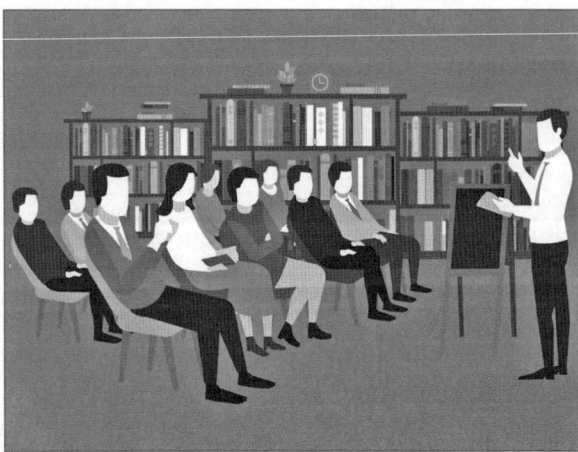

Fig. 9.1: In-service learning experiences.

- The American Nurses Association defined as "Planned education activities intended to build upon the educational and experiential bases of the professional nurse for the enhancement of practice, education, administration, and research or theory development to the end of improving the health of the public".
- In-service education is a planned learning experience provided by the employing agency for employees.
- According to Bagwandeen and Louw (1993), the definition of in-service education and training depends upon, to a large extent, the emphasis that is placed on it in terms of its plans and design. In addition, they also believe that generally, in-service training includes such aspects as updating teacher knowledge and skills.
- Henderson has defined in-service education and training as "In-service education and training may be in most general sense to be taken to include everything that happens to the teacher from the day he takes up his first appointment to the day he retires, which contributes directly or indirectly to the way in which he executes his professional duties".
- According to Brain Cane in Bagwandeen and Louw, "In-service training is taken to include all those courses and activities in which a serving teacher may participate for the purpose of extending his professional knowledge, interest or skill. Preparation for a degree, diploma or other qualification subsequent to initial is included in this definition".
- According to Signe E Froberg, "In-service education is a program of planned learning experiences providing opportunities within a working situation to improve the quality of care provided for patients by correcting information and skill deficiencies of personnel by assisting the inexperienced to acquire needed skills and attitudes, by keeping personnel abreast of changes in health care, and by stimulating the continuous

Chapter 9: In-service Education

Box 9.1: Nature and scope.
• It is a vehicle by which goals and the multiple articulated means available to achieve.
• It aim to developing ability for efficient working and the capacity for learning.
• To improve once competency in life.

development of occupational and personal abilities of each employee." Nature and scope is shown in **Box 9.1**.

PURPOSE, AIMS AND OBJECTIVES (BOX 9.2)

Purpose

- Helps to improve professional competence.
- Keep the nursing personnel abreast of the latest trends and development of new techniques.
- Helps to update the knowledge and skills at all levels.
- Nurses can update the knowledge regarding current research and development.
- Develops interest and job satisfaction among the staff.
- Encourage the employees in achieving staff development and self-confidence.
- Develops leadership skills, motivation and better attitudes

Aims

- The primary objective of in-service education is the improvement of professional practice, development of person as an individual and a responsible citizen.
- It keeps enthusiasm in their learning and makes them to seek latest knowledge.
- It enables to implement the knowledge with skill and ability.
- It improves the health care delivery to the public thus enhancing the quality of effective nursing practice.
- It develops interest and job satisfaction.
- By acquiring current and up to date knowledge, confidence is developed among them.
- Cost consciousness of nursing services in relation to all the programs.
- In-service education is designed to retrain people, to improve their performance and their communicative ability and it is designed to get them started on the never ending continuum education.
- To discover potentialities, to alert personnel in working environment.
- It reduces the turnover and absenteeism.
- To observe and bring changes in staff behavior.
- To maintain high standards in nursing.
- Improves the staff member's chances for promotion.

SCOPE OF IN-SERVICE EDUCATION

- Maintenance of familiarity with new knowledge and subject matter.
- Increased skill in providing service
- Improved attitudes and skills
- Greater skill in utilizing community resources and in working with adults.
- Development and refinement of common values and goals.

NEED FOR IN-SERVICE PROGRAM (BOX 9.3)

- Need for in-service education (ISE) for professional nurses is influenced by research and advances in health care. In the current health environment, the quality appropriateness and effectiveness of interventions assume increasing importance.
- In-service education program for the nursing staff are frequently planned by the nursing service administration.
- The most effective programs give emphasis on outcome rather than on staff development. If result is considered valuable the individual's participation will be active.
- Some hospitals have found that staff development, personal and professional reaches its highest level when members work together to achieve a common purpose.
- Even when the hospital has not in-service program, it would be better for the staff to have such program it would be better for the staff to have such Programs within their wards.
- Well qualified staff nurses can make a worthy contribution to the students education both by assisting in the planned program and by their, e.g., as nurses.
- The head nurse can help medical students in their adjustment to the hospital wards by holding orientation conferences and teaching them some of the fundamentals of nursing care.
- The increased knowledge owing to this program assists in maintaining an efficient ward. Housekeeping workers will also be taught on the ward.

Box 9.2: Objectives.
• To provide incentives to the teachers
• To help the teachers to know their problems
• To solve them by pooling their resources and wisdom
• To employ more effective methods of teaching
• To get acquainted with modern techniques in education
• To broaden the mental outlook of the teachers
• To upgrade the teachers knowledge and understanding of the contents
• To increase the professional efficiency of the teacher

Box 9.3: Need for ISE.
• Increased knowledge and expanding technology
• Nurse's role expansion
• Gain in professional status
• Job satisfaction
• Pop mobility—increased turn over
• Changing role of hospital (curative to preventive and promotive)
• Changing nature of nursing
• Clinical content (technological advances)
• Need for gain in professional status

IMPORTANCE OF IN-SERVICE EDUCATION

- Education for the educator continuous all throughout his professional career in a planned manner.
- Educational extension will contribute to the qualitative improvement of education.
- The ill-service training provided to the nurse is not adequate for the rest of his professional career for discharging his duties effectively.
- It is bringing the required changes in education.
- It is necessary to improve the competence of the nurse in terms of knowledge, skills, interest and aptitude.
- It is helping these individuals in meeting their academic needs and in solving their academic problems.
- It is an essential means for improving education.

PRINCIPLES OF IN-SERVICE EDUCATION

Principles for developing an in-service education program:
- Have the organizational structure for in-service education program as simple as possible.
- Not to include many things at a time.
- Avoid being involved in complex and long-term projects.
- Start with those problems which disturb the personnel most.
- Work with the personnel and give them time to grow.
- Keep flexibility in in-service education program.
- Move step by step, from simple to complex.
- Start in-service education for personnel in a simple and easy way so that they can remember that exists among change.
- A scientific approach, humanism, democracy, unity, inclusiveness, differentiation, integration, continuity, modularity, personalization, end through nature.
- Compliance with state regulation of educational standards.
- In-service education is one of the categories of adult education.
- The specific objectives serve as a guide line in developing in-service education program and activities.

CHARACTERISTICS OF GOOD IN-SERVICE EDUCATION

An in-service education program is considered to be good and effective if it involves the following characteristics:
- In-service education activities are based on real and specific problems of workers or patients.
- It has involved all the personnel in planning, all in-service education activities.
- The in-service educator has developed an insight and thinking in all the members participating in in-service education program. It has resulted in self-improvement from within.
- The learning principles are utilized. Learning is growth, growth is personal and gradual. Growth takes place in a climate favoring the development of new perceptions that can be translated into actual practice.
- In-service education Program is an integral part of working program and time, money, etc., are provided for proper functioning of program.
- Participation and cooperation with the community and educational faculties are included in the activities.

FACTORS AFFECTING IN-SERVICE PROGRAM

The economic, social, medical and technological sciences which affect that society will affect nursing in-service education. The related factors affect the in-service education programs are:
- Cost of health care in-service education program may increase the efficiency of nursing services, but it adds additional expenditure on healthcare delivery system.
- Manpower in-service education requires need qualified human resources, leads to increase human resources.
- Changes in nursing practice leads to frequent changes in the programs and in-service education.
- Standards for nursing practice.
- Organization of nursing departmental planned approaches is regular.

COMPONENTS OF IN-SERVICE EDUCATION (FIG. 9.2)

- **Orientation:** The orientation influences the structure and content of individualized orientation of various groups of nursing service people. The goal of the orientation program is to enhance the competencies of nursing service personnel so that employees may continuously improve the quality of care provided to patients.
- **Skill training:** For the new employee skill training provides an idea about how to carry out the assigned function complex ones. It enables to meet the standards established for quantity and quality of the performance and job satisfaction; it improves the new employee's skill in the routine and special procedures.
- **Leadership development:** The staff should have skills in leadership and management in order to guide a new employee in caring outpatient care activities. At present, the hospitals are recognizing the development of leadership and management qualities among the staff

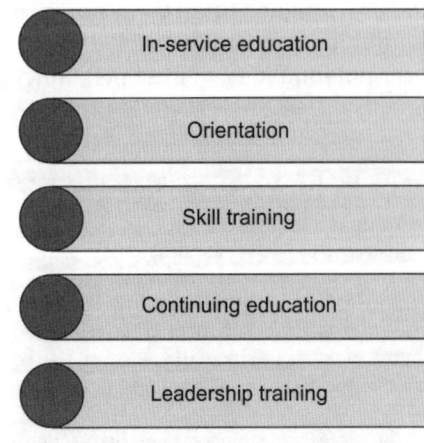

Fig. 9.2: Components of in-service program.

- **Continuing education:** The international council of nurses emphasized the importance of continuing education for nurses in order to ensure safe and effective nursing care; it consists of a large number of educational programs and activities. It is necessary for all the level of nursing personnel to deal with the needs of nursing oneself aware of all the development in the field of the specialization.

APPROACHES TO IN-SERVICE EDUCATION

Whether the pattern of in-service education desired to be centralized, decentralized or coordinated approach will directly affect the organization policies and practices.

Centralized Approach

- The centralized approach has its origin in the belief that the in-service curriculum ought to emanate from and be conducted by nursing personnel in the central administration of the agency.
- None of the learners are consulted or participate in planning learning experiences and yet are expected to attend an in-service offering.
- Centralized approach to in-service education leads to in reducing spontaneous.
- Some of the advantages to administrator of centralized approach are found where budget control and evaluation of the programming are facilitated, when use of resources, people, places and things are decided, and then committees are directed to work on specific problems identified by administration.

Decentralized Approach

- The decentralized approach is based on a conviction that the in-service curriculum for nursing personnel should be the responsibility, in large measure, of the practicing nurse with whom the personnel work.
- Decentralized in-service education is planned by and conducted for the employees of one or more units.
- The employees may be expected to keep administration informed of their activities and possibly consult with administration when help is wanted, but the employees are expected to develop and direct their own learning experiences.
- With a decentralized approach, control in planning for in-service is a responsibility of employees.
- Initiative and participation are qualities which are valued; they may be fostered by decentralized approach.
- The hazards decentralized approach are: lack of leadership, conflicts, inefficiency, less or no budget will be expected.
- The advantages of decentralized approaches lie in those individuals, who work on the same unit and confront problems in common, share the responsibilities for meeting in-service needs which planning and implementation of program. Proper contribution of the participants is also expected.

Coordinated Approach

- The coordinated approach is a compromise between the centralized and decentralized patterns in that, while the practicing nurse does indeed carry large measures of responsibility for the in-service curriculum, the central administration of nursing personnel of the agency is responsible for a broad program which is of importance to all nursing personnel.
- In this way, coordination is improved, duplication is avoided, and unity of efforts is maintained. An added advantage of coordinated approach is that realistically, people will tend to lend support to an effort in which they personally participate or contribute; this approach involves both nursing administrators and practitioners in complementary way.
- Coordinated approach provides for mutual cooperation and assistance to central administration and unit personnel in the agency.
- For the in-service education curriculum, a central planning group, comprised of elected representatives from categories of personnel and the in-service staff which is in a staff rather than line capacity, formulates short and long range goals and plans for the agency.
- An administrative advisory group comprised of chiefs in the agency serves as a consultative, informational resource to the planning group and as facilitator and expediter where and when cooperation needed. **Figure 9.3** shows steps in developing in-service program.

ORGANIZATION OF IN-SERVICE EDUCATION

Orientation (Fig. 9.4)

The orientation program usually includes a tour of the physical setting as well as information on the philosophy goals and structure of the overall hospital and the department of nursing team. Under normal circumstances it takes only a few days to orient new employees to the work situation and setting.

- The new nursing personnel require help and inspiration during their first difficult days in the field.
- They need assistance in nursing procedures, records and reports with which they may not be familiar and above all they need a welcome from all as well as a feeling of security.
- The program of introduction will depend on the staff's preparation, her experience and interest in the program.
- The nursing procedure, standing instructions and manual of policies should be explained to the staff and also demonstrated whenever indicated.
- Arrangement should be made with senior and experienced staff for observation of nursing activities in home, school and community.

Objectives of Orientation

- To support the new employee during the transition period to the assigned area.
- To assist the new employee in identifying individual strength and weakness.

Chapter 9: In-service Education

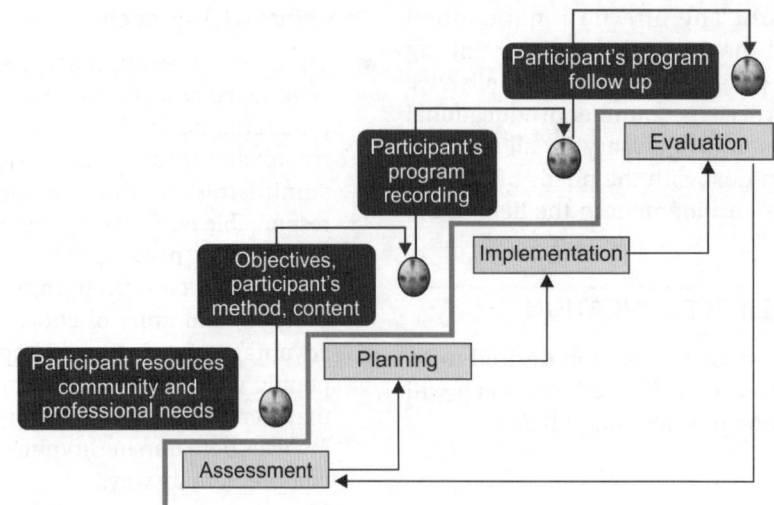

Fig. 9.3: Steps in developing in-service program.

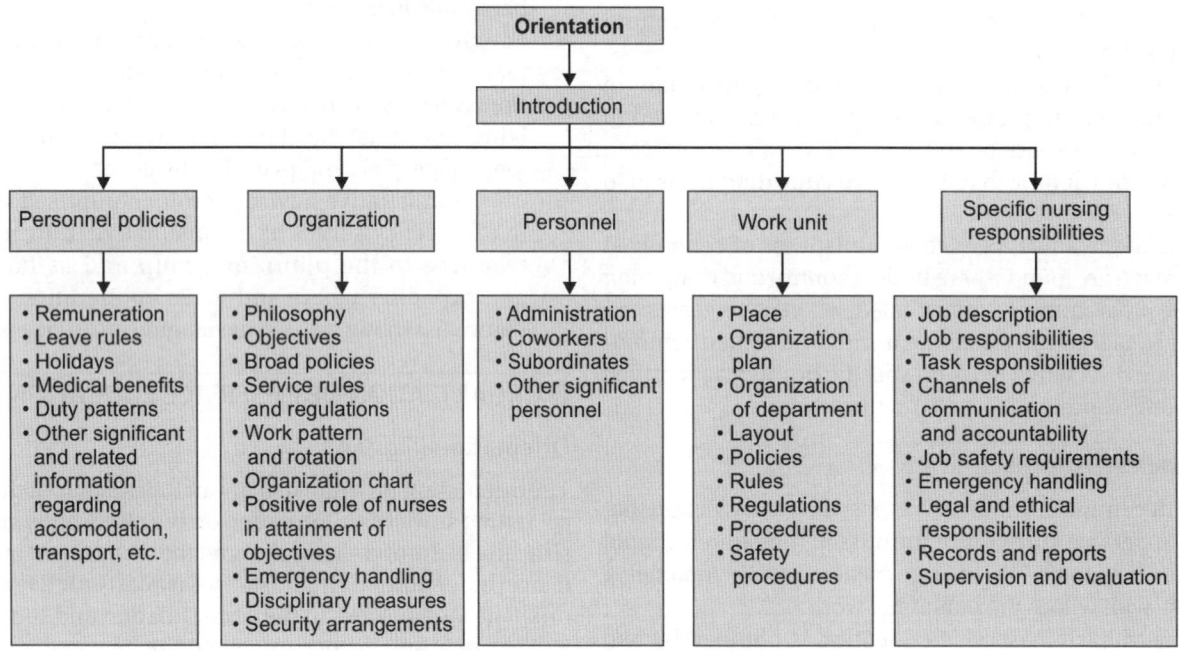

Fig. 9.4: Orientation in in-service program.

- Provide ongoing appraisal of the new employee's performance during orientation via the regularly scheduled meetings.
- Provide an introduction, review of basic skills and selected learning experiences based upon individual needs.
- Act as a liaison between the employee and the staff, assisting and encouraging the staff to participate in teaching the new employee.

Purposes
- To acquire knowledge their relationship and function
- To know organizational set up, history of the hospital including policies, routines of the hospital
- To understand the job description of the different categories of the employees
- To know the staffing patterns with new strategies, salary facilities and residential facilities

Components
There are two types of components: 1. Centralized orientation, 2. Decentralized orientation

- **Centralized orientation:** This includes general orientation, orientation to hospital and aid orientation to nursing.
  - **General orientation:** Physical set up, policies, purposes, schedule and role of employees.
  - **Orientation to the hospitals:** Organizational setup of the hospital history, and philosophy of the hospital, practice of the hospital, resources available like library, basic safety of the patients.
  - **Orientation to nursing department:** Organization of nursing department, resources available to nursing development. Special program or ward activities, such as ward conferences, presentations.
- **Decentralized orientation:** This includes orientation to the nursing unit and orientation to the nursing team.

- **Orientation to nursing unit:** Ward routine, duties taking and handing over charges, clinical activity like providing patient care, admission and discharge procedure, providing for investigations controlling cross infections.
- **Orientation to the nursing team:** Duties, responsibilities and functions of each team member, methods and tool for report and challenging patient care information, evaluation other orientation areas and orientation programs.

Orientation Skill Training Program

- Orientation training program introduces a new employee to these basic aspects of her job.
- In hospital field, if any new nurses are appointed, first the supervisor has to discuss with them the job chart, polices, procedures, and fulfillment of objectives, standing orders, policies of institution.
- If she is well-oriented to her working situation, she will be getting adjusted to the new environment very easily and do the work effectively.
- Orientation skill training has to be given for development of knowledge and skills (cognitive, psychomotor and affective domains).
- In community filed orientation training. Camps will be organized to school teachers, village leaders and MPAW by the health personnel about the concept of health and illness, etiological factors for disease, identification of case, prevention and treatment in order to reach Health for All (HFA) by 2000 AD.

The major benefits of an effective orientation program are:
- Orientation can create in the new employee a favorable impressing with respect to the work and the organization.
- Orientation can help to relieve the new employee's anxiety about the job and help him or her to become comfortable in the position.
- Orientation can help provide critical information concerning the job and organization. In the process, it helps the employee develop more realistic job expectations.
- Orientation can save time and effort during the critical learning process.

Skill Training

A skill is a great ability or proficiency. The skill training provides how and why to the new employer in carrying out the assigned functions. Skill training may range from simple to complex or general to specific.
- The importance of skill training and orientation to new employee providing close relationship between good nursing care and good ward management.
- Skill training helps the new employee to develop new knowledge and skill required to do particular task, e.g., a hospital acquiring new equipment, such as cardiac monitor or a new incubator to care low birth weight infant.

Objectives of Skill Training

- It enhances the employee standard of working performance
- It lessens the direct supervision needed by the employer
- Reduces friction
- Provides the job satisfaction
- Provides to perform correct method
- Lessen the wrong method being carried out
- Understand 'how' and 'why'

Leadership and Management

Leadership and management are important because the nurse is expected to function with the help of auxiliary members of nursing staff. Her competence in such areas in writing care plans, conducting conference, giving transfer reports, supervising and directing nonprofessional staff will he large measure which determines the degree of the nurse success in a charge as team leader role.

- The growing complexities of hospital staff today make it imperative for many people to have skills in leadership management in order to guide a diverse staff in carrying out patient care responsibilities.
- More and more hospitals are recognizing the special abilities of leadership and management and are eager to cultivate these qualities among appropriate staff.

Objectives

- Decentralize leadership management competency and spread this among personnel
- Permit increased delegation of authority
- Promote good morals among administrative personnel which in turn influence staff morale
- Aid in reducing costly turn over in top positions
- Level up appreciation of service and objectives of hospital.
- Assist the individual to project her own personality in the job using desirable concepts of leadership and management.
- Lessen amount of direct supervision and guidance needed

Management skills and leadership training: For the administrators and the senior personnel, for the persons who possess higher qualifications, who is having the chances for promotion and the supervisors the authorities will give in-service training to obtain management skill and leadership skills in order to supervise the institution to achieve the targets by reaching goals and preparing the persons to solve their problems if any need arises and to have smooth environment in their working areas.

Continuing Education

- Continuing education means the phenomenon of ever learning which does not stop at any particular stage.
- It includes all learning opportunities which would be taken up after full time education has stopped.
- It is the resumption of the process of studying or learning which might have interrupted because of some economic, professional and personnel compulsion of the individual.
- The American Nurses Association (ANA) has defined continuing education as "learning activities", intended to build upon the education and experience basis of the professional nurse for the enhancement of practice

education, administration, and research or theory development.
- Continuing education program provide teaching and learning strategies that are based upon the learning theory which states that adult learners should participate in the development of their learning objectives.

Need for Continuing Education (Box 9.4)

- Kothari Education Commission also suggested that education institutions should arrange courses which will make people to understand and solve their problems in life and to train wider knowledge and experience.
- Learning through continuing education is also essential for the rural people, who must acquire full knowledge about rapid advancement of agricultural and economic techniques just as urban people have to acquire commercial techniques.
- Indian Education Commission has rightly stated about it, "Education does not end with school, but it is a lifelong process."
- Continuing education program provide teaching and learning strategies that are based upon learning theory which states that adult learners should participate in the development of their learning objectives.
- Continuing education is the most essential requirement of the adult today. He can enjoy a better, healthier and more successful life only if he continues his education up to end of his life.

Types (Fig. 9.5)

- **Centralized in-service training:** In nursing service department, one department will held responsibility for improvement of knowledge, skills, practice of their nursing staff. They will devote full time for in-service education program and its activities.
- **Decentralized in-service education:** This is planned for staff members who work together, giving care for clients with similar conditions and share common nursing goals. Programs are planned around the special relevant interests of the employees, e.g., TRR, ICCU units.

Box 9.4: Need.

- Rapid technological advances related to knowledge explosion have greatly altered the practice of nursing
- The gap between scientific knowledge and its application grows wider each year as a result of multiple influences
- Elimination of certain illnesses, particularly the communicable diseases
- New drugs to cure some illnesses and alter the course of many
- Surgeries are being performed successfully in areas that would not have been attempted 10–20 years ago
- Organ transplants are no more a novelty
- Complex and intricate machinery can extend lives
- All these advances require more highly skilled nursing care in a great variety of settings
- Continuing education is an accepted way of life

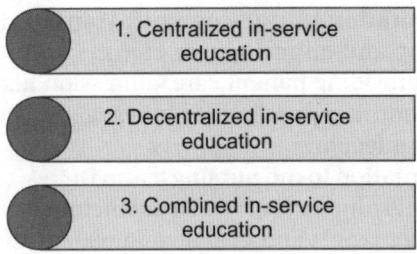

Fig. 9.5: Types.

- **Combined or coordinated in-service education approach:** There will be a central nursing in-service education department consists of nurse in each division, who holds leadership responsibility for staff development activities, whose time is devoted fully for teaching-learning situations. They plan, conduct, evaluate the program and further plan their programs basing on the need arises.

EVALUATION METHODS USED

Questionnaires and Inventories

- The advantages of some sort of pencil-and-paper response procured some time after training are roughly parallel to those of written RMRs immediately after training.
- Questionnaires and inventories have the added advantage of the relatively systematic planning and coverage that a good instrument involves.
- Hypotheses of an "explanatory," as contrasted with a purely summary-descriptive, nature can be tested, as, for example, "Did people with the strongest initial interest tend to feel they learned the Most?"
- The resulting data can be used to get answers to questions formulated before any training sessions are held

Interviews

- Talking with group members or co-workers some time after training, either individually or in groups, gets helpful and thorough data again the more valuable because a systematic pre planned set of questions can be answered by careful inquiry.
- Interviews share the advantages and are advantages of oral evaluation suggested above.
- They take practicing if they are to get evidence that can be counted on; and careful recording is important.
- The processing and analysis of interview data is extremely time-consuming.
- An added advantage, however, is that most people are not ordinarily listened to very much in our culture, and interviews are not only ego involving but fun (and even flattering) for the interviewee so data are easier to get.

Observation of behavior in the in-service program:

- We have saved until last the evaluation method that most people find most effective for judging the consequences of training for in-service program skills.

- The basic question is: Are members doing any better what they originally were worried or concerned about?
- From this point of view, members, the trainer(s), and co-workers not involved in the training are all looking at in-service performance with a keenly pragmatic eye to see whether the program is going any more smoothly.

PROBLEMS RELATED TO IN-SERVICE EDUCATION (BOX 9.5)

- Lack of incentives
- Lack of motivation
- Lack of interest
- In appropriate method and tech ii questions
- Inadequate evaluation technique
- Inappropriate curriculum and courses
- Inadequate training of teacher educators
- Administration problems
- Organization problems
- Functional problems
- Lack of specification in objectives
- Lack of follow up programs
- Lack of relationship and type of in-service education programs.

SUGGESTIONS FOR IMPROVEMENT

Suggestion for the improvement of in-service education program:

- A large scale and coordinated program of continuing education for nurses of all levels should be organized by instruction and trained nurses association.
- Visualizing our limit resources is advisable to arrange for each nurse in initial stage program at the rate of 3 months continuing education in every five years of completed service.
- A fundamental policy may be evolved at national level to make adequate to involve every nurse in their professional growth.
- The program of in-service education should be varied in nature to meet the needs of nurses belonging to different categories.
- Planning of in-service education should follow a comprehensive approach based on understanding needs of nursing.
- There is a need of developing community education through deeper thinking and pooling of ideals.
- Success of in-service education will depend largely on the ability and competence of experts.

Box 9.5: Problems related to in-service education.
- Lack of incentives
- Lack of motivation
- Lack of interest
- Inappropriate methods and techniques
- Inadequate evaluative techniques
- Inappropriate curriculum and courses
- Inadequate facilities or resources problems
- Inadequate training of teacher education

NURSING IN-SERVICE EDUCATION

A need was felt by the nursing administrators that a planned nursing in-service education needs to be started so as to increase the knowledge base of practicing nurses in order to improve and maintain high standard of nursing care in the hospital.

Aims/Objectives

- To increase the existing knowledge base of nurses practicing clinical nursing.
- To improve and maintain high standard of nursing care to patients, which would increase the satisfaction level of patients/relatives.
- To improve communication skills among nursing personnel.
- To update knowledge regarding handling/upkeep of latest and sophisticated instruments and gadgets.
- To enable nurses to secure credit points for renewing their nursing license by the DNC. **Figure 9.6** shows concept of in-service program.

Common Topics

Classes for sister in charges/ANS/DNS/NS/CNO
- Human relations in nursing
- Materiel management
- Ethical and legal issues in clinical nursing
- Conflict management
- Stress management
- Nursing administration

Classes for bedside nurses
- Patient safety
- Nursing process
- Human relations in nursing
- Ethical and legal issues in clinical nursing
- Pre- and postoperative nursing management
- Stress management
- Medication administration safety

Needs for in-service education in nursing:
- Needs for development of manual, behavioral and communication skills essential for execution of their jobs.
- Needs for development of decision making and managerial skills.

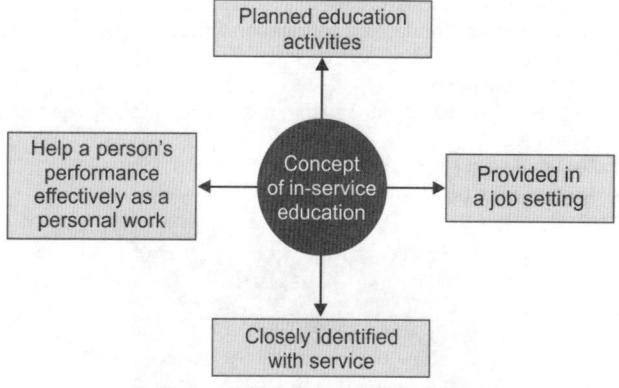

Fig. 9.6: Concept of in-service program.

- Needs for introduction to their routine job, which are expanding new, higher, complicated. Needs for development of leadership skills
- Needs for development of analytical and innovative thinking for investigating the potentialities and efficiency of their job.

ADULT EDUCATION/LEARNING

Adult education is concerned not with preparing people for life, but rather with helping people to live more successfully. Thus, if there is to be an overarching function of the adult education enterprise, it is to assist adults to increase competence, or negotiate transitions, in their social roles (worker, parent, retiree, etc.), to help them gain greater fulfilment in their personal lives, and to assist them in solving personal and community problems **(Fig. 9.7)**.

Definition

- Adult learning is defined as 'the entire range of formal, non-formal and informal learning activities which are undertaken by adults after a break since leaving initial education and training, and which results in the acquisition of new knowledge and skills.
- The European Commission defines adult learning as, 'all forms of learning undertaken by adults after having left initial education and training, however far this process may have gone (e.g., including tertiary education).'

Characteristics of Adult Learner (Box 9.6)

Adult learners have characteristics that set them apart from 'traditional' school or college learners. All adults come to courses with a variety and range of experiences, both in terms of their working life and educational backgrounds. This impacts on how and why they participate in learning. While each student has individual learning needs, there are some characteristics that are common to adult learners.
- **Adults have accumulated life experiences:** Adults come to courses with experiences and knowledge in diverse areas. They tend to favor practical learning activities that enable them to draw on their prior skills and knowledge.

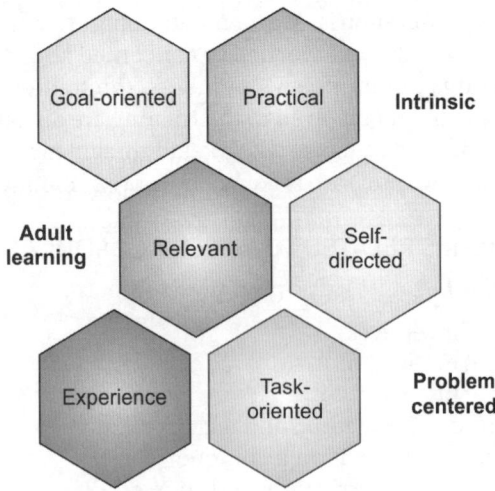

Fig. 9.7: Adult learning.

Adults are realistic and have insights about what is likely to work and what is not. They are readily able to relate new facts to past experiences and enjoy having their talents and knowledge explored in a teaching situation.
- **Adults have established opinions, values and beliefs** which have been built up over time and arrived at following experience of families, relationships, work, community, politics, etc. These views cannot be dismissed and must be respected.
- **Adults are intrinsically motivated:** Learners increase their effort when motivated by a need, an interest, or a desire to learn. They are also motivated by the relevance of the material to be addressed and learn better when material is related to their own needs and interests. For learners to be fully engaged in learning their attention must be fully focused on the material presented.
- **Individual differences:** Adults learn at various rates and in different ways according to their intellectual ability, educational level, personality and cognitive learning styles. Teaching strategies must anticipate and accommodate differing comprehension rates of learners.
- **Adults learn best in a democratic, participatory and collaborative environment:** Adults need to be actively involved in determining how and what they will learn, and they need active, not passive, learning experiences.
- **Adult students are mature people** and prefer to be treated, as such being 'lectured at' causes resentment and frustration.
- **Adults are goal-oriented/relevancy-oriented:** Adults need to know why they are learning something. Adults have needs that are concrete and immediate. They can be impatient with long discussions on theory and like to see theory applied to practical problems. They are task or problem-centered rather than subject-centered. Adults tend to be more interested in theory when it is linked to practical application.
- **Adults are autonomous and self-directed:** They are self-reliant learners and prefer to work at their own pace. Individuals learn best when they are ready to learn and when they have identified their own learning needs.

> **Box 9.6:** Characteristic of adult learning.
> - Adult are autonomous and self directed
> - Adult have accumulated a foundation of life-experience and knowledge
> - Adult are goal-oriented
> - Adult are relevancy oriented so they must see a reason for learning something
> - Adult are practical
> - Adult need to be shown respect

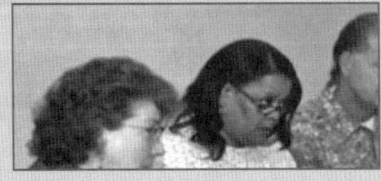

Where a student is directed by someone else to attend a course, e.g., by an employer, then that individual may not be ready to learn or may not see the value in participating on that course. This can lead to a mismatch of goals between all parties—student, employer and trainer.

- **Adults are practical and problem-solvers:** Adults are more impatient in the pursuit of learning objectives. They are less tolerant of work that does not have immediate and direct application to their objectives. Problem based learning exercises are welcomed as they build on prior experience and provide opportunity for practical application of materials/theories covered.
- **Adults are sometimes tired when they attend classes:** Many students are juggling classes with work, family, etc. They, therefore, appreciate varied teaching methods that add interest and a sense of liveliness to the class.
- **Aging concerns:** Adults frequently worry about being the oldest person in a class and are concerned about the impact this may have on their ability to participate with younger students. Creating an environment where all participants feel they have a valuable contribution can work to allay such concerns.
- **Adults may have insufficient confidence:** Students come to class with varying levels of confidence. Some may have had poor prior experiences of education leading to feelings of inadequacy and fear of study and failure. This can manifest itself in many ways, as indicated in the next section.

Characteristics of Adult Learning (Box 9.7)

- **Persistence:** Persevering when the solution to a problem is not readily apparent.
- **Decrease impulsivity:** Think before speaking or doing.
- **Listen:** Listen to others with empathy and understanding.
- **Flexibility in thinking:** Consider other options—there's never one right way to do everything.
- **Metacognition:** Try to be aware of your own thinking.
- **Check for accuracy and precision:** Revise, revise and revise.
- **Questioning and problem posing:** Be critical in your questioning.
- **Use past knowledge:** Draw on what you know and apply it to new situations.

Box 9.7: Characteristics of adult learners.

- **Autonomous and self-directed:** An adult learner prefers to be actively involved in their own learning, and in directing their own learning goals.
- **Bring life experiences and knowledge:** An adult leaner will have past experiences, knowledge, opinions and learning that they bring to the placement.
- **Goal-oriented:** Students are motivated to learn when they can see the need to acquire knowledge to address a real life problem or situation.
- **Relevancy-oriented:** An adult learner will learn best when they can relate the learning task to their own goals and what they want to achieve.

- **Precise language and thought:** Use more descriptive language to communicate more precisely.
- **Use all the senses:** Utilize as many sensory pathways as possible—visual, tactile, kinesthetic, auditory, olfactory, and gustatory.
- **Creativity:** Use your ingenuity, originality, and insightful—we are all creative beings.
- **Be curious:** Work on your sense of wonderment and inquisitiveness—learn to enjoy problem solving and develop a sense of efficacy as a thinker.

Scope of Adult Education

- The scope of adult education is very comprehensive. Social education covers all those topics that are not touched by education in general at school.
- Topics, such as religion, politics and family planning can now be discussed with adults who have a mature understanding. Moreover, it aims at giving a new orientation to the outlook of adults to suit the dynamic world.
- Then, the growth grooves of each individual are different from those of others.
- Social education harmonizes differences in growth and it also provides an opportunity for growth to those who have not been able to grow properly or completely earlier.
- Happily, greater emphasis has been laid on Adult Education in the Seventh Five-Year Plan. The tenth point in Prime Minister Rajiv Gandhi's 20-Point Programme—'Expansion of Education'—also makes special mention of stimulating adult literacy.
- Sizeable funds have been allocated and separate staff, including the block and Aanganwari people has been deployed to foster adult education.
- Adult education officers have been appointed in each college and they supervise the running of adult schools by student volunteers.

Factors Influencing Adult Learning (Fig. 9.8)

There are numerous factors which motivate adult learning and sometimes it is a combination of issues which lead them to make that decision.

- **Personal advancement:** This is the most common reason given for adults who want to learn. It can encompass the opportunity to gain promotion in their current workplace and, therefore, to increase the income. It can facilitate a career change or may be motivated by keeping ahead of competitors by taking a particular course.
- **Self-improvement:** Learning will increase the knowledge which, for many, will also improve self-confidence. The self-esteem will go up as a result of proving the abilities in completing a course successfully
- **Stimulation and escape:** Learning in itself is an opportunity to break free from any rut might have found yourself in. You may have become bored with the current routine, either within your personal or professional life (or both), and learning will often be the kick-start you have been looking for to motivate yourself again and can

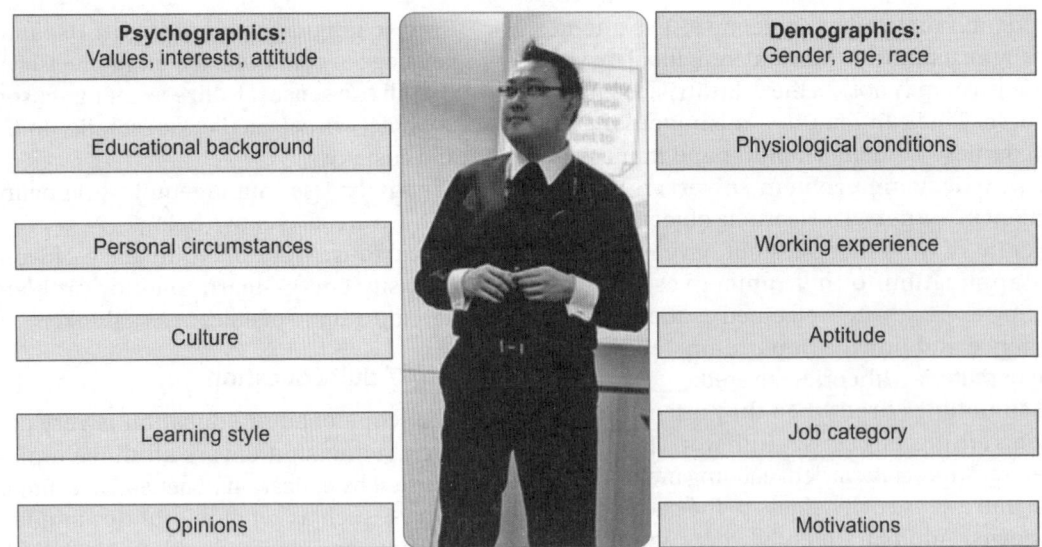

Fig. 9.8: Factors that affect adult learning.

also offer an 'escape' from the daily humdrum which you might feel you are experiencing
- **Increasing your social relationships:** Whether you have a number of good, loyal friends or you feel you have become a bit isolated, many adults choose to return to learn as it will widen their social network in terms of creating new, additional friendships or will offer them the possibility of making new friends with whom they might share some common ground.
- **External influences:** Sometimes you will find adults who would not otherwise necessarily choose to return to learn but are doing so as it is expected of them by others. By this, it means that it could be your employer who requires you to go on a course or, in some cases, if you have been unemployed for quite some time, it may be that you are asked to choose a course of learning in order to remain eligible to continue to receive state benefits.
- **Cognitive interest:** Many adults choose to return to learn simply because they have an enquiring mind and a mental 'thirst' to absorb more knowledge about a particular subject they are interest in. This would also include people who wish to pursue a particular hobby but need to understand more about it first and also those who may have undergone lifestyle changes. A good example here would be retirees who are looking for something to fill their time in order to make their lives more meaningful.

Principles of Adult Learning (Fig. 9.9)

Adults are Internally Motivated and Self-directed

Adult learners resist learning when they feel others are imposing information, ideas or actions on them. The role is to facilitate a students' movement toward more self-directed and responsible learning as well as to foster the student's internal motivation to learn. As clinical educator you can:
- **Set up a graded learning program** that moves from more to less structure, from less to more responsibility and from more to less direct supervision, at an appropriate pace that is challenging yet not overloading for the student.
- **Develop rapport** with the student to optimize your approachability and encourage asking of questions and exploration of concepts.
- **Show interest** in the student's thoughts and opinions. Actively and carefully listen to any questions asked.
- **Lead the student toward inquiry** before supplying them with too many facts.
- **Provide regular constructive** and specific feedback (both positive and negative)
- **Review goals** and acknowledge goal completion
- **Encourage use of resources,** such as library, journals, internet and other department resources.
- **Set projects or tasks for the student** that reflects their interests and which they must complete and "tick off" over the course of the placement. For example: to provide an in-service on topic of choice; to present a case-study based on one of their clients; to design a client educational handout; or to lead a client group activity session.
- **Acknowledge the preferred learning style** of the student. A questionnaire is provided below that will assist your student to identify their preferred learning style and to discuss this with you.

Adults bring Life Experiences and Knowledge to Learning Experiences

- **Adults like to be given opportunity** to use their existing foundation of knowledge and experience gained from life experience, and applies it to their new learning experiences. As a clinical educator you can:
- **Find out about your student:** Their interests and past experiences (personal, work and study related)
- **Assist them to draw on those experiences** when problem-solving, reflecting and applying clinical reasoning processes.
- **Facilitate reflective learning opportunities** which Fidishun (2000) suggests can also assist the student to examine

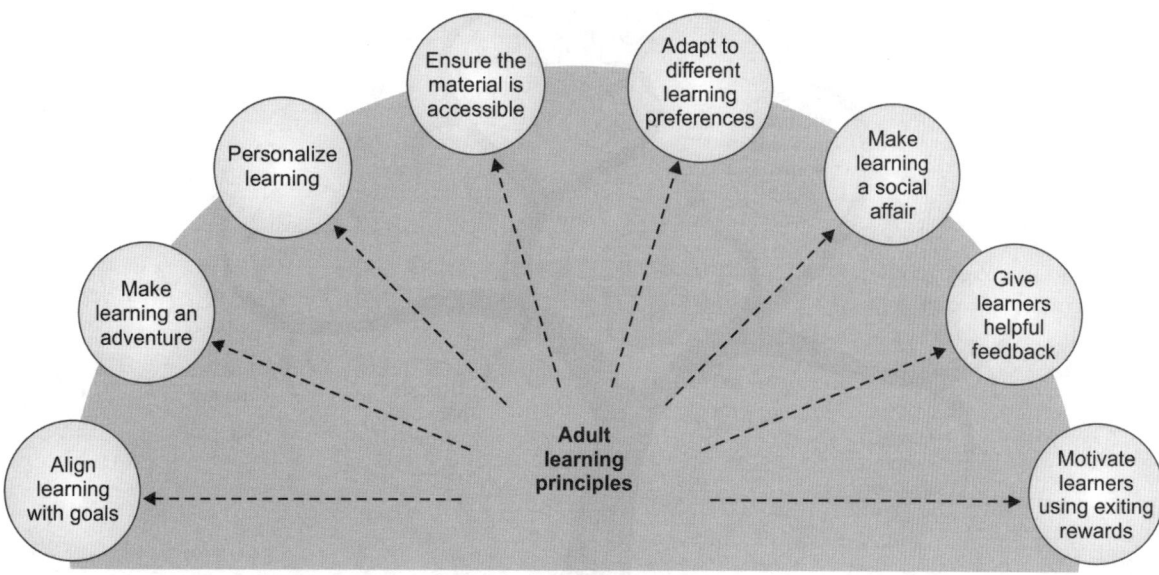

Fig. 9.9: Adult learning principles.

existing biases or habits based on life experiences and "move them toward a new understanding of information presented".

Adults are Goal-oriented
Adult students become ready to learn when "they experience a need to learn it in order to cope more satisfyingly with real-life tasks or problems". The nurse role is to facilitate a student's readiness for problem-based learning and increase the student's awareness of the need for the knowledge or skill presented. As educator, you can:
- Provide meaningful learning experiences that are clearly linked to personal, client and fieldwork goals as well as assessment and future life goals.
- Provide real case-studies (through client contact and reporting) as a basis from which to learn about the theory, OT methods, and functional issues implications of relevance.
- Ask questions that motivate reflection, inquiry and further research.

Adults are Relevancy-oriented
Adult learners want to know the relevance of what they are learning to what they want to achieve. One way to help students to see the value of their observations and practical experiences throughout their placement is to:
- Ask the student to do some reflection on for example, what they expect to learn prior to the experience, on what they learnt after the experience, and how they might apply what they learnt in the future, or how it will help them to meet their learning goals.
- Provide some choice of fieldwork project by providing two or more options, so that learning is more likely to reflect the student's interests.
- "Students really benefit from regular 'teaching sessions'— time spent going through assessments, such as how to do a kitchen assessment, and having in-services presented on specific topics, such as Cognition or Perception" "I find they understand more about a topic when it is directly relevant to the work context. This is invaluable as it ties theory to practice".

Adults are Practical
Through practical fieldwork experiences, interacting with real clients and their real life situations, students move from classroom and textbook mode to hands-on problem solving where they can recognize firsthand how what they are learning applies to life and the work context. As a clinical educator you can:
- Clearly explain your clinical reasoning when making choices about assessments, interventions and when prioritizing client's clinical needs.
- Be explicit about how what the student is learning is useful and applicable to the job and client group you are working with.
- Promote active participation by allowing students to try things rather than observe. Provide plenty of practice opportunity in assessment, interviewing, and intervention processes with ample repetition in order to promote development of skill, confidence and competence.

Adult Learners like to be Respected
Respect can be demonstrated to your student by:
- Taking interest
- Acknowledging the wealth of experiences that the student brings to the placement
- Regarding them as a colleague who is equal in life experience
- Encouraging expression of ideas, reasoning and feedback at every opportunity.

It is important to keep in mind that the student is still developing occupational therapy clinical practice skills. However, with the theory and principles of adult learning in mind, you can facilitate the learning approach of the

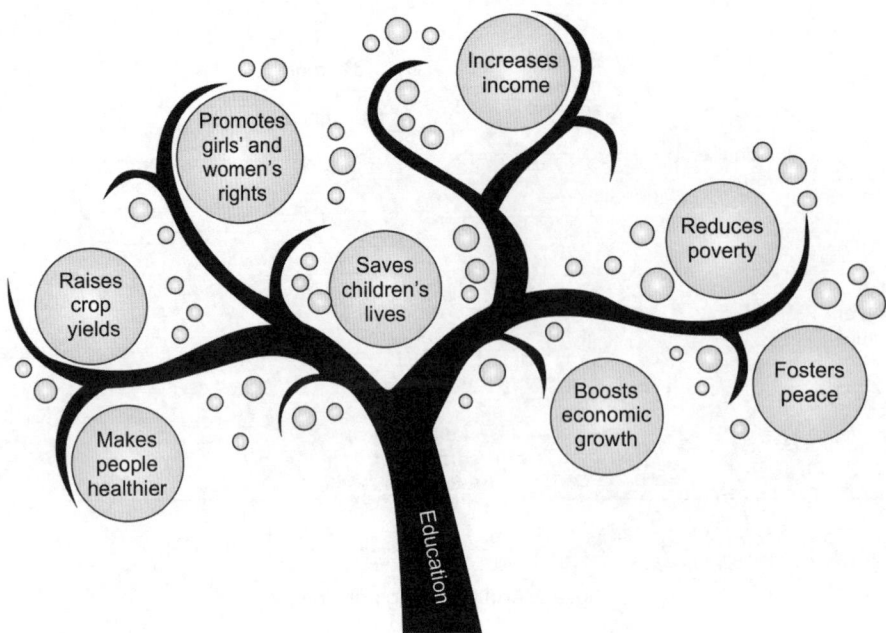

Fig. 9.10: Importance of adult learning.

student to move from novice to more sophisticated learning methods.

Importance of Adult Education (Fig. 9.10)

Adult education, as the term signifies, is the education of grown-up men and women who are above eighteen years. Bryson says, "Adult education includes all activities with an educational purpose, carried on by people, in the ordinary business of life that uses only part of their energy to acquire intellectual equipment."

- Teachers, government servants, NSS and other volunteers, social education workers, etc.
- Regular educational institutions, such as schools, colleges, rural colleges, community centers, agriculture extension groups, worker's educational associations and voluntary organizations.
- Informal educational devices, such as forums, study circles, group discussions, listening groups, camps.
- Recreational, educational bodies, such as theaters, cinemas, clubs, societies, fairs, melas, nautanki, etc.
- Institutions whose primary aim is not education, such as religious bodies, the army, parents associations, co-operative societies and other government departments.

CONCLUSION

In-service education is the vehicle by which goals and the multiple articulated means available to achieve them can be explored. It can be used to consider and solve problems, institutes and advance learning, elicit and analyze and systematize individual ideas for group; develop the idea of the hospital as another community agency; and struggle to understand ourselves, other and inherent relationships. Continuing education consists of all opportunities and facilities for personal and professional growth outside of formal education programs that lead to degree or certificate.

REVIEW QUESTIONS

Long Essays

1. Define in-service education; explain the principles of in-service education.
2. Discuss in detail about approaches to in-service education.
3. Define adult education; explain the characteristics and scope of adult education.

Short Essays

1. Need for in-service program.
2. Importance of in-service education.
3. Characteristics of good in-service education.
4. Components of in-service education.
5. Organization of in-service education.
6. Orientation skill training program.
7. Factors influencing adult learning.
8. Principles of adult learning.

Short Answers

1. Scope of in-service education.
2. Orientation.
3. Objectives of skill training.
4. Leadership development.
5. Centralized approach.
6. Decentralized approach.
7. Coordinated approach.
8. Problems related to in-service education.
9. Self-improvement.
10. Personal advancement.
11. Importance of adult learning.

BIBLIOGRAPHY

1. Battistoni RM. Civic Engagement across the Curriculum: A Resource Book for Service Learning Faculty in all Disciplines. Providence: Campus Compact; 2002.
2. Brandsford JA, Brown L, Cocking RR. How People Learn: Brain, Mind, Experience, and School. Washington, DC: National Academy; 2000.
3. Ojo MO. Quality teacher education. The Pivot of National Development: Nigeria Journal of Professional Teacher. 2006;1(2): 158-70.
4. Stoops S, Rafferty M, Johnson R. Handbook of educational administration: A guide for practitioners, Boston: Allyn and Bacon, Inc.; 1981.
5. Taylor J. The resident professors: A leadership role for connecting theory and practice Motor Skills: Theory into Practice. 1980; 4:51-8.
6. Wilson S. Current trends in staff development. In: Rubin L (Ed). Curriculum handbook, London, Allyn and Bawn Inc.; 1977.

CHAPTER 10

Material Management

LEARNING OBJECTIVES

- Meaning of Material Management
- Goals, Aims, Purpose, Objectives and Scope of Material Management
- Principles of Purchasing and Material Management
- Material Management Process
- Functions of Materials Management
- Procurement
- Procurement Cycle Steps
- Inventory Management
- Advantages of Material Management
- Inventory Control

INTRODUCTION

Material management is an approach for planning, organizing, and controlling all those activities principally concerned with the flow of materials into an organization. The scope of materials management varies greatly from company to company and may include material planning and control, production planning, purchasing, inventory control, in-plant materials movement, and waste management **(Fig. 10.1)**.

It is a business function for planning, purchasing, moving, storing material in an optimum way which helps organization to minimize the various costs, such as inventory, purchasing, material handling and distribution costs. Materials management is part of business logistics and refers to overseeing the location and movement of physical items or products. There are three main elements associated with such management: spare parts, quality control, and inventory management. Materials management is important in large manufacturing and distribution environments, such as warehouses, where there are multiple parts, locations, and significant money invested in these items.

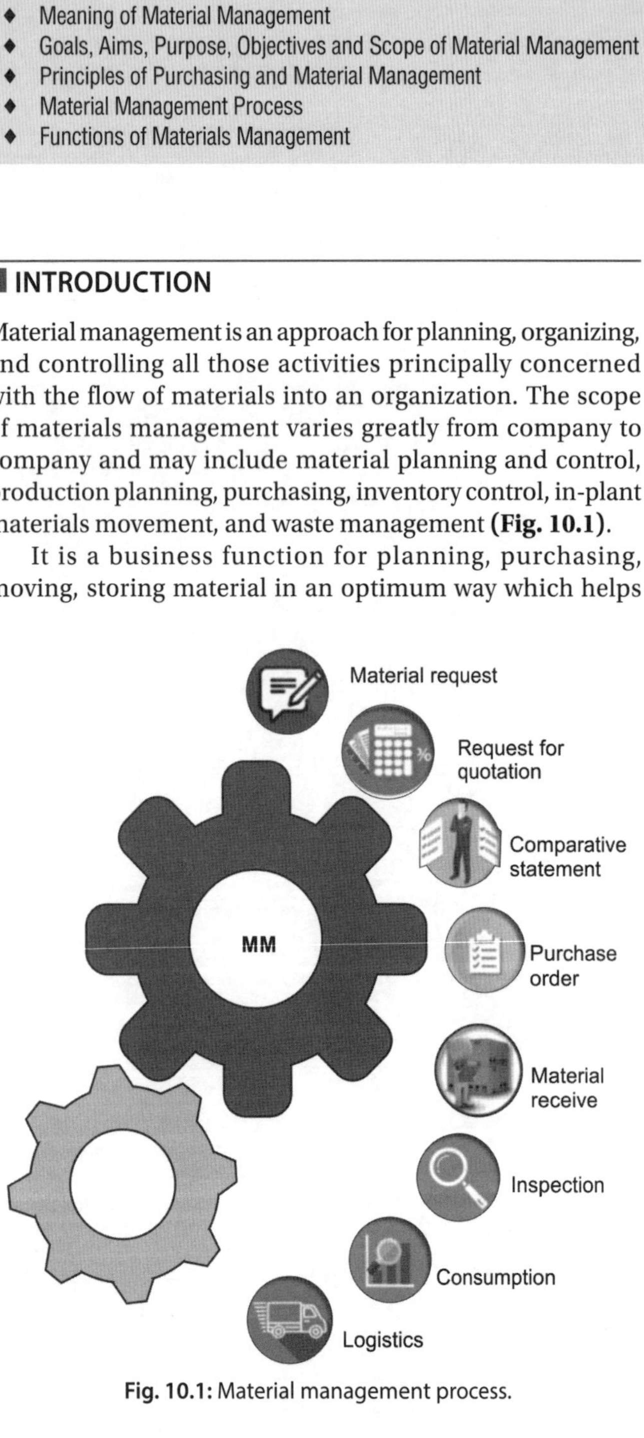

DEFINITION

In the health service organizations material management includes the complete supply process from purchase distribution.

- Material is defined as equipment, apparatus and supplies used by an organization or institution. Material is an essential resource to achieve the objectives of health organization.
- Material management is management and control of goods, services and equipment from the acquisition to disposition. It is concerned with providing the drugs, supplies and equipment needed by the health personnel to deliver health services.
- Material management is a scientific technique, concerned with planning, organizing and controlling the flow of materials from their initial purchase through internal operations to the service point through distribution.
- "Management of goods services and equipment from acquisition to disposition." —*Housely*
- "Material management is the integrated function of an organization dealing with supply of materials and allied activities in order to achieve the maximum coordination and optimum expenditure on materials."

—*Khare and Monga*

Fig. 10.1: Material management process.

- According to Judith and Maradole, as applied to nursing services, "the management and control of medical, surgical and clerical, inter-department services and equipment from acquisition on floor to disposition of patient care."
- According to the International Federation of Purchasing and Materials Management, "Materials management is a total concept having its definite organization to plan and control all types of materials, its supply, and its flow from raw stage to finished stage so as to deliver the product to customer as per his requirements in time. This involves materials planning, purchasing, receiving, storing, inventory control, scheduling, production, physical distribution and marketing."
- "Material management is the integrated functioning of the various sections of an organization dealing with the supply of materials and allied activities in order to achieve maximum coordination." — *NK Nair*

MEANING OF MATERIAL MANAGEMENT

- It is planning, directing, controlling and coordinating all those activities concerned with material and inventory from the inception to their introduction into the manufacturing processes.
- It includes all the activities of store from stage of forecasting of requirements to utilization to the final disposal. Store required by the hospital varies from simple housekeeping materials to sophisticated equipment.
- It is concerned with providing the drugs, supplies and equipment by the personnel to deliver healthcare services.
- It is also viewed as a scientific technique concerned with planning, organizing and controlling the flow of materials from their initial purchase, internal operations to the distribution at service point.
- According to Judith A, material management is the management and control of medical, surgical, clerical, interdepartmental services and equipment from acquisition on floor to disposition.
- Housely defined material management as 'the management and control of goods, services and equipment from acquisition to disposition'.

PURPOSE OF MATERIAL MANAGEMENT

- To gain economy in purchasing
- To satisfy the demand during period of replenishment
- To carry reserve stock to avoid stock out
- To stabilize fluctuations in consumption
- To provide reasonable level of client services

AIM OF MATERIAL MANAGEMENT

The aim of material management is to bring about control over acquisition, storage, retrievability, distribution, use and disposal of supplies and equipment in order to carry the primary responsibilities of an organization in an efficient, effective and economical manner. Material management seems to ensure availability of:

- The right material
- The right quality
- Right quantity of supplies
- At the right time
- At the right place
- For the least cost

GOALS OF MATERIAL MANAGEMENT (BOX 10.1)

'Materials Management' is a term used to connote "controlling the kind, amount, location, movement and timing of various commodities used in production by industrial enterprises".

- The goal of materials management is to provide an unbroken chain of components for production to manufacture goods on time for the customer base.
- The materials department is charged with releasing materials to a supply base, ensuring that the materials are delivered on time to the company using the correct carrier.
- Materials is generally measured by accomplishing on time delivery to the customer, on time delivery from the supply base, attaining a freight budget, inventory shrink management, and inventory accuracy.
- The materials department is also charged with the responsibility of managing new launches.
- In some companies materials management is also charged with the procurement of materials by establishing and managing a supply base.
- In other companies the procurement and management of the supply base is the responsibility of a separate purchasing department.
- The purchasing department is then responsible for the purchased price variances from the supply base.
- In large companies with multitudes of customer changes to the final product over the course of a year, there may be a separate logistics department that is responsible for all new acquisition launches and customer changes.
- This logistics department ensures that the launch materials are procured for production and then transfers the responsibility to the plant materials management.

SCOPE OF MATERIAL MANAGEMENT (FIG. 10.2)

The scope is vast. Its sub-functions include materials planning and control, purchasing, stores and inventory management besides others. Basically, under its scope are:
- Emphasis on the acquisition aspect
- Inventory control and stores management
- Material logistics, movement control and handling aspect
- Purchasing, supply, transportation, materials handling, etc.

Box 10.1: Material management goal.

- Optimum materials acquisition
- Optimum inventory turnover rate
- Good vendor relationship
- Material cost control
- Effective issue and distribution
- Elimination of losses and pilferage

Chapter 10: Material Management

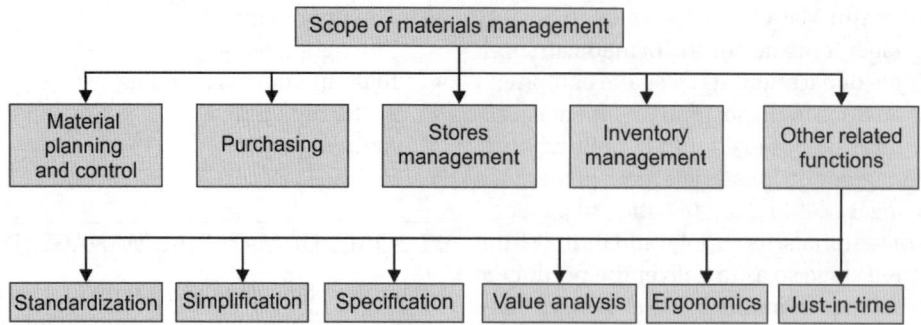

Fig. 10.2: Scope of material management.

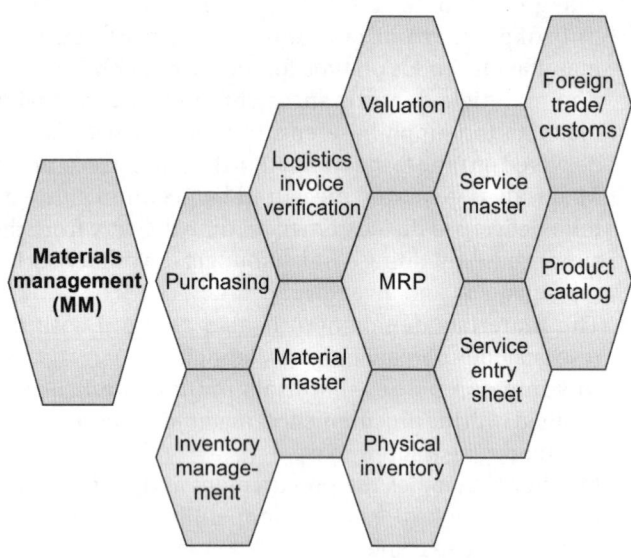

Fig. 10.3: Components of material management.

- Supply management or logistics management
- All the interrelated activities concerned with materials.

Figure 10.3 shows components of material management.

OBJECTIVE OF MATERIAL MANAGEMENT

- To buy at the lowest price, consistent with desired quality and service
- To maintain a high inventory turnover, by reducing excess storage, carrying costs and inventory losses occurring due to deteriorations, obsolescence and pilferage
- To maintain continuity of supply, preventing interruption of the flow of materials and services to users
- To maintain the specified material quality level and a consistency of quality which permits efficient and effective operation
- To develop reliable alternate sources of supply to promote a competitive atmosphere in performance and pricing
- To minimize the overall cost of acquisition by improving the efficiency of operations and procedures
- To hire, develop, motivate and train personnel and to provide a reservoir of talent
- To develop and maintain good supplier relationships in order to create a supplier attitude and desire furnish the organization with new ideas, products, and better prices and service
- To achieve a high degree of cooperation and coordination with user departments
- To maintain good records and controls that provide an audit trail and ensure efficiency and honesty
- To participate in make or buy decisions

The objectives and functions of materials management can be categorized in two ways as follows (**Box 10.2**):

I. **Primary objectives:** Which can be classified as:
   1. Efficient materials planning
   2. Buying or purchasing
   3. Procuring and receiving
   4. Storing and inventory control
   5. Supply and distribution of materials
   6. Quality assurance
   7. Good supplier and customer relationship
   8. Improved departmental efficiency

II. **Secondary objectives:** There can be several secondary objectives of materials management. Some of them are given below:
   1. Efficient production scheduling
   2. To take make or buy decisions
   3. Prepare specifications and standardization of materials
   4. To assist in product design and development
   5. Forecasting demand and quantity of materials requirements
   6. Quality control of materials purchased
   7. Material handling
   8. Use of value analysis and value engineering
   9. Developing skills of workers in materials management
   10. Smooth flow of materials in and out of the organization

---

Box 10.2: Functions of materials management.

- **Materials planning:** Estimating requirements—preparing MRP—forecasting inventories—scheduling of orders—monitoring production
- **Materials sourcing:** Identifying suppliers—choosing the right supplier—planning supply chain systems—estimating transportation costs—scheduling-follow up
- **Inventory control:** Planning of control systems—exercise control through control systems—maintain the inventory levels
- **Budgeting:** Estimating working capital requirements
- **Stores management:** Physical control of materials—stores maintenance—minimize obsolescence—disposal of waste—maintenance of records-stock control

Material Planning

- "Material planning is the scientific way of determining the requirements that goes into meeting production needs within the economic investment policies".
  —*Gopalakrishnan and Sunderasan*
- It is done at all stages and all levels of management. Material planning is based on certain feedback information and reviews.

Aim of Material Management Planning

To get:
- The right quality
- Right quantity of supplies
- At the right time
- At the right place
- For the right cost

Purpose of Material Management Planning

- To gain economy in purchasing
- To satisfy the demand during period of replenishment
- To carry reserve stock to avoid stock out
- To stabilize fluctuations in consumption
- To provide reasonable level of client services

Basic Principles of Material Management Planning

- Planning
- Organizing
- Staffing
- Directing
- Controlling
- Reporting
- Budgeting
- Sound purchasing methods
- Skillful and hard poised negotiations
- Effective purchase system
- Should be simple
- Must not increase other costs
- Simple inventory control program

Elements of Material Management Planning

- Demand estimation
- Identify the needed items
- Calculate from the trends in consumption
- Review with resource constraints

PRINCIPLES OF PURCHASING AND MATERIAL MANAGEMENT (FIG. 10.4)

Purchasing is the most important function in the field of materials management. Correct purchasing influences the profitability of an organization to a great extent. Correct purchasing or efficient purchasing is possible only if the fundamental principles of scientific purchasing are followed. The fundamental principles of scientific purchasing are:

- **Principle of right quality:** Materials of right quality are to be purchased for the job so that quality of the products can be maintained.

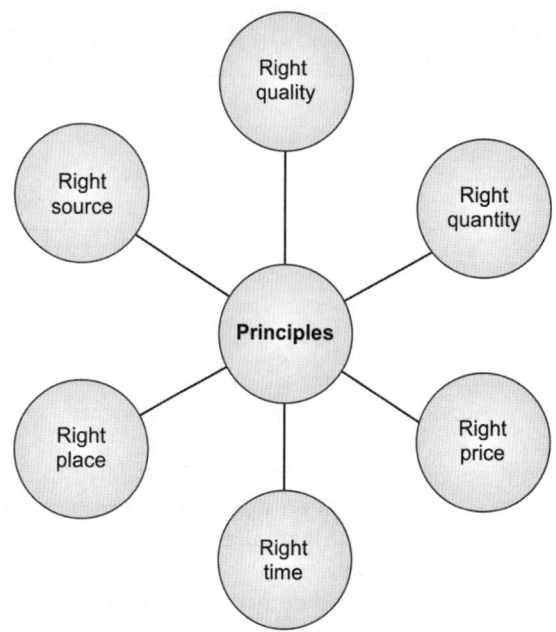

Fig. 10.4: Principles of purchasing.

- **Principle of right time:** Materials should be purchased in right time so that production will not be held up due to want of materials.
- **Principle of right quantity:** Materials should be purchased in right quantity so that wastages and losses due to overstocking can be avoided. Interruption in production due to shortage of materials can also be avoided by purchasing the right quantity of materials.
- **Principle of right source:** The right source of purchase will help to select the supplier who can offer to supply materials on favorable terms and conditions at an economical price and also in right time and quantity.
- **Principle of right price:** Materials should be purchased at right price by inviting quotations from different suppliers and making comparison. Principle of right price will help to keep the material cost under control.
- **Principle of right place:** This principle requires that the required materials should be received from the supplier at a place which is near to the store or the production department requiring those materials or at some other convenient place. This will help to avoid the unnecessary consumption of time and money in carrying the materials from the place of supply to the place of requirement.

MATERIAL MANAGEMENT PROCESS (FIG. 10.5)

The following is the general process of material management:

- **Material determination:** Material determination is done either by the concerned departments or through the planning and control of materials. This can cover both MRP and goods demand with the approach based on inventory control. The regular monitoring of stock levels of materials is defined in the master records. You can enter your requests for purchase, or they can be generated automatically by the materials planning and control.
- **Source determination:** The purchasing component allows you to identify potential sources of supply

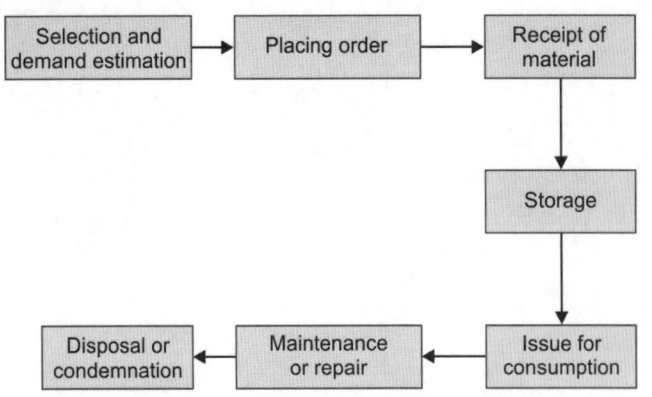

Fig. 10.5: Process of material management.

Box 10.3: Functions.
- Material planning and programming
- Purchasing and outsourcing
- Inventory control
- Storekeeping and warehousing
- Standardization and evaluation of all products
- Transportation and material handling
- Inspection and quality control
- Cost reduction through value analysis
- Disposal of surplus/obsolete material
- Distribution

based on existing orders and longer-term purchase agreements. This speed up the process of creating requests for quotation (requests) that can be sent to vendors electronically.
- **Vendor selection and comparison of estimates:** The system is capable of simulating scenarios of pricing, so you can compare a number of citations.
- **Order processing system** adopts the acquisition of information in demand and supply to help you create a purchase order. As with purchase requisitions, you can generate own or planning and controlling system generates it automatically.
- **Order tracking:** The system checks the reminder periods you have specified and—if necessary—automatically prints reminders or expediters at predefined intervals. It also offers an update on the status of all purchase requisitions, quotations, and purchase orders.
- Receipt of goods and inventory management of goods receipt staff is able to confirm receipt of goods simply by entering the number of purchase orders by specifying permissible tolerances.
- **Invoice verification:** The system supports control and matching of invoices. Accounts payable is informed of the quantity and price changes because the system has access to PO and goods receipt data. This speeds up the verification process and compensation for the payment of invoices.

FUNCTIONS OF MATERIALS MANAGEMENT (BOX 10.3)

Materials management is concerned with the costs of materials, supply and use. The following areas are involved, such as production control, shipping, receiving and stores which we will explain below:
- **Production and control of materials:** The preparation of schedules is very important to carry out in order to hit the results. The requirements of parts or materials are determined according to the production schedules. This is prepared with orders that are requested by customers in advance. This is how production can be carried out without any problems.
- **Purchasing:** This is the purchase of the materials needed in the entire production process. The objective of this department is to maintain the flow of materials and services needed to operate in the company. To keep investments and losses in inventory to a minimum. Choose the sources of supply, finalize the terms of purchase and their follow-up, maintain the relationships with the suppliers, approve payments for the suppliers, evaluate and qualify the development of the suppliers. This department fulfils the function of buying quality products at reasonable prices.
- **Stores:** When the material is delivered, physical control, conservation and maintenance of records, proper location and storage is done in the stores.
- **Transport:** It is important to be able to move the materials from the point of purchase to the company or to the customers or to the place where they are going to be stored. Ideally, you should hire cheap and fast transportation according to how often you need to move production materials around.
- **Material handling:** It is the follow-up of the material process, to know that everything has the flow that is needed in the production of the products.
- **Receiving:** The reception is responsible for unloading the materials, counting the units and sending them to the stores.

PROCUREMENT

The process of buying in goods or services from an external provider. Covers everything from determining the need for new goods to buying, delivering and storing them **(Fig. 10.6)**.
- Procurement is the sourcing and purchasing of goods and services for business use.
- It is the acquisition of goods or commodities by a company, organization, institution, or a person. This simply means the purchase of goods from suppliers at the lowest possible cost.
- It is also defined as the process of obtaining goods and services from preparation and processing of a requisition through to receipt and approval of the invoice for payment.
- According to Defense Acquisition University, It is the act of buying goods and services for the government.

Objectives
- Acquire needed supplies
- Obtain high quality supplies
- Assure prompt and dependable delivery

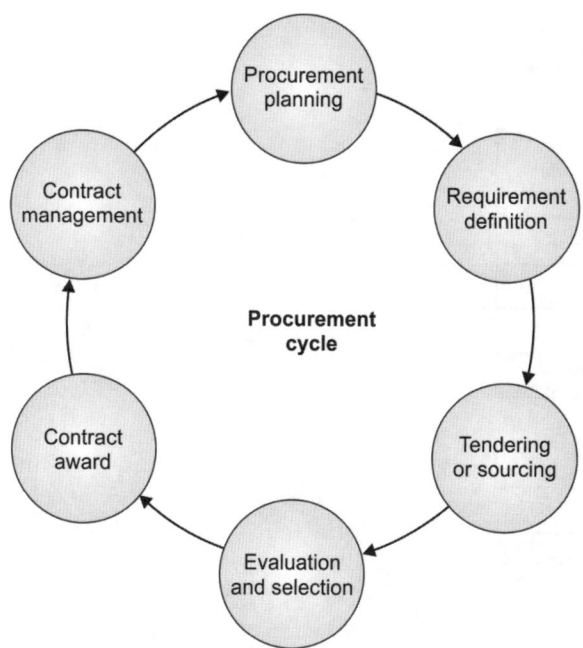

Fig. 10.6: Procurement cycle.

- Distribute the procurement workload
- Optimize inventory management

Objectives of Procurement System
- Acquire needed supplies as inexpensively as possible
- Obtain high quality supplies
- Assure prompt and dependable delivery
- Distribute the procurement workload to avoid period of idleness and overwork
- Optimize inventory management through scientific procurement procedures

Methods in Procurement Process and Negotiation Strategies
- Open tender
- Restricted or limited tender
- Negotiated procurement
- Direct procurement
- Rate contract
- Spot purchase
- Risk purchase
- Many suppliers strategy
- Few suppliers strategy

Points to Remember while Purchasing
- Proper specification
- Invite quotations from reputed firms
- Comparison of offers based on basic price, freight and insurance, taxes and levies
- Quantity and payment discounts
- Payment terms
- Delivery period, guarantee

Procurement of Equipment
- Latest technology
- Availability of maintenance and repair facility, with minimum down time
- Post warranty repair at reasonable cost
- Upgradeability
- Reputed manufacturer
- Availability of consumables
- Low operating costs
- Installation
- Proper installation as per guideline

Storage
- Store must be of adequate space
- Materials must be stored in an appropriate place in a correct way
- Group wise and alphabetical arrangement helps in identification and retrieval
- First-in, first-out principle to be followed
- Monitor expiry date
- Follow two bin or double shelf system, to avoid stock outs
- Reserve bin should contain stock that will cover lead time and a small safety stock. **Figure 10.7** shows steps in procurement and **Figure 10.8** shows procurement strategy.

PROCUREMENT CYCLE STEPS (FIG. 10.9)

Management in any company must understand the art of obtaining products and services. The procurement cycle follows specific steps for identifying a requirement or need of the company through the final step of the award of the product or contract. Responsible management of public and corporate funds is vital when handling this necessary process, whether in strong or weak economic markets. Following a proven step-by-step technique will help management successfully achieve its goals.

Step 1: Need recognition: The business must know it needs a new product, whether from internal or external sources. The product may be one that needs to be reordered, or it may be a new item for the company.

Step 2: Specific need: The right product is critical for the company. Some industries have standards to help determine specifications. Part numbers help identify these for some businesses. Other industries have no point of reference. The company may have ordered the product in the past. If not, then the business must specify the necessary product by using identifiers, such as color or weight.

Step 3: Source options: The business needs to determine where to obtain the product. The company might have an approved vendor list. If not, the business will need to search for a supplier using purchase orders or research a variety of other sources, such as magazines, the Internet or sales representatives. The company will qualify the suppliers to determine the best product for the business.

Step 4: Price and terms: The business will investigate all relevant information to determine the best price and terms for the product. This will depend on if the company needs commodities (readily available products) or specialized

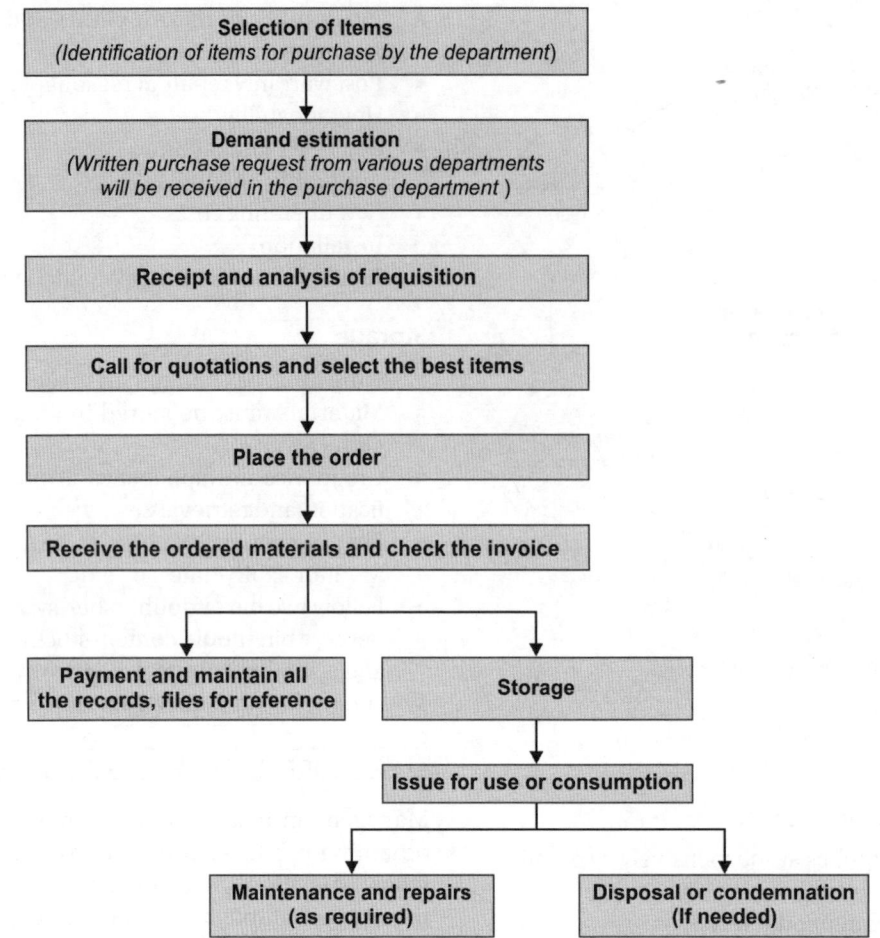

Fig. 10.7: Steps in procurement.

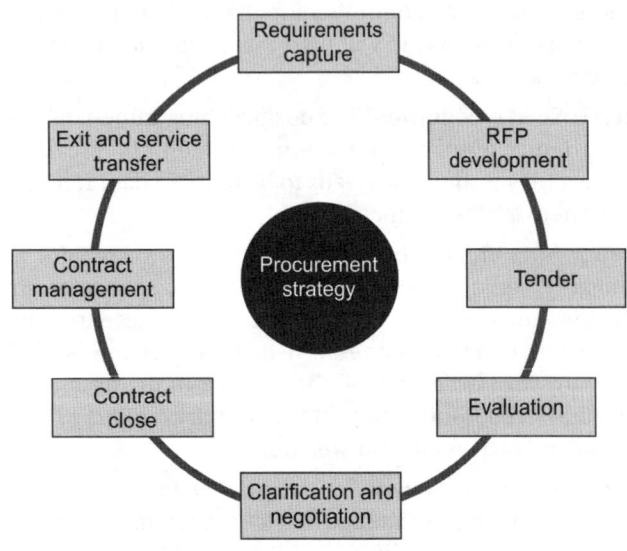

Fig. 10.8: Procurement strategy.

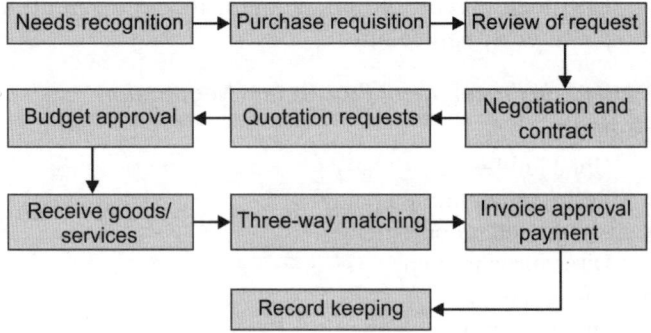

Fig. 10.9: Stage of a procurement process.

materials. Usually, the business will look into three suppliers before it makes a final decision.

Step 5: Purchase order: The purchase order is used to buy materials between a buyer and seller. It specifically defines the price, specifications and terms and conditions of the product or service and any additional obligations.

Step 6: Delivery: The purchase order must be delivered, usually by fax, mail, personally, email or other electronic means. Sometimes the specific delivery method is specified in the purchasing documents. The recipient then acknowledges receipt of the purchase order. Both parties keep a copy on file.

Step 7: Expediting: Expedition of the purchase order addresses the timeliness of the service or materials delivered. It becomes especially important if there are any delays. The issues most often noted include payment dates, delivery times and work completion.

Step 8: Receipt and inspection of purchases: Once the sending company delivers the product, the recipient accepts or rejects the items. Acceptance of the items obligates the company to pay for them.

Step 9: Invoice approval and payment: Three documents must match when an invoice requests payment—the invoice itself, the receiving document and the original purchase order. The agreement of these documents provides confirmation from both the receiver and supplier. Any discrepancies must be resolved before the recipient pays the bill. Usually, payment is made in the form of cash, check, bank transfers, credit letters or other types of electronic transfers.

Step 10: Record maintenance: In the case of audits, the company must maintain proper records. These include purchase records to verify any tax information and purchase orders to confirm warranty information. Purchase records reference future purchases as well.

■ INVENTORY MANAGEMENT (FIG. 10.10)

Companies that store inventory must have a management system to track the materials and products in the organization. Inventory management is a method to meet the needs of the organization while keeping the costs of storing materials to a minimum. The management system the company uses impacts several departments within the organization, such as purchasing, planning, accounting and production.

- Inventory control is the process by which inventory is measured and regulated according to predetermined norms, such as economic lot size for order, safety stock, minimum level, maximum level, order level, etc.
- Inventory control is about product availability and balancing the costs of ownership with the costs of procuring, which includes purchasing, receiving and paying.
- Inventory control is the technique of maintaining the size of the inventory at some desired level keeping in view the best economic interest of an organization.

Objectives

- To supply the materials in time
- To give maximum clients service
- To reduce or minimize investment in inventories
- To minimize idle time
- To avoid shortage of stock
- To minimize the losses
- To meet unforeseen future demand
- To average out demand fluctuations
- To balance various inventory costs

Meet Customer Demand

- The inventory management system ensures the company has the materials available to build product to meet customer demand.
- Accurate quantities in the system allow the company to build the product within the time frame the customer demands as well.
- Inaccuracies in the system can result in shortages of materials or products, which may delay production and delivery times for customers

Reduce Costs

- An accurate inventory management system prevents delays in purchases or over ordering materials for production.
- Excessive amounts of inventory tie up company funds and can result in waste. For example, changes in production or material specifications can cause an abundance of materials held in stock to become obsolete.
- A lean inventory is flexible and can respond faster to material changes.
- Defects found in materials may cause excessive waste when large amounts of inventory are in stock.
- A leaner inventory also reduces the space needed to store materials. Keeping only what is necessary on hand reduces the company's investment in materials until there is customer demand.

Production Planning

- The production planning department relies on accurate inventory quantities to schedule builds or production runs.
- An inaccurate inventory can cause delays in the materials necessary to build products.
- The planning department schedules production to meet the demands of customer orders.
- An inventory management system ensures the smooth flow of materials to production when it is needed to create products for customers.

Purchasing

- The inventory management system provides trigger points for material purchases.
- Inaccuracies in the inventory quantities may result in ordering delays or over ordering materials for production.
- The purchasing department orders materials when the quantity reaches a specific amount.
- Vendor lead times are a factor in determining the quantity necessary to trigger a purchase.

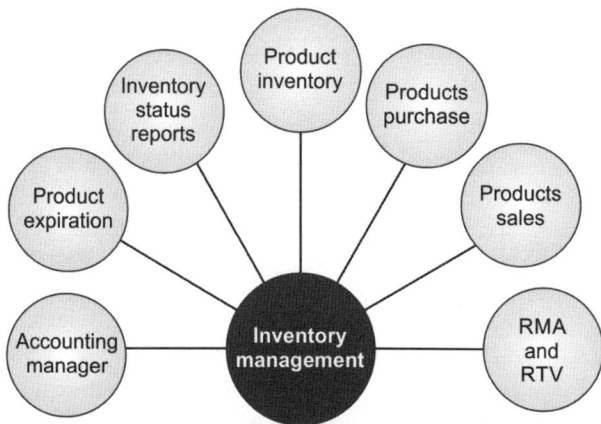

Fig. 10.10: Inventory management.

Importance of Inventory Control

- To provide maximum supply service, consistent with maximum efficiency and optimum investment
- To provide cushion between forecasted and actual demand for a material
- To have optimum level of inventory: not too large, not small.
- To eliminate duplication in ordering
- To take care of fluctuations in demand and lead time
- To take care of increasing price tendency of commodities or rebate in bulk buying
- To increase transportation efficiently
- To minimize the inventory costs
- To minimizing waiting time
- To provide a check against the loss of material
- To better utilization of stocks available
- To facilitate cost accounting activities
- To locate and disposes inactive and obsolete store items.

ROLE OF NURSE MANAGER (BOX 10.4)

- Ensuring regular and adequate flow of supply
- Monitoring quality and safety of the materials
- Indenting, receiving, storing, checking for all necessary equipment and supply
- Maintaining of emergency stocks
- Arranging and assisting in audit
- Participation in policy making for material management
- Evaluating the efficacy of the material management system followed in particular nursing unit.
- Make sure that all the personnel in the ward should be clearly known who may use ward articles and equipment and who assumes responsibility for it.
- The head nurse must be vigilant and prevent waste or misuse by educating the staff in the economical and appropriate use of all equipment and materials.

ADVANTAGES OF MATERIAL MANAGEMENT (BOX 10.5)

Effectual material management system can bring numerous advantages for organization in competitive business, such as reducing the overall costs of materials, better handling of materials, reduction in duplicated orders, materials will be on site when needed and in the quantities required, improvements in labor productivity, improvements in project schedule, quality control, better field material control, better relations with suppliers, reduce of materials surplus, reduce storage of materials on site, labor savings, stock reduction, purchase savings and better cash flow management.

To sum up, materials management thought is to deal with resources in an integrative way for national fiscal development. It is a conceptual frame for thoroughly addressing the movement of materials through the economy and the environment from extraction to end point. Material management has created a niche in many organizations, which have implemented the integrated materials management. These organizations usually enjoy the following advantages:

- Better accountability on part of materials as well as other departments as no one can shift blame to others.
- As materials management is handled by single authority, it can result in better coordination, as it becomes the central point for any material related problems.
- Materials management department makes sure that better quality material is supplied timely to the requesting departments. This can result in better performance of the organization.
- A materials management system is typically controlled through an information system, thus, can help in taking decisions related to material in the organization.
- One indirect advantage of material management is that good quality material develops the ethical and moral standard in an organization. However, please note there is no study on this issue.

ROLE OF A NURSE IN MATERIAL MANAGEMENT (BOX 10.6)

The nurse as the user of the material is in the best position to cut the cost of materials in her unit, or to utilize it at its best. Her role as a middle manager is very important in the smooth functioning of the unit. Hence, her role in material management can be summarized as:

- She should have sound knowledge of the requirements and functioning of her unit.
- Must prepare budget for materials required.
- Forecast the demands for smooth running of the unit (less or more supplies will cause mismanagement and poor quality of patient care).

Box 10.5: Advantages of material management.

- Reducing the overall costs of materials
- Better handling of materials
- Reduction in duplicated orders
- Materials will be on site when needed and in the quantities required
- Improvements in labor productivity
- Improvements in project schedule
- Quality control
- Better field material control
- Better relations with suppliers
- Reduce storage of materials on site
- Stock reduction, purchase savings and better cash flow management

---

Box 10.4: Role of head nurse or nurse-in-charge.

- Responsible for keeping an adequate amount of equipment and supplies in the ward
- Make sure that equipment and supplies are in good conditions
- Put in a requisition for necessary equipment for repair and maintenance when needed.
- Make sure that equipment and supplies are conveniently located
- Make sure that all the personnel in the ward should clearly know who may use ward articles and equipment and who assumes responsibility for it.

Box 10.6: Role of nurse.

- Maintain supply
- Readily available
- Good working condition
- First in, first out
- Locked
- Regular and surprise checking
- Delegate responsibility
- Same place
- Proper method
- Follow policies
- Prevent wastage

- Prepares, assists and maintains the policy about purchasing, inventory, maintenance, prevention of pilferage and condemnation of the unserviceable items.
- Exercise her powers to control the inventory in her unit.
- Ensures perfect functioning of the equipment in the unit under her control.
- Should be able to provide feedback about the materials regarding their quality to the purchase department.
- Accurate recording and reporting of the materials required regarding their maintenance and quality.
- Prepares guidelines and ensures that they are followed properly regarding the breakdown of equipment, loss of equipment and avoid mishandling of them.
- Research activities to assess the impact of material management on patient care.
- Evaluation, of the procedures, policy and performance of equipment and feasibility of the policies should be documented.
- Should be able to prevent pilferage and fraud, hence be alarmed at the night time.

INVENTORY CONTROL (FIG. 10.11)

Inventory control means stocking adequate number and kind of stores so that the materials are available whenever and whatever is required. Scientific inventory control results in optimal balance. Inventory control is an important aspect of material management. If the level of inventories goes up the carrying charges also increase but the procurement cost decreases. On the other hand, if we have a similar inventory, turn-over is greater requiring lesser carrying charges but more of procurement costs, as orders have to be repeated more often.

Meaning of Inventory Control

- In healthcare system, material management is concerned with providing the drugs, supplies and equipment needed by health personnel to deliver health services.
- The right drugs, supplies and equipment must be at the right place, at the right time, and in the right quantity in order that health personnel deliver health services.
- Inventory control it is an important aspect of material management.
- Inventory control is a scientific system which indicates as to what to order, when to order, and how much to order, and how much to stock so that purchasing costs and storing costs are kept as low as possible.

Definition

- Inventory control is the process of maintaining the optimum needed quantity that is sufficient for smooth operation of the organization.
- Inventory management can be viewed as the process of maintaining a just adequate supply of something so, that the demand pattern can be satisfied without hiccups.

Objectives of Inventory

- To reduce financial investment
- To facilitate smooth production operation
- If an offer of discount comes for a bulk purchase, to decide whether to go for bulk purchaser not.
- To avoid carrying cost
- To improve quality of care with lesser inventory
- To avoid obsolescence of inventor

Table 10.1 summarizes classifications of inventory.

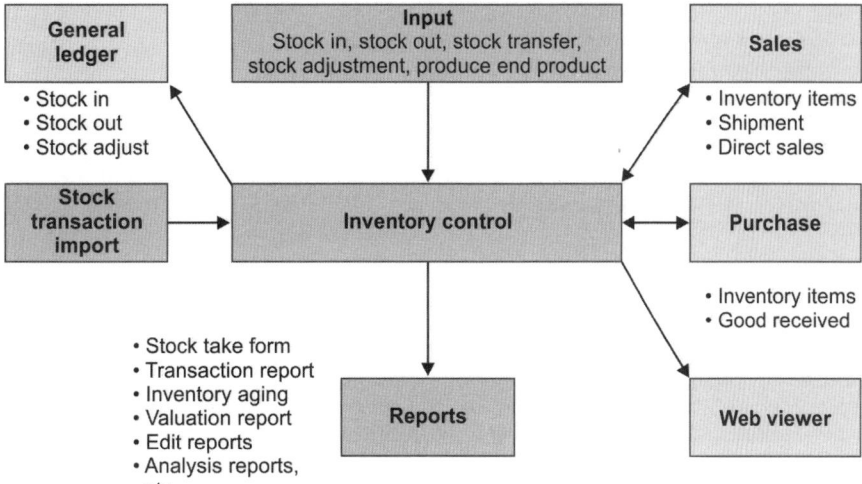

Fig. 10.11: Inventory control.

Table 10.1: Classifications of inventory.

Sl. No.	Types	Description
1.	Raw material inventories	This consists of raw material and semi-finished goods supplied by another firm
2.	Finished goods inventory	Finished goods inventory idling in the stock room waiting for dispatch
3.	In process inventory	They are semi-finished goods undergoing the manufacturing process
4.	Indirect inventory	These consists of lubricants, spare parts, etc., which are necessary for proper operations and maintenance

Steps in Inventory Control

1. Fixing minimum quantities or ordering points and maximum quantities, or amounts to order on all materials.
2. Arranging a method for allocation of material and orders which are in process.
3. Creating stores accounts, which will control the store room.

Functions of Inventory Control

- To provide maximum supply service, consistent with maximum efficiency and optimum investment.
- To provide cushion between forecasted and actual demand for a material.

Selective Controls in Material Management

Techniques in Inventory Control (Table 10.2)

- ABC analysis (Always Better Control)
- VED analysis (Vital, Essential, Desirable)
- HML analysis (High, Medium, Low)
- FSN analysis (Fast, Slow moving and Non-moving)
- SDE analysis (Scarce, Difficult, Easy)

Principles of Inventory Management

- Determination of order quantity
- Determination of reorder point of record level

Advantages of Inventory

- Delivery in time
- Possibility of discount for bulk purchase
- Unforeseen circumstances can be handled to some extent.
- Workers and machinery need not idle.

Disadvantages of Inventory

- Working capital is tied up
- More space required
- Increases insurance charges
- Increased overhead expenses
- Charges of damage, pilferage replacement, etc., is more
- Increase charge for obsolescence

CONCLUSION

Material management is an important management tool which will be very useful in getting the right quality and right quantity of supplies at right time. Having good inventory control and adopting sound methods of condemnation and disposal will improve the efficiency of the organization. Principles of material management and procurement are applicable to every organization as well as individuals. A thorough understanding and use of the techniques of materials management would help

Table 10.2: Techniques in inventory control.

Sl. No.	Types	Description
1.	ABC analysis	It is the process of classifying items by using values as measures. ABC analysis helps us in segregating the items from one another and tells us how much valued the items is and controlling it to what extent is in the best interest of the organization. The main objective of ABC analysis is to frame policy guidelines regarding control of items: • ABC analysis is the analysis of the store items cost criteria • It is a simple approach, which avoids being money wise • The cost of each item is multiplied by the number used in a given period and then these items are tabulated in descending numerical value order • It will be seen that first 10% of items approximately account for 70%, the next 20% for 20% of value and the last 70% account for 10% of value • It has been seen that a large number of items consume only a small percentage of resources and vice-versa • Items represent the high cost center, B items represent the immediate cost centers, and C-items represent low cost centers • A very close control is exercised over A items while less stringent control is adequate for those in the category B, and less attention for category C
2.	VED analysis	The vital items are stocked in abundance, essential items, safety, stocks and very strict control. Essential items are moderate controls, purchase based on rigid requirements and reasonably strict watch. Desirable items are ordinary control, safety stocks it high, purchase based on usage estimate. The stores when subjected to analysis based on their criticality can be classified into vital, essential and desirable stores. This analysis is termed as VED analysis. • **Vital:** items without which treatment comes to standstill, i.e., non-availability cannot be tolerated • **Essential:** Items whose non-availability can be tolerated for 2–3 days, because similar or alternative items are available

Contd...

Contd...

Sl. No.	Types	Description
		• **Desirable:** Items whose non-availability can be tolerated for a long period. Although the proportion of vital, essential and desirable items varies from hospital to hospital depending on the type and quantity of workload, on an average vital items are 10%, essential items are 40% and desirable items make 50% of total items available. Although not included in scientific VED analysis, in some public organizations which are static or inefficiently managed, there is a peculiar category of 'U' items which can be grouped as unnecessary. These unnecessary items get purchased due to the following reasons: • Thoughtless continuation of previous purchase • Indifferent attitude towards hospital formulary • Fear of change • Poor supervision and control • Unfair practice due to vested interest The vital items are stocked in abundance; essential items are stocked in medium amounts, and desirable items we stocked in small amounts. By stocking the items in order of priority, vital and essential items are always in stock which means a minimum disruption in the services offered to the people.
3.	HML analysis	As the name materials are classified to their unit value as high, medium and low
4.	XYZ analysis	X items are those whose stock value are high, while Z items are those values are low. Understandably Y items fall between the two categories

5.	FSN analysis	Movement analysis forms the basis for this classification. The items are classified as fast moving, slow moving and non-moving based on their consumption pattern:
		• It is based on rate of consumption
		• The items can be classified into:
		   – Fast moving
		   – Slow moving
		   – Non-moving
		   – Obsolete
		An understanding of the movement of items helps to keep proper levels of inventories by deciding a rational policy or reordering. This method is based on the fact that some stock items have a much higher annual usage value than others. This after doing a cost analysis, stock items are separated into three classes with the following characteristics.

6.	SDE analysis	Classification methods on source of supply, SED classification is a system where materials are sorted out as scare to obtain, difficult to obtain and easy to obtain. SDE analysis Unit value is the basis of this analysis and not the annual consumption value H—Unit value >1000 (Sanctioned by higher officials) M—Unit value 100 to 1000 L—Unit value <100
7.	GOLF analysis	In the GOLF system, classification is based on the availability and nature of supplies. Government supplies, ordinary suppliers, local suppliers and foreign suppliers
8.	SOS analysis	Raw material can be classified into seasonal or off season items

in ordering the supplies when needed, controlling their use, keeping them safely and in working order. This also prevents chances of non availability of equipment and drugs as being out of stock of these reduces the usefulness of the hospital system.

REVIEW QUESTIONS

Long Essays

1. Define material management; explain the goals, aims, purposes and scope of material management.
2. Define material management planning; explain aims, purposes and principles.
3. Describe the procurement cycle steps in detail.
4. Define inventory control; explain in detail about objectives, steps and functions.

Short Essays

1. Objective of material management.
2. Principles of purchasing and material management.
3. Material management process.
4. Functions of materials management.
5. Procurement, explain the objectives and cycle.
6. Inventory management.
7. Role of a nurse in material management.

Short Answers

1. Materials planning.
2. Materials sourcing.
3. Inventory control.
4. Stores management.
5. Purchasing.
6. Importance of inventory control.
7. Advantages of material management.

BIBLIOGRAPHY

1. Arnold JT, Chapman SN, Clive LM, et al. Introduction to materials management; 2001.
2. Basavanthappa BT. Nursing administration, 1st edition. New Delhi: Jaypee Brother's Medical Publishers (P) Ltd; 2000.
3. Brown RG, Brown VCM, Basler P, et al. Materials Management. New York; 1977.
4. Gopalakrishnan, Sunderasan. Material Management, Prentice Hall of India Pvt Ltd. New Delhi; 1979.
5. Gupta S, Kanth S. Hospital stores management, an integrated approach, 1st edition. New Delhi: Jaypee Brother's Medical Publishers (P) Ltd; 2004.
6. Kini DU. Materials management: The key to successful project management. Journal of Management in Engineering. 1999;15(1): 30-4.
7. Kulkarni GR. Managerial accounting for hospitals. Mumbai: Ridhiraj Enterprise; 2003.
8. Kumar R, Goel SL. Hospital administration and management. Vol 1, 1st edition, New Delhi: Deep and Deep Publications.
9. Lee L, Dobler DW. Purchasing and materials management: Text and cases. New York, NY: McGraw-Hill; 1977.

CHAPTER 11

Nursing Audit

Learning Objectives

- History of Nursing Audit
- Definition, Meaning and Objectives of Learning
- Objectives and Goals of Nursing Objectives
- Steps, Types and Methods of Audit
- Principles and Techniques in Auditing
- Nursing Audit System
- Advantages and Disadvantages in Audit
- Audit Committee
- Procedure for Obtaining Audit Evidence
- Audit Process
- Steps of Audit Cycle
- Nursing as a Total Quality Controls
- Uses of Nursing Audit
- Role and Functions of Nurse Manager for Effective Quality Care

INTRODUCTION

"Audit" is a Latin word, and the verb audio ('hear') indicates both active listening and the action of investigation and interrogation of the judiciary. Transferred to the English vocabulary "audit" takes on a meaning of "an official inspection of an organization's accounts, typically by an independent body".

Audit is the instrument for quantify assurance. It developed in 19th century; the nursing audit is similar to an audit performed by accounting departments. It is a process that offers the nursing personnel in a health agency the opportunity to create and enforce standards of nursing care and to examine their own practice in systematic manner. Audit in nursing management is the professional evaluation of the quality of the patient care, by analyzing through all the facilities, services rendered, measures involved in diagnosis, treatment and other conditions and activities that affect the patients **(Fig. 11.1)**.

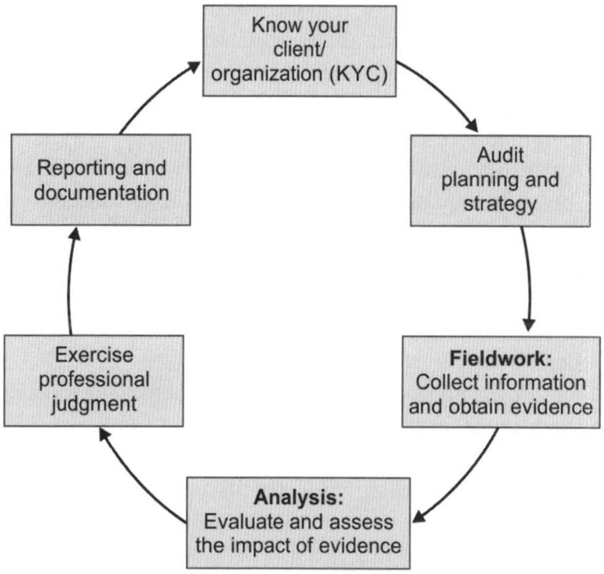

HISTORY OF NURSING AUDIT

- Nursing audit is an evaluation of nursing service. Before 1955 very little was known about the concept.
- It was introduced by the industrial concern and the year 1918 was the beginning of medical audit.
- George Groword, pronounced the term physician for the first time medical audit.
- Ten years later Thomas R Pondon MD established a method of medical audit based on procedures used by financial account. He evaluated the medical care by reviewing the medical records.
- First report of nursing audit of the hospital published in 1955. For the next 15 years, nursing audit is reported from study or record on the last decade.

Fig. 11.1: Audit is an instrument for quantify assurance.

- The program is reviewed from record nursing plan, nurse's notes, patient condition, nursing care.

DEFINITION

- According to Robert H Montgomery, "Audit is a systematic scrutiny of books and record of a commercial undertaking so as to certify its financial process and the findings are reported in this respect."
- According to Charles Worth, "Audit is the process of ascertaining whether the administrator has spent or is spending its fund in accordance with terms of legislature, instrument which appropriated money.

- Nursing audit refers to the assessment of the quality of clinical nursing. —*Elison*
- Nursing audit is the means by which nurses they can define standards from their point of view and describe the actual practice of nursing. —*Goster Walfer*
- Nursing audit is the systematic, critical analysis of the quality of clinical/community care. It is an official examination of nursing records for the purpose of evaluation verification and betterment of nursing care.
- Nursing audit is a systematic formal and written appraisal by nurses of the quality of the content and process of nursing service from care record for discharged patients.
- Nursing audit is the systematic critical analysis of the quality of clinical care. It is an official examination of nursing records for the purpose of evaluation.
- Nursing audit is a process of collecting information from nursing reports and other documented evidence about patient care and assessing the quality of care by the use of quality assurance programmer.

MEANING OF AUDITING

- Auditing is broadly defined as a systematic process of objectively obtaining and evaluating evidence in respect of certain assertions about economic actions and events, to ascertain the degree of correspondence between those assertions and established criteria and reporting the results to interested parties.
- Auditing usually covers a particular period of time. Auditing may be narrowly defined as a written report on the examination of financial statements for a particular period of time.
- Every administrator of a large, medium or small health institution has to be concerned with effectiveness of health care.
- Nursing is an important component of total medical and healthcare services of the institution.
- Public awareness of their rights for safe health delivery system and increase in the cost of medical treatment both necessitate that nurses are accountable for their practices.
- This is the reason that nursing process has become a legal document in many countries for, e.g., in England; the nursing process has been legalized.
- The nurses must decide what is best for their patients and must meet the expectations of patients and medical personnel.
- Excellence of health deliver is determined by the patient's degree of health which is maintained through health activities with existing resources.
- Quality of nursing is difficult to measure both qualitatively and quantitatively but is possible and makes an important component of medical audit which comprises nursing audit also.

OBJECTIVES OF AUDIT (FIG. 11.2)

- To justify the cost incurred on human and material resources.

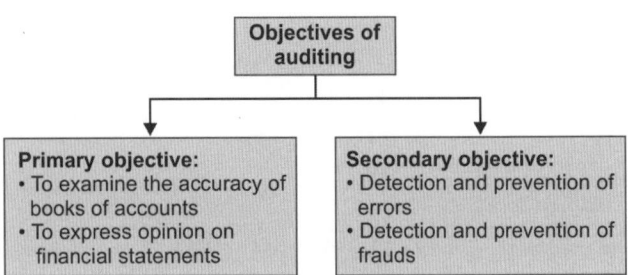

Fig. 11.2: Objectives of auditing.

- To study the quality of patient care against defined criteria.
- To take remedial actions towards cost effectiveness.
- To assess the competence of nursing staff.
- To prevent repetition of mistakes and to bring to notice the deficiencies in hospital care and in correcting the causative factors.
- To bring to notice the overall objective of nursing audit is quality assurance of delivered care in relation to change in the health status of the patient and cost effectiveness.

OBJECTIVES OF NURSING AUDIT

- To evaluate the quality of nursing care given.
- To achieve the desired and feasible quality of care.
- To provide a way for better records.
- To focus on care provided and care provider.
- To provide rationalized care thereby maintaining uniform standards worldwide.
- To contribute to research.

GOALS OF NURSING AUDIT

- Improve quality of health care.
- Promote improved communication among nurses and other health team members.
- Improve quality of nursing care.
- Detect and analyze problems and errors
- Ensure that nurses are accountable or answerable for the care.
- Contribute to research
- For the purpose of reimbursement.

CHARACTERISTICS OF AUDIT

- Audit looks at the entire process of care including administration and not just at clinical management.
- Compares the care which actually is given. Standard procedures are agreed to decide which care should be given.
- Concentrates on finding solutions for the problems identified.

Essential features of audit is shown in **Figure 11.3**.

CHARACTERISTICS OF NURSING AUDIT

- It improve the quality of nursing care.
- It compares actual practice with agreed standards of practice.

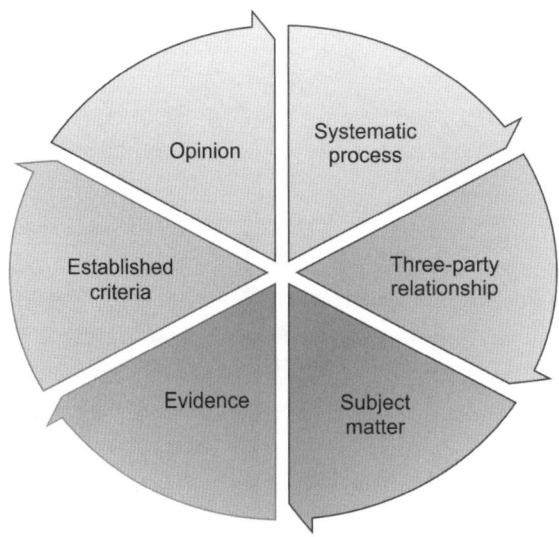

Fig. 11.3: Essential features of audit.

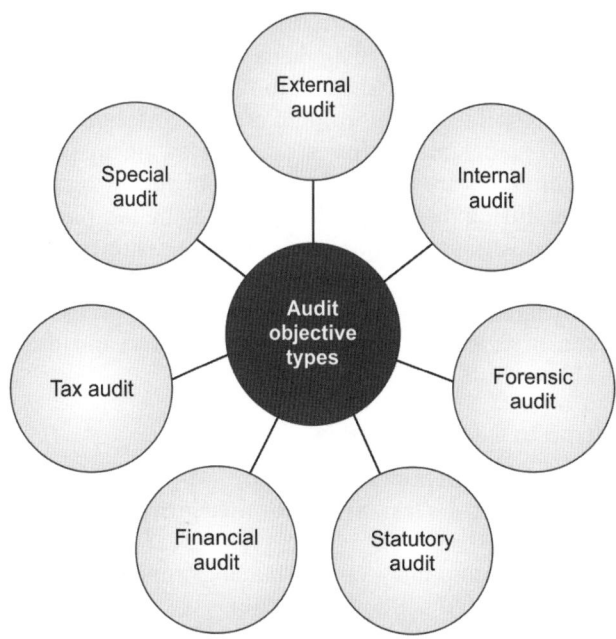

Fig. 11.4: Types of audit.

- It is formal and systemic.
- It involves peer review.
- It requires the identification of variations between practice and standards followed by the analysis of causes of such variations.
- It provides feedback for those whose records are audited.
- It includes follow-up or repeating an audit sometimes later to find out if the practice is fulfilling the agreed standards.

STEPS IN AUDIT PROCESS

- Selection of a topic
- Development of criteria
- Development of performance standards
- Chart preview
- Identification of variation
- Analysis of variation
- Development of solutions to correct poor performance
- Implementation of corrective action
- Evaluation and reaudit

TYPES OF AUDIT

An audit can be retrospective or concurrent or prospective audit **(Fig. 11.4)**.

- **Retrospective audit:** A retrospective nursing audit will identify the specific nurse who is responsible for patients care at various times during hospitalization and deficiencies in performance or charting will be reported back to the nurse.
- **Concurrent audit:** It reviews and evaluates records while persons are receiving care. The advantage is providing opportunities for making changes in the ongoing care program.
- **Prospective audit:** It identifies how future performance will be affected by current interventions. Most frequently used quality control is process audit, structure audit and outcome audit.
- **Process audit:** They are used to measure the process of care and how the care was carried out; and are task oriented and focus on whether or not standards of nursing practice are being met.
- **Structure audit:** These audits assume there is a relationship between setting, quality care, and appropriate structure.
- **Outcome audits:** They are end results of care. It determines what results occurred as a result of specific intervention by nurses for clients.

METHODS OF AUDIT

There are two methods:
1. **Retrospective view:** This refers to an in-depth assessment of the quality after the patient has been discharged, have the patients chart to the source of data. Retrospective audit is a method for evaluating the quality of nursing care by examining the nursing care as it is reflected in the patient care records for discharged patients. In this type of audit specific behaviors are described then they are converted into questions and the examiner looks for answers in the record. For example, the examiner looks through the patient's records and asks:
   a. Was the problem solving process used in planning nursing care?
   b. Whether patient data collected in a systematic manner?
   c. Was a description of patient's prehospital routines included?
   d. Laboratory test results used in planning care?
   e. Did the nurse perform physical assessment? How was information used?
   f. Were nursing diagnosis stated?
   g. Did nurse write nursing orders? And so on.

2. **The concurrent review:** This refers to the evaluations conducted on behalf of patients who are still undergoing care. It includes assessing the patient at the bedside in relation to predetermined criteria; interviewing the staff responsible for this care and reviewing the patient's record and care plan. It is achieved by reviewing patient care during the time of hospital stay by the patient. It includes assessing the patient at the bed-side in relation to predetermined criteria, such as errors, omissions, deficiencies, as well as efficiencies and also excess in the care of patients under them. It involves direct and indirect observation.

Method to Develop Criteria

- Define patient population
- Identify a time framework for measuring outcomes of care
- Identify commonly recurring nursing problems presented by the defined patient population
- State patient outcome criteria
- State acceptable degree of goal achievement
- Specify the source of information
- Design and type of tool

Points to be Remembered

- Quality assurance must be a priority
- Those responsible must implement a program not only a tool.
- A coordinator should develop and evaluate quality assurance activities.
- Roles and responsibilities must be delivered
- Nurses must be informed about the process and the results of the program
- Data must be reliable
- Adequate orientation of data collection is essential.
- Quality data should be annualized and used by nursing personnel at all levels.

PRINCIPLES OF AUDITING

Fundamental principles are those according to which the books of business accounts are audited **(Fig. 11.5)**. These principles can be changed according the desire of the auditor. We discuss the main principles of auditing under these headings:

- **Planning:** It is the basic principle of auditing. The auditor should plan before starting the work. In planning auditor decides accounting about the system and internal control procedure.
- **Honesty:** Honesty and sincerity is the second important principle of auditing. The loyalty of auditor to work and profession must be beyond the doubts.
- **Impartiality:** In case of audit the attitude of the auditor must be impartial. Keeping in view this principle his personal views may not be included in the audit report.
- **Secrecy:** Secrecy must be maintained by the auditor during the process of audit. He cannot disclose any information to the third party.

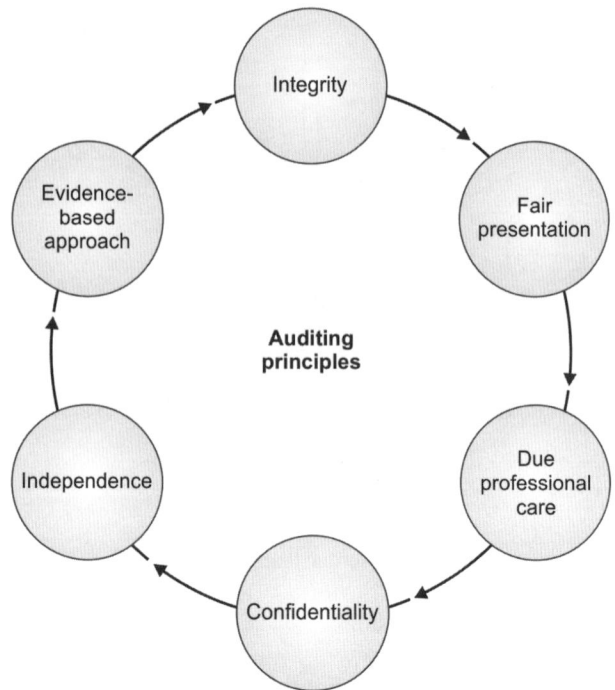

Fig. 11.5: Principles of auditing.

- **Evidence:** During the audit the auditor can collect the evidence through the working papers. He can frame his opinion on the audit evidence. The nature and source of evidence must be kept in view by the auditor.
- **Consistency:** It is an important principle of auditing. In case of selecting the rates of depreciation and valuation of stock the accountant must follow the rates of the coming years. In this regard there should be consistency and changes are not acceptable.
- **Legal framework:** The business activities may run within the rules and legal formalities. To protect the rights of the interested parties rules must be applied.
- **Working paper preparation:** The auditor collect documents providing evidence that audit was carried out according the principles. The auditor prepares the working paper and kept in this custody as a proof.
- **Internal control:** The auditor will examine the accounting system and inter control. To frame his opinion, he keeps in view the evidence obtained from the books.
- **Report:** According the principle of auditing a report will be prepared by the auditor at the end. It may be conditional or unconditional. The auditor can draw conclusion and disclose the facts and figures about the business for general information.

TECHNIQUES OF AUDITING/AUDIT TECHNIQUES

Techniques of auditing mean the procedure and method which is adopted by the auditor in checking the accounts. Following are the important techniques of audit **(Fig. 11.6):**

- **Examination of record:** This technique is commonly used by the auditors; the inspection of books and documents is made to verify the validity of data.

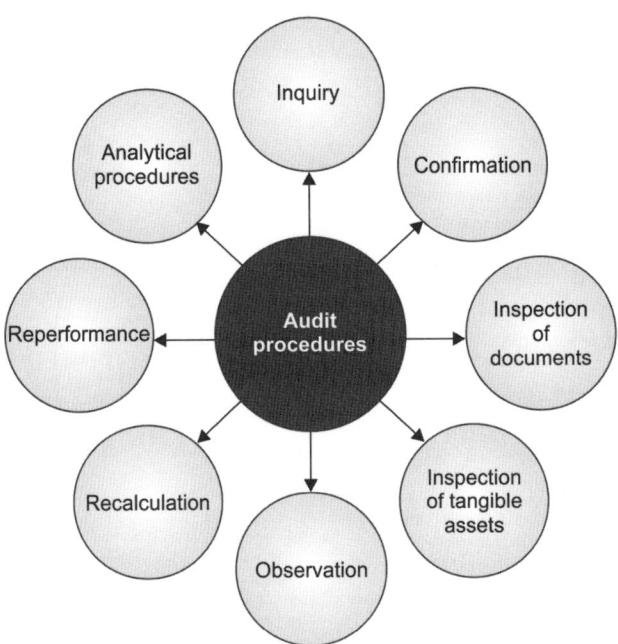

Fig. 11.6: Audit procedures.

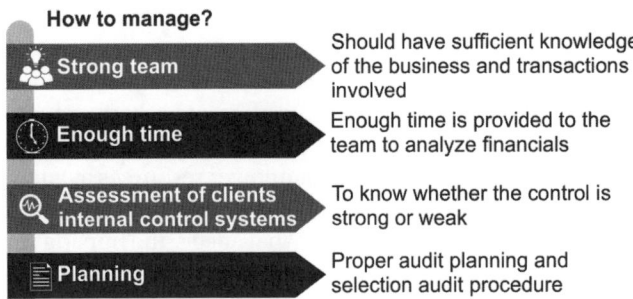

Fig. 11.7: Audit risk.

- **Inquiry:** The auditor can also use the technique of inquiry. He can get the information from resource persons inside or outside the enterprise.
- **Sampling:** Auditor can select few items from whole accounting information. This technique enables the auditor to obtain and evaluate the evidence of some characteristics of the whole class. It is helpful in forming the conclusion.
- **Confirmation:** To ensure the accuracy of the data auditor can collect the information from the debtor. Confirmation is response to an inquiry to prove certain data recorded in the books.
- **Compliance:** To check the arithmetical accuracy of accounting record, the balancing accounts can be compared with the vouchers to test the reliability of data.
- **Compliance test:** These tests are designed to check the effectiveness and compliance of internal control. In obtaining the audit evidence, auditor is concerned with the existence of effective internal control.
- **Use of computer techniques:** There is large number of audit techniques, such as audit software, test packs and mapping which can be used by the auditor to test the accuracy of the data.
- **Substantive test:** These are designed to obtain evidence that data produced by accounting system is accurate or not. It has two kinds: (i) Test of detail transaction. (ii) Test of significant ratios and trends.
- **Dependence on experts and auditors:** The auditor has to rely on the internal and other auditors to complete his work. He has also to rely on other experts, such as lawyers, engineers and doctors for their expert opinion about the business.
- **Analytical review:** It consists of studying significant ratios, trends and investigating different changes. This review procedure is based on the expectations of relationship among the past and present data. **Figure 11.7** shows audit risk.

ETHICAL PRINCIPLES

In carrying out the audit of financial statements, auditors should comply with the ethical guidance issued by their relevant professional bodies. Ethics is more of a norm or a certain code of conduct expected of a group of individuals or a professional body. It dictates some degree of inward values expected of such groups of individuals or body. The ethical principles which govern the auditors' professional responsibilities include:

- Integrity
- Objectivity
- Independence
- Professional competence and due care; professional behavior
- Confidentiality

BENEFITS OF AUDIT

- **Patient:** The fundamental principle behind nursing care audit is to everyone involved in care.
- **Nursing staff:** For nurses, nursing care audit offers the opportunity to concentrate on areas of care where their skills and efforts can have positive outcomes, greater senses of achievement, autonomy, responsibility and provides a means for self-improvement.
- **Community:** The new purchases provides environment in the hospital, which requires practitioners to quantify the work they do nursing care audit allows nurses to measure the more intangible aspects of their work, in particular the quality care and also demonstrate the contribution.

NURSING AUDITOR

- **Internal auditor:** The nursing experts from within the hospital are deputed for internal audit and the auditing is done within the agency or hospital.
- **External auditor:** Nursing and the medical administrations from the ministry and other agencies of professional association, such as Trained Nurses' Association of India (TNAI) undertake the nursing audit in the desired agency or hospital.

NURSING AUDIT SYSTEM

Nursing audit refers to the assessment of the quality of clinical nursing. For nursing auditing, questions are asked such as Is nursing properly practiced? Assessment of structure of care, Are facilities, equipment and manpower resources available conducive to the delivery of quality care. While assessment of outcome care, auditors also asks, what effects, the nursing care have on alteration of the health status of the recipient of care?

ADVANTAGES OF NURSING AUDIT

- A biographical index of quality of nursing
- A patient is assured of good services.
- It will give valuable and pertinent information for the staff.
- It will lead to between cooperation and communication among the nurse and health team.
- It will help each professional nurse for her self-evaluation.
- It helps the administration as better planning.
- It will reduce the incidence of medical legal complication.
- It will broaden and strengthen nursing service.

DISADVANTAGES OF NURSING AUDIT

- Appraises the outcomes of the nursing process, so, it is not so useful in areas where the nursing process has not been implemented.
- Many of the components overlap making analysis difficult.
- Is time consuming.
- Requires a team of trained auditors.
- Deals with a large amount of information.
- Only evaluates record keeping.
- Only serves to improve documentation, not nursing care.

Current challenges of audit is shown in **Box 11.1**.

AUDIT COMMITTEE

Before carrying out an audit, an audit committee should be formed, comprising of a minimum of five members who are interested in quality assurance, are clinically competent and able to work together in a group **(Fig. 11.8)**. It is recommended that each member should review no more than 10 patients each month and that the auditor should.

Responsibilities and Duties of Audit Committee

- Review and safeguard the auditor's performance and independence.
- Continuous monitoring of financial reporting, maintain the accuracy and credibility of the report.
- Review annual financial statement with the company's management before being submitted to the Board
- Review the reason of default by any stakeholder.
- Review all policies related to risk management and financial management of the company.
- Review reports submitted by internal auditors in case of fraud or suspected frauds.

Box 11.1: Current challenges.

Labor
- Excessive labor
- Insufficient training
- Poor layouts/unnecessary handling
- Unbalanced operations
- Unplanned overtime
- Lack of employee involvement
- Poor attendance

Cost
- Downtime
- Cost rising
- Extra equipment
- Excessive capacity
- Unplanned equipment

Delivery
- Poor response
- Premium freight
- Missed shipments/deliveries
- Inconsistent schedules
- Inventory errors
- Unrealistic forecasts
- Lack of customer input concerning requirements

Quality
- Excessive variation
- Warranty cost
- Incapable processes
- Increased inspection

Communication
Poor customer/vendor relation

Inventory
- Additional material handling
- Bottlenecks
- Complex inventory management
- High inventory levels
- Large lot sizes
- Long changeover
- Long lead time
- Unbalanced material flow

Safety
- Safety
- Accidents
- Unsafe work environment

Engineering
- Poor design control
- Lack of cross-functional input
- Uncontrolled changes
- Engineering changes without process changes
- Obsolete technology
- Poor prototype quality/quality control
- Unexpected cost increases
- Poor management of requirements
- Tolerance stack up not in +/−3σ
- Warranty issues due to design

- Approve any legitimate modifications in relation to transaction with related parties.
- Monitor the usage of funds raised through public offerings
- Confirming all compliances with the concerned legal and governmental bodies.
- Recommend the appointment or removal of external auditors if needed.

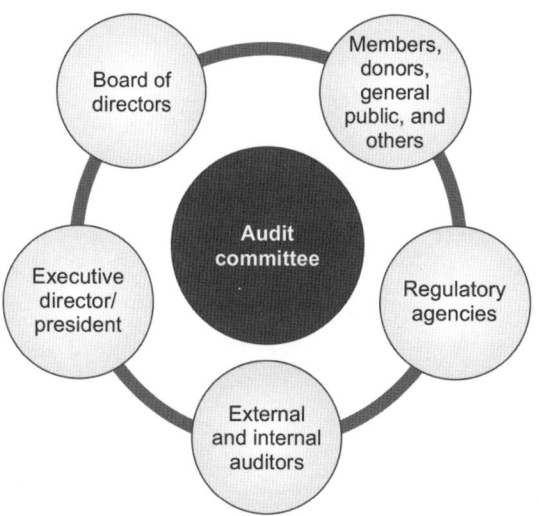

Fig. 11.8: Audit committee.

- Discuss and review the financial situation the firm and report any shortcomings in managerial internal control.
- Review the work, remuneration offered and removal of chief internal auditor.
- Scrutinize all inter-corporate loans
- Evaluation of undertakings by the firm
- To establish a vigil mechanism

RELIABILITY OF AUDIT EVIDENCE

The reliability of audit evidence is influenced by its source which may either be internal or external; and by its nature which may be visual, documentary or oral. The auditor must be aware of the following matters in assessing the reliability of audit evidence (**Box 11.2**):

- Audit evidence from external sources (for example, confirmation received from a third party) is more reliable than that obtained from the entity's records.
- Audit evidence obtained from the entity's records is more reliable when the related accounting and internal control systems operate effectively.
- Audit evidence obtained directly by auditors is more reliable than that obtained by or from the entity.
- Audit evidence in the form of documents and written representations are more reliable than oral representations.
- Original documents are more reliable than photocopies, telexes or facsimiles.

Box 11.2: Reliability of audit evidence.
• Evidence from sources outside an entity is more reliable than evidence obtained solely from within the entity. • Evidence generated internally is more reliable when the internal control structures are effective. • Evidence obtained directly by the auditor is more reliable than evidence obtained from the client. • Evidence in the form of documents or written representations is more reliable than oral representations. • Evidence provided by original documents is more reliable than evidence provided by photocopies or facsimiles.

PROCEDURE FOR OBTAINING AUDIT EVIDENCE

Auditors normally obtain audit evidence by inspection, observation, enquiry, confirmation, computation and analytical procedures (**Fig. 11.9 and Box 11.3**). The choice of one or a combination of the procedures which the auditor may adopt is dependent, in part, upon the period of time during which the audit evidence sought is available and the form in which the accounting records are maintained.

- **Inspection:** Inspection involves the following:
  - Examination of records, documents or tangible assets
  - Provision of audit evidence of varying degrees of reliability depending on their nature and source and the effectiveness of internal controls over their processing. Three major categories of documentary audit evidence are listed below in descending degree of reliability as audit evidence:
    1. Evidence created and provided to auditors by third parties
    2. Evidence created by third parties and held by the entity
    3. Evidence created and held by the entity

  Inspection provides reliable audit evidence about the existence of the tangible assets inspected, but not necessarily as to the ownership or value of such assets.

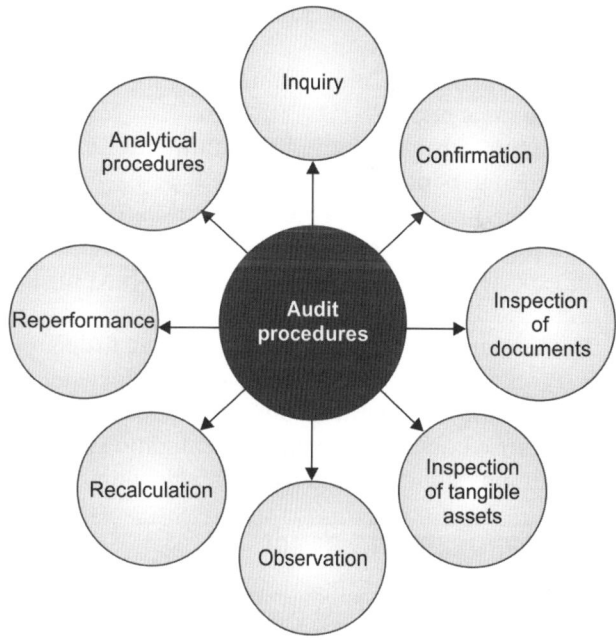

Fig. 11.9: Audit procedure.

Box 11.3: Procedures to obtain audit evidence.

• **Inspection:**
  – Examination of records, documents like annual reports, financial statements, project documents, correspondence, memoranda, reports, directions to staff, internal audit reports.
  – Examining tangible assets WRT existence
• **Confirmation:** Consists of response to an inquiry to corroborate information contained in the records.
• **Direct observation:** Looking at a process or procedure being performed by others

- **Observation:** The auditor by observation looks at a procedure being performed by others. For example, the auditor observes the counting of stock by the entity's staff or the performance of internal control procedures as part of the conduct of an audit.
- **Enquiry and confirmation:** Enquiry involves seeking information within and outside the entity. Enquiry may be formal or informal. Responses to enquiries obtained from third parties may confirm or disprove information previously made available to the auditor.

    Confirmation involves obtaining response to an enquiry to corroborate information previously made available to the auditors in the course of the audit.
    Examples of direct confirmation are as follows:
    - Confirmation of debts by communication with debtors;
    - Confirmation of legal cases by communication with the entity's solicitors; and
    - Confirmation of bank balances by communication with the entity's bankers, etc.
- **Computation:** The auditor uses computation to check the arithmetical accuracy of source documents and accounting records. Computation also involves performing independent calculations.
- **Analytical procedures:** Analytical procedures consist of the analysis of relationship between:
    1. Items of financial data
    2. Items of financial and nonfinancial data, derived from the same period
    3. Comparable financial information deriving from different periods or different entities.

    Analytical procedures are used to identifying consistencies and predicted patterns or significant fluctuations and unexpected relationships, and the results of investigations performed.
- **Documentation:** It is the duty of the auditor to document matters which are important in providing evidence to support the audit opinion and evidence that the audit was carried out in accordance with auditing standards, accounting standards and relevant regulations.

AUDIT PROCESS (FIG. 11.10)

According to Lancaster (1988) there are six steps to conduct an audit.
1. **Selection of a topic for audit:** Before the auditing is done one needs to identify the aspect of care which is to be audited.
2. **Selection of explicit criteria for quality care:** The criteria for assessing the quality care has to be decided. Any type of audit needs to have particular criteria on the basis of which auditing will be done. Each criterion should be clearly phrased in numerical, descriptive or behavioral terms.
3. **Review of records:** If the retrospective kind of auditing is to be done the auditor needs to decide in what particular time he/she wants to review the charts.

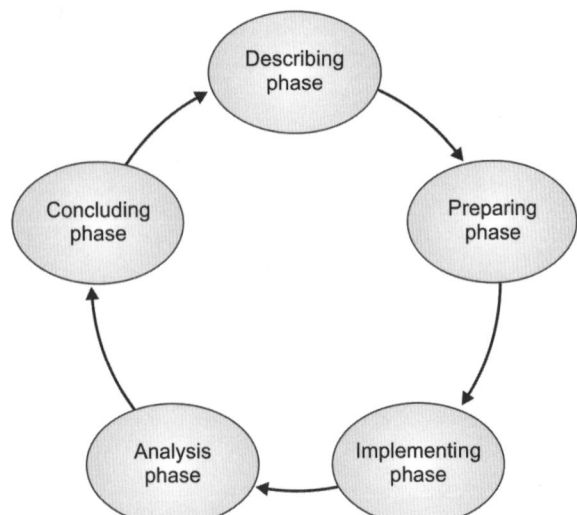

Fig. 11.10: Nursing audit process.

4. **Peer reviews of all cases that do not meet criteria for quality care:** If the criterion set for auditing is not met then peer review is done to find the reasons.
5. **Recommendations to correct deficiencies:** Specific recommendations are given to correct deficiencies like staff development program—in-service education, etc.
6. **Follow-up of the topic:** After giving recommendations, one needs to do a follow-up to assess audit cycle gives series of actualities which when followed eliminate any confusions.

Setting of standards: Minimum standards are set for structure, process and outcome audit.

Observes practice: In observing practice directing a concurrent auditing is done where direct care is given by the care giver whereas records are observed after the patient is discharged.

Compare with standards: All observations whether ongoing or given in the past, are compared with the set.

Implement change: After observing the deficiencies, motivation and education is given to the care givers. So a change can be implemented and again reauditing can be done to evaluate the quality of care.

STEPS OF AUDIT CYCLE (FIG. 11.11)

1. **Identify the need for change:** This may come from personal experience. A problem may be identified from every day practice, and following this there is a feeling that something could or should have been done better. Problems can be identified in three basic areas of practice work:
    i. **Structure:** This refers to the input of care, such as manpower, premises and facilities, e.g., 'Are the numbers of emergency appointments enough to cope with demand?'
    ii. **Process:** This refers to the provision of care (looking at what is done and how it is done), e.g., 'Are all patients on ACEI having urea and electrolytes checked?'

Chapter 11: Nursing Audit

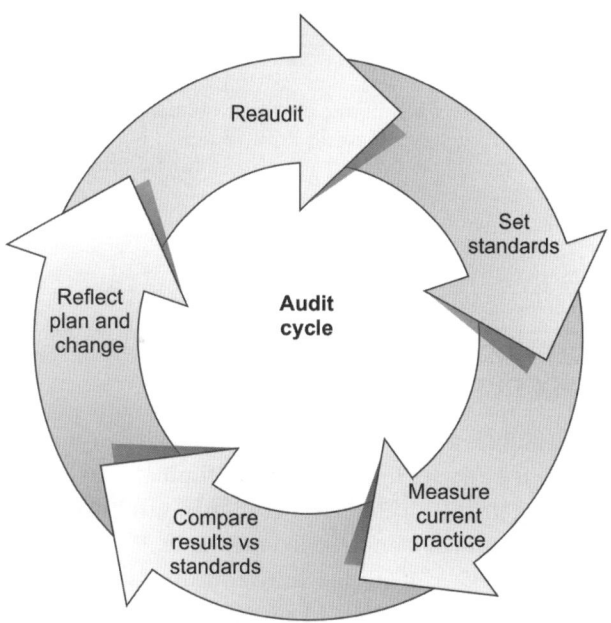

Fig. 11.11: Steps of audit cycle.

iii. **Outcome:** This refers to the result of clinical intervention, e.g., 'Are patients on lipid reducing regimes achieving target cholesterol levels?'

2. **Setting criteria and standards:** This is where you can say what should be happening.
   - **A criterion is an item of care or some aspect** of care that can be used to assess quality.
     The criterion is written as a statement. Below are three criteria one relating to an audit in structure, one an audit in process and one an audit in outcome.
     – All patients requesting an urgent appointment will be seen that day.
     – All patients with epilepsy should be seen at least once a year.
     – All patients on warfarin should have their INR within the recommended limits.
   - **Criteria can be defined from recent medical literature**, and the best experience of clinical practice these are called 'Normative criteria'.
   - **To make the criteria (statement) useful the standard needs to be defined.** A standard describes the level of care to be achieved for any particular criteria, e.g., A standard may state: 98% of patients requesting urgent appointments will be seen the same day. 90% of patients with epilepsy should be seen at least once a year. 100% of patients on warfarin will have their INR within the recommended limits.
   - **Standards must be set.** The level of standard can often be controversial. There are basically three options:
     i. A minimum standard: This describes the lowest acceptable standard of performance. Minimum standards are often used to distinguish between acceptable and unacceptable practice.
     ii. An ideal standard describes the care it should be possible to give under ideal conditions, with no constraints. Such a standard by definition cannot usually be attained.
     iii. An optimum standard lies between the minimum and the idea. Setting an optimum standard requires judgment discussion and consensus with other members of the primary care team. Optimum standards represent the standard of care most likely to be achieved under normal conditions of practice.

3. **Collecting data on performance:** Identify what data needs to be collected, how and in what form it needs to be collected, and who is going to collect it. Remember only collect information that is absolutely essential.

4. **Issues performance against criteria and standards:** With the information collected analysis is possible, and identification of any area of care below the predetermined standard of the criteria can be made. The results can then be used to develop an action plan, i.e., What needs to be done? How it needs to be done? Who is going to do it and When is it going to be done?

5. **Re-evaluation:** The audit cycle is now almost complete, but without re-evaluating the care the practice is giving it is impossible to see if recommendations have been implemented and the level of care improved.

NURSING AS A TOTAL QUALITY CONTROLS

- An audit is a systematic and official examination of a record, process or account to evaluate performance.
- Auditing in health care organization provide managers with a means of applying control process to determine the quality of service rendered.
- Nursing audit is the process of analyzing data about the nursing process of patient outcomes to evaluate the effectiveness of nursing interventions.
- The audits most frequently used in quality control include outcome, process and structure audits.

Outcome Audit

- Outcomes are the end results of care; the changes in the patients health status and can be attributed to delivery of healthcare services.
- Outcome audits determine what results if any occurred as result of specific nursing intervention for clients.
- These audits assume the outcome accurately and demonstrate the quality of care that was provided.
- Example of outcomes traditionally used to measure quality of hospital care includes mortality, its morbidity, and length of hospital stay.

Advantages and disadvantages of audit is shown in **Table 11.1**.

Process Audit

- Process audits are used to measure the process of care or how the care was carried out.
- Process audit is task oriented and focuses on whether or not practice standards are being fulfilled.
- These audits assumed that a relationship exists between the quality of the nurse and quality of care provided.

Table 11.1: Advantages versus disadvantages of audit cycle.	
Advantages	Disadvantages
• Can be used as a method of measurement in all areas of nursing • Seven functions are easily understood • Scoring system is fairly simple • Results easily understood • Assesses the work of all those involved in recording care • May be a useful tool as part of a quality assurance programme in areas where accurate records of care are kept	• Appraises the outcomes of the nursing process, so it is not so useful in areas where the nursing process has not been implemented • Many of the components overlap making analysis difficult, is time consuming • Requires a team of trained auditors • Deals with a large amount information • Only evaluates record keeping. It leading to improve documentation, not nursing care

Structure Audit

- Structure audit monitors the structure or setting in which patient care occurs, such as the finances, nursing service, medical records and environment.
- This audit assumes that a relationship exists between quality care and appropriate structure.
- These above audits can occur retrospectively, concurrently and prospectively.

The seven functions of professional nursing are used as the framework for an audit. These functions are:

1. Nursing care of the patient.
2. Care given by other professionals.
3. Observation of signs, symptoms and reaction.
4. Application and execution of nursing procedures and techniques.
5. Promotion of physical and emotional health by direction and teaching.
6. Reporting and recording.
7. Application and execution of physician's legal orders.

■ USES OF NURSING AUDIT

- **Nursing care services:** It helps in modifying nursing care plans and nursing care process; implementing a program for improving documentation of nursing care through improved charting policies; focusing attention, weaknesses identified; nursing round and term conferences, and designing responsible orientation and in-service education program.
- **Nursing administrator:** Providing evaluation of particular program, such as orientation of personnel or establishment of a patient teaching program; support for financing a particular program; serving as basis for planning new programs; identification of areas of strength and weakness in various settings; determining the influence of varied staffing patterns. For supervisors and head nurses: Identifying areas of needed patient care improvement; providing basis for in-service education program, and identifying needs of staff members who gives direct care to patient.
- **Staff nurses:** It provides a self-examination of care; identifies a particular type of care in which practice may be improved merely by increased attention and identifies types of care on which improvement will depend.

■ ROLE AND FUNCTIONS OF NURSE MANAGER FOR EFFECTIVE QUALITY CARE

Clinical audit is a part of the continuous quality improvement process. It consists in measuring a clinical outcome or a process against well-defined standards, established using the principles of evidence-based medicine. The comparison between clinical practice and standards leads to the formulation of strategies, in order to improve daily care quality. This review examines the basis of clinical audit and the data about the efficacy of this methodology, focusing on nephrology issues. We think that clinical audit could offer to the modern nephrologists a useful tool to monitor and advance their clinical practice.

Roles of Nurse Manager

- Encourages followers
- Clearly communicates standards of care to subordinates
- Encourages the setting of high standards
- Implement quality control proactively
- Uses control
- Positively active in communicating quality control finding
- Acts as a role model

Functions of Nurse Manager

- In conjunctions with other personnel in the organization establishes clear cut, measurable standards of care and determines the most appropriate methods for measuring if those standards have been met.
- Selects and uses process, outcome and structure audits appropriately as quality control tools.
- Assesses appropriate sources of information in data gathering for quality control tools.
- Determines discrepancies between care provided and unit standards and seeks further information regarding why standards were not met.
- Uses quality control findings as a measure of employee performance and rewards, coaches, counsels or disciplines employees accordingly.
- Keeps abreast of current government and licensing regulations that affect quality control.

CONCLUSION

A profession concerns for the quality of its service constitutes the heart of its responsibility to the public. An audit helps to ensure that the quality of nursing care desired and feasible is achieved. This concept is often referred to as quality assurance.

REVIEW QUESTIONS

Long Essays
1. Define audit; explain the objectives, goals and characteristics.
2. Describe the methods of audit.
3. Explain audit process; discuss in detail about the steps of audit process.

Short Essays
1. Types of audit.
2. Principles of auditing.
3. Techniques of auditing.
4. Advantages and disadvantages of auditing.
5. Audit committee role and responsibilities.
6. Nursing as total quality controls.
7. Procedure for obtaining audit evidence.
8. Uses of nursing audit.

Short Answers
1. Steps in audit process.
2. Ethical principles of auditing.
3. Benefits of audit.
4. Nursing auditor.
5. Nursing audit system.
6. Reliability of audit evidence.
7. Process audit

BIBLIOGRAPHY

1. Bjorvell C. Development of an audit-instrument for nursing care plans in the patient record. Qual Health Care. 2000; 9:6-13.
2. BT Basavanthappa. Nursing Administration. New Delhi; Jaypee Brothers; 2002.
3. Cheater FM, Keane M. Nurses' participation in audit: a regional study. Quality in Health Care. 1998;7:27-36.
4. Goel SL, Kumar R. Hospital administration and management. New Delhi: Deep and Deep publishers; 2000.
5. Jamtvedt G. Audit and feedback: effects on professional practice and health care outcomes. J. Quality in Health Care. 2000; 7: 27-36.
6. Jogelkar KS. Hospital word management professional adjustments and trends in nursing. Mumbai: Vora medical publications;1990.
7. Johnston G. Reviewing audit: barriers and facilitating factors for effective clinical audit. Quality in Health Care. 2000; 9:23-36.
8. Marquis BL, Huston C J. Quality control. Audits as a quality control tool. In Leadership roles and management function in nursing: theory and application, 8th edition. Philadelphia, PA: Wolters Kluwer Health. 2015. pp.551-3. (GI)
9. McClelland G. Assessing scrub practitioner non-technical skills: a literature review. Journal of Perioperative Practice. 2014; 25(1-2): 12-8. (RV)
10. Nicholas-Holley J. Auditing the needs of recovery room staff providing care for the child in an acute hospital. Journal of Perioperative Practice. 2016; 26(5):102-5. (GI)

CHAPTER 12

Directing or Leading

LEARNING OBJECTIVES

- Definition, Principles, Elements of Directing
- Supervision and Guidance
- Participatory Management
- Interprofessional Collaboration
- Management by Objectives
- Team Management
- Assignments and Rotations
- Maintenance of Discipline
- Leadership in Management

INTRODUCTION

Directing is said to be a process in which the managers instruct, guide and oversee the performance of the workers to achieve predetermined goals. Directing is said to be the heart of management process. Planning, organizing, staffing has got no importance if direction function does not take place. Directing initiates action and it is from here actual work starts. Direction is said to be consisting of human factors. In simple words, it can be described as providing guidance to workers is doing work. In field of management, direction is said to be all those activities which are designed to encourage the subordinates to work effectively and efficiently. According to Human, "Directing consists of process or technique by which instruction can be issued and operations can be carried out as originally planned". Therefore, Directing is the function of guiding, inspiring, overseeing and instructing people towards accomplishment of organizational goals (**Fig. 12.1**).

DEFINITIONS

Direction has been defined by certain important managerial authorities in the following words:

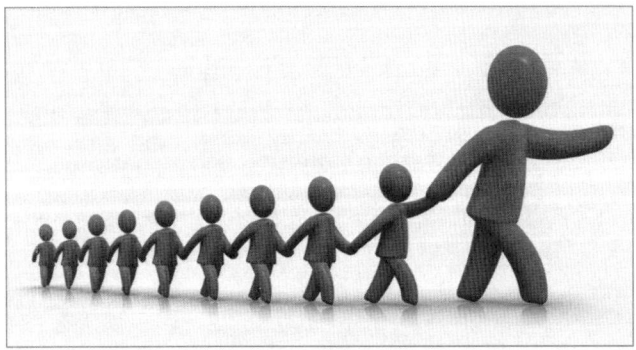

Fig. 12.1: Direction.

- "Activating deals with the steps a manager takes to get subordinates and others to carry out plans".
  —*Newman and Warren*
- "Directing is the inter personnel aspect of managing by which subordinates are led to understand and contribute effectively and efficiently to the attainment of enterprise objectives." —*Koontz and O'Donnell*
- "Directing means moving to action and supplying simulative power to a group of persons". —*GR Terry*
- "Direction is telling people what to do and seeing that they do it to the best of their ability". —*Dale*
- "Directing involves determining the course, giving orders and instructions and providing dynamic leadership". —*Marshall*
- In the words of Ernest Dale, "Direction is telling people what to do and seeing that they do it to the best of their ability. It mistakes are corrected, providing on-the-job instructions and, of course, issuing orders."
- In the words of Theo Haimann, "Directing consists of the process and techniques utilized in issuing instructions and making certain that operations are carried on as originally planned."

MEANING OF DIRECTION

In the words of Theo Haimann, "Management is the art and process of getting things done through and with the people." The managers have, therefore, the responsibility not only of planning and organizing the operations but also of guiding and directing the subordinates. Thus, direction, in simple words, is guiding the subordinates in doing work. In this way, direction is an important managerial function performed by all the managers at all levels of organization. Direction is concerned with directing human efforts towards the achievement of organizational goals and objectives. A superior or boss in an organization gives direction to his subordinates and the subordinates receive directions from their superiors or bosses.

NATURE OF DIRECTION

- **Management function:** Direction is a managerial function performed by all the managers or supervisors at all the levels of an enterprise.
- **Guiding process:** Direction is not limited to the issuing of orders as well as instructions but it also includes the process of guiding and inspiring subordinates.
- **Continuous activity:** Direction is the continuous activity. It start from planning function throughout and there is no end to it and directing function continues at all the levels of the management process till the end.
- **Flow of direction:** The flow of direction in an organization initiates from the top level to the bottom level.
- **Direction has wide dimensions:** It is not concerned with only issue of orders and instructions to the subordinates. It also includes communication, motivation and supervision of subordinates.
- **Readily acceptable:** Direction should be such which is readily acceptable to the subordinates. It should be both oral and written keeping in view the time factor and the capability of subordinates.

CHARACTERISTICS OF DIRECTION

Direction has got following characteristics (**Box. 12.1 and Fig. 12.2**):

1. **Pervasive function:** Directing is required at all levels of organization. Every manager provides guidance and inspiration to his subordinates.
2. **Continuous activity:** Direction is a continuous activity as it continuous throughout the life of organization.
3. **Human factor:** Directing function is related to subordinates and therefore it is related to human factor. Since human factor is complex and behavior is unpredictable, direction function becomes important.
4. **Creative activity:** Direction function helps in converting plans into performance. Without this function, people become inactive and physical resources are meaningless.
5. **Executive function:** Direction function is carried out by all managers and executives at all levels throughout the working of an enterprise, a subordinate receives instructions from his superior only.
6. **Delegate function:** Direction is supposed to be a function dealing with human beings. Human behavior is unpredictable by nature and conditioning the people's behavior towards the goals of the enterprise is what the executive does in this function. Therefore, it is termed as having delicacy in it to tackle human behavior.

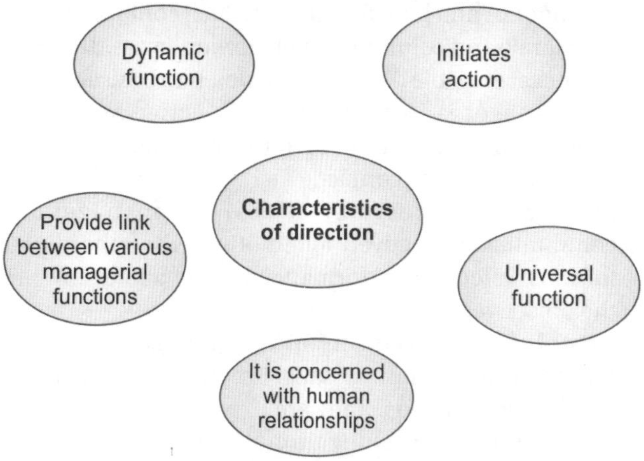

Fig. 12.2: Characteristics of direction.

PRINCIPLES OF DIRECTING

Directing is a complex function as it deals with employees whose behavior is unpredictable. Effective directing is an art which a manager can learn and perfect through practice. Directing has the following principles which make the directing function effective in the organization (**Fig. 12.3**).

- **Principle of leadership:** It is the ability to lead effectively and is essential for the effective directing of the subordinates.
- **Principle of communication:** A good system of communication between the superior and his subordinates helps to improve mutual understanding. Upwards communication helps a manager to understand the subordinates to express their feeling. Through this principle the management recognizes the importance of an informal organization.
- **Principle of direct supervision:** Directing becomes more effective when there is a direct personal contact between

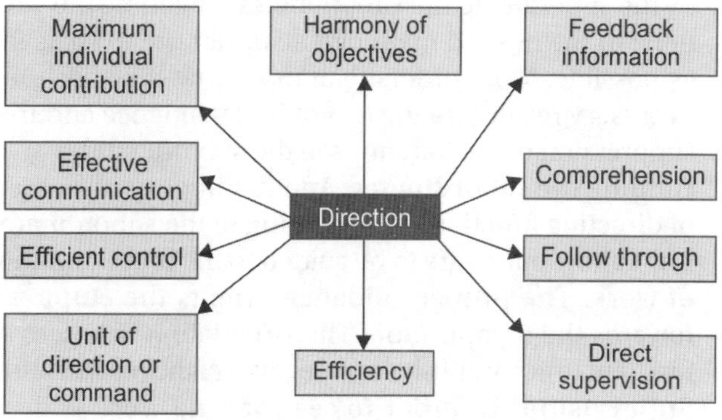

Box 12.1: Nature of direction.

Following are included in the characteristics of direction:
- **An important function of management:** All the functions and achievements of management are depending on proper direction. If proper guidance is not provided to the employees in an enterprise, it cannot be successful in achieving its objects.
- **Continuity:** Direction is a continuous process because it is required at every stage of management. It goes with the work. Where the work is in progress, the direction continues.
- **To order:** Higher officer order their subordinates to do their jobs and the subordinates have to work according to these orders.
- **To coordinate:** The success of direction lies in the coordinated efforts of the employees of the enterprise.

Fig. 12.3: Principles of direction.

the superior and his subordinates. Such contact improves the morale and commitment of the employees. Therefore, whenever possible direct supervision is to be used. Hence the manager is to supplement objective methods of supervision and control with direct personal supervision to ensure personal contact.

- **Principle of direct objectives:** The manager is to communicate effectively and motivate the subordinates for most effective performance for the achievement of the objectives.
- **Principles of harmony of objectives:** Employees join the organization to satisfy their physiological and psychological needs. They are expected to work for the achievement of organizational objectives. They will perform their tasks better if they feel that it will satisfy their personal goals. Therefore, the manager is to guide the subordinates so that their individual interest harmonizes with the organizational interests.
- **Principle of unity of command:** A subordinate is to get orders and instruction only from one superior. If he is made accountable to two superiors simultaneously, there will be confusion, conflict, disorder and indiscipline in the organization. Therefore, every subordinate should be asked to report to only one manager.
- **Principle of managerial communication:** A good system of communication between the superior and his subordinates helps to improve mutual understanding. Upwards communication helps a manager to understand the subordinates to express their feeling. The manager being the principle medium of communication, should keep lines of communication open.
- **Principle of comprehension:** The communication should ensure that the recipients of the information actually comprehend it.
- **Principle of direct communication:** The direct flow of information is most effective for communications.
- **Principle of appropriate techniques:** The manager is to use correct direction techniques to ensure efficiency of directing. The techniques used are to be suitable to the superior, the subordinates and the situation.

ELEMENTS OF DIRECTING (FIG. 12.4)

- **Issuing of orders and instructions:** The first element of directing function is the issuing of orders and instructions by the superiors to the subordinates for getting the work done in the desired manner. The orders are to be as few as possible. More orders than those that are absolutely necessary result into the loss of independence and thus suppression of the initiatives of the subordinates.
- **Guiding the subordinates:** Another important element of directing function is the guiding of the subordinates. The subordinates are to be guided to the proper method of work. The proper guidance orients the employee towards the organization. This orientation is necessary for them to accomplish the objectives of the organization.
- **Supervision:** In order to see that the work is done according to the instructions, the superior must observe

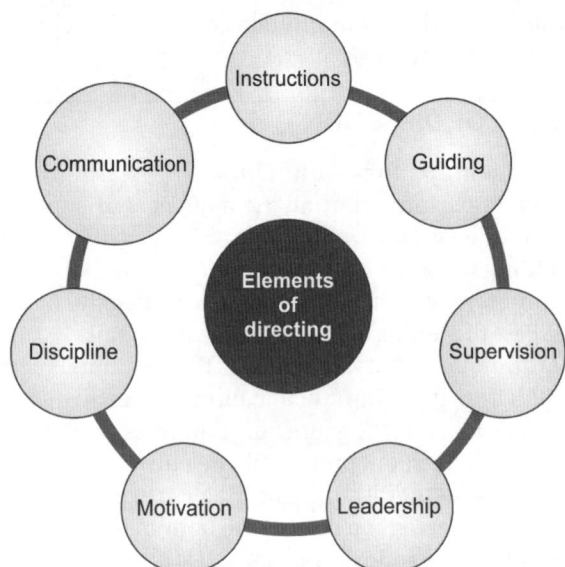

Fig. 12.4: Elements of directing.

the activities of the subordinates. Supervision is an important component of the function of directing.
- **Leadership:** Leadership is the ability to persuade and motivate others to work in a desired way for achieving the goal. Thus, a person who is able to influence others and make them follow his instructions is called a leader. Leadership is the process, which influences the people and inspires them to willingly accomplish the organizational objectives.
- **Motivation:** Motivation is one of the important elements of directing. Motivation of the employees is one of the most challenging problems for the management. It has to induce the employees to utilize their talent and skill to contribute to the organizational goal. It creates in men, the willingness to work whole-heartedly for attaining objectives. Issuance of proper instructions or orders does not necessarily ensure that they will be properly carried out. It requires manager to inspire or induce the employees to act and get the expected result.
- **Maintenance of discipline:** Discipline is an important element of directing function. Proper discipline is required to be maintained in the organization for the orderly behavior of the employees.
- **Communication:** Communication is the core of direction. It is through the communication network that a manager instructs his subordinates as to what they should do and how they should do it. Communication refers to the process by which a person (known as sender) transmits information or messages to another person (known as receiver). Proper communication results in clarity and securing the cooperation of subordinates.

FUNCTIONS OF DIRECTION

The process of directing function involves the following elements: Direction has certain elements. The important elements of direction are:

- **Issuing of order and instruction:** The first element of direction is the issuing of orders and instructions by the superiors to the subordinates for getting the work done in the desired manner.
- **Guiding the subordinates:** Another important element of direction is guiding the subordinates. The subordinates have to be guided to the proper method of work.
- **Supervision:** Supervision is an important component of direction. Supervision implies overseeing the work of subordinates to ensure that the performance of the subordinates conforms to plans and contributes to the attainment of the organizational goal.
- **Leadership:** Leadership influences the work of subordinates. Appropriate and inspiring leadership alone can influence the subordinates to better their performances.
- **Motivation:** Motivation creates in men, the willingness to work whole-heartedly for attaining objectives.
- **Maintenance of discipline:** Discipline is an important element of direction. Proper discipline has to be maintained in the organization for the orderly behavior of the employees.
- **Communication:** Communication is the core of direction. It is through the communication network that a manager instructs his subordinates as to what they should do and how they should do it.
- **Coordination:** Direction implies coordination, so coordination is one of the important elements of direction.

IMPORTANCE OF DIRECTION

Directing various employees in an organization is an important managerial task. It is indispensable for achieving enterprise objectives **(Box 12.2)**.

Effective direction provides the following advantages:
- **Initiates action:** Direction is required to initiate action. The functions of planning, organizing, staffing etc., will be taken up only when direction is given to initiate them. Direction starts the actual work for achieving enterprise objectives.
- **Improves efficiency:** A manager tries to get maximum work from his subordinates. This will be possible only through motivation and leadership and these techniques are a part of direction.
- **Ensures coordination:** Direction helps in ensuring mutual understanding and team work. The individual efforts are directed in such a way that personal performances help in achieving enterprise objectives. The integration of various activities is possible through direction.
- **Helpful in implementing changes:** A business operates in a changing environment. New situations develop every now and then. A proper system of motivation will help employees in taking up new challenges.
- **Provides stability:** Effective leadership, supervision and motivation will help in the smooth growth of an enterprise. A growing concern will provide stability to its activities.
- **Motivation:** Motivation is an important element of direction. Motivation is a factor which encourages persons to give their best performance and help in achieving enterprise goals. A strong positive motivation will enable the increased output of employees. A key element in direction is motivation. It helps in getting willing co-operation of employees.
- **Supervision:** Direction involves giving instructions to employees for undertaking some work. In order to see whether employees are doing the things as per targets or not there is a need for supervision. In supervision all the activities of the employees are controlled and efforts are made to ensure proper achievement of targets.
- **Coordination:** Direction will be effective only when there is a proper coordination. In direction, different persons are asked to perform specific tasks. In order to see that efforts of every employee are in the direction of achieving organizational goals there is a need to coordinate various activities.

TECHNIQUES OF DIRECTING

Directing is an important function carried out by top management. It is the order or instruction to subordinate staff to perform a work or not to perform in a specific way. The techniques of directing are: delegation, supervision, orders and instructions **(Fig. 12.5)**.

Delegation

Delegation is an important mean of directing. The subordinates are assigned tasks and given powers to recruit them. In delegation, a superior assigns some of his work

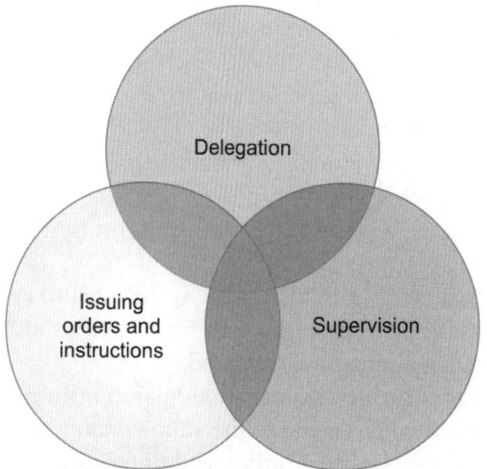

Fig. 12.5: Techniques of directing.

Box 12.2: Importance of direction.
- Initiates action
- Improves efficiency
- Ensures coordination
- Helpful in implementing changes
- Provides stability
- Motivation
- Supervision

to the subordinates and gives those rights or powers. The subordinates are authorized to undertake the assigned work. Delegation is a means of sharing authority with the subordinates and providing them with an opportunity to learn. Delegation as a means of directing may bring out some problems.

- It may be difficult to spell out exact tasks and assignments of the subordinates. There may be some overlapping and uncertainties in job descriptions. The subordinates should learn to adjust them in such situations.
- There may be some contradiction in assignment of task and delegation of authority.
- The subordinates may sometimes act beyond the assigned authority taking it as implied from the superiors. The superiors will have to bear with such situations.
- An indiscriminate delegation may create an imbalance in the organization since every subordinate may not have the same capacity and maturity.
- If the delegation of authority is too rigid then it kills initiative and creativity.

Supervision

- Supervision is a means to oversee the work performed by subordinates. It should be ensured that work is performed as per the plans and guidelines.
- Every superior has to supervise the work of his subordinates. At operative level supervision is the job of a manager.
- A supervisor at the lower level remains in touch with the workers. He guides them for doing the work, maintains discipline and work standards and solves the grievances of workers.
- Supervision at different levels acts as a directing activity.

Issuing Orders and Instructions

- The issuing of orders and instructions is essential to undertake the work for achieving the organizational goals.
- No manager can get a work done without issuing orders and instructions to subordinates. An order, instruction, directing or command is a means of initiating, modifying or stopping an activity.
- In the words of Koontz and O'Donnell has a directional technique, an instruction is understood to be a charge (command) by a superior requiring a subordinate to act or refrain from acting in a given circumstance.
- According to this definition an instruction is always given by a superior to a subordinate directing to undertake a work in a specified manner or prohibit him from some activity.
- The orders and instructions are the primary tools of directing by means of which the activities are started, altered, guided and terminated.
- While issuing an order a manager should be clear in his mind what he wants the subordinates to do or not to do. The clarity of orders will determine the level of performance of subordinates.

A good order has the following characteristics:
- The order should be clear and easily understood.
- The order should be complete in all respects. It should not create doubts in the minds of subordinates.
- It should be compatible with the objectives of the organization.
- There should be specific instructions as to the time by which the order should be executed or completed.
- The order should be so conveyed that it stimulates ready acceptance.
- The order should preferably be in writing.
- The order should be conveyed through proper chain of command and it should also contain the reasons for issuing it.

ADVANTAGES OF DIRECTION

- **Integrative force:** Direction integrates the activities of employees. It is mainly concentrated about what, when, where and who to do the work. Without integration none of the activities can be fulfilled. Effective operation can be achieved only when the efforts of all employees are integrated.
- **Initiate the action:** In direction, a manager motivates the subordinates to perform the activities. When an employee receives the direction, his or her initiative will be started to do work.
- **Improves efficiency:** Direction consists of motivation, leadership and communication. When all these managerial tools are implemented the potentiality of employees is fully utilized from which they perform high performance.
- **Facilitates change:** Change always comes in an organization. Healthy change is important. Some people do not want the condition of change. But change is inevitable. Direction is an important function of management that gives the orders and motivates the personnel for change.
- **Helps in stability and growth:** Direction is an integrated activity of motivation, leadership and communication. These activities help in stability of the organization. When these activities are used, the capabilities are utilized which helps in flexibility and growth of the organization.
- **Helps to achieve the organizational goals:** The manager gives the direction to do work and it gives knowledge, information and goals of the organization. When all people know about the goals it helps on achieving the organizational goals effectively.
- **Means of motivation:** When direction is effective and meaningful, the employees are properly motivated. Direction works for motivating people to contribute maximum efforts. It brings positive feeling towards the organization.

SUPERVISION

Supervision means overseeing the employees at work. It has been defined as the authoritative direction of the work of one's subordinates. It is a necessary concomitant of their hierarchical organization in which each level of subordinate to the one immediately above it and subject to its, orders. Workers at the intermediate levels of the organization supervise as well as are supervised.

Definition

Supervision means observing the subordinates at work to see that they are working according to plans and policies of the organization and keeping the time to educate and to help them solving their work problems.

Objectives of Supervision

- Help the staff to do their job skillfully and effectively to give maximum output with minimum resources cost effectiveness.
- Help the staff develop the individual capacity to the fullest extent with a view to channels the same in favor of work.
- Guide and/or assist in meeting predetermined work objectives or targets. In nursing preventive, promotive, curative and rehabilitative care to people.
- Help to promote effectiveness of the subordinates/staffs. Ensuring that the subordinate staff or supervise does what he/she supposed to do.
- Help to motivate subordinates to maintain high morale, i.e., promotion of motivation and morale among all the nursing staff.
- Help the members of the team to recognize problems, identify solutions and to take action.
- Help to develop team spirit and promote team work for effective functioning.
- Help to improve the attitudes of the members towards the work or program, i.e., bridging the gap between the workers' personal goal and the organizational goal by providing guidance in the right direction.

Importance of supervision is shown in **Figure 12.6**.

Functions of Supervision

- **Orientation of newly posted staff:** Transfers and postings, or new postings of personnel are common in all organizations. All new corners should be informed about their functions, the methods that they should use, the personal with whom they will work and the community wherein they will work, that needs an orientation.
- **Assessment of the workload of individuals and groups:** It must be ensured that the workload is within the physical and mental competence of a worker. Otherwise job should not be assigned to them. A supervisor should not expect from workers a level of effort that is beyond them.
- **Arranging for the flow of materials:** A supervisor must find out the needs for supplies and equipment and arrange for their supply in good time.
- **Coordination of the efforts:** A supervisor coordinates the work of his/her workers and agencies and promotes team work.
- **Promotion of effectiveness of workers:** This may be done through performance evaluation and introducing concepts of staff development.
- **Promotion of social contact within the work team:** Social contacts help to bring the staff together and increase group cohesiveness. A good supervisor should provide opportunity for it.
- **Helping individuals to cope with their personal problems:** Personal problems are likely to come up while dealing with workers. Those may be outside the supervisors' duties but a sympathetic understanding on his part improves the individual morale.
- **Facilitating the flow of communication:** A free flow of communication among members is necessary for team work. Supervisor should encourage free communication among peer, team members.
- **Raising the level of motivation:** All good work should be given due credit through recognition. Supervisor must provide opportunities for growth and achievements.
- **Establishment of confidence:** Supervision is a control measure as well as leadership technique. The supervisor must know what work is being done and with what effectiveness. A number of techniques, such as observation and record review can be used for this purpose.
- **Development of confidence:** Supervisors must know the background of workers and try to develop mutual confidence. There is a need to combine understanding with firmness and to take a personal interest without sacrificing impartiality or discipline.
- **Emphasis on achievement:** It has been proved that the development of a smooth work routine and the improvement of human relations without corresponding emphasis on goal achievement are not likely to increase productivity.

Functions of Supervisor

H Nilsson gives the following list of eleven principal duties of a supervisor:
1. To understand the duties and responsibilities of his own position
2. To plan the execution of the work

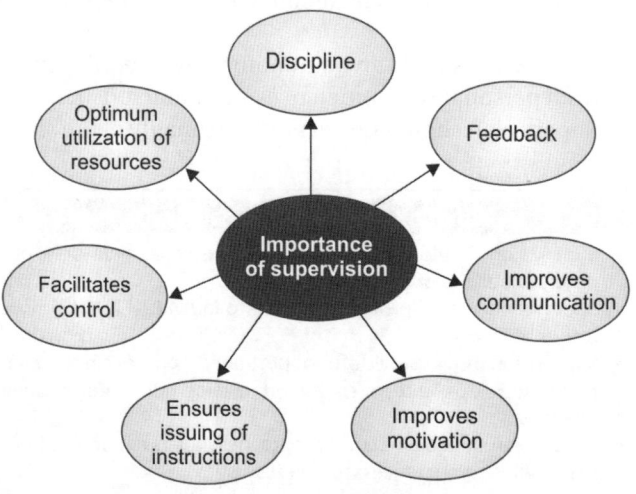

Fig. 12.6: Importance of supervision.

3. To divide the work among subordinates and to direct and assist them in doing it
4. To improve his own knowledge as technical expert and leader
5. To improve his work methods and procedures
6. To train the personnel
7. To evaluate the performance of the employees
8. To correct mistakes, solve employees' problems and develop discipline
9. To keep subordinates informed about policies and procedures of the organization above the changes to be made
10. To cooperate with colleagues and seek advice and assistance when needed
11. To deal with employee suggestions and complaints

Factors Influences Effective Supervision

Factors of effective supervision is shown in **Figure 12.7**.

- **Human relations skill:** Supervision is mainly concerned with instructing, guiding and inspiring human beings towards greater performance. For purposes of direction, the supervisor has to rely on leadership, counseling, communication and other determinants of human relations.
- **Technical and managerial knowledge:** Guidance implies a complete understanding of all work problems, for which: the supervisor should have good knowledge about technical aspect of job and also the managerial aspects.
- **Leadership position:** The authority of supervisors must be made commensurate with their duty so as to make the job of supervision a satisfying, rewarding and challenging one. So, the supervisors are to be vested with necessary authority for enabling them to exercise leadership over the group and influence the employees.
- **Improved upward relations:** To ensure good quality of supervision, the supervisor's upward relations must be well-established, which means to say that supervisors should be regularly allowed to present their views and suggestions to top executives in regard to the personnel and their work performance, for which, the top management must pay adequate attention and thought on supervisory jobs to ensure good quality supervisions.
- **Relief from nonsupervisory duties:** To make the supervisory duties purposeful, the supervisors are to be relieved of many routine activities that divert their attention from the real job.
- **General and loose supervision:** According to some experience, the general and loose supervision is more productive than close supervision. Here the leader must allow freedom and initiative to his followers for pursuing a common course of action.

Principles of Supervision

The principles underlying the concepts of supervision are as follows **(Box 12.3)**:

- Supervision should not be overburdened to any individual or group.
- Supervision causing unreasonable pressure for achievements results in low performance and low confidence in the supervisor.
- Supervise diagnosis; do not overestimate his understanding and memory.
- Human behavior with due consideration to human weaknesses. This should be kept in minds of supervisors.
- Supervisors should create atmosphere of cordiality and mutual trust.
- Supervision should be planned and adopted to the changing conditions. It calls for good planning and organization.
- Supervisors must possess sound professional knowledge.
- Supervision to be exercised without giving the subordinate a sense that they are being supervised.
- Supervision strives to make the unit a good learning situation. It should be a teaching earning process.
- Supervision should foster the ability of each staff-member to think and act for herself/himself.
- Supervision should encourage workers' participation in decision-making.
- Supervision needs good communications.
- Supervision should have strength to influence downwards depends on capacity to influence upwards.
- Supervision is a process of cooperation and coordination.
- Supervision should create suitable climate for productive work.
- Supervision should give autonomy to workers depending from personality, competence and characteristics.
- Supervision should respect the personality of the staff.

> **Box 12.3: Principles of supervision.**
> - Supervision should encourage self-expression so as to draw out potential abilities of a worker.
> - Supervision should provide initiative to individual to take more responsibility.
> - Supervision should provide full opportunity to do work in cooperation to develop the team spirit. And develop good interpersonal relationship.
> - Supervision should give autonomy to the workers depending from personality, competence and characteristics.
> - Supervision interprets policies and give creative instructions.

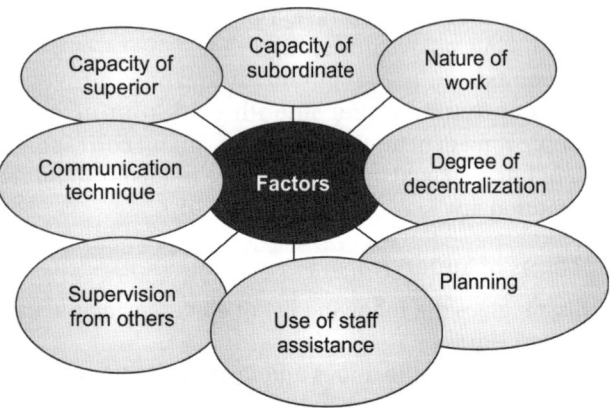

Fig. 12.7: Factors of effective supervision.

- Supervision should stimulate the workers/staff ambitions to grow in effectiveness.
- Supervision should focus on continued staff growth and development.
- Supervision is responsible for checking and guidance.
- Good leadership is part of good supervision.

Qualifications of Supervisor

- Should be trained person—professional training and experience
- Should understand the training background and ability of the supervised
- Should have good knowledge of local practices, cultural patterns health problems in general and available resources of the community.
- Have at least five year experience as community health nurse
- Be intelligent capable of learning readily and of retaining the knowledge.
- Be able to convey knowledge to the others in an understanding and interesting way.
- Through knowledge about administrative regulations.
- Be able when necessary, to show authority without being too demanding and without losing the respect of subordinates.
- Self-confidence and be able to gain the confidence of others.
- Set the climate for cooperation between coworker and shifts for a smoothing running.

Qualities of Supervisor

- Should have human approach to human problems
- Competent to take quick decisions
- Honest in dealing with subordinates
- Should have patience and does not lose temper.
- Should not depend up on his formal authority too much.
- Should be a good leader to guide the subordinates
- Should have sufficient technical skill to perform the jobs to be supervised.
- Maintain interest in good nursing care.
- Be able to promote good public relations.
- Keep up with new trends in nursing and be able to do convey this information to others.

Techniques of Supervision (Fig. 12.8)

Supervision means overseeing the employees at work. It has been defined as the authoritative direction of the work of one's subordinates. Supervision is the art of overseeing, watching and directing with inspecting another's work, evaluating her or his performance and approving or correcting performance.

- Group conference
- Individual conference
- Anecdotal records
- Initial conference
- Control of early experience
- Assistance with bedside care
- Reassurance
- Supervision of nursing procedure
- Conferences—individual group
- Incidental teaching

Supervision Methods

- **Technical vs creative supervision:** Technical methods are some of the basic supervisory skills which need to be trained. Group conferences, group discussions. For example, techniques of service study, record construction, time study, etc. Creative supervision provides maximum adaptation to the situation. For example instead of a orientation period of two weeks for each new staff member, a variable plan in both contents and time according to the needs of each individual should be formulated.
- **Cooperative vs authoritarian supervision:** In cooperative supervision there is a full participation of each member of the group in planning, action and decision whereas in authorities supervision responsibility ventures entirely on the supervisor with the staff following his/her.
- **Scientific vs institutive supervision:** Scientific supervision relies on objective study and measurement than personal judgment or opinion. Whereas inactive supervision needs to maintain the interpersonal relationship.

Difference between direction and supervision is shown in **Table 12.1**.

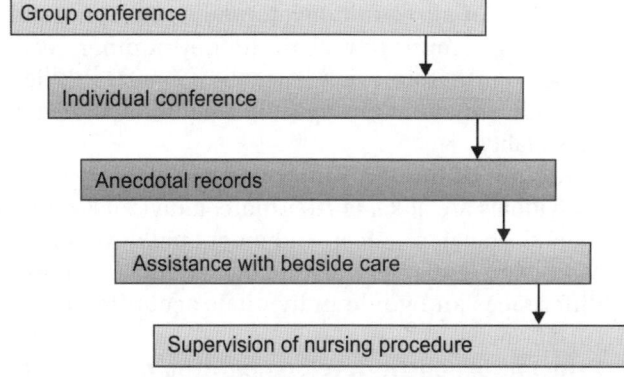

Fig. 12.8: Techniques of supervision.

Table: 12.1: Distinction between direction and supervision.		
Basis	Direction	Supervision
Introduction	Process of guiding, ordering and influencing others to achieve goals	Act of monitoring and observing the performance of others
Nature	Goal-oriented	Task-oriented
Scope	Broader	Limited
Decision making power	Yes	No
Level of management	Top level	Middle and lower level
Face-to-face contact	Not compulsory	Compulsory

GUIDANCE

The guidance refers to advice or information provided by a person of experience, to solve a problem or improve something. The guidance refers to the process of helping individuals to discover and develop their potential. The need of guidance is something that cannot be ignored by anyone.

Definition

- "Guidance is the process of helping individuals through their own efforts to discover and develop this potentialities happiness and social usefulness". —*Morris*
- "Guidance may be defined as assisting individual to prepare for his future life, to fit for his place in Society."
- "Guidance is a process of helping every individual, through his own efforts, to discover and develop his potentialities for his personal happiness and social usefulness." —*Ruth Strang*

Objectives of Guidance

- To help individual to understand and accept the positive and negative aspects of his personality, interests, aptitudes, attitudes, etc.
- Provide a wide choice and opportunities
- Help make adjustment in the new life situation.
- Help in facing the challenges of life and manage tensions by realizing and accepting the facts.
- Help in solving social and personal problems and be able to adjust with oneself and the environment.

Aims of Guidance

- Exploring self
- Determining values
- Setting goals
- Improving efficiency
- Building relationship
- Accepting responsibility for the future

Purpose of Guidance

- To enable the individual or person to be matured, socially responsible, economically self-sufficient and ultimately to be self-directing citizen, for that necessary programs are undertaken for his best development.
- It enables the individual/person to take right decision in each and every stage of his life by overcoming the necessities and incorporating the necessities.
- To achieve of self-sufficiency in each and every aspects of life, the individual/person is helped to analyze his self clearly, i.e., his strength, limitation, interests, aptitudes, abilities, potentialities, etc.
- Guidance is organized with the help of different services to provide realistic information about potentialities of the individual and the opening of the world of work in which he is best fitted for.

Types or areas of guidance services is shown in **Figure 12.9**.

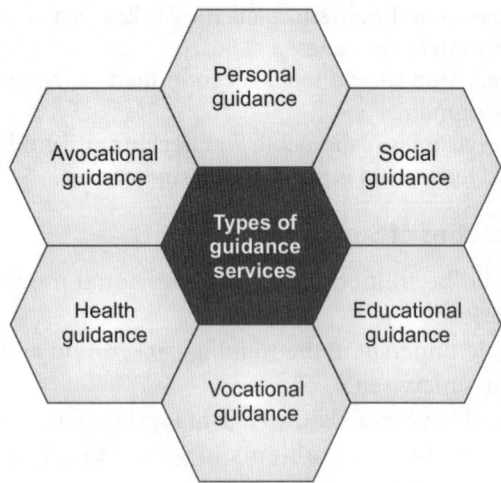

Fig. 12.9: Types/areas of guidance services.

Nature of Guidance

- It is a continuous process
- It is apart from instruction
- Guidance is a process of development rather than direction
- Guidance fulfills some aims of education

Characteristics

- Are identifiable aids to assist individuals
- Are involved in achieving goals of education
- Are supported by functional preparation of teachers in guidance activities
- Provide for competent leadership
- Are based on knowledge of the needs of pupils and upon competencies of the staff members
- Are services made available to all
- Need the cooperation of parents and community
- Are more preventive than curative
- Are founded on the concept of the totality of the individual
- Should be evaluated constantly

Principles of Guidance

The principles of guidance certainly form the basis of the need of guidance. Furthermore, principles of guidance are important principles without which guidance cannot take place. Below are the principles of guidance **(Box 12.4)**:

- **Principle of all-round development:** Guidance must take into account the all-round development of the person. Furthermore, guidance must ensure this desirable adjustment in any specific area of the individual' personality.
- **Principle of human uniqueness:** Certainly no two individuals are alike. Furthermore, individuals differ in mental, social, physical, and emotional development. Moreover, guidance must recognize these important differences and guide individuals according to their specific need.
- **Principle of holistic development:** This principle states that guidance must take place in the context of total

> **Box 12.4:** Principles of guidance.
>
> **According to Crow and Crow:**
> - All-round development of individuals
> - Principles of individual differences
> - Guidance is related to every aspect of life
> - Cooperating among persons
> - Guidance is a continuous and lifelong process
> - Guidance for all
> - Principles of elaboration
> - Responsibility of teachers and parents
> - Flexibility
> - Principles of evaluation
> - Guidance by a trained person
> - Principle of periodic appraisal

personality development. Moreover, a child grows as a whole. Also, if one aspect of personality is in focus, then the other areas of development must be kept in mind. Most noteworthy, these other areas of development indirectly influence the personality.

- **Principle of cooperation:** This principle states that there cannot be any force on any individual regarding guidance. Moreover, the cooperation and consent of the individual is a prerequisite for providing guidance.
- **Principle of continuity:** The principle says that the guidance must take place as a continuous process to an individual. Also, this guidance must take place in different stages of the individual's life.
- **Principle of extension:** In this principle, there should not be a limitation of guidance to a few individuals. Most noteworthy, the extension of guidance must be to all individuals of all ages.
- **Principle of adjustment:** It is certainly true that guidance influences every aspect of an individual's life. However, guidance is chiefly concerned with a person's mental or physical health. Furthermore, this adjustment takes place at school, home, society, and vocation.

Need and Importance of Guidance

Guidance is needed wherever there are problems. The need and importance of guidance are as follows:
- Self-understanding and self-direction: Guidance helps in understanding one's strength, limitations and other resources. Guidance helps individual to develop ability to solve problems and take decisions.
- Optimum development of individual
- Solving different problem of the individual
- Academic growth and development
- Vocational maturity, vocational choices and vocational adjustments
- Social personal adjustment
- Better family life
- Good citizenship
- For conservation and proper utilization of human resources
- For national development

Types of Guidance

Broadly speaking, there are a dozen types of guidance, in accordance with various fields and situations where guidance is needed. The various fields or types are:
- Personal-social guidance
- Educational guidance
- Vocational guidance
- Physical guidance
- Hygiene guidance
- Martial guidance
- Home guidance
- School guidance
- Leadership guidance
- Religious guidance
- Leisure time guidance
- Old-age guidance

PARTICIPATORY MANAGEMENT

Participative (or participatory) management, otherwise known as employee involvement or participative decision making, encourages the involvement of stakeholders at all levels of an organization in the analysis of problems, development of strategies, and implementation of solutions. Employees are invited to share in the decision-making process of the firm by participating in activities, such as setting goals, determining work schedules, and making suggestions. Other forms of participative management include increasing the responsibility of employees (job enrichment); forming self-managed teams, quality circles, or quality-of-work-life committees; and soliciting survey feedback. Participative management, however, involves more than allowing employees to take part in making decisions **(Fig. 12.10)**.

Definition

Participatory management is the practice of empowering members of a group, such as employees of a company or citizens of a community, to participate in organizational decision making.

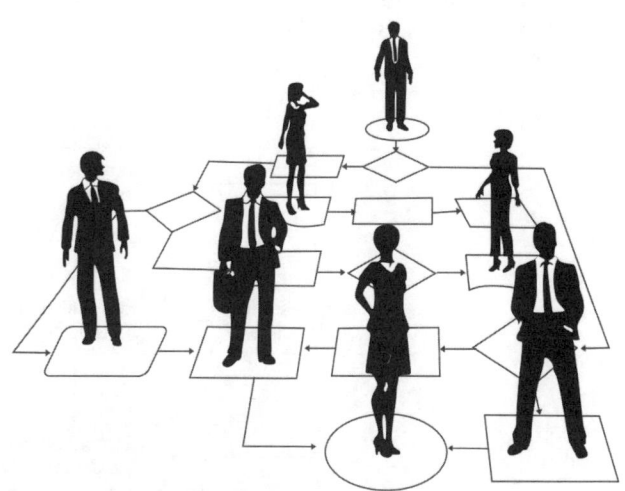

Fig. 12.10: Participative management.

Concept of Participation

- The concept of "Participative Management" is closely related with the concept of industrial democracy. Participative management means involving workers in the decision making process.
- Participative management is based on the concept that when the worker invests his time and ties his fate to the workplace, he should be given an opportunity to participate in the decision making process of the management.
- The employee should be given an opportunity to express his views and due importance should be given to them by the management while framing policies.

Process of Participatory Management

The four processes include:
1. Information sharing, which is concerned with keeping employees informed about the economic status of the company.
2. Training, which involves raising the skill levels of employees and offering development opportunities that allow them to apply new skills to make effective decisions regarding the organization as a whole.
3. Employee decision making, which can take many forms, from determining work schedules to deciding on budgets or processes.
4. Rewards, which should be tied to suggestions and ideas as well as performance. **Figure 12.11** shows universally recognized concept.

Features of Participation

Features of participation provides higher status to employees:
- Employees are given a chance to participate in the decision making process of the organization. This empowers the employees. Provides psychological satisfaction to employees.
- Employees are allowed to express their views and their views are given due consideration. Management even frames some policies according to their expectations.
- Participative management is followed and practiced in many countries. Brings employees and management closer.
- Participative management facilitates meaningful communication and ensures cordial relations. Beneficial to both parties.
- Participative management is beneficial to both parties; organization and employees. Through participative management, both the parties are satisfied.

Participative Management Styles

Information Management

- One style of participatory management is creation of a workplace environment in which information is shared readily with employees.
- This includes financial projections, earnings and operational budgets as well as information related to long-term strategic planning.
- This approach provides transparency in all aspects of business and allows for employee comment, input and suggestions.

Mentoring and Training Management

- A participatory managed work environment provides ongoing training, skills development, professional enrichment and mentoring to employees at all levels.
- Employees regularly take on new or additional responsibilities, cross-train in different areas of business and give their newfound skills a hands-on try under the supervision of a mentor.
- Employees are encouraged to share knowledge and information with the goal being a diversely trained, well-rounded workforce that takes advantage of each employee's most notable skills.

Recognition Management

- Another form of participatory management includes a forum in which employees are recognized regularly for their achievements and contributions.
- The reward approach is designed to increase performance, motivate employees and provide positive reinforcement for a job well done.
- Employees also have the opportunity to see how their contributions directly affect the company in a positive manner.

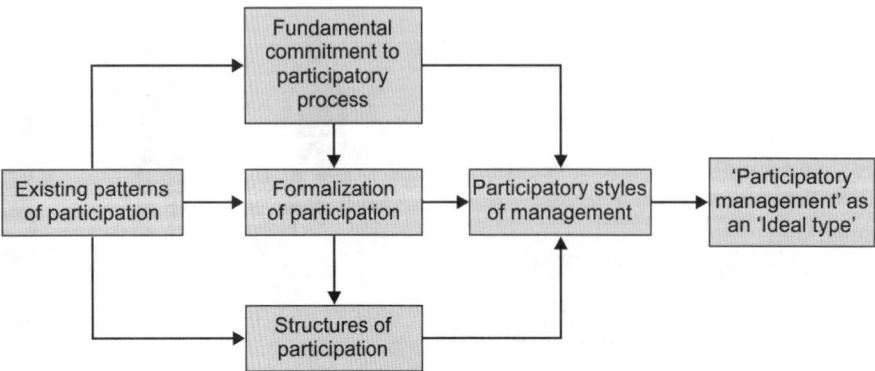

Fig. 12.11: Universally recognized concept.

Teaching Management
- Participatory management often features a teaching component in which employees are guided on the fundamentals of the decision-making process.
- Employees receive insight into a particular problem, issue or strategy and the cognitive tools necessary for breaking down the issue into problem-solving components.
- Using this management style, employees continually enhance their knowledge of how the company operates and are able to bring ever-improving skills to the workplace.

Shared Decision-making Management
- All forms of participatory management include a form of shared decision-making, but this particular style goes even deeper.
- Under shared decision-making management, employees participate in focus group, complete surveys, participate in brainstorming sessions and often work in self-monitored groups on specific tasks and projects.
- Management typically provides parameters for employees to work within and to contribute suggestions and ideas, and many also feature a formal review process to ensure every idea is weighed and vetted carefully.

Advantages of Participative Management

Undoubtedly participative approach to management increases the stake or ownership of employees. But there is more to it. The following points elucidate the same.
- **Increase in productivity:** An increased say in decision making means that there is a strong feeling of association now. The employee now assumes responsibility and takes charges. There is lesser new or delegation or supervision from the manager. Working hours may get stretched on their own without any compulsion or force from the management. All this leads to increased productivity.
- **Job satisfaction:** In lots or organizations that employ participative management, most of the employees are satisfied with their jobs and the level of satisfaction is very high. This is especially when people see their suggestions and recommendations being implemented or put to practice. Psychologically, this tells the individual employee that, 'he too has a say in decision making and that he too is an integral component of the organization and not a mere worker'.
- **Motivation:** Increased productivity and job satisfaction cannot exist unless there is a high level of motivation in the employee. The vice versa also holds true! Decentralized decision making means that everyone has a say and everyone is important.
- **Improved quality:** Since the inputs or feedback comes from people who are part of the processes at the lowest or execution level. This means that even the minutest details are taken care of and reported. No flaw or loophole goes unreported. Quality control is thus begins and is ensured at the lowest level.
- **Reduced costs:** There is a lesser need of supervision and more emphasis is laid on widening of skills, self management. This and quality control means that the costs are controlled automatically.

Disadvantages of Participative Management (Box 12.5)

There is a flip side to everything; participative management stands no exception to it. Whereas this style of leadership or decision making leads to better participation of all the employees, there are undoubtedly some disadvantages too.
- **Decision making slows down:** Participative management stands for increased participation and when there are many people involved in decision making, the process definitely slows down. Inputs and feedback starts pouring from each side. It takes time to verify the accuracy of measurements which means that decision making will be slowed down.
- **Security issue:** The security issue in participative management also arises from the fact that since early stages too many people are known to lots of facts and information. This information may transform into critical information in the later stages. There is thus a greater apprehension of information being leaked out.

Positive Points of Participative Management
- Employees are more involved in their work because they are able to better express and max-out their ideas. They will also be given lots of feedback and directives regarding their actions.
- The motivation is higher in the working groups, indeed this mode of operation is based on the valuation of each one's work, and the employees will do their best to get recognition.
- Engagement is also higher among employees as they will have a greater sense of belonging to the company; through the responsibilities they are given.
- This will result in greater cooperation and knowledge sharing between the teams. There will be a true collaborative culture in the company that will positively impact the company's results.
- There will be greater autonomy among employees; they can go further in their work before consulting their manager.

Box 12.5: Participative management is NOT.

- It is not permissiveness. It holds people responsible.
- It is not weakness. It takes character to apply.
- It is not involvement in trivia. Only significant decisions should go through the process.
- It does not mean giving up authority. We delegate authority with matching amounts of responsibility and accountability.
- It does not mean giving up all decision making. We delegate only the amount of decision making which is appropriate under the circumstances.
- It does not mean postponing action. It should occur quickly and avoid constant fixes.

- The exchanges will be easier thanks to this spirit of collaboration. Employees will be less afraid to suggest new things to their peers and employers.

Benefits of Participative Management

- **Innovation and increased efficiency:** The problem solving process and openness to new ideas can result in innovation. Apart from this as mentioned above there is also knowledge sharing amongst the workers and the managers.
- **Timeliness:** There is improved communication between the managers and the workers and between workers across different units. A loophole or flaw is reported in time.
- **Employee satisfaction and motivation:** Empowering the employees increases their ownership or stake in their work. This increases efficiency and productivity. Consequently there is decreased absenteeism and less employee turnover. This also works in attracting more people towards the organization and the job.
- **Product quality:** A say in decision making means that workers can immediately pin point and suggest remedial measures for improving the efficiency of the process they are apart of. This means that quality control in product or service is exercised for the lowest level.
- **Less supervision requirements:** There is greater focus on management of self with due emphasis of widening one's skill set. One of the major benefits of this is that there is a lesser need of supervision and support staff.
- **Better grievance redressal:** Increased communication paves way for reduced number of grievances and quick and effective resolution of dispute (often on the spot). Union-management relationship is also benefited and strengthened.
- **Hiring flexibility:** Hiring flexibility is increased as a result of cross training. Increased coordination among team members also offers a comfort zone for the newly hired.

INTERPROFESSIONAL COLLABORATION

Interprofessional collaboration (IPC) is defined as "when multiple health workers from different professional backgrounds work together with patients, families, carers (caregivers), and communities to deliver the highest quality of care." It is based on the concept that when providers consider each other's perspective **(Fig. 12.12)**.

Definition

Collaborative practice occurs, according to the World Health Organization, "when multiple health workers from different professional backgrounds provide comprehensive services by working with patients, their families, caregivers and communities to deliver the highest quality of care across settings."

Concept of Interprofessional Collaboration

- Interprofessional collaboration occurs when 2 or more professions work together to achieve common goals and

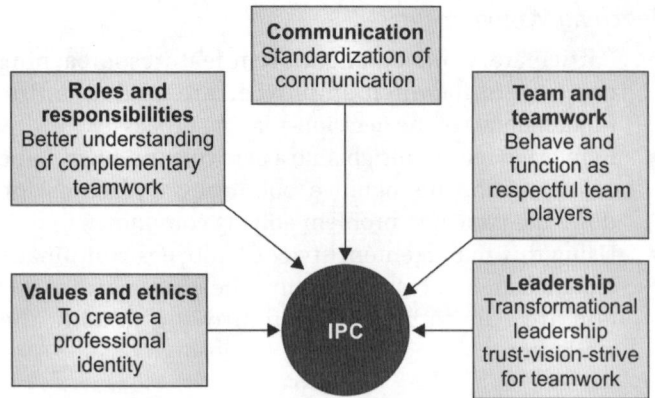

Fig. 12.12: Interprofessional collaboration (IPC).

is often used as a means for solving a variety of problems and complex issues.
- The benefits of collaboration allow participants to achieve together more than they can individually, serve larger groups of people, and grow on individual and organizational levels.

Need of Interprofessional Collaboration

Effective interprofessional collaborative practice (ICP) can lead to:

- Improved access to health interventions and improved coordination between different sectors for individuals and their families with more involvement in decision making.
- A comprehensive, coordinated and safe health system that is responsive to the needs of the population.
- Efficient use of resources.
- Reduced incidence and prevalence of disability. In particular disability associated with noncommunicable diseases when health systems embrace ICP across the full course of the disease (health promotion, illness and injury prevention as well as disease management and cure, and rehabilitation).
- Increased job satisfaction, with reduced stress and burnout of health professionals.

Collaborator in healthcare is shown in **Figure 12.13**.

Health system infrastructures enable ICP:

- There must be a sufficient supply of health professionals to meet population needs.
- Collaborative teams should have appropriate and complementary skills, thus ensuring access to the right professional at the right time in the right place. The skill mix will differ according to the purpose of the team that has been brought together, the characteristics and needs of patients/clients and the practice setting.
- Administrative systems (including human resources and financial planning, budget setting and reimbursement) should all support collaboration.
- ICP should apply across the continuum of health services, including preventive, curative, rehabilitative and palliative professional services.

Chapter 12: Directing or Leading

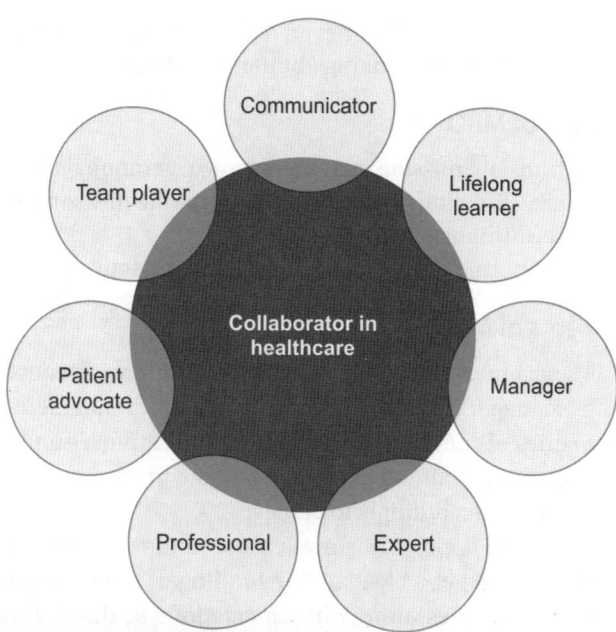

Fig. 12.13: Collaborator in healthcare.

Interprofessional Collaboration Strategies

Interprofessional collaboration strategies include encouraging social interaction through small events, use of team building exercises, rewarding team wins, breaking down office silos with open plan work areas, having leadership encourage open communication and creativity, and through the use of technology platforms built for collaboration. Knowledge sharing and innovation increases with communication, so it's worthwhile to promote teamwork in your organization.

Barriers and recommendations for enhancing interprofessional collaboration is discuss in **Table 12.2**.

Benefits of Interprofessional Collaboration in Healthcare

- **Improve patient care and outcomes:** A patient walks into the emergency department (ED) complaining of chest pains. An ED doctor checks him out, followed by a cardiologist, who orders some tests and waits on the results from the radiologist, who confirms what both doctors suspected: the patient is having a heart attack.
- **Reduce medical errors:** Studies have shown that interprofessional collaboration in healthcare can help to reduce preventable adverse drug reactions, decrease mortality rates, and optimize medication dosages.
- **Start treatment faster:** Interprofessional collaboration bridges the gaps. So does clinical communication technology. It keeps care team members connected.
- **Reduce inefficiencies and healthcare costs:** Interprofessional collaboration in healthcare helps to prevent medication errors, improve the patient experience and deliver better patient outcomes-all of which can reduce healthcare costs. It also helps hospitals save money by shoring up workflow redundancies and operational inefficiencies.
- **Improve staff relationships and job satisfaction:** Every health profession has its own subculture, knowledge base, and philosophy. Interprofessional collaboration levels the playing field and acknowledges that everyone plays a vital role on the care team. That sense of community

Table 12.2: Barriers and recommendations for enhancing interprofessional collaboration.

Barriers	Recommendations
Barriers to evidence-based programs that support transitions to practice: 1. Insufficient residency programs 2. Lack of employer accountability for collaborative academic-practice programs 3. Insufficient research investment 4. Challenges to implementation of BSN-level education	Recommendations for evidence-based programs to support transitions to practice: • Establish a shared commitment for evidence-based programs that are sustainable and cost effective via the collaborative development, implementation, and evaluation of nurse residency programs. • Hold employers accountable to develop and evaluate transition programs in collaboration with academic partners. • Support employers and academic partners to invest in research about transition program designs that includes data related to return on investment (ROI). • Encourage employers to require BSN-level education as a minimum credential for preceptors. • Solicit funding to support BSN level education.
Barriers to culturally competent care: 1. Lack of cultural diversity 2. Insufficient recruitment efforts to achieve diverse workforce 3. Cultural, religious, and racial preferences not respected or understood 4. Desired workforce attributes not include community diversity	Nurse-led initiatives for culturally competent care: • RNs create an environment and practice in a manner congruent with cultural diversity and inclusion principles. • Leaders in academia work to recruit diverse students to achieve a multicultural workforce and develop curricula to promote cultural competence. • RNs promote policies and organizational culture that ensures that cultural, religious, and racial preferences of patients, families and RNs are respected and incorporated into the plan of care. • Employers of nurses should invest in the development of a workforce that reflects the community they serve.
Barriers to effective interprofessional environments: 1. Little or no reflection of interprofessional practice in academic and practice models 2. Few nurse-designed collaborative models 3. Limited access to workforce data	Recommendations for creating/enhancing interprofessional environments: • Leaders in academia and practice should develop and test effective interprofessional practice collaborative models. • Nurses should drive and engage in research to develop and test interprofessional practice and academic collaborative models. • Establish a shared commitment to create infrastructures to collect and analyze data on current and future needs of the RN workforce. • Identify useful workforce data and consider joint collection and analysis of workforce and education data.

and camaraderie can also boost staff retention and recruitment.

MANAGEMENT BY OBJECTIVES

Management by objectives (MBO) can also be referred as Management by Results or Goal Management, and is based on the assumption that involvement leads to commitment and if an employee participates in goal setting as well as setting standards for measurement of performance towards that goal, then the employee will be motivated to perform better and in a manner that directly contributes to the achievement of organizational objectives **(Fig. 12.14)**.

Definition

- John Humble has defined "Management by objectives as a dynamic system which integrates the company's need to achieve its goals for profit and growth with the manager's need to contribute and develop himself."
- Further George Ordiome has also written and stressed the management by objectives is not merely a set of rules, a series of procedures or even a set method of managing, but it is a way of thinking about management.

Purpose of MBO

- To translate mission statements into operational terms
- To give directions and set standards for the measurement of performance.
- To set both long-term and short-term objectives.

Concepts of MBO

- Management by objectives (MBO) is an approach adopted by managers to control their employees by implementing a series of concrete goals that both the employee and the organization aim to accomplish in the immediate future and work accordingly to achieve.
- The MBO approach is implemented to ensure that the employees get a clear understanding of their roles and responsibilities, along with expectations, so that they can understand the relation of their activities to the overall success of the organization.
- If the management by objectives strategy is not adequately set, decided upon, and controlled by organizations, self-centered workers can be likely to misinterpret results, wrongly portraying the achievement of short-term, narrow-minded goals.

Mnemonic SMART (Fig. 12.15)

MBO follows the mnemonic SMART while setting objectives. 'SMART' objectives are:
- **Specific:** Target a specific area for improvement.
- **Measurable:** Quantify or suggest an indicator of progress.
- **Assignable:** Specify who will do it.
- **Realistic:** State what results can realistically be achieved, given available resources.
- **Time-bound:** Specify when the result(s) can be achieved.

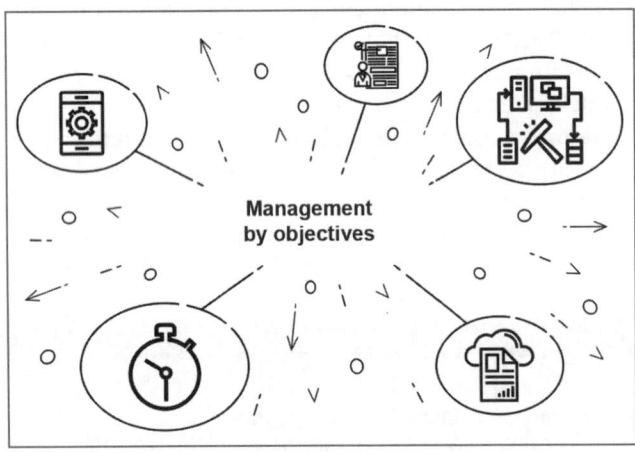

Fig. 12.14: Management by objectives.

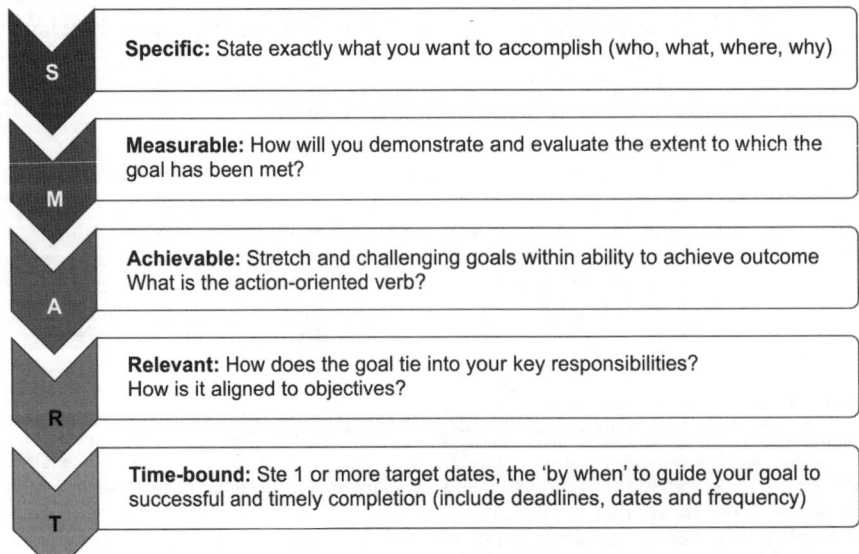

Fig. 12.15: Mnemonic 'SMART'.

Principles of Management by Objectives (Fig. 12.16)

- Cascading of organizational vision, goals and objectives
- Specific objectives for each member
- Participative decision making
- Explicit time period
- Performance evaluation and feedback

MBO Strategy: Three Basic Parts

- All individuals within an organization are assigned a special set of objectives that they try to reach during a normal operating period. These objectives are mutually set and agreed upon by individuals and their managers.
- Performance reviews are conducted periodically to determine how close individuals are to attaining their objectives.
- Rewards are given to individuals on the basis of how close they come to reaching their goals.

Steps in Management by Objectives Process (Fig. 12.17)

- **Define organization goals**: Setting objectives is not only critical to the success of any company, but it also serves a variety of purposes. It needs to include several different types of managers in setting goals. The objectives set by the supervisors are provisional, based on an interpretation and evaluation of what the company can and should achieve within a specified time.
- **Define employee objectives**: Once the employees are briefed about the general objectives, plan, and the strategies to follow, the managers can start working with their subordinates on establishing their personal objectives. This will be a one-on-one discussion where the subordinates will let the managers know about their targets and which goals they can accomplish within a specific time and with what resources. They can then share some tentative thoughts about which goals the organization or department can find feasible.
- **Continuous monitoring performance and progress**: Though the management by objectives approach is necessary for increasing the effectiveness of managers, it is equally essential for monitoring the performance and progress of each employee in the organization.
- **Performance evaluation**: Within the MBO framework, the performance review is achieved by the participation of the managers concerned.
- **Providing feedback**: In the management by objectives approach, the most essential step is the continuous feedback on the results and objectives, as it enables the employees to track and make corrections to their actions. The ongoing feedback is complemented by frequent formal evaluation meetings in which superiors and subordinates may discuss progress towards objectives, leading to more feedback.
- **Performance appraisal**: Performance reviews are a routine review of the success of employees within MBO organizations.

Elements of MBO

MBO includes multiple components which constitute the organizational goals and vision. These elements are as follows (Fig. 12.18):

- **Job-related objectives**: In MBO, employees are briefed out on the common organizational goals along with their individual goals and expectations of the organization.
- **Growth objectives**: Here, the emphasis is on the long-term organizational goals and the expected growth in future. Also, individual growth is linked to organization growth.

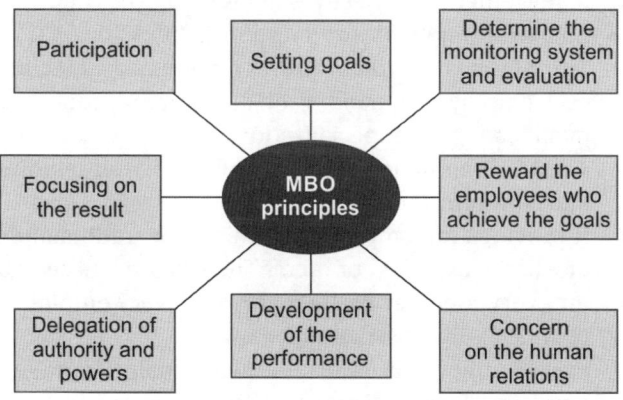

Fig. 12.16: Principles of MBO.

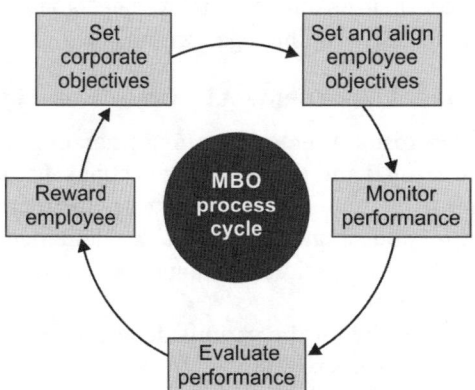

Fig. 12.17: MBO process cycle.

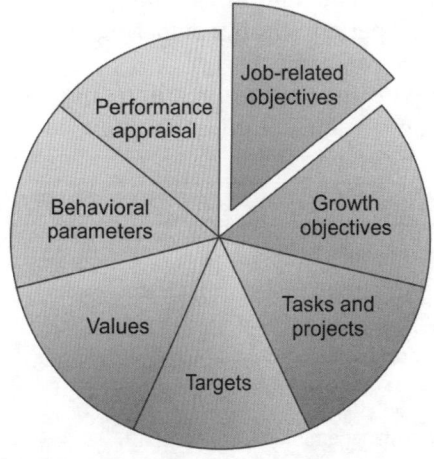

Fig. 12.18: Elements of MBO.

- **Tasks and projects:** This is the part where the roles, responsibilities, duties and projects to be handled by each individual are chalked out.
- **Targets:** The vision of the organization, in the long run, is well-defined, and the individuals are directed to aim at these set objectives.
- **Values:** Another crucial element of MBO is the organizational values, perception, beliefs and business ethics.
- **Behavioral parameters:** The management also defines the individual's code of conduct, attitude and response to a particular situation.
- **Performance appraisal:** MBO also includes the evaluation of individual performance concerning the efforts and contribution made by each employee for the growth of the organization.

Characteristics of MBO

Some may say that MBO is just about framing the business goals and objectives, but it is much more than that. Following features of MBO will broadly enlighten the above statement (Box 12.6):

- **Resource optimization:** MBO ensures the proper utilization of the available resource (i.e., human resources) eliminating the wastage of these resources in terms of time and efforts.
- **Goal orientation:** The initial step in MBO is the goal formation, and all the efforts are directed towards the accomplishment of these set objectives.
- **Multiple accountability:** In MBO, goals are formed for the employees, and therefore, everyone has their course of action for which they are individually accountable.
- **Universally applicable:** The concept of MBO can be applied to almost all the organizations, whether business entities or non-profit organizations.
- **Systems approach:** It is applied to the whole system and thus integrates the efforts of the individual, the organization and its environments in a single direction.
- **Simple and comprehensive:** Since MBO is a non-technical process, it can be easily understood by all types of managers and employees.
- **Operational:** It is practically applicable to the day to day business operations, and the performance can be evaluated periodically by comparing the actual result to the desired outcome.
- **Employee management participation:** The top management does not just set the goals in MBO but involves the active participation of the employees and the managers too.
- **Key result areas (KRA):** The priority zones in the organization which require special attention and are considered to be crucial for the growth and development of the business are termed as KRA. Thus, MBO focuses on this KRA for enhancing the overall performance.

Essential Conditions for Successful Execution of MBO

- Support from all
- Acceptance of MBO program by managers
- Training of managers
- Organizational commitment
- Allocation of adequate time and resources
- Provision of uninterrupted information feedback

Implications of MBO in Nursing

- Measures and judge performance.
- Correlates individual performance to organizational goals.
- Clarifies job responsibilities expected from staff.
- Fosters the increasing competence and growth of subordinates.
- Provides data base for estimating salary and promotion.
- Stimulates the subordinates' motivation.
- Helps in organizational integrating the activities.

Benefits of Management by Objectives

- Management by objectives helps employees appreciate their on-the-job roles and responsibilities.
- The Key Result Areas (KRAs) planned are specific to each employee, depending on their interest, educational qualification, and specialization.
- The MBO approach usually results in better teamwork and communication.
- It provides the employees with a clear understanding of what is expected of them. The supervisors set goals for every member of the team, and every employee is provided with a list of unique tasks.
- Every employee is assigned unique goals. Hence, each employee feels indispensable to the organization and eventually develops a sense of loyalty to the organization.
- Managers help ensure that subordinates' goals are related to the objectives of the organization.

Advantages of Management by Objectives (Fig. 12.19)

- Provides result oriented planning wherein goals can be easily verified and translated into actions. It contributes to improved productivity and better performance.
- It helps subordinates to get positive guidance from the superiors and superiors get willing cooperation from their subordinates.
- The possibility for the various departments working at cross purposes is very less.
- Contributes for effective management by providing lot of clarity in the objectives that is necessary to achieve them.

Box 12.6: Characteristics of MBO.

- Resource optimization
- Goal orientation
- Multiple accountability
- Universally applicable
- Systems approach
- Simple and comprehensive
- Operational
- Employee management participation
- Key result areas

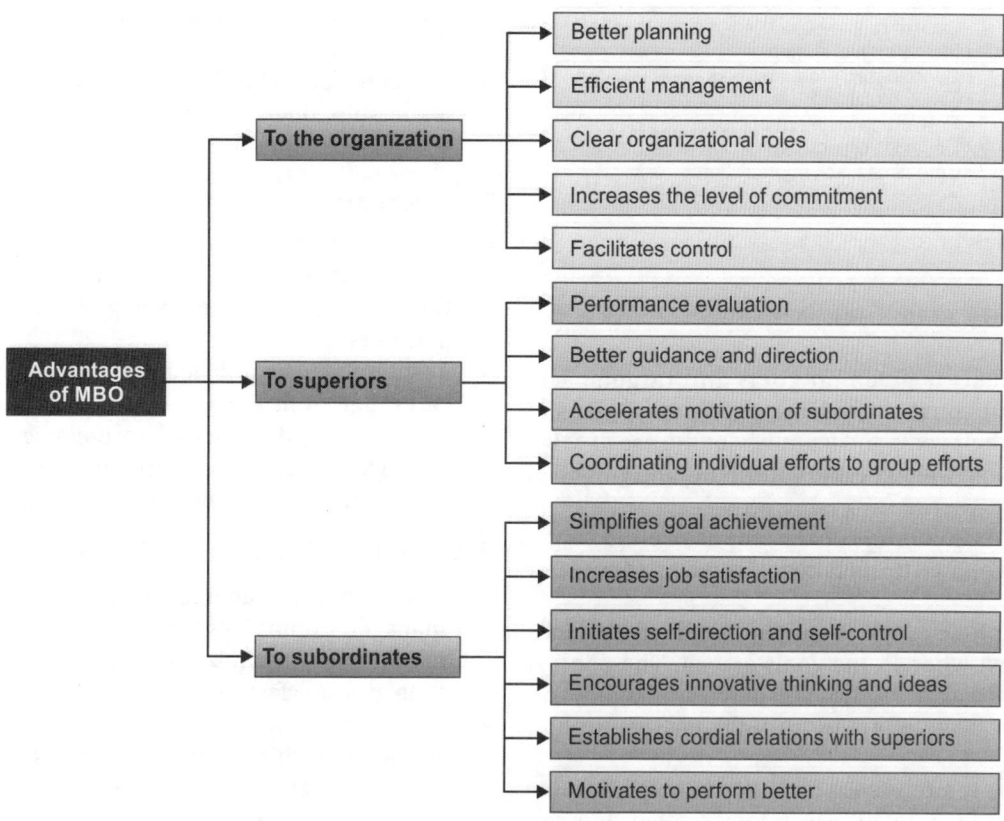

Fig. 12.19: Advantages of MBO.

- Forces the management to plan the activities in a systematic way.
- Facilitates objective performance appraisal. As the goals themselves become the standards against which the actual performance is measured, MBO system itself acts as an effective performance appraisal tool.
- Contributes for the installation of a democratic and participative setup. The interaction that takes place between the superiors and subordinates is a good sign of human resource development in the organization.
- Provides personal satisfaction to the subordinates and makes them more committed towards accomplishment of goals.
- Provides ample scope for flexibility and adaptability.

Demerits of MBO

In spite of many advantages, MBO may not be considered as a panacea for all the evils of the organization.

- **Lack of top management involvement and support:** For an MBO program to succeed, it must have the complete support of top management.
- **Lack of understanding of the philosophy behind MBO:** MBO program in some organizations face the resistance of employees because it is imposed on them as 'control device' to curb their freedom.
- **Difficulty in setting realistic and meaningful objectives:** Some jobs and areas of performance cannot be quantified and hence are not amenable for objective evaluation.
- **Increased time pressure:** To use MBO program, manager must learn to establish priorities and use the time effectively.
- **Lack of relevant skills:** Managers may not have the requisite skills for identifying objectives, communication and interpersonal interaction, such as counseling and giving and receiving feedback.
- **Lack of individual motivation:** The rewards and incentives for superior performance have to be specified clearly. Ambiguity or uncertainty regarding the outcome of the efforts is one of the reasons for the nonperformance.
- **Poor integration with other systems:** The objective setting and review phases must be performed in conjunction with other activities, such as budgeting, forecasting and the like. Often managers are neither taught how to set the objectives nor familiarized with the various plans and policies of the organization. In such cases, each department ends up going its own way, and the results are counterproductive to the overall organization.
- It creates frustration in a manager because when it is not implemented properly there is utter confusion and management is not able to adapt even to the old system.
- It takes time and effort and involves too much paper work.

Limitations of Management by Objectives (Fig. 12.20)

- Management by objectives often ignores the organization's existing ethos and working conditions.

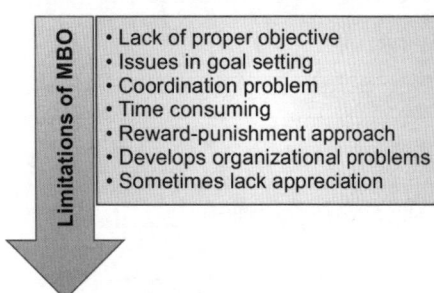

Fig. 12.20: Limitation of MBO.

- More emphasis is given on goals and targets. The managers put constant pressure on the employees to accomplish their goals and forget about the use of MBO for involvement, willingness to contribute, and growth of management.
- The managers sometimes over-emphasize the target setting, as compared to operational issues, as a generator of success.
- The MBO approach does not emphasize the significance of the context wherein the goals are set. The context encompasses everything from resource availability and efficiency to relative buy-in from the leadership and stakeholders.
- Finally, there is a tendency for many managers to see management by objectives as a total system that can handle all management issues once installed. The overdependence may impose problems on the MBO system that it is not prepared to tackle, and that frustrates any potentially positive effects on the issues it is supposed to deal with.

TEAM MANAGEMENT

Team management is a concept where a group or team of individuals performs any given task. Team management is an important concept in every field where individuals with different skills work together to achieve a common goal. In business, team management is the collective effort of all employees to achieve organization objectives (**Fig. 12.21**).

Definition

Team management is the ability of an individual or an organization to administer and coordinate a group of individuals to perform a task. Team management involves teamwork, communication, objective setting and performance appraisals.

Importance of Team Management

- Every organization comprises of many employees who are assigned a particular role in their job.
- Each individual performs their job and tasks as per the requirement. But the collective effort of everyone is what companies want to achieve their business goals. This is where team management and team work are essential.
- Team management is essentially managing a team.
- Team building exercise, any issues among team members have to be resolved, the best skills have to be used and the business goals have to be met as a part of team management.
- The concept is closely interwoven with other skills like leadership, time management, decision making, good governance, communication making, etc.

Team Building
- Team building refers to a wide range of activities, presented to businesses, schools and sports teams, religious or nonprofit organizations designed for improving team performance.
- Team building is pursued via a variety of practices, and can range from simple bonding exercises to complex simulations and multiday team building retreats designed to develop a team (including group assessment and group-dynamic games), usually falling somewhere in between.

Effective Team Management Tips and Strategies

Team management is an important skill which is required by any manager. Companies have to identify leaders who can control, direct and maximize the output of their team. Some tips and strategies for effective team management are (**Fig. 12.21**):

- **Communication:** A good streamlined and honest discussion with team members is essential for effective team management. The team members have to be constantly communicated business ideas and company strategies which the leadership is thinking about so that employees are aware of what the company's vision is.
- **Motivation:** Effective team management requires constant motivation of employees. A strong team requires that all the members are motivated and full of positive energy to complete their tasks.
- **Feedback:** Feedback of employees by seniors as well as peers is important for effective team management. Companies evaluate employees using techniques like 360 degree feedback and help employees improve.
- **Transparency:** Having a transparent organizational structure is critical for time management. Subordinates

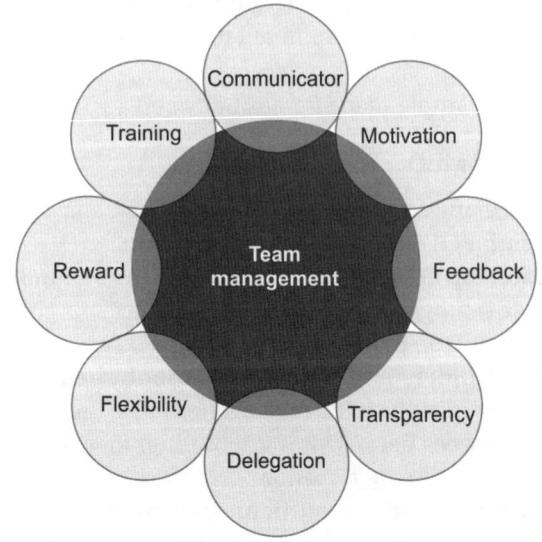

Fig. 12.21: Effective team management tips and strategies.

and team members should have easy access to top management, discuss new ideas, revolt certain wrong practices, employee voice should be heard, etc.
- **Delegation:** Effective team management ensures a team leader uses delegation of authority while giving work to members. This helps in employee's confidence who feel that the manager trusts their work skills and abilities.
- **Flexibility:** Team members who have flexibility at work using methods like work life balance help in their business output, which is important for effective team management.
- **Reward:** Recognizing the efforts of team members through rewards, awards, prizes, promotions, etc., are essential for good team management as this helps in employee confidence.
- **Training:** Updating employee skills with regular training and development helps in strong team management. New skills, tools, learning methodologies, training sessions, etc., help sharpen employee skills and thereby improve team output.

Team Managers

Team managers are responsible for the day-to-day activities and guidance of their team members. The team manager sets targets, implement guidelines, and assist with any issues the employees may have. A team manager has to ensure that all members understand the team's objectives and work together to achieve it. Constant monitoring by the manager helps to ensure that everyone is working towards the same goal.

Team managers should know about team strategies, working with remote teams, using technology, workplace diversity, management styles, mediation, macro, and micro-management. Their roles can be long-term or project based, depending on the duration of a particular assignment.

Team managers:
- **Implement** team goals or objectives
- **Supervise**, train or guide team members
- **Mediate** any interpersonal issues
- **Inspire** and motivate team members
- **Provide** effective feedback
- **Manage** remote teams
- **Utilize** technology effectively
- **Be knowledgeable** about each team members job role

Skills
- Be self-motivated
- Be customer oriented
- Be trustworthy and efficient
- Have prior managerial experience
- Have excellent interpersonal skills
- Have effectual time and project management skills
- Be able to make responsible and effective decisions
- Be able to work on own initiative
- Be able to communicate efficiently—both written and verbally
- Be able to meet targets and handle a high pressure environment
- Be able to lead and manage teams

Team Management Techniques

- **Hire the right people:** Finding the right team members for your team is difficult, but it's also crucial. Having the right talent in your team helps you keep your project's productivity at its highest level.
- **Set achievable goals:** Effective goal-setting should be a crucial part of your team management strategy. Everyone on your team should clearly understand what they are striving for daily. Keep in mind that without clear, concise goals (short-term and long-term), your team is very likely to miss deadlines.
- **Establish a team mission:** Having a good team management strategy is a complete waste is your team does not even feel like a team at all. So, before you assign roles and goals to your team, establish a team mission that brings everyone together.
- **Delegate tasks effectively:** It's easy for a team to fall by the wayside when tasks and responsibilities are not assigned responsibly. With multiple people working on the same project, you have to ensure that you delegate the right roles and responsibilities to the right person.
- **Maintain open communication:** Keeping communication channels wide open is important to the success of any business.
- **Manage time wisely:** Every individual, a manager or a team member, tend to feel like there are never enough hours in the day, making effective time management a matter of great importance. Avoid time-wasting activities like too many meetings; too much social media use, too many phone calls, etc., should be a part of your team management plan.
- **Discuss teamwork in performance reviews:** A team must be held accountable for their roles and responsibilities. Accountability is essential to maintaining an effective work environment for a team.
- **Provide feedback more often:** Hiring the right talent is not enough to make effective team management a reality. You have to keep them motivated at all times. Providing sincere praise is one of the best ways to keep motivation and drive up for your team members.
- **Resolve team issue ASAP:** Teams are expected to work together. Unfortunately, there are often times when teams disagree on things, which can even lead to workplace conflicts. That's what makes conflict resolution an important aspect of your job as a manager.
- **Hold team building events:** If you want to add a bit of fun to the whole team management campaign, team building activities are the perfect way to go. And there is an array of activities that your team can enjoy both inside and outside of the office.
- **Cheer on your team:** As the team manager, you are the team's biggest cheerleader. You are the one who should make the team feel appreciated for all of the hard work they do.
- **Keep positive vibes in the office:** In addition to being the biggest cheerleader for your team, it is important that you uphold a positive vibe in the office. Find ways to promote

a positive work environment where people are willing to work together to the best of their abilities.
- **Celebrate wins:** Achieving success is not enough. If you really want to make your teamwork effectively and efficiently, you have to celebrate their achievements—large or small.

Pros

- A proven system of diverse thinking and behavioral elements that contribute to a broad-based
- Greater possibility for shared and aligned goals and objectives
- Higher degree of collaboration and communication
- Stronger team dynamics as a whole throughout the organization
- Ability to relate to diverse audiences as managers—this is one of the key points of the Fast Company article, in having a team that can relate across generations.
- Boundless innovation stemming from a holistic viewpoint on creativity and results.

Cons

- **Analysis paralysis:** With so many perspectives, there can be a delay in coming to the best idea quickly
- **Need for ultimate consensus:** The Blogging Innovation article cautions against this, stating: "As odd as it may sound, one of the greatest impediments to building productive teams is practicing management by consensus."
- **Watered down solutions:** With a team management approach, each person is coming from their own point-of-view, and the overall solution could get unnecessarily filtered to be everything to everyone.
- **Teams that are too agreeable:** Teams can often follow the personality and approach of the top dog, in this case you just get a bunch of Yes-Men and Yes-Women.
- **Lack of productivity:** Sometimes 5 heads are not better than particularly when it slows down ideas and devolves into self-congratulatory back-patting amongst the leadership team.

■ ASSIGNMENTS

Planning of patient assignment is not a mere matter of dividing up the patients among the available members of the staff, but it is assigning an individual patient or group of patients to nurses according to the patient's nursing care needs and nurses ability to give care to those assigned patients. Methods of patient assignment is given in **Box 12.7**.

> **Box 12.7:** Methods of patient assignment.
> - Case method nursing or total patient care
> - Functional nursing
> - Team nursing or modular nursing
> - Primary nursing
> - Case management or managed care
> - Progressive patient care

Definition of Assignment

- Assignment refers to "a written delegation of duties to care for a group of patients by trained personnel assigned to the unit."
- It refers to the manner in which the total work of the nursing unit is divided up among personnel.

Purposes of Assignment

- To delegate the work to be done to the nursing personnel.
- To gain the cooperation of the nursing personnel by knowing and accepting the acceptance of the work to be done.
- To provide patient with best possible nursing care.
- To provide a well rounded education experience for student nurses
- Suggest appropriate procedures for nursing care, with maximum efficiency with minimum care, with maximum efficiency with minimum effort.
- Gain the cooperation of workers in the acceptance of work to be done.

Objectives

- To promote the patient with the best possible nursing care.
- To plan assignments which are interesting and stimulating to professional growth.
- To provide a broad education and experience for each student nurse.
- To achieve good ward management.

Principles of Personnel Assignment

- Made by the head nurse or nurse in charge for each individual nurse.
- Based on:
  - Nursing needs of each patient and approximate time required to care for him.
  - The capabilities, skill level, previous experience and the interest of the staff members.
  - Job description.
- Planned weekly, and revised daily if necessary to assure continuity of care.
- Take into account all the direct, indirect and unit activities
- Consider the geographical location of the unit and the assigned duties to save nurse's time and effort.
- Must be balanced among nursing staff.
- Never to assign the same task to more than one nurse.

Challenges in patient assignment is discuss in **Box 12.8**.

> **Box 12.8:** Challenges in patient assignment.
> - Problem of personal management
> - Shortage of trained manpower
> - Lack of adequate training
> - No involvement in planning
> - No autonomy in nursing activities
> - Inadequate number of nursing staff

Principles of Patient Assignment

- Equal case load depending on staff ability and hours.
- Patient assignment should be made according to the needs of each patient and of the nurse's ability to give him the care.
- In hospital where student nurses are being educated, assignment must necessarily revolve round the requirements for the student's education.
- For nurses to grow in professional competence, assignments must be varied and challenging to their ability.
- Activities are better performed when each one is made responsible for a single person.
- If there are not enough nurses on duty to carry the nursing load. It is preferable to overload the graduate staff nurses than the students or nonprofessional works.
- Assignments of patients and duties should not be changed frequently than is absolutely essential.
- The care required by all patients in the group assignments to one nurse must be considered when making assignments.
- Assignments planning are closely related to time planning. If patients are to receive good care in the late afternoon and early evening, usually as many nurses are required during these periods as during the morning hours.
- The best use will be made of nurse's time, if the patients assigned to one nurse are geographically close together.

Process of Organizing Patient Care

The head nurse or the nurse in charge should carry out their duties and responsibilities through applying the following steps:

- **Planning:** Is a process of developing a course of action for meeting the needs of patient. In planning, the head nurse decides what should be done, when, how, where, by whom and to whom.
- **Assigning:** Assignment of patient and nursing activities are written in the assignment sheet by the head nurse/nurse in charge, based on the principles of assignment.
- **Leading:** Includes issuing instructions, motivation, and coordination of activities, by making rounds, checking performance and conducting conferences.
- **Evaluating:** By reviewing nursing performance and patient progress to be compared by the assignment and nursing care plan.
- **Reporting:** The head nurse prepares a nursing unit report "e.g., shift report" which includes patient's needs, special observations, census, bed number, all critically ill and post-operative patients, patients needs special preparation on methods of assigning personnel:
  - The traditional methods
    - Case method
    - Functional method
    - Team method
    - Modular nursing
    - Primary nursing method
  - The advanced method

Case Management

- **Case method:** It is the oldest mode of organizing patient care. In this method, nurses assume total responsibility for meeting all the needs of assigned patients during their time on duty. It involves the assignment of one or more clients to a nurse for a specific period of time, such as shift. Complete care, including treatments, medication administration and nursing care planning, is the assigned nurse's responsibility.
- **Functional method:** This method focuses on getting the greatest amount of tasks in the least time. In this method, the nursing care is divided into tasks and each staff member is assigning to perform one or two tasks for all patients in the unit according to the level of skill required for performance as follows.
- **Team nursing:** Team nursing was developed because of social and technological changes in world war-II drew many nurses away from hospitals, learning haps, services, procedures and equipment became more expensive and complicated, requiring specialization at every turn. It is an attempt to meet increased demands of nursing services and better use of knowledge and skills of professional nurses (Box 12.9).
- **Modular nursing:** Modular nursing assignment is used when the nursing staff includes technical and nurse aides, as well as professional nurses. Although two or three persons are assigned to each module, the greatest responsibility for the care of assigned patients falls on the professional nurse. The professional nurse is also responsible for guiding and teaching nonprofessional nurse.
- **Progressive patient care:** Progressive client care is a method in which client care areas or units provide various levels of care, e.g. (1) intensive care unit for the critically ill, (2) post intensive care unit, (3) regular care units, (4) convalescent unit, and (5) self-care unit. Here the clients are evaluated with respect to all level (intensity) of care needed. As they progress towards increased self-care (as they become less ethically ill or in need of intensive care or monitoring) they are marked to units/wards staffed to best provide the type of care needed.
- **Primary nursing method:** This method is the best in an agency with an all-professional nurse staff. It is a

---

Box 12.9: Team nursing.

- Team nursing is based on philosophy in which groups of professional and nonprofessional personnel work together to identify, plan, implement and evaluate comprehensive client-centered care.
- In team nursing an RN leads a team composed of other RNs, LPNs or LVNs and nurse assistants or technicians.
- The team members provide direct patient care to group of patients, under the direction of the RN team leader in coordinated effort.
- The charge nurse delegates authority to a team leader who must be a professional nurse. This nurse leads the team usually of 4 to 6 members in the care of between 15 and 25 patients.
- The team leader assigns tasks, schedules care, and instructs team members in details of care.

comprehensive, continuous and coordinated nursing process for meeting the total needs of each patient.

- **Case management:** Case management is a process of monitoring an individual patient's health care by the case manager, for the purpose of maximizing positive outcomes and containing costs. The case manager has graduate-level preparation or is at an advanced level of nursing practice. The case manager role requires not only advanced nursing skills but also advanced managerial and communication skills.

Need and importance of nursing assignments: Availing nursing assignment help is a true sign to fathom various information and skill about nursing which could eventually help to grow your skills and knowledge. A nursing assignment which is composed by the nursing assignment help experts of LiveWebTutors delivers new information, such as:

- A nursing assignment which is composed by our nursing assignment help experts assists you to distinguish systems of logical and numerical research standards for viable human services application.
- With prominent nursing assignment help, you will be able to fathom how to exhibit the exhaustive use of the basic intuition utilizing the nursing procedure.
- Our nursing assignment help allows you to outline basic speculation to create composed and deliberate segments of the nursing procedure.
- Availing nursing assignment help writing services from the nursing assignment writing experts also show the capacity to apply thorough expert learning about the nursing procedure.
- Our nursing assignment help also assists to utilize the nursing procedure as a deliberate and objective coordinated rule for quality, separately focused care.
- The nursing assignment from the nursing assignment help experts also assists you to exhibit complete comprehension of the way of life of expert perfection in nursing.
- Our nursing assignment help would also assist you to exhibit a far-reaching proficient learning of nursing society norms of magnificence which is conveyed in relation to the topic.
- Our nursing assignment help also assists you to coordinate perception of nursing norms of magnificence inside the setting of nursing aptitudes and practice.
- Our nursing assignment help shows the way of life of expert nursing magnificence accomplished through deep-rooted learning.
- You will be able to perceive the requirement for the progression of expert practice through commitments to instruction, organization, social insurance approach, and information improvement.

ROTATIONS

Job rotation is considered as an effective tool for successful implementation of HR strategy. It is about settling employees at the right place where they can deliver the maximum results. In today's highly competitive world, this can be proved as the best strategy to find the immediate replacement of a high-worth employee from within the organization. Finding the most suitable people and shifting them to take on the responsibilities of a higher level is a tough task. Job rotation helps HR managers determine who can be replaced by whom and create a suitable and beneficial fit.

Master Rotation Plan in Nursing

- Master rotation plan (MRP) is an overall plan which shows rotation of all the students in a particular educational institution.
- Master rotation plan denotes duration of the placement that includes theoretical block, partial block (half clinical, half theory block) and clinical block.

Purposes of MRP

- Availability of an advance plan before implementation of curricular activities during an academic year for the entire program.
- All concerned are aware of the placement of students in clinical fields.
- Coordination becomes more effective when theory, practice correlates, and integrity exist.
- Helps the students and teachers to prepare themselves for working in the areas.
- Any modifications are required based on situations concerned, collaborations between the faculty and service staff can be made for smooth running of organizational activities, and meeting the objectives of educational program.
- Assessment of the curricular program is more effective.
- Plan in accordance with the concerned curriculum plan/syllabus for the entire course/program.
- Plan in advance for all students in all years of program.
- Plan the activities by following maxims of teaching.
- Select areas that can provide expected learning experiences.
- Acquaint the clinical supervisor with clinical objectives and rotation plan.
- Provide each clinical experience of same duration to all the students.
- Rotate each student through each learning experience or block.

Clinical Rotation Plan in Nursing

"Clinical rotation plan is the statement, which explains the order of the clinical posting of various groups of nursing students belonging to different classes in relevant clinical areas and community health settings as per the requirements laid down by the statutory bodies."

In nursing education clinical rotation refers to "regular, successive and recurrent posting of various groups of nursing student belonging to different classes in specific nursing fields, i.e., OPD's, specialty, wards, OT, delivery room, clinics, community health fields-clinics, outreach centers, sub-centers, health centers, schools, etc.

Table 12.3: Benefits and drawbacks of job rotation.

Advantages of job rotation	Disadvantages of rotation of employees
Allows managers to see your hidden talents	Wastage of time and effort
Helps in exploring interests and ideas	Employees take time
Identifies skills and attitudes	Leads to a whole lot of stress and anxiety
Motivates all employees and helps them to deal with new challenges	It does not check the time wasted
Boosts satisfaction and lowers the rate of attrition	Zero results
Helps in aligning all requirements and competencies	
Keeps away all fraudulent practices	

Benefits and drawbacks of Job rotation is shown in **Table 12.3**.

Factors Considered

- The objectives of the course have to be clearly stated.
- Number of students in each class.
- Number and size of department teaching units, or wards where student should be given opportunity for practicing clinical skills/clinical experience.
- The duration of clinical experience in each area as per INC and university/Board norms.
- The number of teaching faculty available for clinical supervision. Adhere to rotation plan.
- The clinical rotation plan must be in accordance with the total curriculum plan.
- It has to be prepared in advance.
- Theoretical instructions should precede as closely as possible with clinical experience.
- The teacher and student ratio will be 1:4 or as prescribed by INC.
- Select the type of learning experience from simple to complex.
- Clinical supervisor must be familiar with the rotation plan.
- Each student should get all the experience on rotation wise.
- All students should enter and leave the clinical area at the same time and they should complete the assignment in time.

Faculty Role in Clinical Posting

- The teacher has to prepare objectives for clinical experience.
- Based on objectives, clinical experience has to be planned in advance to provide specific planned learning experiences.
- If necessary for some of the topics provide spot clinical teaching and such topic has to be repeated to each group of student as they rotate.
- Plan the course outline and so that theory can be correlated to practice.
- Get permission from clinical authority.
- Ensure that each student is aware of the objectives and assignments and criteria for evaluation.
- Place and guide the student to get required clinical experience.
- Orient the student to the clinical area, ward staff, etc., where they are posted.
- Participate in teaching, supervision, and evaluation of students in the ward.
- Arrange ward teaching, ward discussions and case presentation.
- Help the students for effective charting of records and reports.

MAINTENANCE OF DISCIPLINE

The word 'discipline' comes from the Latin term 'disciplina' which means teaching, learning and growing. When employees are unsuccessful in meeting organizational goals, managers must attempt to identify reasons for their failure and counsel employees accordingly. If employees fail because they are unwilling to follow rules or established policies and procedures, or they are unable to perform their duties adequately despite assistance and encouragement, the manager/administrator has an obligation to discipline the employee.

Meaning of Discipline

- Discipline can be defined as a training or molding of the mind and character to bring about desired behaviors. Thus discipline allows one individual to have some control over another.
- It is a necessary and positive tool in promoting subordinate growth. Constructive discipline uses discipline as a means of helping the employees to grow, not as a punitive measure.
- Punishment is frequently included when defining discipline but it also can be defined as training, educating and/or molding.
- The primary emphasis in constructive discipline is assisting employees to behave in a manner that allows them to be self-directive in meeting organizational goals.
- Discipline refers to working in accordance with certain recognized rules, regulations and customs, whether they are written or implicit in character. Human performance is greatly influenced by the state of discipline in any organization.

Advantages of Discipline

The discipline has following advantages for employees as well as an organization.

- Discipline creates a climate under which individual excellence is encouraged, group performance improved and harmonious working is developed.
- Discipline sets a pattern to acceptable behavior and performance on the part of human beings, i.e., it provides a code of conduct for the guidance of the group.

- Good discipline promotes individual growth, develops human capacity and stimulates will to perform effectively, i.e., it helps in morale building.

Causes of Indiscipline in Staffing

- Discipline is imposed when indiscipline steps in the organization. The causes of indiscipline and suggestion are given below. Faulty disciplinary actions taken by the authorities may lead to indiscipline. It has been suggested that disciplinary actions must be consistent enough to provide equal justice to all concerned, for which managerial actions in regard to discipline must be free from any bias, privilege or favoritism.
- Neglect of employee's grievances neglecting or deferring the settlement of employees grievances cause indiscipline, such as strikes, agitation and others. It has been suggested that the grievances of the employees should be settled by enquiring as early as possible. Otherwise it leads to poor performance, poor morale and serious indiscipline.
- Wrong placement and promotions or remunerations also leads to indiscipline. Taking prompt decision for right placement, timely promotion and proper remuneration helps to reduce such indiscipline.
- Deficiency of well-defined code of discipline also leads to indiscipline. The code of discipline should encompass sufficient rules, regulations, customary practices for the guidance and information to employees.

    Hence, proper code of discipline should be formulated and circulated and communicated in clear and simple language to all employees.
- Divide and rule' policy in the organization also leads to indiscipline. This type of behavior on the part of the administration or management should not be practiced at any cost in the interest of the organization.
- Improper attitude towards employee's problem leads to indiscipline. Basically attitudes influence human beings and their activities; moreover discipline itself is a byproduct of attitude. Understanding of the employees' personal problems and individual difficulties helps to maintain discipline.
- Ill-equipped supervisor may cause indiscipline. As the maintenance of discipline is the case of supervisory responsibilities, indiscipline may spring from the want of the right type of supervision.

Dealing with Disciplinary Problems

When dealing with disciplinary problems. It is better to conduct disciplinary conference. While conducting disciplinary conference both directive and nondirective interview techniques can be used. To guide the discussion in the conference, the manager should begin with clear statement of the broken behavior rule, i.e., gives description of the specific rule broken by the employee.

- Should describe corrective action expected by the employees, i.e., action that employee should take to correct the problem.
- Should specify the time allowed to employee to remedy his shortcomings, i.e., amount of time allowed the employee to correct his or her behavior.
- Further discipline to result if specified behavior change is not made.
- See that disciplinary conference documented and included in employment record.

Errors in Discipline

While administering discipline, there are some common management failures come across by the managers refer to errors in discipline as follows:
- Delay in administering discipline.
- Ignoring rule violation in hope that it is an isolated event.
- Accumulation of rule violations causing irritated manager to 'blow up'.
- Administering sweetened discipline.
- Failure to document disciplinary actions accurately.
- Failure to act within time limits set by grievance procedure.
- Imposing discipline disproportionate to the seriousness of the offence.
- Disciplining inconsistently.

As stated above, failure to follow due process in disciplinary procedures results in unfair, inappropriate or ineffectual disciplinary action.

Management in Disciplinary Action

To apply due process in disciplinary actions the manager must ensure that:
- There is an agency rule or standard that governs the behavior under consideration.
- The employee was aware of the rule or standard governing her or his problem behavior.
- The employee did, in fact, violate the agency rule or standard.
- The penalty imposed is appropriate to the rule or standard violated.

In recent days some of the managers in industry and health care have stimulated employees to aim for the 'higher ideal' of organization by employing what is known as 'positive discipline' or discipline without punishment. The positive discipline is based on the assumption that an employee with self- respect, respect for authority and interest in the job will adhere to high quality work standards.

The positive discipline consists of the following steps:
- Friendly oral reminder to employee of first violation.
- For repeated violations, written statement of problem and work goals to employee.
- Development by manager and employee of action plan to improve employees' behavior.
- Repeat violation, one-day paid leave to reflect on commitment to agency goals.
- Submission by employee of written statements of intent to stay and improve or leave agency.
- Employee notified that failure to meet commitments with result in termination. For maintenance of effective

discipline in the organization following four practices are essential.
1. Condonation of past offences.
2. Agreement as to disciplinary rules.
3. The discipline committee.
4. Investigation by the human resource management.

Role and functions of administrator in discipline: The following are the roles and functions of administrator/manager in discipline.
- He or she encourages employees to be self- disciplined in conforming to established rules and regulations.
- Assists employees to identify themselves with organizational goals, their increasing the likelihood that the standards of conduct deemed be accepted by the organization and will be accepted by its employees.
- Humanistically uses discipline as a means of promoting employee growth.
- Periodically assesses the need for existing rules and regulations and suggests modifications as necessary.
- Is self-aware regarding the power and responsibility inherent in having formal authority to set rules and discipline employees?
- Demonstrates sensitivity to the environment in which discipline is given.
- Serves in the role of coach in performance deficiency coaching.
- Ensures that rules and regulations are clearly written and communicated to subordinates.
- Discusses rules and policies with subordinates, explaining the rationale for their existence and encouraging questions.
- Enforces established rules in a fair and consistent manner.
- Judiciously uses formal authority to take progressively stronger forms of discipline when employees continue to fail to meet expected standards of achievement.
- Carefully documents employees behavior(s) that prompts disciplinary action and any attempts to counsel the employee.
- Uses developed communication skills to do the following, Clearly explain the nature or seriousness of disciplinary problems.
  - Allow employees feedback in the disciplinary process. Explain disciplinary actions to be taken and why.
  - Describe expected behavioral changes and what the consequences of failure to change, will be.
  - Reach agreement and acceptance of the disciplinary plan with the employee.
- Disciplines union employees in accordance with the steps, penalties and time frames established in the union contact.
- Advises employees in seeking disciplinary action redress through informal and formal grievance procedure.

LEADERSHIP IN MANAGEMENT

Leadership is the ability to influence an individual or group in order to attain the group's goal, at the same time maintaining

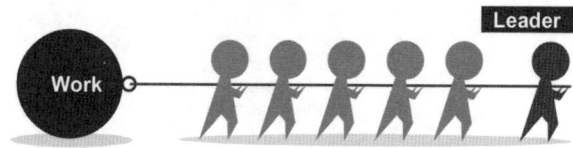

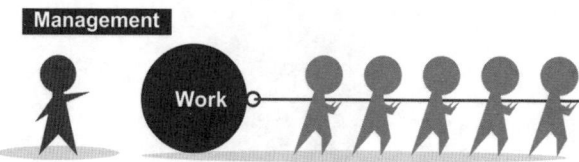

Fig. 12.22: Leadership in management.

Fig. 12.23: Leadership traits.

the morale of the group. As a leader, she is a change agent. Change is all about us, and nursing must change to keep up. The head nurse stimulates her staff to see possibilities for improvement in patient care, helps them decide what they want to do and gives encouragement every step of the way, by and large, leaders are democratic, they set an example in their attitudes towards patients, families, personnel and they plan ahead **(Figs. 12.22 and 12.23)**.

Definition

- Leadership can be defined as a process of influencing the activities of an individual or a group to strive willingly towards goal achievement in a given situation **(Fig. 12.24)**.
- Leadership is defined as the process of influencing others toward a goal. —*Bennie and Nanas*
- A leadership may be defined as the influence, the art or the process of influencing people so that they still strive willingly towards the achievement of group goals.
  —*Chester Koonts and O'Donnell*
- "Leadership refers to the quality of the behavior of individuals nearby they guide people on their activities in an organization". —*Bernard*
- "Leadership is regarded as the form which the authority assures when it rafters into a process".
  —*Mooney and Recley*
- "Leadership is the ability to awaken in others the desire to follow a goal or objective". —*RT Livingston*

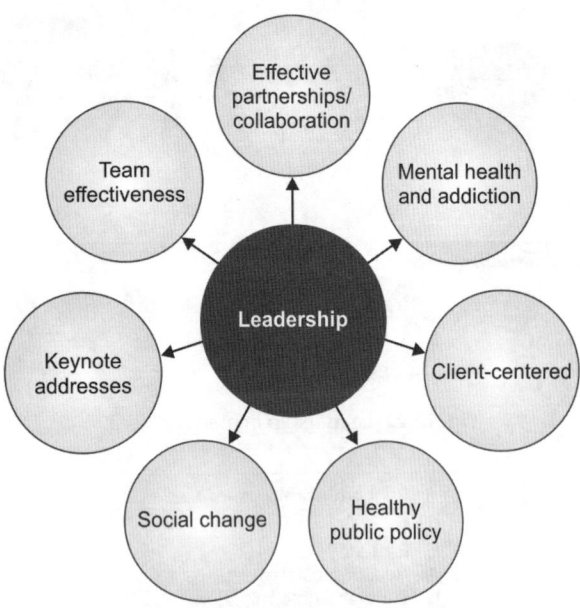

Fig. 12.24: Leadership.

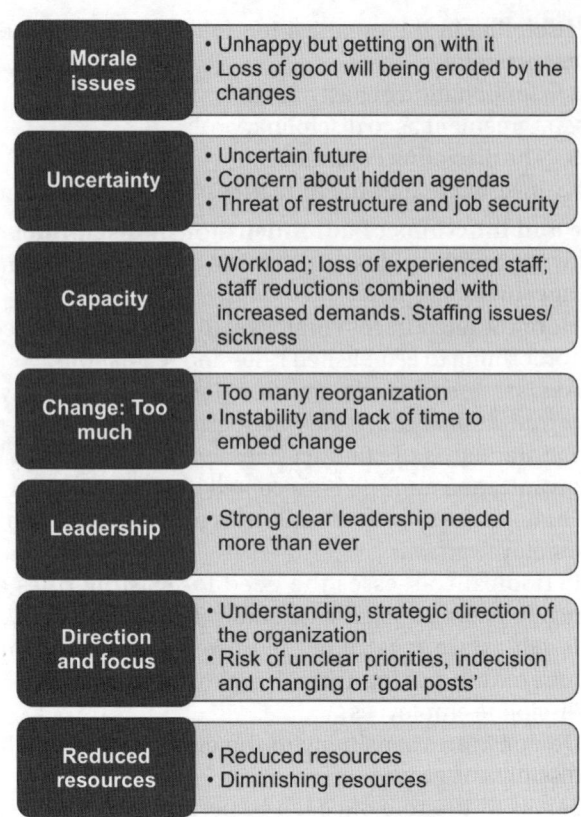

Fig. 12.25: Characteristics of leadership.

Importance of Leadership

- Good leadership is a motivating factor for personnel in an organization. Higher the motivation better would be the performance.
- Good leadership builds morale of the employees, high morale leads to high productivity and organizational stability.
- Good leadership exerts direction and control in the organization for better production.
- Good leadership encourages good interpersonal relationship in the organization.

Characteristics of Leadership (Fig. 12.25)

On the basis of analytical study of above definitions, it may be concluded that leadership is an ability to direct, and motivate other persons of an organization so that they may contribute their efforts towards the success of organization.

- **Followers:** The success of leadership depends upon the number of followers. Larger be the number of followers, more successful will be the leadership. Leadership cannot be thought of in the absence of followers.
- **A personal quality:** Leadership is a personal quality of character and behavior which enables him to influence his men to follow and the followers follow his order and direction.
- **A common goal:** Leadership clusters around the achievement of common goals. There must be some common goals before the leader and his followers. All the activities must be oriented to achieve these goals.
- **Active relations:** Presence of active relations between a leader and his followers are essential for effective leadership. The leader must himself initiate as he wants to be done by his followers.
- **Vitality and endurance:** A good leader is one, who works with courage and patience even in adverse circumstances. He must be capable to face difficult conditions. He must be having sufficient ability to forecast the situation and to take the necessary steps to solve the problems.
- **Decision making power:** Decision making power is an important quality of a leader. A leader has to deal with a group of different nature and different abilities in the process of leadership; he has to take many decisions. The leader must have strong power to take the decision according to the need of circumstances. The decision must be taken at the right time after having a careful thought on the internal and external factors.
- **Initiative:** It is necessary for a successful leader that he should be able in motivating his followers to contribute their efforts to achieve the predetermined objectives of their enterprise. For this, it also becomes necessary that the leader should himself do what he wants to get done by his followers.
- **Analytical capacity:** A successful leader must have analytical capacity also. Analytical capacity means the abilities to work according to the need of circumstatives and to accept the quality.
- **Responsibility:** Feeling of responsibility is a time necessity for a successful leader. If the leader does not feel his responsibility, he cannot, be successful in motivating his followers what he wants to get done by them.
- **Enthusiasm courage, tact and devotion:** A leader it have enthusiasm, courage, tact and devotion. He must be having polite behavior towards his followers. He must be intelligent. If a leader possesses all these above noted qualities, he will be successful in influencing his followers.

Main Functions of Leader

- **To administer:** The main function of a leader is to administer the enterprise successfully. For this he uses the orders and directions to the subordinates, to be considers the utility of orders, practicability and the efficiency of the persons to whom the orders are being used.
- **To get the cooperation:** A leader gets the cooperation of his followers. He should able in convincing his followers that success of enterprises is their own success. If he succeeds in this task, he will be able in getting full co-operation of his followers.
- **To motivate the subordinates:** An important function to leader is to motivate his subordinates to contribute their efforts achieve the objects of enterprise. These motivations may be monetary as well as nonmonetary. These motivations increase to the morale of employees and open the way to achieve their full cooperation.
- **To coordinate:** Establishment of coordination among different activities of the enterprise and the activities of different employees is another important function of a leader. A leader has to see whether all the activities of all the employees are integrated and coordinated. For this he has to coordinate and communicate the orders and directions of top management to the workers and the feelings, problems and suggestions of workers to the top management.
- **To maintain discipline:** Discipline is the force, which directs, regulates and controls the activities of an enterprise. Therefore, the important function of a leader is to maintain discipline in the enterprise. It becomes very easy for the enterprise to achieve its objects. Therefore the leader has to make his best to maintain discipline. For this he has to reward and regard the employees who keep the discipline. Moreover, leader himself should present an ideal to the cause of discipline.
- **To maintain loyalty towards the enterprise:** It is a main function of a leader that he should get the loyalty of his followers towards the enterprise. The workers should feel that they are for the growth and success of enterprise and the enterprise is for them.

Leadership Styles

Leadership styles are the patterns of behavior which a leader adopts in influencing the behavior of his followers (subordinates) in the organizational contact. Based on the type of leader's behavior, leaders may be classified as follows: 1. Autocratic leadership, 2. Democratic leadership, 3. Laissez-faire leadership

Autocratic Style

- Autocratic leader takes all decisions and assigns a responsibility to himself. He is firm, insistent, self-assured and dominating (e.g., Aurangzeb, Tipu, Ashoka and Shahjahan).
- Such a leader stresses prompt, orderly and predictable performance from employees or followers.
- The authoritarian leader may also be "Benevolent autocratic", i.e., paternalistic leader, says often by "You do what I say, I know that is best for you" (which means he is generally having a condescending attitude towards employees, who therefore, tends to be cautious when dealing with this leader). This style of leadership is always present in nursing.
- This is also known as authorization, directive, and stages. In this style a manager centralizes decision-making power in himself.
- He structures the complete work situation for his employees and they do what they are told.
- Here the leadership may be negative, because followers are uniformed, insecure, and afraid of leader's authority.

Democratic Style

- In the democratic style of leadership, the leader values the individual characteristics and abilities of each subordinate.
- Here the leader is a catalyst for group decision making and shared responsibility.
- This style is a people centered approach and allows greater individual participation in decision making process.

Participation Style

- Participation style of leadership is a compromise between autocratic and democratic styles.
- In this style, the manager presents her or his analysis of problems and proposals for action to employees, inviting their criticism and comments.
- Having weighed the subordinates "responses" the manager makes final decisions about the group future activities.
- Here the leader allows subordinates to participate in decision-making; consequently the subordinates have the feeling of satisfaction and freedom.

Laissez-faire Style

- Laissez-faire technique means giving freedom (complete) to subordinate. In this style, the manager once determines policy, programs and limitations for action and the entire process is left to subordinates.
- Group members perform everything and the manager usually maintains contact with outside persons to bring the information and materials which the group needs.
- This type of style is suitable to certain situations where the manager is almost nil.
- It tends to permit different units of organization to proceed at cross-purpose and can rarely in business organizations.

CONCLUSION

Directing is a complex managerial function consisting of all the activities that are designed to encourage subordinates to work effectively. It includes supervision, motivation, communication and leading. The principles which guide effective directing may be classified as principles related to the purpose of directing and principles related to direction process. Directing helps to initiate action by people in the organization towards attainment of desired objectives. For example, if a supervisor guides his subordinates and clarifies their doubts in performing a task, it will help the worker to achieve work targets given to him. Directing integrates employee's efforts in the organization in such a way that every individual effort contributes to the organizational performance. Thus, it ensures that the individuals work for organizational goals.

REVIEW QUESTIONS

Long Essays

1. Define direction; explain the nature and characteristics of direction.
2. Explain the various techniques used in direction.
3. Define supervision; explain the objectives and principles of supervision.
4. Define guidance; explain the objectives, aims and purposes of guidance.
5. Explain the advantages and disadvantages of participative management.
6. Describe the steps in management by objectives process.
7. Define assignment; enumerate the purposes and principles involved in assignment.
8. Define leadership; explain the importance and characteristics of leadership.

Short Essays

1. Explain the principles of direction.
2. Briefly describe the elements of direction.
3. Discuss the functions of direction.
4. Explain the importance of direction.
5. Factors influences effective supervision.
6. Functions of supervisor.
7. Principles of guidance.
8. Process of participatory management.
9. Participative management styles.
10. Benefits of participative management.
11. Interprofessional collaboration: need and strategies.
12. Management by objectives: objectives and principles.
13. Elements of management by objectives.
14. Define team management; discuss the importance and techniques.
15. Principles of patient assignment.
16. Need and importance of nursing assignments.
17. Clinical rotation plan in nursing.
18. Master rotation plan in nursing.
19. Leadership in management.
20. Leadership styles.

Short Answers

1. Advantages of direction.
2. Human relations skill.
3. Need and importance of guidance.
4. Techniques of supervision.
5. Supervision methods.
6. Participative management.
7. SMART.
8. Characteristics of management by objectives.
9. Benefits of management by objectives.
10. Advantages of management by objectives.
11. Limitations of management by objectives.
12. Faculty role in clinical posting.
13. Maintenance of discipline.
14. Case method.
15. Team nursing.
16. Progressive patient care.
17. Rotations.
18. Causes of indiscipline in staffing.
19. Functions of leader.
20. Laissez-faire style.

BIBLIOGRAPHY

1. Agrawal R. Educational, vocational guidance and counseling, New Delhi: Sipra Publication; 2006.
2. Benner P, Sutphen M, Leonard V, Day L. Educating nurses: A call for radical transformation. San Francisco, CA: Jossey-Bass; 2010.
3. Benner P. From novice to expert: Excellence and power in clinical nursing practice. Upper Saddle River, NJ: Prentice Hall Health; 2001.
4. Bernardes A. Implementation of a participatory management model: Analysis from a political perspective. J Nurs Manag. 2015;23 (7): 888-97.
5. Chand S. Guidance and counseling. New Delhi: Rajendra Ravindra Pvt.Ltd; 2008.
6. Coye RW, Belohlav JA. An exploratory analysis of employee participation.Group and Organization Management. 1995; 20(1): 4-17.
7. Greenfield WM. Decision making and employee engagement. Employment Relations Today. 2004; 31(2):13-24.
8. Kaner S, Lind L. Facilitator's guide to participatory decision-making. Gabriola Island, BC, Canada: New Society Publishers; 1996.
9. Keef L. Generating quality interaction. Occupational Health and Safety. 2004;73(5): 30-1.
10. Kinra K. Guidance and counseling. Noida: Dorling Kindersley Pvt.Ltd; 2008.
11. Lofmark A, Smide B, Wikblad K. Competence of newly-graduated nurses-A comparison of the perceptions of qualified nurses and students. J Adv Nurs. 2006; 53(6):721-8.
12. Marion L. Implementing the new ANA standard 8: Culturally congruent practice. Online Journal of Issues in Nursing (in press)
13. McCoyTJ. Creating an open book organization: Where employees
14. think and act like business partners. New York: Amacom; 1996.
15. Pant PR. Principles of management. 2nd edition. Kathmandu: Buddha Academic Publishers; 2010.
16. Robbins SP. Essentials of organizational behavior. 8th edition. Upper Saddle River, NJ: Prentice Hall; 2005.
17. Singh I. Leading and managing in health. Kathmandu: Hisi; 2006.

CHAPTER 13

Leadership

Learning Objectives

- Definition, Concepts, and Theories
- Leadership Principles and Competencies
- Leadership Styles—Situational Leadership, Transformational Leadership
- Methods of Leadership Development
- Mentorship/Preceptorship in Nursing
- Delegation, Power and Politics, Empowerment, Mentoring and Coaching
- Decision-making and Problem-solving
- Conflict Management and Negotiation
- Implementing Planned Change

INTRODUCTION

A nurse manager coordinates and manages a nursing staff. She ensures the staff. Leadership represents an abstract quality in a man. It is a psychological process of influencing followers or subordinates and providing guidance to them. Thus the essence of leadership is follower ship. It is the followers who make a person as leader. An executive has to earn followers. He may get subordinates because he is in authority but he may not get a follower unless he makes the people to follow him only willing followers can and will make him a leader (**Fig. 13.1**).

DEFINITION

- Leadership is the ability to influence other people.
  —*Lansdale*
- Leadership is the ability of a manager to induce subordinate to work with zeal confidence.
  —*Koontz and O Donnell*
- Leadership as the ability to secure desirable actions from a group of followers voluntary, without the use of coercion.
  —*Afford and Beaty*

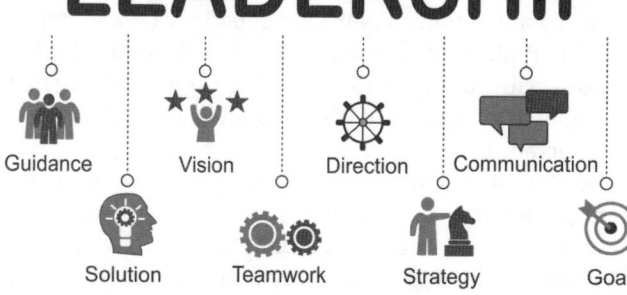

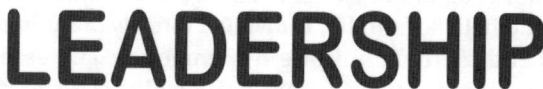

Fig. 13.1: Leadership.

- Leadership is the process of influencing the behavior and work of others in group effort towards the realization of special goal in a given situation.
- Leadership is the activity to persuade others to seek defined objectives enthusiastically. It is the human factor which binds a group together and motivates it towards goals.
  —*Keith Davis*
- Leadership is interpersonal influence exercise in a situation and directed through communication process, towards the attainment of a special goal or goals.

NATURE OF LEADERSHIP (FIG. 13.2)

- Leadership derives from the power and is similar to, yet distinct from, management. In fact, "leadership" and "management" are different. There can be leaders of completely unorganized groups, but there can be managers only of organized groups. Thus it can be said that a manager is necessarily a leader but a leader may not be a manager.
- Leadership is essential for managing. The ability to lead effectively is one of the keys to being an effective manager because she/he has to combine resources and lead a group to achieve objectives.
- Leadership and motivation are closely interconnected. By understanding motivation, one can appreciate better what people want and why they act as they do. A leader can encourage or dampen workers' motivation by creating a favorable or unfavorable working environment in the organization.
- The essence of leadership is followership. In other words, it is the willingness of people to follow a person that makes that person a leader. Moreover, people tend to follow those whom they see as providing a means of achieving their desires, needs and wants.

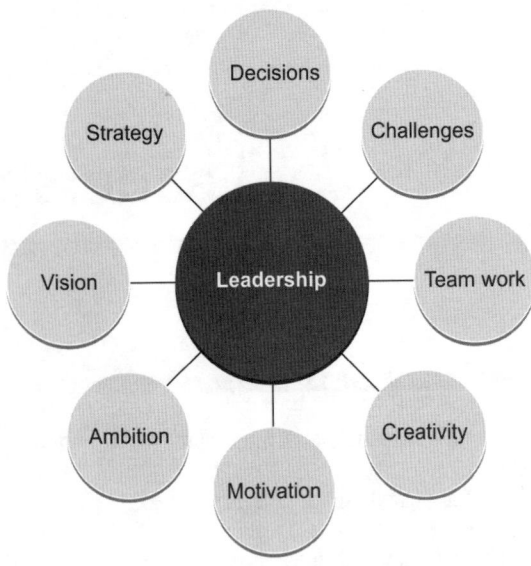

Fig. 13.2: Nature of leadership.

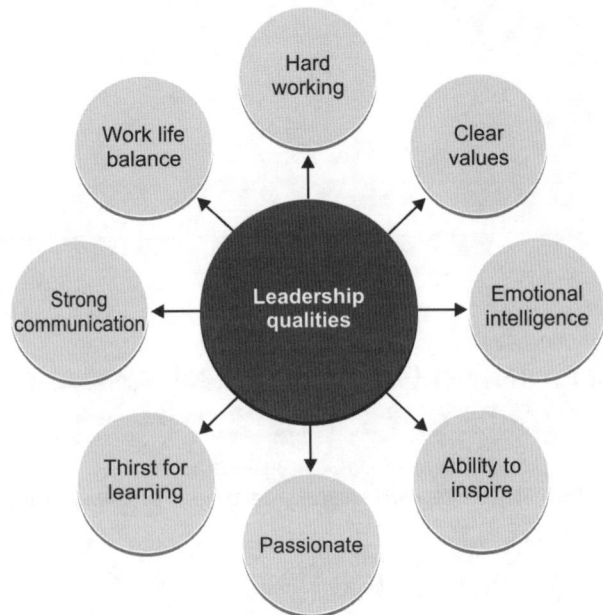

Fig. 13.3: Qualities of leadership.

- Leadership involves an unequal distribution of power between leaders and group members. Group members are not powerless; they can shape group activities in some ways. Still, the leader will usually have more power than the group members.
- Leaders can influence the followers' behavior in some ways. Leaders can influence workers either to do ill or well for the company. The leader must be able to empower and motivate the followers to the cause.
- The leader must co-exist with the subordinates or followers and must have a clear idea about their demands and ambitions. This creates loyalty and trust in subordinates for their leader.
- Leadership is to be concerned about values. Followers learn ethics and values from their leaders. Leaders are the real teachers of ethics, and they can reinforce ideas. Leaders need to make positive statements of ethics if they are not hypocritical.
- Leading is a very demanding job both physically and psychologically. The leader must have the strength, power, and ability to meet the bodily requirements; zeal, energy, and patience to meet the mental requirements for leading. Qualities of leadership is shown in **Figure 13.3**.

ELEMENTS OF LEADERSHIP

- **Ability to delegate tasks:** By delegating tasks to others, the workload is shared and team spirit thrives. Though there is one caveat: the right task must be assigned to the right person, so that it can be completed correctly, effectively, and in a timely manner.
- **Excellent communication:** An effective leader is one who communicates well across a variety of different media—email, telephone, and face-to-face. Staff needs to be able to grasp the purpose, the directions, and the end goal of any project in order for it to be completed successfully. Without excellent communication skills, managers will have an extremely difficult time establishing and maintaining a productive work environment.
- **Confidence:** Leaders are expected to be the company's backbone by being strong and confident. Managers are expected to support and carry an organization through both the good times and the bad, while still displaying an assertive and positive demeanor.
- **Honesty:** An extremely integral aspect of effective leadership is honesty. When a leader makes a statement or takes a particular decision, all team members must be able to believe that the leader will follow through and keep his or her word.
- **Creativity:** Though we all strive to hit targets, sometimes things do not go as planned. Unexpected events occur that require adjustments to be made to previous decisions that were made, or current plans of action. At these times, leaders must be able to step up to the plate quickly, and think creatively to come up with stable solutions, as staff turn to them for support and guidance.

CHARACTERISTICS OF LEADERSHIP (FIG. 13.4)

- **Leadership is a process of influence:** Influence is the ability of an individual to change the behavior, attitude, and belief of another individual directly or indirectly.
- **Leadership is not one-dimensional:** The essence of leadership is followership. Leadership is a systems thinking in multiple dimensions. In terms of systems thinking, the organizational performers (followers) are must in the leadership process. Without followers there can be no leadership.
- **Leadership is multifaceted:** Leadership is a combination of personality and tangible skills (drive, integrity, self-confidence, attractive personality, decisiveness, etc.), styles (authoritarian to laissez-faire), and situational factors (organization's internal and external environment,

Leadership characteristics

- Poised
- Takes initiative
- Skilled communicator
- Respects others
- Works well with others
- Cooperative
- Hard worker
- Good manager
- Dependable
- Democratic
- Confident
- Accepts responsibility
- Neat appearance
- Respected by others
- Open minded well informed
- Courteous
- Visionary
- Thinks ahead
- Punctual
- Service-oriented

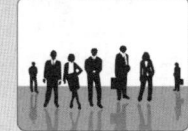

Fig. 13.4: Characteristics of leadership.

> **Box 13.1:** Twelve principles of leadership.
>
> From another perspective, Advanced Rescue Technology (April-May 2005: Volume 8. Number 2) defines 12 principles of leadership vital in mountain rescue. It's not such a stretch to apply these principles to success in an O and P business:
> 1. Know yourself and seek self-improvement;
> 2. Be technically and tactically proficient;
> 3. Know when the situation is dangerous or beyond your capabilities;
> 4. Make sound and timely decisions;
> 5. Set the example;
> 6. Praise in pubic, critize in private;
> 7. Know your rescuers (staff) their capacities and limitations;
> 8. Keep your team members informed;
> 9. Develop a sense of responsibility in your team members
> 10. Ensure the task is understood, supervised, and accomplished
> 11. Train your rescuers (staff) as a team; and
> 12. Stress safety (reason and common sense), balancing the risks with the mission to be accomplished.

objectives, tasks, resources, and cultural values of leaders and the followers).

- **Leadership is goal-oriented:** Leadership is "organizing a group of people to achieve a common goal." Thus, the influence concerns the goals only. Outside the goals, the concerns are not related to leadership.
- **Leadership is not primarily a particular personality trait:** A trait closely linked to leadership is charisma, but many people who have charisma (e.g., movie actors and sports heroes) are not leaders.
- **Leadership is not primarily a formal position:** There have been many great leaders who did not hold high positions, e.g., Mahatma Gandhi, Martin Luther King. On the other hand there are people who hold high positions but are not leaders.
- **Leadership is not primarily a set of important objectives:** It involves getting things done.
- **Leadership is not primarily a set of behaviors:** Many leadership manuals suggest that leadership involves doing things, such as delegating and providing inspiration and vision; but people who are not leaders can do these things, and some effective leaders do not do them at all.

PRINCIPLES OF LEADERSHIP (BOX 13.1)

- **Know yourself and seek self-improvement:** In order to know yourself, you have to understand your be, known, and do, attribute. Seeking self-improvement means to continually strengthen your attributes. This can be accomplished through self-study, formal classes, reflection, and interacting with others.
- **Be technically proficient:** As a leader, you must know your job and have a solid familiarity with your employees' tasks.
- **Seek responsibility and take responsibility for your actions:** Search for ways to guide your organization to new heights. And when things go wrong, they always do sooner or later—do not blame others. Analyze the situation, take corrective action, and move on to the next challenge.
- **Make sound and timely decisions:** Use good problem solving, decision-making, and planning tools.
- **Set the example:** Be a good role model for your employees. They must not only hear what they are expected to do, but also see. We must become the change we want to see.
  —*Mahatma Gandhi*
- **Know your people and look out for their well-being:** Know human nature and the importance of sincerely caring for the workers.
- **Keep your workers informed:** Know how to communicate with not only them, but also seniors and other key people.
- **Develop a sense of responsibility in your workers:** Help to develop good character traits that will help them carry out their professional responsibilities.
- **Ensure that tasks are understood, supervised, and accomplished:** Communication is the key to this responsibility.
- **Train as a team:** Although many so called leaders call their organization, department, section, etc., a team; they are not really teams…they are just a group of people doing their jobs.
- **Use the full capabilities of your organization:** By developing a team spirit, you will be able to employ your organization, department, section, etc., to its fullest capabilities.

Skills and qualities of a good leader is discusses in **Box 13.2**.

LEADERSHIP TECHNIQUES

- Planning and organizing the work schedule according to availability of personal and materials.
- Assigning work to subordinates should be defined and recorded with clear cut directions.
- Proper teaching and guidance to subordinates.
- Good communication is needed for proper understanding, cooperation and unified action.
- Cooperations and coordination between superior and subordinates.
- Identifying talented subordinates and involving them in planning.
- Democratic supervision.

> **Box 13.2:** Skills and qualities of a good leader.
>
> - Different research in leadership studies has explored several skills and qualities of an effective leader. Researchers argued that we cannot mention a particular quality makes a good leader. A good leader is composed of a set of attributes that makes him different from typical people and a manager. These attributes or qualities include the following. (Muteswa, 2016)
> - **Clear vision:** Leaders should have a clear vision. He should transcend the vision to the followers and influence them to achieve the vision.
> - **Confidence:** The leader shows an extreme level of confidence in his action so that the follower can rely on his/her.
> - **Drive and dedication:** Leaders should exhibit a high level of drive, dedication, and commitment to achieve the vision or goals. Leaders try with utmost dedication and full of energy until he reaches the destination.
> - **Honesty and integrity:** Honesty and integrity are very vital qualities of a leader. A leader should act honestly. His duty is to show the right track to the followers not to manipulate them. Leader achieves credibility through honesty and integrity.
> - **Courage to make a decision:** Leaders should have the courage to make critical and tough decisions. Sometimes he has to take decisions with sole responsibility.
> - **Intelligence:** Various research on leadership behavior puts emphasis on the leadership skills of intelligence. A leader requires intelligence to gather, and analyze the abstract and complex situation.
> - **Job-related knowledge:** Robbins and others (Robbins and Coulter, 2017) emphasis on job-related knowledge of the leader. A leader should have sufficient knowledge about the areas he or she works. For example, a leader might be a political leader, in that case, he should have knowledge about political science.

- Evaluation of performance of subordinates and self.
- Awareness of responsibilities and account.

IMPORTANCE OF LEADERSHIP

Leadership is an important function of management which helps to maximize efficiency and to achieve organizational goals **(Fig. 13.5)**. The following points justify the importance of leadership in a concern.

- **Initiates action:** Leader is a person who starts the work by communicating the policies and plans to the subordinates from where the work actually starts.
- **Motivation:** A leader proves to be playing an incentive role in the concern's working. He motivates the employees with economic and noneconomic rewards and thereby gets the work from the subordinates.
- **Providing guidance:** A leader has to not only supervise but also play a guiding role for the subordinates. Guidance here means instructing the subordinates the way they have to perform their work effectively and efficiently.
- **Creating confidence:** Confidence is an important factor which can be achieved through expressing the work efforts to the subordinates, explaining them clearly their role and giving them guidelines to achieve the goals effectively. It is also important to hear the employees with regards to their complaints and problems.
- **Building morale:** Morale denotes willing cooperation of the employees towards their work and getting them into confidence and winning their trust. A leader can be a morale booster by achieving full cooperation so that they perform with best of their abilities as they work to achieve goals.
- **Builds work environment:** Management is getting things done from people. An efficient work environment helps in sound and stable growth. Therefore, human relations should be kept into mind by a leader. He should have personal contacts with employees and should listen to their problems and solve them. He should treat employees on humanitarian terms.
- **Coordination:** Coordination can be achieved through reconciling personal interests with organizational goals. This synchronization can be achieved through proper and effective coordination which should be primary motive of a leader.

Figure 13.6 shows leadership qualities.

LEADERSHIP THEORIES

Interest in leadership increased during the early part of the twentieth century. Early leadership theories focused on what qualities distinguished between leaders and followers, while subsequent theories looked at other variables, such as situational factors and skill level. While many different leadership theories have emerged, most can be classified as one of eight major types **(Fig. 13.7)**:

1. **"Great Man" theories:** Great Man theories assume that the capacity for leadership is inherent—that great

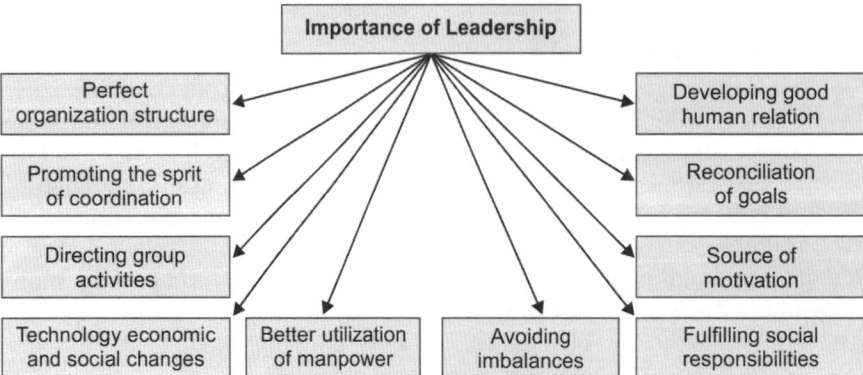

Fig. 13.5: Importance of leadership.

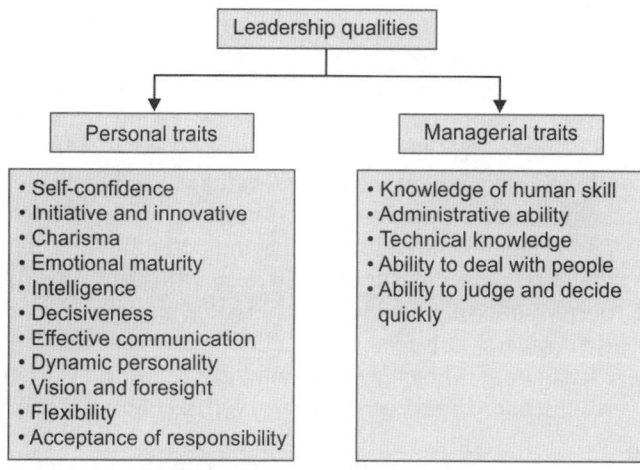

Fig. 13.6: Leadership qualities.

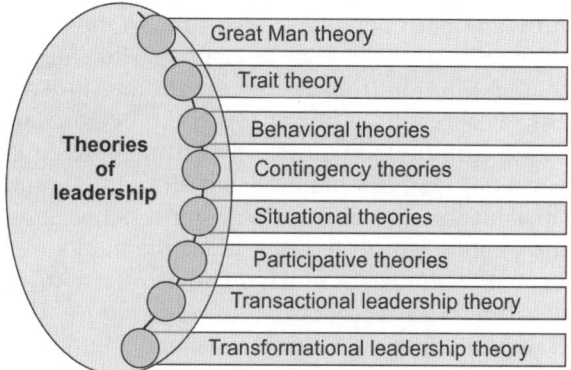

Fig. 13.7: Theories of leadership.

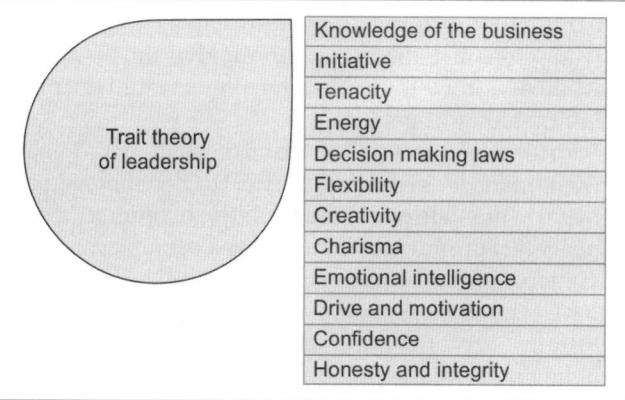

Fig. 13.8: Trait theory of leadership.

leadership, how do we explain people who possess those qualities but are not leaders? This question is one of the difficulties in using trait theories to explain leadership.

3. **Contingency theories:** Contingency theories of leadership focus on particular variables related to the environment that might determine which particular style of leadership is best suited for the situation. According to this theory, no leadership style is best in all situations. Success depends upon a number of variables, including the leadership style, qualities of the followers, and aspects of the situation.

4. **Situational theories:** Situational theories propose that leaders choose the best course of action based upon situational variable. Different styles of leadership may be more appropriate for certain types of decision-making.

5. **Behavioral theories:** Behavioral theories of leadership are based upon the belief that great leaders are made, not born. Rooted in behaviorism, this leadership theory focuses on the actions of leaders, not on mental qualities or internal states. According to this theory, people can learn to become leaders through teaching and observation.

6. **Participative theories:** Participative leadership theories suggest that the ideal leadership style is one that takes the input of others into account. These leaders encourage participation and contributions from group members and help group members feel more relevant and committed to the decision-making process. In participative theories, however, the leader retains the right to allow the input of others.

7. **Management theories:** Management theories (also known as "Transactional theories") focus on the role of supervision, organization, and group performance. These theories base leadership on a system of reward and punishment. Managerial theories are often used in business; when employees are successful, they are rewarded; when they fail, they are reprimanded or punished.

8. **Relationship theories:** Relationship theories (also known as "Transformational theories") focus upon the connections formed between leaders and followers. These leaders motivate and inspire people by helping group members see the importance and higher good of the task. Transformational leaders are focused on the performance of group members, but also want each person to fulfill his or her potential. These leaders often have high ethical and moral standards.

QUALITIES OF GOOD LEADER

- **Integrity:** Integrity is expected of health care professional. Patients, colleagues, and employers all expect nurses to be honest, law-abiding and trust worthy.
- **Courage:** Sometimes, being a leader means taking some risks.
- **Initiative:** Good ideas are not enough. To be leader, you must act on those good ideas. This requires initiative on your part.

leaders are born, not made. These theories often portray great leaders as heroic, mythic, and destined to rise to leadership when needed. The term "Great Man" was used because, at the time, leadership was thought of primarily as a male quality, especially in terms of military leadership.

2. **Trait theories (Fig. 13.8):** Similar in some ways to "Great Man" theories, trait theory assumes that people inherit certain qualities and traits that make them better suited to leadership. Trait theories often identify particular personality or behavioral characteristics shared by leaders. But if particular traits are key features of

- **Energy:** Leadership also requires energy. Both leadership and management are hard satisfying endeavors that require effort on your part.
- **Optimism:** When the work is difficult and one crisis seems to follow another in rapid succession, it is easy to become discouraged. However, it is important not to let discouragement keep you and your coworkers from seeking ways resolve your difficulties.
- **Perseverance:** Effective leaders do not give up easily. In seated, they persist, continuing their efforts when others tempted to give up the struggle.
- **Balance:** In our effort to become the best nurses, we may forget that other aspects of life are equally important.
- **Ability to handle stress:** There is some stress in almost every job.
- **Self-awareness:** People who do not understand themselves are limited in their ability to understand the motivations of other people.

DIFFERENCE BETWEEN LEADERSHIP AND MANAGEMENT

Leadership differs from management in a sense that **(Table 13.1)**:

- While managers lay down the structure and delegates authority and responsibility, leaders provides direction by developing the organizational vision and communicating it to the employees and inspiring them to achieve it.
- While management includes focus on planning, organizing, staffing, directing and controlling; leadership is mainly a part of directing function of management. Leaders focus on listening, building relationships, teamwork, inspiring, motivating and persuading the followers.
- While a leader gets his authority from his followers, a manager gets his authority by virtue of his position in the organization.
- While managers follow the organization's policies and procedure, the leaders follow their own instinct.
- Management is more of science as the managers are exact, planned, standard, logical and more of mind. Leadership, on the other hand, is an art. In an organization, if the managers are required, then leaders are a must/essential.
- While management deals with the technical dimension in an organization or the job content; leadership deals with the people aspect in an organization.
- While management measures/evaluates people by their name, past records, present performance; leadership sees and evaluates individuals as having potential for things that can not be measured, i.e., it deals with future and the performance of people if their potential is fully extracted.
- If management is reactive, leadership is proactive.
- Management is based more on written communication, while leadership is based more on verbal communication.

FACTORS INFLUENCING LEADERSHIP (BOX 13.3)

- Personality is one of five elements that will influence our leadership behavior. According to most studies, personality does not change, but behavior can change. Leadership qualities can be taught and individuals can set personal behavior targets to begin changing counterproductive actions that hinder success into leadership qualities, or new habits, that result in success.
- The situation should determine our response to events and people. However, often times the habits we have formed in the past are what comes out in any given situation. That is reacting, not responding. Leaders understand that it is critical to respond appropriately to each situation and not let our initial reaction dictate our leadership effectiveness.
- Individual needs play into the leadership behavior we exhibit. For example, a need for power would tend to lead someone to be more authoritative and demanding, whereas a need to be liked by others would encourage "going-along-to-get-a-long."
- Perhaps the greatest influence on our leadership behavior is our manager's leadership style. For better or worse, we begin to emulate our manager's style in order to keep the peace, get promoted, be viewed as a team player, or keep our job. As leaders, we need to recognize the influence we have over others and stop and think before responding.
- Finally, the operating environment can effect our behavior. If we are in an environment that encourages risk-taking, we are more likely to take risks for instance. Leaders understand that we have to interpret our operating environment for those around us in a way that is motivating, encouraging creativity and allowing

Table 13.1: Difference between leadership and management.	
Leadership	**Management**
• Setting direction/creating vision • Assembling team • Creating shared values • Knowing skills/motivations of each team member • Adjudicating/resolving conflict • Inspiring/leading by example • Knowing when to devolve power • Changing team to get right chemistry	• Understanding goals of team and company • Creating and prioritizing tasks to be completed (a project) • Assigning tasks to appropriate team member • Motivating and guiding individual contributors (carrot vs stick) • Reviewing work output and quality • Controlling scope of project • Reporting status up, down and to peers

Box 13.3: Factors affecting leadership style.
- Personal value systems
- Manager's experience
- Confidence in subordinates
- Feelings of security
- Nature of the business problems
- Type of organization (size, structure)
- Effectiveness of teams and groups
- Skills and experience of subordinates
- Pressure (time, costs)

appropriate flexibility, rather than with rigidity and inflexibility.

LEADERSHIP STYLES

Different types of leadership styles exist in work environments. Advantages and disadvantages exist within each leadership style. The culture and goals of an organization determine which leadership style fits the firm best. Some companies offer several leadership styles within the organization, dependent upon the necessary tasks to complete and departmental needs (**Fig. 13.9**).

- **Autocratic leaders:** Autocratic leaders are an excessive form of transactional leadership, where a leader makes use of high levels of power over his team members. People within the team are given few opportunities for making suggestions, even if these would be in the team's or organizations interest.
- **Bureaucratic leaders:** Bureaucratic leaders work by the book, ensuring that their staffs follow procedures accurately. This is a very right approach for work involving serious safety risks (such as working with machinery, with toxic substances or at heights) or where large sums of money are involved (such as cash-process).
- **Charismatic leaders:** A charismatic leaders style can appear similar to a transformational leadership style, in that the leader bring in huge doses of enthusiasm into his team, and is very energetic in driving others forward. Charismatic leadership carries great responsibility, and needs long-term commitment from the leader.
- **Democratic leaders:** Even though a democratic leader will make the final decision, he invites other members of the team to contribute to the decision-making process. This not only increases job satisfaction by involving team members in what is going on, but it also helps to develop people's skills. Team members feel in control of their own destiny, and are motivated to work smart by more than just a pecuniary reward.
- **Laissez-faire leaders:** They known as delegative leaders offer little or no guidance to group members and leave decision-making up to group members. While this style can be effective in situations where group members are highly qualified in an area of expertise, it often leads to poorly defined roles and a lack of motivation.

Autocratic Leadership

In this type of leadership, the leader alone determines policies and makes plans. He tells others what to do and how to do it. He demands strict obedience and relies on power. The formula used by him is "Do what I say or else..." meaning thereby that an employee will be punished if he does not follow orders. An autocratic leader may sometimes be paternalistic or benevolent also. The formula used by this type of leader is "Do what I say because I am good to you." Both the forms of autocratic leadership (authoritarian and benevolent) are disliked by employees (**Fig. 13.11 and Box 13.4**).

In one form, the employee remains under constant fear. In other form he remains under constant gratitude. In both the forms, the leader is the key person. The whole operation of the organization depends upon him. In his absence it may function inadequately or not at all.

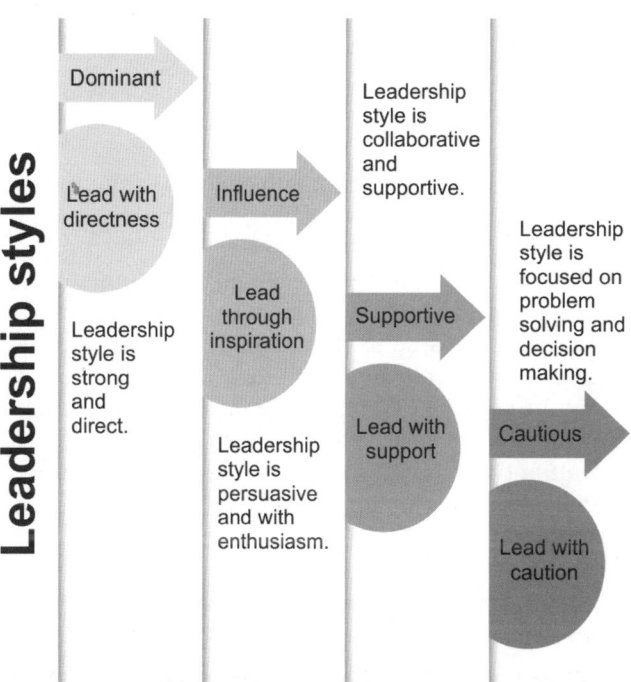

Fig. 13.9: Leadership styles.

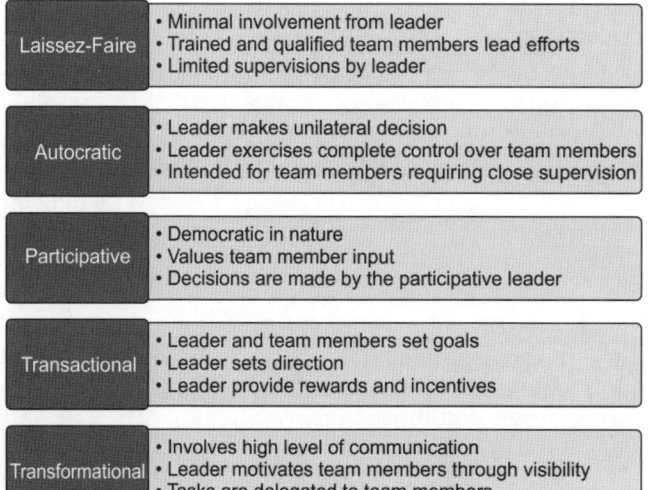

Fig. 13.10: Leadership styles.

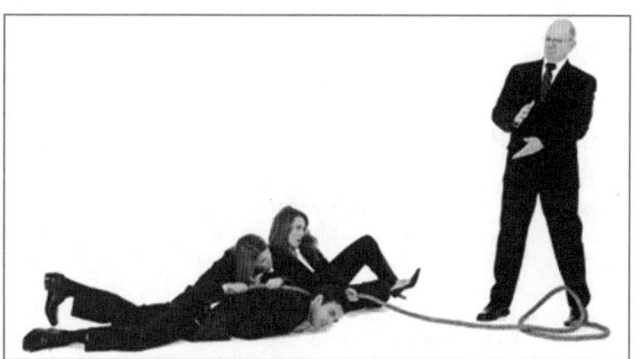

Fig. 13.11: Autocratic leadership

> **Box 13.4:** Autocratic leadership.
>
> *Autocratic leadership*
> - The leaders retains all or most of the authority with himself, very little is delegated to the follower.
> - Tells employees what they want do and how to do it (without getting the advice from others).
> - Generally, this style is not a good way to get the best performance from a team.
>
> *Characteristics*
> - Leader have most authority and control in decision-making
> - Consultation with other is minimum and decision-making becomes a solitary process.
>
> *Benefits*
> - Effective supervision
> - Less time consuming for decision-making
>
> *Disadvantages*
> - Staff become tense, fearful
> - Staff expect their opinion heard
> - Low staff moral, absenteeism

Merits

- This type of leadership, when appropriate, can increase efficiency, save time and get quick results, especially in a crisis or an emergency situation.
- The paternalistic form of this style of leadership works well with employees who have a low tolerance for ambiguity, feel insecure with freedom and even minor decision-making requirements and thrive under clear, detailed and achievable directives.
- Chain of command, and division of work (who is supposed to do what) are clear and fully understood by all.

Difference between transactional and transformational leaders are discuss in **Table 13.2**.

Demerits

- The apparent efficiency of one-way communication often becomes a false efficiency since one-way communication, without feedback, typically leads to misunderstandings, communication breakdowns and costly errors.
- The autocratic manager is alone in his decision-making. He receives little, if any, information and ideas from his people as inputs into his decision-making. This is generally dangerous in today's environment of technological and organizational complexity.
- Today, most people resent authoritarian rule which excludes them from involvement and reduces them to machine-like cogs without human dignity or importance. They express their resentment in the form of massive resistance, low morale and low productivity.

Democratic Leadership

In this type of leadership (also known as participative or person-oriented leadership) the entire group is involved in and accepts responsibility for goal setting and achievement **(Fig. 13.12 and Box 13.5)**.

- Subordinates have considerable freedom of action. The leader shows greater concern for his people than for high production.
- A part of the leader's task is to encourage and reinforce constructive inter-relationships among members and to reduce intra-group conflict and tensions.
- The sociometric pattern for democratic leadership is a network which involves a tight pattern of complete inter-relationships among all members. While the leader is quite an important figure in a democratic situation, he is not the key figure that he is in an authoritarian situation.
- He serves more as a coordinator or agent for the group. Hence the group is not dependent upon him as an individual and can function effectively in his absence.

Merits

- When people participate in and help formulate a decision, they support it (instead of fighting or ignoring it) and

Basis	Transactional	Transformational
Active vs proactive	Leadership is responsive and its basic orientation is dealing with present issues	Leadership is proactive and forms new expectations in followers
Basis of exchange	Rely on standard forms of inducement, reward, punishment and sanction to control followers	Distinguished by their capacity to inspire and provide individualized consideration, intellectual stimulation and idealized influence to their followers
Motivation	Motivate followers by setting goals and promising rewards for desired performance	Motivate followers to work for goals that go beyond self-interest
Performance in action	Depends on the leader's power to reinforce subordinates for their successful completion of the bargain	Arouses emotions in followers
Organizational culture	Works within the organizational culture as it exists	Changes the organizational culture
Position of followers	Relationship with followers based upon levels of exchange. Awards related to productivity	Put followers in front and develop them; take followers' to next level; inspire followers to transcend their own self-interests in achieving superior results
Focus	On the details	On the big picture
Telling or selling	Once the contract is in place, takes a 'telling' style	Has more of a 'selling' style. Transactional leadership
Situation handling	Takes up weakened organization	Takes up stagnated organization

Table 13.2: Difference between transactional and transformational leader.

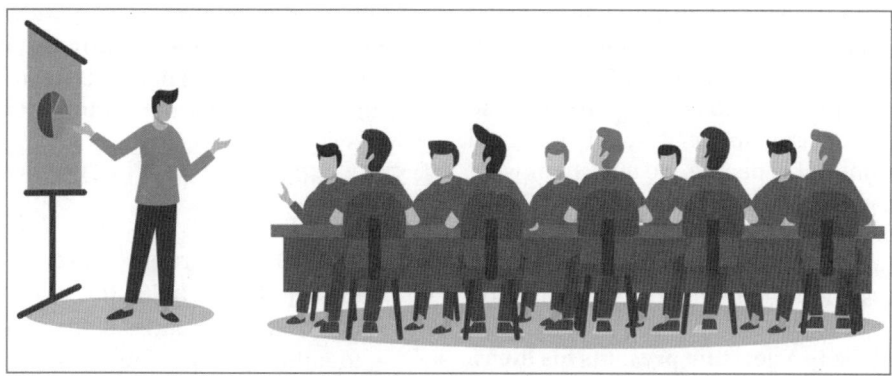

Fig. 13.12: Democratic leadership.

> **Box 13.5:** Democratic leadership.
> - **Leader makes final decision:** Invites other members of the team to contribute to the decision-making process
> - **Increases job satisfaction:**
>   – Involves employees/team members in what's going on
>   – Helps develop people's skills
>   – Employees are motivated to work hard because they feel in control of their own destiny
> - Can lead to things happening more slowly but end result is better
> - Suitable where teamwork is essential and quality is more important than speed

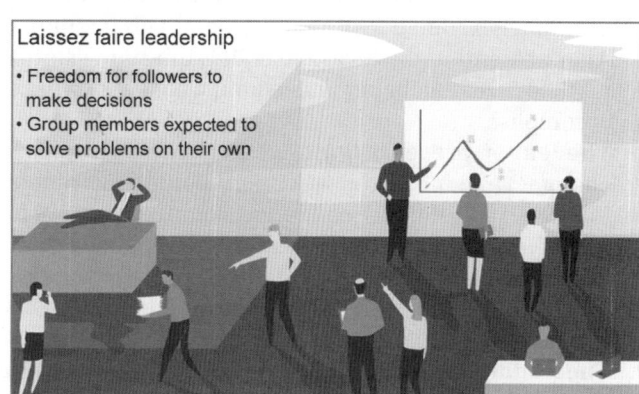

Fig. 13.13: Laissez faire leadership.

work hard to make it work, because it is their idea and, now, a part of their life and their ego. In other words, the participative leader has the critical factor of built-in-personal motivation working for him.

- The leader consistently receives the benefit of the best information, ideas, suggestions, and talent-and operating experience-of his people.
- This style of leadership permits and encourages people to develop, grow and rise in the organization (both in terms of responsibility they can assume and service they can contribute).

Demerits

- The participative style can take enormous amounts of time and, if not exercised properly, may degenerate into a complete loss of leader's control.
- Some leaders may use this style as a way of avoiding responsibility. **Figure 13.13** shows Laissez faire leadership.

Free-rein Style

In this type of leadership, the leader exercises absolutely no control. He only provides information, materials and facilities to his men to enable them to accomplish group objectives. This type can be a disaster if the leader does not know well the competence and integrity of his people and their ability to handle this kind of freedom **(Fig. 13.14)**.

- As the spectrum demonstrates, there are a number of alternative ways in which a leader can relate himself to the group.
- At the extreme left of the spectrum, the emphasis is on the leader-won what he is interested in, how he sees things, how he feels about them.

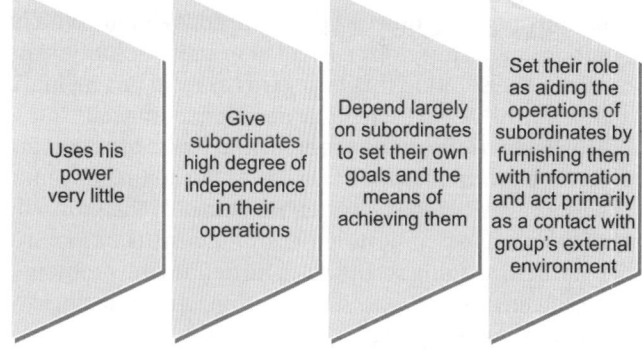

Fig. 13.14: Free-rein leadership style.

- As we move towards the employee-centered end of the spectrum, however, the focus is increasingly on the subordinates—on What they are interested in? How they look at things? How they feel about them?
- The center of the spectrum finds a more equitable balance between the authority exercised by the leader and the amount of participation the group can exercise.
- **The leader makes the decision and announces it:** In this case, the leader who is frankly authoritarian "Tells" people what his decisions are, and demands unquestioning obedience. He does not give any consideration to what they will think or feel about his decisions. A bureaucratic leader who manages entirely by the organization's policies, and rules and permits people little or no freedom falls under this category.

- **The leaders "sells" his decision:** Here the leader behaves like a diplomat. Although like an autocrat he has already taken a decision, he prefers to take the additional step of persuading his subordinates to accept it. In doing so he usually relates his decision to the personal individual needs and aspirations of his people. He tells them what they have to gain from his decision. This style of leadership is indispensable for the "staff" who realize the inadequacy of their real authority and are utterly dependent on the skills of persuasion to get the help and cooperation needed.
- **The leader having made a decision presents his ideas, invites questions:** Here the leader who has arrived at a decision provides an opportunity for his subordinates to get a fuller explanation of his thinking and his intentions. After presenting the ideas, he invites questions so that his associates can better understand what he is trying to accomplish.
- **The leader presents tentative decisions, subject to change:** This kind of a behavior permits the subordinates to exert some influence on the decision. The initiative for identifying and diagnosing the problem remains with the leader. He also arrives at a tentative decision. But before finalizing it, he presents this tentative decision for the reaction of his subordinates.
- **The leader presents the problem, gets suggestions and then makes his decision:** Up to this point the leader has come before the group with the solution of his own. Not so in this case. The subordinates now get the first chance to suggest solutions. The leader's initial role involves identifying the problem. He then in consultation with his subordinates develops a list of alternative solutions and selects the solution that he regards as most promising. In this way he reserves the final decision to himself.
- **The leader defines the problem and limits of action and lets the group make a decision:** At this point, the leader acts as a participative leader. He passes to the group the right to make decisions either by consensus or majority vote. Before doing so, however, he defines the problem to be solved and the boundaries within which the decision must be made.
- **The leader permits the group to make decisions within limits defined by the situation:** This represents an extreme degree of group freedom only occasionally encountered in formal organizations.

SKILLS REQUIRED IN LEADERSHIP

To be an effective leader the nurses need the primary leadership skills that are as follows:
- **Skills of personal behavior:**
  - Is sensitive to feelings of the group.
  - Identifies self with the needs of the group.
  - Does not ridicule or criticize another's suggestions.
  - Helps other feel important and needed.
  - Does not argue.
- **Skills communication:**
  - Listen attentively
  - Make sure everyone understands what is needed and the reason why?
  - Establishes positive communication with the needs of the group as a routine part of that job. Recognizes that everyone's contributions are important.
- **Skills of organization:** The effective leader helps the group to:
  - Develop long and short range objectives.
  - Break big problems into small ones.
  - Share responsibilities and opportunities.
  - Plan act, follow-up and evaluate.
  - Be attentive to details.
- **Skills of self-examination:**
  - Is aware of personal motivations.
  - Is aware of the group members level of hospitals for taking appropriate countermeasures.
  - Helps the group to be aware of their attitudes and values.

Leadership Activities

Leadership includes variation of activities which includes directing, supervising and coordinating.

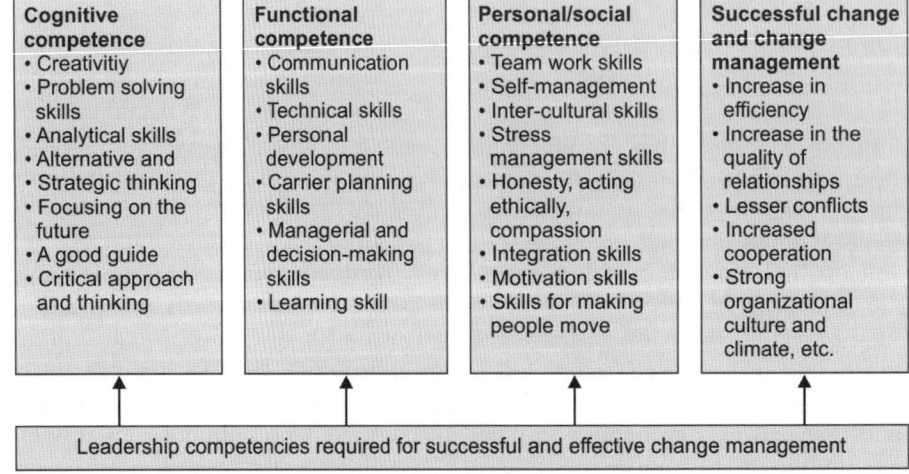

Fig. 13.15: Leadership competencies.

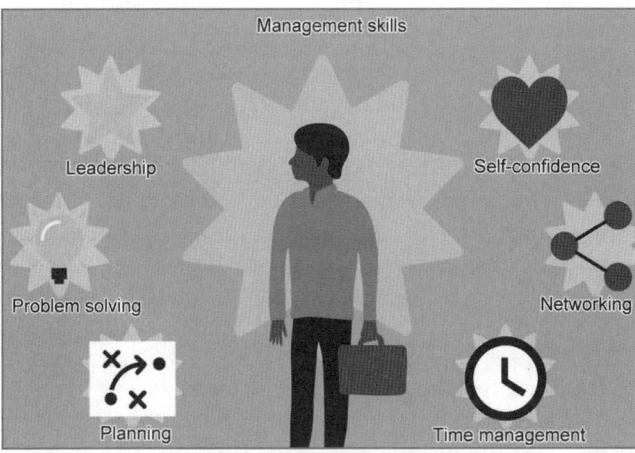

Fig. 13.16: Management skills.

- **Directing:** It is the process by which actual performance of staff and people is guided towards common goals. A leader uses assignments, orders, procedures, rules, regulations, standards, opinions, suggestions and questions to direct subordinate behavior.
- **Supervising:** Supervision is a continuous administrative and educative process which enables the supervisor through the medium of his relationship with the supervisors to contribute towards the continuous growth of the supervision which includes inspecting another's work, evaluating her or his performance, and approving or correcting performance.
- **Coordinating:** Coordination includes all the activities that enable work group members to work together harmoniously.

Management skills is shown in **Figure 13.16**.

LEADERSHIP COMPETENCIES

Leadership competencies are leadership skills and behaviors that contribute to superior performance. By using a competency-based approach to leadership, organizations can better identify and develop their next generation of leaders. Essential leadership competencies and global competencies have been defined by researchers. However, future business trends and strategy should drive the development of new leadership competencies. While some leadership competencies are essential to all firms, an organization should also define what leadership attributes are distinctive to the particular organization to create competitive advantage.

Leading the organization:
- Managing change
- Solving problems and making decisions
- Managing politics and influencing others
- Taking risks and innovating
- Setting vision and strategy
- Managing the work
- Enhancing business skills and knowledge
- Understanding and navigating the organization

Leading the self:
- Demonstrating ethics and integrity
- Displaying drive and purpose
- Exhibiting leadership stature
- Increasing your capacity to learn
- Managing yourself
- Increasing self-awareness
- Developing adaptability

Leading others:
- Communicating effectively
- Developing others
- Valuing diversity and difference
- Building and maintaining relationships
- Managing effective teams and work groups

Global Leadership Competencies

Developing successful global leaders is a competitive advantage for multinational organizations. In addition to essential leadership competencies, global leaders face special challenges that require additional competencies. To address the unique challenges of global leaders, researchers have identified global leadership competencies that can contribute to success. Among these global competencies, developing a global mindset, cross-cultural communication skills and respecting cultural diversity are paramount to succeeding in the global workplace.

Global Executive Competencies

- Open-minded and flexible in thought and tactics
- Cultural interest and sensitivity
- Able to deal with complexity
- Resilient, resourceful, optimistic and energetic
- Honesty and integrity
- Stable personal life
- Value-added technical or business skills

Leadership competencies can be used to effectively select, develop and promote leaders in an organization. Certain factors, such as business strategy and future trends should be taken into account when creating leadership competencies. All business strategies are different and HR practitioners should use the business strategy, including the global business strategy, to drive the use of competencies in selecting and developing leaders. By effectively building a unique set of skills for the organization's leaders, the firm will sustain competitive advantage.

SITUATIONAL LEADERSHIP STYLE

Situational theories of leadership work on the assumption that the most effective style of leadership changes from situation to situation. To be most effective and successful, a leader must be able to adapt his style and approach to diverse circumstances (**Fig. 13.17**).

Meaning of Situational Leadership

- Situational leadership is described as an adaptive style that encourages leaders to take stock of their team members and make adjustments as per their needs and desires.

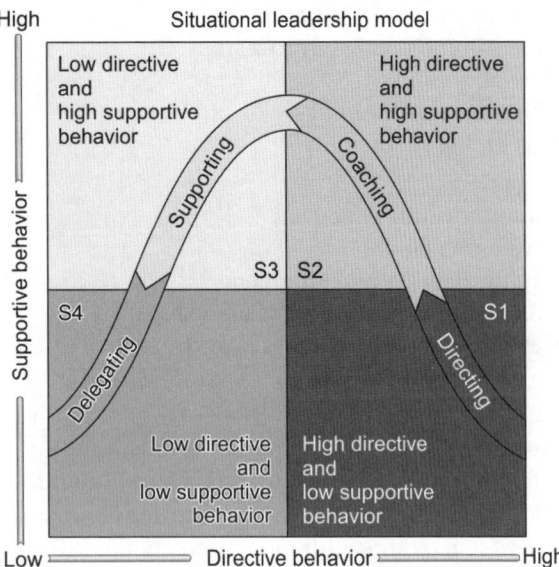

Fig. 13.17: Situational leadership.

- It does not ask the leader to put his onus on workplace factors instead suggests them to adapt their styles as per their follower's ability and style.
- The situational leadership model categorically states that it is impossible to find one leadership style that is better than the other. Hence, it is better to encourage relationship-relevant and task-relevant leadership that is flexible and adaptive.

Hersey and Blanchard's Situational Leadership Theory

The term "situational leadership" is most commonly derived from and connected with Paul Hersey and Ken Blanchard's Situational Leadership Theory. This approach to leadership suggests the need to match two key elements appropriately: the leader's leadership style and the followers' maturity or preparedness levels.

The theory identifies four main leadership approaches:
1. **Telling:** Directive and authoritative approach. The leader makes decisions and tells employees what to do.
2. **Selling:** The leader is still the decision maker, but he communicates and works to persuade the employees rather than simply directing them.
3. **Participating:** The leader works with the team members to make decisions together. He supports and encourages them and is more democratic.
4. **Delegating:** The leader assigns decision-making responsibility to team members but oversees their work.

In addition to these four approaches to leadership, there are also four levels of follower maturity:
1. **Level M1:** Followers have low competence and low commitment.
2. **Level M2:** Followers have low competence, but high commitment.
3. **Level M3:** Followers have high competence, but low commitment and confidence.
4. **Level M4:** Followers have high competence and high commitment and confidence.

Six Styles within Situational Leadership

Daniel Goleman, the author of Emotional Intelligence, defines six styles within situational leadership:
1. **Coaching leaders**, who work on an individual's personal development as well as job-related skills. This style works best with people who know their limitations and are open to change.
2. **Pacesetting leaders**, who set very high expectations for their followers. This style works best with self-starters who are highly motivated. The leader leads by example. This style is used sparingly since it can lead to follower burnout.
3. **Democratic leaders**, who give followers a vote in almost all decisions. When used in optimal conditions, it can build flexibility and responsibility within the group. This style is, however, time consuming and is not the best style if deadlines are looming.
4. **Affiliative leaders**, who put employees first. This style is used when morale is very low. The leader uses praise and helpfulness to build up the team's confidence. This style may risk poor performance when team building is happening.
5. **Authoritative leaders**, who are very good at analyzing problems and identifying challenges. This style is good in an organization that is drifting aimlessly. This leader will allow his or her followers to help figure out how to solve a problem.
6. **Coercive leaders**, who tell their subordinates what to do. They have a very clear vision of the endgame and how to reach it. This style is good in disasters or if an organization requires a total overhaul.

Table 13.3 summarizes pros and cons of situational leadership.

Characteristics

The following are some of the basic characteristics of the situational leadership style. Since the leadership style is flexible, there are no fixed traits that a situational leader exhibits. These attributes may all come into play depending on the situation.

- **Flexibility:** The fundamental idea of situational leadership is that there is no such thing as a single best or fixed type of leadership. Leadership changes according to the requirements of the group or organization, and successful leaders are able to be flexible and adapt their style of leadership to the level of maturity of the group that they are trying to lead.
- **Changes according to the situation:** The leadership style that the situational leader brings into play will be dependent on the situation at hand and the development level of the individuals involved. If the development level is low, the situational leader becomes more task-oriented. If the individuals are sufficiently developed, the leader will be more supportive.
- **Directing:** Situational leadership will be high on the "directive" aspect when the subordinates are not sufficiently developed and need constant supervision. Here, the leader gives specific instructions about what the goals

Table 13.3: Pros and cons of situational leadership.

Pros	Cons
Employee development level: Leaders adjust their behavior according to the skill and motivation level of employees (Kelchnei n.d.)	**Confusion:** As situational leader changes his behavior according to the circumstances, inconsistency leads to confusion among employees regarding the response they shall expect from their manager (Wile n.d.)
Motivation: Support provided to the employees along with proper guidance boost their morale (Kelchner n.d.)	**Leadership or management?** As leader adapts his behavior, this short-term view confuses the leadership style with management technique (Wile n.d.)
Productivity: Supportive environment and high morale increases the productivity at work (Kelchner n.d.)	**Outside factors:** The situation may change itself in response to the behavior adapted by a situational leader (Wile n.d.)
Employee retention: Employees tend to stay with managers who are motivating (Kelchner n.d.)	**Perception:** Employees may perceive the leadership style to be manipulative and resultantly leader loses their trust (Wile n.d.)

are, and exactly how the goals need to be achieved. It is similar to a parent supervising the actions of a toddler.

- **Coaching:** If the situation demands it, the leader will also coach their team. This is an extension of the directive approach; the leader still provides detailed instructions but they also focus on encouraging the subordinates, soliciting inputs, and explaining why they have made certain decisions.
- **Participating:** The situational leader may try to encourage a team to become more independent performing the tasks by letting them take routine decisions. High-level problem-solving is still under their purview, but they allow team members to actively participate in the decision-making process.
- **Delegating:** When dealing with a highly matured and capable team, the situational leader will gradually reduce their supervision and involvement in the daily activities of team members. The leader is involved while discussing the tasks and deciding on the goals to be achieved, but after that team members have complete freedom on how they want to accomplish these goals.
- **Integrity:** The situational leader does not change their approach merely to take advantage of the situation. They simply adapt in a way that is most appropriate considering factors, such as the maturity level of followers, the organizational structure and culture, and the goals to be achieved. They do so with integrity, and are not motivated by a desire to unfairly capitalize on the weaknesses of the team or organization.
- **Courage:** It takes a lot of courage for a leader to try out different leadership approaches and figure out which one is ideal. Most leaders stick to a particular way of doing things—whatever has worked best for them in the past. But situational leader is not afraid to take chances and to adopt a radically different leadership style if the situation demands it.
- **Clear vision:** The situational leader has a clear vision of where the team is going. This is what allows a leader to identify and adopt the most effective behaviors and strategies to get to the goal.
- **Humility:** The situational leader does not claim to know it all. With a group of highly developed and mature followers, they have the humility to accept limitations and seek the higher wisdom of the group.

Advantages of Situational Leadership

The advantages of situational leadership are as follows:
- The situational leader can vary his style as per the need of the hour.
- It is a simple method that involves lots of flexibility and intuitiveness.
- Situational leadership creates a relaxed and comfy environment for the team members.
- It takes into account the various developmental phases
- There is a greater chance of open communication.
- The situational leadership helps in building constructive relationships between the team leader and team members.

Disadvantages of Situational Leadership

The disadvantages of situational leadership are as follows:
- Every manager cannot adapt the mantle of situational leadership with ease because he is not programmed to make changes as per the needs of his workforce.
- Situational leadership puts its focus more on short-term goals and immediate needs rather than long-term goals.
- Defining the maturity levels of all the team members is a complicated task that needs patience, time and lots of effort.
- The situational leadership has proved ineffective in task-oriented environments where you have to follow a specific set of regulations, policies, and rules that are inflexible.
- If a situational leader misreads any situation, the task will crumble down like a house of cards.
- Situation leadership is based on the fact that the leader has to shift his approach as per the need of the hour and it can create confusion.
- It encourages corporate dependency.
- The situational leadership theory is as strong as its leader. If the leader is not up to the task, then it can create chaos in the existing scenario.

■ TRANSFORMATIONAL LEADERSHIP STYLE

Transformational leadership may be found at all levels of the organization: teams, departments, divisions, and organization as a whole. Such leaders are visionary, inspiring, daring, risk-takers, and thoughtful thinkers. They have a charismatic appeal. But charisma alone is insufficient for changing the

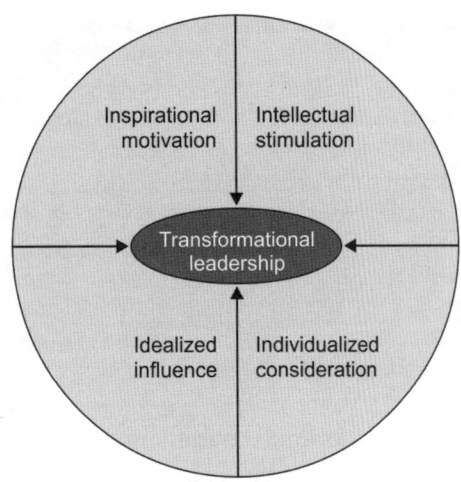

Fig. 13.18: Transformational leadership.

way an organization operates. For bringing major changes, transformational leaders must exhibit the following four factors **(Fig. 13.18)**:

Inspirational Motivation:
- The foundation of transformational leadership is the promotion of consistent vision, mission, and a set of values to the members.
- Their vision is so compelling that they know what they want from every interaction.
- Transformational leaders guide followers by providing them with a sense of meaning and challenge.
- They work enthusiastically and optimistically to foster the spirit of teamwork and commitment.

Intellectual Stimulation:
- Such leaders encourage their followers to be innovative and creative. They encourage new ideas from their followers and never criticize them publicly for the mistakes committed by them.
- The leaders focus on the "what" in problems and do not focus on the blaming part of it.
- They have no hesitation in discarding an old practice set by them if it is found ineffective.

Idealized Influence:
- They believe in the philosophy that a leader can influence followers only when he practices what he preaches.
- The leaders act as role models that followers seek to emulate. Such leaders always win the trust and respect of their followers through their action.
- They typically place their followers needs over their own, sacrifice their personal gains for them, ad demonstrate high standards of ethical conduct.
- The use of power by such leaders is aimed at influencing them to strive for the common goals of the organization.

Individualized Consideration:
- Leaders act as mentors to their followers and reward them for creativity and innovation.
- The followers are treated differently according to their talents and knowledge.

- They are empowered to make decisions and are always provided with the needed support to implement their decisions.

Implications of Transformational Leadership Theory (Fig. 13.19)

- The current environment characterized by uncertainty, global turbulence, and organizational instability calls for transformational leadership to prevail at all levels of the organization.
- The followers of such leaders demonstrate high levels of job satisfaction and organizational commitment, and engage in organizational citizenship behaviors.
- With such a devoted workforce, it will definitely be useful to consider making efforts towards developing ways of transforming organization through leadership.

LEADERSHIP DEVELOPMENT

Leadership development refers to any activity that enhances the capability of an individual to assume leadership roles and responsibilities. Examples include degree programs in management, executive education, seminars and workshops, and even internships. These types of learning opportunities focus on developing knowledge, skills, self-awareness, and abilities needed to lead effectively.

Definition

Leadership development: Any activity that enhances the quality of leadership within an individual or organization.

Successful leadership development is the result of three things:
1. Individual learner characteristics, including willingness and ability to learn
2. The quality and nature of the leadership development program, including its structure and content.
3. Opportunities to practice new skills and receive performance feedback.

Methods of Leadership Development

Leader development takes place through multiple mechanisms: formal instruction, developmental job assignments,

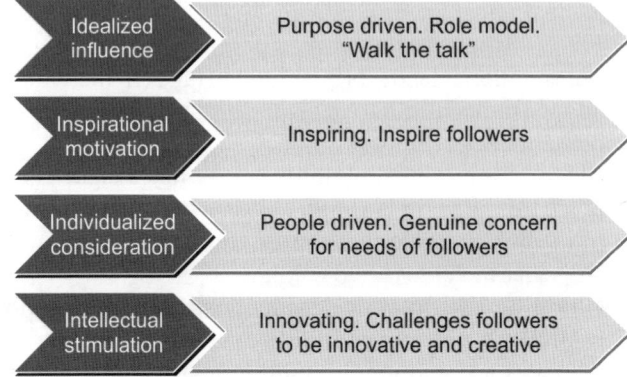

Fig. 13.19: Implications of transformational leadership theory.

Cognitive capacities	Dispositional attributes	Motives/values	Social capacities	Problem-solving skills	Expertise and knowledge
• General intelligence • Cognitive complexity • Creativity	• Adaptability • Extroversion • Risk propensity • Openness	• Need for socialized power • Need for achievement • Motivation to lead	• Social intelligence • Emotional intelligence • Persuasion and negotiation skills	• Metacognition • Problem construction • Solution generation • Self-regulation skills	Expertise and knowledge in specific areas

360-degree feedback, executive coaching, and self-directed learning. These approaches may occur independently but are more effective in combination.

Formal Training

- Organizations often offer formal training programs to their leaders.
- Traditional styles provide leaders with required knowledge and skills in a particular area using coursework, practice, "overlearning" with rehearsals, and feedback (Kozlowski, 1998).
- This traditional lecture-based classroom training is useful; however, its limitations include the question of a leader's ability to transfer the information from a training environment to a work setting.

Developmental Job Assignment

- Following formal training, organizations can assign leaders to developmental jobs that target the newly acquired skills.
- A job that is developmental is one in which leaders learn, undergo personal change, and gain leadership skills resulting from the roles, responsibilities, and tasks involved in that job.
- Developmental job assignments are one of the most effective forms of leader development.
- A "stretch" or developmental assignment challenges leaders' new skills and pushes them out of their comfort zone to operate in a more complex environment, one that involves new elements, problems, and dilemmas to resolve (**Fig. 13.20**).

360-Degree Feedback

- The 360-degree feedback approach is a necessary component of leader development that allows leaders to maximize learning opportunities from their current assignment.
- It systematically provides leaders with perceptions of their performance from a full circle of viewpoints, including subordinates, peers, superiors, and the leader's own self-assessment.
- With information coming from so many different sources, the messages may be contradictory and difficult to interpret.
- However, when several different sources concur on a similar perspective, whether a strength or weakness, the clarity of the message increases.
- For this mechanism to be effective, the leader must accept feedback and be open and willing to make changes.
- Coaching is an effective way to facilitate 360-degree feedback and help effect change using open discussion.

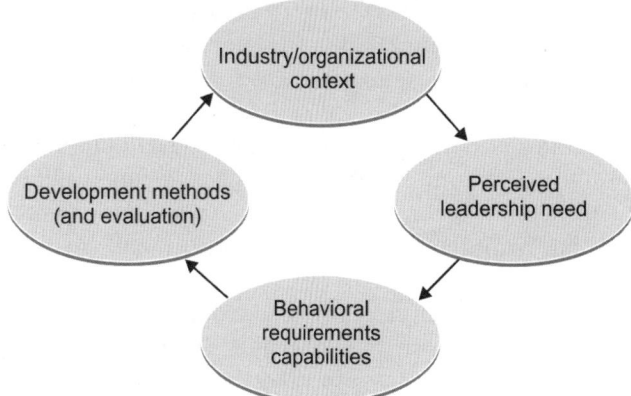

A cluster of five, core enduring themes of leadership

Fig. 13.20: Leadership development—strategy.

Coaching

- Leadership coaching focuses on enhancing the leader's effectiveness, along with the effectiveness of the team and organization.
- It involves an intense, one-on-one relationship aimed at imparting important lessons through assessment, challenge, and support.
- Although the goal of coaching is sometimes to correct a fault, it is used more and more to help already successful leaders move to the next level of increased responsibilities and new and complex challenges.
- Coaching aims to move leaders toward measurable goals that contribute to individual and organizational growth.

Self-directed Learning

- Using self-directed learning, individual leaders teach themselves new skills by selecting areas for development, choosing learning avenues, and identifying resources.
- This type of development is a self-paced process that aims not only to acquire new skills but also to gain a broader perspective on leadership responsibilities and what it takes to succeed as a leader.

Leadership Development Models
- McCauley, Van Veslor, and Ruderman (2010) described a two-part model for developing leaders.
- The first part identifies three elements that combine to make developmental experiences stronger: assessment, challenge, and support.
- Assessment lets leaders know where they stand in areas of strengths, current performance level, and developmental needs.
- Challenging experiences are ones that stretch leaders' ability to work outside of their comfort zone, develop new skills and abilities, and provide important opportunities to learn.

- Support—which comes in the form of bosses, coworkers, friends, family, coaches, and mentors—enables leaders to handle the struggle of developing.
- The second part of the leader-development model illustrates that the development process involves a variety of developmental experiences and the ability to learn from them.
- These experiences and the ability to learn also have an impact on each other: leaders with a high ability to learn from experience will seek out developmental experiences, and through these experiences leaders increase their ability to learn.
- The leader-development process is rooted in a particular leadership context, which includes elements, such as age, culture, economic conditions, population gender, organizational purpose and mission, and business strategy.
- This environment molds the leader development process. Along with assessment, challenge and support, leadership contexts are important aspects of the leader-development model.

General Electric Model of Leadership Development

- Another well-known model of leadership development is used by the General Electric Corporation.
- Managers with high potential are identified early in their careers.
- Their development is monitored and planned to include a variety of job placements to develop skills and experience, a rigorous performance—evaluation process, and formal training programs at the corporate leadership center in Crotonville, New York.
- For top managers, the CEO leads some of the training; the CEO also reviews performance evaluations for high-potential managers during site visits to the various subsidiary divisions.

EFFECTIVE LEADERSHIP IN NURSING

Leadership is critical to advancing the nursing profession. All levels of an organization require strong nursing leadership to establish a healthy work environment. Strong leadership is particularly crucial at the point of care where most front line staff work and patient care is delivered. To develop the leadership skills necessary to support the development of healthy work places, current and future nurses will need guidance and mentoring.

According to the American Association of Colleges of Nursing (AACN), nursing leadership should always be available because nursing leaders play a critical role in helping to give nurses a voice in the development of patient care environments. Leaders can help create a deeply satisfying organizational culture at the unit level by engaging staff in the development of shared values in their work. This demands a pattern shift from a more traditional command-and-control style of staff supervision toward a transformational style of

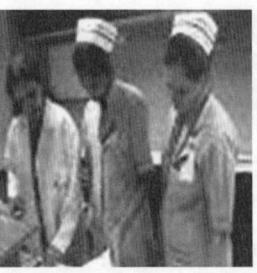

L-lead, love, learn
E-enthusiastic, energetic
A-assertive, achiever
D-dedicated and serious
E-effective, efficient
R-responsible, respectful

Fig. 13.21: Nursing leadership can be best described using the word LEADER.

leadership in which leaders enhance the motivation, confidence and performance of their follower groups **(Fig. 13.21)**.

QUALITIES OF NURSE LEADER

- Knowledge of self, i.e., self-awareness.
- Personal qualities, such as integrity, honesty, ability to co-operate, motivate, enthusiastic and so on.
- Initiative qualities, such as willingness to help and assist self-confidence, courage and decidedness.
- Technical qualities, such as mastery over subject, expert knowledge and expertise to work.
- Teaching abilities, i.e., ability to communicate.
- Administrative abilities, i.e., managing, organizing, co-coordinating, etc.
- Intellectual skills.
- Enthusiasm.
- Tactful ability to win the loyalty and support of others.
- Emotional control.
- Conscientiousness.
- Quality of building human relations.

LEADERSHIP STYLES IN NURSING MANAGEMENT

The way a nurse manager leads her staff not only affects her employees' morale and productivity, it also affects the quality of patient care. At one end of the spectrum, some nurses lead with an authoritarian style, while others put the needs of their employees above all else. However, many find that they can merge strong leadership with an inclusive approach. Five leadership styles for nurses is shown in **Figure 13.22**.

Democratic

- Democratic nurse leaders include their subordinates in goal-setting and decision-making, soliciting their suggestions and feedback.
- Then, they consider this information along with their own research and opinions. However, the leader has the final say.
- This leadership style also encourages the personal and professional development of nurses and allows them some autonomy.
- With its emphasis on individual nurses and their contributions to the team, this style often motivates employees to take initiative and consistently contribute their best efforts.

Five leadership style for nurses
Servant leaders: Develop the skills of individual team members to inspire and motivate them.
Transformational leaders: Unite team members by communicating a shared vision and mission.
Democratic leaders: Focus on improving the system and bringing individuals together.
Authoritarian leaders: Make decisions without input from others and micromanage team members.
Laissez-faire leaders: Use a hands-off, reactive approach instead of actively working to make changes.

Fig. 13.22: Five leadership style for nurses.

Affiliative

- This leadership style puts people first, emphasizing the well-being and job satisfaction of team members.
- Affiliative leaders often take a passive approach to managing their fellow nurses, taking great care not to anger or upset their subordinates.
- They may also hesitate to take a strong stance regarding decision-making, but strive to ensure tasks are completed on time.
- This style can be valuable for boosting morale or bringing together a fractured team, but it inhibits the leader's authority and can interfere with her ability to step in when decisive action is required.
- Without a strong leader to guide the team's efforts, productivity and efficiency can also suffer.

Transformational

- Transformational leaders encourage the personal and professional development of the nurses they manage by promoting teamwork, emphasizing self-esteem and urging employees to participate in the establishment of hospital policies and procedures.
- This leadership style relies on a positive, charismatic approach to managing employees.
- It focuses on strong communication skills, confidence and integrity. Instead of issuing orders and expecting automatic compliance, transformational leaders explain the "how" and "why" of hospital procedures in addition to helping nurses understand the facility's vision.
- They use empathy to understand their employees' needs and motivations, using this insight to tailor their management and communication style to individual employees.

Authoritarian

- Some nurse managers prefer a stricter approach to leadership; they make all the decisions and rarely solicit input or feedback from employees.
- They issue orders and expect employees to carry them out promptly and without question.
- They also closely supervise employees, reducing the amount of autonomy the staff has.
- This leadership style allows for little innovation or flexibility; instead, it requires strict adherence to hospital policies.
- While this strategy often ensures tasks are completed quickly and efficiently, it can also cause discord and job dissatisfaction.

■ MENTORSHIP IN NURSING

Mentoring is a vital process in nursing; it is a means for experienced nurses to orient and to facilitate acclimation of novice nurses to their new role. This process involves the art and science of guiding another through the purposeful actions of inspiring, coaching, teaching, directing, and leading an individual to a new place of cognition (**Fig. 13.23**).

Definition

- A mentor is an experienced practitioner who establishes a caring relationship with a novice nurse as a trusted counselor, guide, role model, teacher, and friend, providing opportunities for personal and career development, growth, and support to the less experienced individual.
- A nurse mentor is a nurse who has more experience in a nursing field than you do and is willing to share their knowledge and time to help you achieve the goals. Mentoring can be done formally or informally.

Character traits and skill of mentor: The best mentors share certain character traits and skill sets that make them right for the task. These traits and skill sets include:

- **Positivity:** Remaining upbeat and undiscouraged, especially in regard to the job of nursing.
- **Tolerance:** Willing to accept all kinds of people.
- **Patience:** Capable of maintaining calm and focus when dealing with difficult challenges.
- **Insight:** Able to assess situations and provide useful solutions and/or advice.
- **Clarity:** Able to clearly communicate information and advice.

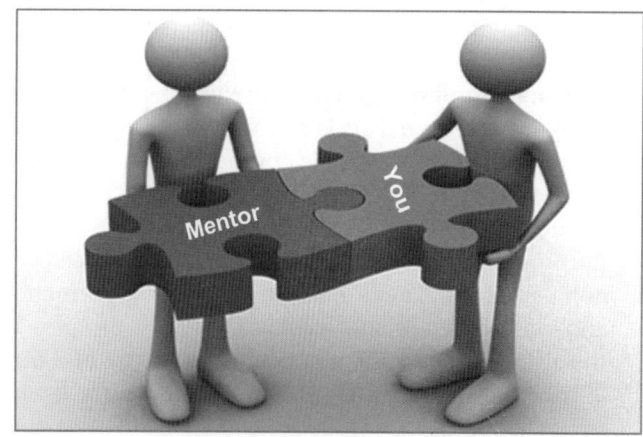

Fig. 13.23: Mentorship in nursing.

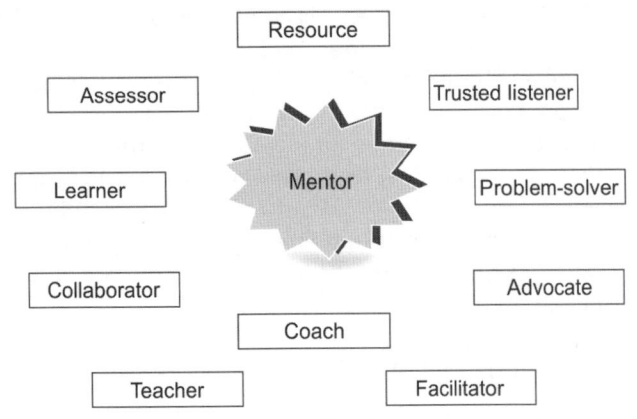

Fig. 13.24: Role of mentor.

- **Commitment:** Possessing an earnest devotion to the job of nursing and the role of nurse mentor. **Figure 13.24** shows role of mentor.

Qualities of an Effective Nurse Mentor

What makes a nurse mentor an effective leader? Mentor-mentee relationships rely on trust, so nurse mentors should know how to establish a rapport of trust between themselves and their mentees. To help ensure a good mentorship relationship, nurse mentors must possess ethical and moral integrity and demonstrate a willingness to share personal and professional stories, including failures. Additional qualities ideal for nurse mentors include the following:

- **Organized manager:** A nurse mentorship, whether formal or informal, should be structured. A competent nurse mentor has strong time management skills to balance clinical responsibilities with scheduled meetings with their mentees to discuss various topics.
- **Advanced professional development:** A knowledgeable nurse mentor can speak to a wide range of topics, from nursing practice and work environment issues to career counseling and personal advice.
- **Persistent:** Practical follow-up skills enable nurse mentors to proactively and regularly check in on their mentees' job satisfaction.
- **Collaborative and goal-oriented:** Both the mentor and mentee should be involved in the development of the mentoring plan, so the ability to establish a vision that sets goals is a crucial competency.
- **Personable and straightforward:** Nurse mentors possess strong interpersonal skills and can communicate with clarity while demonstrating compassion and patience. They are active listeners with strong relationship—building, training, and teaching skills.
- **Encouraging:** Nurse mentors are empathetic, patient, and nonjudgmental. They are skilled in providing affirmation and giving and receiving feedback.
- **Insightful:** Nurse mentors understand the ins and outs of the healthcare system to provide new nurses with strategies for navigating it.

Table 13.4 shows difference between mentor and teacher.

Table 13.4: Difference between mentor and teacher.

Mentor	Teacher
A mentor has greater perspective	A teacher has greater knowledge
Relationship last for long period	Relationship last for specific period
Mentor is more experienced and qualified. Often a senior person who pass on knowledge, experience and open doors to reach opportunities	Teacher does not require to have direct experience as of student aspirational role, unless teaching is skill focused and specific
Mentoring goals are set	The agenda is focused on achieving specific and immediate goals
Mentor does not link own success to that of mentee	Teacher may link own success to that of student
Mentor does not have own personal agenda	Teacher may have own personal agenda
It is more relationship building	Teacher promote skills development and attitude changes

Usefulness of Mentorship

"Mentoring helps cultivate nurse leaders, retain nurses, and diversify the nursing workforce." By strengthening the nursing workforce, nursing mentorship improves the quality of patient care and outcomes. The Foundation identifies three specific benefits:

- Mentoring can foster the leadership skills that nurses need to secure larger roles in developing, designing and delivering health care.
- Mentoring relationships inside healthcare organizations and academic institutions can help those organizations retain nurses and nurse educators, reducing the cost of turnover.
- Mentoring can help diversify the mostly white and female profession by supporting minority and male nurses. This diversification can lead to fewer health disparities within the population by providing diverse role models.

Benefits of taking student nurses are discussed in **Box 13.6**.

Successful Nursing Mentorship

According to mentoring guidelines from the Academy of Medical-Surgical Nurses, "Successful mentoring relationships must be built on trust, openness to self-disclosure, affirmation, and willingness and skill in giving and receiving feedback." The guidelines state the following:

- The mentor and mentee must trust each other.
- They both must be willing to share information about themselves, including unpleasant experiences they have had.
- They both must give constructive feedback—positive and negative.
- Mentors need to let mentees know regularly that they believe the mentee will succeed.

■ PRECEPTORSHIP IN NURSING

Preceptors and preceptorships have been a part of nursing for many years. Preceptors teach students across a variety

> **Box 13.6:** Benefits of taking student nurses.
>
> - Provides professional development opportunity for nurses.
> - Brings enthusiasm and two-way learning into practices.
> - Enables nurses to keep up-to-date with clinical knowledge and skills.
> - Gives student nurses the opportunity to experience a quality placement.
> - Is a great recruitment tool.
> - Helps secure the primary care workforce of the future.

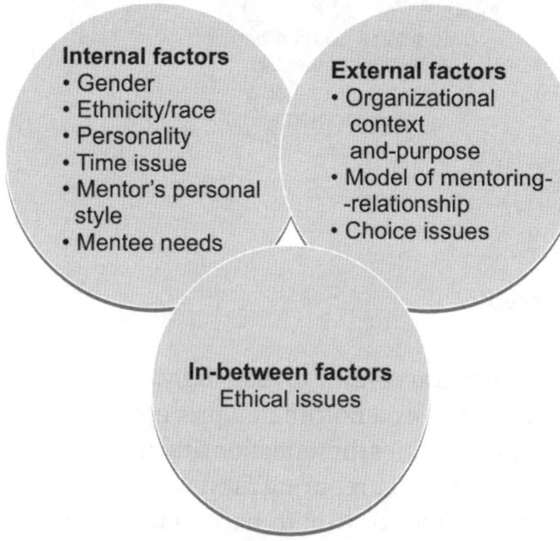

and knowledgeable in their role, both clinically and as an instructor.

Benefits of Preceptorship

Preceptorship helps newly registered professionals have the best possible start as a registered professional. Preceptorship has a variety of benefits for employers and preceptees, among others.

Benefits for nurses, midwives and nursing associates:

- Preceptorship offers the structured support needed to transition their knowledge into everyday practice successfully.
- It provides a lifelong journey of reflection and the ability to self-identify continuing professional development needs.
- A positive preceptorship experience is reported to result in newly registered nurses, midwives and nursing associates having increased confidence and sense of belonging, feeling valued by their employer.

Internal factors
- Gender
- Ethnicity/race
- Personality
- Time issue
- Mentor's personal style
- Mentee needs

External factors
- Organizational context and-purpose
- Model of mentoring-relationship
- Choice issues

In-between factors
Ethical issues

Fig. 13.25: Factors that influence mentoring relationship.

Benefits for Employers

Effective preceptorship outcomes are linked to improved recruitment and retention. Attracting and retaining skilled nurses, midwives, and nursing associates is important for delivering better, safe and effective care.

Principles of Preceptorship

Organizational culture and preceptorship: A period of preceptorship immerses the newly registered nurse, midwife and nursing associate into their professional role and into the ways of working and culture of their new workplace.

A good organizational culture that supports preceptorship will have the following characteristics:

- It is kind, fair, impartial, transparent, collaborative and fosters good interprofessional and multiagency relationships.
- There is an understanding of the importance of having systems and processes in place to support and build confidence of newly registered nurses, midwives and nursing associates.
- There is an approach to preceptorship that prioritizes individual mental and physical health and wellbeing, and promotes accountability, self-reflection and safe practice in accordance with the Code.

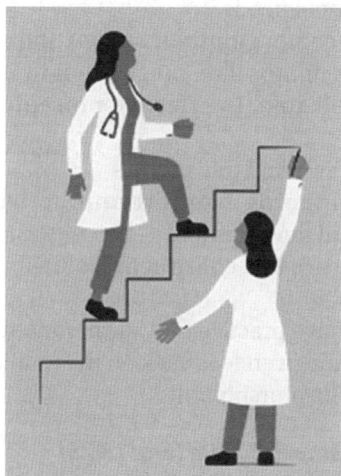

Fig. 13.26: Preceptorship in nursing.

Benefits of being a preceptor is shown in **Figure 13.27**.

Quality and Oversight of Preceptorship (Box 13.7)

Being committed to the Principles of Preceptorship and having preceptorship programs available/running is seen as key activities within the organization. There is evidence of management of the process, and evaluation of its efficacy and outcome.

To ensure effective preceptorship:

- There are processes in place to identify those who require preceptorship.

of acute, community, and continuing care practices. They provide a safety net of experienced staff to answer questions and provide insight. While there are multiple considerations for providing a preceptor experience **(Fig. 13.26)**.

Definition

- A preceptorship is defined as a relationship between an experienced nursing staff member and a newly hired staff member; the length of this relationship depends on the orientation period of the specific nursing unit or clinic.
- Nursing preceptors initiate new staff to the professional environment. To be successful, preceptors must be willing

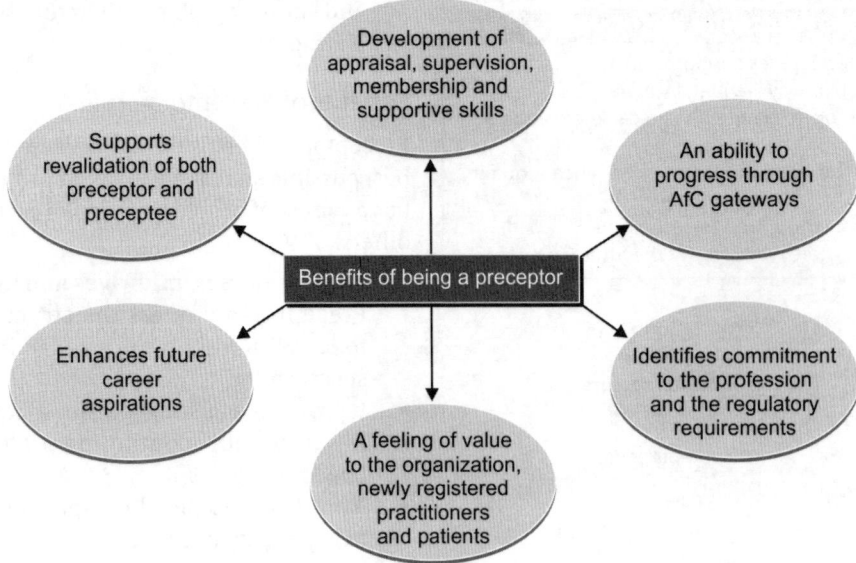

Fig. 13.27: Benefits of being a preceptor.

> **Box 13.7:** Qualities of an effective preceptor.
> - Good communication skills
> - A professional role model
> - Willing to invest time in preceptee
> - A good listener and problem-solver
> - Sensitive to the needs and inexperience of the preceptee
> - Familiar with current theory and practice
> - Competent and confident, in the preceptor role
> - Nonjudgmental attitude to coworkers
> - Assertiveness
> - Flexibility to change
> - Adaptability to individual teaching needs

- There is sufficient preceptor capacity to support all of those who require preceptorship.
- The employer, preceptees and preceptors understand and comply with national and local policies, and the relevant governance requirements required.
- Preceptorship activities should complement the preceptees' induction and orientation into the local workplace.
- There is recognition of the impact of system challenges on effective preceptorship and how to mitigate these.
- Processes are in place to monitor, evaluate and review preceptorship programs.
- There is a governance framework around preceptorship which allows the process to be audited and reported.

Preceptee Empowerment

Preceptorship is tailored to the individual nurse, midwife and nursing associate preceptee's new role and the health or care setting. It seeks to recognize and support the needs of the preceptee to promote their confidence in their professional healthcare role.

In effective preceptorship models, preceptees:
- Are provided with the appropriate resources to enable them to develop confidence as newly registered nurses, midwives and nursing associates.
- Are supported according to their individual learning needs.
- Are supported by a nominated preceptor.
- Have opportunities for reflection and feedback to support their approach to preparing for revalidation.
- Are empowered to work in partnership with preceptors and are able to influence the content and length of their preceptorship program to meet both individual and organizational needs.

Preparing preceptors for their supporting role: Preceptors should receive appropriate preparation to understand and undertake their role. In effective preceptorship models, preceptors:
- Act as professional role models
- Receive ongoing support and actively engage in professional development
- Are supportive and constructive in their approach to the preceptee
- Share effective practice and learn from others
- Seek and are given feedback on the quality of all aspects of their preceptorship role.

The Preceptorship Program (Fig. 13.28)

Preceptorship should take account of the setting in which the individual nurse, midwife and nursing associate is working and providing care.

Preceptorship programs will:
- Be timely and align with the start of a new employment role
- Recognize the knowledge, skills, attributes and competence nurses, midwives and nursing associates have at the point of registration.
- Seek to ensure that activities within the program are agreed with the individual preceptee
- Vary in length and content according to the needs of the individual nurse, midwife and nursing associate and the organization. Individual countries, regions or organizations may set minimum or maximum lengths for preceptorship.

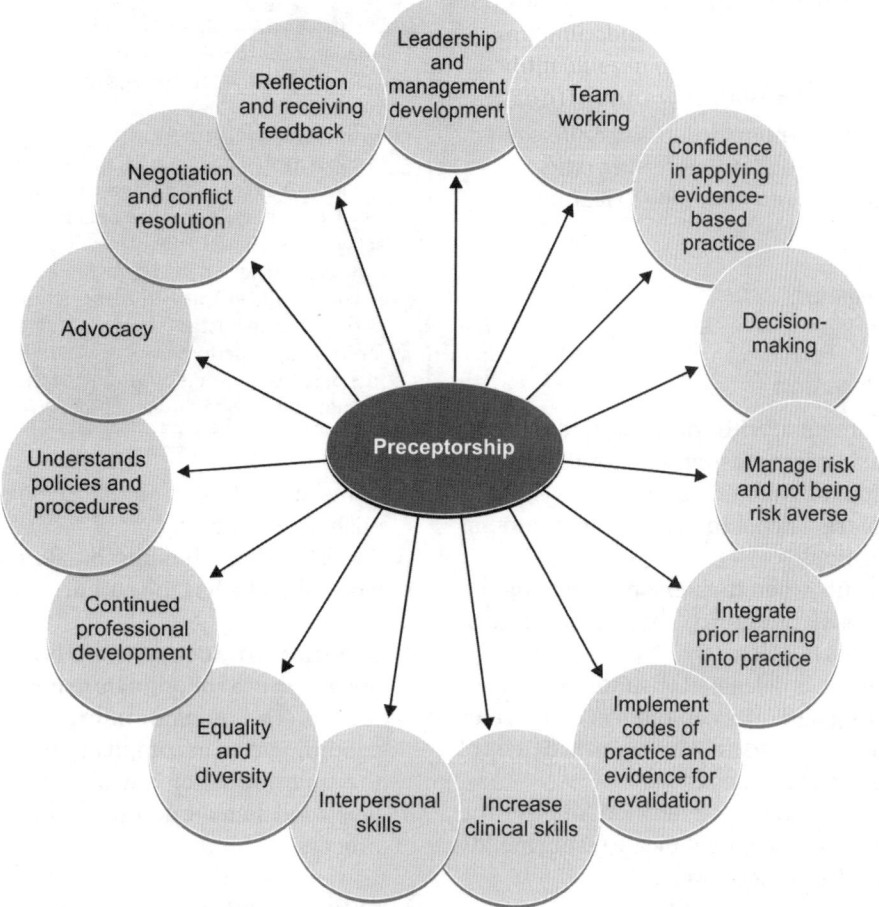

Fig. 13.28: Preceptorship.

- Include activities designed to welcome and integrate the preceptee into the team and place of work.
- Be designed to ensure that it is possible for the preceptee to meet the aims and outcomes of the preceptorship program within the agreed timeframe.

DELEGATION

Delegation is the assignment of authority to another person (normally from a manager to a subordinate) to carry out specific activities. It is the process of distributing and entrusting work to another person. Delegation is one of the core concepts of management leadership **(Fig. 13.29)**.

Definitions

- The entrustment of a part or responsibility and authority to another and the creation of accountability for performance. —*Allen*
- "Delegation takes place when one person gives another the right to perform work on his behalf and in his name, and the second person accepts a corresponding duty or obligation to do what is required of him." —*OS Hiner*
- "Delegation refers to a manager's ability to share his burden with others. It consists of granting authority or the right to decision-making in certain defined areas and charging subordinates with responsibility for carrying through an assigned task." —*Douglas C Basil*

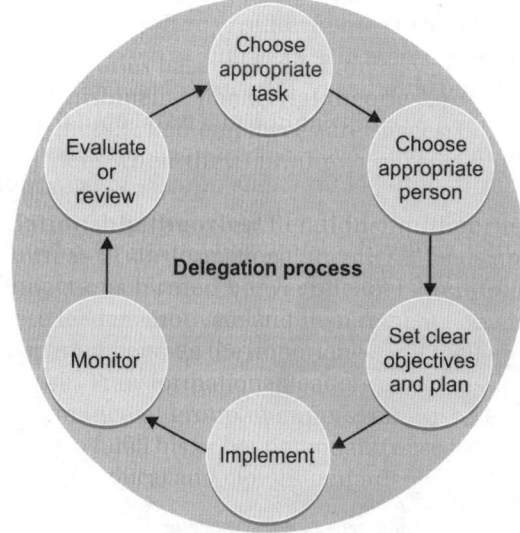

Fig. 13.29: Delegation process.

Purpose of Delegation

The following are five purposes of delegating:
1. Assigning routine tasks
2. Problem solving
3. Changes in the nurse manager's own job emphasis
4. Capability building

5. Assigning tasks for which the nurse manager does not have time.

Principles of Delegation (Box 13.8)

- Select the right person to whom the job is to be delegated.
- Delegate both interesting and uninteresting tasks.
- Provide subordinates with enough time to learn.
- Delegate gradually
- Delegate in advance
- Consult before delegating
- Avoid gaps and overlaps

Characteristics of Delegation

Inclination is the assignment of authority to subordinates in a defined area and making them responsible for the results. Delegation has the following characteristics:

- Delegation takes place when a manager grants some of his powers to subordinates.
- Delegation occurs only when the person delegating the authority himself has that authority, i.e., a manager must possess what he wants to delegate.
- Only a part of authority is delegated to subordinates.
- A manager delegating authority can reduce, enhance or take it back. He exercises full control over the activities of the subordinates even after delegation.
- It is only the authority which is delegated and not the responsibility. A manager cannot abdicate responsibility by delegating authority to subordinates.

Elements of Delegation (Box 13.9)

Delegation involves following three elements:

1. **Assignment of responsibility:** The first step in delegation is the assignment of work or duty to the subordinate, i.e., delegation of authority. The superior asks his subordinate to perform a particular task in a given period of time. It is the description of the role assigned to the subordinate. Duties in terms of functions or tasks to be performed constitute the basis of delegation process.
2. **Grant of authority:** The grant of authority is the second element of delegation. The delegator grants authority to the subordinates so that the assigned task is accomplished. The delegation of responsibility with authority is meaningless. The subordinate can only accomplish the work when he has the authority required for completing that task.
3. **Creation of accountability:** Accountability is the obligation of a subordinate to perform the duties assigned to him. The delegation creates an obligation on the subordinate to accomplish the task assigned to him by the superior. When a work is assigned and authority is delegated then the accountability is the by-product of this process.

Types of Delegation

Delegation may be of the following types:

- **General or specific delegation:** When authority is given to perform general managerial functions, such as planning, organizing, directing etc., the subordinate managers perform these functions and enjoy the authority required to carry out these responsibilities. The specific delegation may relate to a particular function or an assigned task.
- **Formal or informal delegation:** Formal delegation of authority is the part of organizational structure. Whenever a task is assigned to a person then the required authority is also given to him. This type of delegation is part of the normal functioning of the organization. Every person is automatically given authority as per his duties.
- **Lateral delegation:** When a person is delegated an authority to accomplish a task, he may need the assistance of a number of persons. It may take time to formally get assistance from these persons.
- **Reserved authority and delegated authority:** A delegator may not like to delegate every authority to the subordinates. The authority which he keeps with him

---

Box 13.9: The elements of delegation.

Delegation is the process of entrusting and transferring responsibility and authority by the top management to the lowest level. The elements of delegation are the following:

- **Responsibility:** The work or duty assigned to a particular position. Involves mental and physical activities which must be performed to carry out a task or duty. Two categories: management functions which covers POSDICON and operative functions which include all activities that have to do directly with their specialization.
- **Authority:** Refers to the power or the right to be obeyed.
- **Accountability:** This is the answerability of the obligation to perform the delegated responsibility and to exercise the authority for the proper performance of the work. It cannot be delegated. It is given to the person who accepts the responsibility and is accountable only to the extent that he is given the authority to.

Box 13.8: Principles of delegation.

- Principle of delegation by results expected
- Principle of functional definition
- Scalar principle
- Authority principle
- Principle of unity of command
- Principle of absoluteness of responsibility
- Principle of parity of authority and responsibility

Basis	Authority	Responsibility	Accountability
Meaning	It means right to command	It is the obligation to perform an assigned task	It means the answerability for outcome of the assigned task
Delegation	It can be delegated	It cannot be entirely delegated	It cannot be delegated at all
Origin	It arises from formal position	It arises from delegated authority	It arises from responsibility
Flow	It flows downward from superior to subordinate	It flows upward from subordinate to superior	It flows upward from subordinate to superior

is called reserved authority and the authority which is assigned to the subordinates is delegated authority.
- **Prerequisites for delegation:** Every superior tries to retain as much authority as possible. The load of work or circumstances may compel delegation downwards. If the authority is not willingly delegated then it will not bring desired results.
- **Willingness to delegate:** The first prerequisite to delegation is the willingness of the superior to part with his authority. Unless the superior is psychologically prepared to leave his authority, delegation will not be effective.
- **Climate of trust and confidence:** There should be a climate of trust and confidence among superiors and subordinates. The subordinates should be given enough opportunities or real job situations where they use their talent and experience.
- **Faith in subordinates:** Sometimes the superiors do not delegate authority with the fear that subordinates will not be able to handle the job independently. They are not confident of the qualities of subordinates and do not want to take risks. The superior may be over conscious of his skill and competence with the result that he is hesitant to delegate authority.
- **Fear of supervisors:** There is often a fear among superiors that their subordinates may not over take them, once they are given higher responsibility.

Principles of delegation is discuss in **Box 13.9**.

Barriers in Delegation

Delegation barriers many managers experience or **(Fig. 13.30)**.
- **Ego:** I can do it better myself.
- **Time:** Takes too long to explain.
- **Accountability:** I'm accountable if it goes wrong.
- **Skills gaps:** My staff do not possess the technical skills.
- **Authority threat:** Delegation reduces my own authority. Stressed out managers who go from crisis to crisis and spend most of their working day 'fighting fires' are probably failing to delegate. The 'firefighting' is reactive management, not proactive management.

Benefits of Delegating

Delegation of tasks to others offers the following benefits:
- Gives you the time and ability to focus on higher-level tasks
- Gives others the ability to learn and develop new skills
- Develops trust between workers and improves communication
- Improves efficiency, productivity, and time management

Guidelines for Delegating Tasks

Although delegating tasks boosts efficiency and productivity, and improves time management, it is important to delegate tasks correctly. Here are some things to keep top-of-mind:
- Ensure that the objectives are clear and that the person taking on the additional responsibility has the tools to do it well.
- Ask for any concerns and be open to suggestions and ideas.
- Provide a guideline on the amount of time and/or money to be spent on the delegated task.
- Play to the individual's strength–each person has a unique skill-set and talent. Delegate work that is likely result in better overall efficiency.
- For long-term delegated tasks, follow-up to keep your workers on the right track.

Advantages of Delegation (Fig. 13.31)

- **Best use of human resource:** Proper delegation means effective use of work force. Task assigned keeping in mind the skills of an employee often gives good results.
- **More time:** Effective delegating skills work gives managers extra time to do other work that are of more critical nature.
- **Speeds up decision-making:** Empowering subordinates to take decisions in their area of expertise speeds up the work process as they do not have to seek approval at every step.
- **Builds team spirit:** Working together generates team spirit, develops team involvement and understanding of the business.
- **Improves interpersonal and intrapersonal communication:** Employees through daily interaction get

Barriers in the delegate/subordinate
1. Lack of experience
2. Lack of competence
3. Lack of self-confidence
4. Lack of incentives
5. Fear of harsh criticism from supervisor
6. Overdependence on the boss
7. Overload of work

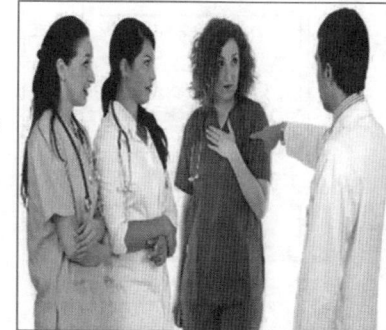

Fig. 13.30: Barriers to delegation.

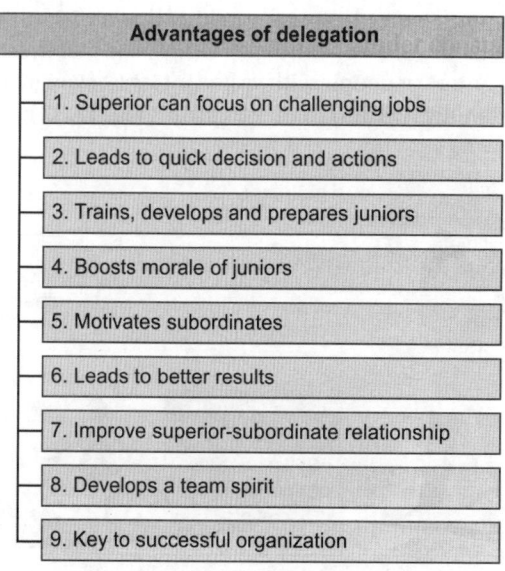

Advantages of delegation
1. Superior can focus on challenging jobs
2. Leads to quick decision and actions
3. Trains, develops and prepares juniors
4. Boosts morale of juniors
5. Motivates subordinates
6. Leads to better results
7. Improve superior-subordinate relationship
8. Develops a team spirit
9. Key to successful organization

Fig. 13.31: Advantages of delegation.

opportunities to learn from each other and reflect on their own work.

- **Inflow of new and innovative ideas:** Different ideas and perspectives inspire people to see things from a different angle, motivate them to explore other areas of development and keep them engaged.
- **Helps build bench strength:** The work environment trains and prepares the employees to face adverse situations so that the work does not get hindered under any circumstances.

Disadvantages of Delegation

Effective delegating work can have a flip side if the responsibilities are over, under or wrongly delegated. To avoid adversities the knowledge of what to delegate, whom to delegate and how much to delegate is extremely important.

- **Lack of knowledge of employees skills:** Wrong delegation of task can prove fatal for a project and business.
- **Lack of trust:** Many managers either lack trust or do not want to trust their subordinates. They try to do everything themselves due to which their work pressure never gets eased out.
- **Lack of interest:** Managers who keep the interesting work to themselves and assign routine and monotonous to others give rise of discontentment and disengagement.
- **Lack of credit:** When multiple people work on a single project the credit of the work often gets distributed. The true contribution of each person is at times not recognized.
- **Lack of authority:** It is also important to delegate sufficient authority along with responsibility. Only then can employees work their full potential.

■ POWER AND POLITICS

Power and politics in organizations are a reality that no organization can ignore. Though the evolution of the modern corporation and the concomitant rise of the managerial class with a professional way of running the firms is touted to be one of the contributory factors for the decline on power politics in organizations, one cannot just simply say that there are no power centers or people with vested interests even in the most professionally run and managed firms **(Fig. 13.32)**.

Definition

- Power refers to a capacity that A has to influence the behavior of B, so that B acts in accordance with A's wishes. This definition implies a potential that need not be actualized to be effective and a dependency relationship.
- Power is frequently defined as the ability to influence the behavior of others with or without resistance.

Bases of Power (Fig. 13.33)

Formal Power

- **Coercive power:** Power that is based on fear.
- **Reward power:** Compliance achieved based on the ability to distribute rewards that others view as valuable.
- **Legitimate power:** The power a person receives as a result of his or her position in the formal hierarchy of an organization.
- **Information power:** Power that comes from access to and control over information.

Personal Power

- **Expert power:** Influence based on special skills or knowledge.
- **Referent power:** Influence based on possession by an individual or desirable resources or personal traits.
- **Charismatic power:** An extension of referent power stemming from an individual's personality and interpersonal style.

Power Tactics

Ways in which individuals translate power bases into specific actions:

- Legitimacy
- Rational persuasion
- Inspirational appeals
- Consultation
- Exchange
- Personal appeals
- Ingratiation
- Pressure
- Coalitions

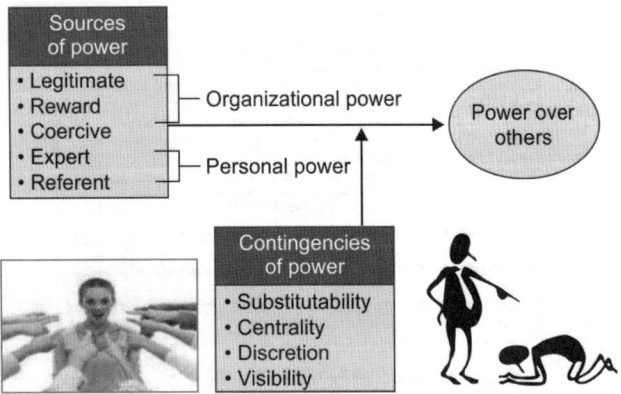

Fig. 13.32: Power and politics.

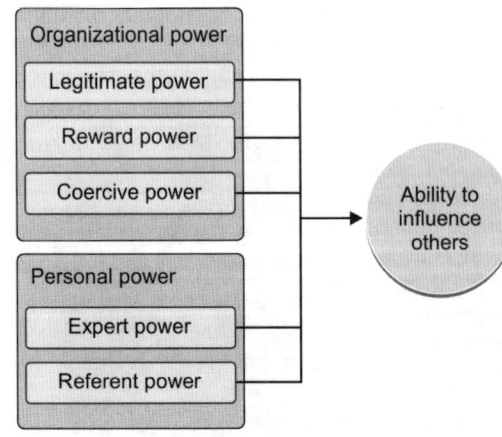

Fig. 13.33: Bases of power.

Power in groups: Coalitions
- Coalition—an informal group bound together by the active pursuit of a single issue
- Coalitions seek to maximize their size = "strength" in numbers

Sexual harassment: Unwelcome advances, requests for sexual favors, and other verbal or physical conduct of a sexual nature. Sexual harassment is about power.

POLITICS

Political behavior are those activities that are not required as part of one's formal role in the organization, but that influence, or attempt to influence, the distribution of advantages and disadvantages within the organization. Legitimate and illegitimate political behaviors are common in organizations. Politics is a fact of life in organizations.

Workplace politics, (office politics or organizational politics) is the use of power and social networking within an organization to achieve changes that benefit the organization or individuals within it. Influence by individuals may serve personal interests without regard to their effect on the organization itself.

Factors Contributing to Political Behavior
- Individual factors (e.g., personality traits, needs)
- Organizational factors (e.g., when organizational resources decline, resources change, low trust exists, high performance pressures, and the opportunity of promotion exists = political behavior is likely)

How do People Respond to Organizational Politics?
- Decreased job satisfaction, increased anxiety, increased turnover, and reduced performance
- Defensive actions: Reactive and protective behaviors to avoid action, blame, or change. **Figure 13.34** shows organization policies that threaten employees.

Types of Politics (Fig. 13.35)
- Attacking and blaming
- Selectively distributing information
- Controlling information
- Forming coalitions
- Cultivating networks
- Creating obligations
- Managing impressions

Impression Management
The process by which individuals attempt to control the impression others form of them. Techniques include conformity, excuses, apologies, self-promotion, flattery, favors, and association.

Implications for Managers
- Power is a two-way street – others are trying to build power along with you.
- Few employees relish being powerless in their jobs and organization.

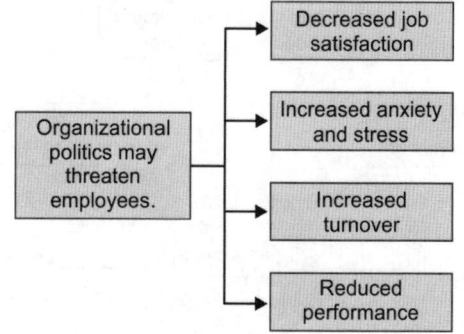

Fig. 13.34: Organization policy threaten employees.

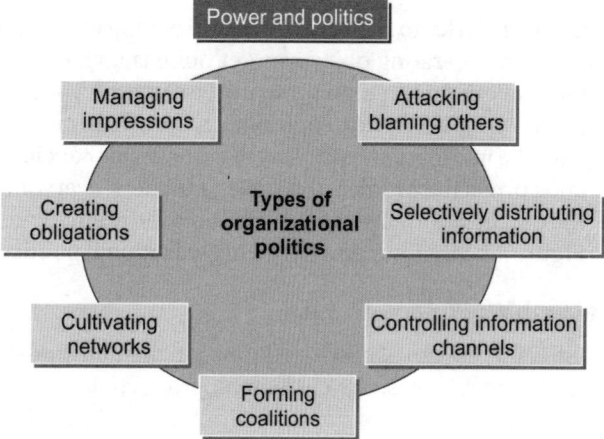

Fig. 13.35: Types of organizational politics.

- People respond differently to various power bases.
- Employees working under coercive managers are unlikely to be committed, and more likely to resist the manager.
- Expert power is the most strongly and consistently related to effective employee performance.
- The power of the boss may also play a role in determining your job satisfaction.
- The effective manager accepts the political nature of organizations.
- Regardless of level in the organization, some people are more politically "astute" than others.
- The politically naive and inept tend to feel continually powerless.

Overcoming Ineffective Politics
- **Create a thematic goal:** The goal should be something that everyone in the organization can believe in, such as, for a hospital, giving the best care to all patients. This goal should be a single goal, qualitative, time-bound, and shared.
- **Create a set of defining objectives:** This step should include objectives that everyone agrees will help bring the thematic goal to fruition.
- **Create a set of ongoing standard operating objectives:** This process should be done within each area so that the best operating standards are developed. These objectives should also be shared across the organization so everyone is aware of them.

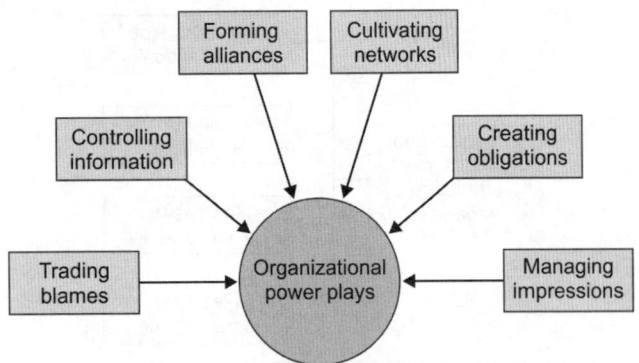

Fig. 13.36: Power and organizational politics.

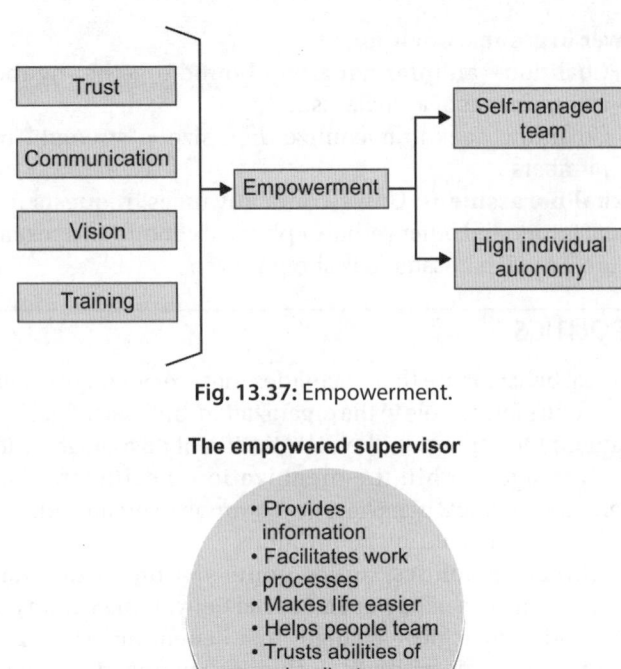

Fig. 13.37: Empowerment.

- **Create metrics to measure them:** Measuring whether the standard operating objectives get done is a vital step in the process. Rather than someone else pointing out what is not working, all the people within the department will have the information necessary to come to this conclusion and correct the problem, because ultimately, everyone in the organization cares about achieving the thematic goal. **Figure 13.36** shows power and organizational politics.

Deal with Workplace Abuse

No one wants abuses of power to happen in their business. It's harmful to employees, the customers, productivity, and the business' overall environment. Preventing it does not always work, as people cannot be fully controlled. If there are abuses of power occurring in your business, here are a few things that can be done:

- **Confront the person:** Best done carefully and in private, confronting the person who is on a power trip or abusing their power is one way of getting them to stop. Someone who has only recently started to become abusive due to their power may not realize that what they are doing is hurtful and unprofessional; power can be an intoxicating force.
- **Document:** It keep track of instances of abuse by documenting it. Write down notes on what happened, when, and where, and take it home with you; never leave it at work where an abusive person may find it and use it as a motive to attack. Check what laws and policies there are regarding recording someone without their permission.
- **Human resources:** A business' human resources department is designed to handle any instance of misbehavior amongst the staff at work. They will have the resources to deal with the situation and will know what can or cannot be done.

■ EMPOWERMENT

In organizations, empowerment means granting employees the autonomy to assume a more active and responsible role. This is accomplished by strengthening their sense of effectiveness as well as by sharing power, information and the responsibility to manage their own work as much as possible. In terms of organizational culture, empowerment is related to the individual autonomy dimension.

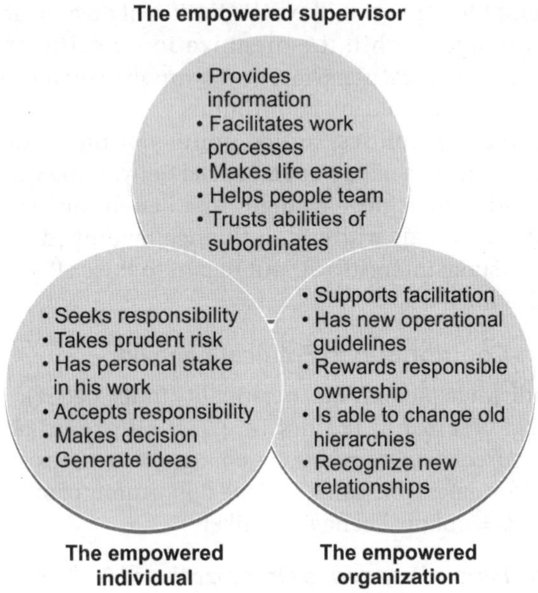

Fig. 13.38: Concepts of empowerment.

Empowerment is the concept in management that if employees are given information, resources, and opportunity at the same time as being held responsible for their job outcomes, then they will be more productive and have higher job satisfaction **(Fig. 13.37)**.

Definition

- Employee empowerment is a management strategy that aims to give employees the tools and resources necessary to make confident decisions in the workplace without supervision. Empowerment is a long-term, resource-intensive strategy that involves significant time and financial investment from the organization's leaders.
- Empowerment refers to the delegation of some authority and responsibility to employees and involving them in the decision-making process, not in mere job activities, but rather at all the levels of management.

Concept of Empowerment (Fig. 13.38)

- Empowerment is the degree of autonomy and self-determination in people and in communities.
- This enables them to represent their interests in a responsible and self-determined way, acting on their own authority.

- It is the process of becoming stronger and more confident, especially in controlling one's life and claiming one's rights.
- Empowerment as action refers both to the process of self-empowerment and to professional support of people, which enables them to overcome their sense of powerlessness and lack of influence, and to recognize and use their resources.

Levels of Empowerment in the Workplace

It is important to understand that empowerment can be developed at three levels:

Organizational Level

An organization that cultivates employee empowerment can better:
- Embrace change, such as digital transformation
- Recognize employees' contribution to the business
- Reward responsible ownership in the workplace
- Support collaboration, including cross-departmental collaboration in the workplace
- Foster a culture of employee engagement
- Retain top talent

Managerial Level

Empowered team leaders can:
- Better support the team and help each team member reach their targets
- Provide the information the teams need when they need it
- Inspire and motivate employees
- Help better connect employees, including the ones working remotely
- Facilitate work processes
- Spread team spirit in the workplace
- Better communicate the business goals and long-term vision
- Make the teams more successful

Individual Level

When employees feel empowered and trusted, they (**Fig. 13.39**):
- Are more willing to go the extra mile for the team and the business
- Take ownership over their work
- Generate ideas
- Know how to take prudent risks to take the business to the next level
- Find meaning and purpose at work
- Feel proud of the company they are working at
- Feel more motivated and engaged

Implementing Empowerment (Fig. 13.40)

By understanding possible barriers to empowerment, here are how empowerment can be implemented in organizations:

At company level:
- Develop a clear mission and communicate it clearly to all employees

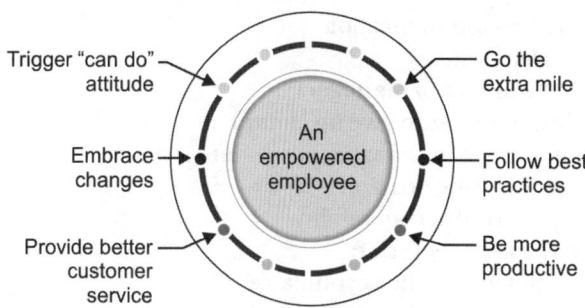

Fig. 13.39: An empowered employee.

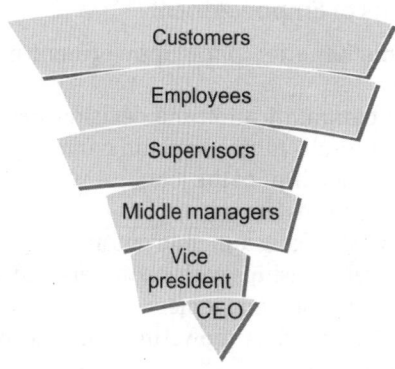

Fig. 13.40: Levels of empowerment in the workplace.

- Build trust within the organization at all levels
- Build an organizational culture that encourage innovation and risk taking
- Provide adequate training so that staff can handle the empowerment
- Replace hierarchical structure with self-managed teams
- Set clear boundaries for authority and accountability

At team level:
- Get staff to involve in selecting their work assignments and the methods for accomplishing tasks
- Create an environment of cooperation, information sharing, discussion, and shared ownership of goals
- Encourage staff to take initiative, make decision, and use their knowledge
- When problems arise, find out what staff think and let them help design the solutions.
- Stay out of the way, give staff the freedom to put their ideas and solutions into practice.
- Maintain high morale and confidence by recognizing successes and encouraging high performance.

Barriers to Empowerment

Here are some barriers that may prevent empowerment to be implemented:

From the aspect of organization:
- Lack of trust between manager and staff
- No clear definition and policy about accountability
- Empowered staff does not receive enough training to be able to handle the empowerment
- No differentiation between staff

- Lack of communication
- Unclear vision

From the aspect of manager:
- Unwillingness to give up control
- Reluctance to change management style
- Fear of losing position
- Cling to old accountability

From the aspect of staff:
- Do not want to be accountable
- Do not realize their values and potentials
- Fear of losing position due to new accountability
- Lack of training

Pros and Cons of Empowerment

Here are some benefits that empowerment may bring to organizations:
- Improves communication and decision-making
- Improves morale, motivation and commitment
- Creates "ownership" of the job
- Increases job satisfaction
- Increases risk-taking and innovation
- Improves relationships with customers and suppliers
- Reduces layers of management

On the other hand, empowerment may also have some negative effects:
- Not everyone wants to be empowered
- We cannot just empower staff and assume that they will assume the empowerment
- Empowerment may not be appropriate for some organizations
- Empowerment actually requires more management effort
- Empowerment means changes and constant changes may keep things unsettled
- There is a risk that empowerment efforts may fail

Enhances empowerment in the workplace:
- Helping employees to stay up-to-date with the company news and industry trends
- Helping employees to get the information they need when they need it so they do not have to spend time looking for it
- Sharing personalized messages with the employees
- Encouraging employees to communicate through their favorite channels.
- Allowing employees to react to the content shared with them and encouraging them to drive discussions in the workplace through questions and comments.
- Allowing employees to personalize their newsfeed so they receive content on the topics they are interested in addition to the content shared within their teams.
- Making it easy for employees to share company news and industry-related content on social media. With Smarp, employees can easily develop their personal brands and position themselves as industry experts through the advocacy amplifier.

■ MENTORING

Mentoring is the employee training system under which a senior or more experienced person (the mentor) is assigned to

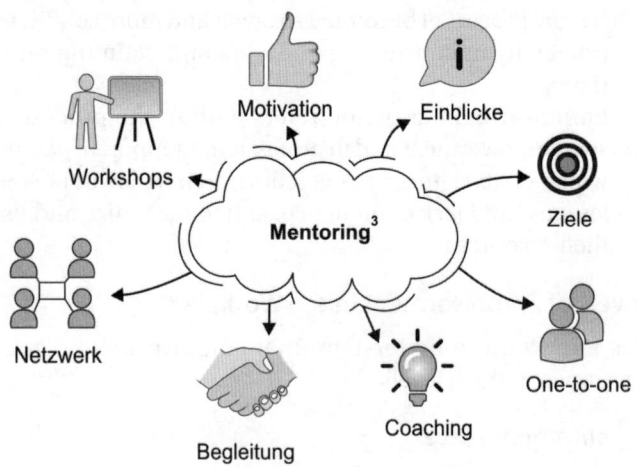

Fig. 13.41: Mentoring.

act as an advisor, counselor, or guide to a junior or trainee. The mentor is responsible for providing support to, and feedback on, the person in his or her charge **(Fig. 13.41)**.

Concept of Mentoring
- Mentoring is an ongoing relationship that is developed between a senior and junior employee.
- Mentoring provides guidance and clear understanding of how the organization goes to achieve its vision and mission to the junior employee.
- Mentoring is a need felt by women recently, when they see the rise of their male counterparts in the workforce. Having a mentor means you have a formally appointed 'guru' at the workplace.

Types
Mentoring can be informal or formal:
- Informal mentoring takes place spontaneously between senior and more junior employees.
- Formal mentoring occurs through a program with an established structure.

Purpose of a Mentorship
- The purpose of a mentorship program is to match up a manager or other experienced employee with someone new to the company or position.
- The mentor takes a mentee, or protégé, under her wing and helps groom his professional career.
- A mentor program can be formal, as in the case of assigning a mentor to a protégé and following specific guidelines for the program, or it can be informal, such as to encourage people to volunteer their services or seek out a mentor and meet on their own terms.
- A successful mentoring program will not only help retain employees, it will assist your training efforts and help boost employee morale.

Key Points on Mentoring
- Mentoring focus on attitude development
- Conducted for management-level employees

- Mentoring is done by someone inside the company
- It is one-to-one interaction.
- It helps in identifying weaknesses and focus on the area that needs improvement.

Ways to become a good mentor at workplace:
Successful people usually attribute a part of their success to their mentors. A good mentor can actually guide and advice a mentee in reaching great professional heights. Here are five ways you can become a great mentor.

1. **Have interest:** Being a great mentor works only when you have genuine interest on your mentee. Choose your mentees well so that you happily invest time in the relationship. Understand the mentee's background and narrative and help him figure out his current situation as well as dreams and aspirations.
2. **Perceive:** Be sensitive to the mentee's environment and situation and use your understanding and personal experience to hear and understand the things that the mentee did not share. Be perceptive in anticipating challenges and share from your life to encourage communication. Maintain confidentiality to increase trust.
3. **Listening and learning:** Have a regular conversation with your mentee. At least once a month works well. Find a common time and informal environment for meeting. Give your mentee undivided attention and ask open ended questions to help the mentee speak freely and openly. For best outcomes, constantly learn from your interactions.
4. **Commitment:** Have an open door policy for your mentees to approach you and seek help whenever required. If they are serious and committed to their personal growth, use your network to make the appropriate connections for them. Be committed to fulfilling your promises to your mentees and hold them accountable too.
5. **Provide feedback:** Ask questions before you advice. Be nonjudgmental and drop biases before you give feedback. Be proactive and assertive in discussing areas of improvement. Figure out how your feedback chats can be structured for maximum effectiveness. Finally, encourage the mentees to take their own decisions.

Responsibilities of a Mentor

The responsibilities of all mentors:
- Assist the employee in developing talents.
- Maintain objectivity and balance.
- Allow the employee to grow and become more independent.
- Foster a sense of risk-taking and independence.
- Balance the responsibilities you take on for the employee.

The additional responsibilities of mentors in a formal program:
- Listen to and acknowledge the employee without undermining the role of the manager.
- Encourage the employee to resolve problems directly with the manager.

Activities of a Mentor

- Attend regular meetings with the mentee, preferably in an informal environment
- Prepare for meetings
- Set the agenda for discussions in collaboration with the mentee
- Allow out of turn meeting with the mentee if the mentee needs one
- Work out plan of action for the mentee in consultation with him
- Maintain dialogue and discussions
- Act as a sounding board
- Observe the mentee and train mentee to observe others
- Provide feedback to mentee
- Acclimatize the mentee with the values, culture, policies and systems of the organization
- Maintain confidentiality befitting mentor-mentee relationship
- Take relevant training to become a better mentor
- Share information with the mentee about continuing professional development and opportunities
- Provide emotional support as needed
- Guard against the exploitation of the mentee by other parties

Mentoring Techniques

The focus of mentoring is to develop the whole person and so the techniques are broad and require wisdom in order to be used appropriately. A 1995 study of mentoring techniques most commonly used in business found that the five most commonly used techniques among mentors were:

1. **Accompanying:** Making a commitment in a caring way, which involves taking part in learning process side-by-side with the learner.
2. **Sowing:** Mentors are often confronted with the difficulty of preparing the learner before him or she is ready to change. Sowing is necessary when you know that what you say may not be understood or even acceptable to learners at first but will make sense and have value to the mentee when the situation requires it.
3. **Catalyzing:** When change reaches a critical level of pressure, learning can jump. Here the mentor chooses to plunge the learner right into change, provoking a different way of thinking, a change in identity or a reordering of values.
4. **Showing:** This is making something understandable, or using your own example to demonstrate a skill or activity. You show what you are talking about, you show by your own behavior.
5. **Harvesting:** Here the mentor focuses on "picking the ripe fruit": it is usually used to create awareness of what was learned by experience and to draw conclusions. The key questions here are: "What have you learned?", "How useful is it?".

Objectives of a Mentoring Program

- To retain and advance talented employees.
- To retain and advance women and minorities.
- To give mentors satisfaction and a rewarding experience.
- To open up new channels of communication, information, and education.
- To demonstrate that the organization invests in people and encourages opportunity for a diverse workforce.
- Non-goal: The program is not intended for sponsoring anyone for a particular position in the organization.

Benefits of Mentorship

To the mentee (a person who is under mentor)
- Makes him feel at home in the organization in a short period of time
- Smoother transition into the work place
- Feeling of having a buddy or friend in the organization in addition to have formal bosses and colleagues
- Availability of support and guidance
- Having a confidant with whom discussions on some specific sensitive issues can be held
- Developmental opportunity
- Having someone who can back you up and sponsor in the organization

■ COACHING

Coaching is a process that is designed to assist motivated individuals in making changes to further their professional development. Human resource management offers coaching services to interested employees. Coaching leadership is when a leader coaches team members to develop them. Coaching leadership focuses on improving employees to become better individuals and professionals in the long term. Coaching leadership can be difficult and time-consuming.

Definition

A coaching style of leadership is characterized by partnership and collaboration. When leaders behave like coaches, hierarchy, command and control give way to collaboration and creativity. Blame gives way to feedback and learning, and external motivators are replaced by self-motivation.

Coaching Focus Areas

- Leadership
- Communication
- Change and transition
- Work/life balance
- Time management
- Meeting facilitation
- Personal organization
- Self management
- Decision-making
- Mission and values
- Strategic planning
- Organizational merges and restructuring
- Team development
- Relationship building

Styles of Coaching

There are three generally accepted styles of coaching in sports: autocratic, democratic and holistic. Each style has its benefits and drawbacks, and it is important to understand all three. For each coach, establishing a personal coaching style will require a firm grasp of their own natural tendencies, and it generally involves incorporating elements that work from each of the three major coaching styles.

I. Autocratic Coaching

- Autocratic coaching can best be summed up by the phrase "My way or the highway." Autocratic coaches make decisions with little to no input from the player or players.
- The coach articulates a vision for what needs to be accomplished by the players, and the players are expected to perform.
- Autocratic coaching is win-focused and typically features inflexible training structures.

II. Democratic Coaching

- Democratic coaching is exactly what it sounds like. Coaches facilitate decision-making and goal setting with input from their athletes instead of dictating to them.
- This style of coaching is athlete-centered, and the athletes shape their own objectives under a framework outlined by the coach.
- Democratic coaches give a lot of autonomy to players and teams, who are active collaborators in their own development and direction.

Difference between coaching and mentoring is shown in **Table 13.5**.

III. Holistic Coaching

- Also known as "laissez-faire" coaching, this style of coaching is founded on the theory that a happy team naturally becomes a successful team.
- Very little is offered in terms of structured training or positive feedback. Instead, the holistic coach works to create an environment where players feel comfortable exploring and pursuing skills development on their own time and in their own way.
- The coach does not act as a central authority, and instead allows the team to set their own agenda.

Elements and Characteristics of Coaching Leadership

Coaching is an art. It is complex and it is easy to fail at. Some key elements and characteristics are required in order to create a platform enabling success. Coaching leadership depends heavily on the leader's ability to direct and support. Furthermore, the cause and effect can be unclear and confusing, making it difficult to calibrate the coaching style quickly.

- **Collaboration:** A coach won't create a successful team if the team does not collaborate. It is less about maintaining

Table 13.5: Difference between coaching and mentoring.

Coaching	Mentoring
• Input based on professional skills and training	• Input based on experience
• Increases performance	• Increases maturity and understanding not skills
• Addresses specific, stipulated needs	• Mentee sets goals
• Designed program	• Mentee responsible for outcomes
• Coach promotes skills development, attitudes change	• Based on relationship building
• Directed and guided by the coach, as appropriate	• No preparation for mentor
• Preparation time required by coach	• Tripartite contract might be necessary if corporate sponsorship (limited to feedback on neutral information, such as attendance, timekeeping, etc.)
• Coach responsible for outcomes	
• Feedback delivered	• No formal assessment at the end of the process
• Tripartite contract if corporate sponsorship	• No formal feedback
• Support work outside session by coach	• No support work outside session

hierarchy and status and more about supporting what's best for the team.

- **Coaching mind-set:** Helping people become their best selves is not a simple task. A coach should think creatively about how to approach the coaching process so that each team member is developed and the team collectively achieves the best result.
- **Scaffolding:** Scaffolding is a term used in education to describe "a variety of instructional techniques used to move students progressively toward stronger understanding and, ultimately, greater independence in the learning process".
- **Feedback:** Team members won't know how well or how poorly they are doing unless they receive feedback. Constructive criticism is necessary for their growth. Coaches know how to use the task behavior component of coaching leadership to appropriately express their feedback.
- **Self-motivation:** Coaching leadership is a two-way street. Coaches should be willing to sacrifice their time to motivate team members to hone their skills and become the best versions of them.
- **Empathy and trust:** As in so many other leadership styles, we come back to empathy being a pillar in leadership. In order to coach well, a leader needs to understand the person being coached on an emotional level.

Pros of Coaching Leadership

- **People enjoy working with coaching leaders:** Coaches help people improve their skills so that they can perform at their best. Therefore, coaching leaders are able to create a work environment where people are highly motivated, eager to learn and willing to collaborate.
- **Coaching leads to clear expectations:** Team members do not have to guess what's required from them. With the coaching leadership style, their coach makes expectations clear and guides the team members towards developing the skills needed to accomplish their tasks as well as their long-term goals.
- **Coaching gives and organization a competitive advantage:** Coaching leadership requires a lot of personal mentorships so that each team member's skills are developed appropriately. They, therefore, become more productive and are more likely to provide mentorship opportunities to others as they climb the corporate ladder.
- **Coaching can identify weaknesses, and transform them into strengths:** It may seem reasonable to argue that it is best to focus on the strengths of a team and use them to the organization's advantage.

Cons of Coaching Leadership

- **Coaching requires a lot of time and patience:** Managers often have too little time to complete their assigned tasks much less to help each team member become skilled at what he or she should do.
- **Coaching is difficult:** Few people are gifted at being effective coaches. It requires confidence, experience and the ability to give meaningful advice.
- **Coaching is a two-way street:** The coaching leadership style will only work if team members are committed to the process. Too much responsibility rests on the leader's shoulders if they aren't.
- **Coaching without good chemistry can impact progress:** The team and leader should work well together in order for the coaching leadership style to be effective. The organization has to consider personality, experience and its most pressing needs before deciding who would be best fit for the role.

■ DECISION-MAKING

Decision-making is a complex, cognitive process often defined as choosing a particular course of action. Decision-making can be regarded as the mental processes (cognitive process) resulting in the selection of a course of action among several alternatives. Every decision-making process produces a final choice (**Fig. 13.42**). The output can be an action or an opinion of choice.

Definition of Decision-making

- Decision-making is the mental process of selecting a course of action from a set of alternatives.
- According to the Oxford Advanced Learner's Dictionary the term decision-making means—the process of deciding about something important, especially in a group of people or in an organization.

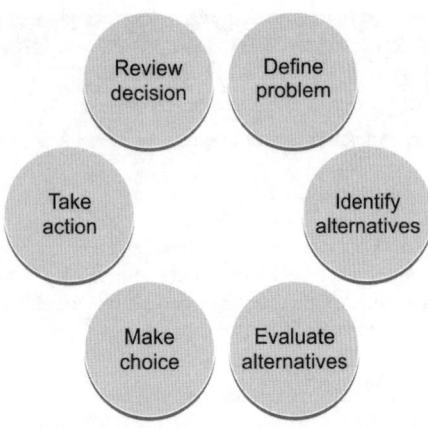

Fig. 13.42: Decision-making process.

Box 13.11: Characteristics of decision-making.

- Decision-maker has freedom to choose an alternative.
- Decision-making may not be completely rational.
- Goal-oriented
- Mental or intellectual process because the final decision is made by the decision-maker.
- Decision may be expressed in words or may be implied from behavior.
- Choosing from among alternative course of operation implies uncertainty about the final result of each possible course of operation.
- Rational, thorough analysis and reasoning and weighing consequences of the various alternatives.

- Trewatha and Newport defines decision-making process as follows: "Decision-making involves the selection of a course of action from among two or more possible alternatives in order to arrive at a solution for a given problem".
- Decision-making is the selection based on some criteria from two or more possible alternatives". —*George R Terry*
- A decision can be defined as a course of action consciously chosen from available alternatives for the purpose of desired result. —*JL Massie*
- A decision is an act of choice, wherein an executive forms a conclusion about what must be done in a given situation. A decision represents a course of behavior chosen from a number of possible alternatives. —*DE Mc Farland*

Characteristics of Decision-making (Box 13.11)

- Decision-making is based on rational thinking.
- It is a process of selecting the best from amongst alternatives available.
- It involves the evaluation of various alternatives available.
- It is the end product because it is preceded by discussions and deliberations.
- Decision-making is aimed to achieve organizational goals.
- It also involves certain commitment.

Elements

Following elements can be derived from the above mentioned definitions:

- Decision-making is a selection process and is concerned with selecting the best type of alternative.
- The decision taken is aimed at achieving the organizational goals.
- It is concerned with the detailed study of the available alternatives for finding the best possible alternative.
- Decision-making is a mental process. It is the outline of constant thoughtful consideration.
- It leads to commitment. The commitment depends upon the nature of the decision whether short term or long term.

Techniques of Decision-making

Table 13.6 summarizes techniques of decision making.

Steps in Decision-making

Decision-making comprises a series of sequential activities that together structure the process and facilitate its conclusion. These steps are:

1. Establishing objectives
2. Classifying and prioritizing objectives
3. Developing selection criteria
4. Identifying alternatives
5. Evaluating alternatives against the selection criteria
6. Choosing the alternative that best satisfies the selection criteria
7. Implementing the decision

Decision-making Styles

There are countless perspectives and tactics to effective decision-making. However, there are a few key points in decision-making theory that are central to understanding how different styles may impact organizational trajectories.

Table 13.6: Techniques of decision-making.		
Types of decision	Traditional	Modern
1. *Programmed* – Routine, repetitive decisions – Organization develops specific processes for handling them	1. Habit 2. Clerical routine: Standard operating procedures (SOPs) 3. Organization structure: Common expectations, a system of subgoals, well defined informational channels	1. Operations research: Mathematical analysis, models, computer simulations 2. Data processing
2. *Nonprogrammed:* – Nonroutine, one-shot, ill-structured, novel policy decisions – Handled by general problem-solving processes	1. Judgement, intuition and creativity 2. Rule of thumb 3. Selection and training of executives	Heuristic problem-solving technique applied to: • Training human decision makers • Constructing heuristic computer programs

Decision-making styles can be divided into three broad categories:
1. **Psychological:** Decisions derived from the needs, desires, preferences, and/or values of the individual making the decision. This type of decision-making is centered on the individual deciding.
2. **Cognitive:** This is an integrated feedback system between the individual/organization making a decision, and the broader environment's reactions to those decisions. This type of decision-making process involves iterative cycles and constant assessment of the reactions and impacts of the decision.
3. **Normative:** In many ways, decision-making (particularly in groups, such as within an organization) is about communicative rationality. This is to say that decisions are derived based on the ability to communicate and share logic, using firms premises and conclusions to drive behavior.

Importance of decision-making in management is shown in **Figure 13.43**.

Scientific Approach to the Decision-making Process

The scientific approach is a formalized reasoning process (**Fig. 13.44**). It consists of the following steps:
Step-1: The problem for analysis is defined and the conditions for observation are determined.
Step-2: Observations are made under different conditions to determine the behavior of the system containing the problem.
Step-3: Based on the observations, a hypothesis that describes how the factors involved are thought to interact or what is the best solution to the problem, is conceived.
Step-4: To test the hypothesis, an experiment is designed.
Step-5: The experiment is executed and measurements are obtained and recorded.
Step-6: The results of the experiment are analyzed and the hypothesis is either accepted or rejected.

Guidelines for Effective Decision-making

The following guidelines may be followed for effective decision-making:
- Define the goals.
- Ensure that the decision will contribute to the goal.
- Adopt a diagnostic approach to decision-making.

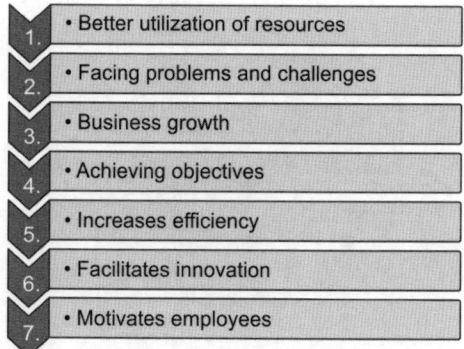

Fig. 13.43: Importance of decision-making in management.

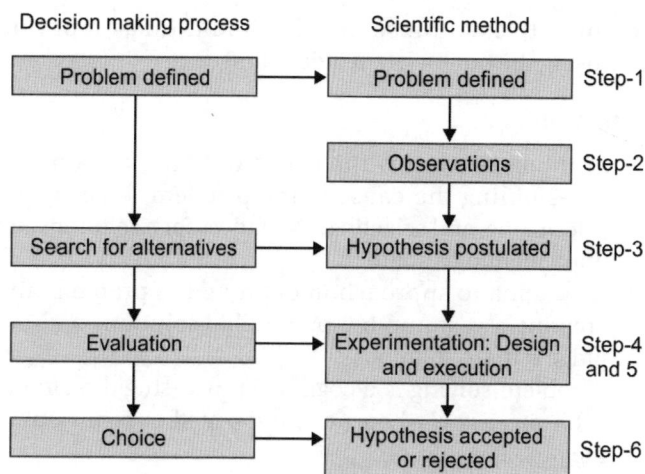

Fig. 13.44: Relationship of the scientific approach to the decision process.

- Involve subordinates in decision-making process.
- Ensure successful implementation of the decision.
- Evaluate the results, and
- Be flexible and revise the decision which does not yield the desired results.

Theories of Decision-making

The major theories of decision-making are:
- **The Intuition Theory or the Traditional Theory:** Decisions are taken by intuition ox hunch without really considering carefully all the alternatives. A person just decides a particular course of action because he feels that, that course is the best one.
- **The Classical Theory:** This is just opposite to Intuition Theory. Here the decision is made rationally, after a careful probing into all the alternatives. It is essentially a theory of decision-making under conditions of certainty which is, of course, a rare phenomenon.
- **The Behavioral Theory:** Decisions are made on the basis of a limited, approximate model of the real situation.

Advantages of Decision-making

- It is characterized by order and direction that enables managers to determine where they are.
- Provide a framework for data gathering which is relevant to the decision.
- Allows application of previous knowledge and experiences that minimize errors and improve quality of patient care and work of an organization.
- Increase manager's confidence and ability to make sound decisions.

■ PROBLEM-SOLVING

Problem-solving and decision-making are important skills for business and life. Problem-solving often involves decision-making, and decision-making is especially important for management and leadership. There are processes and techniques to improve decision-making and the quality of decisions. Decision-making is more natural to certain personalities, so these people should focus more on improving the quality of their decisions.

Definition

1. Problem solving is the act of defining a problem; determining the cause of the problem; identifying, prioritizing, and selecting alternatives for a solution; and implementing a solution.
2. A systematic approach to defining the problem and creating a vast number of possible solutions without judging these solutions.
3. "Problem solving is a cognitive processing directed at achieving a goal where no solution method is obvious to the problem solver".

Problem-solving Skills

Problem-solving skills help you determine the source of a problem and find an effective solution. Although problem-solving is often identified as its own separate skill, there are other related skills that contribute to this ability.

Some key problem-solving skills include:
1. Active listening
2. Analysis
3. Research
4. Creativity
5. Communication
6. Dependability
7. Decision-making
8. Team-building

Scientific Method of Problem-solving

Step 1: Problem awareness: The first step in problem-solving behavior of an individual concerns his awareness of the difficulty or problem that needs a solution.

Step 2: Problem understanding: The difficulty or problem experienced by the individual should be properly identified by a careful analysis. He should be clear about his problem. The problem then should be pinpointed in terms of the specific goals and objectives. Thus all the difficulties and obstacles in the path of the solution must be properly named and identified and what is to be got through the problem-solving efforts should then be properly analyzed **(Fig. 13.45)**.

Step 3: Collection of relevant information: In this step, the individual is required to collect all the relevant information about the problem through all possible sources. He may consult experienced persons, read the available literature, revive his old experiences, think of possible solutions and put in all relevant efforts for widening the scope of his knowledge concerning the problem in hand.

Step 4: Formulation of hypothesis or hunch for possible solutions: In the light of the collected relevant information and nature of his problem, one may then engage in some serious cognitive activities to think of the various possibilities for the solution of one's problem. As a result, he may start with a few possible solutions for his problem.

Step 5: Selection of a proper solution: In this step, all the possible solutions, thought of in the previous step, are closely analyzed and evaluated. Gates and others (1946) have suggested the following activities in the evaluation of the assumed hypothesis or solution:

- One should determine the conclusion that completely satisfies the demands of the problem.
- One should find out whether the solution is consistent with other facts and principles which have been well established.
- One should make a deliberate search for negative instances which might cast doubts on the conclusion.
- The above suggestions can help the individual to consider a suitable solution for his problem out of the many possible solutions.

Step 6: Verification of the concluded solution or hypothesis: Monitor your decision. Assess the results of your solution. Are you satisfied with the results? Did your solution resolve the problem? Did it produce a new problem? Do you have to modify your solution to achieve better results? Are you closer to achieving your goal? What have you learned?

Problem solving skills are shown in **Figure 13.46**.

Problem-solving Strategies

The following techniques are usually called problem-solving strategies:
- **Abstraction:** Solving the problem in a model of the system before applying it to the real system.
- **Analogy:** Using a solution that solves an analogous problem

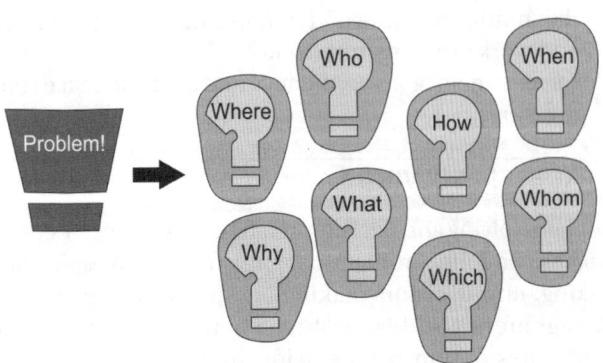

Fig. 13.45: Problem understanding.

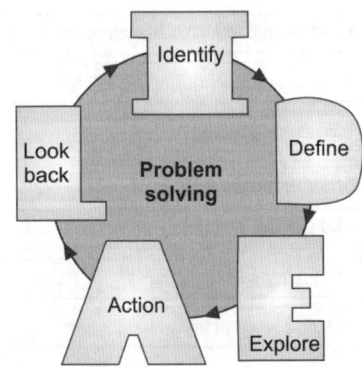

Fig. 13.46: Problem-solving skills.

- **Brainstorming (especially among groups of people):** Suggesting a large number of solutions or ideas and combining and developing them until an optimum solution is found.
- **Divide and conquer:** Breaking down a large, complex problem into smaller, solvable problems.
- **Hypothesis testing:** Assuming a possible explanation to the problem and trying to prove (or, in some contexts, disprove) the assumption.
- **Lateral thinking:** Approaching solutions indirectly and creatively.
- **Means-end analysis:** Choosing an action at each step to move closer to the goal.
- **Method of focal objects:** Synthesizing seemingly nonmatching characteristics of different objects into something new.
- **Morphological analysis:** Assessing the output and interactions of an entire system.
- **Proof:** Try to prove that the problem cannot be solved. The point where the proof fails will be the starting point for solving it.
- **Reduction:** Transforming the problem into another problem for which solutions exist.
- **Research:** Employing existing ideas or adapting existing solutions to similar problems.
- **Root-cause analysis:** Identifying the cause of a problem.
- **Trial and error:** Testing possible solutions until the right one is found.

CONFLICT MANAGEMENT

Conflict management is the process of limiting the negative aspects of conflict while increasing the positive aspects of conflict. The aim of conflict management is to enhance learning and group outcomes, including effectiveness or performance in an organizational setting. Properly managed conflict can improve group outcomes.

Definition

- Conflict management, also known as conflict resolution, involves having a workplace that precludes conflict and a management team that successfully handles and resolves workplace issues.
- Conflict management refers to techniques and ideas designed to reduce the negative effects of conflict and enhance the positive outcomes for all parties involved.

Concept of Conflict Management

- Conflict management is the principle that all conflicts cannot necessarily be resolved, but learning how to manage conflicts can decrease the odds of nonproductive escalation.
- Conflict management involves acquiring skills related to conflict resolution, self-awareness about conflict modes, conflict communication skills, and establishing a structure for management of conflict in your environment.
- All members of every organization need to have ways of keeping conflict to a minimum and of solving problems caused by conflict, before conflict becomes a major obstacle to your work.

Conflict Management Skills

- The aim for professionals in the workplace should not be to avoid conflict, but to resolve it in an effective manner.
- Employees with strong conflict resolution skills are able to effectively handle workplace issues.
- Communicating clearly, empathetically, and patiently leads to favorable outcomes and keeps professional relationships strong.

Conflict Management Styles (Fig. 13.47)

Conflicts happen. How an employee responds and resolves conflict will limit or enable that employee's success. Here are five conflict styles that a manager will follow according to Kenneth W Thomas and Ralph H Kilmann:

1. **An accommodating** manager is one who cooperates to a high degree. This may be at the manager's own expense and actually work against that manager's own goals, objectives, and desired outcomes. This approach is effective when the other person is the expert or has a better solution.
2. **Avoiding** an issue is one way a manager might attempt to resolve conflict. This type of conflict style does not help the other staff members reach their goals and does not help the manager who is avoiding the issue and cannot assertively pursue his or her own goals. However, this works well when the issue is trivial or when the manager has no chance of winning.
3. **Collaborating** managers become partners or pair up with each other to achieve both of their goals in this style. This is how managers break free of the win-lose paradigm and seek the win-win. This can be effective for complex scenarios where managers need to find a novel solution.
4. **Competing:** This is the win-lose approach. A manager is acting in a very assertive way to achieve his or her own goals without seeking to cooperate with other employees, and it may be at the expense of those other employees. This approach may be appropriate for emergencies when time is of the essence.

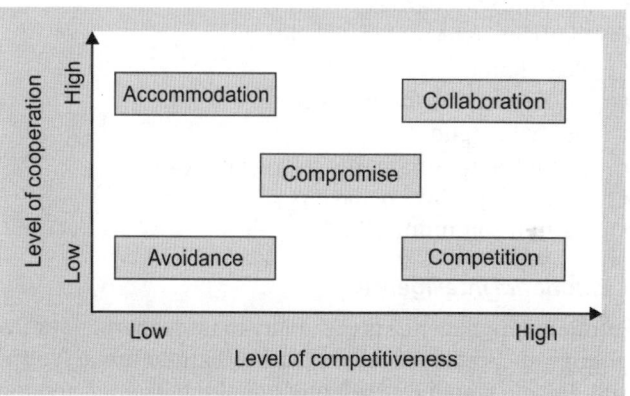

Fig. 13.47: Conflict management styles.

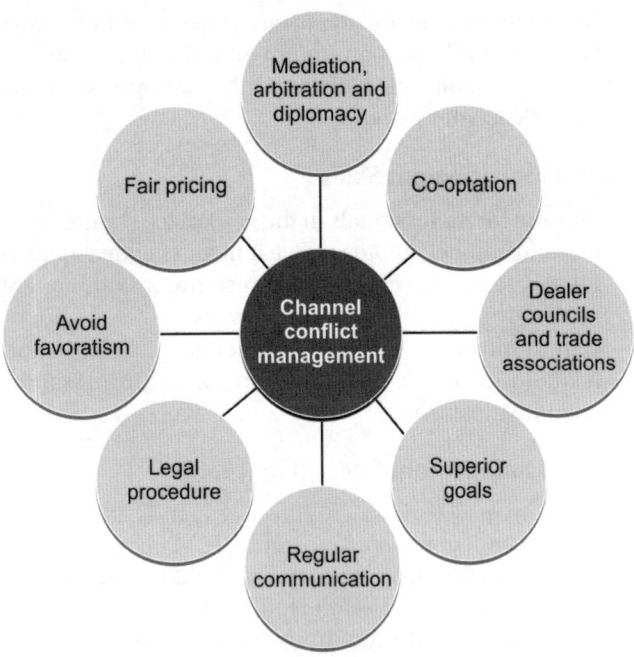

Fig. 13.48: Channel conflict management.

5. **Compromising:** This is the lose-lose scenario where neither person nor manager really achieves what they want. This requires a moderate level of assertiveness and cooperation. It may be appropriate for scenarios where you need a temporary solution or where both sides have equally important goals. **Figure 13.48** shows channel conflict management.

Types of Conflict Management Skills

I. Communication

Much unnecessary conflict can be avoided simply with clear, accurate written and verbal communication; a single lost email could lead to failed plans and fingers pointed. Examples of good communication skills include:
- Quickly addressing problems
- Understanding reluctant participants
- Formalizing agreements
- Active listening
- Leadership
- Mediating
- Meeting with parties
- Modeling reasonable dialogue
- Negotiating
- Nonverbal communication
- Open dialogue
- Suppressing conflict-provoking behaviors
- Teaching positive behaviors
- Written communication

II. Emotional Intelligence

Emotional intelligence is the ability to understand your own feelings and those of others, and to handle those feelings well. People who have high emotional intelligence are good at identifying and meeting the needs of others while taking responsibility for their own needs and feelings. A few ways they do this are:
- Being adaptable
- Being analytical
- Asserting feelings
- Compromising
- Showing curiosity
- Forgiving transgressions
- Helping others
- Identifying triggers
- Recognizing improvements
- Setting ground rules
- Showing respect
- Modifying behavior
- Being motivated
- Being optimistic:
  - Being self-aware
  - Displaying self-regulation

III. Empathy

Empathy means feeling what others feel. The ability to see a situation from someone else's viewpoint, and to understand their needs, motivations, and possible misunderstandings, is critical to effective conflict management.
Hallmarks of empathy include:
- Accountability
- Asking for feedback
- Building trust
- Showing compassion
- Embracing diversity and inclusion
- Giving constructive feedback
- Handling difficult people
- Managing emotions
- High emotional intelligence
- Identifying nonverbal cues
- Recognizing differences
- Understanding different viewpoints
- Good interpersonal skills
- Ability to recognize problems
- Good self-control
- Ability to embrace different opinions

IV. Creative Problem Solving

Understanding and communication are all very well and good, but do not help much if you do not have a solution for the underlying problem, whatever that problem may be. Examples of problem-solving conflicts in the workplace include:
- Conflict analysis
- Brainstorming solutions
- Collaborating
- Verbal communication
- Convening meetings
- Creativity
- Decision-making
- Designating sanctions
- Nonverbal communication
- Problem solving

- Sense of humor
- Goal integration
- Monitoring compliance
- Reconfiguring relationships
- Fair resolution

Conflict Management Strategies to Resolve Issues

Conflict happens when two different groups perceive some incompatibility between themselves, which can lead to conflict. How a manager reacts and deals with that conflict will have a large impact on the outcome. There are many different strategies to deal with conflict. One of the more common strategies was developed by Maccoby and Studder. They determined it was best to prevent conflict from ever taking place. Below are Maccoby and Studder's five strategies to resolve conflict before it happens:

1. **Anticipate:** Take time to obtain information that can lead to conflict
2. **Prevent:** Before conflict occurs, develop strategies
3. **Identify:** If it is interpersonal or procedural, move quickly to manage it
4. **Manage:** Remember, conflict is emotional
5. Resolve: React without blaming and you will learn through dialogue

NEGOTIATION

Negotiation is a method by which people settle differences. It is a process by which compromise or agreement is reached while avoiding argument and dispute. In any disagreement, individuals understandably aim to achieve the best possible outcome for their position (or perhaps an organization they represent). However, the principles of fairness, seeking mutual benefit and maintaining a relationship are the keys to a successful outcome **(Fig. 13.49)**.

Definition

- Negotiation is the process of conferring to arrive at an agreement between different parties, each with their own interest and preferences.
- A give and take decision-making process involving interdependent parties with different Preferences.

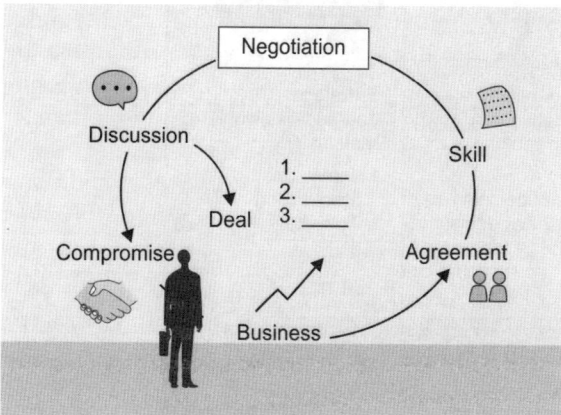

Fig. 13.49: Negotiation.

P's of Negotiation

Like P's of marketing, essentials of negotiation are called as P's of negotiation. They are as follows:

- **Purpose:** Aim is required otherwise it will result in wastage of money, manpower and time.
- **Plan:** Main agenda on which negotiation is to be carried on.
- **Pace:** Main points should be covered in discussions; also proper breaks must be introduced to maintain interest of peoples involved.
- **Personalities:** Negotiator initiating negotiation must have convincing power, effective communication skills, can influence people and process of negotiation.

Factors Affecting Negotiation

- **Place:** Familiarity with surrounding helps in boosting confidence.
- **Time:** Time should be adequate for smooth exchange of ideas and securing agreement before it is too late.
- **Attitude:** Attitude of both parties should be positive, i. e, willingness to make an agreement or deal.
- **Subjective factors:** Like relation of two parties involved, status difference, information and expertise.

Principles of Negotiation

Four principles of best practice negotiation

1. **Preparation:** Understanding the issues and the people and equipping the team for the process.
2. **Relationship:** Developing a strategy for maintaining the relationship before, during and after negotiations.
3. **Communication:** Building trust by applying an open communication style.
4. **Problem-solving:** Exploring options and strategies for reaching agreement.

Stages of Negotiation

In order to achieve a desirable outcome, it may be useful to follow a structured approach to negotiation. For example, in a work situation a meeting may need to be arranged in which all parties involved can come together **(Box 13.12)**.

The process of negotiation includes the following stages:

- **Preparation:** Before any negotiation takes place, a decision needs to be taken as to when and where a meeting will take place to discuss the problem and who will attend.

Box 13.12: Stages of negotiation.

In order to achieve a desirable outcome, it may be useful to follow a structured approach to negotiation. For example, in a work situation a meeting may need to be arranged in which all parties involved can come together. The process of negotiation includes the following stages:
- Preparation
- Discussion
- Clarification of goals
- Negotiation towards a win-win situation
- Agreement
- Implementation of a course of action

Setting a limited time-scale can also be helpful to prevent the disagreement continuing.
- **Discussion:** During this stage, individuals or members of each side put forward the case as they see it, i.e., their understanding of the situation.
- **Clarifying goals:** From the discussion, the goals, interests and viewpoints of both sides of the disagreement need to be clarified.
- **Negotiate towards a win-win outcome:** This stage focuses on what is termed a 'win-win' outcome where both sides feel they have gained something positive through the process of negotiation and both sides feel their point of view has been taken into consideration.
- **Agreement:** Agreement can be achieved once understanding of both sides' viewpoints and interests have been considered.
- **Implementing a course of action:** From the agreement, a course of action has to be implemented to carry through the decision.

Negotiation Skills (Fig. 13.50)

Negotiation skills are qualities that allow two or more parties to reach a compromise. These are often soft skills and include abilities, such as communication, persuasion, planning, strategizing and cooperating. Understanding these skills is the first step to becoming a stronger negotiator.

I. Communication
- Essential communication skills include identifying nonverbal cues and expressing yourself in a way that is engaging.
- It is important to understand the natural flow of conversation and always ask for feedback.
- Active listening skills are also crucial for understanding the other party. By establishing clear communication, you can avoid misunderstandings that could prevent you from reaching a compromise.

II. Persuasion
- The ability to influence others is an important skill for negotiation.
- It can help you define why your proposed solution is beneficial to all parties and encourage others to support your point-of-view.

III. Planning
- In order to reach an agreement that benefits both parties, it is crucial you consider how the consequences will impact everyone in the long-term.
- Planning skills are necessary not only for the negotiation process but also for deciding how the terms will be carried out.

IV. Strategizing
The best negotiators enter a discussion with at least one backup plan, but often more. Consider all possible outcomes, and be prepared for each of these scenarios.

Types of Negotiation

Most negotiation outcomes will fall into one of two categories: "win-win" or "win-lose." By understanding the different types of negotiations you may encounter, you can determine the most relevant skills for your role and work to improve them. Here are forms of negotiation:

I. Distributive Negotiations
- Also called distributive bargaining, this form of negotiation occurs when there is a limited amount of resources and each party assumes if they lose something, the other party will gain something.
- Instead of each party attempting to come to an agreement based on their interests and needs, each party is working to get more than the other party.
- For example, a client may feel if a provider does not lower the price for a service, they will be paying too much, and

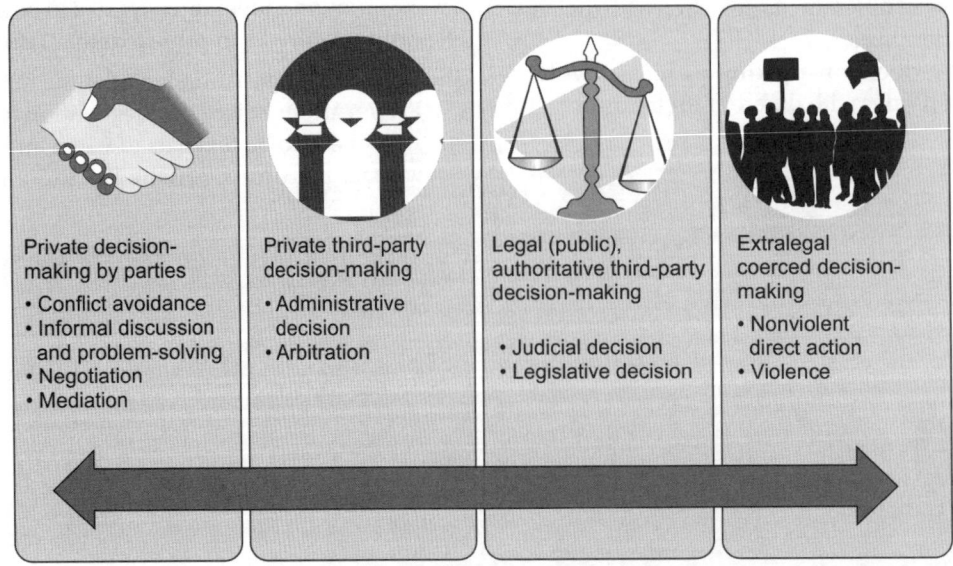

Fig. 13.50: Negotiation skills.

the service provider may feel if they decrease their price, they will lose money.

II. Integrative Negotiations

- Often referred to as a "win-win," an integrative negotiation occurs when everyone benefits from the agreement.
- In order to come to an integrative agreement, each party receives some value.
- The integrative negotiation process may take longer because both parties have to feel fully satisfied before coming to an agreement.

III. Management Negotiations

Negotiating with management can be stressful. In some cases, employees may feel uncomfortable sharing their wants and needs with someone in a more senior position.

IV. Coworker Negotiations

Depending on your job, you may have to negotiate with your coworkers. Many positions require close teamwork and without strong negotiation skills, you may face imbalances in work distribution.

V. Vendor Negotiations

Some employees manage external vendors, and their performance rating may be affected by how they negotiate. Also, the ability to reach an agreement with service providers can affect your professional relationships and general business success.

Tips to Improve your Negotiation Skills

Not all forms of negotiation are effective, and measuring success can be challenging. To evaluate your effectiveness, it is wise to identify how well your intended outcome aligns with the final agreement. Follow these tips to improve the negotiation skills:

1. Identify the final goal
2. Practice building rapport
3. Be willing to compromise
4. Consider imposing time restrictions
5. Take the multiple offer approach
6. Exercise confidence
7. Don't take "no" personally
8. Understand your weaknesses
9. Practice

Negotiation Process Offer Counter Agreement

- **Offer:** First proposal made by one party to another in the negotiation stage.
- **Counter offer:** Offer made by second party to first party, or proposing their offer against first party offer.
- **Concession:** Increase or decrease made in the offer or change in the idea.
- **Compromise:** Sacrifice made by both or one party.
- **Agreement:** Point where both parties agrees, which is beneficial to both.

■ IMPLEMENTING PLANNED CHANGE

Planned change is the process of preparing the entire organization, or a significant part of it, for new goals or a new direction. This direction can refer to culture, internal structures, processes, metrics and rewards, or any other related aspects. While constant change is the new normal and the best companies embrace it, not all change is planned. On occasion, organizations will suddenly adapt to new market demands and heightened competition.

Planned Change Models

I. Kurt Lewin's three-step Change Model

Lewin's change model provides a general framework for planned change which includes three basic steps **(Fig. 13.51)**:

1. **Unfreezing** or reducing forces that keep things within an organization the way they are. Unfreezing happens through so-called "psychological disconfirmation." For example, running an organization-wide innovation survey and evaluating the results.
2. **Moving** or shifting the organization's behavior. This involves an intervention.
3. **Refreezing** or stabilizing the organization in a new state of equilibrium. This step is not possible without support mechanisms. For example, building a solid corporate innovation capability.

II. Action Research Model

Also known as participatory action research, action learning, action science, or self-design model, the action research model is also prominent among organizational change specialists. Action researches activities are typically top-down and happen in iterative cycles of research and action. Consequently, they require considerable collaboration between staff and externals. Some other important features of the model include:

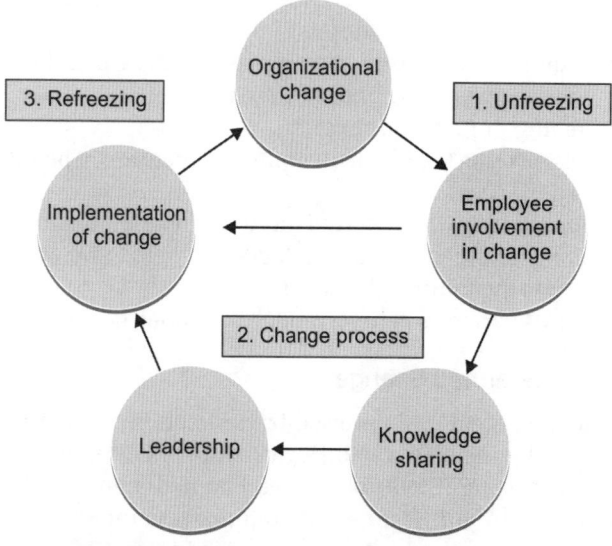

Fig. 13.51: Kurt Lewin's three-step change model.

Chapter 13: Leadership

1. Heavy emphasis on data gathering and diagnosis before action and planning, e.g., using big data to solve (big) problems.
2. Used to enact change at the unit level and even the organizational level; it is also a popular model in developing nations (applied to international settings); used to promote social change and innovation.

8 Main steps of the action research model:
1. Problem identification—typically by an executive
2. Consultation with behavioral science expert—like Dan Ariely
3. Data gathering (interviews, observation, questionnaire, performance data) and preliminary diagnosis
4. Feedback to key client/group
5. Joint diagnosis of a problem
6. Joint action planning
7. Action (the actual "moving" from one state to another)
8. Data gathering after action (often leads to re-diagnosis and new action)

III. Positive Model

A third important model is the positive model. This model represents a notable departure from both Lewin's model and the specifics of action research. While the latter are "deficit"-based (they focus on problems/scarcity), the positive model focuses on what the organization is doing right and how existing capabilities can be used to help the organization reach new heights.

The positive model is also about:
- Positive expectations that create anticipation that directs behavior towards making things happen.
- Applying a process called appreciative inquiry. This process infuses a positive value orientation into analyzing and changing organizations.
- Promoting member involvement and creating a shared vision; the shared appreciation acts as a guide of what the organization could be.

5 Main steps of the positive model:
1. Initiating the inquiry, i.e., the issues the organization has the most energy to address
2. Inquiring into existing best practices—here, members of the organizations conduct interviews
3. Telling "innovation stories"
4. Discovering the themes (common dimension of peoples' experiences)
5. Envisioning the preferred future via possibility propositions and relevant stakeholders and delivering ways to create the future ("the action" itself).

Figure 13.52 shows general model of planned change.

Steps in Planned Change

Once managers and an organization commit to planned change, they need to create a logical step-by step approach in order to accomplish the objectives. Planned change requires managers to follow an eight-step process for successful implementations, which is illustrated in **Figure 13.53**.

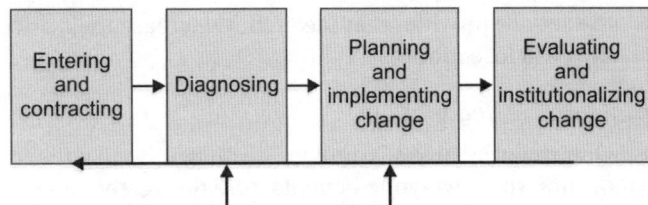

Fig. 13.52: General model of planned change.

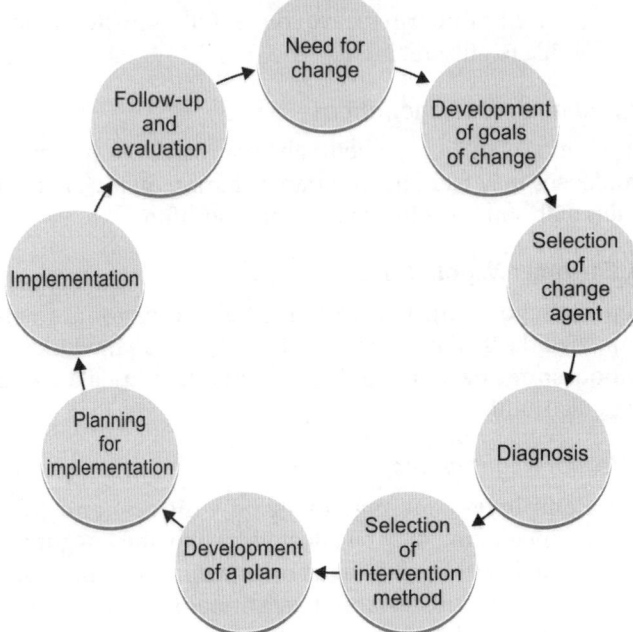

Fig. 13.53: Stages of planned change.

Step 1: Recognize the need for change. Recognition of the need for change may occur at the top management level or in peripheral parts of the organization. The change may be due to either internal or external forces.

Step 2: Develop the goals of the change. Remember that before any action is taken, it is necessary to determine why the change is necessary. Both problems and opportunities must be evaluated. Then it is important to define the needed changes in terms of products, technology, structure, and culture.

Step 3: Select a change agent. The change agent is the person who takes leadership responsibility to implement planned change. The change agent must be alert to things that need revamping, open to good ideas, and supportive of the implementation of those ideas into actual practice.

Step 4: Diagnose the current climate. In this step, the change agent sets about gathering data about the climate of the organization in order to help employees prepare for change. Preparing people for change requires direct and forceful feedback about the negatives of the present situation, as compared to the desired future state, and sensitizing people to the forces of change that exist in their environment.

Step 5: Select an implementation method. This step requires a decision on the best way to bring about the change. Managers can make themselves more sensitive to pressures for change by using networks of people and organizations with different perspectives and views, visiting other organizations exposed to new ideas, and using external standards of performance, such as competitor's progress.

Step 6: Develop a plan. This step involves actually putting together the plan, or the "what" information. This phase also determines the when, where, and how of the plan. The plan is like a road map. It notes specific events and activities that must be timed and integrated to produce the change. It also delegates responsibility for each of the goals and objectives.

Step 7: Implement the plan. After all the questions have been answered, the plan is put into operation. Once a change has begun, initial excitement can dissipate in the face of everyday problems. Managers can maintain the momentum for change by providing resources, developing new competencies and skills, reinforcing new behaviors, and building a support system for those initiating the change.

Step 8: Follow the plan and evaluate it. During this step, managers must compare the actual results to the goals established in Step 4. It is important to determine whether the goals were met; a complete follow-up and evaluation of the results aids this determination. Change should produce positive results and not be undertaken for its own sake.

■ CONCLUSION

Leadership is a process of social influence, which maximizes the efforts of others, towards the achievement of a goal. Notice key elements of this definition: Leadership stems from social influence, not authority or power. Leadership requires others, and that implies they do not need to be "direct reports." A leader is someone who can see how things can be improved and who rallies people to move toward that better vision. Leaders can work toward making their vision a reality while putting people first. Just being able to motivate people is not enough—leaders need to be empathetic and connect with people to be successful. Leaders do not have to come from the same background or follow the same path. Future leaders will actually be more diverse, which brings a variety of perspectives. Of course, other people could disagree with my definition. The most important thing is that organizations are united internally with their definition of leadership.

■ REVIEW QUESTIONS

Long Essays

1. Define leadership; explain the nature and elements of leadership.
2. Discuss techniques and importance of the leadership.
3. Describe the various theories of leadership.
4. Enumerate different types of leadership styles.
5. Define delegation; explain the principles and characteristics of delegation.
6. Define negotiation; explain the factors, principles and step in detail.

Short Essays

1. Characteristics of leadership.
2. Explain the principles of leadership.
3. Difference between leadership and management.
4. Factors influencing leadership.
5. Difference between transactional and transformational leader.
6. Skills required in leadership.
7. Situational leadership style.
8. Methods of leadership development.
9. Effective leadership in nursing.
10. Leadership styles in nursing management.
11. Mentorship in nursing.
12. Preceptorship in nursing.
13. Power and politics in nurse.
14. Empowerment in the workplace.
15. Mentoring techniques.
16. Elements and characteristics of coaching leadership.
17. Characteristics of decision-making.
18. Techniques of decision-making.
19. Theories of decision-making.
20. Scientific method of problem-solving.
21. Conflict management styles.
22. Types of negotiation.
23. Implementing planned change.

Short Answers

1. Qualities of good leader.
2. Charismatic leaders.
3. Bureaucratic leaders.
4. Free-rein leadership style.
5. Leadership activities.
6. Leadership competencies.
7. Advantages of situational leadership.
8. Inspirational motivation.
9. Coaching.
10. Self-directed learning.
11. Leadership development models.
12. Qualities of nurse leader.
13. Qualities of an effective nurse mentor.
14. Usefulness of mentorship.
15. Benefits of preceptorship.
16. Principles of preceptorship.
17. Elements of delegation.
18. Types of delegation.
19. Barriers in delegation.
20. Advantages of delegation.
21. Factors contributing to political behavior.
22. Types of politics.
23. Empowerment.
24. Pros and cons of empowerment.
25. Decision-making styles.
26. Problem-solving skills.
27. Problem-solving strategies.
28. Types of conflict management skills.
29. Creative problem solving.

BIBLIOGRAPHY

1. Allen S. Mentoring: The magic partnership. Canadian Operating Room Nursing Journal. 2006;24(4):30.
2. Alper S, Tjosvold D, Law KS. Conflict management, efficacy, and performance in organizational teams. Personnel Psychology. 2000; 53 (3):625-42.
3. Anderson L. A learning resource for developing effective mentorship in practice. Nursing Standard. 2011; 25(51):48-56.
4. Barker E R. Mentoring -a complex relationship. Journal of the Academy of Nurse Practitioners. 2006;18:56-61.
5. Benner P. Using the Dreyfus model of skill acquisition to describe and interpret skill acquisition in nursing practice and education. Bulletin of Science Technology & Society. 2004;24(3):188-99.
6. Billings D, Kowalski K. Developing your career as a nurse educator: The importance of having (or being) a mentor. The Journal of Continuing Education in Nursing. 2008; 39(11):490-1.
7. Blauvelt M, Spath M. A faculty mentoring program: At one school of nursing. Nursing Education Perspectives. 2008;29(1):29-33.
8. Darling L. What to do about toxic mentors. The Journal of Nursing Administration. 1985;5:43-4.
9. Feeg V. Mentoring for leadership tomorrow: Planning for succession. Pediatric Nursing. 2008;34(4): 277-8.
10. Holmes D, Hodgson P, Simari R, Nishimura R. Mentoring: Making the transition from mentee to mentor. Circulation. 2010;121: 336-40.
11. Jacobson S, Sherrod D. Transformational mentorship models for nurse educators. Nursing Science Quarterly. 2012; 25(3):279-84.
12. McCloughen A, O'Brien L, Jackson D. Esteemed connection: creating a mentoring relationship for nurse leadership. Nursing Inquiry. 2009;16(4):326-36.
13. Metcalfe S. Educational innovation: Collaborative mentoring for future nursing leaders. Creative Nursing. 2010;16(4):167-70.
14. Mijares L, Baxley S, Bond M. Mentoring: A concept analysis. The Journal of Nursing Theory. 2013;17(1):23-8.
15. Riley M, Fearing A. Mentoring as a teaching-learning strategy in nursing. MEDSURG Nursing. 2009;18(4):228-34.
16. Wilson V, Andrews M, Leners D W. Mentoring as a strategy for retaining racial and ethnically diverse students in nursing programs. The Journal of Multicultural Nursing & Health. 2006;12(3):17-23.

CHAPTER 14

Controlling

LEARNING OBJECTIVES

- Implementing Standards, Policies, Procedures, Protocols and Practices
- Nursing Performance Audit, Patient Satisfaction
- Nursing Rounds, Documentation-Records and Reports

INTRODUCTION

Controlling is one of the managerial functions, such as planning, organizing, staffing and directing. It is an important function because it helps to check the errors and to take the corrective action so that deviation from standards are minimized and stated goals of the organization are achieved in a desired manner. According to modern concepts, control is a foreseeing action whereas earlier concept of control was used only when errors were detected.

Control in management means setting standards, measuring actual performance and taking corrective action. Controlling consists of verifying whether everything occurs in conformities with the plans adopted, instructions issued and principles established. Controlling ensures that there is effective and efficient utilization of organizational resources so as to achieve the planned goals. Controlling measures the deviation of actual performance from the standard performance, discovers the causes of such deviations and helps in taking corrective actions **(Fig. 14.1)**.

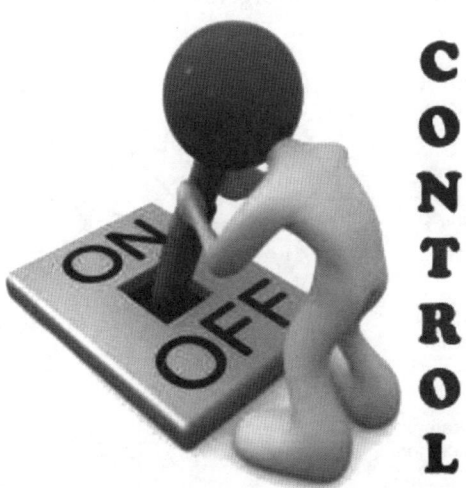

Fig. 14.1: Control as a managerial function.

DEFINITIONS

- **According to EFL Breach:** Control is checking current performance against pre-determined standards contained in the plans, with a view to ensure adequate progress and satisfactory performance.
- **According to Harold Koontz:** Controlling is the measurement and correction of performance in order to make sure those enterprise objectives and the plans devised to attain them are accomplished.
- **According to Stafford Beer:** Management is the profession of control.
- **According to Brech:** "Controlling is a systematic exercise which is called as a process of checking actual performance against the standards or plans with a view to ensure adequate progress and also recording such experience as is gained as a contribution to possible future needs."
- **According to Terry and Franklin:** "Controlling is determining what is being accomplished—that is, evaluating performance and, if necessary, applying corrective measures so that performance takes place according to plans".
- **According to Dale Henning:** "Control is the process of bringing about conformity of performance with planned action."

FEATURES OF CONTROLLING FUNCTION

Following are the characteristics of controlling function of management:

- **Controlling is an end function:** A function which comes once the performances are made in conformities with plans.
- **Controlling is a pervasive function:** which means it is performed by managers at all levels and in all type of concerns.
- **Controlling is forward looking:** because effective control is not possible without past being controlled. Controlling

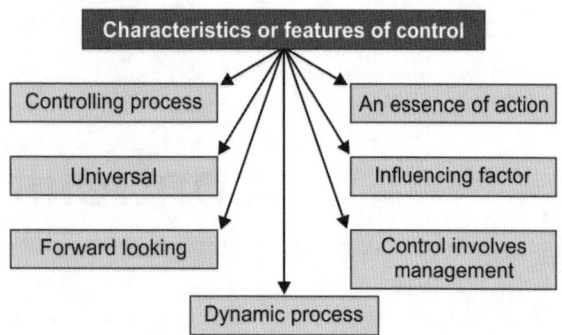

Fig. 14.2: Characteristics or features of control.

always looks to future so that follow-up can be made whenever required.
- **Controlling is a dynamic process:** Since controlling requires taking reviewal methods; changes have to be made wherever possible.
- **Controlling is related with planning:** Planning and Controlling are two inseparable functions of management. Without planning, controlling is a meaningless exercise and without controlling, planning is useless. Planning presupposes controlling and controlling succeeds planning. **Figure 14.2** shows characteristics or features of control

NEED OF CONTROLLING FOR ORGANIZATIONS

Controlling, in simple words, checks for mistakes and informs an organization about current and new challenges. Controlling is important for all organizations and explained in following points:
- **Accomplishing organizational goals:** One of the most significant steps in controlling involves determining possible deviations caused when the actual operations under perform vis-a-vis desired performance levels.
- **Judging accuracy of standards:** Corrective actions mean the process of identifying and eliminating the causes of problems or possible variations thus preventing its recurrence. As mentioned earlier, controlling can lead to changes in plans for an organization.
- **Facilitating coordination in action:** Controlling ensures that everything works in accordance to the plans set in an organization. It focuses on building equilibrium between efforts and desired results or output.
- **Decision-making:** Controlling process is complete when decisions on corrective actions are undertaken. These decisions are directed towards making improvements or adjustments, which are consistent with organization's mission and goals.
- **Improving employee motivation:** Controlling makes superiors/supervisors to continuously monitor, supervise and motivate their employees during work. They set the standards for their employees and cross-check through performance appraisals whether the employees have been able to meet them and advise them to perform effectively.
- **Ensuring order and discipline:** Controlling encourages distribution of powers from the superiors at the top management level to the subordinates at the middle-level who act as a link between top management and employees at the bottom level management.
- **Efficient use of resources:** Controlling enables efficient use of human and physical resources by avoiding possible delays, wastage or spoilage.

ELEMENTS OF AN EFFECTIVE CONTROL SYSTEM (FIG. 14.3)

Control is an essential feature of successful management much of precision of a managerial education is focused on the improvement of control techniques. Control is a process that guides activity towards some pre-determined goal. To achieve the desired one, the following are the important requirements for making any control system effective:
- **Direct control:** Modern system of control is employee-oriented rather than work-oriented. Control should be exercised on people who had machine and materials. People generally oppose the control measures, so their attitude should be made to change by proper education about control and its significance.
- **Control by objectives:** The control must be goal oriented and by objectives. As objectives clarify the expected results in meaningful and realistic terms, they provide the control standards with which actual performance can be measured. The control system should be according to the nature and needs of organizations.
- **Control should be forward looking:** Control must be forward looking in character. It should bring out the deviation in light at an earliest. It must focus on strategic points with exceptions.
- **Control should be simple and balanced:** Control must be simple and balanced in nature. A control device that is not intelligible cannot be practiced by the manager. So control tools must be simple and intelligible to both—controller and controlled.
- **Managerial self-control:** Control is effected through managerial positions in the organization structure. So each managerial position must be vested with adequate authority for exercising control. Allocation of fixed duties and responsibilities goes a long way towards securing effective control in the organization.

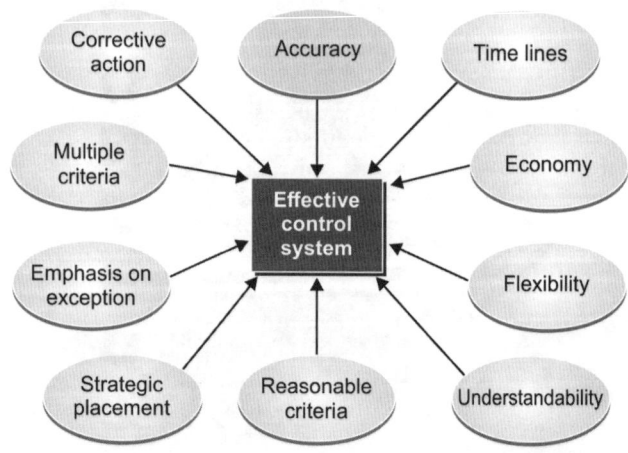

Fig. 14.3: Effective control system.

- **There should be flexibility in control:** Control system should provide for some change but its basic structure must be retained. It has been seen that even the best plans and other predetermined criteria need to the changed from time to time.
- **Economy in control:** Economy is an important requirement of any control system. It is a truism to state the control must be worth its results. A simple control procedure proves too economical.
- **Feedback system:** Feedback is the process of adjusting future actions based upon information about past performance. Recently the concept has received attention very much. It shows the worth and utility of control process.
- **Control should not be negative:** It must be positive and constructive. It must be helpful. Control is not a command. It is guidance. The management should recognize the importance of human beings in control systems.

PROCESS OF CONTROLLING

Control process involves the following steps as shown in the **Figure 14.4**:

- **Establishing standards:** This means setting up of the target which needs to be achieved to meet organizational goals eventually. Standards indicate the criteria of performance. Control standards are categorized as quantitative and qualitative standards. Quantitative standards are expressed in terms of money.
- **Measurement of actual performance:** The actual performance of the employee is measured against the target. With the increasing levels of management, the measurement of performance becomes difficult.
- **Comparison of actual performance with the standard:** This compares the degree of difference between the actual performance and the standard.
- **Taking corrective actions:** It is initiated by the manager who corrects any defects in actual performance.

Controlling process thus regulates companies' activities so that actual performance conforms to the standard plan. An effective control system enables managers to avoid circumstances which cause the company's loss.

IMPORTANCE OF CONTROLLING (FIG. 14.5)

After the meaning of control, let us see its importance. Control is an indispensable function of management without which the controlling function in an organization cannot be accomplished and the best of plans which can be executed

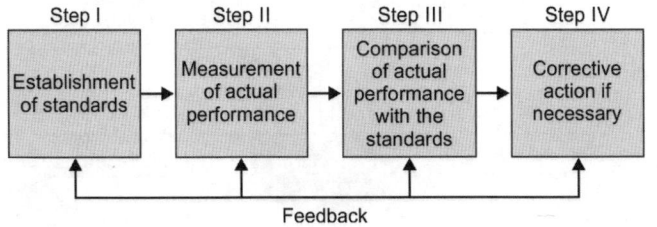

Fig. 14.4: Process of controlling.

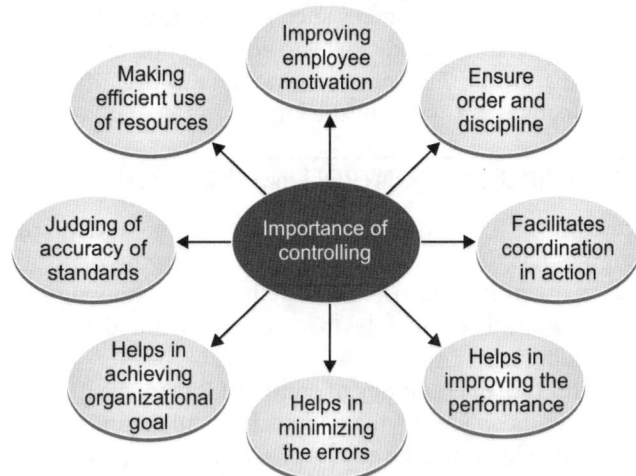

Fig. 14.5: Importance of controlling.

can go away. A good control system helps an organization in the following ways:

- **Accomplishing organizational goals:** The controlling function is an accomplishment of measures that further makes progress towards the organizational goals and brings to light the deviations, and indicates corrective action. Therefore, it helps in guiding the organizational goals which can be achieved by performing a controlling function.
- **Judging accuracy of standards:** A good control system enables management to verify whether the standards set are accurate and objective. The efficient control system also helps in keeping careful and progress check on the changes which help in taking the major place in the organization and in the environment and also helps to review and revise the standards in light of such changes.
- **Making efficient use of resources:** Another important function of controlling is that in this, each activity is performed in such manner so an in accordance with predetermined standards and norms so as to ensure that the resources are used in the most effective and efficient manner for the further availability of resources.
- **Improving employee motivation:** Another important function is that controlling help in accommodating a good control system which ensures that each employee knows well in advance what they expect and what are the standards of performance on the basis of which they will be appraised. Therefore, it helps in motivating and increasing their potential so to make them and helps them to give better performance.
- **Ensuring order and discipline:** Controlling creates an atmosphere of order and discipline in the organization which helps to minimize dishonest behavior on the part of the employees. It keeps a close check on the activities of employees and the company can be able to track and find out the dishonest employees by using computer monitoring as a part of their control system.
- **Facilitating coordination in action:** The last important function of controlling is that each department and

employee is governed by such predetermined standards and goals which are well versed and coordinated with one another. This ensures that overall organizational objectives are accomplished in an overall manner.

PRINCIPLES OF CONTROLLING (BOX 14.1)

Controlling is a procedure of ensuring that satisfactory progress has been made in accordance with the plans and noting down the experience benefited for achieving forth coming goals. The principles of management function control are as follows:

- **Principle of efficiency of controls:** Efficiency of control depends on identifying approaches and techniques and also highlighting the causes of possible or real deviations from plans by minimizing the costs or other unwanted consequences.
- **Principle of affirmation of the objectives:** Identifying potential or deviations from plans must be controlled earlier by allowing remedial actions in order to achieve the objectives.
- **Principle of control responsibility:** The manager who is given the charge of completing the plans is mainly responsible for exercising control.
- **Principle of direct control:** There is no need for indirect controls if the managers and their subordinates are excellent in quality.
- **Principle of standards:** Efficient control needs accuracy, purpose and aptness.
- **Principle of critical-point control:** Effective control needs attending crucial issues in reviewing performance against an individual plan.
- **The exception principle:** To achieve efficiency in the results of control, it is important for a manager to focus his control on exceptions.
- **Principle of flexible controls:** Flexibility in designing controls is important for them to succeed in spite of failures or unexpected changes in plans.
- **Principle of action:** Proper planning, organizing, staffing and direction is required for justifying control in case there is any deviations from plans.
- **Principle of reflection of plans:** Designing more controls will effectively serve the welfare of the enterprises and its managers and also reflect the structure and nature of plans.
- **Principle of organizational aptness:** Designing more controls will assist in correcting the deviation of events from plans and also reflect its place in the organization which is accountable for action.
- **Principle of individuality of controls:** It is important for individuals to understand the control measures and exercise it in order to be consistent with the position, operational tasks, skill and needs.

LIMITATIONS OF CONTROLLING (FIG. 14.6)

- **Lack of satisfactory standards:** It is quite difficult to fix satisfactory standards for many intangible activities such as results of management, developments, human relations and public relations. Activities of the workers for service of advisory nature and other activities relating to the behavior of the workers do not indicate quantitative output and identify their level of attainment. Therefore, controlling becomes difficult.
- **Effects of external factors:** Internal factors could be checked and put in the right perspective in time, but it is impossible to check and control the external factors. For example, change in the government policy, new inventions or discoveries, changes in the fashions and liking of the consumers, etc., cannot be checked by the control system.
- **Imperfections in management:** Economic consideration is not possible if we measure everything and everybody's work. Intangible performance always brings difficulties and responsible for making the task complicated for the measurement of results. If one fails to measure the performance in quantitative and qualitative terms, the results of behavioral activities have to be evaluated by managers on their own thinking and judgment.
- **Problem in setting of individual responsibilities:** Assignment of individual responsibilities becomes difficult. The effective impact of control in most of the cases depends on how responsible are the workers in the organization.
- **Limitation of corrective actions:** To some extent, it is true that there are certain organizations which have taken

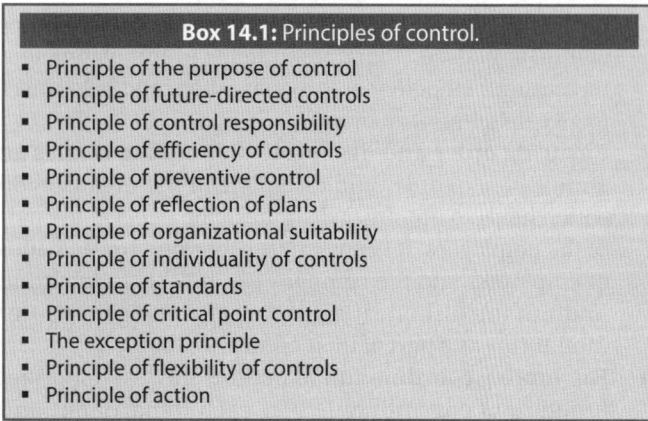

Box 14.1: Principles of control.
- Principle of the purpose of control
- Principle of future-directed controls
- Principle of control responsibility
- Principle of efficiency of controls
- Principle of preventive control
- Principle of reflection of plans
- Principle of organizational suitability
- Principle of individuality of controls
- Principle of standards
- Principle of critical point control
- The exception principle
- Principle of flexibility of Controls
- Principle of action

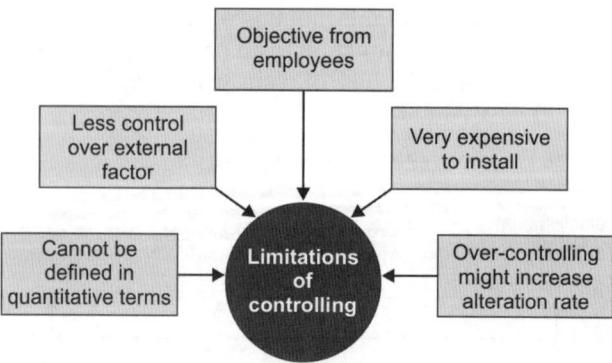

Fig. 14.6: Limitations in controlling.

corrective actions quickly and were successful in avoiding errors. But problems arise where management does not take corrective action in time to avoid deviations.

- **More expansive devise:** To make the control more systematic and effective. It requires careful and timely investigation of different business activities. It requires appointment of more skilled people, which requires more money to reward the workers for their work. Thus, it becomes a costly affair in terms of money and time.
- **Human reactions to control:** Control creates tension in the minds of workers and affects their actions and thinking. The pressure of work gives negative results and reduces the quantity and quality of work. The workers ignore long term goals and gives false reports about the performance.

TRADITIONAL TECHNIQUES OF CONTROL (FIG. 14.7)

- **Direct supervision and observation:** Direct Supervision and Observation' is the oldest technique of controlling. The supervisor himself observes the employees and their work. This brings him in direct contact with the workers. So, many problems are solved during supervision. The supervisor gets first hand information, and he has better understanding with the workers. This technique is most suitable for a small-sized business.
- **Financial statements:** All business organizations prepare Profit and Loss Account. It gives a summary of the income and expenses for a specified period. They also prepare Balance Sheet, which shows the financial position of the organization at the end of the specified period. Financial statements are used to control the organization. The figures of the current year can be compared with the previous year's figures. They can also be compared with the figures of other similar organizations. Ratio analysis can be used to find out and analyze the financial statements. Ratio analysis helps to understand the profitability, liquidity and solvency position of the business.
- **Budgetary control:** A budget is a planning and controlling device. Budgetary control is a technique of managerial control through budgets. It is the essence of financial control. Budgetary control is done for all aspects of a business such as income, expenditure, production, capital and revenue. Budgetary control is done by the budget committee.
- **Break-even analysis:** Break-even analysis or break-even point is the point of no profit, no loss. For example, when an organization sells 50K cars it will break even. It means that, any sale below this point will cause losses and any sale above this point will earn profits. The Break-even analysis acts as a control device. It helps to find out the company's performance. So the company can take collective action to improve its performance in the future. Break-even analysis is a simple control tool.
- **Return on investment (ROI):** Investment consists of fixed assets and working capital used in business. Profit on the investment is a reward for risk taking. If the ROI is high then the financial performance of a business is good and vice-versa. **ROI** is a tool to improve financial performance. It helps the business to compare its present performance with that of previous years' performance. It helps to conduct inter-firm comparisons. It also shows the areas where corrective actions are needed.
- **Management by objectives (MBO):** MBO facilitates planning and control. It must fulfill following requirements:
  - Objectives for individuals are jointly fixed by the superior and the subordinate
  - Periodic evaluation and regular feedback to evaluate individual performance
  - Achievement of objectives brings rewards to individuals.
- **Management audit:** management Audit is an evaluation of the management as a whole. It critically examines the full management process, i.e., planning, organizing, directing, and controlling. It finds out the efficiency of the management. To check the efficiency of the management, the company's plans, objectives, policies, procedures, personnel relations and systems of control are examined very carefully. Management auditing is conducted by a team of experts. They collect data from past records, members of management, clients and employees. The data is analyzed and conclusions are drawn about managerial performance and efficiency.
- **Management information system (MIS):** In order to control the organization properly the management needs accurate information. They need information about the internal working of the organization and also about the external environment. Information is collected continuously to identify problems and find out solutions. **MIS** collects data, processes it and provides it to the managers. MIS may be manual or computerized. With MIS, managers can delegate authority to subordinates without losing control.
- **PERT and CPM techniques:** Program Evaluation and Review Technique (**PERT**) and Critical Path Method (**CPM**) techniques were developed in USA in the late 50's. Any program consists of various activities and sub-activities. Successful completion of any activity

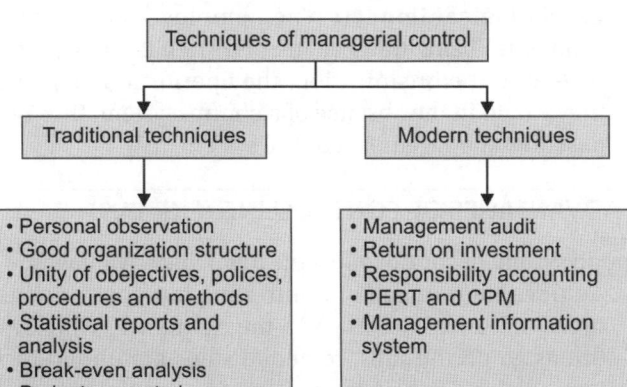

Fig. 14.7: Techniques of managerial control.

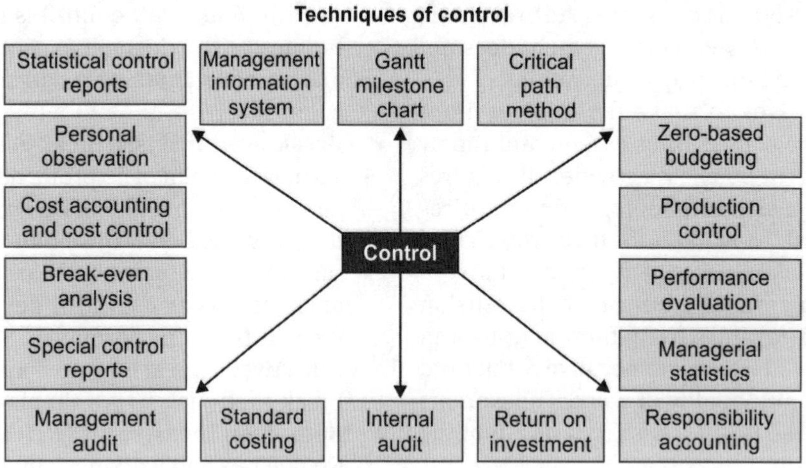

Techniques of control

- Statistical control reports
- Management information system
- Gantt milestone chart
- Critical path method
- Personal observation
- Cost accounting and cost control
- Break-even analysis
- Special control reports
- Management audit
- Standard costing
- Internal audit
- Return on investment
- Zero-based budgeting
- Production control
- Performance evaluation
- Managerial statistics
- Responsibility accounting

(Control)

Fig. 14.8: Techniques of supervision.

depends upon doing the work in a given sequence and in a given time. Importance is given to identifying the critical activities. Critical activities are those which have to be completed on time otherwise the full project will be delayed.

- **Self-control:** Self-control means self-directed control. A person is given freedom to set his own targets, evaluate his own performance and take corrective measures as and when required. Self-control is especially required for top level managers because they do not like external control. The subordinates must be encouraged to use self-control because it is not good for the superior to control each and everything. However, self-control does not mean no control by the superiors. The superiors must control the important activities of the subordinates. **Figure 14.8** shows techniques of supervision.

■ SOUND CONTROL SYSTEM

A sound control system is important for the following reasons:

- **Helps in detecting mistakes:** A continuous control mechanism helps in detecting mistakes at early stages of performance. It saves time, effort and money by not allowing the problems turn into major deviations at later stages. Increasing costs, labor absenteeism and turnover, defective product samples are few of the indications that managers note at the early stage so that production schedule is not disturbed subsequently.
- **Helps in managing complex situations:** In a small-sized organization, managers can personally control various organizational activities but as organizations grow in size, they become complex and managers cannot personally monitor all the activities.
- **Helps managers face change and uncertainty:** Past policies help managers make plans for future. Future being uncertain, planned objectives may not be achieved. Changes in consumer preferences and demand, technological factors, Government regulations, policies of suppliers and competitors can make the plans ineffective.
- **Helps in monitoring the actions of employees:** If employees are sure of not making mistakes, actual results will always be as expected and there will be no need for managers to monitor their activities; but it does not happen.
- **Helps in identifying potential of the organizations:** Control system enables the organization to face challenges and changes as they occur and helps to explore future opportunities which the organizations can venture into.
- **Facilitates delegation:** Managers delegate authority down the scalar chain as organizational workload cannot be handled by them alone. However, the accountability continues to vest with managers. Managers ensure that delegated tasks are effectively accomplished by the subordinates. An effectively designed control system helps managers in this regard.
- **Facilitates decentralization:** Increasingly complex organizations decentralize the activities to effectively achieve their goals. Wide geographical dispersions with respect to production, marketing and research activities make it impossible for the control mechanism to be initiated from the head office.
- **Coordination:** Control provides unity of direction to various organizational activities. It ensures that actions conform to plans and there is complete synchronization between physical, financial and human resources; internal and external environment; and goals at various levels.
- **Psychological impact:** When employees know their actions are being watched, that is, when there is control system in the organization, they perform better than they would in the absence of a control system. **Box 14.2** describes management control system.

■ ADVANTAGES OF CONTROLLING (FIG. 14.9)

A good system of control offers the following advantages:

- **Achievement of goals:** Controlling is a goal-oriented process. It keeps activities on the right track. Whenever things go off the rails, remedial steps are undertaken immediately. Every attempt is made to conform events, to set targets and thereby achieve results efficiently and effectively.

> **Box 14.2:** Management control system.
>
> - **Policies control:** The success of business hangs on formulation of sound policies and proper implementation. There is a great need of control over policies.
> - **Control over organization:** For the control over organization the management uses organization's manual and organizational chart. Designing and organizing various departments for smooth running of business is very essential. If any problem or conflict arises the management control attempts to remove the causes of such frictions and rationalize the organizational structure as to ensure its efficient working.
> - **Control over personnel:** Anything that the business accomplishes is the result of the action of those people who work in the organization. It is people, not figure, that get things done. The personnel manager is responsible to draw a control plan for having control over the personnel of the concern.
> - **Control over wages and salaries:** Control over wages and salaries is sometimes assigned to the personnel department or a specially constituted wages and salary committee.
> - **Control over cost:** The cost accountant who is responsible to control cost set cost standards, labor material and overhead. He makes comparison of actual cost data with standard cost. Cost control is delicate task and is supplemented by budgetary control system.

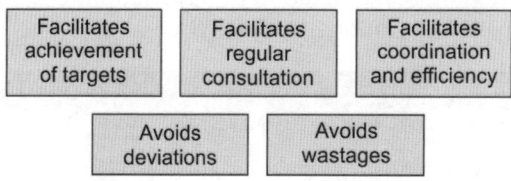

Fig. 14.9: Advantage of controlling.

- **Execution and revision of plans:** It is through controlling appropriate steps are taken to ensure that each plan is implemented in a predetermined way. Controlling measures progress, uncovers deviations, indicates corrective steps and thus keeps everything on track.
- **Brings order and discipline:** In an organization, while pursuing goals managers and their subordinates often commit mistakes. For example, problems are diagnosed incorrectly, lesser quality inputs are ordered, wrong products are introduced, and poor designs are followed, and so on.
- **Facilitates decentralization of authority:** When managers delegate work to lower levels, they must also ensure that the subordinates do not deviate from a predetermined course of action. A system of control ensures this by forcing subordinates to conform to plans.
- **Promotes coordination:** Control facilitates coordination between different departments and divisions by providing them unity of direction. Individuals and their activities are tied to a set of common objectives. Such a unified focus ensures accomplishment of results efficiently and effectively.
- **Cope with uncertainty and change:** The environment in which organizations operate is complex and ever changing. New products emerge, innovations come up, and new regulations are passed, and so on.

STANDARDS

A standard is a means of determining what something should be. In nursing education, the standard refers to the established criteria for the provision of nursing education. In case of nursing practice, standards are the established criteria for the practice of nursing. Standards are having permanent value. A nursing standard can be a target. Standard is an established rule as basis of comparison in measuring or finding capacity, quality context and value of objects in the same category. Standard is a broad statement of quality. It is a definite level of excellence as adequately required, aimed at or possible. Standard is a predetermined baseline condition as level of excellence that comprises a model to be followed and practiced. It is used as a measurement tool.

Definitions

- "A standard is a model of established practice which has general recognition and acceptance among registered professional nurses and is commonly accepted as correct standards of practice are agreed on levels of competence as determined by the ANA and specially nursing organizations".
- "Standards are defined as authoritative statements that describe a common level of care as performance by which the quality of practice can be determined or measured. Standard helps define professional practice".

Meaning of Standards

- Standards are as broad statement of quality. It is a definite level of excellence or adequately required, aimed at possible.
- It agreed upon achieved level of performance, considered proper and adequate for a specific purpose against which actual performance is compared.
- Standard is an acknowledge measure of comparison for quantities or qualitative value, criterion, norm.
- Standard are established rules or basis of comparison in measuring or judging capacity, quality context and value of objects in the same category. **Figure 14.10** shows management standards.
- The term norm is frequently used synonymously with standard in the literature. Selected standards are reliable and relevant for the category being compared.

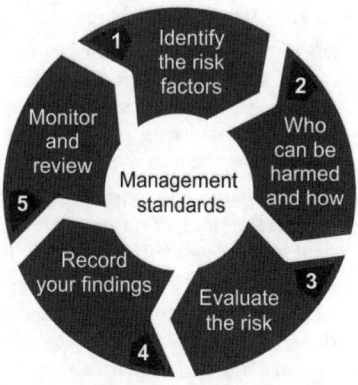

Fig. 14.10: Management standards.

Chapter 14: Controlling

Purposes of Standards

In order to provide a high quality of nursing education is necessary that nurse educators develop standard education and appropriate evaluation tools.

- Standards give direction and provide guidelines.
- Standards provide a baseline for evaluating quality cr nursing education and thereby quality care.
- It helps to plan for the faculty recruitment, development of infrastructure and others.
- It aids in curriculum planning, implementation are evaluation.
- It assists in planning for student welfare activities are staff welfare activities.
- Standards help improve quality of nursing care increase effectiveness of care and improve efficient.
- A standard may help to improve documentation c nursing care.
- Standards may help to determine the degree to which standards of nursing care maintained.
- Standards help supervisors to guide nursing staff improve performance.
- Standards may help to improve basis for decision-making
- Standards may help justify demands.
- Standards may help clarify nurse's area of accountability.
- Standards may help nursing to define clearly different levels of care.

Important of Standards

- It is an authoritative statement by which the quality nursing practice, service and education can be judged.
- In nursing practice, standards are established for the practice of nursing.
- It is a guideline, a recommended path to safe conand and aid to professional performance.
- It provides a baseline for evaluating quality of nurse care, increases effectiveness of care and improve efficiency.
- Standards, help supervisors to guide nursing staff improve performances.
- Standards may help to clarify nurses' area of accountability.
- Standards may help nursing to clearly define different levels of care.
- Standard is a device for quality assurance as quality control.

Table 14.1 describes Joint Commission of American Hospital (JCAH) nusing services standards.

Sources of Nursing Standards

- Professional organization or association, e.g., Trained Nurses' Association of India (TNAI)

Table 14.1: Joint Commission of American Hospital (JCAH) nursing services standards.

Standards	Emphasis
Standard I	• The nursing department/service shall be directed by a qualified nurse administer and shall be appropriately integrated with the medical staff and with other hospital staffs that provide and contribute to patient care • The administrator of the nursing department/service shall be a qualified, Registered nurse with appropriate education, experience, and licensure and demonstrated ability in nursing practice and administration
Standard II	• The nursing department/service shall be organized to meet the nursing care needs of patients and to maintain established standards of nursing practice • The nursing department/service shall have a written organizational plan that delineates lines of authority, accountability and communication. The manner in which the nursing department/service is organized shall be consistent with the variety of patient services offered and the scope of nursing care activities • Reviewing and approving policies and procedures • Establishing standards of nursing care accounting for professional and administrative nursing staff activities. Implementing the approved policies of the nursing department/service. Appointing committees as needed. Encouraging nursing staff personnel to participate in staff education programs
Standard III	• Nursing department/service assignments in the provision of nursing care shall be commensurate with the qualifications of nursing personnel and shall be designed to meet the nursing care needs of patient • A sufficient number of qualified registered nurses shall be on duty at all times to give patients the nursing care that requires the judgment and specialized skills of a registered nurse
Standard IV	• Individualized, goal-directed nursing care shall be provided to patients through the use of the nursing process • The nursing process (assessment, planning, intervention, evaluation) shall be documented for each hospitalized patient from admission through discharge
Standard V	• Nursing department/service personnel shall be prepared through appropriate education and training programs for their responsibilities in the provision of nursing care • Education/training programs for nursing department/service personnel shall be ongoing and designed to augment their knowledge of pertinent new developments in patient care and to maintain current competence. The scope and complexity of program shall be based on the documented educational needs of nursing staff personnel and the resources available to meet those needs
Standard VI	• Written policies and procedures that reflect optimal standards of nursing shall guide the provision of nursing care • Written standards of nursing practice and reflected policies and procedures shall define and describe the scope and conduct of patient care provided by the nursing staff. These standards, policies and procedures shall be reviewed at least annually, revised as necessary, dated to indicate the time of the last review, signed by the responsible reviewing authority and implicated
Standard VII	• As part of the hospitals quality assurance program, the quality and—appropriateness of the patient care provided by the nursing department/service are monitored and evaluated and identified problems are resolved • The nursing department/service has a planned and systematic process for monitoring and evaluation of the quality and appropriateness of patient care and for resolving identified problems

Box 14.3: Characteristics of standard.

- Statement must be broad enough to apply to a vide variety of settings must be realistic, acceptable, attainable.
- The nurse care must be developed by members of the nursing profession, preferable nurses practising that the direct care level with consultation of experts in the domain.
- Should be resembled in positive terms and indicate acceptable performance, i.e., good, excellence, etc.
- The nursing care must express what is desirable optional level must be understandable and stated in unambiguous terms.
- Must be based on current knowledge and scientific practice must be reviewed and revised periodically.
- May be directed towards an ideal, i.e., optional standards or may only specify the minimal care that must be attained, i.e., minimum standard.
- Standards that work are objective, acceptable, achievable and flexible.

- Licensing bodies, e.g., statutory bodies, INC, SNC, etc.
- Universities and Boards, e.g., The TN Dr MGR Medical University.
- Institutions/healthcare agencies, e.g., University Hospitals, Health centers.
- Department of institutions, e.g., Department of Nursing.
- Patient care units, e.g., specific patients' unit.
- Government units at National, State and local level.
- Individual standards, e.g., personal standards.

Characteristics of Standards (Box 14.3 and Fig. 14.11)

- Statement must be broad.
- Must be realistic, acceptable and attainable.
- Standards of nursing care must be developed by members of the nursing profession, preferably nurses practicing at the direct care level with consultation of experts in the domain.
- It should be phrased in positive terms.
- Must be understandable and stated in unambiguous terms.
- Must be reviewed and revised periodically.
- May be directed towards an ideal, i.e., optional standards or only specify the minimal care that must be attained, i.e., minimum standard.
- And one must remember that standards that are workable are objective, acceptable, achievable and flexible.

Purposes of Standard Education

The purposes of publishing, circulating and enforcing nursing standards in education are to:
- Improve the quality of nursing education
- Decrease the cost of nursing education
- Ultimately to improve the patient care

Classification of Standards

Nursing care standards can be divided into ends and means standards. The ends standards are patient oriented, they describe the change as desired in a patient's physical status or behavior. The means standards are nursing oriented, they describe the activities and behavior designed to achieve the ends standards. Ends standards require information about the patients. A means standard calls for information about the nurse's performance.

Standards are expected to understand achievable and measurable. Standards can be classified and formulated according to frames of references relating to nursing structure, process and outcome, because standard is a descriptive statement of desired level of performance against which to evaluate the quality of service structure, process or outcomes.

Structure Standard

- The structure is related to the framework, that is care providing system and resources that support for actual provision of care.
- Evaluation of care concerns nursing staff, setting and the care environment.

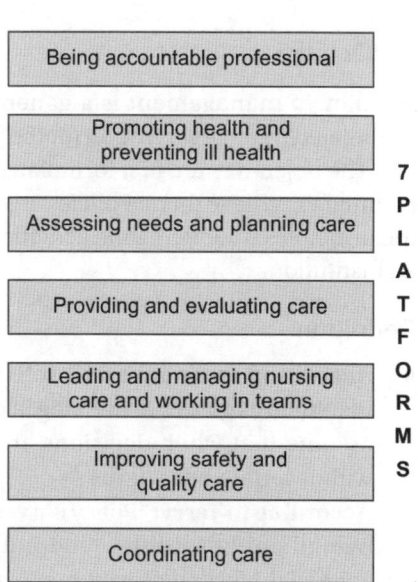

Fig. 14.11: Characteristics of standards.

Chapter 14: Controlling

- The use of standards based on structure implies that if the structure is adequate reliable, and desirable, standard will be met or quality care will be given.

Process Standards

- Process standards describe the behaviors of the nurse at the desired level of the performance.
- The criteria that specify desired method for specific nursing intervention process standards.
- A process standard involves the activities concerned with delivering patient care.
- In process standard, there is an element of professional judgment, i.e., determining the quality of the degree of skill. It includes nursing care techniques, procedures, regimens, processes.

Outcome Standards

- Descriptive statements of desired patient care results are outcome standards, because patient's results are outcomes of nursing interventions.
- Here outcome as a frame of references for setting of standards refers to description of the results of nursing activity in terms of the change that occur in the patient.
- An outcome standard measures change in the patient health status. In quality assurance outcomes are stated in positive terms as the nursing goal is to improve the health status of client.

Classification of Standards in the Hospital

Nursing care standards in hospital can be divided into ends and means standards.

End standards: The end standards are patient oriented; they describe the change as desired in a patient's physical status or behavior.

Mean standards:

- The mean standards are nursing oriented, they describe the activities and behavior designed to achieve end standards.
- End standards require information about the patients. A mean standard calls for information about the nurses' performance.
- Nursing care standards can be classified according to frame of references, relating to nursing structure, process and outcome.

Structure standard:

- A structural standard involves the set-up of the institution. The philosophy, goals and objectives, structure of the organization, facilities and equipment and qualifications of employees are some of the components of the structure of the organization.
- For example, recommended relationship between the nursing department and other departments in a healthy agency are structural standards, because they refer to the organizational structure in which nursing is implemented.
- It includes people, money, equipment, staffing policies, etc. The use of standards based on structure implies that if the structure is adequate, reliable and desirable, standard will be met and quality care will be given.

Process standard:

- Process standards describe the behaviors of the nurse at the desired level of performance.
- A process standard involves the activities concerned with delivering patient care. These standards measure nursing action involving patient care.
- The standards are stated in action verbs that are in observable and measurable terms. For example, "the patient demonstrates."
- The focus is on what was planned, what was done and what was communicated as recorded.
- In process standard, there is an element of professional judgment, i.e., determining the quality as the degree of skill. It includes nursing care technique, procedures, regimens, and processes.

Outcome standards:

- Descriptive statements of desired patient care results are outcome standard, because patients results are outcome of nursing intervention.
- An outcome standard measures changes in the patient health status. This change may be due to nursing care, medical care or as a result of variety of services offered to the patient.
- Outcome standards reflect the effectiveness and results rather than the process of giving care.
- Thus, structural standards are agency or group oriented process standards are nurse oriented and whereas outcome standards are patient results oriented.
- Normative standards describe practices considered 'good' or 'ideal' by some authoritative group.
- Empirical standards describe practices actually observed in a large number of patient care settings.

POLICIES

A policy in management is a general statement which is formulated by an organization for the guidance of its personnel. The objectives are first formulated and then policies are planned to achieve them. Policies are a mode of thought and the principles underlying the activities of an organization or an institution.

Definition

- **According to Koontz and O'Donnel:** "Policies were identified as guides to thinking in decision-making. They assume that when decisions are made, these will fall within certain boundaries."
- **According to Terry:** "Policy is a verbal, written or implied overall guide setting up boundaries that supply the general limits and direction in which managerial action will take place."

Meaning of Policy

- Policies do not require action, but are intended to guide managers in their decision commitments when they do not make decisions.
- Policies acting as principles provide rules of action for achieving organization's specific objectives. The coordinating links in the organization are provided by policies.
- They govern and guide the actions of an organization's overall performance and its objectives in the various areas of operation—production, finance, marketing and personnel.
- The clear formulation of policies helps the executives to plan every operational aspect of the enterprise. This considerably helps them in their decision making.
- Policy gives guidelines and leaves scope for interpretation for the person implementing them. This means that a policy has the flexibility for interpretation. A rigid policy becomes a rule.

Purposes of Policy

The policies are formulated for the following purposes (Fig. 14.12):

- The main purpose of policies is to ensure that there is no deviation from the planned course of action. The framework is set within which everybody is expected to work. Policies ensure that the broad guides for action are adhered to.
- Since policies chalk out a framework for each and every person, it ensures proper delegation of authority also. A manager knows the extent of authority required by a subordinate to undertake the work allotted to him. Policies serve the purpose of delegating adequate authority downwards.
- Policies allow the scope for interpretation. The main aspects are given in a policy but the actual mode of implementation is decided by the concerned person.
- Policies are helpful for future planning also. The impact and influence of policies help in thinking about the future.
- Policies also ensure consistency of action. The guidelines are similar for everybody and actions must conform to the broad outlines.

Formulation Policy

- To facilitate uniformity in actions.
- To set boundaries that provides basic limits and directions for managerial actions.
- To ensure quick decision making.
- To assist in coordinating the efforts of the employees.
- To ensure that goals are achieved as planned.
- To ensure effective delegation of authority, as it sets limits for the decisions taken by the subordinates.

Characteristics of a Sound Policy

Policies are formed to smoothen the working of an organization for achieving its goals. A sound policy will be one which helps in achieving its objectives. Following are the characteristics of a sound policy:

- It should be comprehensive in scope and flexible for its implementation.
- It should ensure good understanding and harmony among different departments.
- It should be based on facts and sound judgments.
- It should be uniform for its application.
- It must reflect its intended objectives,
- It should be clear, definite and positive,
- It should be properly communicated and clearly understood.
- It must be in writing so as to avoid misinterpretation.
- It must be reasonable, permanent and stable.
- It should be periodically reviewed to check up its effectiveness.
- It should incorporate all possible contingencies.

Process of Policy Formulation

Policy formulation is an important aspect of planning. The smooth working of an organization requires the formulation of policies. A well thought exercise is essential to formulate sound policies.

Following process should be followed for formulating a policy:

- **Defining policy area:** The area for which a policy is to be framed should be defined. The objectives and needs of the organization should be kept in mind while specifying the policy area.
- **Identifying policy alternatives:** The second step in policy formulation is the identification of policy alternatives. The alternatives should be decided on the basis of an analysis of external and internal environment.
- **Evaluating alternatives:** All the alternatives are evolved in the light of organizational objectives. It should be analyzed as to what contribution these alternatives will make in helping the organization for achieving its objectives.
- **Selection of a policy:** After proper evaluation, most appropriate alternative is selected. The selection of a policy is a long-term commitment. In case, the

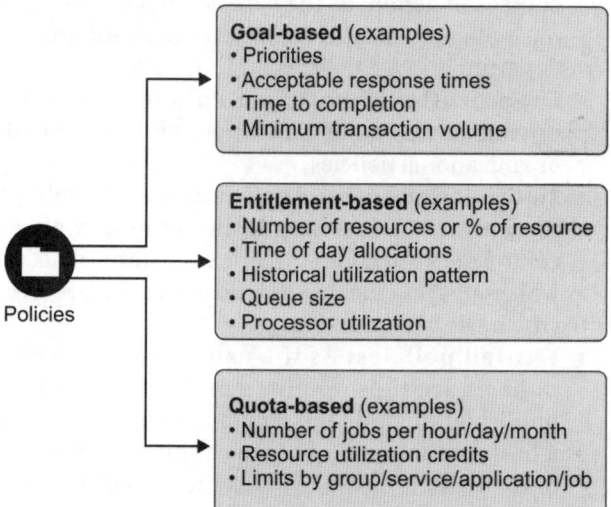

Fig. 14.12: Purposes of policies.

alternatives do not look satisfactory then efforts should be made to develop other alternatives.

- **Trial run of a policy:** The policy should be implemented on a trial basis. It should be assessed if the policy is achieving the desired objectives. There may be suggestions during the test run; these should be used to modify the policy.
- **Implementing policy:** If the policy is finally alright it should be implemented. The policy should be explained to those who are to implement it.

Factors Influencing Policies

Policies are framed to help in smoothening the operations of a business. They are influenced both by internal and external factors. Some of these factors are discussed here:

1. **Objectives and strategies of the organization:** All policies are framed to facilitate the achievement of objectives. The objectives and strategies fix the parameters within which the policies will operate.
2. **Organizational structure:** Organizational structure determines the levels of positions and fixes authority and responsibility of employees.
3. **Available resources:** The availability of resources such as human, financial, physical facilities will influence the formulation of a policy.
4. **Managerial values:** Managers are the persons who are the prime movers of policies. The ethics and value systems of managers have a direct influence on the formation and implementation of policies.
5. **Social factors:** A number of social factors also have an influence on the policies of the organization.
6. **Political factors:** Political factors have a great influence on the policies of an organization. The framework of business is determined by the party in power. The thinking of a political party will certainly be reflected in the industrial, fiscal and monetary policies of the government.

Classification of Policies

The policies are classified as **(Fig. 14.13)**:
 I. **On the basis of origin/source:**
   - **Originated policies:** Policies which are framed by the top executives, and directs the employees about what decisions they can take in a particular situation. Hence, the employees are supposed to follow them strictly.
   - **Appealed policies:** If a subordinate is confused regarding if he/she possesses sufficient authority to look after the situation or not, in that case, the subordinate may seek an order from the superior. This order is said to be appealed authority.
   - **Imposed policies:** Imposed policies are the ones imposed on the business, by the external agencies like government, suppliers, trade unions, industry associations, creditors, etc.
 II. **On the basis of level:**
   - **Basic policies:** Those policies of the firm which are pursued by the top management level are regarded as basic policies.

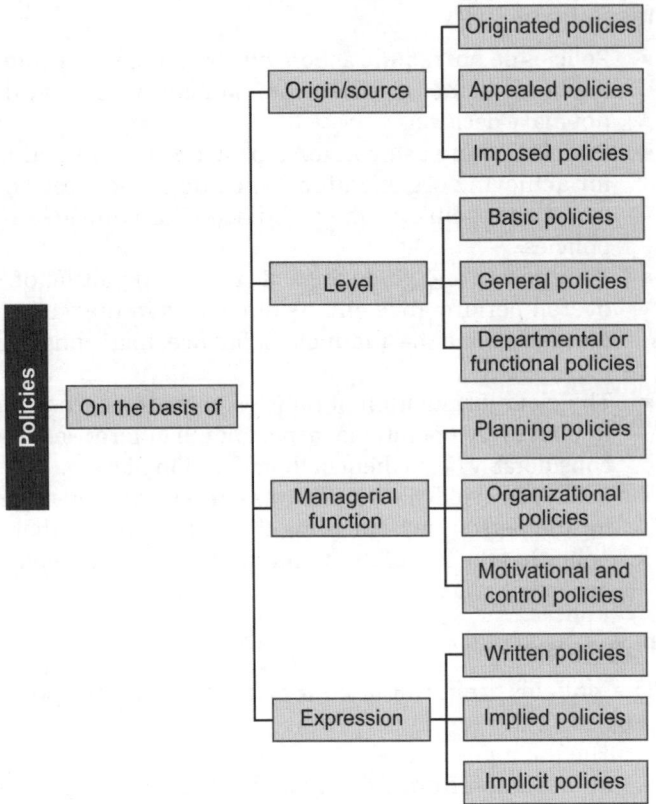

Fig. 14.13: Classifications of policies.

   - **General policies:** General Policies are for middle-level management, as they are related to the company's day to day operations and dealings.
   - **Departmental policies:** Departmental policies are specific in nature as they are framed for the particular department only. For instance marketing policies, production policies, personnel policies, purchase policies, finance policies, research and development policies.
 III. **On the basis of managerial function:**
   - **Planning policies:** Such policies embraces future courses of action, as they are formulated to achieve business targets. These can be organization-wide or department-wide policies.
   - **Organizational policies:** Policies concerning organizational goals and objectives are termed as organizational policies.
   - **Motivation and control policies:** Policies established to motivate or encourage employees as well as to control their activities, so as to lead the firm's objectives, while satisfying the personal goals of the employees.
 IV. **On the basis of expression:**
   - **Written policies:** As the name suggests, written policies are those policies of the firm which are published to guide the employees and also to have a basic understanding of the company's rules. Some of the written media, where written policies can be found are—bulletins or notice boards, news releases, handbooks, booklets or manuals.

- **Implied policies:** Policies which emerges from the conduct are implied policies. It emanates in the area where existing policies are not in force.
- **Implicit policies:** Policies communicated by word of mouth by the key people in the organization are called implicit policies.

Policies the basic set of rules which the employees are required to follow at the time of working and responding. It embraces the 'how' facet of planning. It defines as well as confines the limit of the behavior of employees and so the employees have to work within the periphery of policies.

Advantages of Policies

The advantages of policies are as follows:
- Policies ensure uniformity of action in respect of various matters at various organizational points. This makes actions more predictable.
- Policies speed up decisions at lower levels because subordinates need not consult their superiors frequently.
- Policies make it easier for the superior to delegate more and more authority to his subordinates without being unduly concerned because he knows that whatever decision the subordinates make will be within the boundaries of the policies.
- Policies give a practical shape to the objectives by elaborating and directing the way in which the predetermined objectives are to be attained.

Limitation of Policies

Policies are the guidelines which may help the managers in their day-to-day working. Policies do not provide ready-made answers to every problem. They suffer from the following limitations:
- **No universal solutions:** Policies do not offer universal solutions to all problems. Policies are framed under particular situations and remain suitable under those circumstances only.
- **No instant solutions:** Policies do not provide instant solutions to problems. These are only guidelines for the decision-makers.
- **Dampen human initiation:** Too many policies kill the initiative of managers. They become habituated to act according to policies and do not try to their judgment. Policies also leave little room for individual initiative.
- **No substitute for human judgment:** Policies do not provide standard solution to various problems. They are only guidelines which help managers in taking decisions.

PROCEDURES

A "procedure" is a term used in a variety of industries to define a series of steps, taken together, to achieve a desired result. Procedures explain how to accomplish a task. A procedure is sometimes called a work instruction. A procedure is a sequence of steps for completing a given activity. A procedure may outline the manner in which a particular policy is to be implemented, but it cannot take the place of that policy. Recall that a good policy is inviolate, that is, policies change slowly and infrequently if at all. Procedures, on the other hand, change often as dictated by any number of factors such as staffing, equipment, space, and technology. An earlier procedure related to a given policy may have required a number of steps which can now be eliminated as a result of new technology.

Definition

- A procedure is a document that instructs workers on executing one or more activities of a business process. It describes the sequence of steps, and specifies for each step what needs to be done, often including when the procedure should be executed and by whom
- A procedure is an established method of accomplishing a task, usually with steps that are performed in a prescribed order.

Meaning of Procedure

- The ultimate goal of every 'Procedure' is to provide the reader with a clear and easily understood plan of action required to carry out or implement a policy.
- A well-written procedure will also help eliminate common misunderstandings by identifying job responsibilities and establishing boundaries for the jobholders.
- Good procedures actually allow managers to control events in advance and prevent the organization (and employees) from making costly mistakes.
- Procedure, refers to a comprehensive set of instructions that prescribes a certain way of performing a process, or part of a process, in relation to time.
- It states a chronological sequence for undertaking activities, so as to achieve the objectives.

Features of Procedures

Some important features of procedures are (**Fig. 14.14**):
- They are a guide to action.
- They are generally meant for repetitive work so that some steps are followed every time that activity is accomplished.

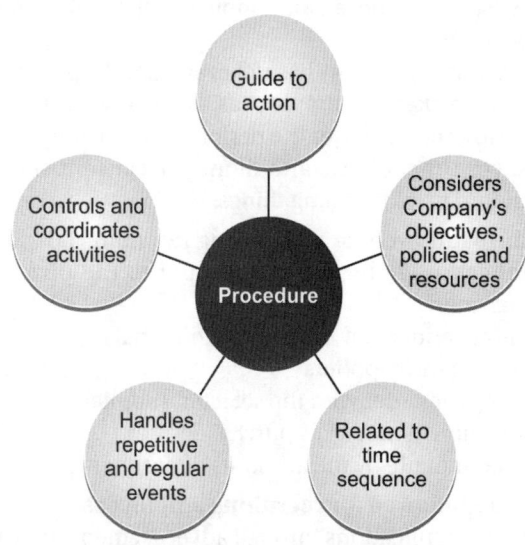

Fig. 14.14: Features of procedure.

This is the reason why 'procedures' are also called 'repetitive use plans.'
- Procedures are established in keeping with the objectives, policies and resources position.
- They are concerned with establishing the time sequence for work to be done.

Differentiating between Policies and Procedures

Policies
- Are general in nature
- Identify company rules
- Explain why they exist
- Tells when the rule applies
- Describe who it covers
- Shows how the rule is enforced
- Describes the consequences
- Are normally described using simple sentences and paragraphs

Procedures
- Identify specific actions
- Explain when to take actions
- Describe alternatives
- Shows emergency procedures
- Includes warning and cautions
- Gives examples
- Shows how to complete forms
- Are normally written using and outline format

Importance of Procedure
Upcoming points will discuss the importance of procedures:
- It defines the manner in which work is to be carried out and eliminate all the irrelevant or repetitive steps.
- It ensures a high level of uniformity in tasks, and consistency in the decisions which helps in avoiding chaos.
- To undertake any task in an effective manner, the procedure suggests the ideal ways and methods.
- It facilitates in eliminating or reducing errors or accidents.
- It assists in the successful completion of the work assigned in a timely manner.
- Procedures specify the base for evaluating the performance of the workers or employees. In this way, it ensures executive control over the performance of employees.
- It saves time, efforts and money because it states the standard ways for doing things.

Procedure followed for purchasing raw materials:
- Request made by the storekeeper to the purchasing department
- Inviting tenders for purchase of materials
- Selecting the suppliers
- Placing the order with the selected suppliers
- Inspection of materials purchased
- Payment made by the accounts department

Procedure followed for recruiting employees:
- Inviting applications through advertisements on various platforms.
- Screening of the employees, through the CV or resume, received for the post.
- Shortlisting the candidates and inviting them.
- Conducting a written test.
- Conducting an interview for the candidates who clear the written test.
- Medical test for those who are selected in the interview round.
- Candidates who pass the medical test successfully are sent joining letter.

Limitations of Procedure
As every coin has two sides, the procedure also has some limitations. As a standard way is prescribed for performing the task, it constrains the scope for innovation or improvement in performing the work.

■ PROTOCOLS

A protocol is a standard set of rules that allow staff to communicate with each other. These rules include what type of data may be transmitted, what commands are used to send and receive data, and how data transfers are confirmed. A protocol may describe mandatory nursing assessments, behaviors, and documentation for establishing and maintaining invasive appliances; methods of administering specific drugs; special-care modalities for patients with certain disorders; other components of patient care; lines of authority.

Definition
A nursing protocol is considered to be a set of predetermined criteria that define appropriate nursing interventions that articulate or describe situations in which the nurse makes judgments relative to a course of action for effective management of common patient care problems.

Meaning of Protocol
- Basically, a protocol is a document that is developed to guide decision-making around specific issues, whether it is how to diagnose, treat and care for someone with a specific condition, what procedures to follow to halt the spread of infection, or how to report that a specific event has taken place.
- The protocol sets out in a step-by-step way what actions should be taken, explaining the reason and justification for each action as it goes.
- It is like a 'guidebook' for health are staff, helping them to make sure they are taking the right action to get the best outcomes and avoid any possible problems.

Constitutes a good protocol:
- Clearly documented lines of accountability
- Specific referral criteria
- Clarity
- Brevity
- Fit with professional guidelines

Importance of Nursing Protocols

- Provide direction and guidance
- Perform with consistency and efficiency
- Avoid conflict and misunderstanding
- Act as a communication and teaching tool
- Define the condition
- Subjective (show history and symptoms)
- Objective (describe findings from physical exam)
- Client education/Counseling (patient education materials)
- Follow-up and consultation/Referral (more specialized care?)

Use of Protocols

The use of protocols serves several general purposes:

- Ensuring that educators remain focused on the specific, agreed-upon objectives and goals for a professional conversation.
- Building the foundational communication and facilitation skills essential to effective professional collaboration.
- Helping to nurture a culture of collegiality, trust, and mutual appreciation.
- Ensuring everyone in the group has an opportunity to contribute and be heard during a discussion.
- Reducing the tendency toward subjective, digressive, or one-sided conversations.
- Promoting focused substantive, in-depth conversations about a specific topic.
- Encouraging active, respectful listening among all participants.
- Providing a "safe space" for teachers to share their work with colleagues without being concerned about negative criticism.
- Allowing difficult questions or issues to be raised in constructive ways.
- Eliminating unhelpful excuses, complaints, or comments about student behavior from professional discussion.
- Keeping conversations focused on goals, solutions, and results.

Nursing Protocols

- The development of comprehensive nursing protocols is basic to a nursing quality control program.
- Most nursing tasks are carried out at the initiative of the nurses rather than in direct response to a physician order.
- The physician makes the medical decisions about medications, diet, and so on; but he nurses must fill in the details to ensure that the patient receives comprehensive nursing care.
- The nursing staff must also ensure that nursing services are rendered if the physician is derelict in writing basic orders.
- While a careful nursing staff will quickly call this problem to the attention of the attending physician, this can delay the patient's care.
- Since a principal goal of a legally effective quality control program is to reduce litigation through increased patient satisfaction, the delay poses a problem, since, it will reduce patient satisfaction even if it does not result in an injury.

Protocol application in nursing: Nursing protocols often deal with procedures that are matters of medical opinion. A physician may order that a gram of penicillin be given the patient in one liter of 5 percent dextrose. The nurse will decide on the type of intravenous (IV) fluid set to use the size and type of needle to use, and the location of the vein to be used. These decisions should be part of the nursing protocol. This will not create a problem unless the protocol that is followed is in opposition to a physician's order.

Advantages of using Protocols

- Framework for a complex, specialized sequence of activities.
- Provides increased autonomy with a focus to shape future work.
- Ensures consensus within the primary care team.
- Legal protection
- Identifies training needs
- May facilitate change

Disadvantages of using Protocols

- Stifles individual care management
- May reduce need for qualified staff
- Require regular review
- Compliance may be problematic
- Restricts clinical discretion

NURSING PERFORMANCE

Nursing performance is an important measure of work productivity and patient safety. At the bedside, nurses are responsible for assessing and monitoring patients' changing conditions, coordinating their care, administering medications precisely, and communicating with the patients and their families

Definition

Nursing performance has been defined as a set of nursing activities or behaviors that are performed by nurses and directed toward the recovery and well-being of the patients assigned to their care. The main purpose is to meet the needs and expectations of the patients through this set of activities.

Concept of Performance

- Nurses spend more time with patients than do any other healthcare providers and patient outcomes are affected by nursing care quality. Thus, improvements in patient safety can be achieved by improving nurse performance.
- Nursing performance, including cognitive, physical, and organizational factors that affect such performance, focusing on research studies that reported original data from nurse participants.
- Nurses monitor the patient over time through direct (physical assessment) and indirect (charting, reviewing

laboratory results) care processes. Active creation of patient information (notes, flow sheets) helps nurses maintain that situation awareness.

Types of Performance

To manage healthcare, nurses perform numerous and diverse tasks that are not limited to direct contact with the patient. Further, RNs also perform activities that do not require RN training, such as housekeeping. Nursing tasks have been classified into three categories: direct patient care, indirect patient care, and nonnursing tasks or tasks unrelated to nursing

- **Direct patient care:** Direct patient care involves tasks performed at the bedside, such as establishing intravenous access and administering medication. Studies indicated that nurses spent 26% to 31% of their time on direct patient care.
- **Indirect patient care:** Patient care is not limited to nursing at the bedside. Indirect patient care, which takes place away from the bedside, also is important. Indirect patient care includes charting, preparing medications, and coordinating care.
- **Nonnursing tasks:** Nurses also perform nonclinical activities that can be performed by other staff. Nonnursing tasks include searching for equipment or supplies and walking. The amount of time spent on nonnursing tasks is important because it is time not spent on patient monitoring. Nurses must maintain situation awareness of a patient's health status. Based on their understanding of the patient's current health status and treatment plan and the typical trajectory of illness, nurses are able to anticipate the patient's short-term health needs and adjust treatment accordingly.

Measurement of Competences

- Competencies are assessed when nurses are first licensed and periodically thereafter to ensure that nurses maintain their proficiencies and remain abreast of current healthcare issues.
- Generally, competencies are the effective application of knowledge, judgment, and skills expected of a nurse. However, the competencies required for a nurse depend on several factors, including education (e.g., vocational nurse vs. baccalaureate degree), role (e.g., provider of care vs. coordinator of care), and unit (e.g., surgical vs. neonatal).
- Although state boards ensure nursing knowledge and safety through administration of the National Council Licensure Examination prior to approving a nursing license, hospitals in all states must continue to ensure staffing competencies as a condition for Joint Commission accreditation.
- Nursing-sensitive quality indicators (NSQIs) refer to the impact that nursing care has on patient outcomes. An example of an NSQI is a hospital-acquired infection.
- Nursing behaviors affect the rate of infections because nurses change dressings, maintain catheters and chest tubes, and practice hand washing. Higher rates of infections are considered indicators of lower-quality nursing care.

Ways to Improve Work Performance as a Nurse:

- **Look into the future:** Set some professional goals. Start with one year from now, where the target could merely be to perfect your skills on the unit. Then, think about three years from now—maybe you can get certified in your field of work.
- **Build upon your weaknesses:** Hands-on clinical skills are taught in nursing school and built upon after graduation. Some areas of nursing use specific skills more than other areas. Seek out opportunities, even if you are scared to build up your weak areas.
- **Join committees:** Joining a committee can improve work performance because it broadens the background as a nurse.
- **Know your limitations:** Gaining an understanding of the limits is sometimes accomplished when you are drowning in work. Try not to take on too much to be a "super nurse."
- **Boost your self-esteem:** Boosting your self-esteem can impact the way you work. Jazz up your scrubs with a new pin, get a massage or buy a new pair of shoes to make yourself feel better.
- **Exercise before work:** Next time you work, take a 15-minute brisk walk before you start your day. It will boost your work performance because you can concentrate better and focus on your tasks.
- **Make a list:** When you are at work, take a few minutes before you assess your patients to prioritize your assignments. Try using a task list and prioritizing as nursing school taught you.
- **Avoid distractions:** If you can, hide at work. As a charge nurse, I have to go into hiding. Constant little distractions or interruptions every time I step out of a room can ruin my daily workflow.
- **Finish what you start:** If there is one thing I tell my new nurses that I train it's, "chart as you go." I work in labor and delivery, which often acts as an ER. It is always changing in pace, making it critical to keep up with documentation in real-time.
- **Learn something new each day:** Always learn something new. When evaluation time comes, create goals to achieve for the next year.

Common problems-related performance: The nursing shortage and inefficiencies in the nursing work system result in task overload for nurses. Nurses work long shifts, often without breaks. Their time is not used efficiently. Examples of the latter include excessive documentation, waiting, and searching. Completion of such tasks results in less time spent on patient monitoring, which is needed to maintain situation awareness.

AUDIT

Audit is the instrument for quantify assurance. It developed in 19th century; the nursing audit is similar to an audit performed by accounting departments. It is a process that offers the nursing personnel in a health agency the opportunity to create and enforce standards of nursing care and to examine their own practice in systematic manner.

Meaning of Auditing

Auditing is broadly defined as a systematic process of objectively obtaining and evaluating evidence in respect of certain assertions about economic actions and events, to ascertain the degree of correspondence between those assertions and established criteria and reporting the results to interested parties. Auditing usually covers a particular period of time. Auditing may be narrowly defined as a written report on the examination of financial statements for a particular period of time.

Definition

- **Nursing audit** is the systematic, critical analysis of the quality of clinical/community care. It is an official examination of nursing records for the purpose of evaluation verification and betterment of nursing care.
- **Nursing audit** is a systematic formal and written appraisal by nurses of the quality of the content and process of nursing service from care record for discharged patients.
- **Nursing audit** is the systematic critical analysis of the quality of clinical care. It is an official examination of nursing records for the purpose of evaluation.
- **Nursing audit** is a process of collecting information from nursing reports and other documented evidence about patient care and assessing the quality of care by the use of quality assurance programmer.

Objectives of Nursing Audit

- To justify the cost incurred on human and material resources.
- To study the quality of patient care against defined criteria.
- To take remedial actions towards cost effectiveness.
- To assess the competence of nursing staff.
- To prevent repetition of mistakes and to bring to notice the deficiencies in hospital care and in correcting the causative factors.

To bring to notice the overall objective of nursing audit is quality assurance of delivered care in relation to change in the health status of the patient and cost effectiveness.

Types of Auditing

- **Nursing management audit:** This type is more structure oriented focusing on administrative aspects of the nurse's responsibilities and nurses that the health facilities are suitably equipped to provide care.
- **Retrospective audit:** This is the evaluation of nursing care by examining the records and charts of discharged patients.
- **Concurrent audit:** It is the evaluation of the nursing care by the observation and retrospective method during the delivery of care. The best method of audit depends on the objective of audit.

Characteristics of Audit

- Audit looks at the entire process of care including administration and not just at clinical management.
- Compares the care which actually is given. Standard procedures are agreed to decide which care should be given.
- Concentrates on finding solutions for the problems identified. **Figure 14.15** shows six principles of auditing.

Principles of Auditing

Fundamental principles are those according to which the books of business accounts are audited. These principles can be changed according the desire of the auditor. We discuss the main principles of auditing under these headings:

- **Planning:** It is the basic principle of auditing. The auditor should plan before starting the work. In planning auditor decides accounting about the system and internal control procedure.
- **Honesty:** Honesty and sincerity is the second important principle of auditing. The loyalty of auditor to work and profession must be beyond the doubts.
- **Impartiality:** In case of audit, the attitude of the auditor must be impartial. Keeping in view this principle his personal views may not be included in the audit report.
- **Secrecy:** Secrecy must be maintained by the auditor during the process of audit. He cannot disclose any information to the third party.
- **Evidence:** During the audit, the auditor can collect the evidence through the working paper. He can frame his opinion on the audit evidence. The nature and source of evidence must be kept in view by the auditor.
- **Consistency:** It is an important principle of auditing. In case of selecting, the rates of depreciation and valuation of stock the accountant must follow the rates of the coming years. In this regard there should be consistency and changes are not acceptable.

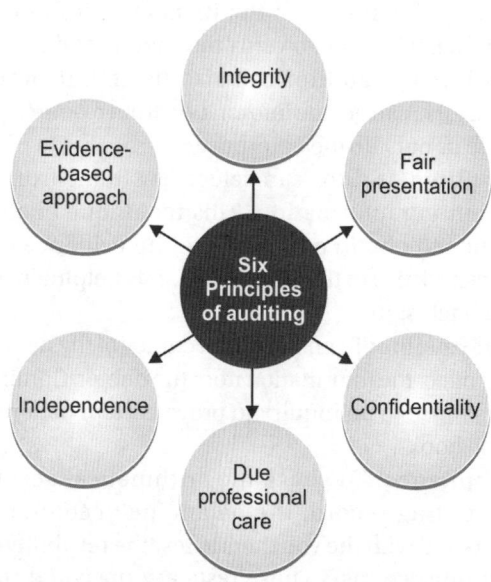

Fig. 14.15: Six principles of auditing.

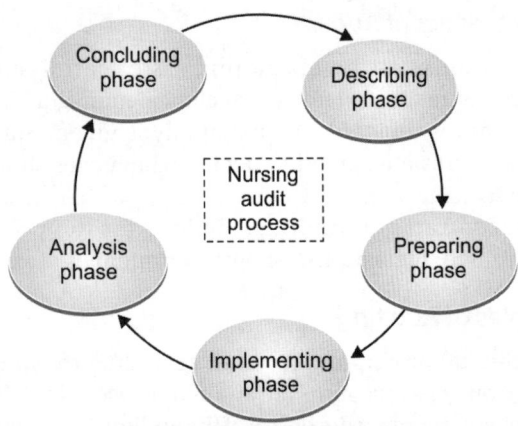

Fig. 14.16: Nursing audit process.

- **Legal framework:** The business activities may run within the rules and legal formalities. To protect the rights of the interested party's rules must be applied.
- **Working paper preparation:** The auditor collect documents providing evidence that audit was carried out according the principles. The auditor prepares the working paper and kept in this custody as a proof.
- **Internal control:** The auditor will examine the accounting system and inter control. To frame his opinion, he keeps in view the evidence obtained from the books.
- **Report:** According the principle of auditing a report will be prepared by the auditor at the end. It may be conditional or unconditional. The auditor can draw conclusion and disclose the facts and figures about the business for general information. **Figure 14.16** shows nursing audit process.

Techniques of Auditing

Techniques of auditing mean the procedure and method, which is adopted by the auditor in checking the accounts. Following are the important techniques of audit:

- **Examination of record:** This technique is commonly used by the auditors; the inspection of books and documents is made to verity the validity of data.
- **Inquiry:** The auditor can also use the technique of inquiry. He can get the information from resource persons inside or outside the enterprise.
- **Sampling:** Auditor can select few items from whole accounting information. This technique enables the auditor to obtain and evaluate the evidence of some characteristics of the whole class. It is helpful in forming the conclusion.
- **Confirmation:** To ensure the accuracy of the data auditor can collect the information from the debtor. Confirmation is response to an inquiry to prove certain data recorded in the books.
- **Compliance:** To check the arithmetical accuracy of accounting record, the balancing accounts can be compared with the vouchers to test the reliability of data.
- **Compliance test:** These tests are designed to check the effectiveness and compliance of internal control. In obtaining the audit evidence, auditor is concerned with the existence of effective internal control.
- **Use of computer techniques:** There are large number of audit techniques, such as audit software, test packs and mapping which can be used by the auditor to test the accuracy of the data.
- **Substantive test:** There are designed to obtain evidence that data produced by accounting system is accurate or not. It has two kinds:
  1. Test of detail transaction.
  2. Test of significant ratios and trends.
- **Dependence on experts and auditors:** The auditor has to rely on the internal and other auditors to complete his work. He has also to rely on other experts, such as lawyers, engineers and doctors for their expert opinion about the business.
- **Analytical review:** It consists of studying significant ratios, trends and investigating different changes. This review procedure is based on the expectations of relationship among the past and present data.

Benefits of Audit

- **Patient:** The fundamental principle behind nursing care audit to everyone involved in care.
- **Nursing staff:** For nurses, nursing care audit offers the opportunity to concentrate on areas of care where their skills and efforts can have positive outcomes, greater senses of achievement, autonomy, responsibility and provides a means for self improvement.
- **Community:** The new purchases provides environment in the hospital requires practitioners to quantity the work they do nursing care audit allows nurses to measure the mole intangible aspects of their work, in particular the quality care and so demonstrate the contribution. **Figure 14.17** shows methods of evaluating internal control system.

Nursing Auditor

- **Internal auditor:** The nursing experts from within the hospital are deputed for internal audit and the auditing is done within the agency or hospital.

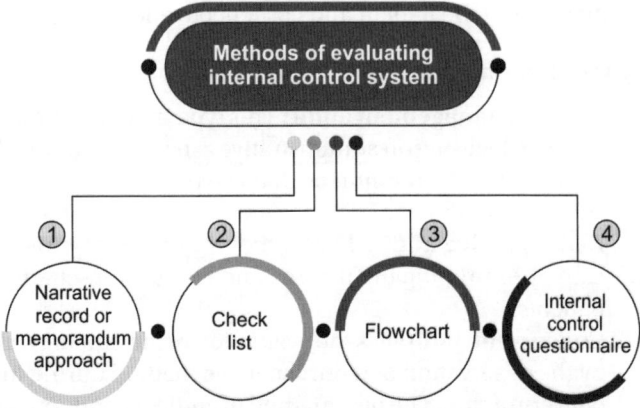

Fig. 14.17: Methods of evaluating internal control system.

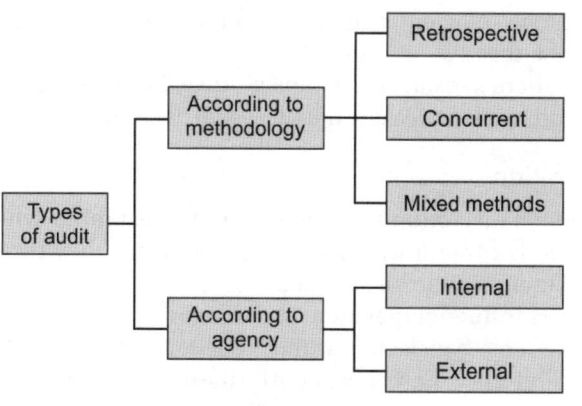

Fig. 14.18: Types of audit.

- **External auditor:** Nursing and the medical administrations from the ministry other agencies of professional association like TNAI undertake the nursing audit in the desired agency or hospital. **Figure 14.18** shows types of audit.

Nursing Audit System

Nursing audit refers to the assessment of the quality of clinical nursing. For nursing auditing, questions are asked such as Is Nursing properly practiced? Assessment of structure of care, Are facilities, equipments and manpower resources available conducive to the delivery of quality care. While assessment of outcome care, auditors also asks, what effects, the nursing care have on alteration of the health status of the recipient of care. **Table 14.2** describes advantages and disadvantages of nursing audit.

Advantages of Nursing Audit

- Can be used as a method of measurement in all areas of nursing.
- Several functions are easily understood.
- Scoring system is fairly simple.
- Results are easily understood.
- Assesses the work of all those involved in recording care.
- It is a useful tool as part of a quality assurance program in areas where accurate' records of care are kept.

Table 14.2: Advantage and Disadvantages of nursing audit.

Advantage	Disadvantage
• Can be used as a method of measurement in all areas of nursing • Seven functions are easily understood • Scoring system is fairly simple • Results easily understood • Assesses the work of all those involved in recording care • May be a useful tool as part of a quality assurance program in areas where accurate records of care are kept	• Appraises the outcomes of the nursing process, so it is not so useful in areas where the nursing process has not been implemented • Many of the components overlap making analysis difficult, is time consuming • Requires a team of trained auditors, deals with a large amount information • Only evaluates record keeping It leading to improve documentation, not nursing care

Disadvantages of Nursing Audit

- Appraises the outcomes of the nursing process, so, it is not so useful in areas where the nursing process has not been implemented,
- Many of the components overlap making analysis difficult.
- Is time consuming.
- Requires a team of trained auditors.
- Deals with a large amount of information.
- Only evaluates record keeping.
- Only serves to improve documentation, not nursing care.

Audit Committee

Before carrying out an audit, an audit committee should be formed, comprising of a minimum of five members who are interested in quality assurance, are clinically competent and able to work together in a group. It is recommended that each member should review no more than 10 patients each month and that the auditor should

Reliability of Audit Evidence

The reliability of audit evidence is influenced by its source which may either be internal or external; and by its nature which may be visual, documentary or oral. The auditor must be aware of the following matters in assessing the reliability of audit evidence:

- Audit evidence from external sources (for example, confirmation received from a third party) is more reliable than that obtained from the entity's records;
- Audit evidence obtained from the entity's records is more reliable when the related accounting and internal control systems operate effectively;
- Audit evidence obtained directly by auditors is more reliable than that obtained by or from the entity;
- Audit evidence in the form of documents and written representations are more reliable than oral representations; and
- Original documents are more reliable than photocopies, telexes or facsimiles.

Procedure for Obtaining Audit Evidence

Auditors normally obtain audit evidence by inspection, observation, enquiry, confirmation, computation and analytical procedures. The choice of one or a combination of the procedures which the auditor may adopt is dependent, in part, upon the period of time during which the audit evidence sought is available and the form in which the accounting records are maintained.

   I. **Inspection:** Inspection involves the following:
   - Examination of records, documents or tangible assets;
   - Provision of audit evidence of varying degrees of reliability depending on their nature and source and the effectiveness of internal controls over their processing; three major categories of documentary audit evidence are listed below in descending degree of reliability as audit evidence:
     – Evidence created and provided to auditors by third parties;

- Evidence created by third parties and held by the entity; and
- Evidence created and held by the entity.

Inspection provides reliable audit evidence about the existence of the tangible assets inspected, but not necessarily as to the ownership or value of such assets.

II. **Observation:** The auditor by observation looks at a procedure being performed by others. For example, the auditor observes the counting of stock by the entity's staff or the performance of internal control procedures as part of the conduct of an audit.

III. **Enquiry and confirmation:** Enquiry involves seeking information within and outside the entity. Enquiry may be formal or informal. Responses to enquiries obtained from third parties may confirm or disprove information previously made available to the auditor. Confirmation involves obtaining response to an enquiry to corroborate information previously made available to the auditors in the course of the audit. Examples of direct confirmation are as follows:
- Confirmation of debts by communication with debtors;
- Confirmation of legal cases by communication with the entity's solicitors; and
- Confirmation of bank balances by communication with the entity's bankers, etc.

IV. **Computation:** The auditor uses computation to check the arithmetical accuracy of source documents and accounting records. Computation also involves performing independent calculations.

V. **Analytical procedures:** Analytical procedures consist of the analysis of relationship between:
- Items of financial data;
- Items of financial and non-financial data, derived from the same period;
- Comparable financial information deriving from different periods or different entities.

Analytical procedures are used to identifying consistencies and predicted patterns or significant fluctuations and unexpected relationships, and the results of investigations performed.

VI. **Documentation:** It is the duty of the auditor to document matters which are important in providing evidence to support the audit opinion and evidence that the audit was carried out in accordance with auditing standards, accounting standards and relevant regulations.

■ PATIENT SATISFACTION

Patient satisfaction is the extent to which patients are happy with their healthcare, both inside and outside of the doctor's office. A measure of care quality, patient satisfaction gives providers insights into various aspects of medicine, including the effectiveness of their care and their level of empathy.
- Patient satisfaction is an important and commonly used indicator for measuring the quality in healthcare.
- Patient satisfaction affects clinical outcomes, patient retention, and medical malpractice claims. It affects the timely, efficient, and patient-centered delivery of quality healthcare.
- Patient satisfaction is thus a proxy, but a very effective indicator to measure the success of doctors and hospitals.

Definition

Patient satisfaction is a measure of the extent to which a patient is content with the healthcare which they received from their healthcare provider.

Factors influencing patient satisfaction:
- Patients' satisfaction with an encounter with healthcare service is mainly dependent on the duration and efficiency of care, and how empathetic and communicative the healthcare providers are.
- It is favored by a good doctor-patient relationship.
- Also, patients who are well-informed of the necessary procedures in a clinical encounter, and the time it is expected to take, are generally more satisfied even if there is a longer waiting time.
- Another critical factor influencing patient satisfaction is the job satisfaction experienced by the care-provider.

Patient as a Consumer

The word "consumer" is derived from the Latin word "consumere" which literally means one who acquires commodities or services. Similarly, the word customer is also defined as "a person who purchases goods or services." Today the patient sees himself as a buyer of health services. Once this concept is accepted, then there is a need to recognize that every patient has certain rights, which puts a special emphasis on to the delivery of quality healthcare, the higher patient satisfaction leads to benefits for the health industry in a number of ways, which have been supported by different studies:
- Patient satisfaction leads to customer (patient) loyalty.
- Improved patient retention—according to the Technical Assistant Research Programs (TARPs), if we satisfy one customer, the information reaches four others.
- They are less vulnerable to price wars. There is sufficient evidence to prove that organizations with high customer loyalty can command a higher price without losing their profit or market share.
- Increased staff morale with reduced staff turnover also leads to increased productivity.
- Reduced risk of malpractice suits—an inverse correlation has been reported for patient satisfaction rates and medical malpractice suits.
- Accreditation issues—it is now universally accepted that various accreditation agencies, such as International Organization for Standardization (ISO), National Accreditation Board for Hospitals (NABH), Joint Commission on Accreditation of Healthcare Organizations (JCAHO), etc., all focus on quality service issues.
- Increased personal and professional satisfaction—patients who improve with our care definitely make us happier. The happier the doctor, the happier will be the patients. **Box 14.4** describes causes of patients dissatisfaction.

> **Box 14.4:** Causes of patients dissatisfaction.
> - Long queue
> - Delay of the appointment
> - Patient queries are not answered by medical staff
> - Short consultation time
> - Unnecessary lab investigation complaint not addressed timely

Service Excellence

Service excellence revolves around three factors: doctor, patient, and organization. **Figure 14.19** shows reasons for reduced quality care.

I. Doctors

The physician has twin responsibilities of giving the best healthcare to the patient, and leading the team or the organization in attaining the goal of satisfying the patient.

- **Break the ice:** Make eye contact, smile, call people by name, express with words of concern.
- **Show courtesy:** Kind gestures and polite words make a patient very comfortable.
- **Listen and understand:** Encourage patients to tell their problem. Invite and answer their questions.
- **Inform and explain:** It promotes compliance. People are less anxious when they know what is happening.
- **See the whole person:** See beyond illness the whole person.
- **Share the responsibility:** Risks and uncertainty are facts of life in medical practice. Acknowledging risks builds trust.
- **Pay undivided attention:** This reduces distractions and interruptions as much as possible.
- **Secure confidentiality and privacy:** Watch what you say, where you say, and to whom you say.
- **Preserve dignity:** Treat the patient with respect. Respect modesty.
- **Remember the patient's family:** Families feel protective, anxious, frightened, and insecure. Extend yourself, reassure, and inform.
- **Respond quickly:** Keep appointments, return calls, and apologize for delays.

II. Patient

A patient's liking the doctor has a lot to do with the patient getting better. A patient's expectations of a good service depend on age, gender, nature of illness, hour of the day, his or her attitude toward the problem and the circumstances.

Understanding a patient: Certain tips can help a doctor or a hospital to understand the patients better:

- Recognize that patients expect a personal relationship that shows compassion and care.
- Recognize that the patient has got certain rights. Various regulatory authorities and hospitals have drawn a charter of rights for the patients.
- Make sure a patient has got a good first impression of you and your set up.
- Step into your patients' shoes; see through their eyes and hear through their ears.
- Minimize the patient's waiting time to the least possible.
- Try to make your problem-solving system to be functional.
- Always obtain feedback from your patients and correct shortcomings, if any.

III. Hospital

Many a times, it happens that with a competent doctor and a compliant patient, the problems persist because of the policies, work culture, and attitude shown by the hospital. Traditionally, hospitals have had discrete functional services such as house-keeping, dietary services, pharmacy, laboratory, etc.

NURSING ROUNDS

There are several methods that can be used effectively in clinical teaching. Nursing rounds are conducted by the head nurse/nurse teacher for the members of her staff/students. To be successful every nurse must be prepared to participate in the discussion of nursing care (**Fig. 14.20**).

Definition

- Nursing rounds are conducted by the head nurse/nurse teacher for the members of her staff/students for a clear understanding of the disease process and the effect of nursing care for each patient.

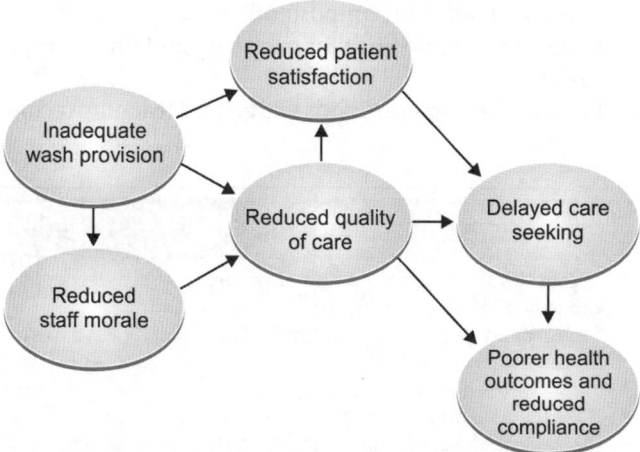

Fig. 14.19: Reasons for reduced quality care.

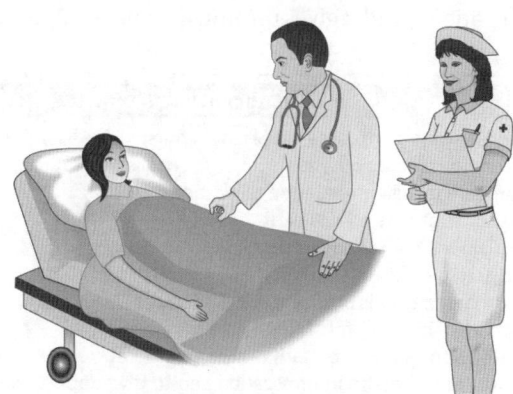

Fig. 14.20: Nursing rounds.

- A nursing round is one which presents an overview of certain aspects of the nursing or medical care of all patients on the ward or of selected patients".

Purposes of Nursing Rounds (Box 14.5)

The purpose for ward rounds includes:
- To observe the physical and the mental condition of the patients and the progress made day to day.
- To observe the work of staff.
- To make specific observation of the patient and to give report to doctor, e.g., wound, drainage, bleeding etc.
- To introduce the patients to the personnel and vice versa.
- To carry out the plan made for the care of the patients.
- To evaluate the results of treatment and the satisfaction of the patient with his care.
- To ensure the safety measures employed for the patient and personnel.
- To orient the nurse/student in handing over/taking over regarding patient's treatment, care done, care yet to be completed and condition of the patient.
- To teach the nursing students and the hospital aids regarding specific conditions.
- To check any preventable conditions present in the patient such as bedsore, foot drop, etc.
- To cheek the emergency equipment kept near the patient and to cheek their safety and working order.
- To compare the clinical manifestation of the patients having some disease so that the student understand in a better manner and gain better insight.
- To prescribe any modification in nursing action.

Types of Nursing Rounds

There are four types of rounds, matrons rounds, nurse management rounds, patient comfort rounds and teaching rounds.

Matrons' Rounds

- Matrons' rounds, which can provide senior nurses with the opportunity to achieve key aspects of their role.
- These include ensuring professional and clinical nursing standards, improving infection control

Nurse Management Rounds

- This round involves the nurse in charge of the shift seeing each patient. And it gives the nurse manager an overview of the condition and needs of all the patients on the wards and the ability of staff to meet these needs.
- Also these rounds have potential benefits for patients, relatives, for the nursing team and for other healthcare professionals.

Patient Comfort Rounds

- They are an important part of maintaining and monitoring the fundamental aspects of individual patient care.
- They should be carried out at 2-hour intervals whenever possible, commencing after lunchtime and continuing for the rest of the day.
- At night time, patient comfort rounds should be carried out before patients go to sleep and again in the early morning.
- It may be necessary to carry out more regular care to some patients.
- The purpose of patient comfort rounds is to maintain a regular review of the patient nursing needs, support the nursing process and evaluate nursing care.

Teaching Rounds

- Nurses learn in a variety of ways: through courses and accredited programs, seminars, conferences, self-directed study and so on.
- One of the most effective ways, however, is to participate in special clinical teaching rounds.
- These are aimed at all learners, whether pre-registration students or qualified staff.
- Teaching round is to learn from direct patient contact with facilitation from an experienced nurse teacher. Also to teach and evaluate nursing care.
- It is useful in developing clinical practice, evidence-based care

Factors to be kept in mind when planning nursing rounds (Box 14.6):

- To consult students previous clinical experience to avoid repetition and to add to earlier experience.
- Keep in mind the probable value and availability of clinical material.
- Explain the plan to the patient.
- Introduce the patient to the group.
- Make the patient feel important.
- Have a post-conference for summary and further explanation.
- Records the nursing rounds in the ward teaching records.

Box 14.5: Purposes of nursing rounds.

- To demonstrate symptoms important in nursing.
- To clarify terminology used.
- To compare the clients reaction to disease.
- To demonstrate the effects of drugs.
- To explain the plan to the patient.
- To illustrate skillful nursing care.
- To compare methods of meeting the needs.
- Instructional purpose for student nurses.
- To learn about disease, pattern of care, treatment.
- To illustrate successful improvization and to give opportunity for the use of different application.

Box 14.6: Factors to be kept in mind when planning nursing rounds.

- To consult students previous clinical experience to avoid repetition and to add to earlier experience.
- Keep in mind the probable value and availability of clinical material.
- Explain the plan to the patient.
- Introduce the patient to the group.
- Make the patient feel important.
- Have a post-conference for summary and further explanation.
- Records the nursing rounds in the ward teaching records.

Steps involved in Rounds

- The entire clinical group of students is assembled at the bedside of a preselected patient who has agreed to participate and who has been briefed before hand as to his role in the learning experience.
- The instructor of the student who is caring for the patient briefs the nursing care.
- The staff nurses of the ward are also allowed to contribute certain genuine points regarding patient care.
- Background information of the patient can be provided away from the bedside.
- The main focus is made on nursing care and only important aspects of the care are discussed.
- At the end, the instructor concludes the discussion by giving her opinion, guidance and relevant instructions.
- The patient is finally briefed up on the conclusions reached following discussion.
- The staff nurse on duty records all the instructions and suggestions given by the instructor and a register (providing the information) is maintained in the ward.

Importance of Nursing Rounds

- In nursing rounds the patient's history and the medical aspects of his care are included only as a background for the understanding of the nursing care.
- The nurse/teacher who have been caring for the patient during the week may present the background information and tell the points in nursing care which she considers to be most essential.
- She is then responsible for answering the questions of the class including these of the head nurse.
- In another method of conducting rounds, the head nurse/teacher may involve any nurse in the group to tell what she knows about the patient and his nursing care; other students make addition and suggestions and help to answer the questions.
- This method is a means of testing the student's knowledge and acquaintance with all the patients on the floor.
- Students prepare by studying indications and actions of drug.
- Students are told prior to rounds so that they may prepare themselves.

Role of Head Nurse in Nursing Rounds

- In preparing for rounds, the nurse selects the patients who are to be discussed in relation to the time which has been set aside for the purpose.
- Rounds should properly not last longer than 20 minutes.
- The head nurse needs to read the patient's progress and prognosis, their nursing care and its effectiveness.
- She should post the time for rounds at least a week in advance and indicates the type of preparation the nurse is to make, i.e., whether she is to know thoroughly the history, care and progress of her own patients or briefly that of all patients in the ward.
- Patient with similar diagnosis but with differing history, treatment, and prognosis may be selected or varied conditions existing in the same ward also can selected for teaching purpose.
- Rounds for staff nurses should be held separately from those for students since the background of the 2 groups vary widely.
- Rounds for students in their first clinical term may need to be held separately. **Figure 14.21** shows potential benefits of nursing grand rounds.

Advantage of Nursing Rounds (Box 14.7)

- This method is a means of testing the student's knowledge and acquaintance with the entire patient's on the floor.
- The students, who are informed prior to rounds, benefit the maximum in real life teaching method.
- No other type of rounds is a substitute for nursing rounds.
- It is always be very valuable for the head nurse to go on regular nursing rounds with clinical instructor.
- An intelligent nurse with creative abilities may find many other ways of successfully assisting student nurses to develop nursing skills.
- Helps in orienting a new nurse/student to the patients.
- An interesting strategy involving the student, teacher and the patient.
- It offers a real life learning situation.
- Evaluation of nursing activity, hurdles faced by nurses in implementing or success nursing care can be appraised.

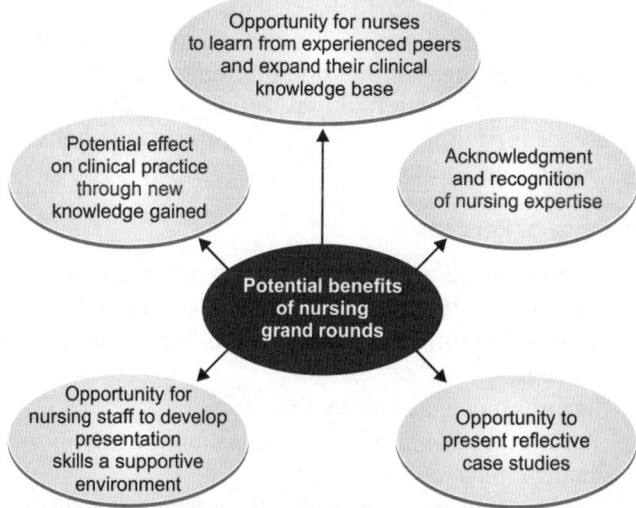

Fig. 14.21: Potential benefits of nursing grand rounds.

Box 14.7: Advantages of nursing rounds.

- Response of the patient is more natural
- Students can select patients with specific problems and plan proper nursing care.

The way of conducting nursing rounds are:
a. Patients are selected with nursing problems to reinforce their theoretical knowledge.
b. The group observes the behaviors of the patient at the bedside and make proper comments.
   - The group observes the equipments and articles under use.
   - The student return to classroom to discuss the nursing diagnosis and needed nursing care for patient.

Disadvantages of Nursing Rounds

- The confidentiality of the patient is hampered.
- The patient may over hear the discussion and he may not like the thought that he is being talked about if he cannot hear.
- If the group is large the teacher may not able to speak loudly enough to be heard, in which case the attention of individuals who are on the fringes is lost.
- Distractions are present in ward.
- An unprepared nursing round has little teaching-learning value.
- Quality of nursing rounds on the quality and presentation of the nurse teacher/head nurse.

DOCUMENTATION—RECORDS AND REPORTS

All professional persons need to be accountable for the performance of their duties to the public. Since nursing has been considered as profession, nurses need to record their work on completion. A record is a permanent written communication that documents information's relevant to a client's healthcare management.

- A record is a clinical, scientific, administrative and legal document relating to the nursing care given to individual family or community.
- The records are a practical and indispensable aid to the doctor, nurse and paramedical personnel in giving the best possible service to their clients.
- Recorded facts have a value and scientific accuracy for more than mere impression of memory and there are guidelines for better administration of health services. Records are the means of communications between health workers and their clients.

Purpose of Records

- Records provide data for program planning and evaluation.
- Records are the tools of communication between the health workers, the family and other development personnel.
- Records indicate plans for the future.
- Records provide baseline data to estimate the long-term changes related to the services.
- Records provide an opportunity for evaluating the services.
- Records help in the research for improvement of nursing care.

Every institution keeps some kinds of records. The hospital is no exception. The patients clinical record is a brief account of the of the patient, results of diagnostic tests, findings of medical examination, treatment and nursing care daily progress notes and advice on discharge.

Importance of Records

- Record provides an accurate and detailed account of treatments and care given to the patient. Therefore, it serves as a guide for follow up of the course of disease and future care.
- The record provides accurate information of the results of medication and treatments given to the patient. So, through the records the physician gets accurate information about the patient's conditions from day to day.
- Records are of great value in the diagnosis, treatments and nursing care.
- A record of illness and treatment saves duplication of work in the future care especially when the patient is transferred from one department to another or from one institution to another or when an attending physician is transferred and other person takes charge. In such situations, it helps the patient to get prompt treatment.
- A well-written record has legal value. The records safeguard the patients, nurses, doctors and the hospital. It serves as evidence that the patient care is intelligently managed.
- Records are tools of communication among the members of the health team. It is of great value for the doctors and nurses at the shifting of duty hours.
- Records help the medical and nursing students in the clinical experience and provide data for care studies.
- Records serve as a reference material for research work.
- The patients record, registers and reports furnish the vital statistics and give information needed to evaluate the service rendered by hospital to the community.
- Data taken from the patient's record points out the health problems of the country and it also provides a base line in which local, state, national and international health services are planned.

Principles of Record Writing

- Since the clinical record is a legal document, it is essential that they should be written clearly, accurately, appropriately and legibly.
- The individual who writes them should sign all entries.
- Care to be taken not to make any error on the records. If anything is crossed out, it should be dated and initialed.
- All records should be written with black ink or typed for better legibility.
- Records should be written in chronological order as to date and time. When recording medications and treatments, note exact time and date on which they are carried out
- Records are written continuously with no blank spaces. If any space is left out, it should be crossed out, dated and signed.
- Lengthy corrections of records are written as amendments.
- Each page of the record should be properly identified with the name, age, IP no., OP no. date, etc.
- Use only standard abbreviations.
- Records should be truthful, brief and complete. It should include all the services given to the patients, the observations made on the patient from day to day and the results of treatments, etc.

Types of Records

- Outpatient and in-patient records
- Nurse's recording
- Doctor's order sheet
- Graphic charts of TPR
- Reports of laboratory examinations
- Diet sheets
- Consent form for operations and anesthesia
- Intake and output chart
- Reports of anesthesia, physiotherapy and other special treatment
- Registers

General Rules of Recording

- Keep separate records or charts for each individual patient.
- It is a legal document; write it, in English, clearly, accurately, appropriately and legibly.
- Name, age, ward, date and in-patient number should be written on each page.
- All entries should be signed by the individual who makes the entry.
- All entries should be written in blue or black ink.
- Chart nursing-care and medications and other treatments only after giving them.
- It should be reliable and accurate.
- Information about patients and their care must be factual.
- Correct spelling is also important for accurate recording.
- Nurses should not allow others to record for her.
- Use only standard abbreviations.
- Do not use ditto marks or chemical formula in charting.
- Each patient should have a daily note, written by nurses on all shifts.
- The information within a record should be complete.
- Concise data are easy to understand.
- Lengthy notes are difficult to read.
- Record immediately after performing nursing activities. It should have correctness.
- It should be organized in a logical format or order.
- Nurses should maintain confidentiality of patents' record.
- Do not use blank space in the record. Keep it crossed.

Nurses Responsibility in Recording

- Generally, nurses' notes contain the following information:
- Treatment and nursing care given by various members of the health team.
- Doctor's orders carried out by nurses.
- Nursing needs met by nurses as per doctor's order.
- Observations, e.g., vital signs, physical signs and behavioral patterns of patient.
- Response of patient to treatment and nursing care.
- Health advice given by nurses and other staff
- Independent nursing functions are also recorded.

Purpose of Reports

Reports are oral or written exchanges of information shared between caregivers or workers in a number of ways. A report summarizes the services of the person or personnel and of the agency. Reports are usually written daily, weekly, monthly or yearly.

- To show the kind and amount of services rendered over a specified period,
- To illustrate progress in reaching goals,
- As an aid in studying health conditions,
- As an aid in planning,
- To interpret the services to the public and to the other interested agencies.

Probably no other single factor is more vital for good administration than prompt and complete reports. They save duplication of efforts and eliminate the need for investigation to learn the facts in situation.

Types of Reports

Reports may be classified as oral and written **(Fig. 14.22)**.

- **Oral report:** Oral reports are given when the information is for immediate use and not for permanency. For example, oral report is made by the nurse who is assigned to patient care, to another nurse who is planning to relieve her, and some of the oral reports may be made to charge nurses and nurse supervisors and also doctors. Reports are to be written when the information is to be used by several personnel, which is more or less of permanent value, for example day and night reports, census, interdepartmental reports and other special reports, needed according to situation, events and conditions.

    The reports used in Hospital setting usually are change-of-shift reports, transfer reports, incident reports, day, evening and night reports, legal reports.

- **Change-of-shift reports** These may be given orally in person by audio taping, recording, or during rounds at the clients' bedside some of the points to be kept in mind while giving such reports are as follows:
    - Provide only essential background information about client (name, sex, age, diagnosis and medical history) but do not review all routine care procedures or tasks.
    - Identify clients' nursing diagnosis or healthcare problems and other related causes but do not review all biographical information on case sheets.
    - Describe objective measurements or observations about clients 'condition and response to health

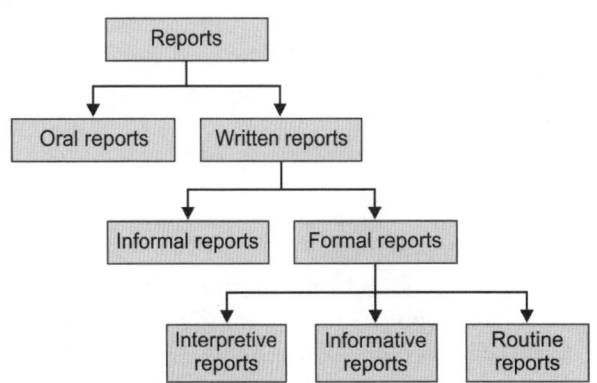

Fig. 14.22: Types of reports.

problem. Stress recent change, but do not use critical comment about clients' behavior.
- Share significant information about family members, as it relates to clients' problems do not make any assumptions about relationship between family members.
- Continuously review ongoing discharge plan. Do not engage in idle gossip.
- Relay to staff significant changes in the way therapies are given. Do not describe basic steps of a procedure.
- Describe instruction given in teaching plan and clients' response. Do not explain detailed content unless staff members ask for clarification.
- Evaluate results of nursing or medical care measures. Do not simply describe results as good or poor. Be specific.
- Be clear on priorities to which oncoming staff must attend. Do not force oncoming staff to guess what to do first.

■ **Transfer-reports:** Patients will frequently be transferred from one unit to another to receive different levels of care. A transfer report involves communications of information about clients from the nurse on sending unit to the nurse on the receiving unit. When giving transfer request, nurse should include the following information:
- Client's name, age, primary doctor, and medical diagnosis
- Summary of medical progress up to the time of transfer
- Current health status—physical and psychosocial
- Current nursing diagnosis or problems and care plan
- Any critical assessment or interventions to be completed shortly
- Needs for any special equipment, etc.

■ **Incident reports:** Nurses usually become involved in client-related incidents as some point in their careers. They must understand the purpose of incident reports and the correct way to report information. While incident reporting, the following points are to be kept in mind:
- The nurse who witnessed the incident or who found the client at the time of incident should file the report.
- The nurse describes in concise what happened specifically objective terms, etc.
- The nurse does not interpret or attempt to explain the cause of the incident.
- The nurse describes objectively the clients, conditions when the incident was discovered.
- Any measures taken by the nurse, other nurses, or doctors at the time of the incident are reported.
- No nurse is blamed in an incident report.
- The report is submitted as soon as possible to the appropriate authority.
- The nurse should never make photocopy of the incident report.

■ **Legal reports:** Incident reports and reports on accidents, mistakes and complaints are legal in nature. There are times when a hospital is criticized for what is claimed to

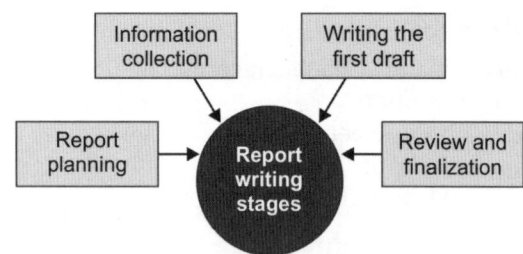

Fig. 14.23: Report writing stages.

be negligence or poor care because of a condition that resulted in discomfort and perhaps serious harm to a patient or client. In such reports, the content is stated briefly and objectively giving all pertinent information. Accuracy, timeliness, completeness and relevancy to the problems are maintained promptly while making such reports. **Figure 14.23** shows report writing stages.

Principles of Record Keeping

Records and reports must be functional, accurate, complete, current organized and confidential.
- **Fact:** Information about clients and their care must be functional. A record should contain descriptive, objective information about what a nurse sees, hears, feels and smells. In the same way, anything happens during the managing the affairs in the institutions/hospital, manager should document inferences or construction with functional information to avoid misleading, misinterpretation and any error in administration.
- **Accuracy:** A client record must be reliable. In other words, information must be accurate so that health team members have confidence in it. The use of correct measurements ensures that a record is accurate.
- **Completeness:** The information within a recorded entry or a report should be complete, containing concise and thorough information's about a client care or any event or happening taking place in the jurisdiction of manager.
- **Correctness:** Delays in recording or reporting can result in serious omissions and untimely delays for medical care or action legally, a late entry in a chart may be interpreted on negligence.
- **Organization:** The nurse or nurse manager communicates information in a logical format or order. Health team members understand information better when it is given in the order in which it occurred.
- **Confidentiality:** Nurses are legally and ethically obligated to keen information about client's illnesses and treatments confidential. In the same way, certain information in management also should be kept confidential.

Any information about clients care or event taking place in the healthcare agencies should be communication with careful thought. All members of health team depend on recorded and reported information. Accurate information ensures continuity and quality of care, and also smooth running of administration.

Nurses Responsibility in Record Keeping

- Nurses have legal responsibility for accurately reporting and recording patient's conditions, treatments and responses to care.
- The medical record is a written or computerized account of a patient's illness and treatment that includes information submitted by all members of the patient healthcare team.
- The medical record is an information source document that should be used to plan care, evaluate care, allocate costs, educate personnel, research care measure and substantiate legal claims.
- Court decisions have stated that the patient's medical record is essential to proper care and the medical record is the property of the health agency.
- The patient has a property right to information contained in the report, the patient has a right to inspect and copy the record after being discharged. However, it is unadvisable to allow a patient to review his/her medical record without medical supervision and explanation because a patient is likely to misunderstand certain record notations.
- Failure to record significant patient information on the medical record makes a nurse guilty of negligence when the patient is injured because of a doctor's ignorance of significant information about medical history, signs and symptoms.
- The medical record must be accurate to provide a sound basis for care planning. Therefore, errors in nurses charting must be corrected promptly in a manner that leaves no doubt about the facts.
- Every health agency should have a policy and protocol that directs that an erroneous chart entry be crossed through labeled as erroneous signed by the employee who corrects the error, and retained in the patient's record.
- Correct information should then be documented to replace the erroneous and corrected entries should never be destroyed.
- Nurses who conspire with doctors and others to falsify a patient's record for purposes of concealing a criminal violation may be found criminally liable.
- Generally, the person who makes reports required by statute is immune from suit under the doctrine of the public's right to know. In many countries, there are statutes that require health personnel to report instances of child abuse, ophthalmic neonatorum, communicable diseases, and births out of wedlock, gunshot wounds, suicide, rape, and use of unperceived narcotics.
- In reporting information about criminal acts obtained during patient care, the nurse must reveal such information only to the police, because it is considered a privileged communication.
- Several aspects of statutory, case, and administrative law control nursing practice and nursing management.

CONCLUSION

Control is the management function in which performance is measured and corrective action is taken to ensure the accomplishment of organizational goals. Control includes coordination of numerous activities: decision making related to planning and organizing activities and information from directing and evaluating each worker's performance. Control is also viewed as being concerned with records, reports, organizational progress toward aims, and effective use of resources. Control uses evaluation and regulation; controlling is identical to evaluation.

REVIEW QUESTIONS

Long Essays

1. Define controlling; explain the need, features and elements.
2. Define standards; enumerate the purposes and importance of standards.
3. Define policy; explain the purpose and policy process.
4. Define nursing performances; explain the types.
5. Define auditing; explain the principles, types and techniques of auditing.
6. Define nursing rounds; explain the purposes and types.

Short Essays

1. Process of controlling.
2. Importance of controlling.
3. Principles of controlling.
4. Traditional techniques of control.
5. Sound control system.
6. Sources of nursing standards.
7. Classification of standards.
8. Characteristics of a sound policy.
9. Define procedures discuss the purposes and importance.
10. Define protocols; explain the purposes and uses.
11. Patient as a consumer.
12. Protocol application in nursing.
13. Principles of record writing.
14. Principles of record keeping.

Short Answers

1. Limitations of controlling
2. Management audit.
3. Management information system.
4. Advantages of controlling.
5. Characteristics of standards.
6. Classification of standards in the hospital.
7. Factors influencing policies.
8. Advantages of policies.
9. Differentiating between policies and procedures.
10. Advantages of using protocols.
11. Common problems-related performance.
12. Objectives of nursing audit.
13. Causes of patients dissatisfaction.
14. Advantage of nursing rounds.
15. Types of reports.

BIBLIOGRAPHY

1. Berman-Rubera S. Leading and embracing change. Business/Change-Management. Retrieved August 20, 2008.
2. Bilchik GS. Are you the problem? Hospitals and Health Networks Magazine. 2002;38-42.
3. Cameron KS, Quinn QE. Diagnosing and Changing Organizational Culture. NY: Jossey-Bass; 2006.
4. Engle Bright JD, Franklin M. Managing a new medication administrative process. Journal of Nursing Administration. 2005;35(9): 410-13.
5. Hunter JC. The World's Most Powerful Leadership Principle: How to Become a Servant Leader. NY: Crown Business; 2004.
6. Lewin K. Field Theory in Social Science: Selected Theoretical Papers. NY: Harper and Row; 1951.
7. Lichiello P, Madden CW. Context and catalysts for change in health care markets. Health Affairs. 1996;15(2):121-29.
8. Maslow AH. Motivation and Personality. N.Y.: Harper and Row; 1970.
9. McCarthy JE. Five concepts for creating change. Nursing Management. 2005;36(5):20-2.
10. Parker M, Gadbois S. Building community in healthcare workplace. Part 3: Belonging and satisfaction at work. Journal of Nursing Administration. 2000;30:466-73.
11. Tappen RM. Nursing Leadership and Management: Concepts and Practice. Philadelphia: FA Davis; 2001.

CHAPTER 15

Total Quality Management

LEARNING OBJECTIVES

- Total Quality Management—Quality Assurance, Quality and Safety
- Performance Appraisal [Program Evaluation Review Technique (PERT)]
- Benchmarking, Activity Plan (Gantt chart)
- Critical Path Analysis

INTRODUCTION

The term 'total' means the entire organization—all teams, departments and functions—is involved in quality management. The 'system' refers to the managerial and technological methods to achieve quality requirements and business objectives throughout an entire organization. Although, it may go by various names, Juran believes 'enterprise excellence' to be a more appropriate name for TQM.

MEANING OF TOTAL QUALITY MANAGEMENT

Total quality management (TQM) is a structured approach to overall organizational management. The focus of the process is to improve the quality of an organization's outputs, including goods and services, through continual improvement of internal practices **(Fig. 15.1)**.

- Total quality management is an ongoing process of detecting and reducing or eliminating errors.
- It is used to streamline supply chain management, improve customer service, and ensure that employees are trained.
- The focus is to improve the quality of an organization's outputs, including goods and services, through continual improvement of internal practices.

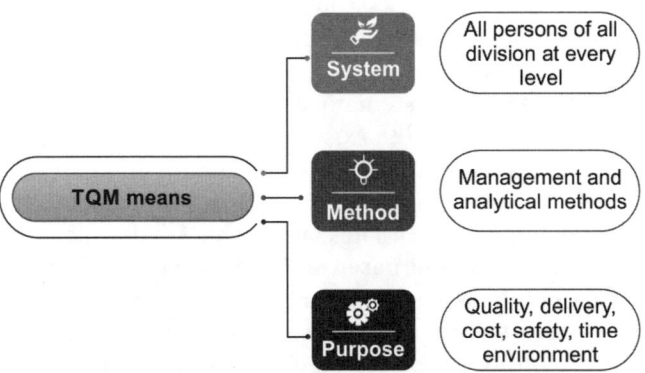

Fig. 15.1: Total quality management.

- Total quality management aims to hold all parties involved in the production process accountable for the overall quality of the final product or service.

HISTORY OF TOTAL QUALITY MANAGEMENT

- Total quality management (TQM) is a term that originated in the 1950s and is today used mainly in Japan.
- TQM was developed by William Deming, a management consultant whose work had a great impact on Japanese manufacturing.
- It is the equivalent of what other countries or organizations may call a company-wide quality management system, enterprise quality management system, or integrated quality management system, to name a few.

DEFINITION

- Total quality management (TQM) refers to management methods used to enhance quality and productivity in business organizations. TQM is a comprehensive management approach that works horizontally across an organization, involving all departments and employees and extending backward and forward to include both suppliers and clients/customers.
- TQM is a management philosophy that seeks to integrate all organizational functions (marketing, finance, design, engineering, and production, customer service, etc.) to focus on meeting customer needs and organizational objectives. **Figure 15.2** shows six Cs of total quality management.

CONCEPT OF TOTAL QUALITY MANAGEMENT

Total quality management is the optimization and integration of all the functions and processes of a business in order to provide for excited customers through a process of continuous improvement. The concept of TQM can be understood by understanding the three terms that make the concept. These are:

Chapter 15: Total Quality Management

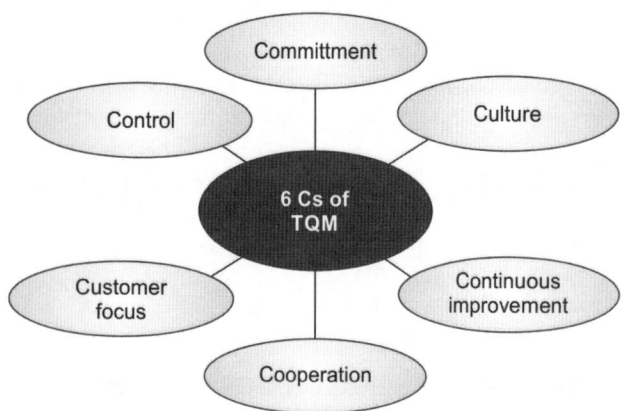

Fig. 15.2: Six Cs of total quality management (TQM).

1. **Total:** Everyone associated with the company is involved in continuous improvement including customers and suppliers.
2. **Quality:** Customers' stated and implied requirements are fully met.
3. **Management:** Executives are fully committed.

TQM is facilitated through clear understanding of the term 'Quality Control':

Q—Quality first
U—User is the king
A—Avoid defects
L—Long-term vision
I—Innovation error proofing
T—Training for all
Y—Yearning for facts
C—Cost consciousness
O—Optimal tolerance
N—Nip the vital few
T—Team work
R—Respect humanity
O—Operator in state of self-control
L—Leadership from top

OBJECTIVES OF TOTAL QUALITY MANAGEMENT

- Process improvement
- Defect prevention
- Priority of effort
- Developing cause-effect relationships
- Measuring system capacity
- Developing improvement checklist and check forms
- Helping teams make better decisions
- Developing operational definitions
- Separating trivial from significant needs
- Observing behavior changes over a period of time

PRINCIPLES OF TOTAL QUALITY MANAGEMENT

Total quality management has a number of key principles which—when implemented together—can move any organization towards business excellence **(Fig. 15.3)**.

- **Customer focus:** Central to all successful TQM systems is an understanding that quality is determined by the customer. No matter what measures you introduce to improve the quality of your products and services, the only way of knowing if they have been successful is customer feedback, whether in the form of reviews, return rates, or satisfaction surveys.

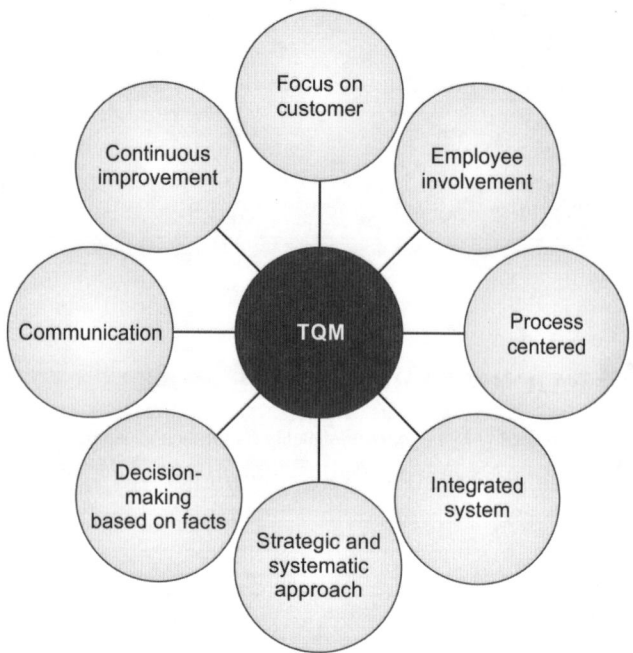

Fig. 15.3: Principles of TQM.

- **Employee involvement:** Every person in an organization-from entry-level workers to management-has a responsibility for the quality of products and services. However, employees can only be invested if they feel empowered to make their own decisions, something that depends on management creating the right workplace environment.
- **Centered on process:** A TQM system will fail without a clear focus on processes and process-led thinking. A process fault is ultimately the cause of most problems, which is why effective monitoring of every single step is an essential part of assessing, maintaining and improving quality.
- **Integrated system:** An organization should have an integrated system that allows for effective total quality management. This may be a bespoke system, or one based on a quality standard, such as ISO 9001, but it should be understood and applied across all functions and departments.
- **Strategic and systematic approach:** Critical to quality management is the existence of a strategic plan that outlines how an organization intends to achieve its mission and business goals. It goes without saying that quality should be a core component of such a plan.
- **Decision-making based on facts:** Business performance can only be assessed using the available facts, such as sales data, revenue figures, and customer retention rates. The opinions of customers, employers and suppliers should never be used to inform decisions.

Chapter 15: Total Quality Management

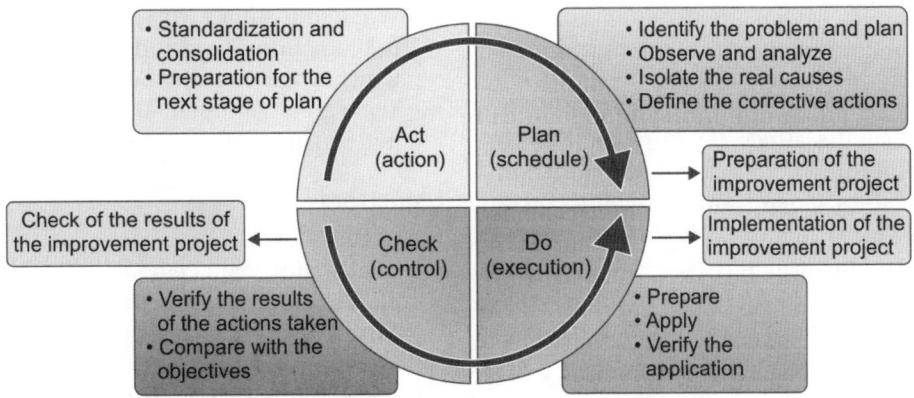

Fig. 15.4: Phases of total quality management.

- **Communication:** Effective communication is essential when an organization is implementing significant changes for the sake of business improvement. Every member of staff should be made aware of the strategy, the timescales involved, and the reasons for implementing it.
- **Continuous improvement:** Applying the principles of DMAIC and Lean Six Sigma will instill an organization with a culture of continuous improvement, driving all employees to constantly seek new ways to be more competitive and deliver high-quality products for all stakeholders.

PHASES OF TOTAL QUALITY MANAGEMENT

Total quality management ensures that every single employee is working towards the improvement of work culture, processes, services, systems and so on to ensure long-term success **(Fig. 15.4)**. Total quality management can be divided into four categories: (Also referred to as PDCA cycle)
1. Plan
2. Do
3. Check
4. Act

Planning phase: Planning is the most crucial phase of total quality management. In this phase, employees have to come up with their problems and queries which need to be addressed. They need to come up with the various challenges, they face in their day-to-day operations and also analyze the problem's root cause. Employees are required to do necessary research and collect relevant data which would help them find solutions to all the problems.

Doing phase: In the doing phase, employees develop a solution for the problems defined in planning phase. Strategies are devised and implemented to overcome the challenges faced by employees. The effectiveness of solutions and strategies is also measured in this stage.

Checking phase: Checking phase is the stage where people actually do a comparison analysis of before and after data to confirm the effectiveness of the processes and measure the results.

Acting phase: In this phase, employees document their results and prepare themselves to address other problems.

ELEMENTS OF TOTAL QUALITY MANAGEMENT

Quality is an essential parameter which helps organizations outshine their competitors and survive the fierce competition **(Figs. 15.5 and 15.6)**. The success of total quality management depends on following eight elements which are further classified into following four groups:
I. Foundation
II. Building bricks

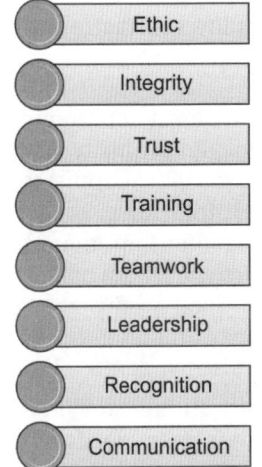

Fig. 15.5: Elements of TQM.

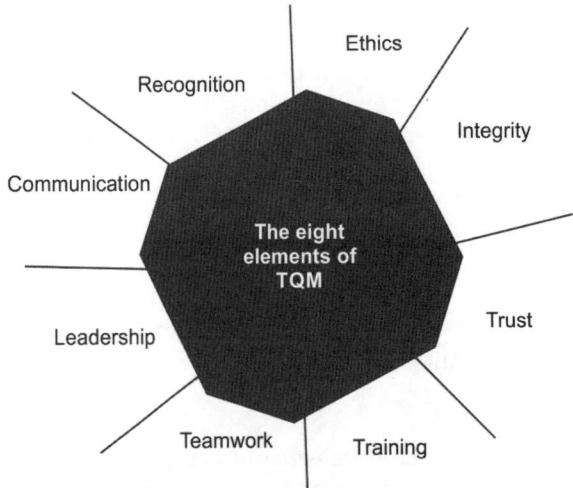

Fig. 15.6: Eight elements of total quality management.

III. Binding mortar
IV. Roof

I. Foundation

Foundation further includes ethics, integrity and trust the entire process of total quality management is built on a strong foundation of ethics, integrity and trust. Total quality management involves every single employee irrespective of his designation and level in the hierarchy.

Ethics

- Ethics is an individual's understanding of what is good and bad at the workplace.
- A thin line of difference does exist between good and bad, which is for you to decide.
- Ethics teach an individual to follow code of conduct of organization and adhere to rules and regulations.

Integrity

- Integrity refers to honesty, values and an individual's sincerity at workplace.
- You need to respect your organization's policies.
- Avoid spreading unnecessary rumors about your fellow workers.
- Total quality management does not work in an environment where employees criticize and backstab each other.

Trust

- Trust is one of the most important factors necessary for implementation of total quality management.
- Employees need to trust each other to ensure participation of each and every individual.
- Trust improves relationship among employees and eventually helps in better decision making which further helps in implementing total quality management successfully.

II. Bricks

Bricks are placed on a strong foundation to reach the roof of recognition. The foundation needs to be strong enough to hold the bricks and support the roof.

Training

- Employees need to be trained on total quality management. Managers need to make their fellow workers aware of the benefits of total quality management and how would it make a difference in their product quality and eventually yield profits for their organization.
- Employees need to be trained on interpersonal skills, the ability to work as a team member, technical know-how, decision making skills, problem solving skills and so on.
- Training enables employees to implement TQM effectively within their departments and also make them indispensable resources.

Teamwork

- Teamwork is a crucial element of total quality management. Rather than working individually, employees need to work in teams.
- When individuals work in unison, they are in a position to brainstorm ideas and come up with various solutions which would improve existing processes and systems.
- Team members ought to help each other to find a solution and put into place.

Leadership

- Leadership provides a direction to the entire process of total quality management.
- Total quality management needs to have a supervisor who acts as a strong source of inspiration for other members and can assist them in decision making.
- A leader himself needs to believe in the entire process of TQM for others to believe in the same.
- Proper downloads, briefs about TQM must be given from to time to employees to help them in its successful implementation.

III. Binding Mortar

Binding mortar binds all the elements together.

Communication

- Communication binds employees and extracts the best out of them. Information needs to be passed on from the sender to the recipient in its desired form.
- Small misunderstandings in the beginning lead to major problems later on.
- Employees need to interact with each other to come up with problems existing in the system and find their solutions as well.

  Three types of communication takes place between employees:
  1. **Downward communication:** Flow of information takes place from the management to the employees
  2. **Upward communication:** Flow of information takes place from the employees to the top level management
  3. **Sideways communication:** Communication also takes place between various departments.

IV. Roof

Recognition

- Recognition is the final element of total quality management.
- Recognition is the most important factor which acts as a catalyst and drives employees to work hard as a team and deliver their lever best.
- Every individual is hungry for appreciation and recognition.
- Employees who come up with improvement ideas and perform exceptionally well must be appreciated in front of all.
- They should be suitably rewarded to expect a brilliant performance from them even the next time.

■ COMPONENTS OF TOTAL QUALITY MANAGEMENT

The major process components of TQM are policy management, daily management and team activity. Some companies include vendor quality also in this process since their quality depends upon vendor's products and services.

Policy Management

- It can also be referred to as policy deployment, management by policy, etc.
- Policy management is a systematic process used to direct corporate resources towards solving problems and making improvements in selecting high priority areas.
- Policy management is essential for executing corporate strategy.
- There should be a total commitment from top management and other employees for policy management.

Daily Management

- Daily management process is to ensure that overall operations are improved and the things done as per planning.
- Daily management is a means both to control and to improve day-to-day operations.
- Day-to-day management problems are solved by daily management process.
- Top management ensures that processes for satisfying customer needs are in place.
- The managers and supervisors are responsible for actual execution and checking of TQM system.

Team Activity

- Team activity is essential to achieve organizational goals and helping in quality improvement.
- The team characteristics may differ depending on the type and nature of problem to be solved.
- A work atmosphere must be developed where managers and workers listen to and respect each other's ideas.
- This type of atmosphere can be developed only when there is a commitment to achieve objectives.
- The team approach is a better way of building trust and respect.

TOTAL QUALITY MANAGEMENT TOOLS

TQM can be put to practice by adopting TQM methods. Adopting the right method is important as success of TQM largely depends upon selection of the method, its suitability for quality management problems and effective implementation by effective leaders. Some of the commonly adopted tools are discussed below (**Figs. 15.7 and 15.8**):

- **Benchmarking:** Benchmarking helps organizations move from introspective to externally focused areas of business operations.
- **Deming wheel:** It refers to plan, do, check and action and helps in developing a new product based on requirements of the customers.
- **ISO-9000:** It aims at providing consistent quality to customers.
- **Just-in-time:** This method aims at delivering the raw materials and components to the production line just-in-time when they are needed.
- **Quality circles:** This method of TQM develops the quality of products and also the individuals.
- **Critical path analysis:** The benefit of this method underlies the fact that it allows the effects of different courses of action to be determined at the planning stage thereby allowing the best overall approach to be decided about the completion of the project.
- **Failure mode and effect analysis (FMEA):** This method helps in designing foolproof products and processes by detecting problems at early stage in a structured manner.

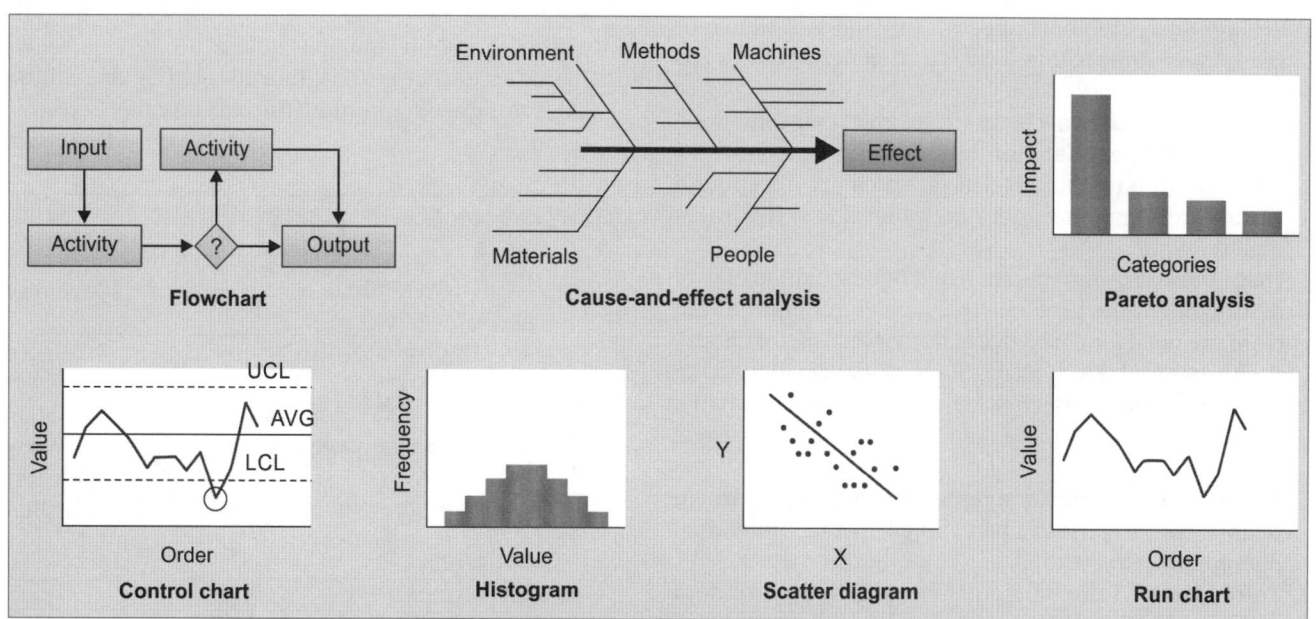

Fig. 15.7: Total quality management tools.
(UCL: upper control limit; LCL: lower control limit; AVG: average)

Chapter 15: Total Quality Management

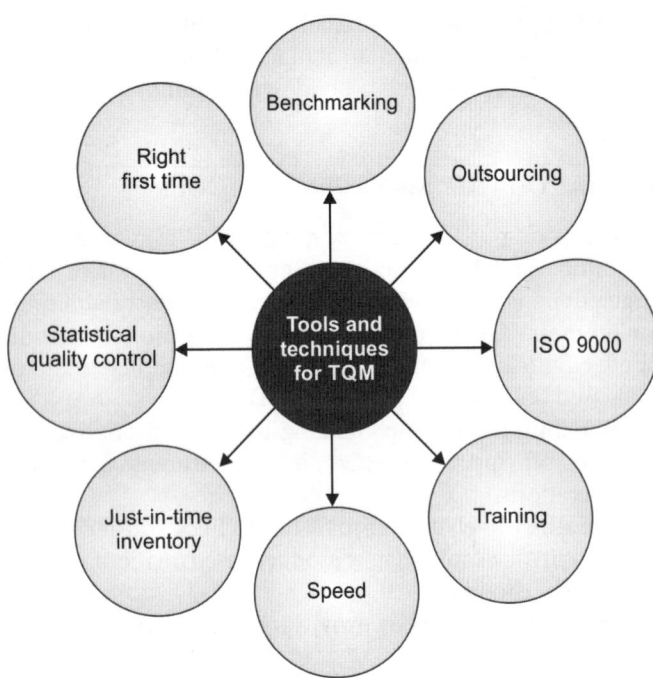

Fig. 15.8: Tools and techniques for total quality management (TQM).

- **Force-field analysis:** It helps managers identify the forces which have maximum impact on implementation of change and, therefore, concentrate their efforts in those areas.
- **Brainstorming:** This method breaks barriers between the departments and the levels of hierarchy and encourages everyone to develop collaborative behavior which strengthens their groups skills.
- **Nominal group technique:** The nominal group technique is "a way of generating ideas from a group and identifying the level of support within the group for those ideas".
- **Suggestion schemes:** Suggestion schemes aim to generate new ideas for moving to continuous improvement through incremental changes. It provides substance to the quality improvement plan and generates ideas to keep it going.
- **C-charts:** The control charts are graphic representations where managers set standards of expected normal variation due to chance causes which are acceptable within the range of upper quality level and the lower quality level.
- **Histograms:** Histograms are visual representation of data that highlight the problem areas which pinpoint to the team the need for corrective action or analysis of data.
- **P-charts:** Similar to C-charts, P-charts help in identifying the percentage of defective items in a sample of variable size which varies by more than 25% of the mean sample size.
- **Pie charts:** It is a pectoral representation of data where relative size, in terms of percentage, of each individual part is shown to the total.
- **Tally charts:** Tally bars are a simple method of data collection and interpretation which can be applied in office and work areas. It helps people of all areas to deal with problems related to quality improvement.

FUNCTIONS OF TOTAL QUALITY MANAGEMENT

Though the chief function of TQM is emphasis on quality, but its works is multidirectional. Some common functions of TQM are:
- Quality policy and its communication
- Team work and participation
- Problem solving tools and technique
- Standardization
- Quality system
- Quality costs and management
- Process control
- Customer-supplier integration
- Education and training
- Quality audit and review

QUALITY ASSURANCE (FIG. 15.9)

Quality assurance (QA) is a managerial tool that encompasses all the systematic actions required for providing sufficient confidence, that a product will meet the requisite quality. Here, the confidence is bifold, as in internally to the company's management and externally to the stakeholders, such as customers, creditors, clients, society, government agencies, third parties, etc.

Quality assurance is a way of preventing mistakes and defects in manufactured products and avoiding problems when delivering products or services to customers; which ISO 9000 defines as "part of quality management focused on providing confidence that quality requirements will be fulfilled".

Definitions

- Quality assurance is an on-going, systematic, comprehensive evaluation of healthcare services and impact of those services on healthcare services. —*Kozier*
- Quality assurance is defined as all activities undertaken to predate and prevent poor quality. —*Neetvert*
- Quality assurance is a program adopted by an institution that is designed to promote the best possible care. —*Delaughery*

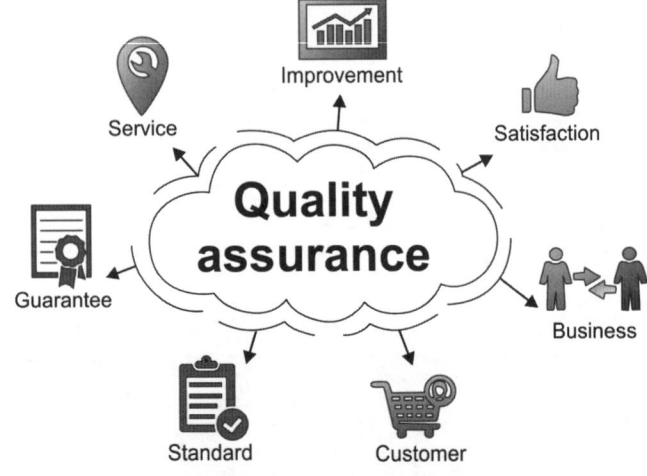

Fig. 15.9: Quality assurance.

- Quality assurance is the process of establishing a target degree of excellence for nursing intervention and taking action to ensure that each patient receives the agreed upon-level of care.
- Quality assurance is a judgment concerning the process of care based on the extent to which that tare contributes to valued outcomes. —*Donabedian 1982*
- Quality assurance is the measurement of provision against expectations with declared intention and ability to correct any demonstrated weakness. —*Shaw*

Concept of Quality Assurance

- Quality assurance is a way of preventing mistakes or defects in manufactured products and avoiding problems when delivering solutions or services to customers.
- Quality assurance is applied to physical products in pre-production to verify what will be made meets specifications and requirements, and during manufacturing production runs by validating lot samples meet specified quality controls.
- Quality assurance is also applied to software to verify that features and functionality meet business objectives, and that code is relatively bug free prior to shipping or releasing new software products and versions.
- Quality assurance refers to administrative and procedural activities implemented in a quality system so that requirements and goals for a product, service or activity will be fulfilled.
- It is the systematic measurement, comparison with a standard, monitoring of processes and an associated feedback loop that confers error prevention.
- This can be contrasted with quality control, which is focused on process output

Meaning of Quality Assurance

- Quality is defined as the extent of resemblance between the purpose of healthcare and the truly granted care. —*Donabedian 1986*
- Quality assurance originated in manufacturing industry "to ensure that the product consistently achieved customer satisfaction".
- Quality assurance is a dynamic process through which nurses assume accountability for quality of care they provide.
- It is a guarantee to the society that services provided by nurses are being regulated by members of profession.
- "Quality assurance is a judgment concerning the process of care, based on the extent to which that cares contributes to valued outcomes".
- "Quality assurance as the monitoring of the activities of client care to determine the degree of excellence attained to the implementation of the activities".

Objectives

- To ensure the delivery of quality client care.
- To demonstrate efforts of health care providers to provide good results.
- To formulate plan of care.
- To evaluate achievement of nursing care.
- To support delivery of nursing care with administrative and managerial services.
- To explain quality assurance models as pre-requisite for quality nursing care.
- To state code of ethics and professional conduct for nurses in India.
- To appreciate importance of practicing standard safety measures.
- Plan and conduct patient teaching sessions.
- To identify appropriate management techniques to be used for managing resources in given situation.

Purposes

- It is required to introduce code of ethics and professional conduct for nurses in India.
- To prepare staff nurse for implementation quality assurance model in nursing.
- To provide best care to patients by maintaining standards.

Purposes and need of Quality Assurance in Nursing

The main purpose of quality assurance is a way of preventing mistakes and to assure the public that the services provided by nurses are committed to continuing competence and quality improvement in order to meet the expectations of receiver, management and regulatory body. In a nursing process, the quality assurance will assess what are the healthcare service are in place and what else needed to improve the quality.

Principles (Box 15.1)

- Quality assurance should include regular evaluation of institutions, their programs or their quality assurance systems by external monitoring bodies or agencies.
- External monitoring bodies or agencies carrying out quality assurance should be subject to regular review.
- Quality assurance should include context, input, process and output dimensions, while giving emphasis to outputs and learning outcomes.
- Quality assurance systems should include the following elements:
  - Clear and measurable objectives and standards, guidelines for implementation, including stakeholder involvement appropriate resources
  - Consistent evaluation methods, associating self-assessment and external review

---

Box 15.1: Principles of quality assurance.

- Customer focus
- Leadership
- Involvement of people
- Process approach
- System approach to management
- Continual improvement
- Factual approach to decision making
- Mutually beneficial supplier relationship

- Feedback mechanisms and procedures for improvement, widely accessible evaluation results.
- Quality assurance initiatives at international, national and regional level should be coordinated in order to ensure overview, coherence, synergy and system-wide analysis.
- Quality assurance should be a cooperative process across education and training levels and systems, involving all relevant stakeholders, within member states and across the community.
- Quality assurance orientations at community level may provide reference points for evaluations and peer learning.

Factors Affecting Quality Assurance in Nursing Care (Box 15.2)

- **Lack of resources:** Insufficient resources, infrastructure, equipment, money for recurring expenses and staff make it impossible for output of a certain quality.
- **Personnel problem:** Lack of trained, skilled and motivated employees, staff in discipline, etc., affects the quality of care.
- **Unreasonable patients and attendants:** Illness, anxiety absence of immediate response to treatment, unreasonable and uncooperative attitude which in turn affects the quality care.
- **Improper maintenance:** Building equipment requires proper, maintenance for efficient use.
- **Absence of well-informed populace:** To improve quality nursing care, it is necessary that the people become knowledgeable and assert their rights to quality care.
- **Absence of accreditation laws:** There is no organization strictly empowered legislation to lay down standards for nursing and medical care so as to regulate the quality of care.
- **Inspect hospitals and ensure that basic requirements are met:** Enquire into major incidence of negligence and take action against health professional involved in malpractices.
- **Lack of incident review procedures:** During a patient's hospitalization several incidents may occur which has a bearing on the treatment and the patient's final recovery.
- **Delayed attendance by physician/nurse:** Incorrect medication burns arising out of faulty procedures, death in a corridor with no nurse/physician accompanying the patient care.
- **Lack of good hospital information system:** A good management information system is essential for the appraisal of quality care.

- **Absence of conducting patient satisfaction surveys:** Surveys to be carried out through questionnaires, interviews, etc., by social worker, hospital management trainees and consultant groups.
- **Lack of nursing care records:** Nurses should use the problem-oriented record system or use nursing process while recording the care given.
- **Miscellaneous:** Lack of good supervision absence of knowledge about the philosophy of nursing care, lack of policy and administrative manual lack of procedure manual, substandard education and training, inadequate quality and number of professionals, lack of evaluation techniques, lack of coordination between and within departments, lack of written job descriptions and job specifications, lack of in service and continuing educational programs.

Approaches to Quality Assurance

There are three approaches from which nursing care can be evaluated to assure quality nursing practice:
1. Structure,
2. Process, and
3. Outcome

Since each of these interaction elements contributes to the quality of nursing care delivered, an improvement in any of the three tends to produce favorable change in the other two.

1. **Structural element:** It includes the physical setting, instrumentality and conditions through which nursing care is administered, such as philosophy, objectives, policies, procedures, records, organizational structures, financial resources, equipment and expectations and attitudes of patients and employees.
2. **Process element:** It includes steps of the nursing process itself- assessment, diagnosing, planning, implementation and evaluation and all subsystems within the nursing process, such as taking a health history, performing a physical examination, making a nursing diagnosis, determining nursing care goals, writing a nursing care plan, performing each care, cure and coordination of tasks prescribed by the care plan, measuring patient care outcome and recording and reporting patient's response to treatment. It is the criteria for measuring nursing care to determine if nursing standards of practice are being met, so they are task oriented.
3. **Outcome element:** It includes changes in patient health systems that result from nursing interventions. For example, modification in signs and symptoms, knowledge, attitudes satisfaction, skill level and compliance with treatment regimen, and established patient outcome criteria.

Quality Assurance Model (Fig. 15.10)

- **Donabedian Model (1985):** It is a model proposed for the structure, process and outcome of quality. This linear model has been widely accepted as the fundamental structure to develop many other models in QA.

Box 15.2: Factors affecting quality assurance in nursing practice.
- Lack of resources
- Personnel problem
- Improper maintenance
- Unreasonable patients and attendants
- Absence of well-informed population
- Absence of accreditation laws
- Lack of incident review procedure

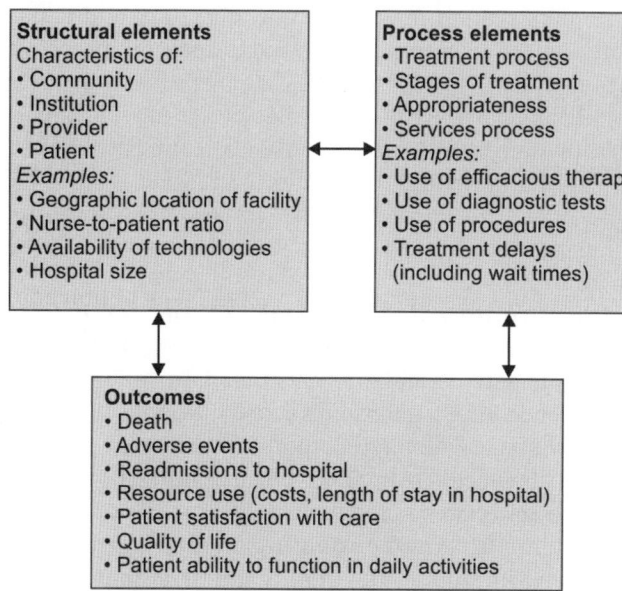

Fig. 15.10: Quality assurance model.

2. **Measure:** Key processes are identified and data are collected.
3. **Analyze:** Data are converted to information; causes of process variation are identified.
4. **Improve:** This stage generates solutions and make and measures process changes.
5. **Control:** Processes that are performing in a predictable way at a desirable level are in control.

Quality Assurance Cycle (Fig. 15.11)

In practice, QA is a cyclical, iterative process that must be applied flexibly to meet the needs of a specific program. The process may begin with a comprehensive effort to define standards and norms as described in Steps 1–3, or it may start with small-scale quality improvement activities (Steps 5–10). Alternatively, the process may begin with monitoring (Step 4). Some teams may even choose to simultaneously begin in two places. For instance, comprehensive monitoring and focused problem solving may start as a coordinated, parallel effort. The ten steps in the QA process are discussed in the following section.

1. **Planning for quality assurance:** This first step prepares an organization to carry out QA activities. Planning begins with a review of the organizations scope of care to determine which services should be addressed.
2. **Setting standards and specifications:** To provide consistently high-quality services, an organization must translate its programmatic goals and objectives into operational procedures. In its widest sense, a standard is a statement of the quality that is expected. Under the broad rubric of standards, there are practice guidelines or clinical protocols, administrative procedures or standard operating procedures, product specifications, and performance standards. For some programs, setting standards and specifications involves a simple review of current guidelines and standard operating procedures to ensure that they are up-to-date.
3. **Communicating guidelines and standards:** Once practice guidelines, standard operating procedures, and

- **ANA Model:** This first proposed and accepted model of quality assurance was given by Long and Black in 1975. This helps in the self-determination of patient and family, nursing health orientation, patient's right to quality care and nursing contributions.
- **Quality Health Outcome Model:** The uniqueness of this model proposed by Mitchell and Co is the point that there are dynamic relationships with indicators that not only act upon, but also reciprocally affect the various components. **System** (Individual, Group/organization) Intervention **Outcome Client** (Individual, Family and Community)
- **Plan, Do, and Study, Act cycle:**
  - It is an improvement model advocated by Dr Deming, which is still practiced widely that contains a distinct improvement phase.
  - Use of PDSA model assumes that a problem has been identified and analyzed for it is most likely causes and that changes have been recommended for eliminating the likely causes.
  - Once the initial problem analysis is completed, a **Plan** is developed to test one of the improvement changes.
  - During the **Do** phase, the change is made, and data are collected to evaluate the results.
  - **Study** involves analysis of the data collected in the previous step. Data are evaluated for evidence that an improvement has been made.
  - The **Act** step involves taking actions that will hardwire 'the change so that the gains made by the improvement are sustained over time.
- **Six Sigma:** It refers to six standard deviations from the mean and is generally used in quality improvement to define the number of acceptable defects or errors produced by a process. It consists of 5 steps: define measure, analyze, improve and control (DMAIC).
  1. **Define:** Questions are asked about key customer requirements and key processes to support those requirements.

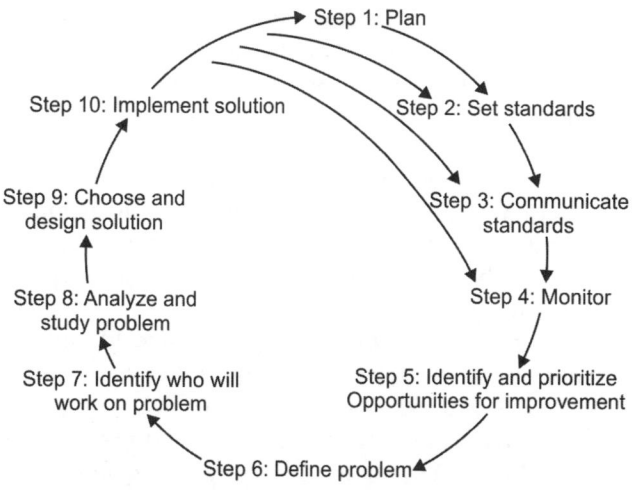

Fig. 15.11: Quality assurance cycle.

performance standards have been defined, it is essential that staff members communicate and promote their use. This will ensure that each health worker, supervisor, manager, and support person understands what is expected of him or her. This is particularly important if ongoing training and supervision have been weak or if guidelines and procedures have recently changed. Assessing quality before communicating expectations can lead to erroneously blaming individuals for poor performance when fault actually lies with systemic deficiencies. Additionally, QA efforts that begin with a surprise examination are likely to cause suspicion rather than support.

4. **Monitoring quality:** Monitoring is the routine collection and review of data that helps to assess whether program norms are being followed or whether outcomes are improved. By monitoring key indicators, managers and supervisors can determine whether the services delivered follow the prescribed practices and achieve the desired results.

5. **Identifying problems and selecting opportunities for improvement:** Program managers can identify quality improvement opportunities by monitoring and evaluating activities. Other means include soliciting suggestions from health workers, performing system process analyses, reviewing patient feedback or complaints, and generating ideas through brainstorming or other group techniques. Once a health facility team has identified several problems, it should set quality improvement priorities by choosing one or two problem areas on which to focus. Selection criteria will vary from program to program.

6. **Defining the problem:** Having selected a problem, the team must define it operationally—as a gap between actual performance and performance as prescribed by guidelines and standards. The problem statement should identify the problem and how it manifests itself. It should clearly state where the problem begins and ends, and how to recognize when the problem is solved. Developing a problem statement is a crucial step in the QA process, and its apparent simplicity is deceptive.

7. **Choosing a team:** Once a health facility staff has employed a participatory approach to selecting and defining a problem, it should assign a small team to address the specific problem. The team will analyze the problem, develop a quality improvement plan, and implement and evaluate the quality improvement effort. The team should comprise those who are involved with, contribute inputs or resources to, and/or benefit from the activity or activities in which the problem occurs. This ensures the involvement of those most knowledgeable about the process.

8. **Analyzing and studying the problem to identify the root cause:** Achieving a meaningful and sustainable quality improvement effort depends on understanding the problem and its root causes. Given the complexity of health service delivery, clearly identifying root causes requires systematic, in-depth analysis. Analytical tools, such as system modeling, flow charting, and cause-and-effect diagrams can be used to analyze a process or problem.

Analytical tools alone will not always provide enough information. A problem-solving team may need to conduct an in-depth examination. Such studies can be based on clinical record reviews, health center register data, staff or patient interviews, service delivery observations.

9. **Developing solutions and actions for quality improvement:** The problem-solving team should now be ready to develop and evaluate potential solutions. Unless the procedure in question is the sole responsibility of an individual, developing solutions should be a team effort. It may be necessary to involve personnel responsible for processes related to the root cause.

10. **Implementing and evaluating quality improvement efforts:** Implementing quality improvement requires careful planning. The team must determine the necessary resources and time frame and decide who will be responsible for implementation. It must also decide whether implementation should begin with a pilot test in a limited area or should be launched on a larger scale. The team should select indicators to evaluate whether the solution was implemented correctly and whether it resolved the problem it was designed to address. In-depth monitoring should begin when the quality improvement plan is implemented. It should continue until either the solution is proven effective and sustainable, or the solution is proven ineffective and is abandoned or modified. When a solution is effective, the teams should continue limited monitoring.

JCAHO Quality Assurance Guideline/Steps

- **Assign responsibility:** According to the Joint Commission, the nurse administrator is ultimately responsible for the implementation of a quality assurance program. Completing step one of the Joint Commission's ten step process require writing a statement that described who is responsible for making certain that QA activities are carried out in the facility. Assigning responsibility should not be confused with assuming responsibility.
- **Delineate scope of care and services:** Scope of care refers to the range of services provided to patients by a unit or department. To delineate the scope of care for a given department personnel should ask themselves, 'what is done in the department?'
- **Identify important aspects of care and services:** Important aspects of nursing care can best be described as some of the fundamental contribution made by nurses while caring for patients. They are the most significant or essential categories of care practiced in a given setting. There is no prescribed list of important aspects of care that every organization must monitor.
- **Identify indicators of outcome (no less than two; no more than four):** A clinical indicator is a quantitative

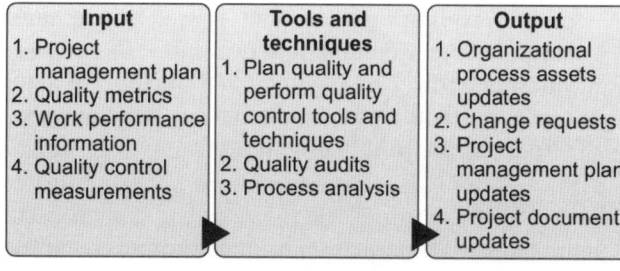

Fig. 15.12: Perform quality assurance.

measure that can be used as a guide to monitor and evaluate the quality of important patient care and support service activities. Indicators are currently considered as being of two general types, i.e., sentinel events and rate-based. Indicators also differ according to the type of event they usually measures (structure, process or outcome).

- **Establish thresholds for evaluation:** Thresholds are accepted levels of compliance with any indicators being measured. Thresholds for evaluation are the level of or point at which intensive evaluation is triggered. A threshold can be viewed as a stimulus for action.
- **Collect data:** Once indicators have been identified, a method of collecting data about the indicators must be selected. Among the many methods of data collection is interviewing patient/family, distributing questionnaires, reviewing charts, making direct observation, etc.
- **Evaluate data:** When data gathering is completed in the process of planning patients care, nurses make assessments based on the findings. In the QA process as a whole, when data collection has been completed and summarized, a group of nurses makes an assessment of the quality of care.
- **Take action:** Nurses are action-oriented professionals. For many nurses, the greater portion of every day is spent on patient's intervention. These actions and interventions conducted by nurses promote health and wellness for patients. Converting nursing energy into the QA process requires formulating an action plan to address identified problems.
- **Assess action taken:** Continuous and sustained improvement in care requires constant surveillance by nurses of the intervention initiated to improve care.
- **Communicate:** Written and verbal messages about the results of QA activities must be shared with other disciplines throughout the facility.

Areas of Quality Assurance

Areas of QA the assurance in various key areas are:
I. **Outpatient department:** The points to be remembered are:
   - Courteous behavior must be extended by all, trained or untrained personnel.
   - Reduction of waiting time in the OPD and for lab investigations by creating more service outlets.
   - Provide basic amenities, such as toilets, telephone, and drinking water, etc.
   - Provision of polyclinic concept to give all specialty services under one roof.
   - Providing ambulatory services or running day care centers.
   - Emergency medical services

   Services must be provided by well trained and dedicated staff, and they should have access to the most sophisticated life-saving equipment and materials, and also have the facility of rendering pre-hospital emergency medical aid through a quick reaction trauma care team provided with a trauma care emergency van.
II. **In-patient services:** Provide a pleasant hospital stay to the patient through provision of a safe, homely atmosphere, a listening ear, humane approach and well behaved, courteous staff.
III. **Specialty services:** A high tech hospital with all types of specialty and superspecialty services will increase the image of the hospital.
IV. **Training:** A continuous training program should be present consisting of on the job training, skill training workshops, seminars, conferences, and case presentations.

Development of a Quality Assurance Program

This program is a carefully planned, phased process, or it may be implemented in one step as part of a fundamental organizational change:

- **Foster commitment of quality:** This process must continue throughout the life of a project and at all levels of the organization. Commitment can be done through awareness-raising seminars, special planning meetings, or one-to-one discussion with an organizations leader.
- **Conduct a preliminary review of quality—related activities:** It is important to conduct an initial review of the organization and to develop a general description of the existing system.
- **Develop the purpose and vision for the quality assurance effort:** Purpose is to build consensus between managers and to set boundaries for the quality assurance effort. The vision will help the staff to understand how their day-today wok relates to quality improvement.
- **Determine level and scope of initial quality assurance activities:** It depend on the resources available, the implementation time frame and the receptivity of management and program staff to the idea of quality assurance, The effort can be implemented at national, regional and district level or within a single health facility.
- **Assign responsibility for quality assurance:** An Existing committee or management body will take on responsibility for quality assurance, integrating it into the general management structure.
- **Allocate resources for quality assurance:** Local resources must be allocated to quality assurance program to become a permanent part of a healthcare organization. It may depend on outside technical and financial assistance.
- **Develop a written quality assurance plan:** This plan is a written document that describes the program objectives

and scope, defines lines of responsibility and authority, and puts forth implementation strategies. The plan helps the staffs to relate quality, goals and objectives to their routine activities.

- **Critical management system:** Quality assurance efforts will focus three critical management systems: Supervision, training and management information systems.
- **Disseminate quality assurance experience:** Dissemination strategy should be devised to share experience inside and outside the organization. Conferences which conduct at local, regional, national and international level will reinforce success encourage dialogue and creativity.
- **Manage change:** A careful, phased approach to change is required and an open and trusting environment must be cultivated.

Approaches for Quality Assurance Program

Approaches of quality assurance are divided into two types:
1. General approach, 2. Specific approach

- **General approaches (Fig. 15.13):** It involves large governing of official body's evaluation of person's or agency's ability to meet standard at a given time.
  - **Credentialing:** It is process of determining and maintaining nursing standards. Functional components of credentialing process according to Hinsvark, credentialing process has four functional components:
    1. To produce a quality product
    2. To confer a unique identity
    3. To protect provider and public
    4. To control the profession
  - **Licensure:** Individual licensure is a contract between profession and state in which profession is granted control over entry into and exists from profession and over quality of professional practice.
  - **Accreditation:** Accreditation is the act of granting credit or recognition especially to an educational institution that maintains suitable standards.
  - **Certification:** Certification is usually a voluntary process within the professions. A person's educational achievement, experience and performance on examination are used to determine person's qualification for functioning in an identified specialty area.
- **Specific approaches:** Quality assurances are methods used to evaluate identified instances of provider and client interaction.
  - **Peer review committee:** These are designed to monitor client specific aspects of care appropriate for certain levels of care. The audit is used by peer review committee to ascertain quality of care.
  - **Nursing audit:** Nursing audit is evaluation of patient care through analysis of written records maintained by nurses in patient's treatment profile.

Role of a Nurse

- Role of nurse is to participate in quality improvement team.
- Properly supervises and check whether patient is receiving proper care or not.
- Contribute innovation and improvement of patient care.
- Participating in improvement projects andpatient safety initiatives.
- Participating in CNE programs and in-service education programs.
- Periodic and continuing appraisal and evaluation of health care situation of patient.
- Participate in research works related to quality assurance.
- Nurse identifies area where need improvement in delivery of care

Benefits of Quality Assurance

Quality assurance enables:
- Bring internal benefits to the university/faculty/department/school/program and the staff
- Bring external benefits to the students and the reputation of the institution
- Continuously improve themselves, the students and the work of the university. Continuous improvement is both the medium and outcome of quality assurance
- Serve accountability and accreditation requirements
- Enhance the reputation of the faculty/department/school/university, and meet external demands for demonstrating quality, quality assurance and quality enhancement. **Table 15.1** describes quality assurance versus quality control.

Challenges of Nurses in Providing Quality Care

- Providing a quality care to patients with lack of resources, such as infrastructures, equipment, and patient's financial status all these are a major concern in today's health care environment.
- The challenges are due to personnel problems, such as lack of skill and training, staff indiscipline.
- The unreasonable and uncooperative attitude of the patients and their family members due to illness, anxiety,

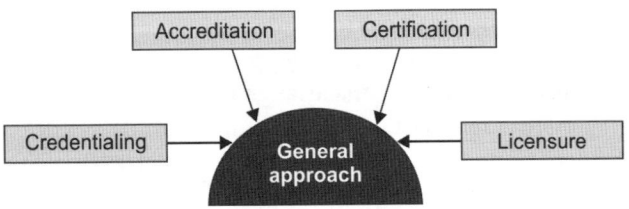

Fig. 15.13: General approach.

Table 15.1: Quality assurance v/s quality control.

Quality assurance	Quality control
Focus on processes	Focus on outputs
Achieved by improving production processes	Achieved by sampling and checking (inspection)
Targeted at the whole organization	Targeted at production activities
Emphasizes the customer	Emphasizes required standards
Quality is built into the product	Defect products are inspected out

absence of immediate response to treatment, ignorance about prognosis, late attendance, etc.
- There is lack of regulatory bodies empowered by legislation to appraise the standards in nursing and medical care to regulate the quality care.
- No proper maintenance of institutional building and equipment's used, so these equipment cannot be used in giving nursing care, so it is necessary to ensure adequate after sale service.
- To improve quality of nursing care the nurses apply their knowledge, skills and experience to provide right care and ensure the patients will get benefited from the quality care. Continuous educational program is important to achieve this.
- Due to shortage they may chance for errors, negligence and health professionals may involved in malpractice.
- The nonavailability of essential drugs and supplies, adulterated and substandard drugs, improperly sterilized or pyrogenic materials this lead to poor quality care.
- Inadequate support services for nurses, such as ward aid, helper, etc., in hospitals and the nursing budget is not separately sanctioned. Nursing posting not upto the ratio as per the norms defined by nursing council.
- Lack of hospital information systems, this play a vital role in effective management for the appraisal of quality care.

Role of Nurses in Quality Assurance

- They should start with establishing their goals and objectives of their practice and review it regularly and maintain excellent safety standards.
- Nurses play a key role in hospitals to promote high quality care cost-effective outcomes and better patient safety by interpreting and applying the policies and procedure guidelines as per the standards.
- Nurses should identify and coordinate the needs of patients and their family members from preadmission to till discharge based on age and cultural and individual patient needs. They should acts as good communicator with the organization, providers and patients and they should helpful for collection of patient information data.
- The nurses usually evaluate their work and behavior from the data collected from patients and collaborate with physicians and other health professionals to develop patient-care guidelines and this help to implement if they need any change to improve patient care. By monitoring themselves and their colleagues, they ensure qualitative requirements are met as per standards.
- They train and educate other nurses for the best practices and help them to improve quality of work.
- They are responsible for taking new initiatives and assist in quality improvements. They should actively monitor the progress of patient care processes by using the spreadsheets, flow diagrams, computer programs, and control charts for recording and monitoring data.
- They create systems using the observations, surveys made in daily clinical practice help to conduct a health

> **Box 15.3:** Benefits and disadvantages of quality assurance.
> **Benefits of quality assurance are:**
> - Final costs reduction
> - Enhanced motivation
> - No barriers between workers and managers
> - Competitive advantages
>
> **Disadvantages of quality assurance are:**
> - Time-consuming (it requires a lot of time to train the staff to perform QA)
> - High initial costs

record audit and compare the care provided to standards of quality care. Benefits and disadvantages of quality assurance is described in **Box 15.3**.

Role of a Nurse Administrator

A nursing administrator has to develop a formalized quality program.
- Review organizational, personnel and environment.
- Focus on standards of nursing care and methods of delivering nursing care.
- Focus on the outcome of care

The concept of quality assurance refers to the accountability of the health professions to the society for the quality, quantity, appropriateness and costs of health services provided. In addition to the development of outcome indicators the agenda for change focus on continuous improvement. Total quality management may be one of the factors guaranteeing the survival of the fittest in the future. Fr the evaluation of care, an ongoing system of quality control was necessary in each hospital.

QUALITY AND SAFETY

The Occupational Health and Safety Administration, or OSHA, protect workers on the job and require employers to provide safe work environments through education, training and government assistance. Safety, quality, and environmental protection constitute a mutually interrelated whole. The primary objective of workplace safety is preventing workplace injuries, illnesses and fatalities. Employers develop detailed plans that provide guidance in the event of an accident, fire, natural disaster or other emergency. Workplace safety plans also identify the roles and responsibilities of employers and employees when responding during incidents.

Definition

- A safety management system (SMS) is a systematic approach to managing safety, including the necessary organizational structures, accountabilities, policies and procedures.
- Safety management system (SMS)—a systematic and explicit approach defining the activities by which safety management is undertaken by an organization in order to achieve acceptable or tolerable safety.
- Risk management is the process by which vulnerabilities are identified and changes are made to minimize the

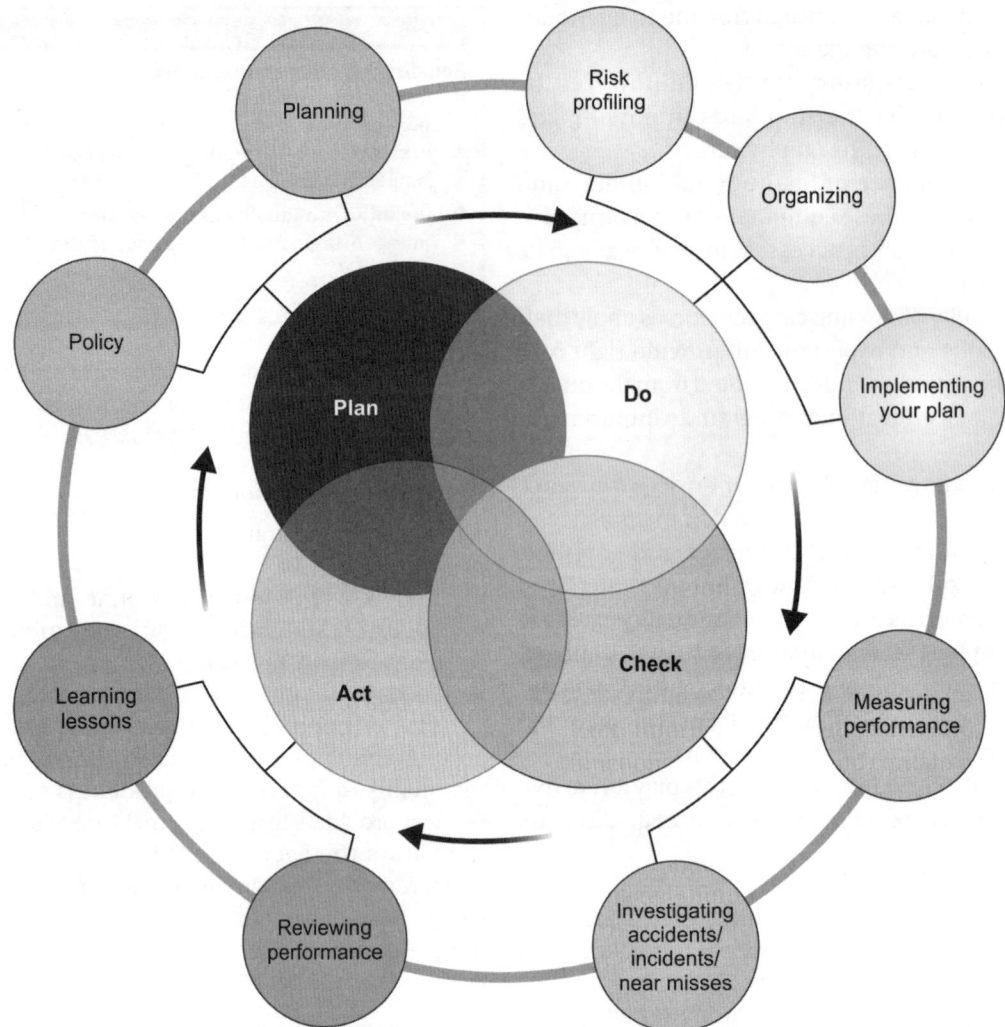

Fig. 15.14: Principles of effective safety management.

consequences of adverse patient outcomes and liability. Related clinical initiatives to reduce risk and harm should be part of a larger organizational commitment to patient safety.

Objective

The objective of a safety management system is to provide a structured management approach to control safety risks in operations. Effective safety management must take into account the organization's specific structures and processes related to safety of operations.

The principal objectives are:
- Nuclear safety
- Radiation protection
- Technical safety
- Fire protection
- Physical security of nuclear materials and nuclear installations
- Occupational safety and health
- Environmental protection

General Principles of Effective Safety Management

Four key stages (Fig. 15.14)
1. **Planning:** Setting policy and formulating a safety plan
2. **Doing:** Delivering safety plan
3. **Checking:** Measuring performance, i.e., monitoring
4. **Acting:** Reviewing performance and acting upon lessons learnt to feedback into Step 1.

Ten Principles of Safety Management

1. Establish and observe a written corporate safety policy.
2. Create an independent safety review process.
3. Identify and evaluate the severity and foresee ability of product hazards.
4. Conduct a design review assessing the risk of injury by considering the hazards, the environment, and foreseeable use.
5. First attempt to eliminate hazards. If not possible, then reduce the opportunity for injury by guarding against the hazards.
6. Warn users of product dangers and motivate them to avoid injury.
7. Promote only the safe use of a product.

Table 15.2: Phases of safety management.

Phase 1: Planning and preparation	Phase 2: Identification and assessment	Phase 3: Execution and improvement
1. Gain executive-level commitment	1. Identify the organization's safety and health strengths and weaknesses	1. Establish, train, and activate improvement project teams
2. Establish the TSM committee	2. Identify safety and health advocates and resistors	2. Activate the feedback loop
3. Mold the committee into a team	3. Benchmark initial employee perceptions concerning the work environment	3. Establish a TSM culture
4. Give the committee safety and health awareness training	4. Tailor implementation to the organization	
5. Develop the organization's safety and health vision and guiding principles	5. Identify specific improvement projects	
6. Develop the organization's safety and health mission and objectives		
7. Communicate and inform		

Note: Phase 2: Identification and assessment phase: This phase consists of developing safety goals and objectives, management training, and strategic decision making on safety management techniques.

8. Maintain safety-related records during the useful life of the product.
9. Continuously monitor safety performance of the product in the hands of users.
10. Promptly notify product users and institute recall procedures where necessary to substantially reduce or eliminate injury. **Table 15.2** describes phases of safety management.

Safety and Environmental Protection Policy

- Place protection of human life and health before all other interests.
- Pursue safety and environmental protection as integral parts of management.
- Comply with laws, regulations, and our public obligations, and we take note of recognized practices.
- Continually improve safety and environmental protection.
- Regularly assess risks and either prevent them, eliminate them, or reduce their impact to an acceptable level.
- Ensure that plant and equipment complies, long-term, with all technical, safety, and economic criteria.
- In selecting and evaluating suppliers, we take into account their attitudes toward safety and the environment.
- Communicate openly and effectively on safety-related topics.
- Secure sufficient numbers of high quality, motivated employees and suppliers.
- Manage key knowledge

Quality-of-Management Policy

- Treat our partners and customers with respect.
- Conduct our planning in accordance with our strategic objectives.
- Standardize and describe our best practices.
- Complete work assignments flawlessly on the first try.
- Perform checks, and respond immediately to shortcomings.
- Take decisions based on knowledge of the matter and verified facts.
- Improve things, and we make changes flexibly and safely.

Safety Management System

A safety management system (SMS) is a systematic approach to managing safety through organizational structures, accountabilities, policies, and procedures.

Four Pillars of SMS

1. **Safety policy and objectives:** This is a statement that establishes senior management's commitment to continuously improve safety and health. It defines the methods, processes, and organizational structures needed to meet safety and health goals.
2. **Safety risk management:** It determines the need and adequacy of new or revised risk controls based on the assessment towards an acceptable risk.
3. **Safety assurance:** It evaluates the continued effectiveness of implementing these control strategies to support the identification of new hazards. Continual improvement practices are also part of this. The role of the quality management system (QMS) is to ensure the quality of our safety performance by identifying the substandard performance of SMS activities and its causes.
4. **Safety promotion:** It is an element that includes training, communication, promotion and education, and other actions to create a positive safety culture within all levels of the workforce.

The role of safety promotion is to:

- Encourage a positive safety culture
- Create an environment where safety objective can be achieved
- Develop awareness in the workforce that gains support for the SMS
- Foster improve communication

Health and Safety Management in Healthcare

- The health and safety policy confirming the employer and management commitment to ensuring safety, health and welfare at work.
- The duties of employers and employees with regard to safety, health and welfare. The responsibilities of key

personnel (include names and where applicable job title/position) with regard to safety, health and welfare, e.g., the responsibilities of the senior manager/director of nursing, etc.
- It is important to ensure that there are clear lines of responsibility and good awareness of responsibilities allocated.
- The arrangements for consultation with employees and arrangements for communicating health and safety information. Include emergency plans, such as evacuation procedures, incident reporting arrangements, etc.
- A written risk assessment, this is the key part of the safety statement where the work related hazards have been identified and the associated risks have been assessed and documented.
- The control measures to eliminate or reduce the risk must also be identified.
- Any other arrangements for securing safety, health and welfare at work and the resources provided, such as arrangements for occupational health expertise, immunization arrangements for employees and health surveillance, arrangements for working with contractors and/or others who share the building, etc.

Safety Management in Nursing

- The safety of nurses from workplace-induced injuries and illnesses is important to nurses themselves as well as to the patients they serve.
- The presence of healthy and well-rested nurses is critical to providing vigilant monitoring, empathic patient care, and vigorous advocacy.
- Many workplace stressors that can produce diseases and injuries are present in nursing work environments.
- These stressors include factors related to the immediate work context, characteristics of the organization, and changes that are occurring external to the organization but throughout the healthcare industry.
- The hazards of nursing work can impair health both acutely and in the long term.
- These health outcomes include musculoskeletal injuries/disorders, other injuries, infections, changes in mental health, and in the longer term, cardiovascular, metabolic, and neoplastic diseases.
- These stressors include aspects of the way work is organized in nursing (e.g., shift work, long hours, and overtime) and psychological job demands, such as work place.

PROGRAM EVALUATION AND REVIEW TECHNIQUE

The program (or project) evaluation and review technique (PERT), commonly abbreviated PERT, is a statistical tool, used in project management, which was designed to analyze and represent the tasks involved in completing a given project. First developed by the United States Navy in the 1950s, it is commonly used in conjunction with the critical path method (CPM).

Definition of PERT

The Program Evaluation Review Technique, or PERT, is a visual tool used in project planning. Using the technique helps project planners identify start and end dates, as well as interim required tasks and timelines. The information is displayed as a network in chart form.

Creating a PERT Chart (Fig. 15.15)

A flowchart is used to depict the Project Evaluation Review Technique. Nodes represent the events, indicating the start or end of activities or tasks. The directorial lines indicate the tasks that need to be completed, and the arrows show the sequence of the activities. There are four definitions of time used to estimate project time requirements:

1. **Optimistic time:** The least amount of time it can take to complete a task.
2. **Pessimistic time:** The maximum amount of time, it should take to complete a task
3. **Most likely time:** Assuming there are no problems, the best, or most reasonable, estimate of how long it should take to complete a task.
4. **Expected time:** Assuming there are problems, the best estimate of how much time will be required to complete a task.

History

- PERT was developed by the US Navy in the 1950s to help coordinate the thousands of contractors it had working on myriad projects.
- While PERT was originally a manual process, today, there are computerized PERT systems that enable project charts to be created quickly.
- The only real weakness of the PERT process is that the time required for completion of each task is very subjective and sometimes no better than a wild guess. Frequent progress updates help refine the project timeline once it gets underway.

Description of PERT Chart

- A PERT chart is a graph that represents all of the tasks necessary to a project's completion, and the order in which they must be completed along with the corresponding time requirements.
- Certain tasks are dependent on serial tasks, which must be completed in a certain sequence.

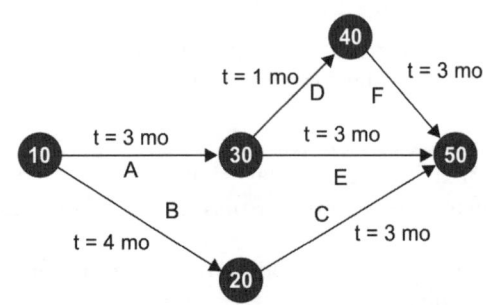

Fig. 15.15: PERT chart.

- Tasks that are not dependent on the completion of other tasks are called parallel or concurrent tasks and can generally be worked on simultaneously.
- PERT charts are preferable to Gantt charts because they more clearly identify task dependencies; however, the PERT chart is often more challenging to interpret. As such, project managers frequently employ both methodologies.

The Three Chances

There are three estimation times involved in PERT; Optimistic Time Estimate (TOPT), Most Likely Time Estimate (TLIKELY), and Pessimistic Time Estimate (TPESS). In PERT, these three estimate times are derived for each activity. This way, a range of time is given for each activity with the most probable value, TLIKELY. Following are further details on each estimate:

1. **TOPT:** This is the fastest time an activity can be completed. For this, the assumption is made that all the necessary resources are available and all predecessor activities are completed as planned.
2. **TLIKELY:** Most of the times, project managers are asked only to submit one estimate. In that case, this is the estimate that goes to the upper management.
3. **TPESS:** This is the maximum time required to complete an activity. In this case, it is assumed that many things go wrong related to the activity. A lot of rework and resource unavailability are assumed when this estimation is derived.

Meaning of PERT

- Program evaluation and review technique (PERT) is a technique adopted by organizations to analyze and represent the activity in a project, and to illustrate the flow of events in a project.
- PERT is a method to evaluate and estimate the time required to complete a task within deadlines.
- PERT serves as an management tool to analyze, define and integrate events.
- PERT also illustrates the activities and interdependencies in a project.
- The main goal of PERT is to reduce the cost and time needed to complete a project.

Terminology in PERT

- **PERT event:** A point that marks the start or completion of one or more activities. It consumes no time and uses no resources. When it marks the completion of one or more activities, it is not "reached" (does not occur) until all of the activities leading to that event have been completed.
- **Predecessor event:** An event that immediately precedes some other event without any other events intervening. An event can have multiple predecessor events and can be the predecessor of multiple events.
- **Successor event:** An event that immediately follows some other event without any other intervening events. An event can have multiple successor events and can be the successor of multiple events.
- **PERT activity:** The actual performance of a task which consumes time and requires resources (such as labor, materials, space, machinery). It can be understood as representing the time, effort, and resources required to move from one event to another. A PERT activity cannot be performed until the predecessor event has occurred.
- **PERT subactivity:** A PERT activity can be further decomposed into a set of sub-activities. For example, activity A1 can be decomposed into A1.1, A1.2 and A1.3. Subactivities have all the properties of activities; in particular a subactivity has predecessor or successor events just like an activity. A subactivity can be decomposed again into finer-grained subactivities.
- **Optimistic time (O):** The minimum possible time required to accomplish a task, assuming everything proceeds better than is normally expected.
- **Pessimistic time (P):** The maximum possible time required to accomplish a task, assuming everything goes wrong (but excluding major catastrophes).
- **Most likely time (M):** The best estimate of the time required to accomplish a task, assuming everything proceeds as normal.
- **Expected time (T_E):** The best estimate of the time required to accomplish a task, accounting for the fact that things do not always proceed as normal (the implication being that the expected time is the average time the task would require if the task were repeated on a number of occasions over an extended period of time).

$$T_E = (O + 4M + P) \div 6$$

- **Float or slack** is a measure of the excess time and resources available to complete a task. It is the amount of time that a project task can be delayed without causing a delay in any subsequent tasks (free float) or the whole project (total float). Positive slack would indicate ahead of schedule; negative slack would indicate behind schedule; and zero slack would indicate on schedule.
- **Critical path:** The longest possible continuous pathway taken from the initial event to the terminal event. It determines the total calendar time required for the project; and, therefore, any time delays along the critical path will delay the reaching of the terminal event by at least the same amount.
- **Critical activity:** An activity that has total float equal to zero. An activity with zero float is not necessarily on the critical path since its path may not be the longest.
- **Lead time:** The time by which a predecessor event must be completed in order to allow sufficient time for the activities that must elapse before a specific PERT event reaches completion.
- **Lag time:** The earliest time by which a successor event can follow a specific PERT event.
- **Fast tracking:** Performing more critical activities in parallel
- **Crashing critical path:** Shortening duration of critical activities

The PERT Process

PERT has a set series of steps in mapping out a complex project, which include:
- List all the tasks and milestones (a.k.a. events) required for completion of the project
- Determine the required sequence of tasks
- Design a chart to visually display all the steps
- Estimate the time required for each task
- Identify the critical path—the longest series of tasks in the project
- Adjust the chart to reflect progress made once the project starts

A PERT chart uses numbered circles or rectangles to represent milestones and straight lines with arrows at the end to represent tasks to be completed. The direction of the arrows, and the numbers, indicate the required sequence. Typically, the numbers increase by 10 at each milestone, so that new tasks can be added along the way without requiring the whole chart to be redrawn and numbered.

PERT Planning Steps

PERT was developed in 1950 by the US Navy during the Cold War and is intended for large projects, which are:
1. Complex
2. Require a series of sequential tasks
3. Performed in parallel with other projects

PERT planning usually involves the following steps:
1. **Identifying tasks and milestones:** Every project involves a series of required tasks. These tasks are listed in a table allowing additional information on sequence and timing to be added later.
2. **Placing the tasks in a proper sequence:** The tasks are analyzed and placed in a sequence to get the desired results.
3. **Network diagramming:** A network diagram is drawn using the activity sequence data showing the sequence of serial and parallel activities.
4. **Time estimating:** This is the time required to carry out each activity, in three parts:
    a. **Optimistic timing:** The shortest time to complete an activity.
    b. **Most likely timing:** The completion time having the highest probability.
    c. **Pessimistic timing:** The longest time to complete an activity
5. **Critical path estimating:** This determines the total time required to complete a project. **Box 15.4** describes application of PERT in nursing.

PERT not only determines the time to complete a specific software development activity, but also determines the cost.

To implement a PERT chart:
- Identify the different tasks needed to complete a project. Make sure to add these in the right order and indicate the duration of each task.
- Create a network diagram. Use arrows to represent the activities and use nodes as milestones.
- Determine the critical path and possible slack. **Figure 15.16** shows differences between PERT and CPM.

Box 15.4: Application of PERT in nursing.

Nurse managers use the PERT system for controlling.
- It forces planning and shows how pieces fit together.
- It does this for all nursing line managers.
- It establishes a system for periodic evaluation and control at critical points in the program.
- It reveals problems and is forward-looking.
- PERT is generally used for complicated and extensive projects or programs.
- Many records are used to control expenses and otherwise conserve the budget.

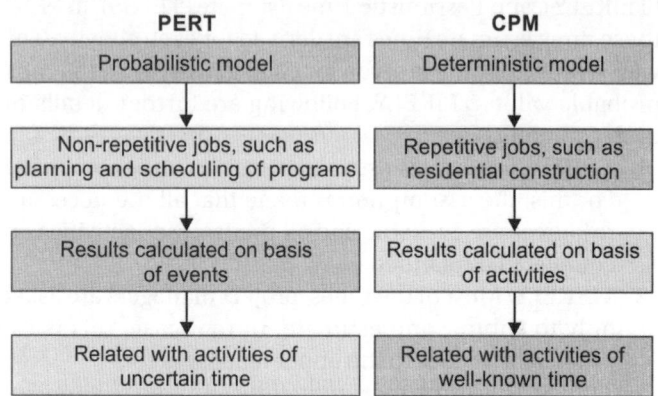

Fig. 15.16: Differences between PERT and CPM.

Advantages of PERT

- PERT chart explicitly defines and makes visible dependencies (precedence relationships) between the work breakdown structure (commonly WBS) elements.
- PERT facilitates identification of the critical path and makes this visible.
- PERT facilitates identification of early start, late start, and slack for each activity.
- PERT provides for potentially reduced project duration due to better understanding of dependencies leading to improved overlapping of activities and tasks where feasible.
- The large amount of project data can be organized and presented in diagram for use in decision making.

Disadvantages of PERT

- There can be potentially hundreds or thousands of activities and individual dependency relationships.
- PERT is not easily scalable for smaller projects.
- The network charts tend to be large and unwieldy requiring several pages to print and requiring specially sized paper.
- The lack of a timeframe on most PERT/CPM charts makes it harder to show status although colors can help (e.g., specific color for completed nodes).

BENCHMARKING

Benchmarking is the practice of comparing business processes and performance metrics to industry bests and best practices from other companies. Dimensions typically measured are quality, time and cost. Benchmarking is used to measure performance using a specific indicator (cost per unit of measure, productivity per unit of measure, cycle time of x per unit of measure or defects per unit of measure) resulting in a metric of performance that is then compared to others.

Also referred to as "best practice benchmarking" or "process benchmarking", this process is used in management in which organizations evaluate various aspects of their processes in relation to best-practice companies' processes, usually within a peer group defined for the purposes of comparison.

Definition

- Benchmarking is a process of finding what best practices are and then proposing what performance should be in the future. The three principles of benchmarking are maintaining quality, customer satisfaction and continuous improvement.
- "Benchmarking is an ongoing outreach activity; the goal of the outreach is identification of the best operating practices that, when implemented, produce superior performance". —*Bogan and English*

Concept of Benchmarking

- Benchmarking is a valuable technique for quickly lifting the performance of an organization.
- Benchmarking activity is not only about auditing practice to ensure practice is achieving required measurable outcomes but supports open comparison and sharing to allow continuous improvement and development.
- The modern health service is being encouraged to ensure uniform provision of high quality health care. Benchmarking pushes the boundaries of best practice ever onwards. Practitioners, aware of developments elsewhere, can develop practice with minimal effort, concentrating resources on new areas for practice.
- Benchmarking often refers to the comparison of indicators in a time-limited approach. It is not yet often perceived as a tool for continuous improvement and support to change.
- Benchmarking's key characteristic is that it is part of a comprehensive and participative policy of continuous quality improvement. Indeed, benchmarking is based on voluntary and active collaboration among several organizations to create a spirit of competition and to apply best practices.

Types

- The benchmarking literature can be mainly separated into two parts: internal and external benchmarking.
- Competitive, functional and generic benchmarking is classified under external benchmarking. The process is essentially the same for each category. The main differences are what are to be benchmarked and with whom it will be benchmarked.

Internal Benchmarking

- Internal benchmarking covers two way communication and sharing opinions between departments within the same organization or between organizations operating as part of a chain in different countries.
- Once any part of an organization has a better performance indicator, others can learn how this was achieved. Findings of internal benchmarking can then be used as a baseline for extending benchmarking to include external organizations.

Advantages of internal benchmarking:
- Ability to deal with partners who share a common language, culture and systems.
- Easy access to data, and giving a baseline for future comparisons.
- The outcomes of an internal benchmarking can be presented quickly.

External Benchmarking

- External benchmarking requires a comparison of work with external organizations in order to discover new ideas, methods, products and services.
- The objective is continuously to improve one's own performance by measuring how it performs, comparing it with that of others.

Competitive Benchmarking

- Comparison with direct competitors only. This is the most sensitive type of benchmarking activity because it is very difficult to achieve a healthy collaboration and cooperation with direct competitors and reach primary sources of information.
- It is believed to be more rational for larger organizations than smaller ones, as they have the infrastructure to support quality and continuous improvement.

Generic Benchmarking

- Refers to the comparisons of business function that are same regardless of business.
- This means that a hotel organization's accounting department would look at the accounting department of a manufacturing organization that has been identified as having the fastest operations.

Functional Benchmarking

- Refers to comparative research and attempts to seek world class excellence by comparing business performance not only against competitors, but also against the best businesses operating in similar fields and performing similar activities or having similar problems, but in a different industry.
- For instance, British Rail Network South East employed a benchmarking process to improve the standard of cleanliness on trains.
- British Airways was selected as a partner because a team of 11 people cleans a 250 seat jumbo aircraft in only 9 minutes.

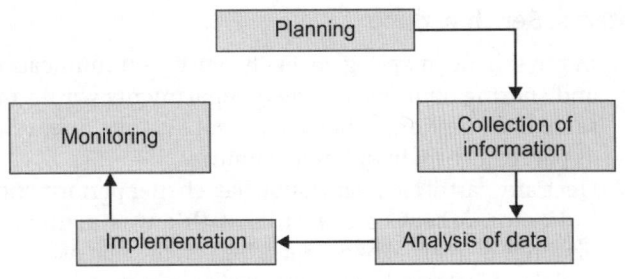

Fig. 15.17: Benchmarking process.

- After the benchmarking exercise, a team of ten people was able to clean a 660 seat train in 8 min.

Benchmarking Process (Fig. 15.17)

- **Plan:** Select the process—form team—understand and document process—establish performance measure
- **Search:** Listing criteria for partner selection—conduct general/secondary research—decide the level to benchmark—identify potential partners and contact.
- **Observe:** Questionnaire sent to partner—telephone contact—direct observation/site visit
- **Analyze:** Sort information and data—quality control information and data—normalize data, if necessary—identify gaps in performance level—identify causes for gaps.
- **Adapt:** Identify improvement opportunities—set target for improvement—develop implementation plan, monitor the progress—write final report.

Guidelines for Successful Benchmarking

Successful benchmarking requires the following:
- Thorough understanding of one's own processes.
- Emphasis on industry best practices.
- Selection of appropriate benchmarking partners and techniques.
- The benchmarking partner's willingness to share information
- Maintaining confidentiality of critical information
- Involvement of management and employees in the analysis of best practices.
- Emphasis on practices and processes not on end results.
- Benchmarking should be a continuous process as the competition is always changing.
- Commitment towards the adoption and implementation of best practices.
- Selection and empowerment of benchmarking teams.
- Willingness to change as per the findings of the benchmarking study.
- The adaptability of the practices should be tested and the implementation results should be verified.
- Strict adherence to the benchmarking. **Table 15.3** describes principles of benchmarking.

Types of Benchmarking (Fig. 15.18)

Benchmarking can be internal (comparing performance between different groups or teams within an organization)

Table 15.3: Principles of benchmarking.

Principle	Comment
Relevant	The benchmark is meaningful for the target domain
Understandable	The benchmark is easy to understand and use
Good metrics	The metrics defined by the benchmark are linear, orthogonal and monotonic
Scalable	The benchmark is applicable to a broad spectrum of hardware and software configurations
Coverage	The benchmark workload does not oversimplify the typical environment
Acceptance	The benchmark is recognized as relevant by the majority of vendors and users

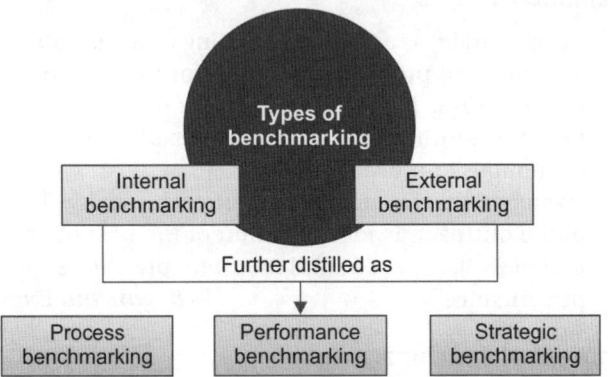

Fig. 15.18: Types of benchmarking.

or external (comparing performance with companies in a specific industry or across industries).

These can be further detailed as follows:

1. **Process benchmarking:** The initiating firm focuses its observation and investigation of business processes with a goal of identifying and observing the best practices from one or more benchmark firms. Activity analysis will be required where the objective is to benchmark cost and efficiency; increasingly applied to back-office processes where outsourcing may be a consideration.
2. **Financial benchmarking:** Performing a financial analysis and comparing the results in an effort to assess your overall competitiveness and productivity.
3. **Benchmarking from an investor perspective:** Extending the benchmarking universe to also compare to peer companies that can be considered alternative investment opportunities from the perspective of an investor.
4. **Benchmarking in the public sector:** Functions as a tool for improvement and innovation in public administration, where state organizations invest efforts and resources to achieve quality, efficiency and effectiveness of the services they provide.
5. **Performance benchmarking:** Allows the initiator firm to assess their competitive position by comparing products and services with those of target firms.
6. **Product benchmarking:** The process of designing new products or upgrades to current ones. This process can sometimes involve reverse engineering which is taking apart competitors products to find strengths and weaknesses.

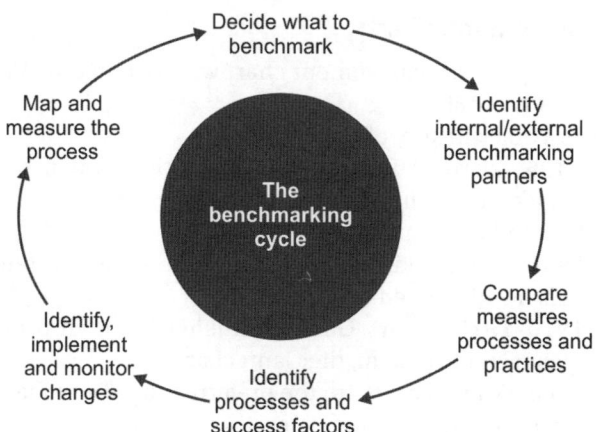

Fig. 15.19: Benchmarking cycle.

7. **Strategic benchmarking:** Involves observing how others compete. This type is usually not industry specific, meaning it is best to look at other industries.
8. **Functional benchmarking:** A company will focus its benchmarking on a single function to improve the operation of that particular function. Complex functions, such as Human Resources, Finance and Accounting and Information and Communication Technology are unlikely to be directly comparable in cost and efficiency terms and may need to be disaggregated into processes to make valid comparison.
9. **Best-in-class benchmarking:** Involves studying the leading competitor or the company that best carries out a specific function.
10. **Operational benchmarking:** Embraces everything from staffing and productivity to office flow and analysis of procedures performed.
11. **Energy benchmarking:** Process of collecting, analyzing and relating energy performance data of comparable activities with the purpose of evaluating and comparing performance between or within entities. Entities can include processes, buildings or companies. Benchmarking may be internal between entities within a single organization, or—subject to confidentiality restrictions—external between competing entities. **Figure 15.19** shows benchmarking cycle.

Cost of Benchmarking

- **Visit cost:** Hotel rooms, travel cost, meals, gift, lost labor time.
- **Time cost:** Members of team will be investing time in researching problems, finding exceptions companies to study, visit, and implementation. And additional staff may also be required.
- **Benchmarking database cost:** Create and maintain database of best practices.
- The cost of benchmarking and be substantially reduced through utilizing may internet resources which are quick and cheaper.

Benefits

Benchmarking has several other benefits as well:

- **Improved quality:** Benchmarking helps organizations to continuously improve the quality of their products and services. Organizations observe the current standard, and then try to surpass that.
- **Better performance:** Benchmarking helps organizations overcome complacency. They continuously strive to improve their performance standards in order to stay relevant in the market.
- **Cost efficiency:** Benchmarking provides organization with valuable data on the last technology, and processes followed in the business environment. These are aimed at increasing productivity while reducing cost. For example, a manufacturing company might learn about a certain machine used by its competitor, which can do the work for five workers. This company might also adopt similar technology to lower its labor cost.
- **Prioritizing areas of improvement:** While organizations understand the importance to develop continuously, they might be unsure at times about where to start the improvement from. Benchmarking helps organizations to identify the areas where the gap between their standard and that of the industry is the largest. This helps organizations to prioritize the areas that they need to work on.
- **Leveraging strength areas:** Benchmarking can also throw light on the areas where the organization is doing much better than what is observed in the market.

Limitation to Benchmarking

- Benchmarking is a tough process that needs a lot of commitment to succeed.
- It is a time consuming and expensive.
- More often than not benchmarking processes end with the "they are different from us" syndrome or competitive sensitivity that prevents the free flow of necessary information.

Benchmarking in Health Systems

1. All professionals involved in health care are under a duty of care, which involves ensuring the uniform provision of a high quality health service. A widely accepted.
2. Benchmarking made its first appearance in the healthcare system in 1990 with the requirements of the Joint Commission on Accreditation of Healthcare Organizations (JCAHO) in the United States, which defined it as a measurement tool for monitoring the impact of governance, management and clinical and logistical functions.

In practice, benchmarking also encompasses:
1. Regularly comparing indicators (structure, activities, processes and outcomes) against best practitioners.
2. Identifying differences in outcomes through inter-organizational visits.
3. Seeking out new approaches in order to make improvements that will have the greatest impact on outcomes; and monitoring indicators.

Chapter 15: Total Quality Management

Common Pitfalls in Benchmarking
- Lack of management commitment and involvement
- Not applied to critical areas first
- Inadequate resources
- No involvement of the line organization.
- Scope not well defined
- To many performance measures
- Critical success factors and performance drivers not understood or identified
- Potential partners ignored
- Poorly designed questionnaires
- Inappropriate data collection method
- Too much and inconsistent data
- Analysis paralysis; excess precision
- Management resistance to change
- No repeat benchmarking

ACTIVITY PLAN (GANTT CHART)

A Gantt chart is a type of bar chart that illustrates a project schedule, named after its inventor, Henry Gantt (1861-1919), who designed such a chart around the years 1910-1915. Modern Gantt charts also show the dependency relationships between activities and current schedule status **(Fig. 15.20)**.

Definition
1. According to Wikipedia, "A Gantt chart is a type of bar chart that illustrates a project schedule and shows the dependency relationships between activities and current schedule status."
2. A Gantt chart is a useful graphical tool which shows activities or tasks performed against time. It is also known as visual presentation of a project where the activities are broken down and displayed on a chart which makes it is easy to understand and interpret.

History of Gantt Charts
The first project management chart was invented by Karol Adamiecki in 1896.
Here's a quick history of Gantt charts:
- **1896:** Karol Adamiecki creates the first project management chart: the Harmonogram, a precursor to the modern Gantt chart.
- **1931:** Adamiecki publishes the Harmonogram (but in Polish with limited exposure).
- **1910-1915:** Henry Gantt publishes his own project management system, the Gantt chart.
- **Today:** Gantt charts are the preferred tool for managing projects of all sizes and types.

Key Parts of a Gantt Chart
A Gantt chart is made up of several different elements. So let's take a quick look at 8 key components so you know how to read a Gantt chart:
1. **Task list:** Runs vertically down the left of the Gantt chart to describe project work and may be organized into groups and subgroups.
2. **Timeline:** Runs horizontally across the top of the Gantt chart and shows months, weeks, days, and years.
3. **Dateline:** A vertical line that highlights the current date on the Gantt chart.
4. **Bars:** Horizontal markers on the right side of the Gantt chart that represent tasks and show progress, duration, and start and end dates.
5. **Milestones:** Yellow diamonds that call out major events, dates, decisions, and deliverables.
6. **Dependencies:** Light gray lines that connect tasks that need to happen in a certain order.
7. **Progress:** Shows how far along work is and may be indicated by % complete and/or bar shading.
8. **Resource assigned:** Indicates the person or team responsible for completing a task.

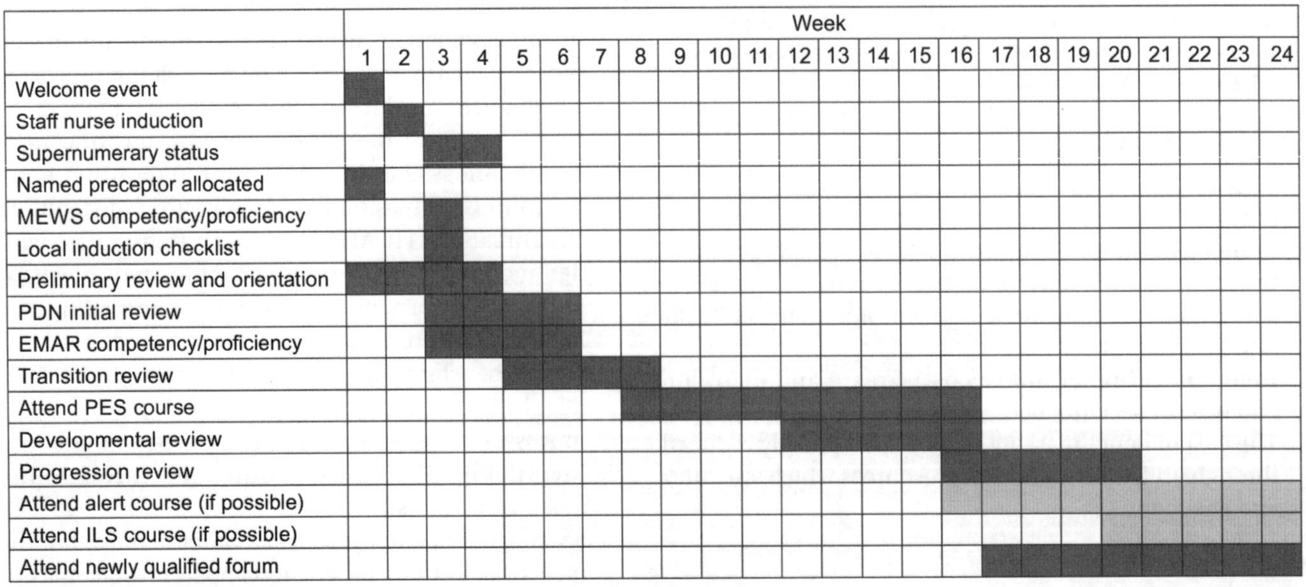

	Week																							
	1	2	3	4	5	6	7	8	9	10	11	12	13	14	15	16	17	18	19	20	21	22	23	24
Welcome event																								
Staff nurse induction																								
Supernumerary status																								
Named preceptor allocated																								
MEWS competency/proficiency																								
Local induction checklist																								
Preliminary review and orientation																								
PDN initial review																								
EMAR competency/proficiency																								
Transition review																								
Attend PES course																								
Developmental review																								
Progression review																								
Attend alert course (if possible)																								
Attend ILS course (if possible)																								
Attend newly qualified forum																								

Fig. 15.20: Gantt chart.

Purpose of a Gantt Chart
- To illustrate the relationship between project activities and time.
- To show the multiple project activities on one chart
- To provide a simple and easy to understand representation of project scheduling

Creating a Gantt Chart
There are two methods to creating a Gantt chart.
1. Using a forward schedule: starting with the list of activities and a given start date (6th Sept in previous example) follow them forwards in time until you hit given deadline.
2. Using a backward schedule: look at the deadline, from that date work in the logical list of activities. Both of these methods allow you to ensure that all necessary activities can possibly be completed within the given project time frame.

Steps to Creating a Gantt Chart
1. Determine project start date and deadline.
2. Gather all information surrounding the list of activities within a project—the work breakdown structure may be useful for this.
3. Determine how long each activity will take
4. Evaluate what activities are dependent on others
5. Create graph shell including the timeline and list of activities.
6. Using either forward scheduling or backward scheduling, begin to add bars ensuring to include dependencies and the full duration for each activity.

Progress Gantt Charts
- In a progress Gantt chart, tasks are shaded in proportion to the degree of their completion: a task that is 60% complete would be 60% shaded, starting from the left.
- A vertical line is drawn at the time index when the progress Gantt chart is created, and this line can then be compared with shaded tasks.
- If everything is on schedule, all task portions left of the line will be shaded, and all task portions right of the line will not be shaded.
- This provides a visual representation of how the project and its tasks are ahead or behind schedule.

Advantages
- A useful tool for displaying time-based information within a project.
- Very simple to create
- They provide a useful overview of project activities, a good starting point for project planning.
- The charts are widely used and understood.
- There exist several PC software packages that allow you to build Gantt charts.

Limitations
- The Gantt chart does not explain the reasoning behind the chosen duration of each activity.
- The Gantt chart is very difficult to update when changes to the project plan take place. This makes it time consuming and results in long-term planning being very difficult.
- Gantt charts encourage a one-step approach to planning- this prevents flexibility in project planning.
- Modern day Gantt charts, using PC software, can look very professional without actually having meaning, preventing project teams from challenging their content. This can lead to difficulties later in the project.
- As Gantt charts are difficult to update manually, they can often become obsolete.
- The charts do not consider project costs or resources.

CRITICAL PATH ANALYSIS

Critical path analysis (CPA) is a project management technique that requires mapping out every key task that is necessary to complete a project (**Fig. 15.21**). It includes identifying the amount of time necessary to finish each activity and the dependencies of each activity on any others.
- Critical path analysis is a project planning method that focuses on identifying tasks that are dependent on other tasks for their timely completion.
- Understanding the dependencies between tasks is key to setting a realistic deadline for a complex project.
- Critical path analysis is used in most industries that undertake highly complex projects.

Definition
- Critical path analysis ("CPA") CPA is a project analysis and planning method that allows a project to completed in the shortest possible time.
- Critical path is a sequence of activity between a project's start and finish that takes the longest time to complete.

History
The critical path method (CPM) is a project modeling technique developed in the late 1950s by DuPont, and was first used in missile—defense construction projects of US Navy. Critical path analysis is commonly used with all forms of projects, including construction, aerospace and defense, software development, research projects, product development, engineering, and plant maintenance, among others. Any project with interdependent activities can apply this method. The first time CPM was used for major skyscraper development was in 1966 while constructing the former World Trade Center Twin Towers in New York City.

Components
The essential technique for using CPM: is to construct a model of the project that includes the following:
- A list of all activities required to complete the project (typically categorized within a work breakdown structure),
- The time (duration) that each activity will take to complete,
- The dependencies between the activities and,
- Logical end points, such as milestones or deliverable items.

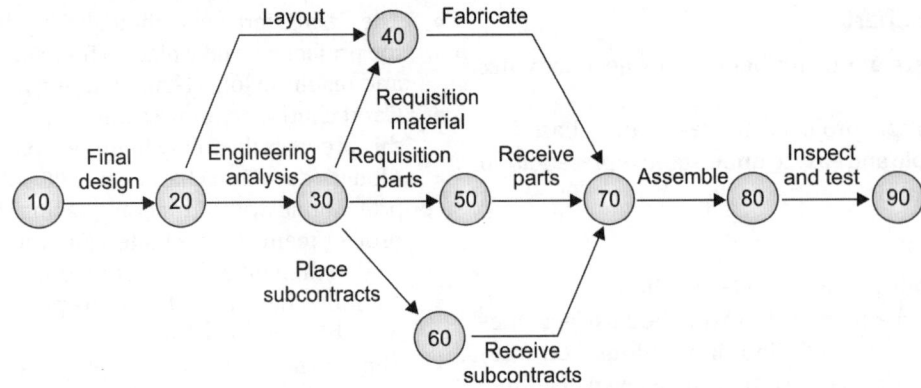

Fig. 15.21: Critical path analysis model.

Terminologies used in CPM

In order to explain the purpose, structure and operation of CPM, it is helpful to define the following terms: Activity—an activity carries the arrow symbol. This represents a task or subproject that uses time or resources

- **Event:** A node (an event), denoted by a circle, marks the start and completion of an activity, which contain a number that helps to identify its location.
- **Dummy activity:** An activity, which is used to maintain the pre-defined precedence relationship only during the construction of the project network, is called a dummy activity. Dummy activity is represented by a dotted arrow and does not consume any time and resource
- **Parallel activity:** There are two activities which being at same event and end at same event. These activities are called parallel activity.
- **Path:** A path is a series of adjacent activities leading from one event to another.
- **Critical path:** A critical path is the sequence of critical activities that forms a continuous path between the start of a project and its completion.
- **Forward pass:** The early start and early finish time calculated by moving forward through the network.
- **Backward pass:** The latest start and latest finish time calculated by moving backward through the network.
- **Float activity:** Float activity for an activity is the difference between its earliest and latest start time or earliest and latest finish time.

Critical Path Method Steps

Step 1: Make the WBS (work break-down structure) or identify the activities that form the project, and their respective durations.

Step 2: Establish an activity sequence, clearly identifying which activity precedes which ones, and what activities can be completed simultaneously.

Step 3: Develop the network diagram. Project network is basically making a WBS of the project, modeled to represent the precedence of activities, where the arcs represent the precedence and the nodes represent the activities.

Step 4: Identifying the critical path—for this step, we need to determine following four time factors for each activity:

1. Earliest Start Time (ES): The earliest an activity can start once all the predecessor activities are over.
2. Earliest Finish Time (EF) = ES + Activity Duration
3. Latest Finish Time (LF): the latest an activity can finish that ensure project completion on time.
4. Latest Start Time (LS) = LF – Activity Duration

   Based on these parameters, activity slack can be calculated, Slack = LS – ES = LF – EF

   If Activity Slack = 0, the activity is a critical activity; otherwise it is a non-critical activity.

   For calculating ES (early start) of an activity:

5. Take the maximum of the predecessor activities' EF (early finish) time, as an activity can start the earliest only when all the predecessor activities end.

   For calculating the LF (late finish) times:

6. The LF of an activity is the minimum of all the following activities' LS (late start) times, as an activity can latest finish only before the first following activity starts.

Step 5: Calculate the project duration, based on the duration of critical path, by adding the duration of the critical activities.

Step 6: Update the network diagram throughout the project implementation process based on the actual project progress to refine the activity and project predictions.

Critical Path Method

- It is an incredibly common and powerful tool used across the garment industry today.
- But it is only as powerful as the data entered into it
- if estimations are off, if resources are not calculated correctly, the entire project may fail.
- Take ample time to identify the critical activities of the project, in the project planning phase itself.

Benefits of CPM

- Useful at many stages of project management
- Mathematically simple
- Give critical path and float time
- Provide project documentation
- Useful in monitoring costs
- Visual representation

Limitations to CPM

- Specified precedence relationship
- Activity time estimates are subjective and depend on judgment
- Can be more difficult understand ten Gantt charts
- The time needed for tasks is not as clear as with Gantt charts

■ REVIEW QUESTIONS

Long Essays

1. Define total quality management; explain the objectives and principles.
2. Define quality assurance; explain purposes, objectives and principles.
3. Define PERT; explain the process and steps.
4. Define benchmarking; explain the purposes, steps, advantages and disadvantages.
5. Define Gantt chart; explain the parts and advantages.
6. Define Critical path analysis (CPA); explain the components, steps and benefits.

Short Essays

1. Phases of total quality management.
2. Elements of total quality management.
3. Components of total quality management.
4. Total quality management tools.
5. Factors affecting quality assurance in nursing care.
6. Approaches to quality assurance.
7. Quality assurance model.
8. Quality assurance cycle.
9. JCAHO quality assurance guideline/steps.
10. Approaches for quality assurance program.
11. Role of nurses in quality assurance.
12. Principles of safety management.
13. Safety management in nursing.

Short Answers

1. Policy management.
2. Team activity.
3. Functions of total quality management.
4. Brainstorming.
5. Nominal group technique.
6. C-charts.
7. Tally charts.
8. Areas of quality assurance.
9. Benefits of quality assurance.
10. Functional benchmarking.
11. Principles of benchmarking.
12. Limitations to CPM.

■ BIBLIOGRAPHY

1. Anthony MK, Theresa, Hertz, Judith. Factors Influencing Outcomes after Delegation to Unlicensed Assistive Personnel. JONA. 2000; 30(10):478-18.
2. Baker S, Campbell GM, Kim B. The Complete Idiot's Guide to Project Management. Alpha Books;2003.
3. Basavanthappa BT. Nursing Administration, 1st edition. New Delhi: Jaypee Brothers; 2000.
4. Cheryl LP, Seagull FJ, Xiao Y. Coordination challenges in operating-room management: an in-depth field study. Amia Annu Symp Proc; 2003.
5. Douglass LM. The effective nurse-leader and manager, 5th edition. Mosby: St. Louis; 1996.
6. Ellis JR, Hartley CL. Managing and Co-ordinating nursing care, 3rd edition. Lippincott: Philadelphia; 1995.
7. Johnson M, Closkey JC. The Delivery of Quality Health Care Series on Nursing Administration. London: Mosby; 1992.
8. Kerzner, Harold. Project Management: A Systems Approach to Planning, Scheduling, and Controlling. John Wiley and Sons; 2003.
9. Koch MW, Fairly TM. Integrated Quality Management: The Key To Improving Nursing Care Quality. Edition, St. Louis, Missouri: Mosby Publications; 1993.
10. Marquis BL, Hutson CJ. Leadership roles and management functions in nursing—Theory and application, 5th edition, Philadelphia: Lippincott Williams and Wilkins; 2006.
11. Morrison M. Professional skills for leadership. Mosby: US; 1993.
12. Punmia BC, Khandelwal K. Project Planning and Control PERT and CPM: For Degree Classes. Laxmi Publications; 2006.
13. Ward MJ, Price SA. Issues in nursing administration. St. Louis: Mosby; 1991.

CHAPTER 16

Organizational Behavior and Human Relations

LEARNING OBJECTIVES

- Concepts and Theories of Organizational Behavior
- Group Dynamics
- Review: Interpersonal Relationship
- Human Relations
- Public Relations in the Context of Nursing
- Relations with Professional Associations and Employee Unions
- Collective Bargaining
- Review: Motivation and Morale Building
- Communication in the Workplace—Assertive Communication
- Committees—Importance in the Organization, Functioning

INTRODUCTION

Organizational behavior (OB) is the study of factors that affect how individuals and groups act in organizations and how organizations manage their environments. The study of organizational behavior is very interesting and challenging too. It is related to individuals, group of people working together in teams. The study becomes more challenging when situational factors interact. The study of organizational behavior relates to the expected behavior of an individual in the organization (**Fig. 16.1**).

DEFINITION

- Organizational behavior is the field of study that investigates how organizational structures affect behavior within organizations.
- The study and application of knowledge about human behavior related to other elements of an organization, such as structure, technology and social systems.
  —*LM Prasad*
- Stephen P Robins defines "Organizational behavior as a systematic study of the actions and attitudes that people exhibit within organizations."
- OB is a systematic study of the actions and reactions of individuals, groups and subsystems.
- OB is the systematic study and careful application of knowledge about how people—as individuals and as members of groups—act within organizations. It strives to identify ways in which people can act more effectively.
- OB is a field of study that investigates the impact that individuals, groups and structures have on behavior within organizations for the purpose of applying such knowledge towards improving an organization's effectiveness.

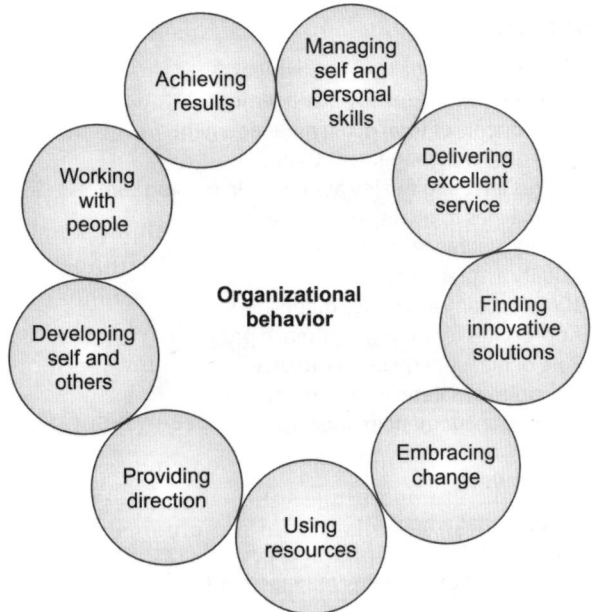

Fig. 16.1: Organizational behavior.

- OB is the study and understanding of individual and group behavior, patterns of structure in order to help improve organizational performance and effectiveness
- "Organizational behavior is directly concerned with the understanding, production and control of human behavior in organizations." —*Fred Luthans*
- "Organizational behavior is a subset of management activities concerned with understanding, predicting and influencing individual behavior in organizational setting."
  —*Callahan, Fleenor and Kudson*
- "Organizational behavior is a branch of the Social Sciences that seeks to build theories that can be applied" to predicting, understanding and controlling behavior in work organizations." —*Raman J Aldag*

Chapter 16: Organizational Behavior and Human Relations

OBJECTIVES OF ORGANIZATIONAL BEHAVIOR (FIG. 16.2)

- To analyze different perspective and potentialities to create and develop the ethical values in an organization,
- To analyze the potentialities towards the ways and means to conduct and organize the systems, methods and approaches for organization development in an organization,
- To analyze the potentialities to develop process, methods and approaches of formal and informal patterns of organization and society,
- To analyze how to make perspective methods and process of effective communication to formulate ethical norms in an organization,
- To analyze various aspects and factors affecting the group cohesiveness,
- To analyze the ways and means to develop different ethical aspects for group dynamism,
- To analyze the mutual interest of individual and group. Mutual interest is represented by the statement 'Organization needs people, and people also need organization',
- To analyze and evaluate the role of different key elements, such as people, structure, technology interactive behavior and environment, etc.
- To analyze and evaluate the behavioral approaches in organization. In context of that all of them are based on 'Art' and 'science'
- To analyze different aspects of work environment which duly affects the behavioral patterns and attitudes of persons?

MEANING OF ORGANIZATIONAL BEHAVIOR

Organizational behavior is "the study of human behavior in organizational settings, the interface between human behavior and the organization, and the organization itself." OB can be divided into three levels: the study of (a) individuals in organizations (micro-level), (b) work groups (meso-level), and (c) how organizations behave (macro-level).

- Organization behavior is a study of the way people interact within groups.
- Normally, this study is applied in an attempt to create **more** efficient business organizations.
- The central idea of the study of organizational behavior is that a scientific approach can be applied to the management of workers.

- Organizational behavior theories are used for human resource purposes to maximize the output from individual group members
- Organizational behavior studies organizations from multiple viewpoints and levels, including behavior within the organization and in relation to other organizations.
- Micro organizational behavior refers to individual and group dynamics in an organizational setting.
- Macro organizational theory studies whole organizations and industries, including how they adapt, and the strategies, structures, and contingencies that guide them.

NATURE OF ORGANIZATIONAL BEHAVIOR (FIG. 16.3)

Different leading authorities in the field of 'the organizational behavior' have defined the nature and scope of this subject in different terms. There is no unanimity of opinion in the matter. However, students of an introductory course in the subject need not be bogged down by this multiplicity of views. Following discussion is enough to understand the basic nature and scope of this discipline.

- **The organizational behavior personified** has a nature, just as any human being has a peculiar nature or the psychological tendency. It is a science, art and philosophy by nature. So, it follows that the subject of the organizational behavior is a science, art and philosophy, too.
- **It is a science:** Because it follows the scientific methods of the observation, the collection of the data, the hypothesis, the theory and the model building ever open to the scientific scrutiny in terms of the relationship among variables under the study and the validity of such a relationship.

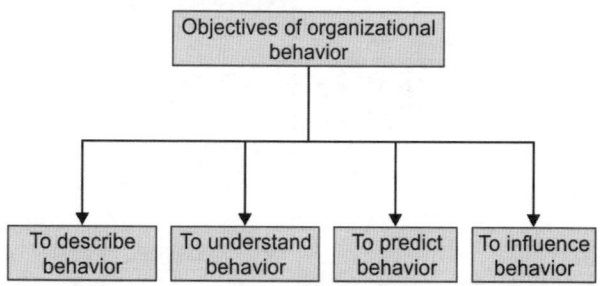

Fig. 16.2: Objectives of organizational behavior.

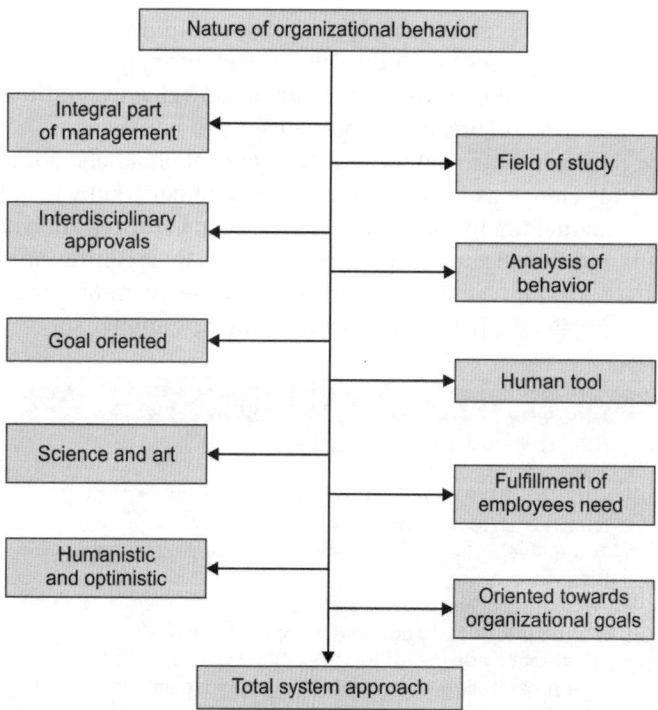

Fig. 16.3: Nature of organizational behavior.

3. **It is an art:** Since, it involves quite a subjective approach, too in terms of the skilful organization of the field studies, the collection of the data and the interpretation of the results by human beings who generally are more subjective than objective in their approach.
4. **It is a philosophy:** Too, in terms of ever trying to philosophize the questions of human beings and the organization's relationship in the behavioral terms. It tries to frame postulations as to what, why, how, and where a particular kind of human behavior takes place in an organization in a particular corner of the globe or the universe along with the other relevant aspects like its impact or effects?

CHARACTERISTICS OF ORGANIZATIONAL BEHAVIOR (BOX 16.1)

- **Behavioral approach to management:** Organizational behavior is that part of whole management which represents the behavioral approach to management. Organizational behavior has emerged as a distinct field of study because of the importance of human behavior in organizations.
- **Cause and effect relationship:** Human behavior is generally taken in terms of cause and effect relationship and not in philosophical terms. It helps in predicting the behavior of individuals. It provides generalizations that managers can use to anticipate the effect of certain activities on human behavior.
- **Organizational behavior is a branch of social sciences:** Organizational behavior is heavily influenced by several other social sciences viz. psychology, sociology and anthropology. It draws a rich array of research from these disciplines.
- **Three levels of analysis:** Organizational behavior encompasses the study of three levels of analysis namely individual behavior, inter-individual behavior and the behavior of organizations themselves.
- **A science as well as an art:** Organizational behavior is a science as well as an art. The systematic knowledge about human behavior is a science and the application of behavioral knowledge and skills is an art. Organizational behavior is not an exact science because it cannot exactly predict the behavior of people in organizations.
- **A body of theory, research and application:** Organizational behavior consists of a body of theory, research and application which helps in understanding the human behavior in organization. All these techniques help the managers to solve human problems in organizations.
- **Beneficial to both organization and individuals:** Organizational behavior creates an atmosphere whereby both organization and individuals are benefitted by each other. A reasonable climate is created so that employees may get much needed satisfaction and the organization may attain its objectives.
- **Rational thinking:** Organizational behavior provides a rational thinking about people and their behavior. The major objective of organizational behavior is to explain and predict human behavior in organizations, so that result yielding situations can be created.

ELEMENTS OF ORGANIZATIONAL BEHAVIOR (FIG. 16.4)

Organizational behavior is also based on certain key elements also called 'fundamental concepts or assumptions'. There are key elements in OB.

1. **People/employee:** The employee is one of the very important parts of an organization. There is no any alternative in an organization without employee/people. You know, there may be many parties in an organization. Some party may be formal and some may be informal.
2. **Structure:** This is the second steps of organizational behavior. Actually, structure means the formal relationship with on the job employee of an organization. There is created different types of position for doing work nicely in the organization.
3. **Technology:** Technology is a very important primary aspect of organizational structure in the modern age. Technology supplies essential resource and equipment to the employee for doing their work efficiently.
4. **Social system:** Everything around us is society and everyone in the social lives together. The social system determines the organizational work environment and from which the organization can operate. As people cannot live alone just like organization cannot run alone its job. The organization has to do its activity with the help of the employee.

> **Box 16.1:** Characteristics of organization behavior.
> - Action and goal oriented discipline.
> - Science as well as art.
> - Multidisciplinary Integrated approach.
> - It is a human tool for human benefits.
> - Three levels of analysis—Individual, group and organization behavior.
> - Wholistic concept of whole system.
> - Mutual interest of people and organization. Individuals view organization as a means to achieve their goals while at the same time organization wish that individuals must work towards the achievement of organizational goal.

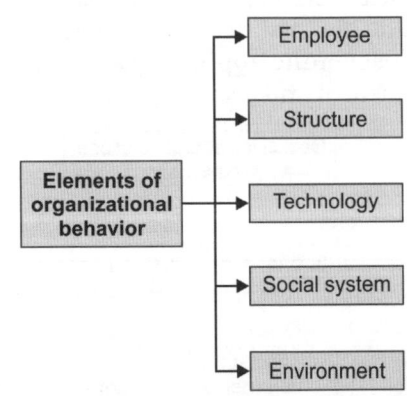

Fig. 16.4: Elements of organizational behavior.

5. **Environment:** There is no any organization where they can survive alone. Every organization has to work on the internal and external environment. Management has to come near to all the staff to maintain a good working environment.

LEVELS OF ORGANIZATIONAL BEHAVIOR

There are three levels of organizational behavior:
1. **Individual level:** Organization behavior views the organization as an individual's behavior. It studies the individual behavior of people how they react to organizational plans, policies, etc. Psychological theories, such as learning, motivation, and leadership are also considered to the study of the behavior of an individual.
2. **Group level:** The organization consists of a group, teams that work together in full cooperation and coordination of each other. OB at the group level focuses on group interaction among members. It is highly concerned with social psychology theories working in a group as it studies.
3. **Organizational level:** Organizational behavior has tried to analyze how organizational structure designs technology influences organizational effectiveness. It tries to focus on the relationship between the organization and the environmental factors that directly or indirectly affect the organization.

There are many levels and class of organizational behaviors. From organization hierarchical stand point, there are three levels of behaviors **(Fig. 16.5)**:
1. **Top level behaviors:** These are the behaviors of the top management executives. They are the leaders and managers. They do the strategic planning, most often concern on the long term focus. They get the biggest pie.
2. **Middle level behavior:** These are the controllers and supervisors. They are the instruction takers, task conveyors and executive doers. They concern on current management issues and middle term vision and focus. They are the second company graders.
3. **Bottom level behaviors:** They are the down liners, the soldiers, the operators and the followers. They are the bottom line doers who get the less pay.

PRINCIPLES OF ORGANIZATIONAL BEHAVIOR

The principles of OB are as follows:
- The productivity of employees can be managed for improved performance.
- Specific techniques are most helpful in producing improved performance, given the organization, industry, and global location.
- Performance can be accurately assessed, even those behaviors not readily observable
- Employees improve performance when (a) they know exactly what is needed (b) have all the resources needed to succeed (c) receive periodic feedback to know if still on course (d) are exposed to new challenges and opportunities to grow (e) seek ways to increase quality and productivity (f) partner with management to find solutions
- Variables change both the behaviors to observe and means of changing. Some outcomes are easy to monitor, such as clinical outcomes. But more often in the 21st century, humans are engaged in knowledge work, the things machines cannot accomplish.
- We continue to learn from experience what works and what does not, until something changes and the outcomes are less predictable.

FACTORS INFLUENCE ORGANIZATIONAL BEHAVIOR

The most important factors that influence organizational behavior **(Fig. 16.6)**:
- Culture, however, it is defined in the organization
- Leadership and how it is implemented in every level
- **Personal accountability and integrity:** The way by which individuals show up everyday into the context of the organization.
- **Communication:** How people communicate information and knowledge with each other and between divisions.
- **Alignment:** How align everyone in the organization with the true goals and objectives of the organization.

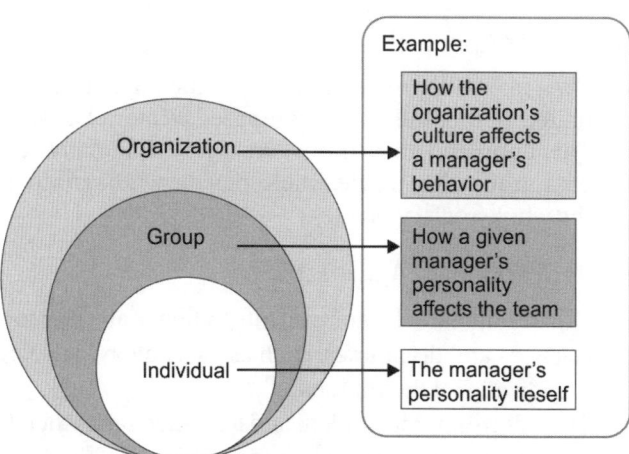

Fig. 16.5: Three levels of analysis.

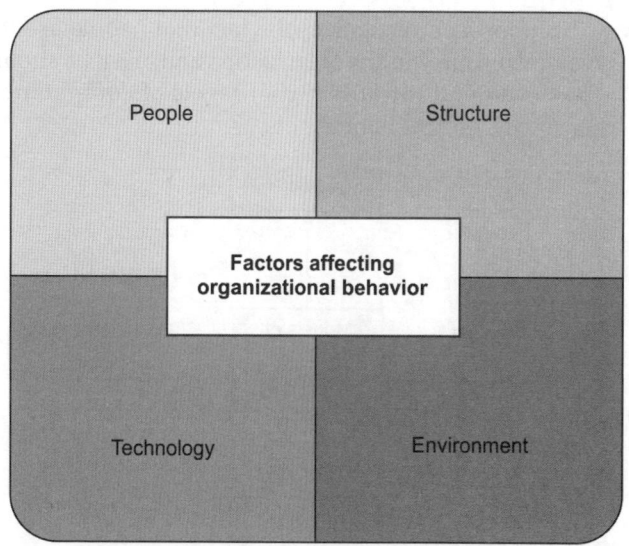

Fig. 16.6: Factors affecting organizational behavior.

- Mission, vision, strategic objectives and how clear they are to everyone
- Relationships between the people of the organization, with other organizations and the market
- Organizational values and how they align with individual values
- Brand identity, external and internal
- Rules, laws, beliefs, theories, processes and procedures

ORGANIZATIONAL BEHAVIOR MODEL (FIG. 16.7)

There are four major models or frameworks that organizations operate out of, Autocratic, Custodial, Supportive, and Collegial (Cunningham, Eberle, 1990; Davis, 1967):

- **Autocratic:** The basis of this model is power with a managerial orientation of authority. The employees in turn are oriented towards obedience and dependence on the boss. The employee need that is met is subsistence. The performance result is minimal.
- **Custodial:** The basis of this model is economic resources with a managerial orientation of money. The employees in turn are oriented towards security and benefits and dependence on the organization. The employee need that is met is security. The performance result is passive cooperation.
- **Supportive:** The basis of this model is leadership with a managerial orientation of support. The employees in turn are oriented towards job performance and participation. The employee need that is met is status and recognition. The performance result is awakened drives.
- **Collegial:** The basis of this model is partnership with a managerial orientation of teamwork. The employees in turn are oriented towards responsible behavior and self-discipline. The employee need that is met is self-actualization. The performance result is moderate enthusiasm.

APPROACHES TO ORGANIZATIONAL BEHAVIOR (FIG.16.8)

I. Human Resources Approach

- This approach recognizes the fact that people are the central resource in any organization and that they should be developed towards higher levels of competency, creativity, and fulfillment.

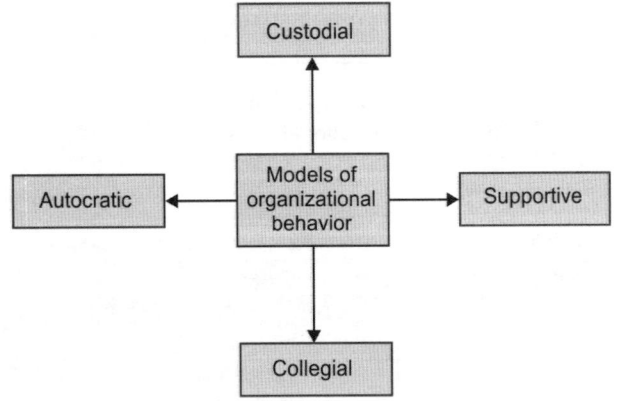

Fig. 16.7: Organizational behavior models.

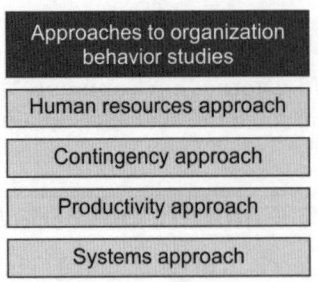

Fig. 16.8: Approaches to organization behavior studies.

- People thus contribute to the success of the organization.
- The human resources approach is also called as the supportive approach in the sense that the manager's role changes from control of employee to active support of their growth and performance.

II. Contingency Approach

- The contingency approach (sometimes called the situational approach) is based on the premise that methods or behaviors which work effectively in one situation fail in another.
- For example; organization development (OD) programs, way work brilliantly in one situation but fail miserably in another situation.
- The contingency approach is also more interdisciplinary, more system-oriented and more research-oriented titan any other approach.

III. Productivity Approach

- Productivity which is the ratio of output to input is a measure of an organization's effectiveness. It also reveals the manager's efficiency in optimizing resource utilization.
- The higher the numerical value of this ratio, the greater the efficiency.
- Productivity is generally measured in terms of economic inputs and outputs, but human and social inputs and outputs also are important.
- For example, if better organizational behavior can improve job satisfaction, a human output or benefit occurs.

IV. Systems Approach

- The systems approach to OB views the organization as a united, purposeful system composed of interrelated parts.
- This approach gives managers a way of looking at the organization as a whole, whole, person, whole group, and the whole social system.

V. Interdisciplinary Approach

- Organizational behavior is an integration of all other social sciences and disciplines, such as psychology, sociology, organizational theories, etc.
- They all are interdependent and influence each other. The man is studied as a whole and therefore, all disciplines concerning man are integrated.

SCOPE OF THE ORGANIZATIONAL BEHAVIOR

The scope of the organizational behavior is as under:
- Impact of personality on performance
- Employee motivation
- Leadership
- How to create effective teams and groups
- Study of different organizational structures
- Individual behavior, attitude and learning
- Perception
- Design and development of effective organization
- Job design
- Impact of culture on organizational behavior
- Management of change
- Management of conflict and stress
- Organizational development
- Organizational culture
- Transactional analysis
- Group behavior, power and politics
- Job design
- Study of emotions

IMPORTANCE OF ORGANIZATIONAL BEHAVIOR (BOX 16.2)

- **Skill improvement:**
  - Study of organizational behavior helps to improve skills.
  - This includes the ability of employees and use of knowledge to become more efficient.
  - It also improves managers, as well as other employees, work skill.
- **Understanding consumer buying behavior:** It also an important part to improve the marketing process by understanding consumer (buying) behavior.
- **Employee motivation:** OB helps to understand the basis of motivation and different ways to motivate employees properly.
- **Nature of employees:**
  - Understanding of personnel and employee nature is important to manage them properly.
  - With the help of OB, we can understand whether employees or people are introvert, extrovert, motivated, dominating, etc.
- **Anticipating organizational events:**
  - The scientific study of behavior helps to understand and predict organizational events.

Box 16.2: Importance of organizational behavior.
- OB provides a road map to our lives in organizations.
- OB uses scientific research to understand and make organization life, as it helps to predict what people will do under various conditions.
- It helps to influence organizational events—to understand and predict events.
- It helps individual understand herself/himself in better fashion.
- It helps manager to manage human resources effectively. For example, motivation.
- It helps organizations for maintaining cordial industrial relations.
- It is also useful in the field marketing.

- For example, annual business planning, demand management, product line management, production planning, resources scheduling, logistics, etc.
- **Efficiency and effectiveness:** Study of organizational behavior helps to increase efficiency and effectiveness of the organization.
- **Better environment of organization:** OB helps to create a healthy, ethical and smooth environment in an organization.
- **Optimum or better utilization of resources:**
  - Study of OB helps to understand employees and their work style and skill better way.
  - By understanding this, management can train and motivate employees for optimum utilization of resources.
- **Importance of OB in the goodwill of organization:** Organizational behavior helps to improve goodwill of organization.

LIMITATIONS OF ORGANIZATIONAL BEHAVIOR

- **Behavioral bias:** It further causes dependence, discontentment, indiscipline, and irresponsibility.
- **Law of diminishing returns:** It says that beyond a certain point, there is a decline in output even after each additional good or positive factor.
- **Unethical practices and manipulation of people:** Knowledge of motivation and communication acquired can be used to exploit subordinates in an organization by the manipulative managers.

GROUP DYNAMICS

The word dynamics means 'force'. Group dynamics means the study of forces within a group. Since human beings have an innate desire for belonging to a group, group dynamism is bound to occur. In an organization or in a society, we can see groups, small or large, working for the well-being. Group dynamics (GD) is concerned with the interactions and forces

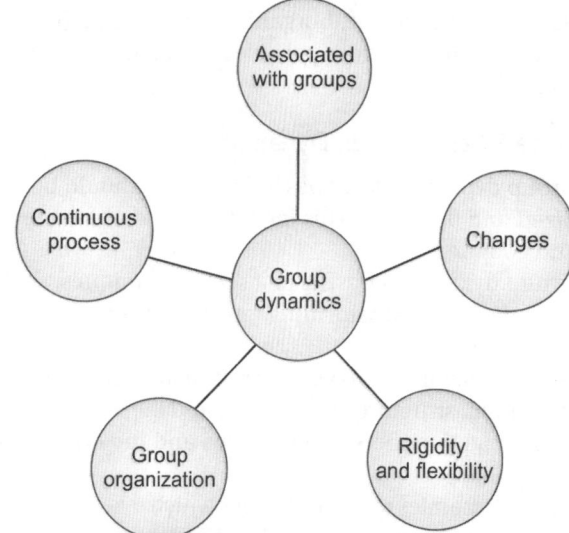

Fig. 16.9: Group dynamics.

between group members in a social situation. When the concept is applied to the study of organizational behavior, the focus is on the dynamics of members of formal or informal groups in the organization, i.e., it is concerned with the gaining knowledge of groups, how they develop, and their effect on individual members and the organizations in which they function. Human being exhibits some characteristic behavior patterns in groups (**Fig. 16.9**).

Definition

- Group as a unit of analysis in group dynamics is of utmost importance. It is a social unit which has been variously defined.
- A group is two or more people who share a common definition and evaluation of themselves and behave in accordance with such a definition.
- A group is a collection of people who interact with one another; accept rights and obligation as members and who share a common identity.
- Cattell defines it as a collection of organizations in which the existence of all is necessary to the satisfaction of certain individual needs in each.
- According to Humans, a group is a number of persons who communicate with one another, often over a span of time, and who are few enough so—that each person is able to communicate with all the others, not at second hand, through other people, but face to face.
- Two or more people who interact personally, or through communication networks, with each other and who come together to achieve particular goals in view.

Objectives

- Identify and analyze the social processes that impact on group development and performance.
- Acquire the skills necessary to intervene and improve individual and group performance in an organizational context.
- Build more successful organization by applying techniques by that provides positive impact on goal achievement.

Characteristics of Group Dynamics

- Group dynamics describes how a group should be organized and operated. This includes pattern of leadership and cooperation.
- Group dynamics consists of a set of techniques, such as role playing, brainstorming, group therapy, sensitivity training, etc.
- Group dynamics deals with internal nature of groups, their formation, structure and process, and the way they affect individual members, other groups and the organization as a whole.
- Group dynamics refers to changes which take place within groups and is concerned with the interaction and forces obtained between group members in a social setting.

Features of Group

- The term group refers to two or more individuals who bear an explicit psychological relationship to one another.
- The group consists of two or more individuals and possesses some cohesiveness. It reveals some amount of interaction among its members who have definite ideas of their position and role in it.
- Relationships concentrating on status and roll along with common values or norms are characteristics features of the group.
- As the group operates on a common task, common attitudes develop and members become aware that they are part of it.

Classifications of Group (Box 16.3)

Groups may be classified in different ways, based on purpose or goal, extent of structuring, legal organization or setting, etc., they are,

I. Formal Groups (or Requires System)

Formal groups are deliberately created with structural associations and are formed to accomplish specific goals and carryout specific tasks which are clearly related to the total organizational mission.

- **Command group:** It is composed of subordinates who report directly to a given boss.
- **Task group:** It represents a group working together to complete a project or a job. Task group's boundaries are not defined by its immediate hierarchical superior.
- **Permanent formal groups:** These bodies, such as top management team, work units in various departments of the organization. Staff groups providing specialized services to the work organization, permanent committee, etc.
- **Temporary or momentary groups:** These are task forces or committees, constituted for temporary period.

II. Informal Groups

The informal groups consist of group of people, in an organization, who relate to each other spontaneously for purposes of mutual benefit and achievements. There are numerous informal groups in an organization.

- **Interest group:** Comes into being for the purpose of achieving some common objectives.
- **Friendship groups:** Are social allegiances which frequently extend outside a work situation.

Box 16.3: Classification of groups.

- Primary and secondary groups
- Formal and informal groups
- Membership and reference groups
- Small and large groups
- Organized and unorganized groups
- In and out-going groups
- Accidental and purposive groups
- Open and closed groups
- Temporary and permanent groups
- Nominal and non-performing groups

- **Membership group:** A membership group is one to which one may consciously belong but with which one has no more than a minimal relationship.
- **Reference group:** These groups to which one may belong and allow oneself to be influenced its member's behavior.

According to their purposes, groups may be classified into the following:
1. Vocational groups
2. Instructional groups
3. Governmental groups
4. Religious groups
5. Fraternal groups
6. Recreational groups
7. Social groups

Based on intimacy, there are two types of groups:
1. **Primary group:** It is characterized by intimate face-to-face association and coordination.
2. **Non-primary or secondary groups:** These are those where the interrelationships are more general and remote. The membership to such group is generally voluntary and easily withdraw able.

Dalton has identified three different kinds of informal which are found in organization: 1. Horizontal cliques, 2. Vertical cliques, 3. Mixed or random cliques.

Principles of Group Dynamics (Fig. 16.10)

The group dynamics is all about how a group behaves and acts in a specific situation. Let us now enlist some of the crucial requirements for standardizing the actions of a group:
- Each of the group members should regard and value the thoughts, status or prestige of the other members.
- The members of a group should develop a feeling of unanimity and maintain coordination within the team.
- A group encounters the entry and exit of members and also reformations and dissolution to meet the purpose of the organization.
- The group members need to stick to the norms or rules formed by them collectively.
- Together as a group, the members have the power to achieve the goals more efficiently.
- Everyone in a group aims at a collective objective of task accomplishment, i.e., the group goal.
- The group norms, composition, authority and objectives are altered and redefined to implement the change.
- The group members should ensure that the activities are performed uninterruptedly.
- The actions and duties of the members are directed towards the group goal or objective.

Stages of Group Development

Bruce Tuckman (1965) developed a model of group development **(Fig. 16.11)**. He labeled the stages, Dr Suess-style:
1. **Forming:** The group comes together and gets to initially know one other and form as a group.
2. **Storming:** A chaotic vying for leadership and trialing of group processes
3. **Norming:** Eventually agreement is reached on how the group operates (norming)
4. **Performing:** The group practices its craft and becomes effective in meeting its objectives. Tuckman added a 5th stage 10 years later:
5. **Adjourning:** The process of "unforming" the group, that is, letting go of the group structure and moving on.

Factors Affecting Group Dynamics (Fig. 6.12)

According to Malcolm and Hudla Knowles, the following four eminent aspects influence the group dynamics significantly:
1. **Psychological forces:** The psychology or desires of the individuals revolve around their need for status, security, recognition, experience and belongingness. All this affects their adaptability to the group.
2. **Past experience:** An individual's behavior in a group depends upon his/her learning from the past events of life comprising of the habits, values, attitude, perception, etc.
3. **Goals and ideology:** Another essential component is the individual's goals and beliefs which may/may not align with that of the whole group, leading to disagreement and unwillingness to perform.
4. **Associational forces:** The associational factors, i.e., the impact of family, geographical habitation, peers group, traditions, customs and religion on the individual; direct his/her actions in a group.

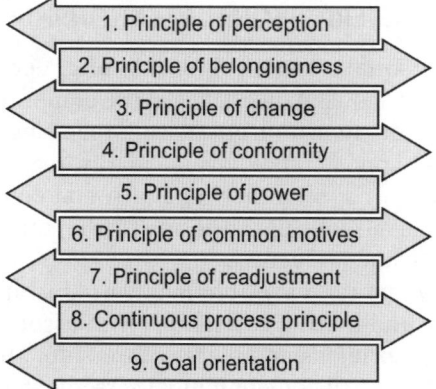

Fig. 16.10: Principles of group dynamics.

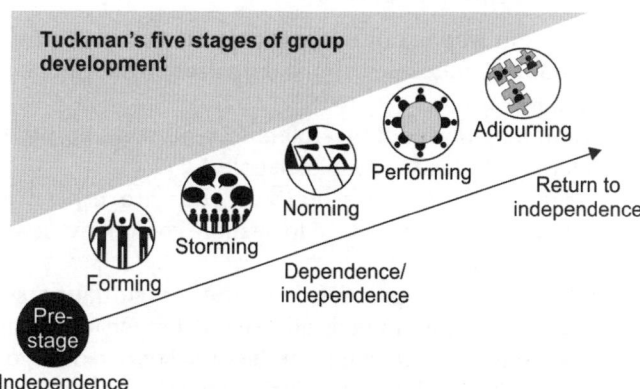

Fig. 16.11: Tuckman's five stages of group development.

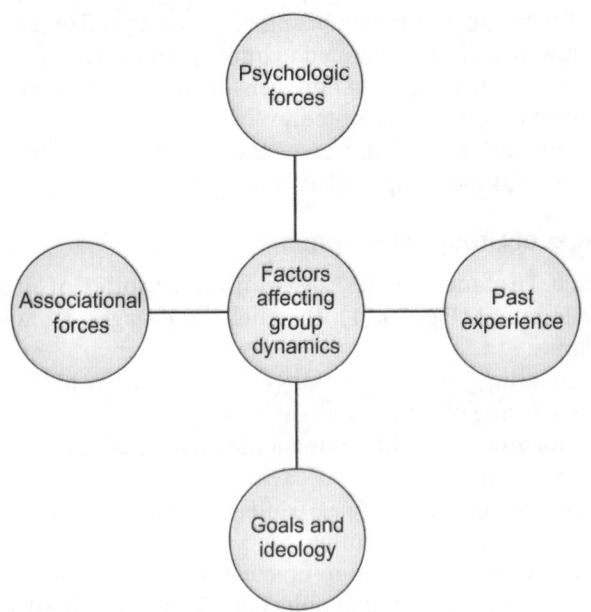

Fig. 16.12: Factors affecting group dynamics.

Importance of Group Dynamism

- The group can influence the thinking of its members. The members are always influenced by the interactions of other members in the group.
- A group with a good leader performs better as compared to a group with weak leader.
- The group can give the effect of synergy, that is, if the group consists of positive thinkers then its output is more than the double every time.
- Group dynamism can give job satisfaction to the members.
- The group can also bring team spirit among the members.
- Even the attitude, perceptions, and ideas of members depend on group dynamism. For example, the negative thinkers can be converted to positive thinkers with the help of the facilitator.
- If the group works as a cohesive group, the cooperation and convergence can result in maximization of productivity.
- Lastly, group dynamism can reduce the labor unrest and labor turnover due to emotional attachment among the group members.

Role of the Group Leader

- A person who is not in a position of authority, who is outranked and is new to the organization, can still be a leader.
- Managing or Leading—refers to a person's ability to successfully lead a group of people.
- Organizations have realized that more leading characteristics are needed to be more competitive in the work world.
- Success of an organization or the individual person (nurse) can be examined and fostered through mentoring other nurses in reaching a professional or personal goal (i.e., furthering their education or obtaining certifications in specialized procedures or areas of nursing), in attaining a leadership role (i.e., charge nurse or supervisor) or being rewarded in performance (recognition or raises)
- The nurse leader provides an atmosphere that allows open communication members.
- Group size, gender composition, race, ethnicity and age among group.
- Cohesion—refers to the degree of attraction and motivation to stay in the group.
- Commitment—refers to a person's feelings and how they identify and are attached to the group's goals or activities.

Role of Nurse Manager in Group Dynamics

- Knowledge of group dynamics is needed by nurse managers to improve leadership competencies and facilitates group discussions and communication.
- Groups are a common feature of a majority of experiences of all nurses in such roles is outcome management, team coordination and teaching of students, patients and families.
- The nurse leader provides an atmosphere that allows open communication members.
- Group size, gender composition, race, ethnicity and age among group.
  - Cohesion—refers to the degree of attraction and motivation to stay in the group.
- Commitment—refers to a person's feelings and how they identify and are attached to the group's goals or activities.

The nurse manager usually has following role in group dynamics:

- Supervise and manage the overall performance of staff in department.
- Analyzing, reporting, giving recommendations and developing strategies on how to improve quality and quantity of nursing care.
- Achieve business and organization goals, visions and objectives.
- Involved in employee selection, career development, succession planning and periodic training.
- Working out compensations and rewards.
- Responsible for the growth and increase in the organizations' finance and earning.
- Identifying problems, creating choice and providing alternative courses of actions.

REVIEW: INTERPERSONAL RELATIONSHIP

An interpersonal relationship is a strong, deep, or close association or acquaintance between two or more people that may range in duration from brief to enduring. This association may be based on inference, love, solidarity, regular business interactions, or some other type of social commitment. Interpersonal relationships are formed in the context of social, cultural and other influences.

The context can vary from family or kinship relations, friendship, and marriage, relations with associates, work, clubs, neighborhoods and places of worship. They may be regulated by law, custom, or mutual agreement, and are the basis of social groups and society as a whole.

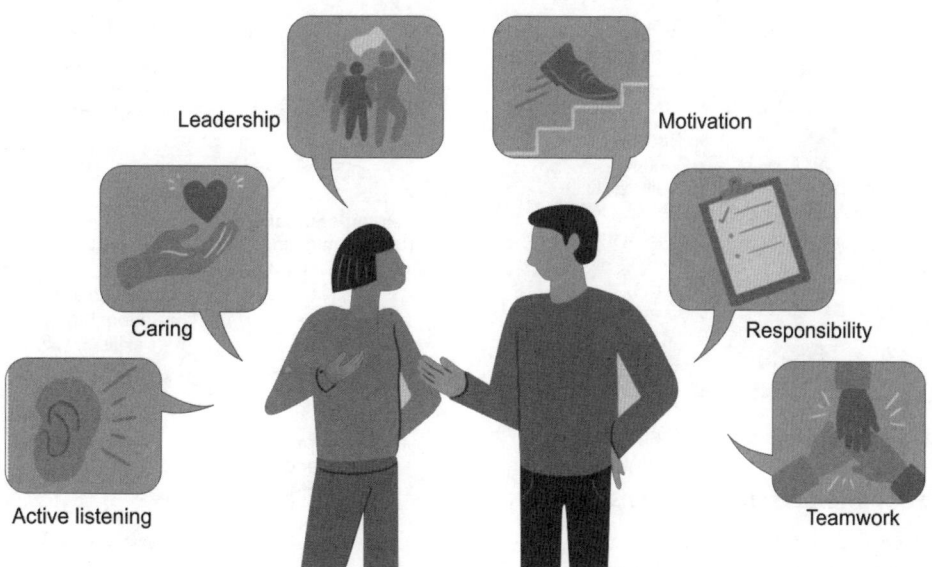

Fig. 16.13: Need for interpersonal relationship.

Definition

- "A healthy interpersonal relationships is one in which the individuals involved, experiences intimacy with each other while maintaining separate identities". According to Sullivan,
- 'Intimacy' is characterized by sensitivity to needs of the other person and mutual validation of personal worth.

Nature of Interpersonal Relationship

An interpersonal relationship is the nature of interaction that occurs between two or more people. People in an interpersonal relationship may interact overtly, covertly, face-to-face or even anonymously. Interpersonal relationships occur between people who fill each other's explicit or implicit physical or emotional needs in some way.

- Interpersonal relationships refer to reciprocal social and emotional interactions between two or more individuals in an environment.
- It is a close association between individuals who share common interests and goals.
- It is the learning experience whereby two people interact to face an immediate health problem, to share, if possible, in resolving it and to discover ways to adapt to the situation.

Figure 16.13 shows need for interpersonal relationship.

Factors affecting Interpersonal Relationship (Fig. 16.14)

- **Compatibility:** Two individuals in a relationship must be compatible with each other. Individuals from similar backgrounds and similar goals in life do extremely well in relationships. People with different aims, attitudes, thought processes find it difficult to adjust and hence fail to carry the relationship to the next level.
- **Communication:** Communication plays a pivotal role in all types of relationships whether it is personal or professional. Feelings must be expressed and reciprocated in relationships. Individuals need to communicate with each other effectively for better understanding.

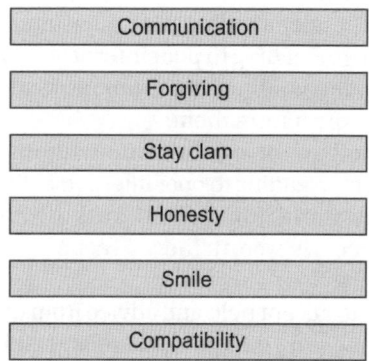

Fig. 16.14: Factors affecting interpersonal relationship.

- **Honesty:** Be honest in relationships. Do not lie or hide things from your partner. Remember every problem has a solution. Think before you speak. Transparency is important in relationships.
- **Stay calm:** Do not overreact on petty things in relationships. Stay calm. Be a little more adjusting. Be the first one to say "Sorry". It will solve half of your problems.
- **Forgiving:** An individual needs to be a little more forgiving in relationships. Do not drag issues unnecessarily. Fighting over small issues is foolish and makes the situation all the more worse.
- **Smile:** As they say "Smile is a curve that makes everything straight." Flash your smile more often. It works. Take care of your facial expressions while interacting with the other person.
- **Time:** Time plays an important role in relationships. Individuals in love must spend adequate time to know each other better. Frustrations arise when people do not have time to meet or interact with each other. Even in organization, individuals must spend quality time with their co-workers to strengthen the bond amongst themselves.

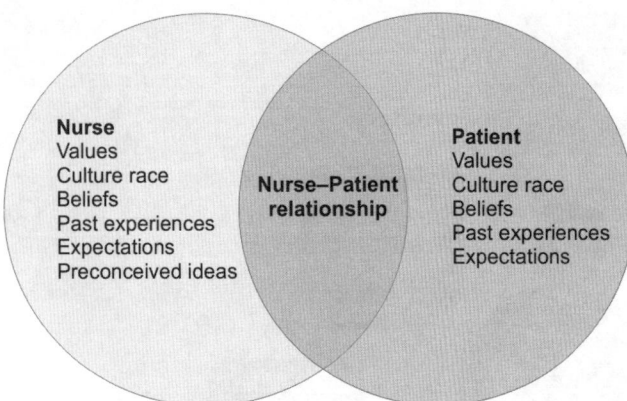

Fig. 16.15: Peplau's theory of interpersonal relationships.

Factors Leading to Poor Interpersonal Relationships

The following factors can lead to poor IPR:
- Lack of interest in work in some personnel may burden the other person which may spoil the friendly environment of the department.
- Lack of self-understanding and understanding of others is another factor leading to poor interpersonal relationship.
- Lack of understanding "how" you respond to others and what you expect from them.
- Deliberately ignoring someone without any cause is another factor leading to poor interpersonal relationships.
- Embarrassment for oneself and others from non-acceptance also contributes to poor interpersonal relationship.
- Unwilling to accept help and advice from others may also lead to unhealthy interpersonal relationships.
- There may be personality clash among people working in a unit. The clashes are usually caused by difference in styles of working.
- Conflicting ideas might arise from different backgrounds and lead to poor interpersonal relationships.

Figure 16.15 shows Peplau's theory of interpersonal relationships.

Theories of Interpersonal Communication

I. Social Exchange Theory

Social Exchange Theory was proposed by George Casper Homans in the year 1958.
- According to Social Exchange Theory "give and take" forms the basis of almost all relationships though their proportions might vary as per the intensity of the relationship.
- In a relationship, every individual has expectations from his/her partner. A relationship without expectations is meaningless.
- According to Social Exchange Theory feelings and emotions ought to be reciprocated for a successful and long lasting relationship.

II. Uncertainty Reductions Theory

Both Charles R Berger and Richard J Calabrese proposed Uncertainty Reductions Theory to explain the relationship

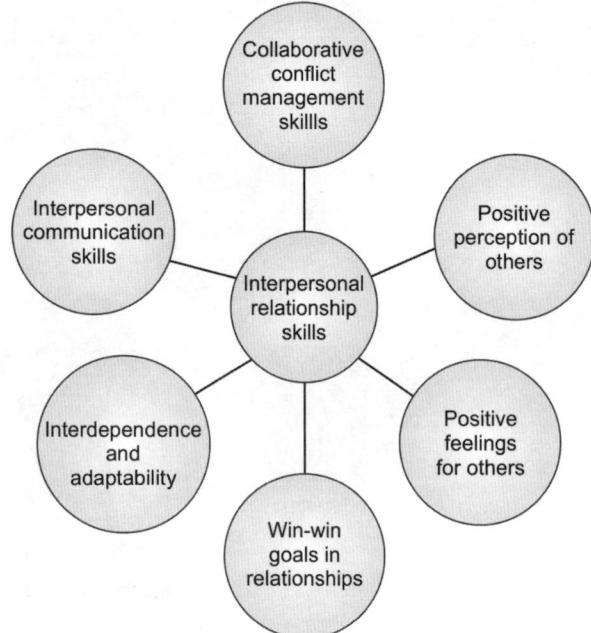

Fig. 16.16: Interpersonal relationship skills.

between individuals who do not know each other much and are complete strangers.
- According to Uncertainty Reductions Theory, two unknown individuals meeting for the first time go through various stages to reduce the level of uncertainty between them and come closer to each other.
- Strangers must communicate well to know each other better and find out their compatibility level.

Following are the stages individuals go through to reduce the level of uncertainty in relationships.

a. **Entry stage:**
   i. The entry stage is characterized by two individuals trying to know each other better. Each one tries to find out the other person's background, family members, educational qualification, interests, and hobbies and so on.
   ii. Each one discloses his/her likes and dislikes to strengthen the bond and take the relationship to the next level.

b. **Personal stage:**
   i. In the second stage or the personal stage, individuals try to find out more about their partner's attitude and beliefs.
   ii. Individuals try to know more about the other person's ethics, values, behavior and nature on the whole.
   iii. Individuals who are no longer strangers learn more about each other's personality traits in the personal stage.

c. **The exit stage:** The personal stage decides the fate of the relationship. Individuals comfortable in each other's company decide to enter into long term commitments i.e., either formally get married or stay together forever.

Stages in Interpersonal Relationships (Fig. 16.17)

It takes time for a relationship to grow and pass the test of time. There are two possibilities in a relationship:

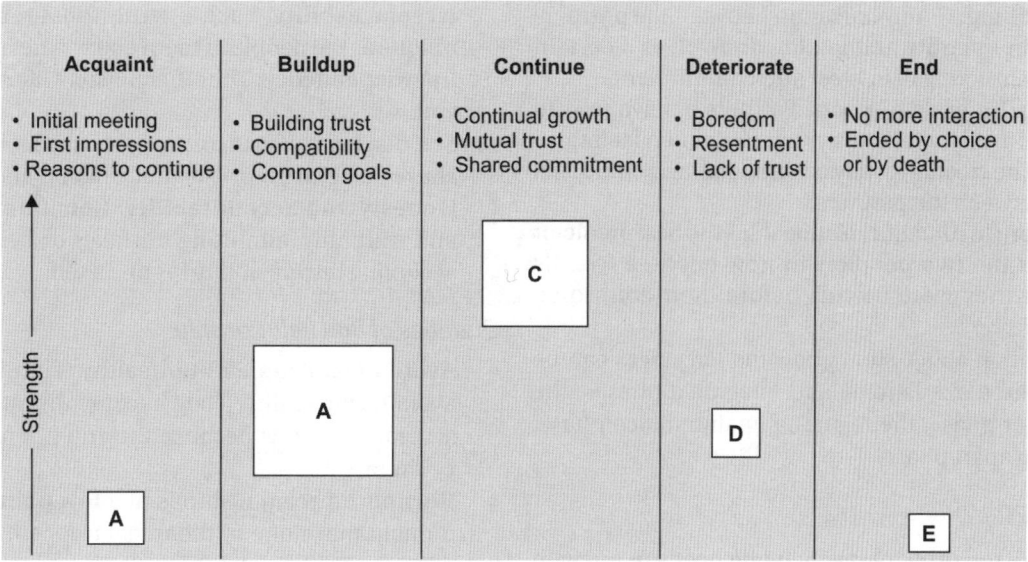

Fig. 16.17: Stages of relationships.

- **Possibility-1:** Two people might start a relationship as mere strangers. They get to know each other slowly and become emotionally and mentally attached to their partners gradually. Such relationships often lead to lasting commitments where individuals decide to be with each other until death separates them.
- **Possibility-2:** Two people might start off well but soon face problems. Troubles in relationship start when people have different opinions, views and fail to reach to a mutually acceptable solution. In such cases individuals decide to move on from a relationship for a fresh start.

According to famous psychologist George Levinger, every relationship goes through following five stages.
- **First stage-acquaintance:** Acquaintance refers to knowing each other. To start relationship individuals need to know each other well. Two individuals might meet at some place and instantly hit it off. People feel attracted to each other and decide to enter into a relationship.
- **Second stage-the buildup stage:** This is the stage when the relationship actually grows. Individuals are no longer strangers and start trusting each other.

    Individuals must be compatible with each other for the relationship to continue for a longer period of time. Individuals with similar interests and backgrounds tend to gel with each other more as compared to individuals from diverse backgrounds and different objectives.
- **Third stage-continuation stage:** This is the stage when relationship blossoms into lasting commitments. It is when people after knowing each other well decide to be in each other's company and tie the knot. Trust and transparency is essential for the charm to stay in relationship forever.
- **Fourth stage-deterioration:** Not all relationships pass through this stage. Lack of compatibility, trust, love and care often lead to misunderstandings and serious troubles in relationship.

Individuals sometimes find it extremely difficult to adjust with each other and eventually decide to bring their relationship to an end.
- **Fifth stage—the termination stage:** The fifth and the last stage is the end of a relationship. Relationship terminates due to any of the following reasons:
    – Death of any one partner
    – Divorce
    – Separation

An ideal relationship results in lasting commitments and marriages whereas there are some relationships which do start on a positive note but end abruptly.

Stages of Relationship Formation

Knapp's model of relational stages
1. **Initiating:** Expressing interest in making contact and showing that you are the kind of person worth getting to know.
2. **Experimenting:** The process of getting to know others and gaining more information about them.
3. **Intensifying:** An interpersonal relationship is now beginning to emerge. Feelings about the other person are now openly expressed, forms of address become more familiar, commitment is now openly expressed, and the parties begin to see themselves as "we" instead of separate individuals.
4. **Integrating:** Identification as a social unit. Social circles merge. Partners develop unique, ritualistic ways of behaving. Obligation to the other person increases. Some personal characteristics are replaced and we become different people.
5. **Bonding:** The two people make symbolic public gestures to show society that their relationship exists (rings, friendship bracelets, gifts, commitment).
6. **Differentiating:** The need to re-establish separate identities begins to emerge. The key to successful differentiation is maintaining a commitment to the relationship while creating the space for autonomy and individuality.

7. **Circumscribing:** Communication between the partners decreases in quantity and quality. It involves a certain amount of shrinking of interest and commitment.
8. **Stagnating:** No growth occurs. Partners behave toward each other in old, familiar ways without much feeling.
9. **Avoiding:** The creation of physical, mental, and emotional distance between the partners.
10. **Termination:** In romantic relationships the best predictor of whether the two people will now become friends is whether they were friends before their emotional involvement.

The illustration above shows how the ten stages can be grouped into three overlapping and integrated phases: the coming together phase, the relational maintenance phase, and the coming apart phase.

Principles of IPR

Given below are the principles which one needs to apply in establishing and maintaining interpersonal relationships:
- Principles of recognition
- Principles of mutual understanding
- Principles of inculcation of common interests
- Principle of respect for human dignity
- Principle of personality development
- Principle of stimulation, motivation and encouragement
- Principle of incentives/rewards for good accomplishment
- Principle of honesty, punctuality and trust worthiness.

Characteristics of Good Relationship

Some qualities of a good relationship may be evident from the moment we meet a person. Other traits develop along with the relationship, giving the relationship strength and stability. These are some of the common characteristics of a good relationship:
- **Rapport:** Where you feel comfortable or at ease with the other person. This can be automatic or it could take time to develop.
- **Empathy:** Refers to the ability to see the world through another person's eyes, understanding his/her feelings and actions.
- **Trust:** Means that you can depend on the other person. When you trust another person you expect acceptance and support from him/her.
- **Respect:** Involves accepting and appreciating the other person for who he/she is.
- **Mental expectations:** Are seen as relationships grow; partners should have the same mutual expectations for it. The relationship should be headed toward the same purpose or goals for both people.
- **Flexibility:** Good relationships are flexible and can adapt to change. Circumstances change and you cannot always carry through on plans you have made together. You sometimes have to make compromises and reassess your goals.
- **Uniqueness:** The relationship stands out or is in some way special or different.
8. **Irreplaceability:** Each interpersonal relationship is as unique as the people in them and can never be recreated.
9. **Interdependence:** The other person's life concerns effects you.
10. **Self disclosure:** In an interpersonal relationship, **people share** and entrust private information about them
11. **Honesty and accountability:** Communicating openly and truthfully, admitting mistakes or being wrong, and accepting responsibility for one's self.

Qualities of Bad Relationship

- **Avoidance:** People in unhealthy relationships simply avoid facing reality. They become distant and will miss several occasions because they do not feel the need to be there.
- **Burnout:** A relationship is at a **low point** or "burnout", it might make one of them feel trapped, tired, helpless, depressed or let down.
- **Compatibility issues:** Incompatibility will make the relationship unhealthy, because you are not compatible, **constant** negativity will hinder intimacy. This will lead to sad relationships in constant conflict.
- **Devotional void:** A lack of commitment can make for unhealthy relationships. For example, when you treat your spouse as a roommate or friend, this does not necessarily mean you have to be in **love** 24/7.
- **Enthusiasm dwindles:** If a relationship is not spontaneous and becomes predictable it itself will not be as exciting as it used to be.
- **Forgiveness void:** Those unwilling or unable to forgive are expected to have unhealthy relationships in the future.
- **Just say yes:** Those that feel that they cannot say no to draw boundaries and sustain limits will make their spouse less of a priority.

Elements of Nurse-client Relationship

- **Contract-setting:** The time, place and purpose of meetings as well as conditions for termination are established between the nurse and client.
- **Boundaries:** Roles of participants are clearly defined, the nurse is defined as a professional helper, the client's needs and problems are the focus of the interaction.
- **Confidentiality:** The nurse should share information only with professional staff that needs to know. The nurse should obtain client's written permission to share information with others outside the treatment team.
- **Therapeutic nurse behaviors:** (a) self-awareness; (b) genuine, warm and respectful; (c) empathy; (d) cultural sensitivity; (e) collaborative goal setting; (f) responsible, ethical practice.

Phases of Nurse-Patient Relationship

Kapoor, Balm (1994) has identified four phases of nurse-patient relationship: (i) preinteraction phase; (ii) introductory or orientation phase; (iii) working phase; (iv) termination phase **(Table 16.1)**.

Chapter 16: Organizational Behavior and Human Relations

Table 16.1: Nurse's tasks in each phase of the relationship process.

Phase	Tasks
Preinteraction	Explore own feelings, fantasies, and fears analyze own professional strengths and limitation gather data about patient when possible plan for first meeting with patient
Introductory, or orientation	• Determine why patient sought help • Establish trust, acceptance, and open communication • Mutually formulate a contract • Explore patient's thoughts, feelings, and actions • Identify patient's problems • Define goals with patient
Working	• Explore relevant stressors • Promote patient's development of insight and use of constructive coping mechanisms. Overcome resistance behaviors
Termination	Establish reality of separation. Review progress of therapy and attainment of goals. Mutually explore feelings of rejection, loss, sadness, and anger and related behaviors

The preinteraction phase begins when the nurse is assigned a patient to develop therapeutic relationship with him/her till, she goes to the patient for interaction:

- The tasks are that nurse explores her/his own fears and anxiety
- Sets objectives for interaction phase

Introductory/orientation phase: It begins when the nurse goes to the patient and introduces herself/himself to the patient:

- The tasks are that the nurse introduces herself/himself to the patient
- Talks with the patients

Working phase: Working phase of the nurse-patient relationship starts when the nurse and patient start interacting with each other and nurse collect the data from primary and secondary sources.

- Assists the patient to identify his/her problem
- Plan the nursing intervention

Termination phase is also called as resolution phase. It begins with orientation phase itself when nurse explains to the patient the purpose of care to the patient. The tasks of nurse would be to help the client:

- To make best use of the services available
- Get prepared for discharge
- Get informed about rehabilitation and follow up

Establishment of IPR

The head nurse is in key position for the establishment of good interpersonal relationship among the personnel in her department. This will also involve communication system existing between and within the hospital departments. A warm, friendly attitude of nurses is reflected in the clients and other employees. The following points will help to establish good interpersonal relationship among the personnel.

- Every member should be kept informed about the job, any changes that are taking place from day to day.
- Give personal reorganization to everyone by giving praise and showing concern whenever they deserve.
- Known each personnel working with you and accept them with their abilities and limitations.
- Any grievances should be dealt with promptly and appropriately.
- Do not that do or say anything that will lower the status of the members in your team.
- Plan, organize and coordinate the activities of your team so that everything gets done in the proper time and in the correct way.
- Remember that every member in your team is working with you and not for you or under you.
- Try to create we feeling in your subordinates.
- Give each person, time and opportunity to plan his work and make sure that everyone understands the work assigned to him/her.
- Provide adequate supplies and equipment needed in the client care.
- Except in case of emergency, avoid interrupting the personnel while they are at work.
- Plan for frequent staff conferences.

Problems of Improper IPR

Poor organization often leads to inefficiency, misunderstanding or actual conflict among the personnel. Any conflict, however slight in the staff, is sensed by the patient and makes him feel insecure.

- Insecurity causes him to increase complaints, and it slows down recovery. The aim of the healthcare team is to restore the health of patient.
- The technical skill must be added with the warmth of human feeling and compassion.
- It is expedient to examine not only the behavior of the patient, but also the atmosphere in which he is being treated.
- These problems can develop at any level of an organization and result in an inability to solve human relations problems.

I. **Symptoms of organizational dysfunction frequently observed are:**
  - Little personal investment by the staff in organizations' objectives and goals.
  - Policies, directives, and orders not being carried out as intended.
  - Competition between staff rather than cooperation or collaboration.

- Failure of staff to report problems although they see anything wrong.
- Staff blames others for problems instead to taking responsibility and seeking solutions.
- Staff taking refuge in procedures and policies instead of searching for better alternatives.

II. **Some selected causes of organizational dysfunction are as follows:**
- Tight control over decision making with little staff participation allowed.
- Staff judgment not being respected by administrative and supervisory personnel.
- Rejection of the experience of others.
- Lack of positive feedback on good performance.
- Lack of corrective feedback on poor performance.
- Tradition encouraged; innovation discouraged for fear of making a mistake.
- Inadequate mechanisms for communication up, down, and sideways in the organization.
- Insufficient direct observation by supervisors.

III. **Within the formal social system:**
- Individuals, professional and nonprofessional groups and departments compete for status, recognition, and privileges focusing on the mission of the patient care.
- The formal structure is often supported or subverted by the informal social relationship that emerges among personnel.
- These traditional groupings, norms, and goals are often informally developed in order to get the job done faster.
- From these nonofficial groupings emerge attitudes towards staff and toward patients that can be either detrimental to the efficiency of medical teamwork, or can help to create a positive atmosphere for achieving the formal goals of the hospital.

HUMAN RELATIONS (FIG. 16.18)

A human relation is the relationship between human resources of the organization. It incorporates management-employees, employees-employees relationship. It also consists of relationship between the organization's human resource and outsiders (such as clients, suppliers). Human resource is one of the important assets of an organization. Hence, healthy human relations lead to increased productivity and efficiency. It also plays crucial role in growth and success of the organization.

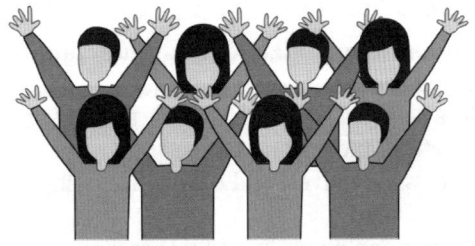

Fig. 16.18: Human relations.

Definition (Fig. 16.19)

- Human relations are the study and practice of utilizing human resources through knowledge and through an understanding of the activities, attitudes, sentiments and interrelationships of people at work. —*DE MacFarland*
- Human relations are the integration of people into a work situation is that it motivates them to work together productively, cooperatively and with economic, psychological and social satisfaction.   —*Keith Devis*

Philosophy of Human Relations

The philosophy of human relations is expressed in the following ten basic tenets:
- The relationship of the individual with the enterprise is a basic one irrespective of whether there is or is not a trade union in the plant. The policies and activities of government, of labor unions, or of a management in the field of industrial relations must be judged in the light of whether they promote or jeopardise this basic relationship.
- An individual enterprise, in its operation, must take full account of the social, spiritual, and economic needs of the individual as an employee, as a stockholder, as a consumer, and as a member of society.
- The industry exists for the individual and not the individual for the industry.
- Loyalty is not an "either-or" proposition. There is no basic in consistency or in compatibility between an employee's interest in his unit and his acceptance of a trade union membership.
- Employers should, as far as it lies within their control, work for and provide the maximum degree of economic security for their employees.
- Sound company personnel policies and practices must be designed to safeguard and promote the rights, interests and welfare of employees as persons.
- No policy, whether it is of the management or of labor, which violates or affronts the rights and freedoms of the individual, can long survive in a free society.
- The cooperation of the individual in the productive process must be won and deserved. It cannot be forced.
- The individual employee, in respect of his status, rights, prospects for advancement, and his economic well-being, is inescapably linked with the success of the enterprise by which he is employed.

Characteristics of Human Relations

The main characteristics of human relations are as follows:
- Human relations are an important process through which an individual's attitude and work are integrated with a view to achieving a willing cooperation on their part in the achievement of the interests of an organization as a whole.
- Members of the organization contribute their bit to get individual and group satisfaction.
- The satisfaction desired by employees may be economic, social and psychological.

Chapter 16: Organizational Behavior and Human Relations

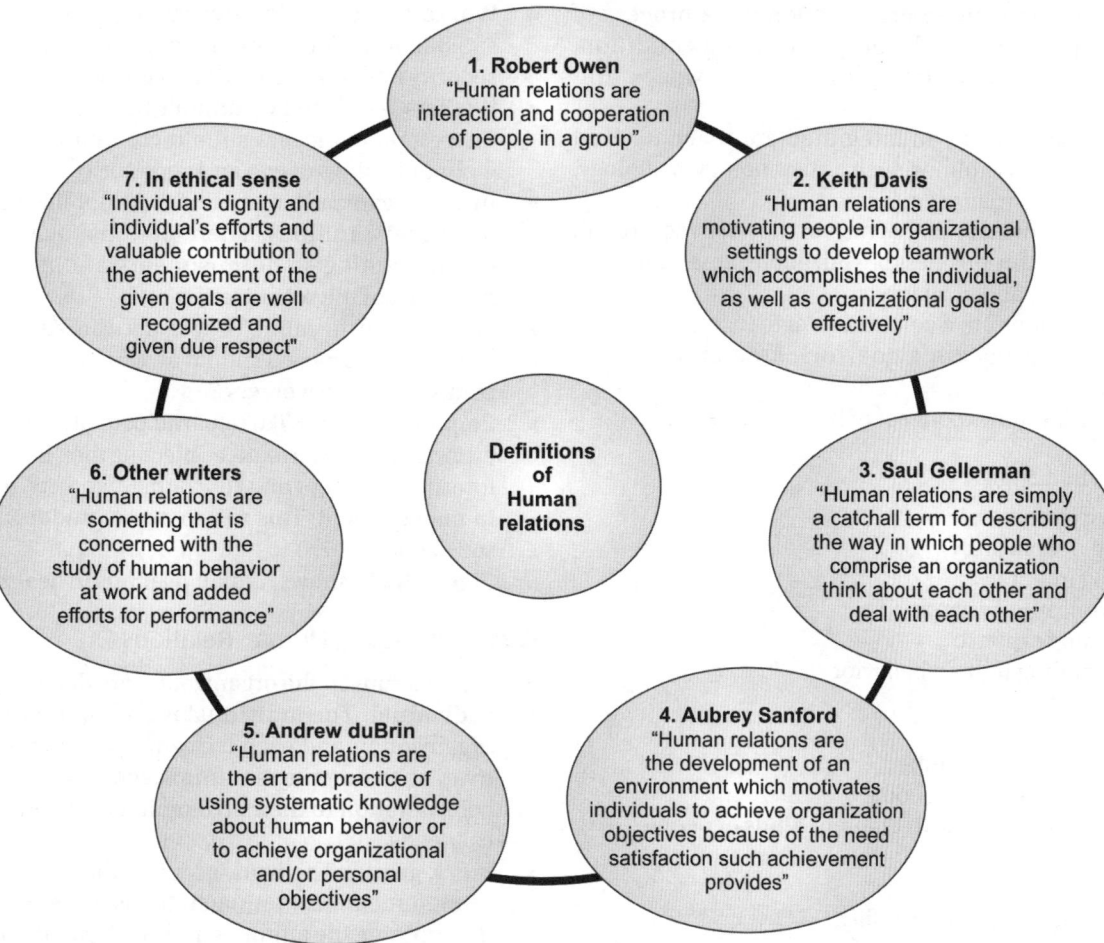

Fig. 16.19: Definitions of human relations.

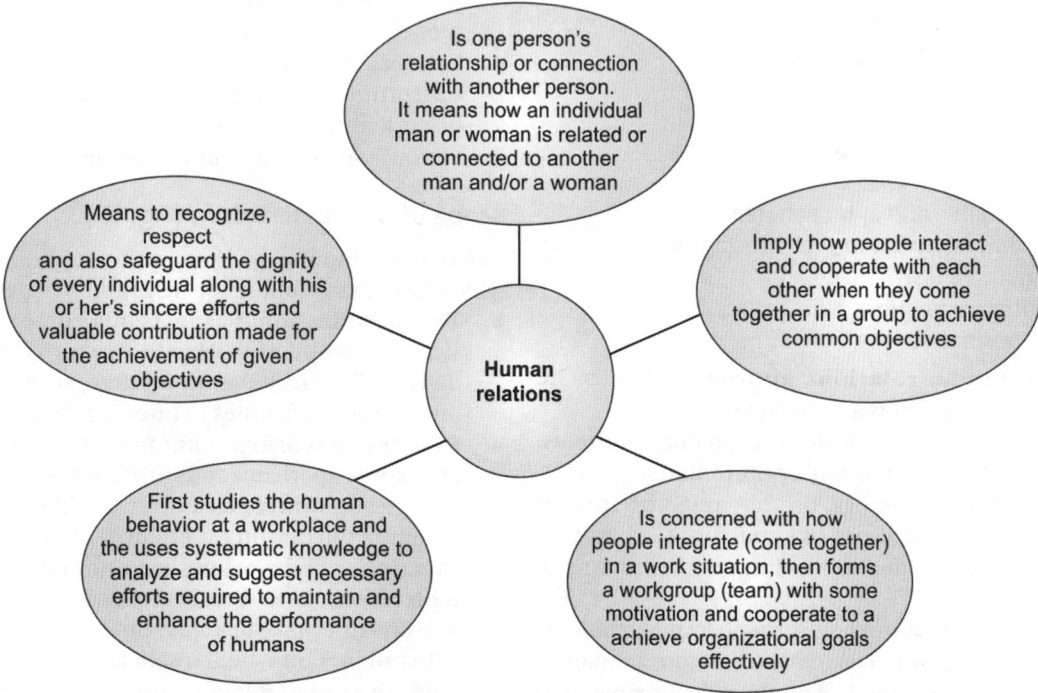

Fig. 16.20: Concept of human relations.

- Human relations in an organization are a process of improving motivation by proper working condition, training programs, timely payment of wages and incentives, etc.
- Human relations are an integrated approach derived from different disciplines, such as psychology, sociology, economics and management.
- Human relations are all pervasive; they are required in business and non-business organizations, small and large organizations, and at all levels.
- Human relations are a continuous activity.
- Human relations are a goal-oriented and focused approach.

Figure 16.20 shows concept of human relations.

Human Relation Skills

- Sensitivity to others
- Treating people fairly
- Listening intently
- Communicating warmth
- Establishing rapport
- Understanding human behavior
- Empathy
- Tactfulness
- Cooperative team member
- Avoiding stereotyping people
- Feeling comfortable with different kinds of people
- Fun person to work with
- Treating others as equals
- Dealing effectively with conflict

Principles of Human Relations

- H-Have self confidence
- U-Understand the view point of others
- M-Make yourself friend of all
- A-Admit it if you are wrong
- N-Never make promises you cannot keep
- R-Respect and courtesy are important
- E-Explain thoroughly
- L-Look, Listen and Learn (L3)
- A-Avoid argument
- T-Try to be sociable and approachable
- I-Insist on selfless service to your community
- O-Others first, self last
- N-Never criticizes in public
- S-Stress on positive always

Principles of human relations approach: The basic principles of human relations approach are:

- Human beings are not interested only in financial gains. They also need recognition and appreciation.
- Workers are human beings. So they must be treated like human beings and not like machines. Managers should try to understand the feelings and emotions of the workers.
- An organization works not only through formal relations, but also through informal relations. Therefore, managers should encourage informal relations in the organization along with formal relations.
- Workers need a high degree of job security and job satisfaction. Therefore, management should give job security and job satisfaction to the workers.
- Workers want good communication from the managers. Therefore, managers should communicate effectively without feelings of ego and superiority complex.
- In any organization, members do not like conflicts and misunderstandings. Therefore, managers should try to stop conflicts and misunderstandings among the members of the organization.
- Workers want freedom. They do not want strict supervision. Therefore, managers should avoid strict supervision and control over the workers.
- Employees would like to participate in decision making, especially, in those matters affecting their interests. Therefore, management must encourage workers' participation in management. This will increase productivity and job satisfaction.

Figure 16.21 shows human relations in health care team.

Factors Affecting Human Relations

Human relations in the organization are determined by:
- **Individual:** The individual is an important part of the organization and each individual is unique. While motivating the employees, management should give due consideration to their economic, social and psychological needs.
- **Work group:** The work group is the centre of focus of human relations approach. It has an important role in determining the attitudes and performance of individual workers.
- **Work environment:** It is important to create a positive work environment where organizational goals are achieved through satisfaction of employees. In general, when employees' needs are satisfied, the work environment is termed positive.
- **Leader:** The leader must ensure complete and effective utilization of all organizational resources to achieve organizational goals. They must be able to adjust to various personalities and situations.

Scope of Human Relations (Fig. 16.22)

The scope of human relations springs up from the problems which have many different causes and perspectives.
- **The organizational aspects of a company**, such as its size, the scope of work and the activity in each work division. These frequently arbitrary structural definitions often cause difficulties in human relations.
- **Every person brings a unique set of talents**, ambitions and work experience to as job. These personal attributes change over time, often as a result of the degree of success or failure the person experiences in the work world.
- **Inexperienced workers may not be able to perform their roles** or tasks in work groups in a competent manner. The time they take to adjust cannot only create problems with production schedules, but can also create particular kinds of human relations problems between them and their co-workers and supervisors.

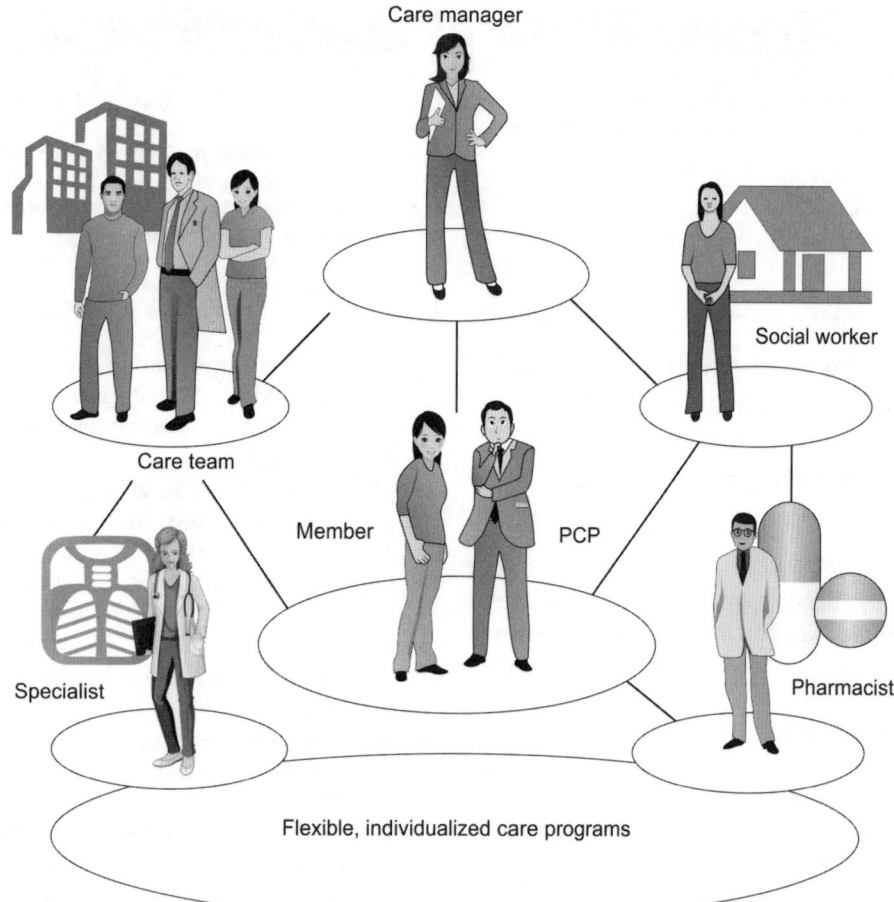

Fig. 16.21: Human relations in health care team.

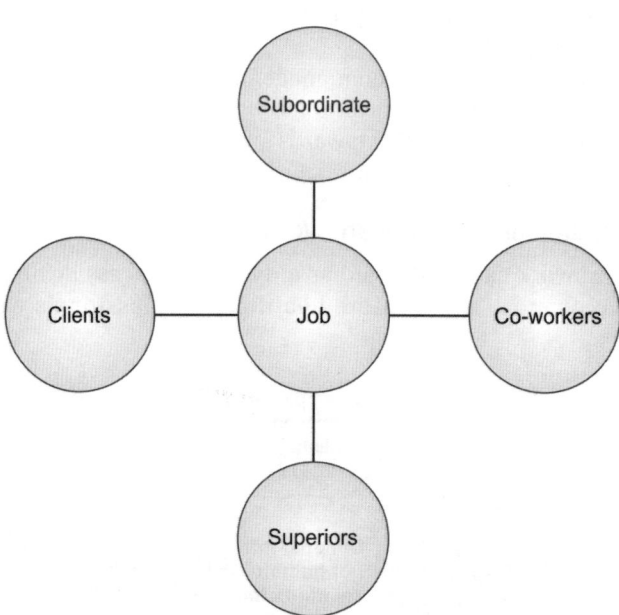

Fig. 16.22: Scope of human relations.

management and create intense problems in human relations.

- **Promotion of individuals to positions of greater responsibility** and authority generally creates a need for changed behavior patterns between the new supervisors and their former peers which, in time can create human relations problems.

Importance of Human Relations Skills (Box 16.4)

- Human rights today, managers and employees have a greater awareness of the rights of employees. This awareness calls for more skillful relations among employees, using tact, trust, and diplomacy with greater skill.
- The global marketplace Improved interpersonal skills are a critical factor in any country's gaining a competitive edge in the world marketplace.
- Growing emphasis on human resources the most important resource in any organization is the human resource
- Renewed emphasis on working groups today's employees tend to like teamwork and participative decision-making in the workplace
- Diversity in the workplace today' workplace contains an unpredicted mixture of racial, cultural, and gender backgrounds.

- **Innovations in technology and production methods** generally require the restructuring of job roles and responsibilities. Radical changes in basic organizational structure can cause severe strains between workers and

Chapter 16: Organizational Behavior and Human Relations

Box 16.4: Importance of human relations.
- Human relations skills needed by managers and leaders.
- Human relations: The way people get along with each other.
- There are five human relation skills needed by leaders and managers:
  1. Self-understanding
  2. Understanding others
  3. Communication
  4. Team building
  5. Developing job satisfaction

Box 16.5: Human relations in nursing.
- Human relation in nursing refer to the relationship of nurses with colleagues and other department personnel and of nurses with patient.
- It is interdepartmental, interdepartmental and interpersonal relationship to provide the quality care to their patients.
- Human relations in nursing also develop when two healthcare personnel interact with each other to achieve the primary goal of maximum patient satisfaction and health promotion irrespective of their field of work.

Suggestions to Improve Human Relations and its Policy

Some of such suggestions are as follows:
- A sound organizational structure clearly specifying—
  - Duties, functions and responsibilities,
  - Authority and
  - Accountability

  Of every one engaged in the organization so that everybody in the organization knows who is who, who is to do what and where, what is the relationship between two individuals and so on. For this, there should be an organizational chart.
- Adequate conditions of employment, such as—
  - Fair wages and
  - Good working conditions.
- Suitable policies for:
  - Scientific and methodical recruitment and selection,
  - Placement and
  - Induction.
- Education, training and development programs for all.
- Real and equal opportunities for advancement to all.
- Promotion from within as far as possible.
- Suitable policy for job termination.
- Respect for the personality of workers—treating the subordinates as respectable human beings, appreciating their emotions and sentiments, and recognizing their personality. The commodity approach or a factor of production approach has become outdated. It is now a well-accepted fact that subordinates deserve human respect, and their dignity should be maintained by the management.
- Personal knowledge about the subordinates.
- Fairness, impartiality and frankness in the management's approach.
- Frankness in dealing
- Direction without commanding
- Keeping promise
- Understanding other's point of view
- Equal weightage for both workers and employers.
- Employers must have a reputation for complete honesty, intelligence, flexibility and consistency of purpose.
- Adequate provision for incentives and fringe benefits.
- Positive approach towards collective bargaining, WPM, profit-sharing and labor co-partnership.
- **Development of personal and social forces:** The Hawthorne experiments has proved that socio-psychological variables play a more prominent role in increasing efficiency and motivating the employees. The management should try to create a friendly atmosphere, exercise democratic style of supervision and emphasize the need of goal congruence.
- **Due recognition to groups and informal relations:** In the organizations, individuals tend to create groups. Often workers tend to react as members of groups and not as individuals. The group determines their norms of behavior.
- **Communication:** The Hawthorne experiments have proved that communication in the organization is very important.
- **Personnel counseling:** The management can establish a system of personnel counseling in the organization.
- **Supervision:** The supervisory climate also has an important role to play in determining and improving human relations. Friendly, attentive and genuinely concerned supervisors affect the human relations favorably.
- **Introducing suggestion scheme:** The suggestion from the workers can be invited relating to various problems, such as production process, difficulties in production and facilities.
- Mutual faith between management and workers.
- Positive role by trade unions.
- Suitable state policy towards labor.

Box 16.5 describes human relations in nursing.

Human Relations in Team Work

Teamwork can be defined as a dynamic process involving two or more two or more healthcare professionals with

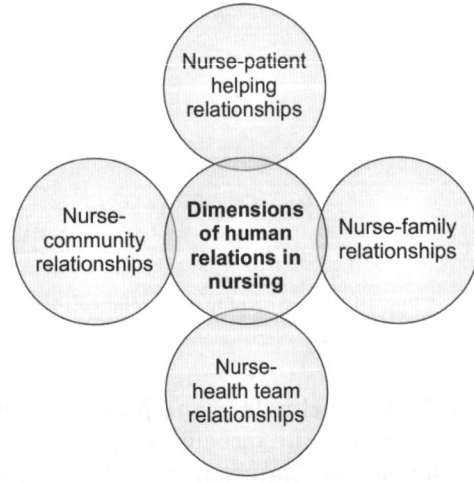

Fig. 16.23: Dimensions of human relations in nursing.

complementary background and skills, sharing common health goals and exercising concerted physical and mental effort in assessing, planning or evaluating patient care in healthcare.

Advantages of Teamwork

- It gives a better end result with high-quality performance from each team member.
- It involves every person and his expertise and responsibilities.
- The execution of new ideas can be more effective and efficient through teamwork.
- It increases ownership with wider communication.
- It leads to information sharing and increases learning in the team and the organization.
- It provides more security and develops personal relationships.
- A particular problem can easily solve in team.
- It helps provide a variety of solutions.
- It increases the willingness of every member to take more risk.
- A team can handle more difficult and complex problem in the workplace.
- A team increases the accuracy of problem solving

Disadvantages of Teamwork

- It may lead to unequal participation of members in a team.
- Some individuals may be good workers; they may not be good team payers.
- It may limit creative thinking
- A team can sometimes take longer to produce desire results.
- Team can also result in added expenses
- It may face some inherent conflict
- Peer pressure

Human Relations in the Context of Nursing (Fig. 16.23)

- Nursing profession is considered as humanity because nurses deal with the human beings in hospital as well as in the community setting.
- Community health nurses conduct home visits and health teaching sessions in the community to make people aware about diseases, their risk factors, and preventive strategies.
- In every professional encounter, nurses have to deal with human beings whether they are patients or their relatives or healthcare team members which may be individual or a group of people at a given time.
- Therefore, it is expected from the nurse that she should be skilled in interpersonal relationship skills because these skills are essential for initiating and maintaining interpersonal relationship.
- Professional relationships are created through the nurse's application of knowledge and understanding of human behavior, communication of social attitude, motives, and commitment to ethical behavior.
- Having a philosophy basis of caring and respect for others will help the nurse to be more successful in establishing relationships of this nature.

Need of Human Relations

- Human relation in nursing refers to the relationship of nurses with colleagues and other department personnel and of nurses with patient.
- It is interdepartmental, interdepartmental and interpersonal relationship to provide the quality care to their patients.
- Human relations in nursing also develop when two healthcare personnel interact with each other to achieve the primary goal of maximum patient satisfaction and health promotion irrespective of their field of work.

Nurse-Patient Helping Relationship

- Helping relationships are the foundations of clinical nursing practice. The nurse assumes the role of a professional helper in such relationships and comes to know patient's health needs.
- The nurse's therapeutic use of communication helps patients overcome their problems by achieving optimum health.
- In therapeutic relationships, nurse often encourage patients to share personal stories, which are called narrative interactions.

Nurse-Family Relationships

- Many nursing situations, especially those in community and home care setting, require the nurse to form helping relationships with the patient's entire family.
- The same principles that guide one-to-one helping relationships also apply when the patient is a family unit; communication within families requires additional understanding of the complexities of family dynamics, needs and relationships

Nurse-Health Team Relationships

- A nurse's functions or roles require interaction with multiple health team members.
- Communication in such relationships may be geared towards team building, facilitating the group process, collaboration, consultation, delegation, supervision, leadership and management.
- Both social as well as therapeutic interactions are needed between the nurse and health team members to build morale and strengthen relationships within the work setting

Nurse-Community Relationships

- Many nurses from relationships with community groups by participating in local organizations, volunteering for community service or by becoming politically active nurses in a community-based practice.
- They must be able to establish relationships with their community to be effective change agents.

- Communication within the community take place through channels, such as neighborhood, newsletters, public bulletin boards, newspapers, radio, television and electronic information sites.

Importance of Human Relations

- Human relation is important as it gives satisfaction, gives a sense of belongingness, boosts morale, and motivates and increases productivity.
- Human relations recognize the dignity of the individual as a human being.
- The concept of being "self" is developed throughout the life of a person.
- George Herbert Head (1964) defined self as "the sum total of people's conscious perception of their own identity as distinct from others. It is not a static phenomenon, but continues to develop and change throughout our lives."

Nurses Role in Human Relations

Human relation refers to the science of applying principles of social psychology in improving the working of an organization and to make it more productive and the worker happier to improve efficiency and job satisfaction. In industrial setting, human relations means the systematic body of knowledge used to explain the behavior of people at work.

- **Care giver:** The caregiver role traditionally included those activities that assist the patient physically and psychologically while preserving the patient's dignity.
- **Care giving encompasses** the physical, psychological, developmental, cultural and spiritual levels.
- **Communicator:** In the role of communicator, nurses identify patient's problems and then communicate these verbally or in writing to other members of the health team. The nurse must be able to communicate clearly and accurately in order for a client's healthcare needs to be met.
- **Teacher:** As a teacher, the nurse helps the client learn about their health and the healthcare procedures they need to perform to restore or maintain their health. The nurse assesses the client's learning needs and readiness to learn, sets specific learning goals in conjunction with the client, enacts teaching strategies, and measures learning.
- **Client advocate:** A client advocate acts to protect the client. In this role the nurse may represent the client's needs and wishes to other health professionals, such as relaying the client's wishes for information to the physician.
- **Counselor:** The nurse counsel's primarily healthy individual with normal adjustments difficulties and focuses on helping the person develop new attitudes, feelings and behaviors by encouraging the client to look at alternative behaviors, recognize the choices, and develop a sense of control.
- **Change agent:** The nurse acts as a change agent when assisting others that is clients, to make modifications in their own behavior, nurses also often act to make changes in a system, such as clinical care, if it is not helping a client return to health. Nurses are continually dealing with change in the healthcare system.
- **Leader:** The leader role can be employed at different levels individual client, family, groups of clients, colleagues or the community.
- **Manager:** The nurse manager also delegates nursing activities to ancillary workers and other nurses, and supervises and evaluates their performance.
- **Case manager:** Nurse case managers work with the multidisciplinary healthcare team to measure the effectiveness of the case management plan and to monitor outcomes. Each agency or unit specifies the role of the nurse case manager.
- **Research consumer:** Nurses often use research to improve client care. In a clinical area, nurses need to (a) have some awareness of the process and language of research, (b) be sensitive to issues related to protecting the rights of human subjects, (c) participate in the identification of significant researchable problems, and (d) be a discriminating consumer of research findings.
- **Expanded career roles:** Nurses are fulfilling expanded career roles, such as those of nurse practitioner, clinical nurse specialist, nurse midwife, nurse educator, nurse researcher and nurse anesthetist.

PUBLIC RELATIONS IN THE CONTEXT OF NURSING

Public relations commonly referred as PR is a modern phenomenon, which goes a long way in building the image of Nursing as a profession. Consequently public relation is an important adjunct of nursing administration as a good public relations will contribute towards a better nursing administration run-in thereby improved quality of nursing care services **(Fig. 16.24)**.

Definition

- Public relation are knowing what the public expects and explaining how administration is meeting these desire.
  —*John Millet*

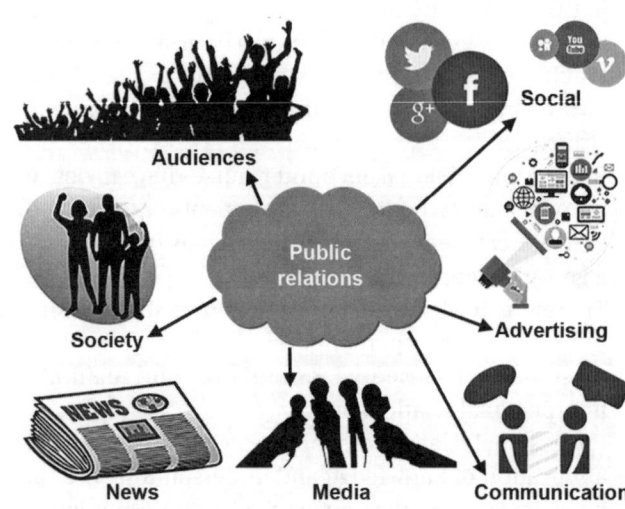

Fig. 16.24: Public relation.

Chapter 16: Organizational Behavior and Human Relations

- Public relation in government is the composite of all the primary and secondary contacts between the bureaucracy and citizens and all the interactions of influences and attitudes established in these contracts. —*JL MeCamy*
- Public relation means the development of cordial, equitable and therefore mutually profitable relations between a business industry organization and the public it serves. —*WT Parry*
- Public relations are the process whereby an organization analyses the needs and desires of all interested parties in order to conduct itself more responsively towards them. —*Rex Harlow*

Meaning of Public Relations

- Public relation is an essential and integrated component of public policy or service.
- The professional public relation activity will ensure the benefit to the citizens, for whom the policies or services are meant for.
- Effective public relations can create and build up the image of an individual or an organization or a nation.
- At the time of adverse publicity or when the organization is under crisis an effective public relations can remove the "misunderstanding" and can create mutual understanding between the organization and the public.

Aims and Objectives of Public Relations

Aims and objectives of educational administrator public relations:

- To provide efficient social life to the students and to prepare them in the art of living together
- To bring school or college and community closes to each other
- To prepare the students for some vocation or profession which according to their interest and ability
- To help the students in unfolding and blossoming of their personality
- To enable the students to have the right type of philosophy of life
- To help in educational exports according to their saluted vocation or profession
- To bring harmony between plans and tasks
- To provide healthy atmosphere for experimentation and research
- To train his faculties to widen his outlook
- To cultivate his mind to form and strength his character
- To build up mind and body and give health and strength

Need of Public Relations

- Keeping the health consumers informed about the availability of the range and types of healthcare services.
- Giving the clientele information on the procedural aspects of healthcare.
- Informing the clientele about the hospital medical and nursing service profile.
- Informing the nursing staff members about hospital's role in their welfare.

Well-executed public relations will:

- Increase visibility for the hospital, employees, programs and services.
- Position the hospital as a healthcare leader and authority within the community or region.
- Expand awareness of the hospital's entire range of programs and services.
- Enhance the hospital's image.
- Aid in recruitment and retention of employees.
- Support efforts to raise funds for new programs and services or assist with the passage of levies and bonds.
- Act as a foundation when negative news about the hospital occurs.
- Boost employee morale

Functions of Public Relations

- Public relation is establishing the relationship among the two groups (organization and public).
- Art or Science of developing reciprocal understanding and goodwill.
- It analyses the public perception and attitude, identifies the organization policy with public interest and then executes the programmes for communication with the public.

Elements of Public Relations (Fig. 16.25)

- A planned effort or management function.
- The relationship between an organization and its publics.
- Evaluation of public attitudes and opinions.
- An organization's policies, procedures and actions as they relate to said organization's publics.
- Steps taken to ensure that said policies, procedures and actions are in the public interest and socially responsible.
- Execution of an action and or communication program.

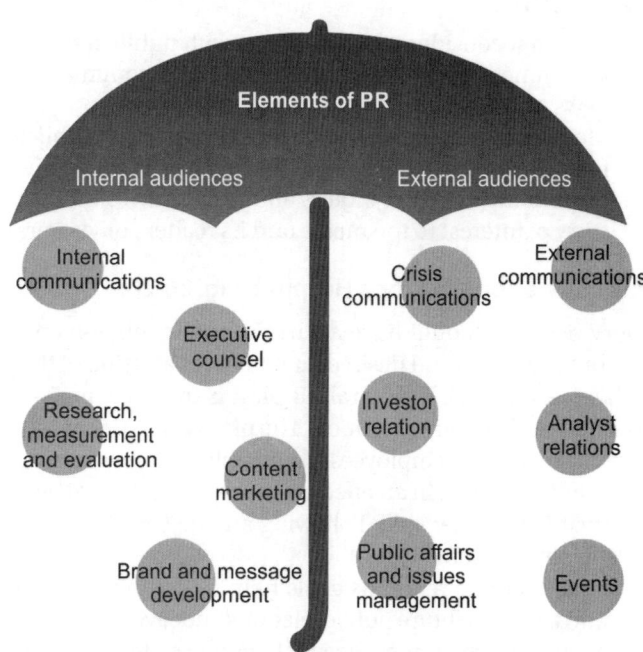

Fig. 16.25: Elements of public relations.

- Development of rapport, goodwill, understanding and acceptance as the chief end result sought by public relations activities.

Forms of Public Relation

Public relation is a general term that may include many other-relations with different audiences, strategies and tactics. For example:

Employee Relations

- It is a function of public relations that includes responding to employee concerns and informing and motivating staff.
- Some tactics used for employee relations may include new employee education, employee award programs and recognitions, new-hire press releases and newsletters to name a few.

Community Relations

- It is the function of actively planning and participating with and within a community for the benefit of the community and the hospital.
- Tactics within this category include community events, volunteer activities and co-sponsorship opportunities with other community organizations.
- Community relations may also include fundraising and development activities.

Government Relations

- It is a function of relating to government officials and agencies about issues that impact the hospital and its audiences.
- Hill climb events in Olympia, letter writing campaigns, and op-ed placements in the newspaper are often part of government relations.

Media Relations

- It is often considered synonymous with public relations, is the function of working with the media to communicate news.
- Media relations can be active- seeking positive publicity for a newsworthy topic at the hospital- or reactive- responding to a news inquiry about a positive or negative story of interest to the media and its readers or viewers.

Public Relation Plan for a Hospital (Fig. 16.26)

Every hospital should have a current public relations plan that outlines goals and desired outcomes for a period of three to five years. Once a general PR plan is in place, periodic planning and updating is critical. The plan and its updates will not only help guide employees responsible for public relations work, but will result in an effective tool to communicate with the board and other staff. Following are the key elements of an effective PR plan:

- **Goals:** Public relations goals help direct the strategies and tactics in future public relations endeavors. The goals should clearly support hospital mission statement. While a mission statement may include what the hospital wants

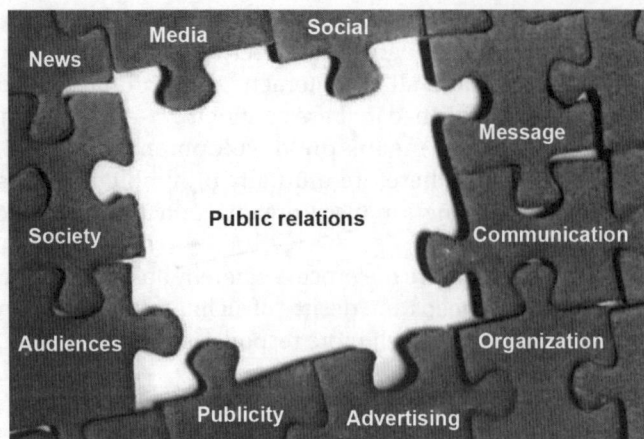

Fig. 16.26: Public relations in hospital.

to accomplish, a public relations goal should be focused on what you want the public to think and know about the hospital

- **Objectives:** Objectives help determine specific outcomes from your public relations efforts. Objectives should be clear and concise, and include timing. **Examples**:
  - Increase awareness of the technology and medical advances used at the hospital within Evergreen County over the next six months.
  - Build the reputation of the hospital in the next three to four years as a cornerstone of the community that provides healthcare services, jobs and community leadership.
  - Encourage renewed interest in specialty hospital services, such as childbirth classes over the next two years.
- **Target audiences:** Detail the groups of people that are important to inform or influence, and why.
  Examples:
  - **Patients:** They purchase healthcare services and generate revenue for the hospital.
  - **Physicians:** They use hospital facilities and generate revenue for the hospital. They control where patients go for care in the hospital or outside of the community.
  - **Media:** They write both positive and negative stories about the hospital, its staff and services. They have considerable influence and access to all of the hospital's target audiences.

  Other audiences to consider may include employees, board members, community leaders, local government officials, state legislators, vendors and suppliers.
- **Tactics:** It is easy for busy hospital professionals to think about tactics first, but it is critical to have a solid strategy in place. Only pursue the tactics that will help achieve the goals. Here are some—best uses for specific tactics.
  - **Brochure/collateral:** To inform patients and community members about programs and services provided at the hospital for promotional use only. It may be provided to media for background, but not to be used instead of effective media tools, such as press releases or fact sheets.

- **Direct mail:** To help create awareness for programs or services with target audiences. Message is controlled.
- **Letters:** Good for personal or business communication. Adjustable length (1–2 pages).
- **Postcards:** Good for event invitations or welcome cards. Inexpensive postage.
- **Direct mail packages:** Good for inclusion in new neighbor welcome packages or community coupon envelopes. Consider including brochures or inserts. Costs are typically part of an advertising or sponsorship package. Production of materials likely not included.
- **Specialty mailings:** Good for awareness efforts, such as a child safety campaign sponsored by the hospital. Mailing may include a magnet with safety tips and local emergency contact information.
- **Distribution methods:** How you distribute materials is often as important as what the organization send. It is a good idea to know which methods the target audiences, especially reporters, prefer.
    - **Mail:** Good to use when timing is less sensitive (one to three days). Good for newsletter mailings, new neighbor welcome packets, media kits, and other materials that are difficult to fax or e-mail. Mail can also be certified to verify receipt or insured to avoid loss.
    - **Fax:** Good for timely communication (faster than mail). Good for press releases, event reminders, and some forms of newsletters (such as weekly news notices). Less effective for documents with images or graphics.
    - **E-mail:** Good for timely and direct communication with an individual. Good for press releases, media reminders, media personnel questions, and pitch letters. Access to e-mail and electronic document size can be limitations.
    - **Face-to-face meetings:** Best way to make a personal connection. It allows for detailed explanation of a point-of-view or complicated subject. Best way to demonstrate excitement, concern, tolerance, empathy, etc.
    - **Phone conference call:** Allows for personal contact when face-to-face is not possible. Good for back-and-forth communication. Inexpensive method for communicating with large groups in different locations (cities/states).
    - **Website:** Web pages allow interested parties to pull information thereby facilitating distribution. Directing people to a website may be done through mailings, publicity or other notices.
    - **Newsletter:** To regularly update a variety of target audiences about the happenings at the hospital. Good way to establish and maintain community support for the hospital and services.
    - **Public service announcement (PSA):** To create awareness of a problem or issue through radio or television.
    - **Press release:** To distribute straightforward news to the media.
    - **Press kit:** To provide extensive information about a topic. It may precede an event or new program launch.
    - **Press conference:** To disseminate time sensitive and critical news to multiple media contacts at once. It should be rarely used.
    - **Special event:** To make a personal connection with target audiences in a positive environment. It is good way to recognize people for good work or launch new programs of facilities.
    - **Speaking engagement:** To reach a target audience, establish the speaker as an expert and build credibility for the speaker and the hospital.
    - **Video:** To communicate messages with emotion through visuals. It is good for town meetings, new employee education, fundraising projects, special events, etc.
    - **Web site:** To provide 24-hour access to information about the hospital. It may include health information or links to health information depending on site design. It is good for general information about the hospital, its services and staff.

Method of Improving Public Relation in Hospital

There are certain other aspects which need careful consideration which are described in brief as under.

- **General:** High quality patient care by the hospital is the theme of any public relation program. No amount of smile, cheers and propaganda will compensate for bad administration and poor professional care in the hospital. **Physical facilities:** Well planned hospital with sufficient waiting area for the patient and its relation in the hospital, optimum floor space for each department of t e hospital, logical layout of the department and work areas, provision of adequate facilities, such as toilets, public utility services, such as canteen, drinking water facility and so on go a long way in improving the image of the hospital.
- **Staff:** In a hospital, the staff consists of variety individuals drawn from different status of the society with different levels of education and background. Imbibing a team spirit in all these groups of people for the patient care will lead to a general satisfaction foe the patients in the hospital.
- **Name labels and uniform:** All functionaries should wear uniforms and name labels. This creates initial good impression on patients and reflects good administration. It also infuses among the employees a pride and sense of belonging to the institutions. These also help in identifying the staff by name and their status. These are particularly useful in OPD and ancillary departments.
- **Importance of color:** Color affects many of our moods and emotions. Proper choice of color can transform depressing and monotonous atmosphere into pleasing and exciting one. It stimulates employee's productivity. Hospital is one area where color can be used with measured success not only in appearance but for the psychological uplifting which it brings to patients.
- **Operating facility:** The operating efficiency in an organization, such as, hospital is the outcome of its soundness of objectives, policies, procedures, programs

and standing orders. The clear cut policy and procedure in writing and their periodic promulgation to the staff specially, clear order regarding organizational structure, defining their duties, authorities and accountability of the staff.

- **The specialty clinics:** The specialty clinics if located proximally are one of the concentrated areas of the OPD services. It will facilitate mutual interaction of the functionaries and effective protocol among the various specialties and will in turn save great deal of effort for the patient to move around for multiple consultations, as and when necessary.
- **Waiting time:** The waiting time in the OPD is invariably the sore point of public grievances. Introduction of appointment system, staggering of OPD timings for the registration, punctual attendance by doctors are some of the remedies which can be introduced to reduce waiting time and have successfully been implemented in many hospitals.
- **Delay in admission**: Anxiety and distress is the result of delays in admission due to long waiting list. In allotting priorities for admission, hospitals consider the physical state of the patients, but forget the social background and as a result, social emergencies have to wait. Adequate facilities in efficient use of present resources can resolve this problem to some extent.
- **Ward reception:** Patients are generally vulnerable to anxiety and fear on arrival in the ward. The reception they get tends to leave a deep impression. Prompt reception improves the morale of the patients.
- **Privacy:** It is normally observed that majority of the patients are dissatisfied with the type of privacy provided in the ward. Provision of screens around each bed would afford greater privacy. To have the privacy and at the same time provide the advantage of companionship of other patients in the ward would go a long way in creating a feeling of warmth and understanding.
- **Food:** Good food, well prepared and attractively served to patients, makes a very favorable impression. Presence of dietician or a nurse at the time of service creates good impact on the patients.
- **Cleanliness:** Cleanliness is much a desired thing in a hospital. It not only enhances the image of the hospital but also helps in controlling hospital infection. Frequent cleaning and liberal use of detergents and deodorants eliminates the stink which is most dissatisfying.
- **Information about illness:** The most important thing to a patient is to know as to what is wrong with him and how long will it take to recover. Information in this respect will always be associated with fear, anxiety and thus, will help in building patients confidence. A doctor or a nurse should be available in the ward during visiting hours to furnish information regarding illness of the patients to their relatives.
- **Visitors:** Relatives and friends come rushing to the hospital the moment they learn about the illness of their near and dear one. This is to show their loyalty, affection

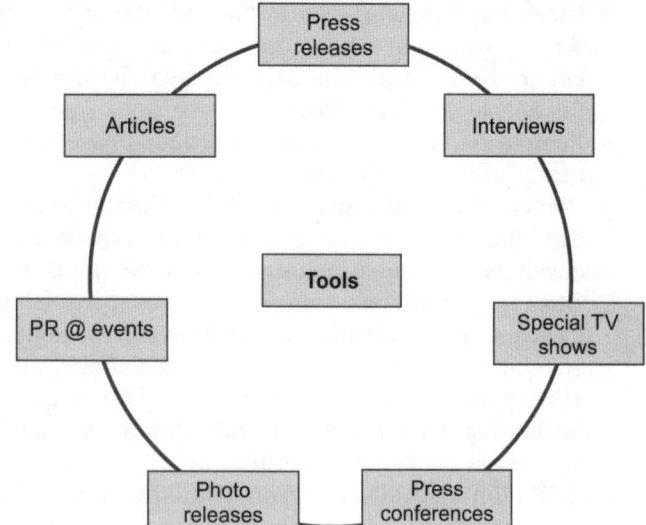

Fig. 16.27: Tools used in public relations.

and strength of ties. It also satisfies emotional needs of the patient. The relatives, etc., are allowed to visit their patients for a short while. The visiting hour policy should be more liberal for the visitors to the serious patients and relatives coming from distant places. Too rigid visiting policy makes the public critical of the hospital.

- **Complaints and suggestions**: The best way to deal with complaints is to do everything possible to avoid getting them by anticipating the problems. In spite of the best intentions of everyone and as it happens everywhere else, sometimes things go wrong. Any complaint and suggestions should receive prompt attention and wherever possible remedial actions be taken. Equally important is that whatever action is taken, the same is communicated to the complaint.
- **Mortuary and chaplain facility:** The disposal of the dead is influenced by religion, social and cultural beliefs and practices. It is necessary to provide within the hospital or its premises a place to which a dead body can be moved quietly so that other patients do not get upset. Disposal of dead has a great bearing on public relations of the hospital. This is a sensitive area for the relatives and friends. Even unintentional neglect or delay may carry unpleasant impression about the hospital. Utmost care is needed by all members of the staff to ensure that prompt and proper disposal of the dead is arranged.

Figure 16.27 shows tools used in public relations.

Need for Public Relation in the Community

- The main goal is to raise the standard of care to the highest level.
- To improve the existing channels of communication and to establish new ways of setting-up of two-way communication.
- To provide the community with the concept of what a hospital and a health center are.
- To ensure financial support
- To create mutual understanding and goodwill through proper communication.

- To provide extra services of volunteers
- To keep in touch with the community to assess their needs.
- To interpret the expectation of the community, their opinion and impression of the hospital to the top level management.
- In large hospitals relationships can become very impersonal. Project a good image of the hospital through effective staff performance.
- Public relationship is all about relationships efforts, commitment and activities, which go into building. The right sort of relationships where there is good public relations, the hospital and healthcare are functioning at its best and contribute maximum to which it serves.

Methods of Maintaining Public Relation in the Community

There are mainly two methods:
1. Operative methods
2. Communicative methods

I. Operative Methods

These methods are essentially connected with every aspect of community operations including those are carried out by such workmen as health personnel, office personnel, enquiry, media personnel, etc. The fundamental ingredients of community operation are:
- Cheerful and courteous behavior
- Prompt and efficient treatment
- Clear surroundings and well appearance of the workers.

Some operations of improving operation of primary healthcare in the community level are:
- A high quality patient care is the key of good public relation
- Adequate physical facility with good functional layout. Waiting room with benches or chairs, water, refreshment facility in the outpatient department.
- To make others happy one must be happy himself. Good morale of workers not only increases efficiency, but workers with high morale interact in a positive manner with one another and also with the patients in the community.
- Operating efficiency with effective coordination among all clinical departments and other supportive services stem from good administration, organization structure, policies, procedures and authority and accountability should be clearly understood by each staff.

II. Communicative Methods

These methods employ means of communication in all possible forms to enable the primary health center to convey its message to the public. Some of these are also intermixed in a way with intra-mutual functions of the hospital or health centers and the operative methods may be used in the following ways:
- Making the available appropriate information to the patients, their relatives and visitors.
- A provision to listen to verbal complains instead of insisting on written one.
- Prompt reply to questions.
- Provision of suggestion box at appropriate place.
- Visual communication, film shows, exhibitions and hospital Boucher are to be displayed.
- Hospital tours can be conducted by the school teachers, students, housewives and members of women's organization and religious leaders.
- Holding an annual hospital day or open day house where public can be shown every aspect of the hospital operation including some of the highly technical functions.
- Using mass media would be helpful to improve public relation.

Qualities of public relation staff:
- Warm and friendly with good common sense
- Good organizing ability
- Good judgment, creativity and then critical ability
- Imagination and appreciate others
- Calm and not excitable person
- Ability to take pains
- Lively and inquisitive minds
- Willingness to work long and in constraint atmosphere, whenever necessary especially in pulse polio campaigns.
- Resilient and a sense of humor
- Flexibility and ability to deal with many problems
- Ability to communicate in any languages
- Capable of correcting and subediting others communication
- Loyalty to the organization

Indicators for assessing public relation in the community:
- Patient-satisfaction surveys
- General opinion pool
- Quality of care using checklist
- Number of complain received
- Extent of voluntary efforts by the community
- Turnover of the health staffs
- Consistency of the attendance of the patients in clinics and health centers
- Donations
- Inpatients leaving against medical advice
- Good recovery: achievement of the health activities
- Poor recovery and high death rate
- Vital rates, such as IMR, MMR, BR and DR in the area
- Incidence and prevalence rate of the communicable diseases in the community

Public Relation in an Educational Institution

Steps followed in public relation: The followings are the steps followed in public relation campaign in an educational institution.
- **Listing and prioritizing of information is to be disseminated:** May wish to inform the public:
  - The new policy of the government or organization
  - The change in the existing policy
  - The new scheme promoted
  - The change in the existing scheme. Public relations activity starts with identifying the message to be disseminated and prioritized.

- **Ascertaining the existing knowledge level or understanding the perceptions of the public:** The organization can check a quick survey among the target group of the public to ascertain the knowledge level of the issue for which the organization is planning to initiate public relations process and in case of the image it is essential to know whether the image is positive, neutral or negative in terms of the assessment or in terms of the organization or both.
- **Communication objectives and prioritize:** Based on the knowledge level or image factor, a communication objective is to be established which is possible to evaluate and the top management approval is required. For example, communication objective instead of using the term increasing awareness level about the scheme, it should be specific "By 2005, in the number of families where of the scheme be at least one lakh" so that we can evaluate the impact.
- **Message and media:** After choosing the objective, the content of the message need to be developed. While developing the message, we should keep in mind the media in which we are going to use for disseminating that message. TV/Visual media may be effective for showing the demonstrating awareness. Training media may be effective whether the recipient may wish to keep the gap or further reference.
- **Implementation of message and media:** Based on the expected reaching level and target group, the budget is to be prepared and message is transmitted through the appropriate media.
- **Impact assessment:** After release of the message, it is essential to study the impact at interval by interacting with the target group.
- **Message redesigned:** In case, the interaction of the target group reveals the message did not reach as expected the modification in message or media need to be done and the revised message should be disseminated.

Types of Public Relation

Advertising: The main forms of advertising are:
1. Brochures or flyers
2. Direct mail
3. E-mail messages
4. Magazines
5. Newsletters
6. Newspaper (major)
7. Online discussion and chat groups
8. Posters and bulletin boards
9. Radio and television announcements

- **Publicity:** Publicity is the spreading of information to gain public awareness for a product, person, service, cause or organization, and can be seen as a result of effective PR planning.
- **Propaganda:** Propaganda is a form of communication that is aimed at influencing the attitude of a community toward some cause or position. Propaganda, in its most basic sense, presents information primarily to influence an audience and change in their attitude.
- **Public diplomacy:** Public diplomacy, broadly speaking, is the communication with foreign publics to establish a dialogue designed to inform and influence. It is practiced through a variety of instruments and methods ranging from personal contact and media interviews to the Internet and educational exchanges.
- **Campaign:** Effective public relations require a knowledge, based on analysis and understanding, of all the factors that influence public attitudes toward the organization. While a specific public relations project or campaign may be undertaken proactively or reactively to manage some sort of image crisis.
- **Promotion:** Commercialization of publicity.
- **Annual reports**: They are ripe with information if they include an overview of your year's activities, accomplishments, challenges and financial status.
- **Collaboration or strategic restructuring:** If you are organization is undertaking these activities, celebrate it publicly.
- **Presentations:** Find ways to give even short presentations, for example, at local seminars, conventions, seminars, etc. It is amazing that one can send out 500 brochures and be lucky to get 5 people who respond. Yet, you can give a presentation to 30 people and 15 of them will be very interested in staying in touch with you.

Qualities of PR in Educational Institution

- Abundant common sense
- First class organizing capacity
- Good judgment and objectivity
- Imagination ability and ability to appreciate
- Infinite capacity for taking pain
- Willingness to work long
- Be realistic and sense of humor
- Ability to write and speak English correctly
- Pleasant voice and ability to speak in public
- Innovative in ideas
- Basic understanding about the profession
- Building abilities
- Intelligence, foresight, result-oriented approach
- Media specialization
- Editorial expertise
- Insight in research

Nursing Service in Public Relations

Involvement of Nursing Service Department in Public Relations: Nursing Service Administration department acts as a liaison between the nursing staff and the hospital management as well as a communicator for the clientele on behalf of the administration. This requires good public relations. There are some essential features, which a nurse administrator as a public relation person must follow. These are:
1. He/she should have a thorough knowledge about the hospital-its philosophy, objective commitments, obligations and policies.

- He/she should be a good and able communicator with knowledge about PR techniques,
- He/she should be sensitive and alert to consumer needs in terms of health and to the healthcare delivery trends.

Tools and Techniques of Public Relations

There can be possibly no exhaustive list of tools; instrumentalities and techniques of maintain good public relations. Time, place and persons always make a difference. Among the normal tools may be listed publicity, advertising, personal contact, public speech and direct mail.

Publicity: It is the most important aspect of public relations, and has become a must for every large organization, including the government. Both democratic and totalitarian regimes make full use of this powerful weapon of influencing and molding public opinion. Publicity means to make public or to disseminate knowledge of facts. It has been defined as the art of dealing with the people in the mass. The principal media of modern publicity are of three type's visual, auditory and telecasts. The various activities of the ministry and the important services rendered by it can be briefly described under the following heads:
- All India Radio
- Doordarshan
- Press Information Bureau
- Publications
- Directorate of Advertising and Visual Publicity
- Films division
- Research and reference division
- Directorate of field publicity

Aims and Objectives of Educational Administrator Public Relations

- To provide efficient social life to the students and to prepare them in the art of living together
- To bring school or college and community closes to each other
- To prepare the students for some vocation or profession which according to their interest and ability
- To help the students in unfolding and blossoming of their personality
- To enable the students to have the right type of philosophy of life
- To help in educational exports according to their saluted vocation or profession
- To bring harmony between the plans and task
- To provide healthy atmosphere for experimentation and research
- To train his faculties to widen his outlook
- To cultivate his mind to form and strength his character
- To build up his mind and body and give him health and strength

Bulletin as a Tool in Public Relations

Institutions of nursing also require public relation in relating with the students, the parents of students the hospital it is attached to, and the community at large. The public relations person users various aids to promote relations they are newspaper, radio, TV, bulletins, bulletin boards.
- Below the title side a brief description about the specified subject of the display material.
- The height of the bulletin board should be 1 meter above the ground.
- The area where the bulletin board are fixed or placed should be well lighted.

Techniques and Attractive Public Relations

- First level relationship school to community to convey information
- Second level relationship school initiates but community is more active school invites community to visit the school and observe to give a feedback.
- Third level relationship is enables the member of community representations two way communications.
- Fourth level relationship the community is given greater opportunity to participate in planning and decision making process on some areas of school operations.

RELATIONS WITH PROFESSIONAL ASSOCIATIONS AND EMPLOYEE UNIONS

Professionals create organizations to work collectively on behalf of issues that enhance their work and their involvement in communities, ensure continued learning and competence, and use political action to influence policymakers to support mission of organization. Professional organizations offer a supportive way to learn leadership skills, to test ideas, and to follow these ideas to completion. Nursing has a national organization open to all graduate nurses, Indian nursing council, trained nurses association of India.

Definitions

- **Collective bargaining:** Negotiation between organized workers and their employer or employers to determine wages, hours, rules, and working conditions.
- **Assertiveness:** It is demanding what you want in a confident way that harms no one but in the same time preserves your rights.
- **Unions:** A union or labor organization is any organization in which employees participate for the purpose of dealing with their employer about grievances, labor disagreements, wages, hours of work, and conditions of employment.

Meaning

Participation in professional organizations is of profit to you and to profession. The profession provides a means through which united efforts can be made to elevate standards of nursing education and practice. It also offers a means of voicing your opinions, developing your abilities and keeping informed of new trends. Registration is necessary for active nursing practice either here or abroad. This is done through your State Nurses Registration Council. It provides you with legal protection and protects the patient from poor nursing care.

Components of Profession

Nursing pathway to professionalism has not been smooth. For decades an ongoing subject for discussion in nursing circles has been the following question "is nursing a profession". Sociologists do not agree that nursing is a profession. They believe it's an emerging profession. Nursing is rather considered by everyone as a profession now. Nursing complies with all criteria of a profession. It has all greatly changed Now

- Today, there is a body of knowledge that is uniquely nursing's own.
- Nursing is no longer based on trial and error but increasingly relies on theory development and research as a basis for practice. We call it evidence-based practice.
- Nursing is now engaged in an ongoing effort to identify and standardize nursing diagnoses, interventions and outcomes all of which are parts of nursing process.
- Individual accountability has become a part of nursing practice. Now society hold nurses individually responsible for their actions.
- Majority of programs offering basic nursing education are now associate degree and baccalaureate programs located in college and universities.

Various vital components of a profession are:
- Education takes place in a college or university
- Education is prolonged
- Work involves mental creativity
- Decision making is based largely on science or theories
- Values, beliefs and ethics are an integral part of preparation
- Commitment dominates material reward
- Accountability rests with Individual

Trained Nurses Association of India (TNAI) (Box 16.6)

The Trained Nurses Association of India is a national professional association of nurses. The present name and organization were established in 1922.

Aims

Aims center upon needs of the individual member and problems in the nursing profession as a whole. Such aims include (1) Upgrading; (2) Development and standardization of nursing education; (3) Improvement of living and working condition for nurses in India; (4) Registration for qualified nurses.

Activities

- TNAI gives scholarships for nurses who wish to go on for advanced study either here or abroad.
- It helped to remove discrimination against male nurses.
- Initiated much needed study and improvement of economic conditions for nurses.
- The TNAI opposes strikes unless all other means of negotiating have failed to bring about satisfactory working conditions.

Membership

Obtained by application and submission of a copy of your state registration certificate. It is possible to apply for a life membership. The official organ of the TNAI is The Nursing Journal of India which is published monthly. The cost of this is included in the annual subscription for membership in the association.

It helps you to be informed of current events in nursing and offers opportunities to publish articles and voice opinions.

Policies and Practices of TNAI

The Trained Nurses Association of India has for many years been greatly concerned about the economic welfare of nurses and action which may be taken to negotiate for better benefits and working conditions for the profession. The following facts have emerged during this time:

- The TNAI cannot be legally appointed as a negotiating body either at a Local, State or National level.
- The advice of the TNAI is listened to, with respect, and sometimes acted upon. But such advice is given on the initiative of the TNAI, but the TNAI does not have the right of representation in negotiations.
- The TNAI as a national body can give a broad support to local or state organizations of nurses.

The organization of the TNAI makes it possible for all nurses to participate at some level. Beginning with the local unit, which is usually made up of personnel in a specific institution, the level of organization moves to the district, state and national levels. Members of the TNAI are usually most active on the level of the local unit. Activities and conferences, however, are planned regularly by the state branches and provide opportunities for valuable professional participation and development of the individual member.

International Council for Nurses (ICN) (Box 16.7)

It was formed in 1899. It is an international association for all nurses in the world. Great emphasis has been on non-discrimination.

Objectives

- Promote the development of strong national nurses associations.

Box 16.6: Trained Nurses Association of India.
- Formed in 1908 at Delhi, India.
- It is a national body of practitioners of nursing at various levels.
- It is a professional association of nurses.

> **Box 16.7:** International Council of Nurses.
> - Founded in 1899, headquartered in Geneva, Switzerland
> - World's first largest international organization for health
> - Represents 16 million international nurses
> - 130 national nurses organization

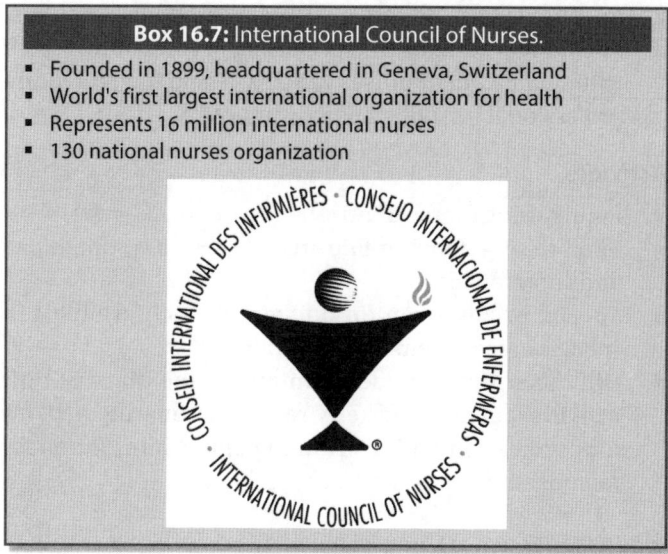

> **Box 16.8:** Function of Indian Nursing Council.
> - Recognizes nurses as separate branch in health services.
> - Regulates nursing training throughout the country.
> - Recognizes qualifications.
> - Seeks information on course of study and training and examination from any states
> - Inspect Schools and Colleges of Nursing.

- Assist national nurses association to improve the standards of nursing and the competence of nurses.
- Assist national nurses associations to improve the status of nurses within their countries.
- Serve as the authoritative voice for nurses and nursing internationally.

Activities
- Makes policy statements on health and social issues.
- Offers a great variety of seminars
- Maintaining and improving the status of nursing around the world

Membership
All nurses can become members of the ICN but not as individuals. The individual nurse becomes a member if his/her national nurses association is a member of ICN. Nurses in India become members of ICN when they become members of the TNAI.

The Commonwealth Nurses Federation
The Commonwealth Nurses Federation was formally organized in 1973 and operates in six regions of the world which are East, Africa, Atlantic, Australia, Pacific, South Asia and Europe. The TNAI is also affiliated with the Commonwealth Nurses Federation. It is made up of nurses associations from commonwealth countries.

Aims
- Promote sharing, better communications and closer relationships between its member associations.
- Provides expert professional advice
- Scholarships for advanced study
- Financial assistance for professional meetings and seminars
- Running an office through which funds can be received and dispersed for the benefit of nursing in countries which are represented.

The Indian Nursing Council (INC)
The Indian Nursing Council, which was authorized by the Indian Nursing Council Act of 1947, was established in 1949.

Purpose
Providing uniform standards in nursing education and reciprocity in nursing registration throughout the country. Nurses registered in one state were not necessarily recognized for registration in another state before this time. The condition of mutual recognition by the state nurses registration councils, which is called reciprocity, was possible only if uniform standards of nursing education were maintained. **Box 16.8** describes function of INC.

Responsibilities
- Prescribes curricula for nursing education in all the states.
- Refuses or Recognizes Programmes of Nursing Education according to standards required.
- Support high standards in nursing.
- Providing registration for foreign nurses.
- Maintenance of the Indian Nurses Register. This register contains the names of all nurses, midwives, auxiliary nurse midwives who are enrolled on all state registers.

Red Cross Society (Fig. 16.28)
- It follows the directions of the Geneva conventions in an effort to protect victims of armed conflict. Its headquarters is in Geneva, Switzerland.
- They delegate visit and inspect prisoner of war camps. They arrange for delivery of mail and food packages to the prisoners.

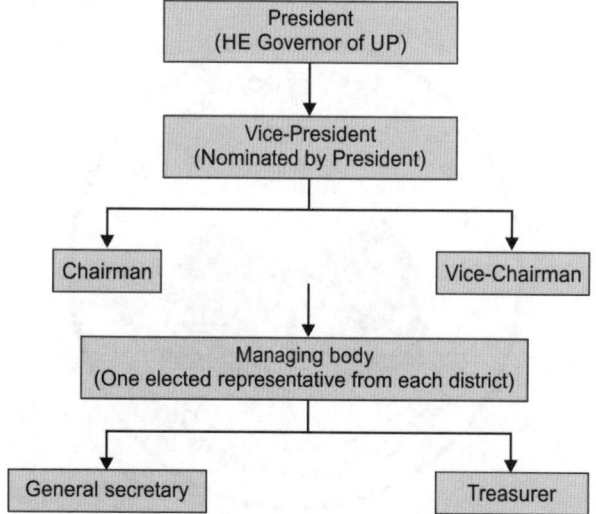

Fig. 16.28: Red Cross Society body members.

- They also offer emergency relief by providing food and medical supplies. A very valuable service is that of a central tracing agency which helps to locate prisoners of war and missing persons long after a conflict is over.
- At times of armed conflict or natural disaster within country these help to give comprehensive care to the affected.

The World Health Organization

- The World Health Organization, commonly called the WHO is also a specialized agency of the United Nations.
- It was organized in 1948 for the purpose of helping to achieve the highest possible level of health for all people
- The WHO has been active in nursing education and practice in a number of ways in India.
- It has offered guidance in setting up programs of Nursing Education. The WHO promotes public health in many ways around the world.
- It is currently known for the declaration of working towards "Health for all by 2000 AD".
- This declaration has given a tremendous push to developing primary healthcare and recognizing the very essential role of nursing in healthcare system.

The Student Nurses Association (SNA) (Fig. 16.29)

The Student Nurses Association organized in 1920, is associated with and under jurisdiction of the TNAI. In addition to providing a means of personal and professional development for the nursing student. The assistant secretary of the TNAI serves as advisor for the SNA.

Purpose and Functions

- Help student nurses learn how the professional organization serves to uphold the dignity and ideals of the nursing profession.
- Promote a close rapport with other student nurses.
- Furnish student nurses advice in their courses of study leading up to professional qualifications.
- Encourages leadership ability and help students to gain a wide knowledge of the nursing profession in all of its different branches.

- Encourage both professional and recreational meetings,
- Encourage students nurses develop a cooperative spirit with other student nurses which will help them in future professional relationships.

Activities

- Fund raising for the TNAI.
- Fund raising done for fine arts and sports competitions and conferences.
- Special prizes given for outstanding achievement in specific areas of nursing education.
- Unit activities include maintaining the diary of unit activities, giving quarterly reports, preparing articles for publication and distributing application forms for membership in the TNAI.

Membership

Fees are minimal and easily met by the nursing student. Nursing students who participate in the Student Nurses Association have a valuable opportunity to begin to develop leadership skills, competitive skills and an interest for the profession as a whole.

The Nurses League of the Clinical Medical Association

The Nurses League of the Clinical Medical Association of India was founded in 1930. It became affiliated to the TNAI in 1936 and promotes membership in this organization.

Objectives

- Promote cooperation and encouragement among Christian nurses.
- Promote efficiency in nursing education and service.
- Secure the highest standards possible in Christian nursing education through the Christian schools of nursing.
- Considering the special work and problems of Christian nurses wherever employed

Activities

- Activities include national and area conferences and retreats for its members.
- Development of leadership abilities is encouraged by participation in these meetings.
- Each meeting also allows for sharing of problems common to the Christian nurse.
- Provides expert professional advice.
- Provides scholarships for advanced study.
- Provides financial assistance for professional meetings and seminars

Membership

Membership fees are required and a life membership is available. Nursing students may become associate members of the league. Membership in the Nurses League may be a requirement for certain nursing positions under control of Christian employing authorities.

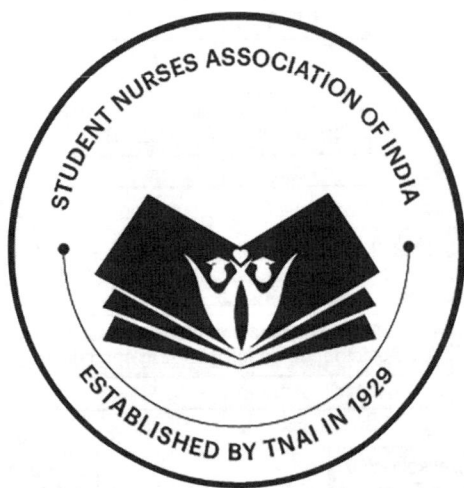

Fig. 16.29: Student Nurses Association of India.

The Christian Medical Association of India (CMAI)

The CMAI began in 1905 as a fellowship of Christian missionary doctors to provide spiritual sharing and support. It gradually developed into a larger organization which included other Christian health professionals and health institutions

Functions

- To provide professional training through formal and informal education, publication of textbooks and other materials and scholarships.
- To encourage community health work through training, advisory services and technical support.
- To assist and support churches and health institutions with study and training.
- To disperse health-related information which will help with health education and lean towards a more healthy and just society?

Membership

Membership is open to doctors, registered nurses and ANM/Health workers, all health professionals. Students in health professional courses may also become members

International Organizations

All nurses work with the treatment of patients, but they often specialize in a specific field. Some of these specialties that nurses may focus on include mental health issues, holistic treatments, female patients or forensics. Professional nurses associations are designed to help these nurses thrive in the nursing specialties by giving them access to the latest research and training.

International Association of Forensic Nurses

- Forensic nurses help investigators solve crimes by treating victims of sexual assault and collecting evidence that can be used in the case.
- They also work in death investigations and treat patients who have been involved in natural disasters.
- The International Association of Forensic Nurses, or IAFN, represents these nurses who contribute to the criminal justice system.
- To help forensic nurses perform the duties of their jobs, the IAFN offers continuing education programs to its members.
- Nurses who pursue these programs can receive certificates in subjects, such as legal nurse consulting, clinical forensics and medicolegal death investigations.

Association of Women's Health, Obstetric and Neonatal Nurses

- The Association of Women's Health, Obstetric and Neonatal Nurses, or AWHONN, is dedicated to nurses who care for women and newborn babies.
- Members of the organization benefit from access to other professionals who work in this field of nursing; the association's publication (The Journal of Obstetric, Gynecologic and Neonatal Nursing) and other publications; and events, such as conventions and education programs.
- In addition, members of AWHONN receive discounts for health, dental and disability insurance plans; financial services, such as tax preparation and financial planning; hotel rooms; entertainment, such as movies and live shows; and car rental services.

American Holistic Nurses Association

- Since 2006, the field of holistic nursing has been recognized as a nursing specialty by the American Nurses Association.
- Nurses who practice this specialty focus on patients' mind, body and spirit when providing treatment.
- The American Holistic Nurses Association, also called the AHNA, services the needs of holistic nurses and has 5,000 members throughout its 160 chapters around the world.
- Members of the AHNA can attend national and local association events; receive publications, such as Journal of Holistic
- Nursing and Connections in Holistic Nursing Research; and attend continuing education classes.

American Psychiatric Nurses Association

- The American Psychiatric Nurses Association was founded in 1986 to benefit nurses who specialize in mental health nursing.
- The organization, also called the APNA, has more than 6,000 members who work around the country.
- The APNA offers member benefits, such as a newsletter (APNA News: The Psychiatric Nursing Voice,) and journal (Journal of the American Psychiatric Nurses Association); an annual conference; and the Annual Clinical Psychopharmacology Institute, which is designed for mental health nurses who wish to pursue training in drug therapies.

American Nurses Association

- The American Nurses Association, or ANA, works to promote the nursing profession and improve the care that patients receive.
- The association, which represents more than three million registered nurses, was founded over 100 years ago. Members of the ANA have access to the association's continuing education programs, social networks, publications (such as a newsletter, The Online Journal of Issues in Nursing and The American Nurse) and insurance plans.

■ COLLECTIVE BARGAINING (FIG. 16.30)

An individual is free to bargain for himself and safeguard his own interest. The phrase collective bargaining consists of two words 'collective' which implies-group action through its representative and 'bargaining' which suggests negotiation. The phrase, therefore, implies collective negotiations of a contract between management's representatives on one side and those of the workers on the other.

Chapter 16: Organizational Behavior and Human Relations

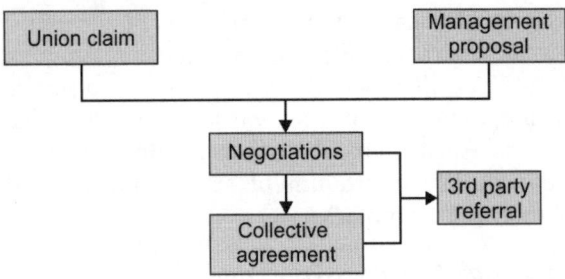

Fig. 16.30: Process of collective bargaining.

This collective bargaining is that arrangement whereby the wages and conditions of the employment of workmen are settled through a bargain between the employer and the workmen collectively, whether represented through their union or by some of them on behalf of all of them.

Definition

According to Marquis and Huston, 2006, collective bargaining may be defined as "activities occurring between organized labor and management that concern employee relations. Such activities include negotiation of formal legal agreements and day to day interactions between unions and management.

Meaning

Collective bargaining is a procedure by which the terms and conditions of employment of workers are regulated by agreements between their bargaining agents and the employers.

Purpose

- The main purpose of collective bargaining is the settlement of industrial disputes or conflicts relating to wages.
- It harmonizes labor relations.
- It promotes industrial enterprise peace by creating equality of bargaining power between the labor and the management.
- It improves working conditions.
- It prevents workers from getting into unfair treatment.

Historical

Nurses in the early 1900s were frustrated by their working conditions. Receiving little support from the established nursing organizations, a few thousand joined trade unions for assistance. In the 1940s nurses in California, Ohio, and Pennsylvania were assisted in the workplaces by the American Nurses Association. One well known independent union is the committee for the recognition of Nursing Achievement at Stanford University in Palo Alto, California formed in 1964; this union has had a successful history of working closely with nursing administration to advance nursing standards and nurse recognition. In the United States, the fraction of all workers represented by a labor organization is declining.

Unions in Bargaining

A union or labor organization is any organization in which employees participate for the purpose of dealing with their employer about grievances, labor disagreements, wages, hours of work and conditions of employment.

Table 16.2 describes advantages and disadvantages of collective bargaining.

Table 16.2: Advantages and disadvantages of collective bargaining.

Sl. No.	Advantages	Disadvantages
1.	Equalization of power between administrators and staff associates can be obtained	Adversary relationship may develop between administration and staff associates
2.	Grievance reporting procedures become possible	Strikes may not be prevented
3.	Staffing for systematic and equitable distribution of work can be established	Unions can interfere with the management of the organization
4.	Professionalism can be promoted	Unionization is considered unprofessional by many nurses
5.	Nurses gain control of practice	Leadership for unions may be difficult to obtain because many professional nurses have little experience in positions of authority

Objectives of Unions

- **Wages:** Employees and their union can be expected to ask for wages which are comparable to those in similar jobs in the local market.
- **Promotions:** Unions will insist that length of service be a factor in promotions.
- **Layoffs:** The union will insist that seniority play a part in regulating layoffs; qualifications being equal, the junior service employees will be paid off first.
- **Discipline:** Employees will be disciplined for just cause; this is standard in all labor agreements.
- **Grievances procedures:** The union will insist that a grievance procedure be established whereby management decisions will be reviewable by representatives of management and the union; if there is still disagreements, the dispute will be referred to arbitration.
- **Fringe benefits:** Pensions, vacations and holidays, social insurance, and general welfare programs will be part of the negotiations, with an attempt to make them comparable to the trend in our society.

Unions in India: Nurses unions or their collective bargaining power is the most vital and indirect determinant of working conditions. Strong union and its bargaining strength determine the conditions and facilities of work.

At present three unions of nurses are working at the central level.
1. All India Government Nurses Federation (AIGNF)
2. Trained Nurses' Union (TNU) and
3. Trained Nurses Association of India (TNAI)

Besides, there are two state level unions, namely,
1. Orissa Nursing Employee's Association (ONEA),
2. Trained Nurses Association of India, Orissa branch.

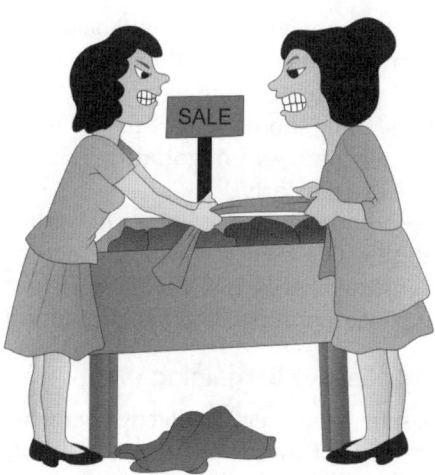

Fig. 16.31: Collective bargaining.

COLLECTIVE BARGAINING (FIG. 16.31)

Collective bargaining is the negotiation between the employer and employee to have smooth functioning of organization. It is important to have control over the demands of employees and autocratic behavior of employer and manager.

Collective bargaining is the way by which employee redress their grievances and asks the employer to fulfill their needs. By this strikes can be avoided. Collective bargaining usually occurs between leaders of association or representatives of employees and the management or employer.

History of Collective Bargaining

- The term "collective bargaining" was first used in 1891 by Beatrice Webb, a founder of the field of industrial relations in Britain.
- It refers to the sort of collective negotiations and agreements that had existed since the rise of trade unions during the 18th century.
- In the United States, the National Labor Relations Act of 1935 made it illegal for any employer to deny union rights to an employee.
- The issue of unionizing government employees in a public sector trade union was much more controversial until the 1950s.
- In 1962, President John F Kennedy issued an executive order granting Federal employees the right to unionize.

Definition

- According to Beach, "Collective Bargaining is concerned with the relations between unions reporting employees and employers (or their representatives).
- According to Stevens to Collective Bargaining as a 'social control technique for reflecting and transmitting the basic power relationships which underlie the conflict of interest in an industrial relations system.'
- According to JH Richardson "Collective bargaining takes place when a number of work people enter into a negotiation as a bargaining unit with an employer or group of employer with the object of reaching an agreement on conditions of the employment of the work people. Collective bargaining is a complex process. It involves psychology, politics and power.
- According to Flippo, "Collective Bargaining is a process in which the representatives of a labor organization and the representatives of business organization meet and attempt to negotiate a contract or agreement, which specifies the nature of employee-employer union relationship".
- Richardson says, "Collective bargaining takes place when a number of work people enter into negotiation as a bargaining unit with an employer or a group of employers with the object of reaching agreement on conditions of the employment of the work people".

Meaning of Bargaining

- The term collective bargaining is made up of two words, 'collective'—which means a 'group action' through representation and 'bargaining', means 'negotiating', which involves proposals and counter-proposals, offers and counter-offers.
- Thus it means collective negotiations between the employer and the employee, relating to their work situations.
- The success of these negotiations depends upon mutual understanding and give and take principles between the employers and employees.
- A process of discussion and negotiation between two parties, one or both of whom is a group of persons acting in concert more specifically it is the procedure by which an employer or employers and a group of employees agree upon the conditions of works.

Objectives of Collective Bargaining (Box 16.9)

Collective bargaining has benefits not only for the present, but also for the future. The objectives of collective bargaining are:
- To provide an opportunity to the workers, to voice their problems on issues related to employment
- To facilitate reaching a solution that is acceptable to all the parties involved
- To resolve all conflicts and disputes in a mutually agreeable manner.

Box 16.9: Objectives of collective bargaining.

Collective bargaining has benefits not only for the present, but also for the future.
The objectives of collective bargaining are:
- To provide an opportunity to the workers, to voice their problems on issues related to employment.
- To facilitate reaching a solution that is acceptable to all the parties involves.
- To resolve all conflicts and disputes in a mutually agreeable manner.
- To prevent any conflict/disputes in the future through mutually signed contracts.
- To develop a conductive atmosphere to foster good organizations relations.
- To provide stable and peaceful organization (hospital) relations.
- To enhance the productivity of the organization by preventing strikes lock-out, etc.

- To prevent any conflict/disputes in the future through mutually singed contracts
- To develop a conductive atmosphere to foster good organizations relations.
- To provide stable and peaceful organization (hospital) relations.
- To enhance the productivity of the organization by preventing strikes lock-out, etc.

Essential Pre-requisites for Collective Bargaining (Boxes 16.10 and 16.11)

Effective collective bargaining requires the following pre-requisites:

- Existence of a strong representative trade union in the industry that believes in constitutional means for settling the disputes.
- Existence of a fact-finding approach and willingness to use new methods and tools for the solution of industrial problems. The negotiation should be based on facts and figures and both the parties should adopt constructive approach.
- Existence of strong and enlightened management which can integrate the different parties, i.e., employees, owners, consumers and society or government.
- Agreement on basic objectives of the organization between the employer and the employees and on mutual rights and liabilities should be there.
- In order that collective bargaining functions properly, unfair labor practices must be avoided by both the parties.
- Proper records for the problem should be maintained.
- Collective bargaining should be best conducted at plant level. It means if there are more than one plant of the firm, the local management should be delegated proper authority to negotiate with the local trade union.
- There must be change in the attitude of employers and employees. They should realize that differences can be resolved peacefully on negotiating table without the assistance of third party.
- No party should take rigid attitude. They should enter into negotiation with a view to reaching an agreement.
- When agreement is reached after negotiations, it must be in writing incorporating all term of the contract.

Features of Collective Bargaining

Some of the salient features of collective bargaining are:

- **It is a group action:** Collective bargaining is a group action as opposed to individual action. Both the parties of settlement are represented by their groups
- **It is a continuous process:** Collective bargaining is a continuous process and does not end with one agreement. It provides a mechanism for continuing and organized relationship between management and trade union. It is a process that goes on for 365 days of the year.
- **It is a bipartite process:** Collective bargaining is a two party process. Both the parties-employers and employees-collectively take some action. There is no intervention of any third party.
- **It is a process:** Collective bargaining is a process in the sense that it consists of a number of steps. The starting point is the presentation of charter of demands by the workers and the last step is the reaching of an agreement, or a contract which would serve as the basic law governing labor-management relations over a period of time in an enterprise.
- **It is flexible and mobile and not fixed or static:** It has fluidity. There is no hard and fast rule for reaching an agreement. There is ample scope for compromise. A spirit of give-and-take works unless final agreement acceptable to both the parties is reached.
- **It is industrial democracy at work:** Collective bargaining is based on the principle of industrial democracy where the labor union represents the workers in negotiations with the employer or employers.
- **It is dynamic:** It is relatively a new concept, and is growing, expanding and changing. In the past, it used to be emotional, turbulent and sentimental, but now it is scientific, factual and systematic.
- **It is a complementary and not a competitive process:** Collective bargaining is not a competitive process, i.e., labor and management do not co-opt while negotiating for the same object.
- **It is an art:** Collective bargaining is an art, an advanced form of human relations.

Box 16.12 describes characteristics of collective bargaining.

Principles of Collective Bargaining (Box 16.13)

For Union and Management

- Collective bargaining should be made an education as well as a bargaining process. It should offer to trade union

---

Box 16.10: Pre-requisites for successful collective bargaining.

- A favorable political climate
- Freedom of association
- Willingness to give and take
- Fair labor practices
- Problem solving attitude
- Continuous dialogue
- Availability of data
- Strong independent and well organized unions
- Recognition of the union as the bargaining agent
- Mutual trust and good faith

Box 16.11: Importance of collective bargaining.

Importance to employees

- Collective bargaining develops a sense of self-respect and responsibility among the employees.
- It increases the strength of the workforce, thereby, increasing their bargaining capacity as a group.
- Collective bargaining increases the morale and productivity of employees.
- It restricts management's freedom for arbitrary action against the employees. Moreover, unilateral actions by the employer are also discouraged.
- Effective collective bargaining machinery strengthens the trade unions movement.

> **Box 16.12:** Characteristics of collective bargaining.
> - **Collective:** Collective bargaining is a two way group process where the employers representative and employees representatives sit together to negotiate terms of employment.
> - **Strength:** Both the parties in collective bargaining are strong and equal.
> - **Voluntary:** Both parties come to the negotiation table voluntarily in order to go in particular negotiation. It is based on discussion, mutual trust and understanding.
> - **Formal:** It is a formal process in which certain employment related issues are to be regulated at national, organization and workplace levels.
> - **Flexible:** It is a flexible and continuous process and not fixed or static.

> **Box 16.13:** Principles of collective bargaining.
> - The management should always deal only with one association or trade union in the organization.
> - The management must have the mutual agreement to the trade union without any conflict.
> - The management should treat the trade union without any partiality.
> - The management should regularly evaluate the rules and regulation to determine the attitude and degree of comfort of its employees.
> - The management should be place vital importance on social consideration.

leaders an opportunity to present to the management the wants, desires, grievances and attitudes of its employees and make it possible for the management to explain to union leaders and through them, to its employees the economic problems which it is confronted with.
- There must be mutual confidence and good faith, and a desire to make collective bargaining effective in practice.
- There should be an honest, able and responsible leadership, for only this kind of leadership make collective bargaining effective and meaningful.
- The management and trade union must look upon collective bargaining as a means of finding the best possible solution, and not as a means of acquiring as much as one can while conceding the minimum. There must be an honest attempt at solving problems.
- Both parties to a dispute should command the respect of each other and should have enough bargaining power to enforce the terms of the agreement that they may arrive at.
- The two parties should meticulously observe and abide by all the national and state laws which are applicable to collective bargaining.
- Both parties must bear in mind the fact that collective bargaining is, in a sense, a form of price fixation and that the success of any collective bargaining depends, in the final analysis, on whether the management and the trade union do a good job of ensuring that the price of labor is properly adjusted to other prices.

For the Management
- The management must develop and consistently follow a realistic labor policy, which should be accepted and carried out by its representatives.
- The management must grant recognition to the trade union without any reservations and accept it as a constructive force in the organization.
- The management should not wait for the trade union to bring employee grievances to its notice but should rather create the conditions in which employees can approach the management themselves, without involving the trade union.
- The management should deal only with one trade union in the organization.
- The management should not assume that employee goodwill will always exist. It should periodically examine the rules and regulations to determine the attitudes and degree of comfort of its employees and gain their goodwill and cooperation.
- The management should extend fair treatment to the trade union in order to make it a responsible and conservative body.
- While weighing the economic consequences of collective. Bargaining, the management should place greater emphasis on social considerations.

Collective Bargaining Process (Fig. 16.32)

The collective bargaining process comprises of five core steps:
1. **Prepare:** This phase involves composition of a negotiation team. The negotiation team should consist of representatives of both the parties with adequate knowledge and skills for negotiation. In this phase, both the employer's representatives and the union examine their own situation in order to develop the issues that they believe will be most important. The first thing to be done is to determine whether there is actually any reason to negotiate at all. A correct understanding of the main issues to be covered and intimate knowledge of operations, working conditions, production norms and other relevant conditions is required.
2. **Discuss:** Here, the parties decide the ground rules that will guide the negotiations. A process well begun is half done and this is no less true in case of collective bargaining. An environment of mutual trust and understanding is also created so that the collective bargaining agreement would be reached.

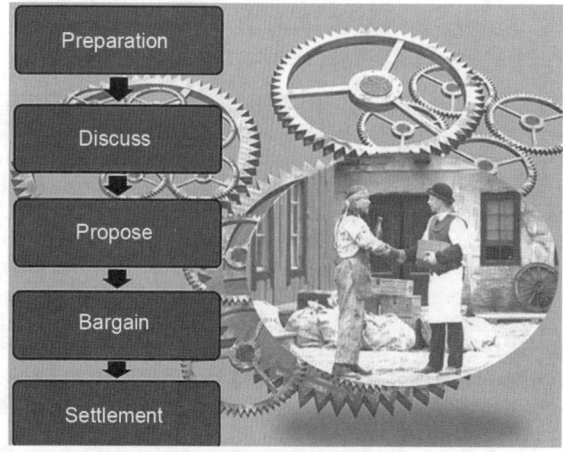

Fig. 16.32: Collective bargaining process.

3. **Propose:** This phase involves the initial opening statements and the possible options that exist to resolve them. In a word, this phase could be described as 'brainstorming'. The exchange of messages takes place and opinion of both the parties is sought.
4. **Bargain:** negotiations are easy if a problem solving attitude is adopted. This stage comprises the time when 'what ifs' and 'supposals' are set forth and the drafting of agreements take place.
5. **Settlement:** Once the parties are through with the bargaining process, a consensual agreement is reached upon wherein both the parties agree to a common decision regarding the problem or the issue. This stage is described as consisting of effective joint implementation of the agreement through shared visions, strategic planning and negotiated change.

Types of Collective Bargaining (Fig. 16.33 and Box 16.14)

- **Distributive bargaining:** Distributive bargaining is defined as a negotiation process by which one party benefits at the others expense. This usually refers to the redistribution of income in the form of higher wages, higher bonuses, or higher financial benefits.
- **Integrative bargaining:** Integrative bargaining is whereby both sides aim to benefit in what is seen as 'win-win' bargaining. Both parties may bring together a list of demands by which an agreement is reached that benefits both parties.
- **Productivity bargaining:** Productivity bargaining involves both parties negotiating around productivity and pay. So unions may suggest that higher salaries would boost productivity. However, this is unknown to the business.
- **Composite bargaining:** Composite bargaining refers to a negotiation that focuses on a number of elements that are not related to pay. They are generally related to employee welfare and job security.
- **Concessionary bargaining:** Concessionary bargaining is based on unions giving back previous benefits to the employer. For instance, trade unions may agree to lower wages in return for job security.

Functions of Collective Bargaining (Box 16.15 and Fig. 6.34)

Professor Butler has viewed the functions as:
1. A process of social change
2. A peace treaty between two parties
3. A system of industrial jurisprudence

I. **Collective bargaining as a process of social change**
   - Collective bargaining enhances the status of the working class in the society. Wage earners have enhanced their social and economic position in relation to other groups.
   - Employers have also retained high power and dignity through collective bargaining.

II. **Collective bargaining as a peace treaty:** Collective bargaining serves as a peace treaty between the employers and employees. However, the settlement between the two parties is a compromise.

III. **Collective bargaining as an industrial jurisprudence:** Collective bargaining creates a system of "Industrial

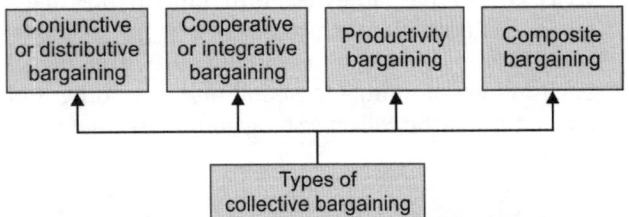

Fig. 16.33: Types of collective bargaining.

> **Box 16.14:** Types of bargaining.
> - **Distributive bargaining:** Under it, the economic issues, such as wages, salaries and bonus are discussed. In distributive bargaining, one party's gain is another party's loss.
> - **Integrative bargaining:** This involves negotiation of an issue on which both the parties may gain, or at least neither party loses.
> - **Attitudinal restructuring:** This involves shaping and reshaping some attitudes, such as trust or distrust, friendliness or hostility between labor and management.
> - **Intra-organizational bargaining:** It generally aims at resolving internal conflicts. This is a type of maneuvering to achieve consensus with the workers and management. Even within the union, there may be differences between groups.

> **Box 16.15:** Function of collective bargaining.
> - Collective bargaining is a process of decision making and mechanism for belonging the power between the employer and employee.
> - Working together, sharing together, deciding together and earning together.
> - It helps to promote the cooperation and mutual understanding between workers and management.
> - It establish uniform condition for employment.
> - It promote stability and prosperity.
> - It increase the economic strength of employee and management.
> - Provide fair rate of wages and amenities for workers.
> - Promote prompt redressal of grievances
> - It provide a solution to industrial sickness.
> - It provide new methods of employment regulatory condition.

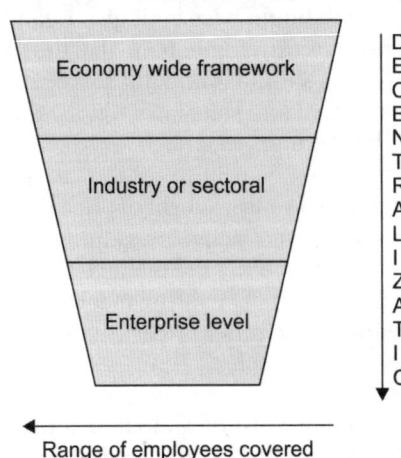

Fig. 16.34: Functions of collective bargaining.

Jurisprudence". It is a method of introducing civil rights into industry. It establishes rules which define and restrict the traditional authority exercised by employers over their employees placing part of the authority under joint control of union and management. In addition to the above, its functions include:
- Increasing the economic strength to employers and employers.
- Improving working conditions and fair wages.
- Maintaining peace in industry
- Prompt and fair redressel of grievances.
- Promoting stability and prosperity of the industry.

Levels of Collective Bargaining

Collective bargaining operates at three levels
1. **National level:** It is a bipartite or tripartite negotiation between union confederations, central employer associations and government agencies. It provides a floor level bargaining on terms of employment, often taken into consideration macroeconomic goals.

    Economy-wide (national) bargaining is a bipartite or tripartite form of negotiation between union confederations, central employer associations and government agencies. It aims at providing a floor for lower-level bargaining on the terms of employment, often taking into account macroeconomic goals.
2. **Sectoral bargaining:** It accounts for standardization of terms of employment in one industry, includes a range of bargaining patterns.
3. **Company level:** This is a supplementary type of bargaining. It emphasizes the point that bargaining levels need not be mutually exclusive.

Advantages of Collective Bargaining

- It is flexible and mobile and not fixed or static.
- It has fluidity or ample scope for compromise.
- It is a complementary process not competitive.
- It helps in achieving better planning.
- It allows smooth functioning of organization.
- It retents the employee in organization.
- It encourages less strike.
- It helps in managing conflicts.

Important Functions of Collective Bargaining

Collective bargaining includes not only negotiations between the employers and unions but also includes the process of resolving labor-management conflicts.

Thus, collective bargaining is, essentially, a recognized way of creating a system of industrial jurisprudence. It acts as a method of introducing civil rights in the industry, that is, the management should be conducted by rules rather than arbitrary decision making. It establishes rules which define and restrict the traditional authority exercised by the management.
- **It is a rule-making or legislative process** in the sense that it formulates terms and conditions under which labor and management will cooperate and work together over a certain stated period.
- **It is also a judicial process,** tar in every collective agreement there is a provision or clause regarding the interpretation of the agreement and how any difference of opinion about the intention or scope of a particular clause is to be resolved. Such interpretation can be left to a joint committee of worker's and management representative or the top level management or to a third party jointly selected by the trade union and the management.
- **It is also an executive process,** for both the management and the trade unions undertake to implement the agreement signed, each accepting a series of obligations under the agreement.

Pros and Cons of Collective Bargaining

Pros

- Can lead to high-performance workplace where labor and management jointly engage in problem solving, addressing issues on an equal standing.
- Provides legally based bilateral relationship.
- Management's rights are clearly spelled out.
- Employers' and employees' rights protected by binding collective bargaining agreement.
- Multi-year contracts may provide budgetary predictability on salary and other compensation issues.
- Unions may become strong allies in protecting higher education from the effects of an economic slowdown.
- Promotes fairness and consistency in employment policies and personnel decisions within and across institutions.
- Employees may choose whether they want union representation.
- A strong labor management partnership may enable the workforce development needed for engaging the technology revolution.

Box 16.16 describes disadvantages of bargaining.

Cons

- Management's authority and freedom are much more restricted by negotiated rules.
- Creates significant potential for polarization between employees and managers.
- Disproportionate effect of relatively few active employees on the many in the bargaining unit. This is particularly the case when collective bargaining involves a system-wide structure of elections.
- Increases bureaucratization and requires longer time needed for decision making.
- Increases participation by external entities (e.g., arbitrators, State Labor Relations Board) in higher education's decision making.

Box 16.16: Disadvantages.
- Reduced individuality.
- Other union members may outvote one's decisions.
- Disputes are not handled with individual and management only.
- Must pay union dues even if one does not support unionization.

- Protects the status quo, thereby inhibiting innovation and change. This is particularly the case when the change involves privatizations.
- More difficult for employees at smaller campuses to have their voices heard.
- Higher management costs associated with negotiating and administering the agreements.
- Eliminates ability of management to make unilateral changes in wages, hours, and other terms and conditions of employment.
- Restricts management's ability to deal directly with individual employees.
- Increased dependence on the private sector for certain services, particularly those requiring technological competence, may be compromised.
- Contract administration is a very difficult process to manage and significantly changes the skill set required of managers and supervisors.

> **Box 16.17:** Key elements of motivation.
> - **Intensity:** Refers to the level of effort provided by the employee in the attempt to achieve the goal assigned to him. Refers to how hard a person tries to do work.
> - **Direction:** Relates to what an individual chooses to do when he is confronted with a number of possible choices.
> - **Persistence:** A dimension of motivation which measures how long a person can maintain effort to achieve the organization's goals.

MOTIVATION

The human behavior is controlled, directed and modified through certain motives, when a person is hungry and is searching for food or constructing a house or mating or learning new skills, we will always be able to trace some such elements which his activities, guide them and his behavior in the lights of his success or failures.

Motivation is that force which impels or incites individual's action, determines the individual's direction of action and his rate of action. When the individual gets any motives, he experiences a tension and disequilibrium and becomes restless. His activities are then initiated. The individual feels a push to behave in a certain direction (**Fig. 16.35**).

Meaning of Motivation

- Motivation is something which prompts, compels and energizes an individual to act or behave in a particular fashion at a particular time for attaining some specific goal or purpose.
- The term 'Motivation' has been derived from the word 'Motive'. A motive is an inner state that activities, energizes or moves an individual and channelizes his behavior towards goals.
- Motivation is the art of understanding these motives and satisfying them to direct and sustain behavior towards the accomplishment of organizational goal.
- Motivation is concerned with how behavior gets started, is energized, sustained, directed and stopped. As motivation is the process of inspiring and impelling people to take required actions by providing stimuli that satisfy their needs and motives.
- Motivation is the complex of forces which propel an individual into action and keep them at work. It reflects the will to work.
- Motivation is defined as the process that initiates, guides and maintains goal-oriented behaviors. Motivation is what causes us to act, whether it is getting a glass of water to reduce thirst or reading a book to gain knowledge.

Definition

- According to Scott, "Motivation means a process of stimulating people to action to accomplish desired goals. It refers to the way in which urges, drives, desires, aspirations, stirrings or needs direct, control or explain the behavior of human being."
- According to Brech, "Motivation is an inspirational process which impels the members of the team to pull their weight effectively, to give their loyalty to the group, to carry out properly the tasks that they have accepted and generally to play an effective part in the job that the group has undertaken.
- Stephen P Robbins, "Motivation is the willingness to exert high levels of effort toward organizational goals, conditioned by the effort's ability to satisfy some individual needs.
- According to the Encyclopedia, "Motivation refers to the degree of readiness of an organism to pursue some designated goal, and implies the determination of the nature and laws of the focus including the degree of readiness.

Nature of Motivation

- Motivation is a psychological concept. It is concerned with the intrinsic forces operating within an individual which impel him or act or not to act in a particular way.
- Motivation is a dynamic and continuous process as it deals with human being which is an ever changing entity modifying itself every moment.

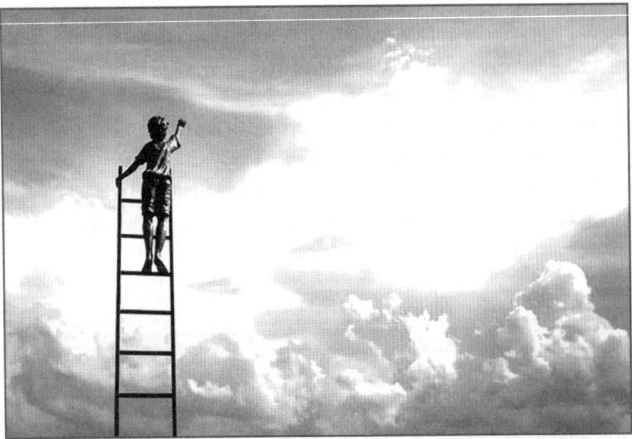

Fig. 16.35: Concept of motivation.

- Motivation is a complex and difficult function. Every person adopts a different approach to satisfy his needs and one particular need may cause different behavior on the part of different people.
- Motivation is a circular process. Feeling of an unsatisfied need causes tension and an individual takes action (drive) to reduce this tension.
- Motivation is different from satisfaction. Motivation is the process of stimulating an individual or a group to take desired action.
- Motivation is the product of anticipated value from a given course of action and the perceived probability that the action will lead to these values.

Elements of Motivation (Box 16.17)

The three key elements in motivation are intensity, direction, and persistence:
1. **Intensity:** It describes how hard a person tries. This is the element most of us focus on when we talk about motivation.
2. **Direction:** High intensity is unlikely to lead to favorable job-performance outcomes unless the effort is channeled in a direction that benefits the organization. Therefore, the quality of effort as well as its intensity matters. Effort directed toward, and consistent with, the organization's goals is the kind of effort once should be seeking.
3. **Persistence:** It measures how long a person can maintain effort. Motivated individuals stay with a task long enough to achieve their goal.

Process of Motivation (Fig. 16.36)

Motivation concerns those processes which produces goal-directed behavior. The basic elements of the process of motivation are:
- **Behavior:** All behavior is a series of activities. Behavior is generally motivated by a desire to achieve a goal. In order to predict and control behavior managers must understand the motives of people.
- **Motives:** Motives prompt people to action. They are the primary energizers of behavior. They are the 'ways' of behavior and mainsprings of action. They are largely subjective and represent the mental feelings of human beings. They are cognitive variables. They cause behavior in many ways. They arise continuously and determine the general direction of an individual's behavior.
- **Goals:** Motives are directed toward goals. Motives generally create a state of disequilibrium, physiological or psychological imbalance, within the individuals. Attaining a goal will tend to restore physiological or psychological balance. Goals are the ends which provide satisfaction of human wants. They are outside an individual; they are hoped for incentives toward which needs are directed. One person may satisfy his need for power by kicking subordinates and another by becoming the president of a company. Thus, a need can be satisfied by several alternate goals.

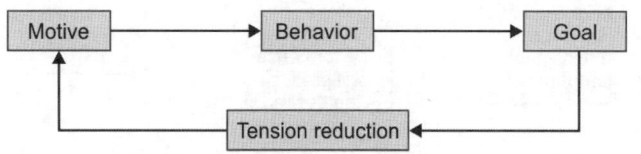

Fig. 16.36: Process of motivation.

Types of Motivation

Motivation may be classified on following bases: 1. Positive or negative, 2. Extrinsic and intrinsic and 3. Financial or non-financial
- **Positive motivation:** It is the process of attempting to influence the employees' behavior through recognition and appreciation of employees' efforts and contribution towards achievement of organizational goal. Examples of positive motivators are—taking interest in subordinate's benefits, appreciation and credit for work done, delegating the authority and responsibility of subordinates, etc.
- **Negative motivation:** It is based upon fear, i.e., demotion, lay off, etc. The fear of punishment affects the behavior towards changes. Though punishment has resulted in controlling the misbehavior and contributed towards positive performance, but it may also lead to poor performance and lower productivity extrinsic and intrinsic motivation.
- **Extrinsic motivation:** It arises away from the job. It does not occur on the job. These factors include wages, fringe benefits, medical reimbursement, etc. Thus, they are generally associated with financial incentives.
- **Intrinsic motivation:** This type of motivation occurs on the job and provides satisfaction during the performance of work itself. Intrinsic or internal motivators include recognition, status, authority, participation, etc., financial and non-financial motivation.
- **Financial motivation:** It is associated with money. It includes wages and salaries, fringe benefits, bonus, retirement benefits, etc.
- **Non-financial motivation:** This type of motivation is not associated with monetary rewards. It includes intangible incentives, such as ego satisfaction, self-actualization and responsibility.

Theories of Motivation (Fig. 16.37)

I. Drive Reduction Theory (Fig. 16.38)
- One of the earlier theories of motivation was the drive reduction theory. It was proposed by Clark Hull.
- This theory proposes that organisms' experiences the arousal of a drive when an important need is not satisfied, and they engage in behavior to reduce the arousal and satisfy the need.
- Primary drives are those that motivate the organism to fulfill some basic need necessary for its survival, such as hunger, thirst or sex.
- An important component of the drive reduction theory is homeostasis. The term homeostasis refers to a state of

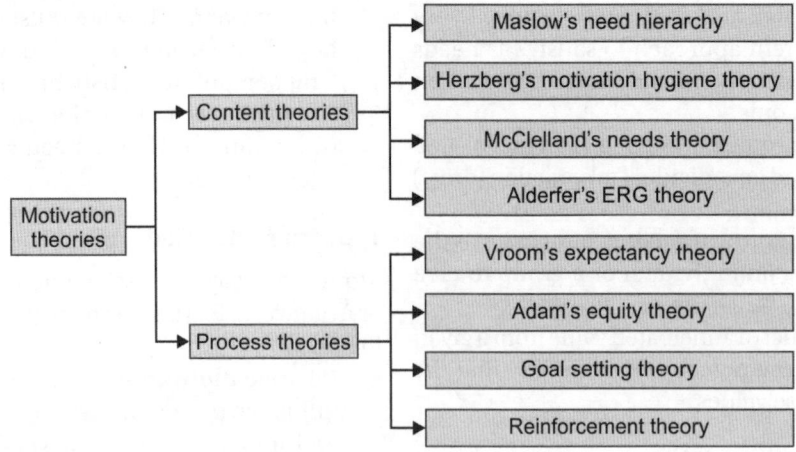

Fig. 16.37: Motivation theories.

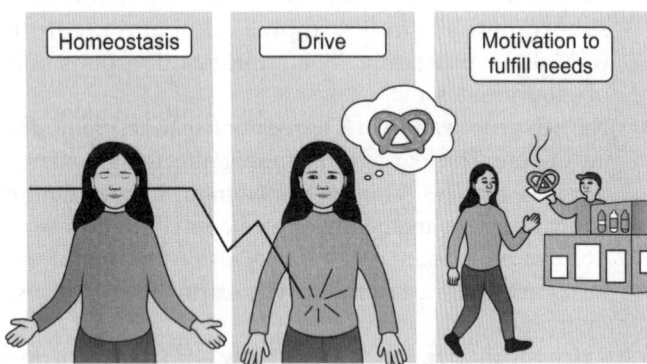

Fig. 16.38: Hull's drive-reduction theory.

balance or equilibrium necessary in many physiological systems.
- Primary drives are biological drives necessary for personal and species survival. Acquired drives develop through learning.
- The drive is the force that motivates an organism to action. Which action the organism finally performs depends on the strength of the organism's habit.
- A habit is a response to some stimulus. The strength of the habit depends on the connection between the stimulus and the response that influences what kind of behavior the drive will energize.

II. Optimum Level of Arousal Theory

- The optimum level of Arousal theory states that drives do not necessarily motivate an organism to seek the lowest level or arousal. Instead they provide motivation to seek an optimum level of arousal.
- Robert Uerles and JD Dodson (1908) conducted an experiment to examine the effects of different arousal levels on learning. They varied arousal levels in mice by changing the intensity of electric shocks and by observing how well the animals performed in simple and complex mazes.
- The Yerkes—Dodson law states that performance on a learning task is related to arousal; the best performance results from intermediate levels of arousal. Performance is also related to the difficulty of the task.

- Yerkes and Dodson found that the mice performed simple tasks better when the stimulation was more intense. For complex tasks, low to intermediate arousal was the best.

III. Cognitive Theories

- A cognitive theory (the word comes from the Latin for knowing) emphasizes some sort of understanding or anticipation of events through perception or thought or judgment as in the estimation of probabilities or in making a choice on the basis of relative value.
- Any organism with memory is capable of recognizing some similarities between the present and the past and hence is able to form some sort of experience with regard to the consequences of its behavior.
- According to a cognitive theory, motivated goal seeking behavior comes to be regulated by these conditions, which are based on the past, modified by circumstances of the present and includes expectations about the future.
- Cognitive Dissonance theory: Festinger (1957) proposed a theory in which certain kinds of unbalanced cognitions are described as dissonant and the subject is under stress to remove this dissonance.

IV. Expectancy Theory (Fig. 16.39)

- Expectancy theory emphasizes the importance of rewards and goals as well as how person's expectations of consequences can influence his behavior. This theory stresses 'pull' rather than 'push'.
- According to expectancy theory, the hunger drive is only part of the reason a hungry rat is motivated to find its way

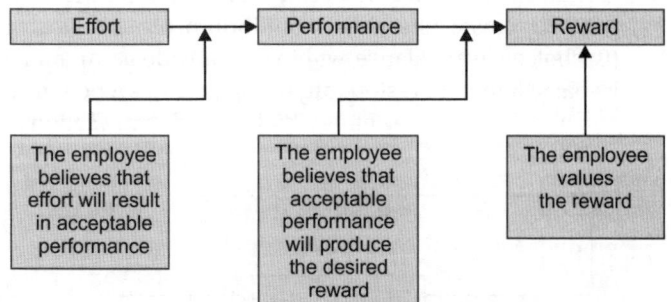

Fig. 16.39: Expectancy theory.

through a maze. It is also motivated because of previous learning experiences in which it has come to expect a bit of food at the end.

- Motivation is composed of two major features: the valence or attractiveness of the goal and the expectancy or the likelihood that its behavior will lead to the goal.
- A simple way of explaining the expectancy theory is to say that; motivation = valence X expectancy. The actions that hungry people take to satisfy their hunger depend very much on valence and expectancy.
- Economic theories assume that the individual can assign value or utility to possible incentives and that he makes his decision according to the risk involved.

V. Psychoanalytic Theory of Modification

- Freud believed that all behavior stemmed from two opposing groups of instincts. The life instincts (Eros) that enhance life and growth and the death instincts (Thanatos) that pushes toward destruction.
- The energy of the life instincts is libido, which involves mainly sex and related activities. The death instinct can be directed inward in the form of aggression towards others. Freud pointed to several forms of behavior:-
  - In dreams, we often express wishes and impulses of which we are unaware.
  - Unconscious mannerisms and slips of speech may reveal hidden motives.
  - Symptoms of illness (particularly symptoms of mental illness) often can be shown to serve the unconscious needs of the person.

VI. Maslow's Hierarchy of Needs

- The behavior of an individual at a particular moment is usually determined by his strongest need. These needs nave a certain priority.
- The lower level needs (e.g., physiological needs) have the highest strength until they are reasonably met. When the lower level needs are met, man goes to satisfy the higher needs.
- The hierarchy needs organized step by step to the satisfaction of other needs—physiological needs, safety and security needs, social needs, esteem needs and self-actualization needs. A satisfied need is no longer a motivator of behavior.

VII. Hertzberg's Two Factor Theory

- According to Hertzberg, there are ten factors called maintenance factors and six factors called motivational factors or satisfactory.
- The absence of maintenance factors cause dissatisfaction in the employees, but their presence may not produce motivation in the employees.
- The presence of motivational factors is necessary to produce motivation and job satisfaction in the individual but their absence may not produce strong dissatisfaction.
- The maintenance factors are—policy and management, supervision, good interpersonal relationship with supervisor, good IPR with peers, and subordinates, fair salary, Job security, personal life, good working conditions and status.
- The motivational factors are achievement, recognition, work itself, advancement, and responsibility.
- The Hertzberg model has given several insights. One of the insights is job enrichment. The idea behind job enrichment is to keep maintenance factors constant or higher while increasing motivational factors by attaching more responsibility satisfying working conditions and power to the job.

Figure 16.40 shows relationship between Hertzberg and Maslow models.

VIII. McClelland's Needs Theory

- McClelland' identified three types of basic motivating needs. They are need for power, need for affiliation and need for achievement.
- Power motive is the need to manipulate others or the drive for superiority over others. Such individuals are generally seeking positions for leadership.
- The affiliation motive is concerned with maintaining pleasant social relationships, sense of intimacy and understanding and enjoy in consoling and helping others who are in trouble.
- Achievement motivated people can be the back bone of most organizations, because they progress faster. They are highly task oriented and work to their optimum capacity.

IX. Carrot and Stick Approach of Motivation

- Carrot and stick approach of motivation comes from the old story that the best way to make a donkey move is to put a carrot out in front of him or beat him with a stick from behind.
- The carrot is the reward for moving and the stick is the punishment for not moving.
- In motivating people for better production in an organization some carrots (rewards) are used, such as money, promotion and other incentives.
- Some sticks (punishments) are used to push the people for desired behavior or to retrain from undesired behavior.

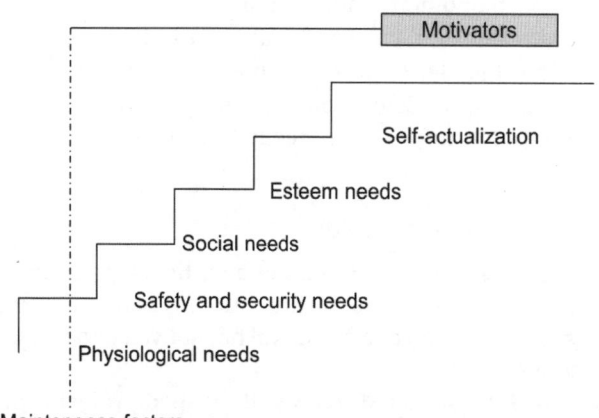

Fig. 16.40: Relationship between Hertzberg and Maslow Models.

Motivational Qualities of Nurse Leader

- **Knowledge and skill, effective communication** of ideas, confidence, commitment, energy, insight into the needs of others and an ability to take the action necessary to achieve goals important to others.
- **Knowledge and skill:** Comes from preparation in the responsibilities of healthcare delivery and organizational duty. This leader has the ability to evaluate the likelihood of success in accomplishing goals, and is able to support or suggest changes.
- **Effective communication of ideas:** Involves the ability to convey ideas clearly and in such a way that they can be heard positively.
- **Confidence:** Comes from an internal sense of security that one is competent to make a statement or take action, and that there is a reasonable chance of success in accomplishing something of value. The motivational leader is secure enough to have a lower need to control and as a result is able to encourage autonomy, participation and the empowerment of staff in decision-making.
- **Commitment:** Is the internalization of an idea and a resulting drive to accomplish specific goals. The mere setting of goals does not indicate leadership that motivates. It is the ability of the leader to translate the importance of the goal (or purpose) to others and to elicit actions from others that support reaching a goal.
- **Energy:** is also needed to empower and fire the imagination of others and constantly invent and move ahead toward future events as well as current needs. Different styles of energy can be motivational. The 'high energy leader' who is effective in one situation may be viewed as 'pushy and aggressive' in another situation.
- **Insight into the needs of others:** is the acute awareness of the reason behind events and an ability to anticipate results of actions. When a leader can put goals into a form that has real or personal value to each person, then motivation will exists.
- **Additional key qualities** of a motivational leader are abilities to listen, reserve judgement, give direct and positive feedback, recognize individual value through respect for others, and use humor.

Professional practice and shared governance depend on the clinical leader to produce an environment that fosters autonomy in decision-making and provides the skills, resources and information needed for others to make this transition.

Seven Rules of Motivation

1. **Set a major goal, but follows a path:** The path has mini goals that go in many directions. When you learn to succeed at mini goals, you will be motivated to challenge grand goals.
2. **Finish what you start:** A half finished project is of no use to anyone. Quitting is a habit. Develop the habit of finishing self-motivated projects.
3. **Socialize with others of similar interest:** Mutual support is motivating. We will develop the attitudes of our five best friends. If they are losers, we will be a loser. If they are winners, we will be a winner. To be a cowboy we must associate with cowboys.
4. **Learn how to learn:** Dependency on others for knowledge supports the habit of procrastination. Man has the ability to learn without instructors. In fact, when we learn the art of self-education we will find, if not create, opportunity to find success beyond our wildest dreams.
5. **Harmonize natural talents with interest that motivates:** Natural talent creates motivation, motivation creates persistence and persistence gets the job done.
6. **Increase knowledge of subjects that inspires:** The more we know about a subject, the more we want to learn about it. A self-propelled upward spiral develops.
7. **Take risk:** Failure and bouncing back are elements of motivation. Failure is a learning tool. No one has ever succeeded at anything worthwhile without a string of failures.

A to Z Steps in Motivation

A—Achieve your dreams. Avoid negative people, things and places. Eleanor Roosevelt once said, 'The future belongs to those who believe in the beauty of their dreams.'

B—Believe in yourself, and in what you can accomplish.

C—Consider things from every angle and aspect. Motivation comes from determination. To be able to understand life, you should feel the sun from both sides.

D—Do not give up and do not give in. Thomas Edison failed once, twice, more than three times before he came up with his invention and perfected the incandescent light bulb. Make motivation your steering wheel.

E—Enjoy! Work as if you do not need money, dance as if nobody's watching, love as if you never cried, and learn as if you will live forever. Motivational momentum takes place when people are happy.

F—Family and Friends—are life's greatest 'F' treasures. Do not loose sight of them.

G—Give more than what is enough. Where does motivation and self improvement take place at work? At home? At school? Always give 110%!

H—Hang on to your dreams. They may dangle in there for a moment, but these little stars will be your driving force. Define your target and hit it, until you hit it!

I—Ignore those who try to destroy you. Do not let other people get the best of you. Stay away from toxic people—the kind of friends who hates to hear about your success. Stay away from negativity!

J—Just be yourself. The key to success is to be yourself. And the key to failure is to try to please everyone.

K—Keep trying no matter how hard life may seem. When a person is motivated, eventually he sees a harsh life finally clearing out, paving the way to self improvement.

L—Learn to love yourself. Now is not that easy?

M—Make things happen. Motivation is when your dreams are put into work clothes.

N—Never lie, cheats or steals. Always play a fair game.

O—Open your eyes. People should learn the horse attitude and horse sense. They see things in 2 ways—how they want things to be, and how they should be.

P—Practice makes perfect. Practice is about motivation. It lets us learn repertoire and ways on how can we recover from our mistakes.

Q—Quitters never win. And winners never quit. So, choose your fate—are you going to be a quitter? Or a winner?

R—Ready yourself. Motivation is also about preparation. We must hear the little voice within us telling us to get started before others will get on their feet and try to push us around. Remember, it was not raining when Noah built the ark.

S—Stop procrastinating. Do not put off until tomorrow what you can do today—we never know what tomorrow will bring!

T—Take control of your life. Discipline and self control jives synonymously with motivation. Both are key factors in self improvement.

U—Understand others. You know how to talk, you should also learn how to listen. Yearn to understand first, and to be understood the second. We have 2 ears and one mouth—use them proportionately!

V—Visualize it. Motivation without vision is like a boat on a dry land. You need to have a crystal clear path.

W—Want it more than anything. Dreaming means believing. And to believe is something that is rooted out from the roots of motivation and self improvement.

X—X Factor is what will make you different from the others. When you are motivated, you tend to put on 'extras' on the life, such as extra time for family, extra help at work, extra care for friends, and so on.

Y—You are unique. No one in this world looks, acts, or talks like you. Value the life and existence, because you only get to spend it once.

Box 16.18 describes motivational theories for better nursing management.

Application of Motivational Theory in Nursing

Motivation theory proposes reasons for behavior. One classic approach is Abraham Maslow's "Toward a Psychology of Being" in 1946. Maslow explains in his later text "Motivation and Personality" in 1954 that individuals move through a hierarchy of motivating needs from physiological to safety, social, esteem and, finally, self-actualization. He suggests that individuals meet each category of needs in that order. Nursing students can identify situations where these needs are met in their practice of nursing.

Role Play Application of Theory

- Teach the students the hierarchy of needs. Ask students to identify an experience to match each level of need. One example is to address the experience of safety in walking across a large hospital parking lot late at night.
- Tell the students to list needs of patients in the same way. An example is the physiological need to address bleeding or pain from an injury.
- Present a scenario of hospital duties that includes a nurse acting to address a need. One example is meeting the need for safety in the intake and medical history process.
- Identify the roles played in the scenario, such as patient, parent and nurse. Assign the roles to students. Ask the role players to act out the scenario. In the discussion of the role play review the hierarchy of needs. Discuss these needs in the areas of physiological, safety, social, esteem and, finally, self-actualization.
- Instruct the other students to assess the nurse's behaviors that met the identified need. Give examples, such as meeting a safety need by asking about allergies to medicines.
- Discuss what needs the nurse may have experienced, such as a need for esteem by being seen as competent

MORALE BUILDING

Morale is a way of describing how people feel about their jobs, employers and companies, and those feelings are tied to the behaviors and attitudes that employees exhibit in the workplace. When employees have good morale, they feel committed to their employers, loyal to their jobs and motivated to be productive.

Definition

- Mooney states, "Morale is the sum total of several psychic qualities which include courage, fortitude, resolution and above all, confidence."
- Davis states, "Organizational morale is basically a mental condition of groups and individuals which determines their attitude."
- Guion defines morale as "The extent to which an individual's needs are satisfied and the extent to which individual perceives that satisfaction as stemming from his total job satisfaction."
- Dr Leighton defined morale as "Capacity of a group of people to pull together persistently and consistently in pursuit of a common purpose."
- In the words of Theo Haimann, "Morale is the state of mind and emotions affecting the attitude and willingness to work, which, in turn affect individual and organizational objectives."

Box 16.18: Motivational theories for better nursing management.
- Need for power
- Need for achievement
- Need for affiliation
- Improving physical working condition
- Increasing the level of training
- Job design
- Work environment
- Positive reinforcement
- Avoidance learning
- Punishment
- Be sure to tell a person he is doing wrong

Meaning

- Morale is the internal feeling of confidence, enthusiasm, zeal, satisfaction, optimism which keeps the frustration level of a person low and he remains satisfied.
- "Morale is a mental condition or attitude of individuals or groups which determines their willingness to cooperate.
- Morale is an important part of organizational climate. It is a vital ingredient of organizational success because it reflects the attitudes and sentiments of organizational members towards the organization, its objectives and policies.
- Employee morale is defined as the attitude, satisfaction and overall outlook of employees during their association with an organization or a business. An employee that is satisfied and motivated at workplace usually tends to have a higher morale than their counterparts.
- Staff morale is the collection of attitudes and feelings an employee has in the workplace.
  Figure 16.41 shows impacts on morale.

Features of Morale

The other features of morale are as follows:
- It is composite of feelings, attitudes and sentiments of the employees.
- It is the degree or enthusiasm and willingness with which the employees contribute their efforts towards the organizational goals.
- It is different from job satisfaction because morale refers to group concept while job satisfaction is an individual concept.
- The degree of morale can be estimated through labor absenteeism and turnover.
- It is both an individual and a group phenomenon. The high moral is reflected in good team and team spirit in case of group morale.
- Morale is the primary concern of the management because high production and productivity of workers are the direct result of high morale.

Importance of Morale

The importance of morale can be studied under the following:
- Higher productivity is the result of the positive attitude of the workers. High morale for this the management should know the impact of its policies and practices on the attitude of the workers.

Feel set up for failure
Feel disconnected
Feel frustrated
Feel uniformed
Feel hopeless
Feel alone
Feel unheard
Feel unsupported
Feel confused
Feel burnt out
Feel like everything is a fight

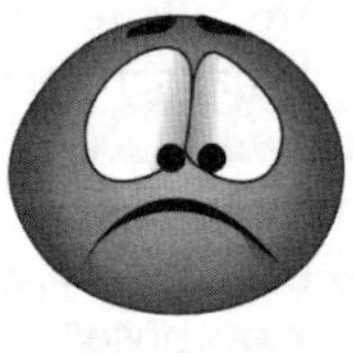

Fig. 16.41: Impacts on morale.

- According to Dale Yoder, "if workers appear to full enthusiastic and optimized about the group activities and mission and friendly to each other, they are described as having good or high morale. If they are dissatisfied irritated, critical, restless and pessimistic, their reactions are described as evidence of poor or low morale."
- The success or failure of the organization very much depends upon the morale of its employee. As per opinion of Keith Davis, "Never under estimate the power of a woman and the same certainly must be said about morale never under estimate the power of morale."
- The high morale is important because it assists management to solve many labor related problems, such as—labor turnover, absenteeism, indiscipline and grievance, etc.
- Government has introduced many labor welfare and social security measures to improve the morale of industrial workers.

It has realized that low morale has long range effects damaging the organization, thus the management has recognize the importance of high morale.

Three-Stage Strategy

I. **Stage one:** "Listen to employees" Leaders should be visible, approachable and well briefed, so they can field questions.
   Listening activities:
   1. Employee survey
   2. Employee discussion/focus groups
   3. Management discussion groups

II. **Stage two:** "Communicate your solutions to business issues and employee concerns" Build a shared understanding of your company's future, including solutions to business issues and progress being made.
   Communication activities:
   1. Public forums:
   2. One-on-One dialogues
   3. Electronic media

III. **Stage three:** "Recognize business and employee accomplishments and successes" Focusing on quick wins and success stories and recognizing employee accomplishments will help keep morale as high as possible
   Recognition activities:
   1. Formal initiatives
   2. Informal gestures
   3. Public recognition

Methods of raising morale: Employees tend to lack motivation to perform their jobs when morale is low. A lack of motivation can also be circular in nature. Management and employees can help increase morale in the workplace by the following means.
- Recognize employees
- Be a respectful manager
- Have one-on-one meetings with employees
- Invest in employees
- Get to know employees
- Pay and reward systems

> **Box 16.19: Factors affecting morale.**
> - The organization
> - The nature of work
> - The level of satisfaction
> - The level of supervision
> - Concept of self
> - Workers perception of reward system
> - The employees age
> - Occupational level

- Job autonomy and discretion
- Support services
- Training

Factors Affecting Employee Morale (Box 16.19)

Employee morale is a complex phenomenon and depends on various factors. Here is the different criterion that affects employee morale:

- **Organization itself:** An organization influences an employee's attitude towards his/her work. The reputation of an organization can certainly build up for better or worse, their attitude towards it.
- **Type of work:** The nature of work an employee is performing at his/her workplace also is greatly responsible to determine the morale.
- **Personal attributes:** Mental and physical health play an important role in determining employee morale. If the employee is not physically or mentally fit, this can be a potential obstacle in their progress and learning at their workplace.
- **Supervision and feedback:** The level of supervision received by an employee is a tremendous factor that affects the morale.
- **Work-life balance:** Most organization fails to recognize the importance of a healthy work-life balance. It is important that the employees have some activities to relax while they are at work.

Ways to Boost Employee Morale

Employee morale is determined by how employees view their work environment and their overall level of satisfaction in their workplace. Employee morale has a direct effect on employee retention. Here are the 4 simple ways of boosting employee morale in your workplace as mentioned by HR leaders across the globe:

- **Streamline work based on skills:** It is important for the Human Resources to recruit and assign people based on their skillset. Make sure you invest in a competent human resources team, so the talent that is acquired performs well and stays happy.
- **Train them well for professional development:** Most organizations fail to understand the importance of training their staff. Be it employee on boarding or any other formal training process, employees should be well-equipped to perform their tasks at work and achieve their goals.
- **Recognize and reward employees:** Employee recognition and reward keeps your workforce motivated. When, as a leader, you create an environment where good work is appreciated, employees feel empowered and take a personal interest in the tasks they are assigned to them.
- **Be open to feedback:** Many organizations today, promote the open door policy, where an employee is free to express what they feel to their superiors or their reporting authority because they are opens to feedback.

Importance of Morale

High morale in the workplace is critical to a business' overall success. Employees who rank high on the morale scale generally exhibit their positive attitude in a number of ways:
1. Better productivity
2. More focused on customers or outcomes
3. Less employee turnover
4. Increased communication between co-workers and management
5. Better work attendance and timeliness
6. Enhanced care about work product
7. Fewer workplace-related injuries or accidents
8. Increased attention to detail

Morale Building Strategies

Various measures can be adopted to improve morale including:
- **Organizational structure:** In tall structures, the distance between managers and workers is relatively more and communication is distorted. Comparatively in flat structures, managers are less distant to workers and effective communication can take place. Such organizational structure increases morale.
- **Job enrichment:** People like to do new, interesting and challenging jobs. Morale of employees increases if they are given opportunities for advancement, recognition and growth. For example, morale of a bank manager will be boosted if he is given the opportunity to manage a branch which the bank is going to open in foreign country.
- **Job security:** Insecurity of job worries the employees, they cannot concentrate on their work, they would be worried about searching for a new job. If employees are given security of their job, they will be able to concentrate on their job and their morale will increase.
- **Effective communication:** Effective communication between manager and employee will help in cooperation and motivation which in turn will help in increasing morale.
- **Worker's participation:** Suggestions of workers should be asked at various times and feasible suggestions should be implemented. There should be participation of workers in decisions involving their interest. If the employees are allowed to participate in decisions affecting them, their morale increases.
- **Employee counselor:** Organizations can take help of psychologists or behavioral scientists to find the reasons of dissatisfaction among employees and finding remedies to it. It will help in increase of morale.

- **Human approach to management:** Employees should be treated like humans, not like other passive factors of production. Their feelings should be respected. Their self-respect and dignity should not be harmed at any cost.
- **Remuneration:** Remuneration is the consideration for the work that employees do in the organization. Employee remuneration should be fair and equitable. It should be justified according to employees' skills and abilities.
- **Grievance redresses:** If the grievances of employees are solved in time, they feel satisfied and their morale increases.
- **Motivation:** Morale of employees can be increased by motivating them. Motivation urges and drives the employees to work. Various persons can be motivated through financial and non-financial motivators.
- **Proper training:** Through training, employees learn new skills and methods to work. By learning new skills, confidence and job satisfaction of employees increases which results in the enhancement of morale.
- **Assigning responsibility:** Morale of employees can be increased by giving them the responsibilities. It is a natural fact that people like to take responsibility so that they can prove their ability; so if employees are trusted and given responsibility, their morale increases.
- **By recognition:** People like to be in limelight; they like to be recognized. If employees are recognized, their morale increases. Employees can be made to realize the feeling of recognition by rewarding performance.
- **Leadership style:** Morale can be improved by adopting a proper leadership style. Positive motivational leadership style and democratic leadership style can be helpful.

COMMUNICATION IN THE WORKPLACE

Communication in the workplace is one of the signs of a high-performance culture. Exchanging information and ideas within an organization is called workplace communication. However, effective communication occurs when a message is sent and received accurately. In every aspect of life (both professional and personal), effective communication is important to success and happiness. Effective communication in the workplace is central to all business goals.

Definition

Workplace communication is the transmitting of information between one person or group and another person or group in an organization. It can include emails, text messages, voicemails, notes, etc.

Nature of Communication

1. Communication serves as the foundation of every facet of a business. Effective communication is communication between two or more persons with the purpose of delivering, receiving, and understanding the message successfully.
2. It is the process of information sharing between team members in a way that keeps in mind what you want to say, what you actually say, and what your audience interprets.

Figure 16.42 shows effective communication skills.

Importance of Communication (Fig. 16.43)

- **Promotes motivation:** Communication promotes motivation by informing and clarifying the employees about

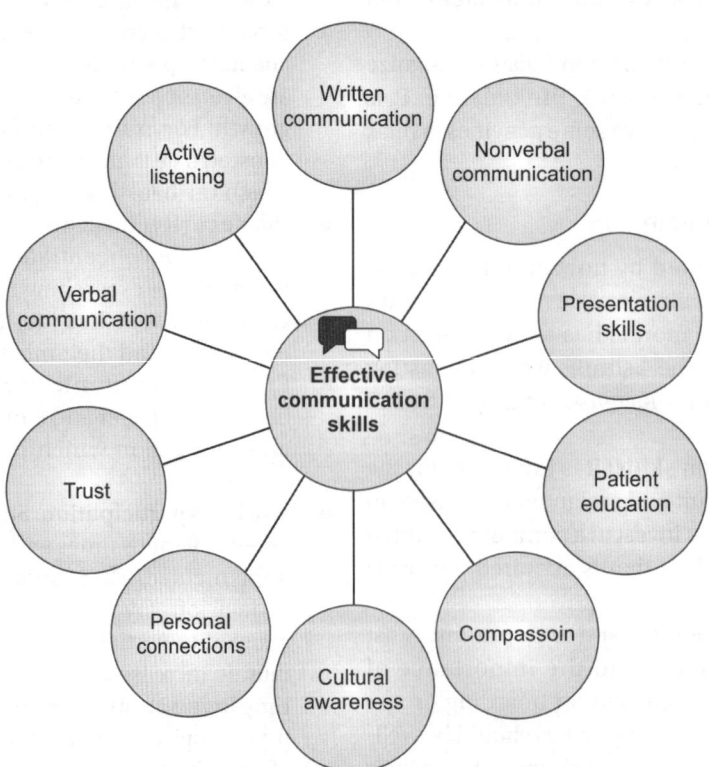

Fig. 16.42: Effective communication skills.

Chapter 16: Organizational Behavior and Human Relations

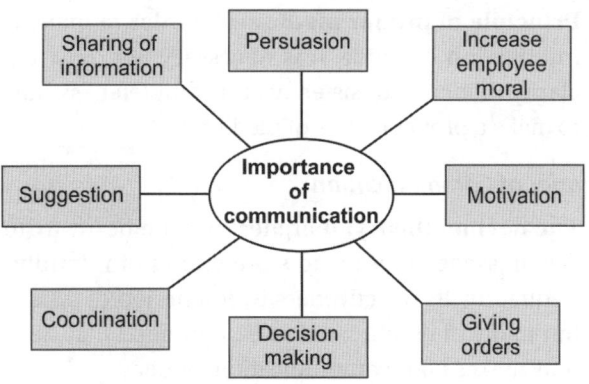

Fig. 16.43: Importance of communication.

the task to be done, the manner they are performing the task, and how to improve their performance if it is not up to the mark.
- **Source of information:** Communication is a source of information to the organizational members for decision-making process as it helps identifying and assessing alternative course of actions.
- **Altering individuals attitudes:** Communication also plays a crucial role in altering individual's attitudes, i.e., a well informed individual will have better attitude than a less-informed individual. Organizational magazines, journals, meetings and various other forms of oral and written communication help in molding employee's attitudes.
- **Helps in socializing:** Communication also helps in socializing. In today's life the only presence of another individual fosters communication. It is also said that one cannot survive without communication.
- **Controlling process:** Communication also assists in controlling process. It helps controlling organizational member's behavior in various ways. There are various levels of hierarchy and certain principles and guidelines that employees must follow in an organization. They must comply with organizational policies, perform their job role efficiently and communicate any work problem and grievance to their superiors. Thus, communication helps in controlling function of management.

Elements of Communication (Fig. 16.44)

- **Source idea:** The Source idea is the process by which one formulates an idea to communicate to another party. This process can be influenced by external stimuli, such as books or radio, or it can come about internally by thinking about a particular subject. The source idea is the basis for the communication.
- **Message:** The Message is what will be communicated to another party. It is based on the source idea, but the message is crafted to meet the needs of the audience. For example, if the message is between two friends, the message will take a different form than if communicating with a superior.
- **Encoding:** Encoding is how the message is transmitted to another party. The message is converted into a suitable form for transmission. The medium of transmission will determine the form of the communication. For example, the message will take a different form if the communication will be spoken or written.
- **Channel:** The Channel is the medium of the communication. The channel must be able to transmit the message from one party to another without changing the content of the message. The channel can be a piece of paper, a communications medium, such as radio, or it can be an email. The channel is the path of the communication from sender to receiver. An email can use the Internet as a channel.

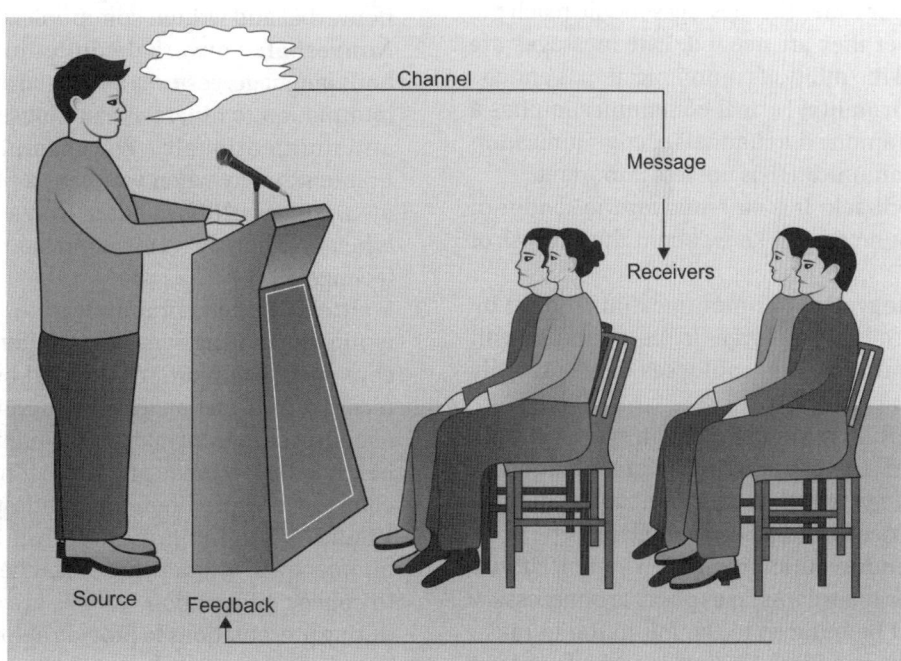

Fig. 16.44: Elements of communication.

- **Receiver:** The Receiver is the party receiving the communication. The party uses the channel to get the communication from the transmitter. A receiver can be a television set, a computer, or a piece of paper depending on the channel used for the communication.
- **Decoding:** Decoding is the process where the message is interpreted for its content. It also means the receiver thinks about the message's content and internalizes the message. This step of the process is where the receiver compares the message to prior experiences or external stimuli.

Feedback: Feedback is the final step in the communications process. This step conveys to the transmitter that the message is understood by the receiver. The receiver formats an appropriate reply to the first communication based on the channel and sends it to the transmitter of the original message.

Principles of Effective Communication

An effective communication system is based on the following principles:

- **Principle of clarity in ideas:** First of all it should be clear in the mind of the sender as to what he wants to say.
- **Principle of appropriate language:** According to this principle, the communication should always be in a simple language. Ideas should be clear and be devoid of any doubt.
- **Principle of attention:** The purpose of communication is that the receiver of information should clearly understand its meaning.
- **Principle of consistency:** According to this principle, communication system should maintain consistency in the objectives of the enterprise, its procedures and processes.
- **Principle of proper time:** The messages should reach the receiver whenever they are needed. Late messages are meaningless and the utility of communication is ended.
- **Principle of informality:** Formal communication has a prominent place among the channels of communication but informal communication is not less important.
- **Principle of feedback:** It is essential for the sender of the message that he should know about the success of the message.
- **Principle of integration:** Communication should be able to introduce all the employees in the enterprise with its objectives so that all the employees move unitedly towards the goal.
- **Principle of flexibility:** Communication system should be able to absorb the changes in the organization. A communication system that cannot absorb changes according to the need becomes meaningless.
- **Principle of economy:** Communication system should not be unnecessarily costly. As far as possible unnecessary messages should be reduced to the minimum to make communication economical. No single employee should be burdened with the work of communication.
- **Principle of proper medium:** In order to make communication effective, it is necessary not only to have clarity of ideas, consistency and completeness but also to make a proper choice of medium.

Theories of Communication

- **The decibel theory:** It argues that the best way to get the message across is to state one's point loudly and frequently. Its effectiveness over a period of time is nil, but many of us still need to be reminded that shouting only makes poor communication louder.
- **The sell theory:** It lays down that the total burden of communication is on the communicator while the receiver is passive and pliable. One of the problem created by this approach is that it tends to increase the barriers between the individuals and thus reduces the chances of hearing each other.
- **The minimet theory:** It assumes that the receiver probably is not much interested in what is being communicated. By telling an individual what he needs to know, he will have little to object and little to question.

Types of Communication in Workplace

There are several different ways we share information with one another. There are four main categories or communication styles including verbal, nonverbal, written and visual:

1. **Verbal:** Verbal communication is the use of language to transfer information through speaking or sign language. It is one of the most common types, often used during presentations, video conferences and phone calls, meetings and one-on-one conversations. Verbal communication is important because it is efficient. It can be helpful to support verbal communication with both nonverbal and written communication.
2. **Nonverbal:** Nonverbal communication is the use of body language, gestures and facial expressions to convey information to others. It can be used both intentionally and unintentionally. For example, you might smile unintentionally when you hear a pleasing or enjoyable idea or piece of information. Nonverbal communication is helpful when trying to understand others' thoughts and feelings.
3. **Written:** Written communication is the act of writing, typing or printing symbols like letters and numbers to convey information. It is helpful because it provides a record of information for reference. Writing is commonly used to share information through books, pamphlets, blogs, letters, memos and more. Emails and chats are a common form of written communication in the workplace.
4. **Visual:** Visual communication is the act of using photographs, art, drawings, sketches, charts and graphs to convey information. Visuals are often used as an aid during presentations to provide helpful context alongside written and/or verbal communication. Because people have different learning styles, visual communication

might be more helpful for some to consume ideas and information.

Skills

- Getting the message across efficiently depends on the skills of the communicator, such as presentation skills, group facilitation skills, negotiation and written communication skills.
- Successful communication also depends upon the capacity of the employees to understand the information.
- This requires providing the employees some basic financial literacy, such as financial statements, sales, profitability, etc.
- When selecting a candidate, most employers seek for those who have strong speaking and writing skills.
- Problem solving and self-motivation are also highly necessary skills among the workplace. These allow rapidly changing environments to become less of a challenge.

Techniques to Improve the Communication

- **Listening:** An active process of receiving information. The complete attention of the nurse is required and there should be no preoccupation with oneself. Listening is a sign of respect for the person who is talking and a powerful reinforce of relationships. It allows the patients to talk more, without which the relationship cannot progress.
- **Broad openings:** These encourage the patient to select topics for discussion, and indicate that nurse is there, listening to him and following him. For example, questions, such as what shall we discuss today?—can you tell me more about that?—and then what happened? from the part of the nurse encourages the patient to talk.
- **Restating:** The nurse repeats to the patient the main thought he has expressed. it indicates that the nurses is listening. It also brings attention to something important.
- **Clarification:** The person's verbalization, especially when he is disturbed or feeling deeply, is not always clear. The patients remarks may be confused, incomplete or disordered due to their illness. So, the nurses need to clarify the feelings and ideas expressed by the patients. The nurses need to provide correlation between the patient's feeling and action. For example, I am not sure what you mean—could you tell me once again? clarifies the unintelligible ideas of the patients.
- **Reflection:** This means directing back to the patient his ideas, feeling questions and content. Reflection of content is also called validation. Reflection of feeling consists of responses to the patient's feeling about the content.
- **Focusing:** It means expanding the discussion on a topic of importance. It helps the patient to become more specific, move from vagueness to clarity and focus on reality.
- **Sharing perceptions:** These are the techniques of asking the patient to verify the nurse understands of what he is thinking or feeling.
- **Theme identification:** This involves identifying the underlying issues or problem experienced by the patient that emerges repeatedly during the course of the nurse-patient interaction. Once we identify the basis themes, it becomes easy to decide which of the patient's feeling and thoughts to respond to and pursue.
- **Silence:** This is lack of verbal communication for a therapeutic reason. Then the nurse's silence prompts patient to talk. For example, just sitting with a patient without talking, non-verbally communicates our interest in the patient better.
- **Humor:** This is the discharge of energy through the comic enjoyment of the imperfect. It is a socially acceptable form of sublimation. It is a part of nurse client relationship. It is constructive coping behavior, and by learning to express humor, a patient learns to express how others feel.
- **Informing:** This is the skill of giving information. The nurse shares simple facts with the patient.
- **Suggesting:** This is the presentation of alternative ideas related to problem solving. It is the most useful communication technique when the patient has analyzed his problem area, and is ready to explore alternative coping mechanisms. At that time suggesting technique increase the patient's choices.

Barriers of Communication at Workplace (Fig. 16.45)

Common barriers to effective communication at workplace:

- **Physical barriers:** Physical structure, location and construction of the workplace acts as a barrier to effective communication. Employees seated remotely from each other hinder effective interaction.
- **Language barriers:** Employees with different native languages will be working in an organization. As everyone in organization are not comfortable with native language of the other person, language acts as a barrier for effective workplace communication. Language barriers, such as differences in slang or register among second language speakers, within a workplace can create issues impeding proper work task completion.

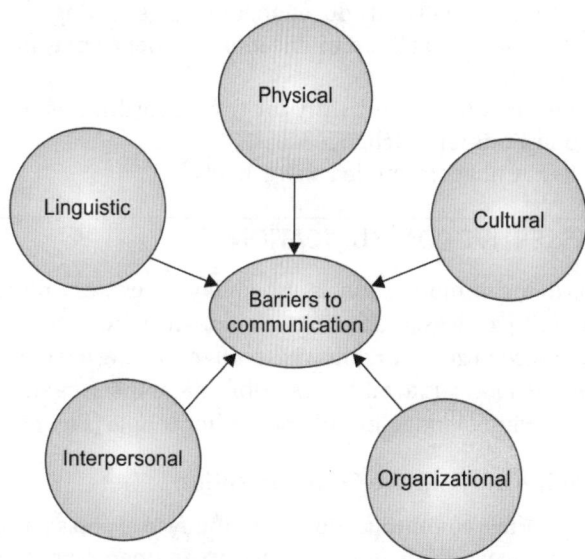

Fig. 16.45: Barriers of communication.

- **Cultural barriers:** Employees from different cultures, following different practices will be working in an organization. This cultural diversity among the employees can act as barrier for effective communication at workplace.
- **Emotional barriers:** Emotional barriers, such as fear, inferiority, shyness, lack of self confidence and skills will stop an employee in communicating effectively with his colleagues.
- **Perception barriers:** Employees will have different experiences, values, preferences and attitudes. These may lead to a variety of assumptions and can act as a communication barrier.

Advantages of Communication

Oral communication:
- It is face-to-face system and hence can be clarified.
- There is an opportunity to ask questions, exchange ideas and clarify meaning.
- It can develop a friendly and cooperative spirit.
- It is easy and quick.
- It is flexible and hence effective.

Written communication:
- It has permanent record for future reference.
- It is less likely to be misunderstood.
- It will have adequate coverage and accuracy.
- Suitable for communicating lengthy messages.
- It is an authoritative communication.

Disadvantages of Communication

Oral communication:
- The spoken words may be misunderstood.
- The facial expression and tone of voice of the communicator may misled the receiver.
- Not suitable for lengthy communication.
- It requires the art of effective specificity
- It has no record for future reference.

Written communication:
- It requires skill and education for understanding.
- It is also one way communication and hence may not be effective.
- There is no opportunity for the subordinates to ask questions and exchange ideas.
- It may not communicate all aspects.

ASSERTIVE COMMUNICATION

Assertive communication is the ability to express positive and negative ideas and feelings in an open, honest and direct way. It recognizes our rights whilst still respecting the rights of others. It allows us to take responsibility for ourselves and our actions without judging or blaming other people **(Fig. 16.46)**.

Meaning of Assertive Communication

- Assertive communication is the ability to express positive and negative ideas and feelings in an open, honest and direct way.

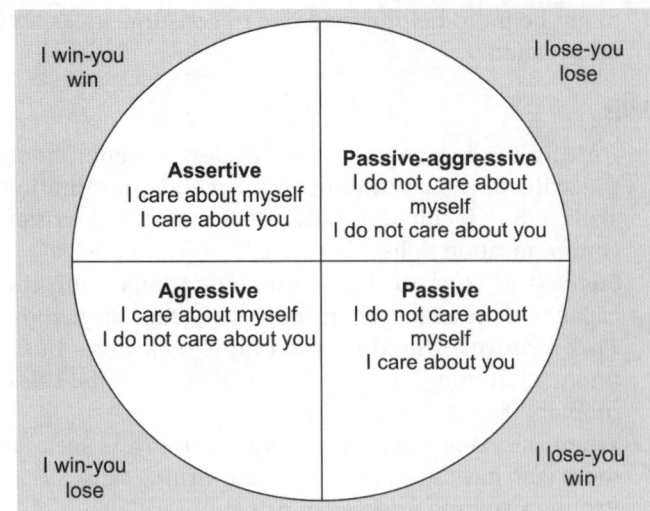

Fig. 16.46: Assertive communication model.

- It recognizes our rights whilst still respecting the rights of others.
- It allows us to take responsibility for ourselves and our actions without judging or blaming other people.
- And it allows us to constructively confront and find a mutually satisfying solution where conflict exists.

Four Behavioral Choices

There are, as I see it, four choices you can make about which style of communication you can employ. These types are:
1. **Direct aggression:** Bossy, arrogant, bulldozing, intolerant, opinionated, and overbearing
2. **Indirect aggression:** Sarcastic, deceiving, ambiguous, insinuating, manipulative, and guilt-inducing
3. **Submissive:** Wailing, moaning, helpless, passive, indecisive, and apologetic
4. **Assertive:** Direct, honest, accepting, responsible, and spontaneous

Characteristics of Assertiveness in Communication

There are six main characteristics of assertiveness skills in communication. These are:
1. **Eye contact:** Demonstrates interest and shows sincerity.
2. **Body posture:** Congruent body language will improve the significance of the message.
3. **Gestures:** Appropriate gestures help to add emphasis.
4. **Voice:** A level, modulated tone is more convincing and acceptable, and is not intimidating.
5. **Timing:** Use your judgment to maximize receptivity and impact.
6. **Content:** How, where and when you choose to comment is probably more important than WHAT you say.

Advantages of Assertiveness Skills in Communication

There are many advantages of assertiveness skills in communication, most notably these:
- Assertiveness helps us feel good about ourselves and others
- Assertiveness leads to the development of mutual respect with others

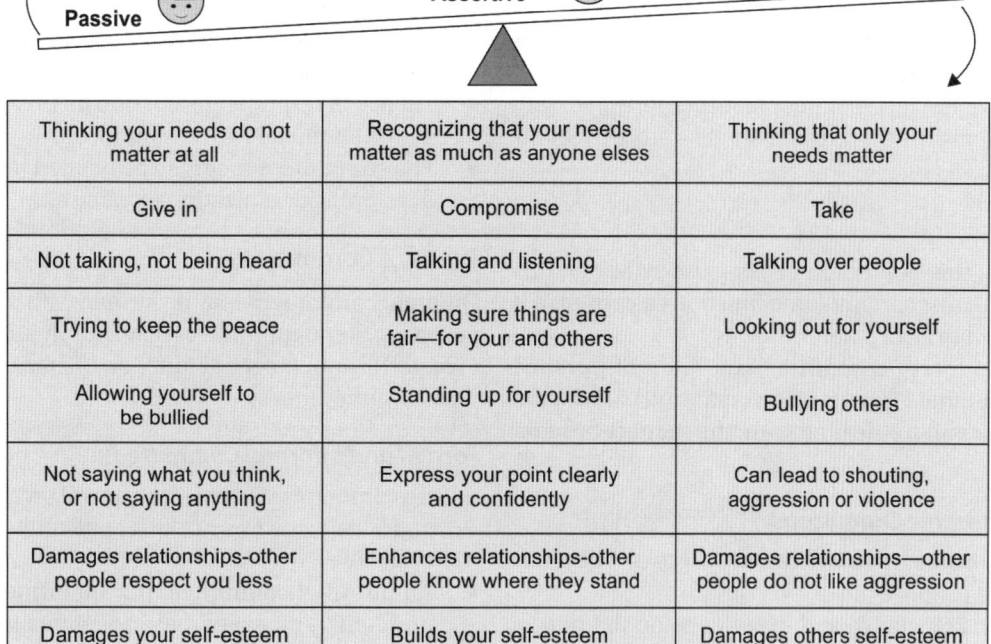

Fig. 16.47: Techniques of assertive communication.

- Assertiveness increases our self-esteem
- Assertiveness helps us achieve our goals
- Assertiveness minimizes hurting and alienating other people
- Assertiveness reduces anxiety
- Assertiveness protects us from being taken advantage of by others
- Assertiveness enables us to make decisions and free choices in life
- Assertiveness enables us to express a wide range of feelings and thoughts

Six Techniques for Assertiveness in Communication

There are six assertiveness techniques—let us look at each of them in turn.

1. **Behavior behearsal:** This is literally practicing how you want to look and sound. It is a very useful technique when you first want to use "I" statements, as it helps dissipate any emotion associated with an experience and allows you to accurately identify the behavior you wish to confront.
2. **Repeated assertion (the 'broken record'):** This assertiveness technique allows you to feel comfortable by ignoring manipulative verbal side traps, argumentative baiting and irrelevant logic while sticking to your point. To most effectively use this assertiveness technique use calm repetition, and say what you want and stay focused on the issue.
3. **Fogging:** This technique allows you to receive criticism comfortably, without getting anxious or defensive, and without rewarding manipulative criticism.
4. **Negative enquiry:** This assertiveness technique seeks out criticism about yourself in close relationships by prompting the expression of honest, negative feelings to improve communication. To use it effectively you need to listen for critical comments, clarify your understanding of those criticisms, use the information if it will be helpful or ignore the information if it is manipulative.
5. **Negative assertion:** This assertiveness technique lets you look more comfortably at negatives in your own behavior or personality without feeling defensive or anxious; this also reduces your critics' hostility.
6. **Workable compromise:** When you feel that your self-respect is not in question, consider a workable compromise with the other person.

Figure 16.47 shows techniques of assertive communication.

COMMITTEES—IMPORTANCE IN THE ORGANIZATION, FUNCTIONING

A committee or commission is a body of one or more persons that is subordinate to a deliberative assembly. Usually, the assembly sends matters into a committee as a way to explore them more fully than would be possible if the assembly itself were considering them. Committees may have different functions and their types of work differ depending on the type of the organization and its needs.

Meaning

- The committee organization is not an independent form of organization but generally functions in conjunction with some other form of organization.

- The formation of committees has become a usual and common feature of modern organizations.
- Committees are found to exist in different areas and at different levels of an organizational structure, in both business and non business organizations.
- It is because of the fact that people react more favorably to a group decision than to the single authority of an individual.

Definition

- A committee has been defined as "a body of persons entrusted with discharging some functions assigned to it as a group and in a corporate capacity".
- According to ferry "committee is a body of persons elected or appointed to meet on an organized basis for the discussion of, and for dealing with, the matters brought before it".

Purposes of Committee Organization

Committees may be created for different purposes. They may be created for the purpose of:
- Pooling facts, knowledge and experience on the part of several executive members of the committees
- Determining broad policies
- Making it possible for employees to participate in decision making
- Securing the facility of communication and coordination between executives
- Giving representations to various groups in an organization
- Making a continuous review and seeking an honest and objective appraisal of the conduct of the business to make sure that all is well in the organization.

Most committees are, however, either decision making or problem solving committees.

Figure 16.48 shows members of committee.

Need for Committees

The main reason for committees is to secure common judgment on administrative matters. The committees are set up for the following reasons:

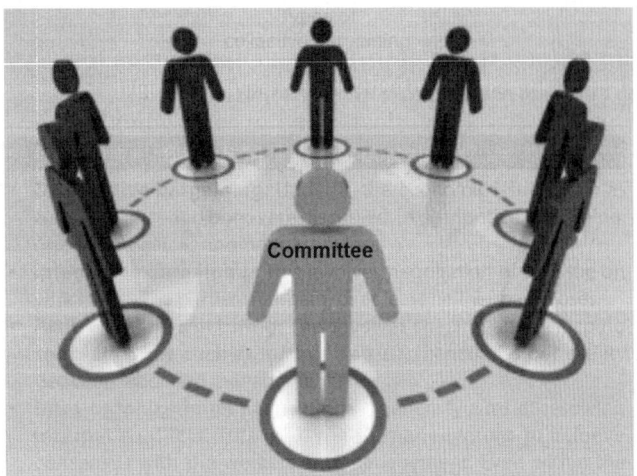

Fig. 16.48: Members of committee.

- The committees provide a forum for exchanging ideas among organizational members.
- The exchange of ideas among members may generate some suggestions and recommendations which may be useful for the organization.
- There can be proper discussion on present problems and efforts are made to find solutions.
- The committees may also be needed in establishing and developing organizational policies.

Types of Committees

Different committees may be formed with different ideas and purposes. Some committees may be only advisory while some may perform managerial functions. There may be following types of committees:

Formal and Informal Committees

- If a committee is formed as a part of organization structure and is delegated some duties and authority, it is a formal committee.
- An informal committee may be formed to tackle some problem. A manager may call some experts to help him in analyzing a problem and suggesting a suitable solution.
- The chief executive may call a meeting of departmental heads and some experts to find out a solution to some problem. In both the cases it is a case of an informal committee.

Advisory Committees

- These are the committees to advice line heads on certain issues. Line officers may refer some problems or issues to a committee for advice.
- The committee will collect information about the problem and recommend solution for the same.
- The line officers have the powers to accept, modify or reject the suggestions of advisory committees.
- These committees have no managerial powers and cannot exert their views on the line executives.

Line Committees

- There may be committees with managerial powers. Instead of giving a work to one person it may be assigned to a number of executives.
- The committees having administrative powers are called line or plural committees.
- Line committees help in planning company policies and programmes and organizing efforts at fulfillment of these plans, etc.
- These committees also direct and control the activities of employees for achieving organizational goals.

Functions

Committees can serve several different functions:
- **Governance:** In organizations considered too large for all the members to participate in decisions affecting the organization as a whole, a smaller body, such as a board of directors, is given the power to make decisions, spend

money, or take actions. A governance committee is formed as a separate committee to review the performance of the board and board policy as well as nominate candidates for the board.

- **Coordination and administration:** A large body may have smaller committees with more specialized functions. Examples are an audit committee, an elections committee, a finance committee, a fundraising committee, and a program committee. Large conventions or academic conferences are usually organized by a coordinating committee drawn from the membership of the organization.
- **Research and recommendations:** Committees may be formed to do research and make recommendations on a potential or planned project or change. For example, an organization considering a major capital investment might create a temporary working committee of several people to review options and make recommendations to upper management or the board of directors.
- **Discipline:** A committee on discipline may be used to handle disciplinary procedures on members of the organization.
- **As a tactic for indecision:** As a means of public relations by sending sensitive, inconvenient, or irrelevant matters to committees, organizations may bypass, stall, or disacknowledge matters without declaring a formal policy of inaction or indifference. However, this could be considered a dilatory tactic.
- **Power and authority:** Generally, committees are required to report to their parent body. Committees do not usually have the power to act independently unless the body that created it gives it such power.

Common Types of Committee

1. **Executive committee:** It is a committee having the power to act, generally or specifically. It is, however more commonly a body with power to govern or administer. It is coupled with the line authority.
2. **Standing committee:** A standing or permanent committee is formed for a specific purpose. It is a committee of a formal type and conducts the routine business delegated to it at regular (weekly or monthly) meetings. Its examples are the finance committee, the transfer committee, the working or consultative committee, etc.
3. **Ad-hoc committee** it is a temporary committee formed for a particular purpose. It stops functioning as soon as its purpose is accomplished. 'Fact-finding' or "exploration" or "investigation" committees usually come under this category. When the purpose of an adhoc committee is accomplished, it reports to the appointing authority and then ceases to exist.
4. **Joint committee:** It is generally formed for the purpose of coordinating the activities, of two or more committees. For instance, a joint consultative committee may consist of representatives of the employer's and employees' committees. A works committee or consultative committee is an example of this type of committee.
5. **Office committee:** Office committees are those committees which are entrusted with the task of office management. These committees may either be executive committees, standing or adhoc committees or joint committees.

Examples of office committees are: the management committee, the finance committee, the audit committee, the office cost control committee, the joint consultative committee, etc. The purpose and functions of an office committee depend upon its nature and the work assigned to it.

Types of Committees in the Industry

The following are some of the important committees of the Board:
- Audit committee
- Shareholders grievance committee
- Remuneration committee
- Risk committee
- Nomination committee
- Corporate governance committee
- Corporate compliance committee
- Ethics committee

Audit Committee

The audit committee shall assist the Board of Directors in the oversight of
- The integrity of the financial statements of the company,
- The effectiveness of the internal control over financial reporting,
- The independent registered public accounting firm's qualifications and independence,
- The performance of the company's internal audit function and independent registered public accounting firms,
- The company's compliance with legal and regulatory requirements,
- The performance of the company's compliance function.

Powers of Audit Committee

The audit committee shall have powers which should include the following:
- To investigate any activity within its terms of reference.
- To seek information from any employee.
- To obtain outside legal or other professional advice.
- To secure attendance of outsiders with relevant expertise, if it considers necessary.

Ethics Committee

The possible roles for an ethics committee are:
- Contribute to the continuing definition of the organization's ethics and compliance standards and procedures.
- Assume responsibility for overall compliance with those standards and procedures.
- Oversee the use of due care in delegating discretionary responsibility.
- Communicate the organization's ethics and compliance standards and procedures, ensuring the effectiveness of that communication.
- Monitor and audit compliance

- Oversee enforcement, including the assurance that discipline is uniformly applied.
- Take the steps necessary to ensure that the organization learns from its experiences.

Advantages of Committees

- A committee may consist of all the departmental heads as members. In the committee meetings, the members are enabled to understand the various problems faced by the other departments in the organization and this promotes better understanding among the departmental heads.
- In committee meetings, decisions are taken after taking into consideration the different views of its members and thus the committee provides a forum for the pooling of knowledge and experience of many persons.
- The committee encourages team spirit and cooperation of various departments in the execution of the plans.
- The committee's work develops awareness of the problem of other departments among the members and this promotes coordination of the various activities of an enterprise.
- In committee meetings, members discuss the various organizational problems, and hence, it can be said that the committee is an excellent means of transmitting information and ideas to the interested organizational members.
- Members of the committee take part in the decision-making process and because of this; they will not resist the implementation of the decisions.

Disadvantages of Committees

- Members with different background and ideals may express different views on the same subject and this may cause delay in taking a decision.
- Committee is an expensive form of organization because of the huge amount to be spent for convening committee meetings.
- In case, there is no mutual confidence among the members, not only will they fail to appreciate each other's views but also misrepresent each other's statements.
- Because of the large number of members in a committee, it is difficult to maintain secrecy regarding the committee's decisions.
- No member can be individually held responsible in case the committee takes incorrect decisions. Because of this, members may not actively participate in the deliberations of the meeting.
- Decision may be arrived at on the basis of compromise among the members or the decisions may reflect accommodation of various viewpoints of the members and because of this, the quality of decision is watered down and not the best from anyone's viewpoint.

CONCLUSION

"Organizational behavior is a field of study that investigates the impact that individuals, groups and organizational structure have on behavior within the organization, for the purpose of applying such knowledge towards improving an organizational effectiveness". The above definition has three main elements; first organizational behavior is an investigative study of individuals and groups, second, the impact of organizational structure on human behavior and the third, the application of knowledge to achieve organizational effectiveness. These factors are interactive in nature and the impact of such behavior is applied to various systems so that the goals are achieved. The nature of study of organizational behavior is investigative to establish cause and effect relationship.

REVIEW QUESTIONS

Long Essays

1. Define organizational behavior; explain the objectives and characteristics.
2. Define group dynamics; explain the features, objectives and types.
3. Define interpersonal relationship; explain the factors affecting interpersonal relationship.
4. Define human relations; explain the characteristics and factors affecting human relations.
5. Explain the relations with professional associations and employee unions.
6. Define collective bargaining; explain the purposes and features and principles.
7. Define motivation; explain the purposes, objectives and types of motivation.
8. Define morale building; explain the features and importance.
9. Define communication; explain the importance, elements and theories of communication.
10. Define committee; explain the purposes, types and advantages of committees.

Short Essays

1. Elements of organizational behavior.
2. Levels of organizational behavior.
3. Principles of organizational behavior.
4. Factors influence organizational behavior.
5. Organizational behavior model.
6. Approaches to organizational behavior.
7. Scope of the organizational behavior.
8. Factors affecting group dynamics.
9. Role of nurse manager in group dynamics.
10. Stages in interpersonal relationships.
11. Phases of nurse-patient relationship.
12. Scope of human relations.
13. Nurses role in human relations.
14. Public relations in the context of nursing.
15. Trained Nurses Association of India.
16. Collective bargaining process.
17. Pros and cons of collective bargaining.
18. Theories of motivation
19. Motivational qualities of nurse leader.
20. Barriers of communication at workplace.
21. Characteristics of assertiveness in communication.

Short Answers

1. Contingency approach.
2. Importance of organizational behavior.
3. Limitations of organization behavior.
4. Stages of group development.
5. Importance of group dynamism.
6. Stages of relationship formation.
7. Principles of IPR.
8. Elements of nurse-client relationship.
9. Problems of improper interpersonal relationships.
10. Human relation skills.
11. Importance of human relations skills.
12. Human relations in team work.
13. Nurse-patient helping relationship.
14. Aims and objectives of public relations.
15. Elements of public relations.
16. Types of public relation.
17. Nursing service in public relations.
18. Collective bargaining.
19. International Council for Nurses
20. Indian Nursing Council
21. Red Cross Society
22. World Health Organization
23. Functions of Collective Bargaining
24. Types of Collective Bargaining
25. Factors Affecting Employee Morale
26. Advantages of Communication
27. Techniques for Assertiveness in Communication

BIBLIOGRAPHY

1. Basvanthappa BT. Nursing Administration, 1st edition, New Delhi: Jaypee Brothers; 2000.
2. Carriers JH. "Cyclical Group Development and Interaction-based Leadership Emergence in Autonomous Teams: An integrated model." Journal of Leadership and Organizational Studies. Summer. 2005.
3. Frey LR, Wolf S. "The Symbolic and Interpretive Perspective on Group Dynamics." Small Group Research. 2004;35(3):277-316.
4. Greenberg J, Baron RA. Behavior in Organizations, 7th edition. Upper Saddle River, NJ: Prentice Hall; 2000.
5. Hellriegel D, Slocum JW, Jr. Organizational Behavior, 10th edition, Thomson South-Western; 2004.
6. Jerald G. Organizational Behavior: The State of the Science. Lawrence Erlbaum Associates; 2003.
7. Katz D, Kahn R. The Social Psychology of Organizations, 2nd edition. New York: John Wiley and Sons; 1978. p 196.
8. Locke EA. The Blackwell Handbook of Principles of Organizational Behavior. Blackwell Publishing; 2002.
9. Luthans F. Organizational Behavior, 10th edition. Boston: McGraw-Hill, 2005.
10. Miner JB. Organizational Behavior: Foundations, Theories, and Analyses. Oxford University Press; 2002.
11. Punnett BJ. International Perspectives on Organizational Behavior and Human Resource Management. ME Sharpe; 2004.
12. Robbins SP. Essentials of Organizational Behavior. Upper Saddle River, NJ: Prentice Hall; 1997.
13. Roger C, Smith T. "Benchmarking Cultural Transition." Journal of Business Strategy; 2000.
14. Samson R. Leadership and management in nursing practice and education. New Delhi: Jaypee Brothers; p. 50-5.
15. Stephen H. "Jam Science: Improvisation is essential for good jazz—and a great tool for effective teams." CMA Management; 2004.

CHAPTER 17

Financial Management

LEARNING OBJECTIVES

- Definition, Objectives, Elements, Functions, Principles and Scope of Financial Management
- Financial Planning (Budgeting for Nursing Department)
- Proposal, Projecting Requirement for Staff, Equipment and Supplies for: Hospital and Patient Care Units and Emergency and Disaster Units
- Budget and Budgetary Process
- Financial Audit

INTRODUCTION

Financial management is a vital activity in any organization. It is the process of planning, organizing, controlling and monitoring financial resources with a view to achieve organizational goals and objectives. It is an ideal practice for controlling the financial activities of an organization, such as procurement of funds, utilization of funds, accounting, payments, risk assessment and every other thing related to money. Financial management is one of the most important aspects in business. In order to start up or even run a successful business, you will need excellent knowledge in financial management.

FINANCIAL MANAGEMENT

Financial management means planning, organizing, directing and controlling the financial activities, such as procurement and utilization of funds of the enterprise. It means applying general management principles to financial resources of the enterprise **(Fig. 17.1)**.

Definition

- "Financial management is the activity concerned with planning, raising, controlling and administering of funds used in the business." —***Guthman and Dougal***
- "Financial management is that area of business management devoted to a judicious use of capital and a careful selection of the source of capital in order to enable a spending unit to move in the direction of reaching the goals." —***JF Brandley***
- "Financial management is the operational activity of a business that is responsible for obtaining and effectively utilizing the funds necessary for efficient operations." —***Massie***

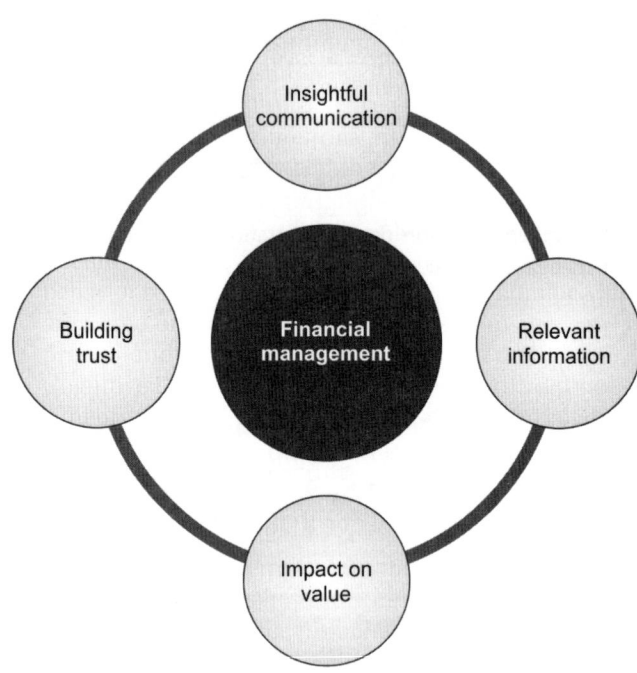

Fig. 17.1: Financial management.

Concept of Financial Management

Financial management refers to the strategic planning, organizing, directing, and controlling of financial undertakings in an organization or an institute. It also includes applying management principles to the financial assets of an organization, while also playing an important part in fiscal management. Take a look at the objectives involved:

- Maintaining enough supply of funds for the organization
- Ensuring shareholders of the organization to get good returns on their investment
- Optimum and efficient utilization of funds

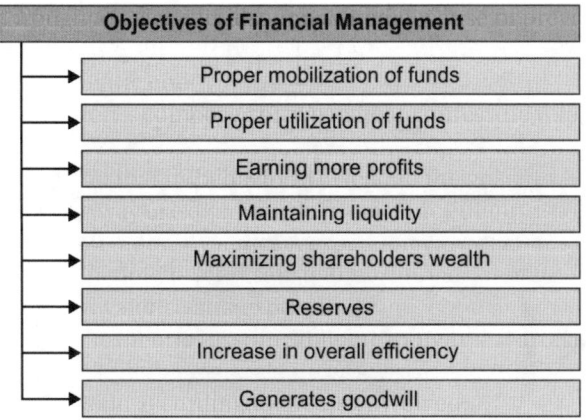

Fig. 17.2: Objectives of financial management.

> **Box 17.1:** Key elements to the process of financial management.
>
> 1. **Financial planning**
>   - Management need to ensure that enough funding is available at the right time to meet the needs of the business.
>   - In the short-term, funding may be needed to invest in equipment and stocks, pay employees and fund sales made on credit.
>   - In the medium and long-term, funding may be required for significant additions to the productive capacity of the business or to make acquisitions.
> 2. **Financial control**
>   - Financial control is a critically important activity to help the business ensure that the business is meeting its objectives.
>   - Financial control addresses questions, such as:
>   - Are assets being used efficiently?
>   - Are the businesses assets secure?
>   - Do management act in the best interest of shareholders and in accordance with business rules?
> 3. **Financial decision-making**
>   - The key aspects of financial decision-making relate to investment, financing and dividends:
>   - Investments must be financed in some way—however there are always financing alternatives that can be considered. For example, it is possible to raise finance from selling new shares, borrowing from banks or taking credit from suppliers.
>   - A key financing decision is whether profits earned by the business should be retained rather than distributed to shareholders via dividends.
>   - If dividends are too high, the business may be starved of funding to reinvest in growing revenues and profits.

- Creating real and safe investment opportunities to invest in.

Objectives of Financial Management

The financial management is generally concerned with procurement, allocation and control of financial resources of a concern. The objectives can be **(Fig. 17.2)**:

- To ensure regular and adequate supply of funds to the concern.
- To ensure adequate returns to the shareholders which will depend upon the earning capacity, market price of the share, expectations of the shareholders.
- To ensure optimum funds utilization: Once the funds are procured, they should be utilized in maximum possible way at least cost.
- To ensure safety on investment, i.e., funds should be invested in safe ventures so that adequate rate of return can be achieved.
- To plan a sound capital structure: There should be sound and fair composition of capital so that a balance is maintained between debt and equity capital.

Principles of Financial Management

Principles mean general guidelines of a firm to perform its activities. The principles of financial management are discussed as follows **(Box 17.2)**:

- **The principle of risk-return trade-off:** Risk and return are closely related with each other. More risk, more return is a common statement. Naturally, an investor expects more return for taking more risk.
- **The principle of net cash flows:** To implement any investment decision, it is important to determine the initial cash outflow to initiate the project and cash inflows received from the project.
- **The principle of internal financing:** It must be preferable to raise funds from the internal sources.
- **The principle of the time value of money:** The value of money changes due to change in time. One must prefer today's one taka (Tk.l) than that of the future.
- **The principle of debt repayment:** It is important to repay the debt capital in time.

> **Box 17.2:** Principles of financial management.
>
> - Trade off risk and return
> - Formation of optimal capital structure
> - Diversification of both investment and borrowing
> - Aware of time value of money
> - Forecast cash flows
> - Take a right insurance plan
> - Concentration on wealth maximization
> - Reinvest rather than consume
> - Determine cost of capital
> - Financial decision align with business life cycle

- **The principle of diversification:** It is not wise to invest the entire fund in a single project. The fund must be diversified to diversify its risk.
- **Principle of liquidity and profitability:** There is a negative relationship between liquidity and profitability.
- **Principle of recovery:** An important principle of business finance is the principle of recovery. It is very much crucial that whether the terms of recovery will be flexible or rigid.
- **The principle of minimum flotation costs:** Flotation costs are needed for external financing. The cost of capital increases due to flotation cost. So, the matter of minimum flotation cost is to be kept in deep concern.
- **Ideal principle of financing:** Ideal principle of raising funds is to run properly. Ideal principles of financing means current assets are to be acquired from short-term fund and fixed assets are to be procured from long-term fund.

- **Principle of recovery:** An important principle of business finance is principle of recovery. It is very much crucial that whether the terms of recovery will be flexible or rigid.
- **The principle of minimum flotation costs:** Flotation costs are needed for external financing. The cost of capital increases due to flotation cost. So, the matter of minimum flotation cost is to be kept in deep concern.
- **Ideal principle of financing:** Ideal principle of raising funds is to be run properly. Ideal principle of financing means current assets is to be acquired from short-term fund and fixed assets are to be procured from long-term fund.
- **Principle of the minimum cost of capital:** Investable funds are not found free of cost. Also cost of capital is not the same for different sources. At this regard, such measures are to be taken which can show the way to lower the cost of capital.
- **Principle of dividend policy:** It is important to the financial manager that what percentage of profit will be distributed to the common shareholders as dividend and what percentage is to be kept as retained earnings for re-investment.
- **The principle of priority:** There may be several project profiles. Among them, which projects are to be given priority bears importance.
- **The principle of firm's goal congruence:** The objective of financing to run projects is to earn some profit. But, the specific goal is to be determined.
- **The principle of the business cycle:** Effective and corrective measures are to be taken at different stages of the business cycle.

Functions of Financial Management (Fig. 17.3)

- **Estimation of capital requirements:** A finance manager has to make estimation with regards to capital requirements of the company. This will depend upon expected costs and profits and future programs and policies of a concern. Estimations have to be made in an adequate manner which increases earning capacity of enterprise.
- **Determination of capital composition:** Once the estimation have been made, the capital structure have to be decided. This involves short-term and long-term debt equity analysis. This will depend upon the proportion of equity capital a company is possessing and additional funds which have to be raised from outside parties.
- **Choice of sources of funds:** For additional funds to be procured, a company has many choices, such as:
  - Issue of shares and debentures
  - Loans to be taken from banks and financial institutions
  - Public deposits to be drawn like in form of bonds.
  Choice of factor will depend on relative merits and demerits of each source and period of financing.
- **Investment of funds:** The finance manager has to decide to allocate funds into profitable ventures so that there is safety on investment and regular returns is possible.
- **Disposal of surplus:** The net profits decision has to be made by the finance manager. This can be done in two ways:

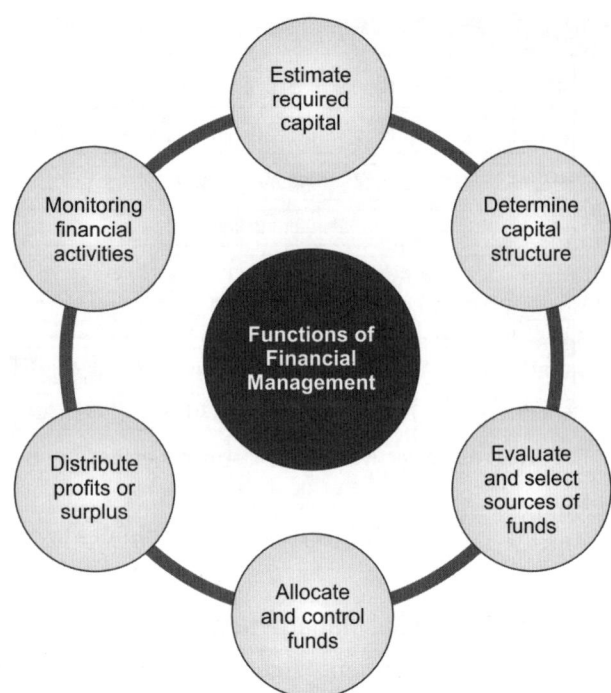

Fig. 17.3: Function of financial management.

1. *Dividend declaration:* It includes identifying the rate of dividends and other benefits like bonus.
2. *Retained profits:* The volume has to be decided which will depend upon expansional, innovational, diversification plans of the company.

- **Management of cash:** Finance manager has to make decisions with regards to cash management. Cash is required for many purposes, such as payment of wages and salaries, payment of electricity and water bills, payment to creditors, meeting current liabilities, maintenance of enough stock, purchase of raw materials, etc.
- **Financial controls:** The finance manager has not only to plan, procure and utilize the funds but he also has to exercise control over finances. This can be done through many techniques, such as ratio analysis, financial forecasting, cost and profit control, etc.

Importance of Financial Management

This form of management is important for various reasons. Take a look at some of these reasons:
1. Helps organizations in financial planning
2. Assists organizations in the planning and acquisition of funds
3. Helps organizations in effectively utilizing and allocating the funds received or acquired
4. Assists organizations in making critical financial decisions
5. Helps in improving the profitability of organizations
6. Increases the overall value of the firms or organizations
7. Provides economic stability
8. Encourages employees to save money, which helps them in personal financial planning.

Scope of Financial Management

The introduction to financial management also requires you to understand the scope of financial management. It is important that financial decisions take care of the shareholders' interests. Further, they are upheld by the maximization of the wealth of the shareholders, which depends on the increase in net worth, capital invested in the business, and plowed-back profits for the growth and prosperity of the organization. The scope of financial management is explained in **Figure 17.4**:

- **Investment decisions** include investment in fixed assets (called as capital budgeting): Investment in current assets is also a part of investment decisions called as working capital decisions.
- **Financial decisions:** They relate to the raising of finance from various resources which will depend upon decision on type of source, period of financing, cost of financing and the returns thereby.
- **Dividend decision:** The finance manager has to take decision with regards to the net profit distribution. Net profits are generally divided into two:
  1. *Dividend for shareholders:* Dividend and the rate of it has to be decided.
  2. *Retained profits:* Amount of retained profits has to be finalized which will depend upon expansion and diversification plans of the enterprise.

FINANCIAL PLANNING

Financial planning is the process of estimating the capital required and determining it is competition. It is the process of framing financial policies in relation to procurement, investment and administration of funds of an enterprise.

Definition

Financial planning is the process of calculating the amount of capital that is required by an organization and then determining its allocation.

Objectives of Financial Planning

Financial planning has got many objectives to look forward to:
- **Determining capital requirements:** This will depend upon factors like cost of current and fixed assets, promotional expenses and long-range planning. Capital requirements have to be looked with both aspects: short-term and long-term requirements.
- **Determining capital structure:** The capital structure is the composition of capital, i.e., the relative kind and proportion of capital required in the business. This includes decisions of debt- equity ratio-both short-term and long-term.
- Framing financial policies with regards to cash control, lending, borrowings, etc.
- A finance manager ensures that the scarce financial resources are maximally utilized in the best possible manner at least cost in order to get maximum returns on investment.

Components of Financial Planning (Figs. 17.5 and 17.6)

Cash Flow Management

- To truly understand your current assets, liabilities, and net worth; it is important to identify – in writing – the status of your personal and professional income and expense balance sheet.

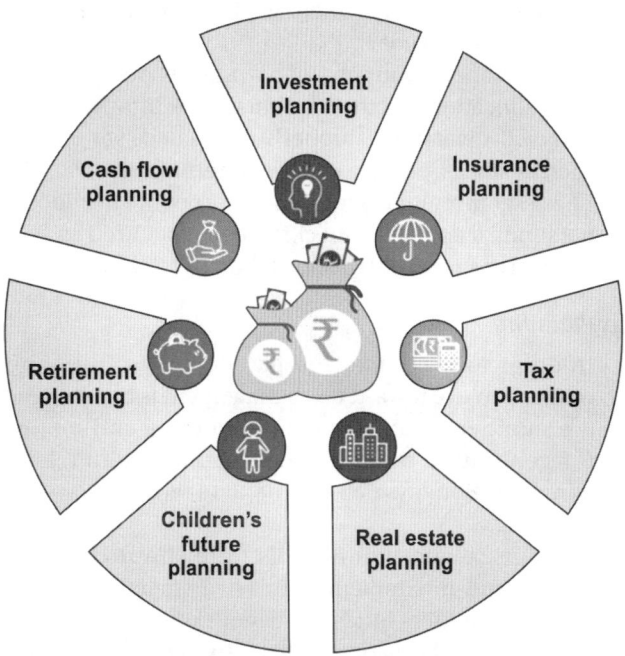

Fig. 17.5: Types of financial planning.

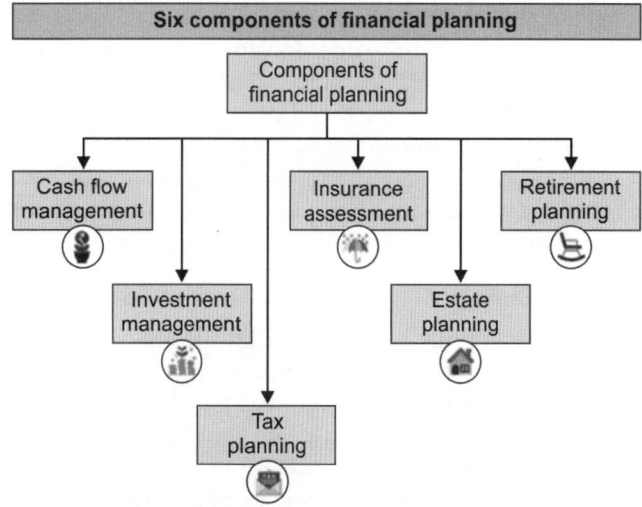

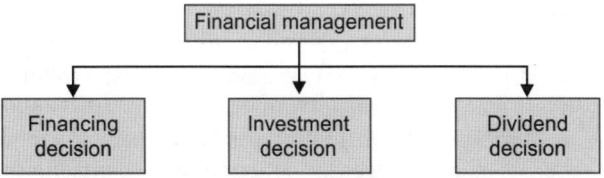

Fig. 17.4: The scope of financial management.

Fig. 17.6: Six components of financial planning.

- We include goal planning as part of this step because setting realistic goals and achieving them is highly dependent on your ability to save for those goals.
- Other aspects of cash flow management include the debt elimination plan, if needed, as well as a comprehensive savings plan.

Investment Management

- When most people think of financial planning, they may think of investing. Many people ask, "What is the latest hot stock?" or "What is the best mutual fund?" Studies have shown that those are bad questions because investing is not about the latest stock or timing the market.
- Investing is a strategy that takes your goals, your risk tolerance, and your timeline into consideration. Then, developing the best investing strategy to meet those goals. Your investing strategy should be the foundation for meeting your retirement goals, education goals and other long-term goals.
- If done properly, your portfolio strategy should include an asset allocation mix that minimizes risk through a global and well-diversified (properly correlated) set of assets, such as stocks, bonds and other alternatives.
- The asset mix and correlation factors of the portfolio are personalized to your specific needs and are key to the long-term success of the portfolio.

Tax Planning

- In order to maximize and preserve your investment returns, an eye toward tax management is crucial. There are number of tax-reduction strategies and methods for generating tax-free income and wealth transfer considerations; which can be achieved by way of tax planning.
- No matter what your age is, one should consider, understand and implement this in a proactive manner.
- For example, debt funds can benefit you more when held for more than 3 years than bank fixed deposits from tax perspective.

Insurance Assessment

- An important and often overlooked component of financial planning is to evaluate the kind of insurance you need to protect yourself and your assets with and your loved ones. Insurance types can include life, disability, health, vehicle and property insurance to name a few.
- Depending on your stage in life, your insurance needs (risk management needs) will change and evolve.

Estate Planning

- No matter your age, estate planning is an integral component of long-term financial planning. You can control the distribution of your assets, both during life and upon death, with the right estate plan structures in place for your unique circumstances and wishes.
- Furthermore, keeping your estate plan current is just as important as creating it in the first place.

Retirement Planning

Retirement planning helps you set a goal for, when you want to retire and your income and lifestyle objectives during retirement. Your advisor can determine, if your current savings are on track and provide guidance on strategies to help achieve those goals.

Importance of Financial Planning

Financial planning is process of framing objectives, policies, procedures, programs and budgets regarding the financial activities of a concern. This ensures effective and adequate financial and investment policies. The importance can be outlined as:

- Adequate funds have to be ensured.
- Financial planning helps in ensuring a reasonable balance between outflow and inflow of funds so that stability is maintained.
- Financial planning ensures that the suppliers of funds are easily investing in companies which exercise financial planning.
- Financial planning helps in making growth and expansion programs which help in long-run survival of the company.
- Financial planning reduces uncertainties with regards to changing market trends which can be faced easily through enough funds.
- Financial planning helps in reducing the uncertainties which can be a hindrance to growth of the company. This helps in ensuring stability an d profitability in concern.

Role of Financial Managers

Financial managers are responsible for the financial health of an organization. They produce financial reports, direct investment activities, and develop strategies and plans for the long-term financial goals of their organization. Financial managers typically:

- Prepare financial statements, business activity reports, and forecasts
- Monitor financial details to ensure that legal requirements are met
- Supervise employees who do financial reporting and budgeting
- Review company financial reports and seek ways to reduce costs
- Analyze market trends to find opportunities for expansion or for acquiring other companies
- Help management make financial decisions.

Important Skills for Financial Managers

- **Analytical skills:** Financial managers increasingly assist executives in making decisions that affect the organization, a task for which they need analytical ability.
- **Communication:** Excellent communication skills are essential because financial managers must explain and justify complex financial transactions.
    Attention to detail. In preparing and analyzing reports, such as balance sheets and income statements, financial managers must pay attention to detail.

- **Math skills:** Financial managers must be skilled in math, including algebra. An understanding of international finance and complex financial documents also is important.
- **Organizational skills:** Financial managers deal with a range of information and documents. They must stay organized to do their jobs effectively.

Types of Financial Management

An organization requires financial management for various activities. For examples: approving loans or credit lines, hiring employees, building customer's relationship, creating company's credit rating, adjustment in budgets, managing cash inflow and outflow activities, risk management and more. One of the essential primary types of financial management decision is to build and increase the valuation of an organization.

Treasury and Capital Budget Management

- Capital budgeting is the planning procedure used to decide if a company's fixed assets, for example, new plant, new machinery; new research projects are worth of allocating funds through the organization capitalization structure (equity, debt or profit earnings).
- Numerous formal strategies are utilized in capital budgeting, for example, profitability index, payback period, net present value, real options valuation, accounting rate of return, internal rate of return, equivalent annual cost and more.

Capital Structure Management

- In corporate finance, capital structure is the manner in which a company finances through a mix of debt or equity securities.
- Debt financing comes as bond issues, while equity comes from retained earnings or as a stock.
- Short-term debt financing, for example, working capital necessities is likewise viewed as a major aspect of the capital structure.
- Here financial management team is responsible for capital structure of a company's short-term debts, long-term debts, equities, preferred stocks and more.

Working Capital Management

- Working capital management of an organization refers to managing bookkeeping methodology and accounting strategies intended to keep track of current assets, current liabilities, cash flow, inventory turnover ratio, working capital ratio and much more.
- The basic role of working capital management is to ensure the organization dependably keeps up adequate liquid cash to meet its short-term debts and operational cost.
- This is one of the types of financial management where team need to maintain working capital management to smoother company's operational cycle, and also to improve the company's earnings.

Financial Planning, Analysis and Control Management

- Financial planning is the undertaking of deciding regarding how a business will accomplish its key objectives and targets.
- More often an organization makes a financial plan after the vision and mission have been set.
- The financial plan describes each and every activities and exercises needed to accomplish these goals.
- Financial analysis is the way toward analyzing businesses, budgets, projects and other finance related matters to decide their execution, suitability and performance.
- Regularly, financial examination is utilized to break down whether a company is steady, liquid or sufficiently productive to permit any investments.
- Financial controls are procedures, arrangements and methods that are actualized to manage finances.
- Financial controls framework give an instrument to management to screen the accomplishment of operational goals and objectives. These types of financial management decisions are undertaken by teams who are more often not responsible for the bookkeeping office, the budget division and the audit related work.

Insurance and Risk Management

- Insurance and risk mostly have a similar objective towards minimizing the organization's risk; however distinctive strategies are implemented to accomplish these objectives.
- Risk management team is accountable for minimizing the organization's risk factors that are threat for their business operations.
- **For example:** Flood, fire or any other natural disasters. These types of financial management are mostly responsible to build techniques to enable the organization to stay in profitable without any affect, by natural disaster or changes in the price due to currency difference.

■ STRATEGIC FINANCIAL MANAGEMENT

Strategic financial management means not only managing a company's finances but managing them with the intention to succeed, i.e., to attain the company's goals and objectives and maximize shareholder value over time.

Elements of Strategic Financial Management

A company will apply strategic financial management throughout its organizational operations, which involves designing elements that will maximize the firm's financial resources and using them efficiently. Here a firm needs to be creative, as there is no one-size-fits-all approach to strategic management, and each company will devise elements that reflect its own particular needs and goals. However, some of the more common elements of strategic financial management could include the following.

Planning

- Define objectives precisely.

- Identify and quantify available and potential resources.
- Write a specific business financial plan.

Budgeting
- Help the company functions with financial efficiency, and reduced waste.
- Identify areas that incur the most operating costs, or exceed the budgeted cost.
- Ensure sufficient liquidity to cover operating expenses without tapping external resources.
- Uncover areas where a firm may invest earnings to achieve goals more effectively.

Managing and Assessing Risk
- Identify, analyze, and mitigate uncertainty in investment decisions.
- Evaluate the potential for financial exposure; examine capital expenditures (CapEx) and workplace policies.
- Employ risk metrics, such as degree of operating leverage calculations, standard deviation, and value-at-risk (VaR) strategies.

Establishing Ongoing Procedures
- Collect and analyze data.
- Make financial decisions that are consistent.
- Track and analyze variance, i.e., differences between budgeted and actual results.
- Identify problems and take appropriate corrective actions.

■ BUDGET (FIG. 17.7)

Budget word was first coined by the British Kings in early days from the word 'BOUGETTE'. Budget is essential in every walk of our life-national, domestic and business. A budget is prepared to have effective utilization of funds and for the realization of objective as efficiently as possible. Budgeting is a powerful tool to the management for performing its functions, i.e., formulation plans, coordination activities and controlling operations etc., efficiently. For efficient and effective management planning and control are two highly essential functions.

Important milestones were:
- **1215 AD:** Constitutional exposure
- **1718 AD:** Consolidated fund act passed which considered budget as financial statement of government activities for facilitating accountability of public fund.
- **1882 AD:** Budget entered the parliament for first time seeking advice.

Definition
- Budget is a concrete precise picture of the total operation of an enterprise in monetary. —*HM Donovan*
- According to Taylor "Budget is a financial plan of Government for a definite period."
- Budget is an operational plan, for a definite period usually a year. Expressed in financial terms and based on expected income and expenditure.

  Budget is a concrete precise picture of the total operation of an enterprise in monetary terms.
- **Nursing budget:** A plan for allocation of resources based preconceived needs for a proposed series of programs to deliver patient care during one fiscal year.
- **Hospital budget:** Is a financial plan to meet future service expectations.

Meaning of Budget
- A budget is defined as the formal expression of plans, goals, and objectives of management that covers all aspects of operations for a designated time period.
- The budget is a tool providing targets and direction.
- Budgets provide control over the immediate environment, help to master the financial aspects of the job and department, and solve problems before they occur.
- Budgets focus on the importance of evaluating alternative actions before decisions actually are implemented.
- A budget is a financial plan to control future operations and results. It is expressed in numbers, such as dollars, units, pounds, hours, manpower, and so on.
- It is needed to operate effectively and efficiently. Budgeting, when used effectively, is a technique resulting in systematic, productive management.
- Budgeting facilitates control and communication and also provides motivation to employees.

Objectives of Budgeting (Fig. 17.8)

The main objective of a firm is to make an excess of revenue over expenses to maximize profit. But it is not a matter of a dream or chance. There is no magic formula for boosting the figure of profit overnight. Budgeting can increase the chances of making profits within the given environment. The main objectives of budgets are as follows:
- To provide a realistic estimate of income and expenses for a period and of the financial position at the close of the period.

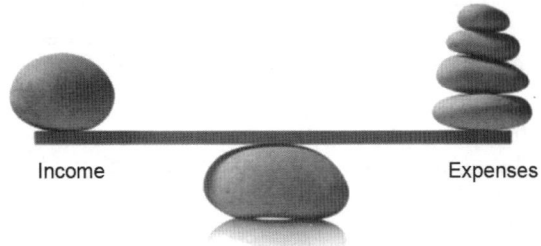

Fig. 17.7: Budget.

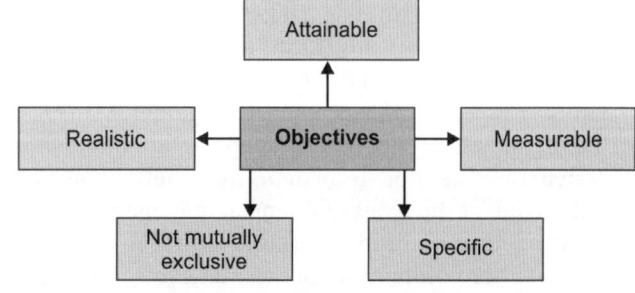

Fig. 17.8: Objectives of budgeting.

- To provide a coordinated plan of action which is design to achieve the estimates reflected in the budget.
- To provide a comparison of actual results with those budgeted and an analysis and interpretation of deviations by areas of responsibility to indicate courses of corrective actions and to lead to improvement in future plans.
- To provide a guide for management decisions in adjusting plans and objectives if there is an uncontrollable change in conditions.
- To provide a ready basis for making forecasts during the budget period to guide management in making day to day decisions.

Purpose of Budget (Box 17.3)

- Budget supplies the mechanism for translating fiscal objective into projected monthly spending pattern.
- Budget enhances fiscal planning and decision-making.
- Budget clearly recognizes controllable and uncontrollable cost areas.
- Budget offers a useful format for communicating fiscal objectives.
- Budget allows feedback of utilization of budget.
- Budget helps to identify problem areas and facilitates effective solution.
- Budget provides means for measuring and recording financial success with the objectives of the organizations.

Primary purpose: To ensure the effective use of scarce financial and nonfinancial resources.

- Budget supplies the mechanism for translating fiscal objective into projected monthly spending pattern.
- Budget enhances fiscal planning and decision-making.
- Budget clearly recognizes controllable and uncontrollable cost areas.
- Budget offers a useful format for communication fiscal objectives.
- Budget allows feedback of utilization of budget.
- Budget helps to identify problem areas and facilitates effective solution.
- Budget provides means for measuring and recording financial success with the objectives of the organization.

Other purposes:
- Coordinating efforts of various departments.
- Establishing a frame of reference for the managerial decision-making.
- Providing a criterion for evaluating managerial performance.

Characteristics of Budget

A budget is a financial document or an action plan which is prepared and used to project future income and expenses. It outlines an organization's financial and operational goals. It can also include nonmonetary information with the monetary information. They need to be made and approved in advance of the year in which they are to be used or implemented.

Following are the characteristics of a good budget:
- It is expressed in quantitative or monetary terms.
- It is prepared for a fixed period of time. It is prepared before the period in which it commences.
- Practical to implement.
- It spells out the objects and the policies to be pursued in order to achieve the objective of the organization.
- Many people are involved in drawing up a budget.
- Flexible enough to allow changes in the changing environment.
- Prepared on the basis of established standards of performance.
- Analysis of cost and revenues.
- On the basis of budget report performance of the organization is constantly monitored.

Principles of Budget (Box 17.4)

- Budget should provide sound financial management by focusing on requirement of the organization.
- Budget requires that program activities planned in advance.
- Budget should focus on objectives and policies of the organization. It must flow from objectives and gives realistic expression to the way of realizing such objectives.
- Setting budget target requires an adequate checks and balance against the adoption of too high or too low estimate. Utmost care is a must for fixing targets.
- Budget period must be appropriate to the nature of business or service and to the type of budget.
- Budgets should ensure the most effective use of scarce financial and nonfinancial resources.
- Budgetary process requires consistent delegation for which fixed duties responsibilities are required to be allocated to managers at different level from framing and executing budget.
- Budgeting should include coordinating efforts of various departments establishing a frame of reference for managerial decision, and providing a criterion for evaluating managerial performance.
- Budget necessitates a review of the performance of the previous year and an evaluation of its adequacy both in quality and in quantity.

Box 17.3: Purpose of budget.

- To control resources
- To communicate plans to various responsibility center managers
- To motivate managers to strive to achieve budget goals
- To evaluate the performance of managers
- To provide visibility into the company's performance

Box 17.4: Principles of budget.

- Provide sound financial management
- Focus on objectives and polices
- Most effective use of finance
- Activities planned in advance
- Delegation of authority and responsibility for execution of budget
- Coordinating efforts of various departments
- Setting targets
- Prepare under the supervision and direction

- While developing a budget, the provision should be made for its flexibility.
- Budget necessitates a review of the performance of the previous year and an evaluation of its adequacy both in quality and in quantity.
- While developing a budget, the provision should be made for its flexibility.
- Budget is prepared under the direction and supervision of the administration or financial officer.
- Budgets are to be prepared and interpreted consistently throughout the organization in the communication of planning process.

Classifications of Budget

Budget consists mainly three sections.
- **Manpower budget:** The manpower budget includes wages and other benefits provided for regular and temporary worker.
- **Capital expenditure budget:** The capital expenditure budget includes purchases of land, buildings and major equipment of considerable expenses and long life.
- **Operating budget:** The operating budget includes the cost of supplies, minor equipment, repairs and overhead expenses.

Types of Budget (Fig. 17.9)

- **Incremental budget** is one based on estimated changes in present operation, plus a percentage increase for inflation, all of which is added to previous year budget.
- **Flexible budget** consists of several financial plans, each for a different level of program activity. It is based on the fact, that operating conditions rarely conform to expectations.
- **Rollover budget** is one that forecasts program, revenues and expenses for a period greater than a year, to accommodate program that are larger than annual budget cycle.
- **Open-ended budget** is a financial plan in which each operating manager presents a single cost estimate for what is considered optimal activity level for each program in the unit, without indicating how the budget should be scaled down if less funding is available.
- **Fixed-ceiling budget** is a financial plan in which the uppermost spending limits are set by the top executive the unit and divisional managers develop budget proposals for their areas of responsibility.
- **Performance budget** is based on functions, which allocate functions, not division's, e.g., direct nursing care, in service education, quality improvement, nursing research.
- **Program budget** is one where costs are computed for a total program, i.e., group total costs for each service program, e.g., maternal child health (MCH), Universal Immunization Program (UIP), Family planning (FP), etc.
- **Production budget** is the budget that aims at securing the economical manufacture of products and maximizing the utilization of production facilities.
- **Revenue and expense budget** is expressed in financial terms and takes the nature of a proforma income statement for the future. It may be prepared in a detail form or in an abstract statement showing the items of profit and loss under classified headings.
- **Capital expenditure budget** is prepared for assuring planned timely capital investment in the business to ensure the availability of capital at the right time over longer period.
- **Zero based budgets** require the nurse manager to examine, justify each cost of every program both old and new, in every annual budget preparation.
- **Sunset budget** is designed to "self destruct" within a prescribed time period to ensure the cessation of spend in by a predetermined date.
- **Sales budget** is the starting point in a budgetary program, since sales are basic activities which give shape to all other activities. Sale budgets are compiled in terms of quality as well as of value.
- **Cash budget** is prepared by way of projecting the possible cash receipts and payments over the budget period.

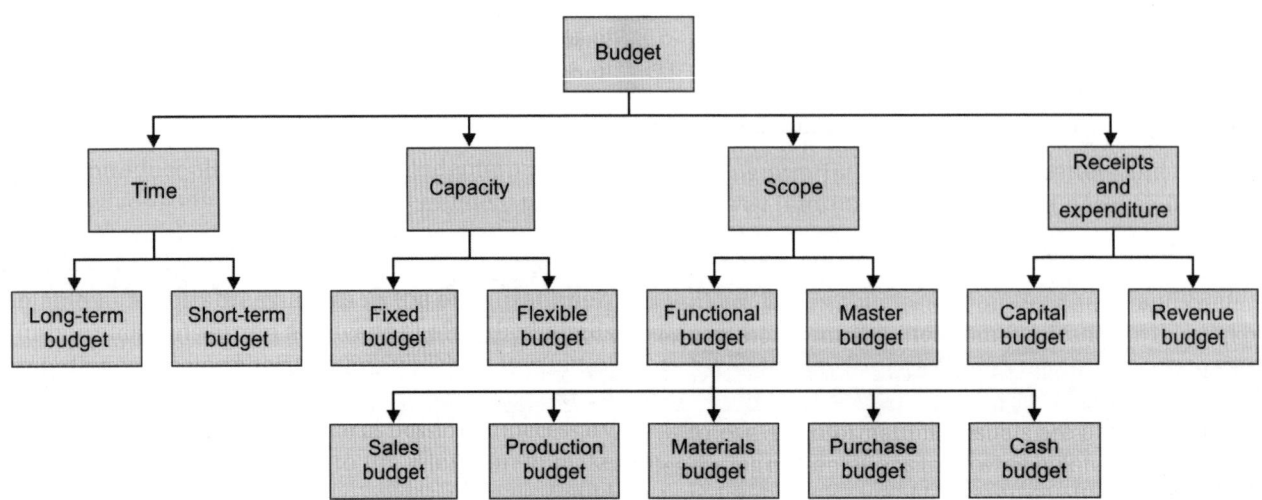

Fig. 17.9: Types of budget.

Steps in the Budgeting Process

Budgeting is a detailed process with several intricate steps leading up to understanding it at large. A step-by-step guide to the budgeting process is given as below.

- **Update budget assumptions:** Budgets are always prepared on certain assumptions. Those assumptions could be related to the sales trends, cost trends or environmental conditions. Before embarking on preparing the budget, these assumptions must be thoroughly reviewed according to the recent environmental conditions.
- **Note available funding:** Limited funding can greatly hinder the growth projects of the business. Therefore, in the preparation of budgets adequate attention has to be given to the available funding as the availability of investable funds will determine the initiation of viable projects.
- **Step costing points:** The business environment is subject to dynamism. Every day it is posed with challenges that can completely change its cost structure. Therefore, in the budgeting process certain factors that can affect the costing for the business should be closely considered. These factors should be identified beforehand in order to make the budget realistic.
- **Create budget package:** In budget package, previous standards related to the budgeting process are taken in order to formulate a budget for the current period. Previous standards are updated according to the recent environmental conditions. Budget package is a kind of outline according to which budget has to be prepared.
- **Obtain revenue forecast:** There is no denying the fact that sales budget is the most crucial budget of all. All the budgets are based on the sales budget. Furthermore, sales budget determines whether the business is generating enough revenue necessary for its survival. Therefore, adequate attention must be given to the preparation of sales budget by forecasting demand accurately.
- **Obtain department budgets:** The department budgets will help to reach a budgeted expenditure for the budgeted period. Each department will prepare its own budget and then all of them will be combined to become a part of the master budget.
- **Validate compensation:** Compensation plans are a significant component of the budgeting process. As compensation is subject to an annual increase, therefore, it should be prepared with great care. The approval for compensation increase should first be taken from the top management, and then it should be augmented in the budgeted compensation plans.
- **Validate bonus plans:** In order to maintain the morale of the employees, bonuses are frequently given to out motivated workers. Bonuses act as an appraisal method. Bonus announcements that are not considered in the budgeting process can create havoc in the profits of the business. Therefore, any bonus plans should be taken into consideration beforehand. The top management should be consulted for any bonus plans.
- **Obtain capital budget requests:** Capital expenditure ensures expansion of the business. It helps the business to avail the opportunities necessary for business growth. Any capital expenditure plans should be taken in advance, and they should be included in the budgeting process accordingly.
- **Update the budget model:** Any changes in the assumptions of the budget model should be updated, and final budget should be prepared accordingly. A delay in this may lead to glitches later on that could cause confusion.
- **Review the budget:** The budget should be reviewed thoroughly once it is prepared in order to correct any flaws. A little decimal placed wrongly can create quite an unbalance in the budget sheet.
- **Obtain approval:** The budget should be presented to the top management. They will evaluate whether it has been prepared according to their requirements.
- **Issue the budget:** The budget should be formally issued after its approval. All the operations there and then will take place according to it.

Skills Needed for Managing a Budget

Many skills make managing a budget easier. These three skills, in particular, make the complex task of budgetary management straightforward.

Budget Preparation

- Preparing a budget for the coming year is a vital skill for managers. When preparing your annual budget, consider things like business objectives and departmental goals.
- Begin by identifying overhead costs that must be paid for the department to function.
- Then you can consider capital investments that could improve the department.
- Taking the time to prepare a detailed and functional budget will make its management much simpler.

Financial Analysis

- Managers must understand how to analyze the financial health of their department, and possibly the entire organization.
- Profits and losses will impact the annual budget.
- An excellent budgetary manager can review financial statements and make informed decisions for their budget based on the information they find.

Financial Forecasting

- Financial forecasting is the process of determining how a business or department will perform at a predetermined future time.
- Budgetary management must include financial forecasting.
- Great managers use financial forecasting to determine where they should invest money and where they should expect additional costs.
- This will help them maintain a balanced budget for the year.

Importance of Budget

Budget is a numerical description of expected income and planned expenditure for an organization for a specified period of time (**Box 17.5**). It is a concrete, precise, picture of the total operation of an enterprise/organization/institution in monetary term, i.e., finance.

The following point serves the importance of budget:
- Budget is needed for planning for future course of action and to have a control over all activities in the organization.
- Budget facilitates co-coordinating operation of various departments and sections for realizing organizational objectives.
- Budget serves as a guide for action in the organization.
- Budget helps one to weigh the values and to make decision when necessary on whether one is of a greater value in the program than the other.

Benefits of Budget (Fig. 17.10)

Budgets are produced in all organizations, whether they are small, large, private or public sector. They are important and are produced for the following reasons:
- To compel planning—by having a formal budgeting procedure, managers are forced to consider business objectives and ways in which those objectives can be achieved.
- To coordinate the activities of the various parts of the business and to ensure that the parts are working together.
- To communicate plans to the various responsibility managers within the enterprise.
- To motivate managers to work towards the business objectives.
- To control activities—the budget provides a yardstick against which the performance of the business can be compared.
- To evaluate the performance of the managers
- The budgeting process helps management learn from past experience. Management can critically look at the success or failure of the past budgets and isolate errors and analyze their causes and establish steps to avoid repetition of the same errors.
- Budgets help in the just measurement of performance. Due to quantification of budgets, the measurement is more objective, thus eliminating biases that might be introduced due to subjective evaluations.
- The budgeting process induces the management to shift attention to the future operations. It forces managers to anticipate and forecast the trends and changes in the external environment.

Limitations of Budget (Fig. 17.11)

Some of the problems associated with budgeting are:
- Budgets are often too rigid and restrictive and supervisors are given little free hand in managing their resources. The budgets may either be changed too often or not at all, making it difficult for employees to meet performance levels.
- Budgets are used to evaluate the performance and results, but the causes of failures and successes are not thoroughly investigated.
- Budgets may be used punitively. The employees may regard budgets simply as rating tools or as a device for catching their mistakes. This will lower their morale and dilute their sense of dedication.
- Budget goals may be conceived as too high. A high production level or sales level may be presented as unrealistic and may create tension and pressures which could very well result in worker inefficiency and create conflict between workers and the management.

Essential Requisition in Budget Preparation

An essential requisition for budget preparation will include:
- **Forecasting:** Sound forecasting may be related to making decisions on purchases, expansion, adverting, services, working capital needs, etc.
- **Accounting:** Well conceived accounting system must be needed to compare the budget information with actual accomplishment. The cost information tells us to how much it will cost to produce or give services.
- **Lines of authority:** Budget preparation, operation and supervision need/require clearly defined lines of authority.

Box 17.5: Importance of the budget.
- Very vital role
- Very complex and lengthy process
- Promoting social welfare activities
- Sound budgeting useful socially, economically and politically
- Indicates shift in government policies and programs
- Budget becomes a tool of planning, articulation of policies, implementation of programs and review of accomplishments

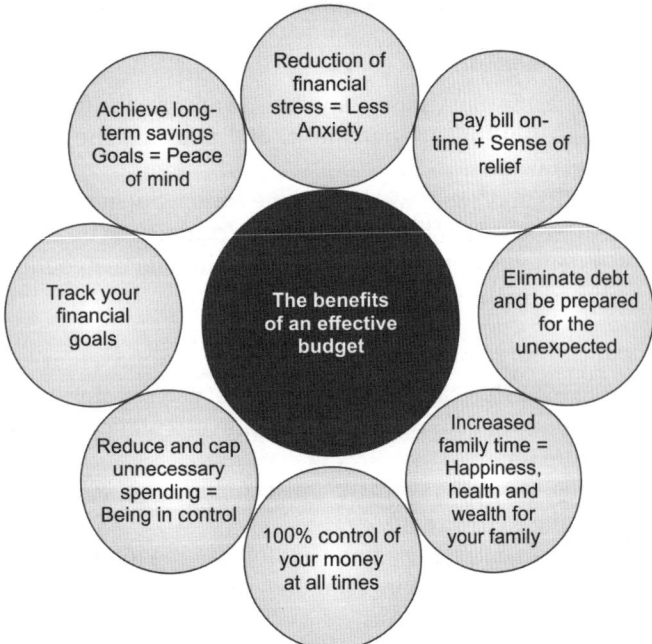

Fig. 17.10: Benefits of an effective budget.

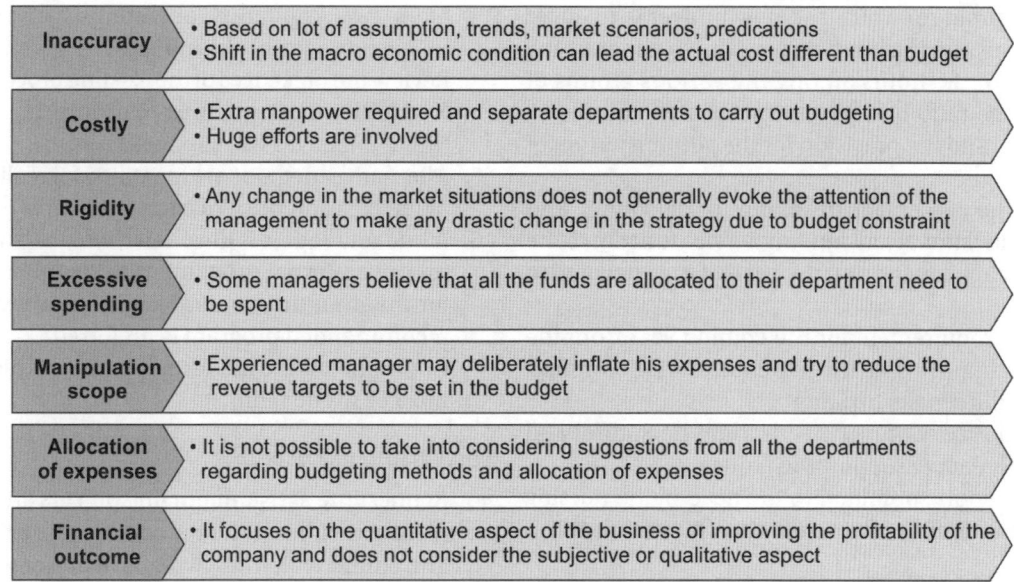

Fig. 17.11: Limitations of budgeting.

- **Budget committee:** Budget needs budget committee in an organization (i) to receive and approve all forecasts, departmental budgets, periodic reports showing comparison of actual, budgeted income and expenditure and (ii) to request for special studies of deviations from the budget and consider revision of budget to meet changed conditions.
- **Business policies:** Clearly defined business policies serve as basis for budget preparations.
- **Statistical information:** In the form of figures, i.e., estimates regarding the budget terms are essential for budget.

Essential Requisition for Budget

- **Forecasting:** Sound forecasting may be related to making decisions on purchases, expansion, advertising, services, working capital needs, etc.
- **Accounting:** Well conceived accounting system must be needed to compare the budget information with actual accomplishment. The cost information tells us to how much it will cost to produce or give service.
- **Lines of authority:** Budget preparation, operation and supervision need/require clearly defined lines of authority.
- **Budget committee:** Budget needs budget committee in an organization (i) to receive and approve all forecasts, departmental budgets, periodic reports showing comparison of actual, budgeted income and expenditure and (ii) to request for special studies of deviations from the budget and consider revision of budget to meet changed conditions.
- **Business policies:** Clearly defined business policies serve as basis for budget preparations.
- **Statistical information:** In the form of figures, i.e., estimates regarding the budget terms are essential for budget.
- Top level management support is essential to ensure successful installation of the budget program.
- **Period of budget:** Length of budget period (usually a year) should be specified.

Steps in Budgeting

While designing and implementing a planning program, the nurse administrator/manager should follow steps as given below.

1. Review the goals of the agency or hospital to identify activities of highest priority, because these are most likely to receive funding.
2. Review the objectives of the existing programs and written for proposed programs to ensure that achievement of these objectives will support agency.
3. Existing programs are revised and proposed programs designed to maximum goal accomplishment.
4. Manpower, capital and operating expenses are computed for each program, old and new.
5. Alternative methods are identified for realizing designated objectives and price of each alternative is determined.
6. Comparisons are made to determine which alternative is most cost-effective.
7. A budget request is developed which details a fiscal plan for the preferred program indicates alternative methods for meeting the same objective, and explains why the recommended program is preferred.
8. Request the assistant nursing officers and supervisors to present their needs for the coming year by a specified date, and confer with those who have presented such need.
9. Review the budget appropriation and actual expenditure for the current year in conjunction with statistical data as to the numbers and distribution of patient, nursing hours, per patient by services, operations and others.
10. Ascertain whether any changes are contemplated, such as opening new facilities for patients or changes in other departments, which affect the nursing services required.

11. Prepare the program which the new budget is to cover in terms of the nursing hours to be given to patients, the distribution of the hours among the various groups of personnel, the ratio of supervisors and head nurses to patients' care and the provision for the administration of nursing unit.
12. Determine the percentage of salaries of personnel who have both educational and nursing service function to be allocated to each function on the basis of time devoted to each.
13. Estimate the requirement for the coming year from the information supplied as the expenditure for supplies, equipment and repairs to date.
14. Prepare a summary of new needs, both personnel and material with data to support the request.

The budget report submitted to the head of the nursing department after carefully reviewed by her/his associates.

Budget as a Tool for Effective Administration

When budget becomes really an effective tool of administrative management the executive must have adequate powers. Facilities and discretion in budgetary matters with following principles.

- **Executive program:** Budget should go hand in hand with programming under the direct supervision of chief executive.
- **Flexibility in timing:** Budget should have provisions to accommodate necessary changes in the light of changing economic situations.
- **Executive responsibility:** The chief executive must see that the departmental programs fulfill the intent of the legislature and due economy is observed in the execution of the program.
- **Multiple procedures:** The methods of budgeting may vary according to the nature of operation. Executive direction: Appropriation should be made for broadly defined function of the department.
- **Reporting:** Budgetary process like preparation of estimates, legislature action and the budget execution must be based on full financial and operating reports coming from all levels of administration.
- **Adequate tool:** Chief executive must have an adequately equipped budget office attached to him and authority to earmark monthly or quarterly allotment of appropriation.
- **Two-way budget organization:** Traffic between central office and the agency offices responsible for budgeting and programming should move in two-way rather than one-way street.

Nurse Manager Role in Budgeting

Steps in budgeting for the nurse manager or administrator:
1. Review the goals of the agency or hospital to identify activities of highest priority because these are most likely to receive funding.
2. Existing programs are revised and proposed programs design to maximum goal accomplishment.
3. Manpower, capital and operating expenses are computed for each program, old and new.
4. Review the objectives of the existing programs and written for proposed programmer to ensure that achievement of these objectives will support agency.
5. Alternative methods are identified for realizing designated objectives and price of each alternative is determined.
6. A budget request is developed which details a fiscal plan for the preferred program indicates alternative methods for meeting the same objective, and explains why the recommended program is preferred.
7. Comparisons are made to determine which alternative is most cost-efficient.

For Nursing in Hospital

- Request the assistant nursing officers and supervisors to present their needs for the coming year by a specified date, and confer with those who have presented such need.
- Ascertain whether any changes are contemplated, such as opening new facilities for patients or changes in other departments, which affect the nursing services required.
- Review the budget appropriation and actual expenditure for the current year in conjunction with statistical data as to the numbers and distribution of patient, nursing hours, per patient by services, operations and others.
- Prepare the program which the new budget is to cover in terms of the nursing hours to be given to patients, the distribution of the hours among the various groups of personnel, the ratio of supervisors and head nurses to patients' care and the provision for the administration of nursing unit.
- Estimate the requirement for the coming year from the information supplied as the expenditure for supplies, equipments and repairs to date.
- Determine the percentage of salaries of personnel who have both educational and nursing service function to be allocated to each function on the basis of time devoted to each.
- Prepare a summary of new needs, both personnel and material with data to support the request. The budget report submitted to the head of the nursing department after carefully reviewed by her/his associates.

Budgeting for Nursing Department

Developing a nursing unit budget can be challenging. However, it's necessary to ensure the unit has everything they need to provide the best quality patient care. Taking the time to create a strong plan, and then monitoring it consistently, is the best way to ensure your nursing unit budget is a success.

Nursing unit budget is a plan that outlines a particular unit's goals and objectives, as well as planned expenses and revenues, in relation to the organization. It also provides guidance on how to best use human and material resources. Budget planning requires the delicate balance of meeting financial goals while ensuring patients receive high-quality care.

Purposes of Budgeting

Budgeting serves a number of purposes:
- **Planning:** A budgeting process forces the business to look into the future. This is essential for survival since it stops management from relying on ad hoc or poorly co-ordinated planning.
- **Control:** Actual results are compared against the budget and action is taken as appropriate.
- **Communication:** The budget is a formal communication channel that allows junior and senior staff to converse.
- **Coordination:** The budget allows coordination of all parts of the business towards a common corporate goal.
- **Evaluation:** Responsibility accounting divides the organization into budgetcentres, each of which has a manager who is responsible for its performance. The budget may be used to evaluate the actions of a manager within the business in terms of costs and revenues over which they have control.
- **Motivation:** The budget may be used as a target for managers to aim for. Rewards should be given for operating within or under budgeted levels of expenditure. This acts as a motivator for managers.
- **Authorization:** The budget acts as a formal method of authorization for a manager for expenditure, hiring staff and the pursuit of plans contained within the budget.
- **Delegation:** Managers may be involved in setting the budget. Extra responsibility may motivate managers. Management involvement may also result in more realistic targets.

Purpose Nursing Budget

- To plan the objectives, programs and activities of nursing services and the fiscal resources to accomplish them.
- To motivate nurse managers and nursing workers through analysis of actual experiences.
- To evaluate the performance of nurse administrators and managers and increase awareness of the costs.

Types of Budget Handled

- **Capital budget:** A capital budget deals with long-term investments for the organization, such as building or remodeling facilities and purchasing medical equipment. This is typically handled at higher levels of the organization instead of at the level of individual nursing units.
- **Operating budget:** An operating budget deals with the day-to-day expenses and revenues of the organization. Within a health care organization, each unit typically has its own operating budget. Some items commonly listed in the operating budget include anticipated daily activities, resources, personnel, supplies, and any short-term or rented medical equipment.
- **Fixed or static budget:** A traditional fixed or static budget is designed to remain constant, regardless of any changes to the organization's needs or operations. Creating a fixed budget is typically a more straightforward process than creating a flexible one. However, a static budget does not accommodate for changing or unexpected needs.
- **Flexible budget:** In contrast to a fixed budget, a flexible budget is designed to change alongside variables like volume, labor costs, and capital expenditures. Due to its dynamic nature, a flexible budget is often more complicated to create than a static one, but this flexibility can be a huge asset when considering the ever-changing needs of a health care organization.

Expenses to Consider for a Nursing Unit Budget

- **Staff:** An operating budget typically lists the number of employees in each category (e.g., RNs, LPNs, and nursing aides), as well as a breakdown of salary and benefit costs for each. It also includes the costs of new hires, current staff salaries, per diem staffing, and any professional development or continued training.
- **Equipment:** This category includes any medical, office, and personal hygiene supplies your unit uses. Each equipment expense is typically listed under an appropriate category or line item in the budget. For example, pens would fall under the "office supplies" heading, while IV tubing would fall under "medical supplies."
- **Interdepartmental charges:**
  - Depending on the facility type, the nursing unit may partner with other departments for services and supplies.
  - For example, if you work in a hospital with an on-site pharmacy that supplies your unit with stock medications, you may be charged for those medications and need to log it as an expense.
  - Patients who use those medications would be charged to cover the expense, which would then be logged on the revenue side of your budget.
- **Revenue:**
  - Revenue can stem from patients, grants, donations, and any financial support from your health care company.
  - Each of these revenue streams should have their own line item within the budget.
  - When adding patient revenue lines to the budget, consider that not all individuals pay the same rate for the same services and supplies.
  - Both government and private health insurance companies have different rates they will cover for different services, and they will typically negotiate with healthcare providers regarding payment.
- **Reducing health care costs:** Part of creating a budget means understanding where to reduce costs without reducing the quality of patient care, staff, or supplies. There are several practical ways to streamline your unit's expenses. Some units may benefit from several methods while others may only be able to use one or two. Work with the staff and learn the unit's needs so you can effectively and safely prioritize resources.
  - Monitor the use of supplies and routinely evaluate supplier cost and unit stock
  - Watch for long-term trends in the unit's patient-to-staff ratios to avoid overstaffing or understaffing

- Work with other units and cross-train staff if there are certain times when you may need to float staff
- Know the options for per diem staffing if the unit regularly needs it and budget ahead of time
- Limit excessive use of unscheduled leave
- Educate staff and enforce standards to comply with insurance company requirements
- Identify and resolve issues that contribute to overtime
- Ensure nursing hours do not exceed the target number of hours per patient day (HPPD)
- **Monitoring and evaluating outcomes of a nursing unit budget:** Monitoring the budget closely and continuously is the best way to prevent surprises in the evaluation process.

Role of Nurse Manager (Box 17.6)

- When the budget is approved, it has given authorization to make expenditure and to collect income as indicated in the budget.
- When the budget is adopted, administrator is committed to support the budget.
- Once the budget is approved, it is the responsibility of the administrator to see that expenditures do not exceed the approximates 1 made to the institution.

PROPOSAL, PROJECTING REQUIREMENT FOR STAFF, EQUIPMENT AND SUPPLIES FOR: HOSPITAL AND PATIENT CARE UNITS AND EMERGENCY AND DISASTER UNITS

A budget is a formal written statement of a hospital's plan for the future. The financial budget is a management control tool normally covering a one year period. The essentials of budgeting are to set specific goals for future operations and to have a periodic comparison of actual results with the financial goals established. Many types of budgets can be used, but three which are important to any hospital are the operating budget, capital budget and the cash budget.

Objectives

The objectives of a budget are:
- To provide written terms of the hospital goals
- To provide a basis for the evaluation of financial performance according to the plans
- To provide a tool to control costs
- To create cost awareness hospital wide

Box 17.6: Role of nurse manager.

- The administrator requires sufficient funds to support sound program.
- The administrator submits a budget request and a justification for the proposed expenditures.
- Budget is presented to the president.
- The budget is reviewed, analyzed and modified on the basis of discussions of president and budget committee.
- Once revisions are made, president presents the budget to board of trustees for approval.

Principles of Hospital Budget

The underlying principal upon whom the financial budget for the hospital should be set is that of equity. This is taken to ensure that:
- Budgets are set with a clear aim of establishing an allocation that is fair to all patients, within the constraints of available resources
- Fairness will be demonstrated by an equivalent potential spend per head of covered population taking due regard to the demographic, epidemiological and socioeconomic factors that influence the demands for healthcare
- Where changes are proposed a reasonable period is allowed for transition to allow hospitals and patients to plan for the continuity of services.

Stages of Budget Plan (Hospital)

- Prepare assumptions, in statistical terms about the kind of services (outputs) the hospital expects to provide.
- Prepare the economic forecasts in respect of new developments.
- Outline the budget goals and policies as per the directives of governing board.
- Prepare a budget package incorporating written instructions.
- Each department head to analyze financial and statistical data generated by his department as well as provided to him by the administration on finance department.
- Summary of each department is recorded between the administration and the department head and also includes observation of financial officer.
- The finance officer to develop the department's revenue budget and forward the department's budget hearing summary to the concerned department head
- The finance officer to prepare a preliminary operating revenue budget for the whole hospital by summarizing and collating the individual's department budget.
- Finance officer to summarize the total budget into a proper budget format.
- In the final step, budget is presented by finance officer to the governing board or finance committee for their approval.

Statistical Budget

- The first step in preparing an operating budget is to prepare the statistical budget.
- The objective is to provide a measure of activity in each department for the upcoming budget period.
- Diagnostic departments measure how many procedures will be provided for the upcoming year, while nursing estimates the number of patient days anticipated.
- Knowledge of the past performance of a facility is useful in the forecasting.
- The last five years are an appropriate amount of history to keep on file. This enables management to plan for future operations.

- Comparisons of past performance with current operations may indicate favorable and unfavorable trends.
- For example, it is very helpful to review the past history of full time equivalents (FTEs) for each department in a hospital.

Expense Budget

- This is the second step in preparing an operating budget. After the statistical budget is prepared, each department can then prepare their expense budget.
- The expense budget is the amount of money each department expects to payout.
- These expenses include salaries, supplies, and other various expenses. These are the dollars the departments must stay within.

Salaries

- It is a good idea to give each department manager a worksheet with each of their employees listed with their anniversary date, present hourly pay, and number of hours scheduled to work.
- The department manager can then make corrections as necessary. They can also look at a pay scale and decide what increases the employee will get at their anniversary date.
- This is also a good time to budget for vacancies and make all corrections.

Supplies

Input from the department heads are necessary if there will be price increases from the vendors and what percentage the prices will increase. If expenses go up, the revenue budget should increase proportionately.

BUDGET AUDIT

A financial audit is conducted to provide an opinion whether "financial statements" (the information being verified) are stated in accordance with specified criteria. Normally, the criteria are international accounting standards, although auditors may conduct audits of financial statements prepared using the cash basis or some other basis of accounting appropriate for the organization. In providing an opinion whether financial statements are fairly stated in accordance with accounting standards, the auditor gathers evidence to determine whether the statements contain material errors or other misstatements.

Definition

- Audit is the examination or inspection of various books of accounts by an auditor followed by physical checking of inventory to make sure that all departments are following documented system of recording transactions. It is done to ascertain the accuracy of financial statements provided by the organization.
- A financial audit is an independent, objective evaluation of an organization's financial reports and financial reporting processes. The primary purpose for financial audits is to give regulators, investors, directors, and manager's reasonable assurance that financial statements are accurate and complete.

Meaning of Auditing

Auditing is broadly defined as a systematic process of objectively obtaining and evaluating evidence in respect of certain assertions about economic actions and events, to ascertain the degree of correspondence between those assertions and established criteria and reporting the results to interested parties. Auditing usually covers a particular period of time. Auditing may be narrowly defined as a written report on the examination of financial statements for a particular period of time.

- There are three main types of audits: external audits, internal audits, and Internal Revenue Service (IRS) audits.
- External audits are commonly performed by Certified Public Accounting (CPA) firms and result in an auditor's opinion which is included in the audit report.
- An unqualified, or clean, audit opinion means that the auditor has not identified any material misstatement as a result of his or her review of the financial statements.
- External audits can include a review of both financial statements and a company's internal controls.
- Internal audits serve as a managerial tool to make improvements to processes and internal controls.

Figure 17.12 shows the audit cycle.

Types of Auditing

- **Nursing management audit:** This type is more structure oriented focusing on administrative aspects of the nurse's responsibilities and nurses that the health facilities are suitably equipped to provide care.
- **Retrospective audit:** This is the evaluation of nursing care by examining the records and charts of discharged patients.
- **Concurrent audit:** It is the evaluation of the nursing care by the observation and retrospective method during the delivery of care. The best method of audit depends on the objective of audit.

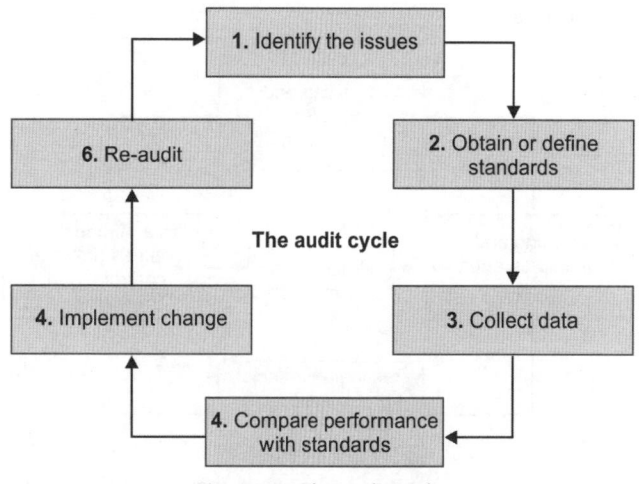

Fig. 17.12: The audit cycle.

Steps in Auditing Process

There are four main steps in the auditing process.
1. The first one is to define the auditor's role and the terms of engagement which is usually in the form of a letter which is duly signed by the client.
2. The second step is to plan the audit which would include details of deadlines and the departments the auditor would cover. Is it a single department or whole organization which the auditor would be covering? The audit could last a day or even a week depending upon the nature of the audit.
3. The next important step is compiling the information from the audit. When an auditor audits the accounts or inspects key financial statements of a company, the findings are usually put out in a report or compiled in a systematic manner.
4. The last and most important element of an audit is reporting the result. The results are documented in the auditor's report.

Basic Procedures for a Financial Audit (Fig. 17.13)

Generally, four key phases are outlined for financial audit process. These phases include planning the audit, determining the working of internal control, testing significant assertions about the data and evaluating compliance, and reporting the evaluations. These phases are explained in **Figure in 17.14**.

Planning

- The process of financial audit begins with a plan that involves the method of collecting data to form an opinion about the organization or company's financial status.
- A way is planned to collect a sample reflecting a point in time in the life of the company or organization.
- The financial transactions and documents are then looked at. It is noteworthy that the sample should show compliance with generally accepted accounting principles (GAAP).

Internal Controls

- The next step involves giving a look at the internal controls.

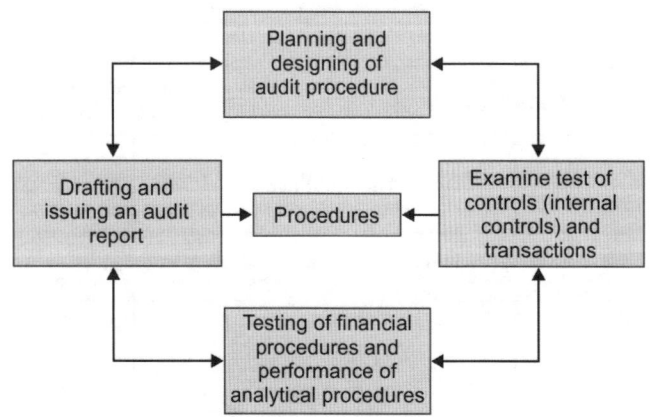

Fig. 17.13: Procedures of financial audit.

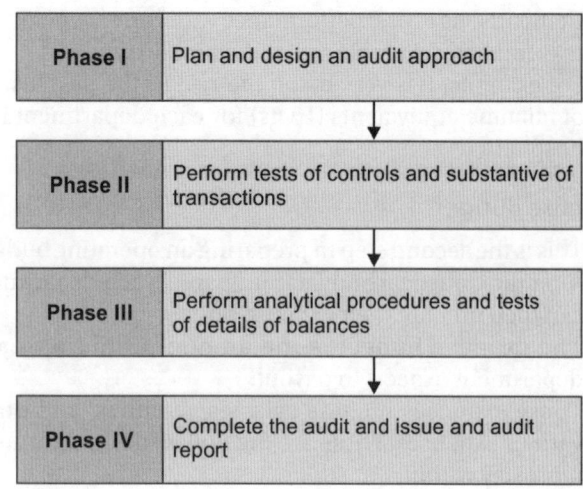

Fig. 17.14: Four phases of a financial statement audit.

- The auditor demands info, looks closely at the records, and watches financial procedures in action.
- Without these steps, the auditor cannot give a statement about the financial status of the organization.

Testing

- Testing implies checking whether the internal controls are working or not.
- An auditor requests more info, returns to the company for more inspections, and watches how financial procedures are being performed.
- If the evidence demonstrates GAAP compliance, the auditor determines that the company successfully detects and prevents the errors.

Reporting

- The final step in financial audit involves giving a conclusion on how the company adheres to accounting standards.
- The audit from a CPA gives the organization an unqualified approval, a qualified approval, a disclaimer, or an adverse finding.
- The unqualified approval is considered as the best result and the adverse finding is considered to be the worst result.

Characteristics of Audit

- Audit looks at the entire process of care including administration and not just at clinical management.
- Compares the care which actually is given. Standard procedures are agreed to decide which care should be given.
- Concentrates on finding solutions for the problems identified.

Audit report examples are shown in **Figure 17.15**.

Principles of Auditing

Fundamental principles are those according to which the books of business accounts are audited. These principles can be changed according to the desire of the auditor. We discuss the main principles of auditing under these headings:

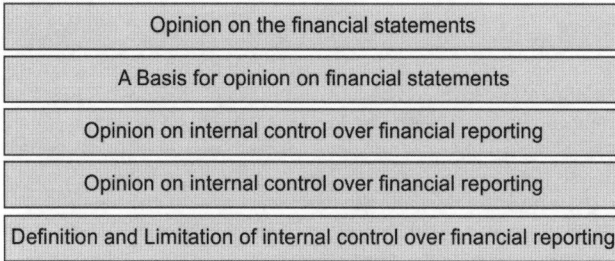

Fig. 17.15: Audit report examples.

> **Box 17.7:** Financial statement audit.
>
> **Basic principles**
> - Integrity, objectivity, and independence
> - Confidentiality
> - Skill and competence
> - Work performed by others
> - Documentation
> - Planning
> - Audit evidence
> - Accounting system and internal control
> - Audit conclusions and reporting

- **Planning:** It is the basic principle of auditing. The auditor should plan before starting the work. In planning auditor decides accounting about the system and internal control procedure.
- **Honesty:** Honesty and sincerity is the second important principle of auditing. The loyalty of auditor to work and profession must be beyond the doubt.
- **Impartiality:** In case of audit the attitude of the auditor must be impartial. Keeping in view this principle his personal views may not be included in the audit report.
- **Secrecy:** Secrecy must be maintained by the auditor during the process of audit. He cannot disclose any information to the third party.
- **Evidence:** During the audit the auditor can collect the evidence. He can frame his opinion on the audit evidence. The nature and source of evidence must be kept in view by the auditor.
- **Consistency:** It is an important principle of auditing. In case of selecting the rates of depreciation and valuation of stock the accountant must follow the rates of the coming years. In this regard there should be consistency and changes are not acceptable.
- **Legal framework:** The business activities may run within the rules and legal formalities. To protect the rights of the interested parties rules must be applied.
- **Working paper preparation:** The auditor collects documents providing evidence that audit was carried out according the principles. The auditor prepares the working paper and kept in this custody as a proof.
- **Internal control:** The auditor will examine the accounting system and inter control. To frame his opinion, he keeps in view the evidence obtained from the books.
- **Report:** According the principle of auditing a report will be prepared by the auditor at the end. It may be conditional or unconditional. The auditor can draw conclusion and disclose the facts and figures about the business for general information.

Financial statement audit is discuss in **Box 17.7**.

■ COST-BENEFIT ANALYSIS

Cost–benefit analysis (CBA), sometimes also called benefit-cost analysis, is a systematic approach to estimating the strengths and weaknesses of alternatives used to determine options which provide the best approach to achieving benefits while preserving savings (for example, in transactions, activities, and functional business requirements).

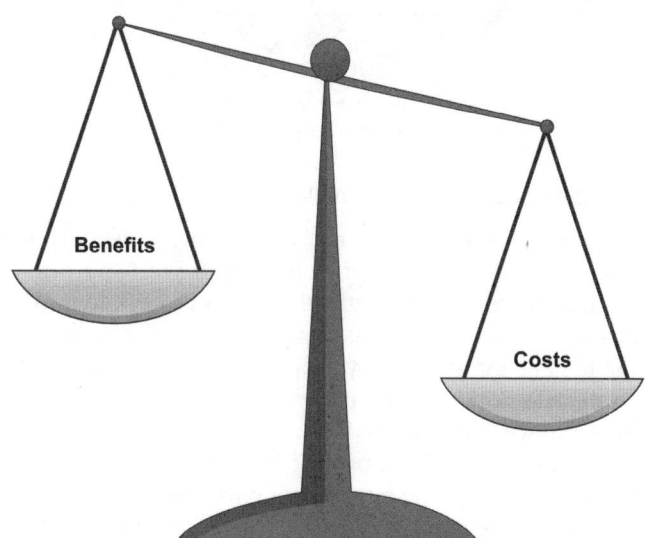

Fig. 17.16: Cost-benefit analysis (CBA)

A CBA may be used to compare completed or potential courses of actions, or to estimate (or evaluate) the value against the cost of a decision, project, or policy. It is commonly used in commercial transactions, business or policy decisions (particularly public policy), and project investments **(Fig. 17.16)**.

Definition

- Cost-benefit analysis (CBA) is a technique for assessing the monetary social costs and benefits of a capital investment project over a given time period.
- A cost-benefit analysis is a process businesses use to analyze decisions. The business or analyst sums the benefits of a situation or action and then subtracts the costs associated with taking that action.

Applications

CBA has two main applications:
1. To determine if an investment (or decision) is sound, ascertaining if – and by how much – its benefits outweigh its costs.
2. To provide a basis for comparing investments (or decisions), comparing the total expected cost of each option with its total expected benefits.

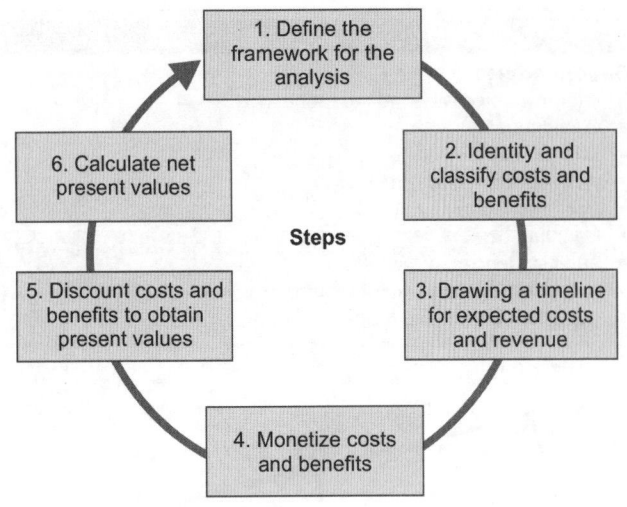

Fig. 17.17: Steps in cost-benefit analysis.

> **Box 17.8:** Eight principles of cost-benefit analysis.
> One of the problems of BCA is that the computation of many components of costs and benefits is intuitively obvious, but there are others for which intuition fails to suggest methods of measurement. The following eight basic principles can help as a guide to cost-benefit analysis (CBA).
> 1. There must be a common unit of measurement and time.
> 2. CBA valuations should represent consumer or producer valuations as revealed by their actual behavior.
> 3. Benefits are usually measured by market choices.
> 4. The analysis of a project should involve a with versus without comparison.
> 5. Some measurements of benefits require the valuation of human life.
> 6. Cost-benefit analysis involves a particular study area (Society or Country).
> 7. Double counting of benefits or costs must be avoided.
> 8. Decision criteria for projects (relate to PDO).

Purpose of Cost-benefit Analysis

The purpose of cost-benefit analysis in project management is to have a systemic approach to figure out the pluses and minuses of various paths through a project, including transactions, tasks, business requirements and investments. Cost-benefit analysis gives you options, and it offers the best approach to achieve your goal while saving on investment. There are two main purposes in using CBA:
1. To determine if the project is sound, justifiable and feasible by figuring out if its benefits outweigh costs.
2. To offer a baseline for comparing projects by determining which project's benefits are greater than its costs.

Process

According to the Economist, CBA has been around for a long time. In 1772, Benjamin Franklin wrote of its use. But the concept of CBA as we know it dates to Jules Dupuit, a French engineer, who outlined the process in an article in 1848.
- What are the goals and objectives of the project? The first step is perhaps the most important because before you can decide if a project is worth the effort, you need a clear and definite idea of what it is set to accomplish.
- What are the alternatives? Before you can know if the project is right, you need to compare it to other projects and see which the best path forward is.
- Who are the stakeholders? List all stakeholders in the project.
- What measurements Are You Using? You need to decide on the metrics you'll use to measure all costs and benefits. Also, how will you be reporting on those metrics? you can create eight different project reports with just one click, including project status reports, variance reports and more.
- What is the outcome of costs and benefits? Look over what the costs and benefits of the project are, and map them over a relevant time period.
- What is the common currency? Take all the costs and benefits you've collected, and convert them to the same currency to make an apples-to-apples comparison.
- What is the discount rate? This will express the amount of interest as a percentage of the balance at the end of a certain period.
- What is the net present value of the project options? This is a measurement of profit that is calculated by subtracting the present values of cash outflows from the present values of cash inflows over a period of time.
- What is the sensitivity analysis? This is a study of how the uncertainty in the output can be apportioned to different sources of uncertainty in its inputs.
- What do you do? The final step after collecting all this data is to make the choice that is recommended by the analysis.

Box 17.8 discuss eight basic principles of cost-benefit analysis.

Principles of Cost-benefit Analysis

The principles of cost-benefit analysis (CBA) are:
- **Appraisal of a project:** It is an economic technique for project appraisal, widely used in business as well as government spending projects (for example, should a business invest in a new information system).
- **Incorporates externalities into the equation:** It can, if required, include wider social/environment impacts as well as 'private' economic costs and benefits so that externalities are incorporated into the decision process. In this way, CBA can be used to estimate the social welfare effects of an investment.
- **Time matters:** CBA can take account of the economics of time—known as **discounting:** This is important when looking at environmental impacts of a project in the years ahead.

Uses of Cost-benefit Analysis

Through the use of cost-benefit analysis in financial services regulation, regulators can determine if their proposals will actually work to solve the problem they are seeking to address. Basing regulations on the best available data is not a legal "hurdle" for regulators to overcome as they draft rules, as some have described it, but rather a fundamental building block to ensure regulations work as intended.

- CBA has traditionally been applied to big public sector projects, such as new motorways, by-passes, dams, tunnels, bridges, flood relief schemes and new power stations.
- The basic principles of CBA can be applied to many other projects or programs. For example, public health programs (e.g., the mass immunization of children using new drugs), an investment in a new rail safety systems, or opening a new railway line.
- Cost-benefit analysis was also used during an inquiry into genetically modified foods.
- Increasingly the principles of cost-benefit analysis are being used to evaluate the returns from investment in environmental projects, such as wind farms and the development of other sources of renewable energy. Financial resources are scarce, CBA allows different projects to be ranked according to those that provide the highest expected net gains in social welfare—this is particularly important given the limitations of government spending.

Main Stages in the Cost-benefit Analysis Approach:

Stage 1a: Calculation of social costs and social benefits. This would include calculation of:

- Tangible benefits and costs (i.e., direct costs and benefits)
- Intangible benefits and costs (i.e., indirect costs and benefits—externalities)

Stage 1b: Sensitivity analysis of events occurring: This relates to an important question - If you estimate that a possible benefit (or cost) is £x million, how likely is that outcome? If you are reasonably sure that a benefit or cost will 'occur' – what is the scale of uncertainty about the actual values of the costs and benefits?

Stage 2: Discounting the future value of benefits: Costs and benefits accrue over time. Individuals normally prefer to enjoy the benefits now rather than later–so the value of future benefits has to be discounted.

Stage 3: Comparing the costs and benefits to determine the net social rate of return.

Stage 4: Comparing net rate of return from different projects—the government may have limited funds at its disposal and therefore faces a choice about which projects should be given the go-ahead.

Barriers of the use of cost-benefit analysis is summarized in **Box 17.9**.

CONCLUSION

Budget and budgetary control provide a set of basic techniques for planning and control. A budget is a quantitative statement, for a defined period of time, which may include planned revenues, expenses, assets, liabilities and cash flows. It is a financial plan outlining how funds will be spent in a given period of time and how these funds will be obtained. The process of preparing a budget is known as budgeting.

Box 17.9: Barriers to the use of cost-benefit analysis.

- **Fundamental barriers**
  - Rejecting the principles of welfare economics
  - Rejecting efficiency as a relevant criterion of desirability
  - Rejecting the monetary valuation of risk reductions
- **Institutional barriers (barriers related to the organization of policy making)**
  - Lack of consensus on relevant policy objectives
  - Formulation of policy objectives inconsistent with cost-benefit analysis
  - Priority given to policy objectives unsuitable for cost-benefit analysis
  - Horse trading/vote trading
  - Political opportunism
  - Unfunded mandates and excessive delegation of authority
  - Abundance of resources
  - Rigidity of reallocation mechanisms
  - Wrong timing of EAT information in decision-making process

REVIEW QUESTIONS

Long Essays

1. Define financial management; explain the objectives and principles.
2. Define financial planning; explain the objectives and importance.
3. Define budget; explain the purposes, objectives and principles.
4. Define auditing; explain the types, steps and principles.
5. Define cost-benefit analysis; explain the purposes, process, principles and uses.

Short Essays

1. Functions of financial management.
2. Importance of financial management.
3. Scope of financial management.
4. Important skills for financial managers.
5. Types of financial management.
6. Elements of strategic financial management.
7. Characteristics of budget.
8. Classifications/types of budget.
9. Steps in the budgeting process.
10. Essential requisition in budget preparation.
11. Budget as a tool for effective administration.
12. Nurse manager role in budgeting.

Short Answers

1. Investment management.
2. Skills needed for managing a budget.
3. Importance of budget.
4. Benefits of budget.
5. Limitations of budget.
6. Lines of authority.
7. Principles of hospital budget.
8. Barriers to the use of cost-benefit analysis.

BIBLIOGRAPHY

1. Brealey RA, Stewart CM. Principles of Corporate Finance, 4th edition. McGraw-Hill, 1991.
2. Dmytrenko A L. "Cost-Benefit Analysis." Records Management Quarterly, 1997.
3. Horngren CT, Gary LS. Introduction to Management Accounting. Prentice-Hall, 1990.

CHAPTER 18: Nursing Informatics/Information Management

LEARNING OBJECTIVES

- Patient Records
- Nursing Records
- Use of Computers in Hospital, College and Community
- Telemedicine and Telenursing
- Electronic Medical Records (EMR), EHR

INTRODUCTION

Nurses has been working in the field of informatics near four decades, the term "nursing informatics" has been considered a specialization in nursing resources since 1984. Many aspects, such as data recovery, ethics, patient care, decision support systems, human-computer interaction, information systems, imaging informatics, computer science, information science, security, electronic patient records, intelligent systems, e-learning and telenursing have been added to the field. Most of nursing professionals believe that it is defined as the integration of information technology and all aspects of nursing, such as clinical nursing, management, research or education.

HISTORY OF HEALTH INFORMATICS

- Initially, the term medical informatics was used to describe "those collected informational technologies which concern themselves with the patient care, medical, decision making process".
- Greenes and Shortliffe (1990) redefined medical informatics as "the field that concerns itself with the cognitive, information processing and communication tasks of medical practice, education and research, including the information science and the technology to support these tasks, an intrinsically interdisciplinary field with an applied focus addressing a number of fundamental research problems as well as planning and policy issues".
- Reston 1984 gave a parallel definition of medical informatics. Since nurses are healthcare practitioners who are involved in patient care decision-making process that uses information technologies, there clearly was a place for nursing in medical informatics.
- Mandil (1991), coined the phrase "health informatics" which he defined as the use of information technology (including both hardware and software) with information management concepts and methods to support the delivery of healthcare.
- Health informatics encompasses medical, nursing, dental, and pharmacy informatics. Health informatics focuses attention on the recipient of care rather than on the discipline of the care giver. **Box 18.1** describes historical perspective.

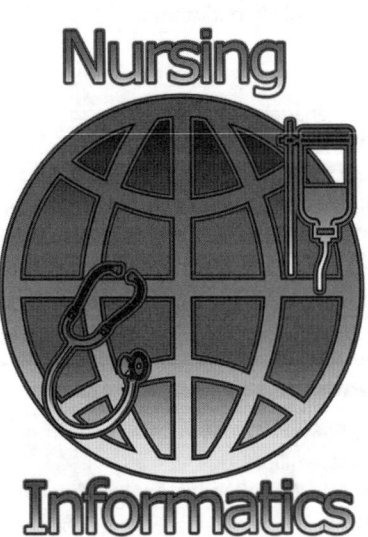

Fig. 18.1: Nursing informatics.

Box 18.1: Historical perspective.

- **1850:** Florence Nightingale emphasized the critical importance of using nursing informatics.
- **Late 1950–1960's:** Hospitals began using computerized information systems
- **1965:** American Hospital Association endorses NI
- **1970s:** Development of the silicon chip
- **1980s:** Usage of computer for diverse hospital functions
- **1990s:** Expanded use of computers to improve patient care and conduct research
- **2001:** Point and click system of healthcare utilized

HISTORY OF NURSING INFORMATICS

- Healthcare began to use computers in the 1950's. Computers, in this era, were typically used in the business office.
- In the 1970's, nursing began to realize the importance of computers to the nursing profession and became involved in the design, purchase, and implementation of information systems.
- In the 1980's, medical and nursing informatics specialties emerged. 1995 saw the first certification exam for NI.
- Hana has defined nursing informatics as the application of IT in the nursing duties including education, management and practice in 1985.
- Integration of information science, computer science and nursing science to support nursing practice and knowledge management was the definition offered in 1989 by Graves and Corcoran.
- The American Nurses Association (ANA) published its aim and standards in 1994-1995 and presented the Nursing Informatics as a specialty that integrates nursing science, computer and information science to provide data communication management, knowledge and nursing work in 2001.
- The post-2000 era saw an unprecedented explosion in the number and sophistication of both computer hardware and software. Telemedicine became possible and was recognized as a specialty in the late 1990's.

DEFINITION

- Hebda (1998), defines nursing informatics as the use of computers technology to support nursing, including clinical practice, administration, education and research.
- Nursing informatics "is the specialty that integrates nursing science with multiple information and analytical sciences to identify, define, manage and communicate data, information, knowledge and wisdom in nursing practice."
- Nursing informatics is the "science and practice (that) integrates nursing, its information and knowledge, with information and communication technologies to promote the health of people, families, and communities worldwide."
- ANA (American Nurses Association) 1994, has defined nursing informatics as the development and evaluation of applications, tools, processes and structures which assist nurses with the management of data in taking care of patients or supporting the practice of nursing.
- "Nursing informatics is defined as combining nursing science, information management science, and computer science to manage and process nursing data, information, and knowledge to deliver quality care to the public."
  —*HRSA, 2008*
- Nursing informatics, as originally defined, refers to the use of information technologies in relation those functions within the purview of nursing, and that are carried out by nurses when performing their duties.
- Nursing informatics is "a combination of computer science, information science, and nursing science designed to assist in the management and processing of nursing data, information and knowledge to support the practice of nursing and the delivery of nursing care.
  —*Graves and Corcoran, 1989*

MEANING OF NURSING INFORMATICS

- Informatics is becoming increasingly present in our profession due to rapidly changing technologic advances. Healthcare systems are assimilating technology into daily practice at a quick pace.
- Nursing informatics is a field of nursing that incorporates nursing, computer, and information sciences to maintain and develop medical data and systems to support the practice of nursing, and to improve patient care outcomes.
- Nurse informaticists work to develop communication and information technologies in healthcare. They also serve as educators, researchers, software engineers, and chief nursing officers.
- Management systems society defines nursing informatics as "a specialty that integrates nursing science, computer science, and information science to manage and communicate data, information, knowledge, and wisdom in nursing practice."

CONCEPT OF NURSING INFORMATICS (FIG. 18.2)

Nursing informatics (NI) centers on the concepts of: 1. Data, 2. Information, 3. Knowledge, 4. Wisdom. These concepts are known as metastructures in nursing informatics **(Fig. 18.3)**.

Data

Raw facts which lacks meaning and described objectively without interpretation, such as:
- Age 15, 19, 23, 60, 70, 190, 110
- Number of patients in ward: 20, 40, 50
- Blood pressure: 120/80, 190/110
- Disease: Diabetes mellitus (DM), hypertension

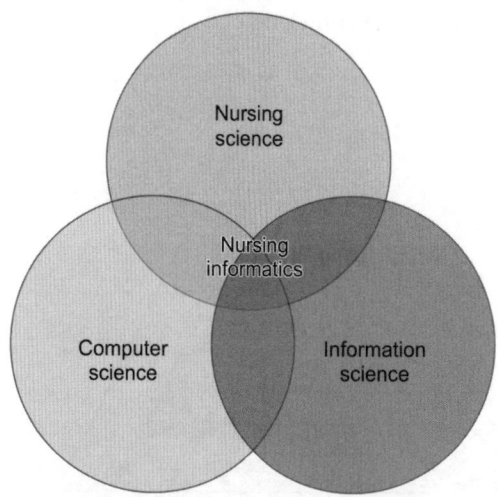

Fig. 18.2: Nursing informatics.

- Weight: 50 kg, 80 kg
- Height: 160 cm, 170 cm

Information

Data that is interpreted, organized, or structured. Data that is processed using knowledge. Data made functional through the application of knowledge, such as:

- Prevalence of patients falls per nursing ward per month—this year compared to last year
- Prevalence of stage 3 cancer patients per year on an Oncology Unit
- Percentage (%) of staff absenteeism on surgical ward among staff nurses per month

Knowledge

Processed information that helps to clarify or explain some aspects of our environment or world that we can use as a basis for action or upon which we can act nursing knowledge: Is defined as information that has been synthesized so that interrelationships are identified and formalized resulting in decisions that guide nursing practice, such as:

- Effectiveness of Patient Monitoring Program in the prevention of patients falls on surgical wards
- Cancer treatment protocols
- Relationship between surgical wards nurse absenteeism and work load and work stress
- Care plans for specific health conditions

Decisions, such as:

- A diagnosis of hypertension or DM
- Using stage 3 cancer protocol to treat this patient
- Refer to hospital management records to identify staff working loads

Nursing and Knowledge

Nurses are:

- **Knowledge workers:** Working with information and generating information and knowledge as a product
- **Knowledge acquirers:** Providing convenient and efficient means of capturing and storing knowledge
- **Knowledge users:** Individuals or groups who benefit from valuable, viable knowledge.

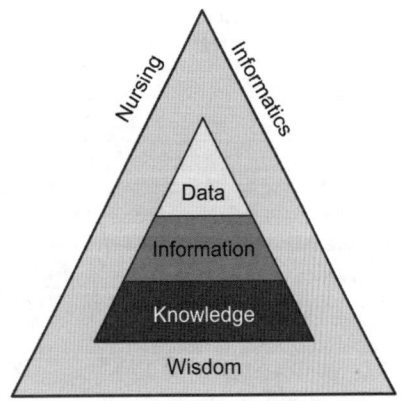

Fig. 18.3: Concepts of nursing informatics.

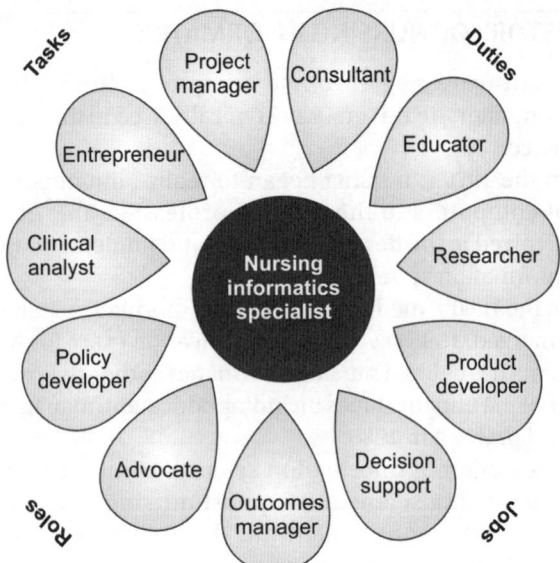

Fig. 18.4: Role of nursing informatics.

- **Knowledge engineers:** Designing, developing, implementing and maintaining knowledge.
- **Knowledge managers:** Capturing and processing collective expertise and distributing it where it can create the largest benefit.
- **Knowledge developers or generators:** Changing and evolving knowledge based on the tasks at hand and information available. **Figure 18.4** shows role of nursing informatics.

GENERAL PURPOSES NURSING INFORMATICS

Nursing's data needs fall into four domains: Nurse need data about client care, provider staffing, administration of care and the organization, and knowledge based research. The first three are distinct areas, whereas research interacts with all of the other three. The four areas and the source for the data are:

1. **Client:** Client care/clinical care and its evaluation, clinical data, and client outcomes. Source: the client record.
2. **Provider:** Professional data, caregiver outcomes, and decision maker variables. Source: personnel records, national data banks, and links to client records.
3. **Administrative:** Management and resource oversight, administrative data, system outcomes, and contextual variables. Source: executive/managerial data and fiscal and regulatory data.
4. **Research:** Knowledge base development. Source: existing and newly gathered data and relational data bases.

SCOPE OF NURSING INFORMATICS (FIG. 18.5)

According to American Nurses Association (ANA), Nursing Informatics is a specialty in nursing that combines nursing science, information science and computer science to distribute and manage data, knowledge and information regarding nursing practice.

This is to provide information and knowledge to patients, nurses and other healthcare providers to be of help in the

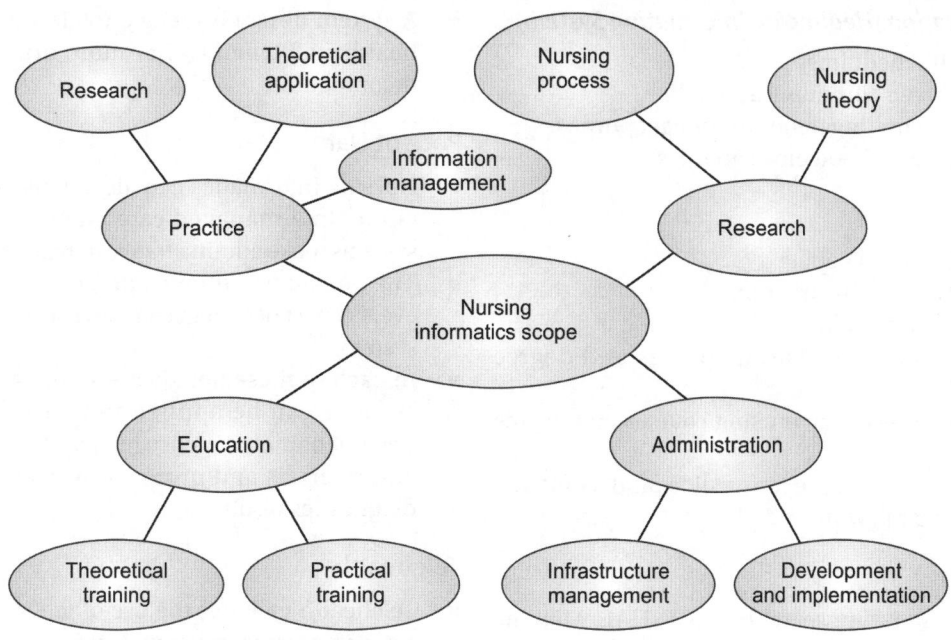

Fig. 18.5: Scope of nursing informatics.

development of health and is attained with the use of the current trends in information technology that distributes knowledge and information, mainly by social media like the internet and the television.

Specifically, the American Nurses Association in the Scope and Standards of Practice has listed the major functional areas for informatics nurses, which include:

- **Administration, leadership and management:** Either directly with clinical informatics departments or in combination with other functional areas, such as serving as project managers
- **Analysis:** Using data to synthesize knowledge, inform decision support, and manage outcomes as well as taxonomies
- **Compliance and integrity management:** Helping make sure organizations are meeting all the national laws and standards, such as HIPAA, FDA, Joint Commission, etc.
- **Consultation:** Serving both internally or externally as a resource
- Coordination, facilitation, and integration—serving as the translator between end-users and IT experts
- **Development:** Translating user requirements into solutions
- **Education and professional development:** Ranges from teaching the end-user to use a device or application to educating the next generation of nurses and the general public
- **Policy development and advocacy:** Being an advocate for consumers, hospital units, and the institution as a whole; also helping shape policies and standards at the state, national and organizational level
- **Research and evaluation:** Conducting research in a variety of informatics topics that impacts both caregivers and consumers

APPLICATION OF NURSING INFORMATICS

Applying Nursing Informatics (Fig. 18.6)

- **Practice:** Knowledge of nursing information systems can be used with nursing practice, such as patient documentation, monitoring devices, developing and implementing care plans and pathways, retrieval of previous records and imaging, use of telehealth, and access to current practice standards.
- **Administration:** Information systems are used with communication, staff scheduling systems, cost and budget analysis, and monitoring of trends with quality and satisfaction data.
- **Education:** Informatics and technology has applications in education, including simulation, electronic learning, teleconferencing, and software availability for educational presentations and programs.
- **Research:** Internet capabilities and electronic databases provide rich access to obtaining, compiling, and conducting research.

—*Baker, 2012*

Nursing Clinical Practice

- Work lists to remind staff of planned nursing interventions.
- Computer generated client documentation.
- Electronic medical record (EMR) and computer-based patient record (CPR).
- Monitoring devices that record vital signs and other measurements directly into the client record (EMR).
- Computer generated nursing care plans and critical pathways.
- Automatic billing for supplies or procedures with nursing documentation.
- Reminders and prompts that appears during documentation to ensure comprehensive charting.

Nursing Administration (Healthcare Information System)

- Automated staff scheduling.
- E-mail for improved communication.
- Cost analysis and finding trends for budget purposes.
- Quality assurance and outcomes analysis.

Nursing Education

- Computerized record keeping
- Computerized assisted instruction
- Interactive video technology
- Distance learning—web-based courses and degree programs.
- Internet resources—formal nursing courses and degree programmes.
- Presentation software for preparing slides and handouts- power points and MS words.

Nursing Research

- Computerized literature searching—CINHAL, Medline and web sources.
- The adoption of standardized language related to nursing terms-NANDA (Formerly the North American Nursing Diagnosis Association), etc.
- The ability to find trends in aggregate data that is data derived from large population groups—SPSS.

Patient Education

- Nursing informatics can be used for symptom management and patient education. The nurse can access the information for the patient or teach the patient where to find appropriate and helpful information.
- For example, on an oncology unit, nursing informatics can be used to teach patients effective symptom management of the treatment modalities which often cause pain, fatigue and poor nutritional status.
- Nursing informatics can also aid in other nursing interventions of the oncology nurse, such as analgesic administration and stress-reduction techniques.

Clinical Alert System

- The computerized clinical alert system can be used in conjunction with the hospital pharmacy.
- A system design is created to alert both pharmacy and health staff when two or more drug prescriptions are incompatible.

Patient Data

- Nursing informatics can also be useful in a physician's clinic. In a managed care environment, information systems make administrative management more efficient.
- The private practitioner, program or facility to manage every aspect of patient care can use one data management system.
- In each of these healthcare settings data management systems can be applied to treatments, diagnostics, documentation, practice management, insurance claims and referrals and protocols as well as treatment and diagnostics results.

Telehealth

- Telehealth includes the use of telephones and sophisticated image transmission systems, such as ECG, faxes and remote camera imaging.
- Telehealth places the ambulance personnel in touch with the Emergency Department and it also operates to put the generalist "nurses and doctors" at the ED in touch with specialists.
- Telehealth is used to evaluate the stroke victims while they are in transit so appropriate therapy can be initiated quickly upon arrival at the ED.
- In similar fashion, a nurse practitioner in a remote ED might be guided via telephone in the proper procedure for inserting chest tubes so a man with a collapsed lung could be stabilized for subsequent transport to a major hospital.
- Finally, nursing informatics can be useful for interdepartmental communication, such as ordering supplies from central supply, lab work, etc.

NURSING INFORMATICS AREAS

Nurse informaticians work as developers of communication and information technologies, educators, researchers, chief nursing officers, chief information officers, software engineers, implementation consultants, policy developers, and business owners, to advance healthcare. Core areas of work include:

Clinical practice	Administration
• Recording of patient assessment data in an electronic health record • Recoding of workload and interventions as a by-product of electronic charting	• Analysis of MIS reports generated from a spreadsheet software application • Review of outcome indicators using a decision-support software application • Recording of workload and interventions as a by-product of electronic charting
Education	**Research**
• Distance learning/teaching via the internet • Recording of workload and interventions as a by-product of electronic charting	• Evaluation of nurse sensitive outcome measures using a standard minimum data set • Use of knowledge bases via the internet • Recording of workload and interventions as a by-product of electronic charting

Fig. 18.6: Sample applications of nursing informatics.

Chapter 18: Nursing Informatics/Information Management

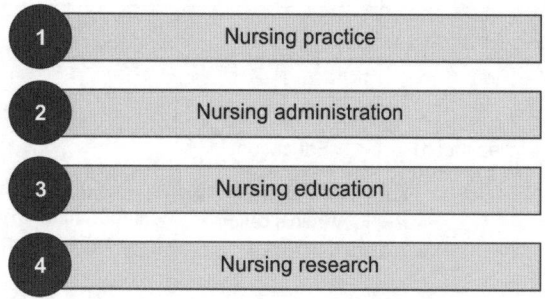

Fig. 18.7: Four major nursing areas.

- Concept representation and standards to support evidence-based practice, research, and education
- Data and communication standards to build an interoperable national data infrastructure
- Research methodologies to disseminate new knowledge into practice
- Information presentation and retrieval approaches to support safe patient centered care
- Information and communication technologies to address interprofessional work flow needs across all care venues
- Vision and management for the development, design, and implementation of communication and information technology
- Definition of healthcare policy to advance the public's health. **Figure 18.7** shows four major nursing areas.

IMPORTANCE OF NURSING INFORMATICS

- Nurses need information to care for patients safely. They need to be able to access medical histories, medication lists, lab and imaging results, and physician/interdisciplinary team notes to get a complete picture of a patient's clinical status.
- They use this information to make decisions efficiently to improve patient care outcomes.
- Nurse informaticists, as well as other healthcare informaticists (pharmacists, physicians, etc.), play a critical role in the continuous development and improvement of healthcare technology.
- Communication is inarguably one of the most important aspects of patient safety.
- The contribution of nurse informaticists in developing and improving technology, such as electronic medical records and computerized provider ordering has been crucial in reducing medical errors, patient care delays, and healthcare costs.

NURSING INFORMATICS INPATIENT CARE

The healthcare information revolution is upon us. Clinicians have more access than ever to electronic health records, diagnostics, and treatment plans. Clinical communication and collaboration platforms are making it easier to manage healthcare workflows, improve coordination, and enhance patient outcomes. Systems integration and data access mean that information and analysis are more vital than ever.

Aligning nursing best practice with clinical workflows and care nursing informatics:

- It is focused on the best ways to achieve good patient outcomes—it is about applying the overall process and best practice to maximize patient care wherever possible.
- Nurse informaticists are often involved in process design, clinical workflow reviews, and new diagnostics and treatment plans.
- They take into account the various options for providing care and use objective facts and analysis to determine the actions that will lead to the most patient-centered, value-based care.

Improving clinical policies, protocols, processes, and procedures data is the lifeblood of nursing informatics:

- The data and information can be used to measure the success of the various protocols, processes, and procedures used in a healthcare organization.
- A nurse informatics will measure and analyze how specific parts of the organization are performing, with a focus on the resulting patient outcomes.

Providing training and learning based on objective:

- Data one of the most valuable ways a nursing informatics can enhance patient outcomes is through providing training to clinical staff.
- They can use data to identify endemic issues in a healthcare organization and consult on the best way to resolve these problems.
- These learning's can be integrated with on boarding new staff, ongoing in-house training, or external education and certification.
- Nursing informaticists can help to create highly-targeted educational programs to deal with specific gaps between ability and provider expectations. **Figure 18.8** shows four major goals.

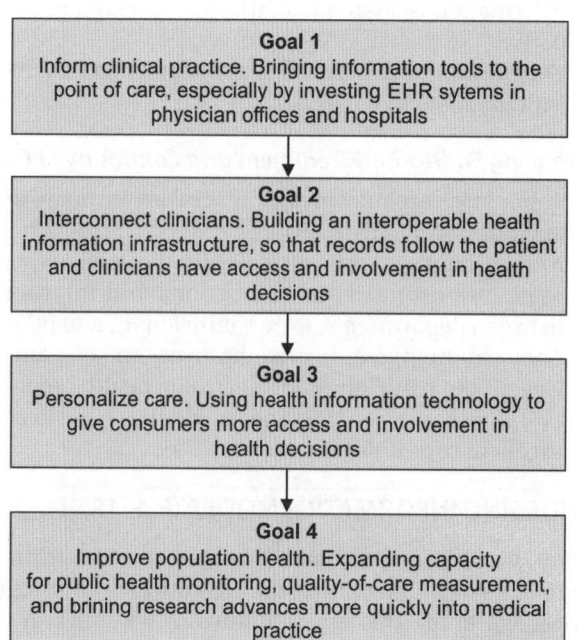

Fig. 18.8: Four major goals.

> **Box 18.2:** Application of nursing informatics/general purpose.
>
> **Nursing clinical practice:**
> - Work lists to remind staff of planned nursing interventions.
> - Computer generated client documentation.
> - Electronic medical record (EMR) and computer-based patient record (CPR).
> - Monitoring devices that record vital signs and other measurements directly into the client record (EMR).
> - Computer generated nursing care plans and critical pathways.
> - Automatic billing for supplies or procedures with nursing documentation.
> - Reminders and prompts that appear during documentation to ensure comprehensive charting.

Box 18.2 describes application of nursing informatics/general purpose.

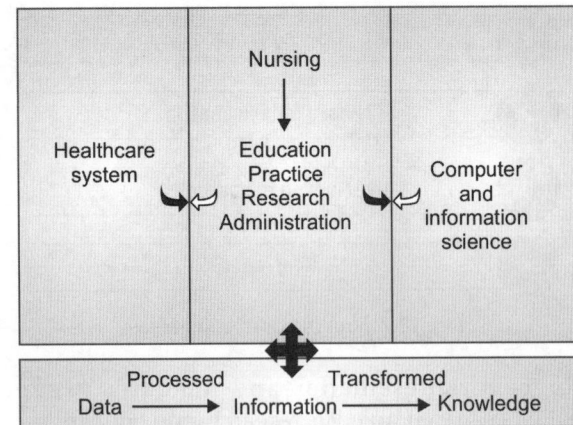

Fig. 18.9: Nursing information model.

Selecting and Testing New Medical Devices Connected
- IoT medical devices can provide vast amounts of health data on patients.
- Nursing informaticists are ideally positioned to understand the true value of that data and provide recommendations on how it can be recorded, accessed, and used.
- Involving informaticists in the selection of medical devices will ensure you have additional criteria for understanding how device data can inform diagnostics, treatment plans, and ultimately patient outcomes.

Reducing Medical Errors and Costs
Nursing informaticists can reduce the chance of medical errors in a healthcare organization, together with associated costs. A combination of staff training, process improvement, and best practice will enhance the quality of care and limit patient risks. There are four main areas that drive medical errors: Communication does not take place when it should
- Incorrect or incomplete information is communicated
- Information is shared with the wrong recipient or third party.
- The message lacks critical facts or is unclear, meaning it isn't understood correctly.

Enhancing End-to-End Treatment and Continuity of Care
- A patient's care may involve several areas, many teams, and dozens of individuals.
- Nursing informaticists can create protocols and processes to ensure proper communications and interactions between departments, teams, individuals, and patients.
- They can help healthcare employees to seek out "one view of the truth" through electronic health records, so everyone has the context and insight they need to ensure excellent continuity of care.

NURSING INFORMATICS MODEL (FIG. 18.9)

Toffler (1990) described the 1990's as a new era for informatics, the process of gaining power through the data-information-knowledge triad. This era continues as we enter the new millennium. The need for nurses to feel comfortable working with computerized data and information is escalating.

- **Health and nursing information science** is the study of how healthcare data is acquired, communicated, stored, and managed, and how it is processed into information and knowledge. This knowledge is useful to nurses in decision-making at the operational, tactical, and strategic planning levels of healthcare.
- **Information systems** used in healthcare include the people, structures, processes, and manual as well as automated tools that collect, store, interpret, transform, and report practice and management information.
- **The realization** that healthcare data and information can be effectively managed and communicated using computer systems, networks, modems and telecommunications has catalyzed the emergence of the science of nursing informatics. As Virginia Saba (1992) predicted, "By the turn of the century, most healthcare delivery systems will function with computers and will be managed by computer literate nurses. I believe, that by the turn of the century, "high tech and high touch" will be an integral part of the healthcare delivery system,".

At present, nursing informatics is an emerging field of study. National nursing organizations support the need for nurses to become computer literate and versed in the dynamics of nursing informatics. We are at a transition period. Becoming educated in nursing informatics is, for the most party, a self-directed and independent endeavor. Programs that offer basic and further education in nursing informatics are beginning to spring up around the globe, but many more are needed to provide easy access for motivated nurses.

COMPETENCIES OF NURSING INFORMATICS

The competency of nursing informatics specialists was determined through studying three categories including computer skills, informatics knowledge and informatics skills. It investigates four levels of nursing practice: beginning nurse, experienced nurse, informatics specialist, and informatics innovator.

Computer Skills

Selected computer skill competencies contain computerized searches and retrieving patient demographics data, the use of telecommunication devices, the documentation of patient care, the use of information technologies for improving nursing care, and the use of networks and computer technology safely.

Informatics Knowledge

- Selected informatics knowledge competencies are the recognition of the use or importance of nursing data for improving practice, and the recognition of the fact that the computer can only facilitate nursing care and that there are human functions that cannot be performed by computers,
- The formulation of ethical decisions in computing, the recognition of the value of clinicians' involvement in the design, selection, implementation, and evaluation of systems in healthcare,
- The description of the present manual systems, the definition of the impact of computerized information management on the role of the nurse and the determination of the limitations and the reliability of computerized patient monitoring systems.

Informatics Skills

- Informatics skills competencies includes the interpretation of information flow within the organization, the preparation of process information flow charts for all aspects of clinical systems, the development of standards and database structures to facilitate clinical care, education, administration or research.
- It also includes the development of innovative and analytic techniques for scientific inquiry in nursing informatics and new data organizing methods and research designs with the aim of examining the impacts of computer technology on nursing, and
- The conducting of basic science research to support the theoretical development of informatics.
- Information literacy skills, competencies, and knowledge are investigated among educators, administrators and clinicians of nursing groups nationally.

■ NURSING CAREER IN INFORMATICS

Nurses at every level now work with informatics through patient records and other technology. However, some nurses choose to specifically focus their career on the intersection of informatics and clinical practice. There are a number of career options available in this lane, including the following:
1. Clinical informatics specialist
2. Nursing informatics specialist
3. Clinical analyst
4. Clinical informatics manager
5. Clinical informatics coordinator
6. Nursing informatics analyst

These roles can be found at every level and facet of healthcare organizations, including leadership and management, advocacy, risk analysis, compliance, consultation, research, evaluation and education. As informatics becomes a more prominent component of the nursing field, job opportunities will likely continue to develop.

- **Informatics nurse specialist (INS):** An RN with formal, graduate education in the field of informatics or a related field and is considered a specialist in the field of nursing informatics.
- **Informatics nurse (IN):** An RN with an interest or experience working in an informatics field. A generalist in the field of informatics in nursing. **Table 18.1** shows TIGER nursing informatics competencies model.

Opportunities

In a world where high technology is rampant, a lot of opportunities await nurse informatics specialists. A career path on nursing informatics can lead to:
- Being hired to assist in implementing a nurse documentation system in a specific organization; and
- Being hired by the owner of the product to install the application to other organizations or healthcare centers in the region, or even in the country.
- With enough experience at multiple sites, the specialist in installation of a specific application may then be able to work for a consulting firm that advises clients on how to implement the application or the system that was installed to different organizations. **Box 18.3** describes nursing informatics functional areas.

Roles of a Nurse Informatics Specialist

In the clinical area, an informatics nurse can work at a hospital and be recognized as a clinical nurse analyst or a clinical informatics specialist. The nurse's responsibilities include the following:
- Data collection
- Creating quality surveys
- Designing and managing clinical databases
- Outcome reporting
- Creating communications using desktop publishing

Table 18.1: TIGER nursing informatics competencies model.		
Component of the model	Standard	Source (Standard setting body)
Basic computer competencies	European Computer Driving License	European Computer Driving License Foundation
Information literacy	Information Literacy Competency Standards	American Library Association
Information management	Electronic Health Record Functional Model—Clinical Care Components	Health Level Seven (HL7)
	International Computer Driving License—Health	European Computer Driving License Foundation

Box 18.3: Nursing informatics functional areas.
- Administration, leadership and management
- Analysis
- Compliance and integrity management
- Consultation
- Coordination, facilitation, and integration
- Development
- Educational and professional development
- Policy development and advocacy
- Research evaluation

- Evaluating and selecting the technology
- Determining end-user requirements and customizing functionality
- Designing forms

Skills of Successful Nursing Informatics Specialists

Nursing informatics is different from traditional nursing, and it might require you to have additional skills and personality traits. Some that can help you succeed include:
- Problem-solving
- Strong interpersonal skills
- Clinical expertise
- Management ability
- Good organization
- Knowledge of technology
- Analytical thinking
- Communication skills
- Leadership experience
- Innovative thinking
- Teaching ability
- Strong information retention

DUTIES OF NURSE IN INFORMATICS

Nurse informaticists play a critical role in not only developing healthcare technology but educating staff and evaluating the results of implementation. Other responsibilities and duties include:
- Assessing and analyzing healthcare technology needs
- Designing systems technology
- Testing systems technology
- Implementing the technology which also includes:
  - Staff training
  - Troubleshooting
  - Escalating issues as needed
- Assisting in the transition from one system's technology to another
- Evaluating the success of implementation; revising as needed
- Serving as project managers
- Assisting in ensuring organizations meet federal healthcare laws, such as The Health Insurance Portability and Accountability Act of 1996 (HIPAA)
- Serving as a resource to staff
- Serving as a liaison between staff and information technology experts
- Assessing user requirements and developing solutions
- Serving as an educator to staff and new nurses
- Developing organizational policies and standards
- Researching different informatics topics that affect healthcare providers as well as patients

BENEFITS OF COMPUTER AUTOMATION IN HEALTHCARE

Electronic Medical Record

- **Improved access to the medical ward:** The EMR can be accessed from several different locations simultaneously, as well as by different levels of providers.
- **Decreased redundancy of data entry:** For example, allergies and vital signs need only be entered once.
- **Decreased time spent in documentation:** Automation allows direct entry from monitoring equipment, as well as point of care data entry.
- **Increased time for client care:** More time is available for client care because less time is required for documentation and transcription of physician orders.
- **Facilitation of data collection for research:** Electronically stored client records provide quick access to clinical data for a large number of clients.
- **Improved communication and decreased potential for error:** Improved legibility of clinician documentation and orders is seen with computerized information systems.
- Creation of a lifetime clinical record facilitated by information systems.

Other Benefits

- Decision support tools as well as alerts and reminders notify the clinician of possible concerns or omissions. An example of this is the documentation of patient allergies in the computer system. The healthcare providers would be alerted to any discrepancies in the patient medication orders.
- Effective data management and trend finding include the ability to provide historical or current data reports.
- Extensive financial information—can be collected and analyzed for trends. An extremely important benefit in this era of managed care and cost cutting.
- Data related to treatment, such as inpatient length of stay and the lowest level of care provider required can be used to decrease costs.

LEGAL ISSUES IN NURSING INFORMATICS

Nursing informatics is a booming and vital profession in healthcare. It requires a solid knowledge base in nursing and its application to the field of informatics. It can be fraught with legal issues as well. The nurse informatics needs to ensure, insofar as is humanly possible, the legal issues inherent in this profession are avoided before they become problems that must be resolved.

- Develop policies and procedures for the use of the health information system utilized in the healthcare facility in which he or she works. Provide training and in-services and be available to healthcare staff as they become familiar with, and continue to use, the health information system;
- Patient safety must be the highest priority in any informatics system when patient care is involved. If the patient is not the center of the system, it will become a liability rather than an asset that helps to improve patient care;
- All health team members must use the system as it is intended to be used. Not entering information into the system or attempting to by-pass it, as examples, will result in a failure of communication among and between health team members;

- Established age-old and proven principles of good documentation from hand-written medical records must be followed when documenting patient care and other necessary communication in the EMR;
- Privacy of patient information held in the system must be as secure as is possible. The use of passwords or codes must be used only by those to whom the password or code is assigned. Print-outs of patient information must be used minimally, not leave the facility, and shredded when their use is no longer needed; and
- Health team members must not allow others to use their code or password to gain entry into the system, to gain information for unauthorized use or to document for person assigned that code. Clear codes of conduct for all health team members prohibiting these actions, and any discipline that can be imposed, must be developed and disseminated to all staff.

CURRENT TRENDS AND ISSUES

- As nurses have been practicing in the automation of healthcare data and the integration of nursing data within information systems, a realization of the need for agreed-on definitions of the appropriate elements describing clients and their care came to light.
- Werely and Lang 1998, have identified and described the need for a standardized data set in nursing, the Nursing Minimum Data Set in Nursing, the Nursing Minimum Data Set (NMDS). Adoption of the NMDS would allow for an ongoing collection of data that can be compared across setting and client populations for clinical and administrative decision making.
- According to the study groups on Nursing Information Systems (1983), computerizing the data facilitates the management and use of the information by standardization, organization and automation to produce timely and comprehensive information. The NMDS provides structure for electronic storage of nursing data, and the unified nursing language provides the substantive data definition to be stored in that structure.

PATIENT RECORDS (FIG. 18.10)

The terms medical record, health record, and medical chart are used somewhat interchangeably to describe the systematic documentation of a single patient's medical history and care across time within one particular healthcare provider's jurisdiction. The medical record includes a variety of types of "notes" entered over time by healthcare professionals, recording observations and administration of drugs and therapies, orders for the administration of drugs and therapies, test results, X-rays, reports, etc. The maintenance of complete and accurate medical records is a requirement of healthcare providers and is generally enforced as a licensing or certification prerequisite.

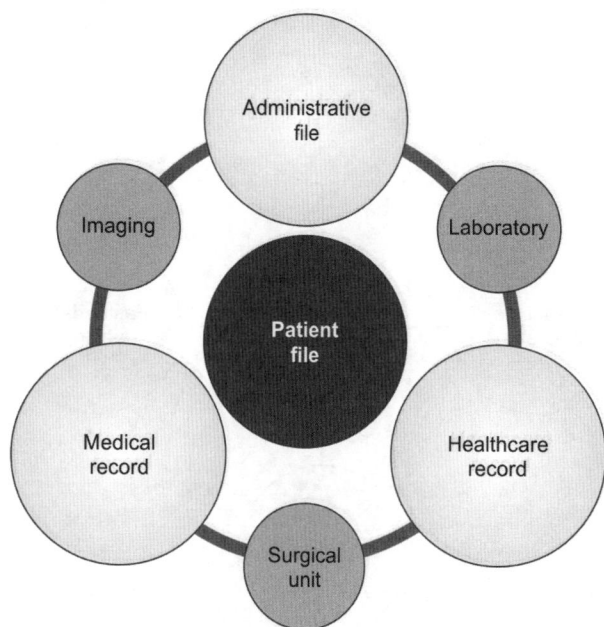

Fig. 18.10: Patient records.

Definition

- **Documentation:** It is the process of communicating in written form about essential fact. Records and reports are essential components of documentation.
- **Records:** It is a written communication that permanently documents the information relevant to a client's healthcare management.
  Record is the valuable sources of data for all members of the healthcare team.
- **Reports:** Reports may be oral or written form of documentation.
  Report is an oral, written or computer-based communication intended to convey information to other.

Purpose of Documentation

- **Communication:** The primary purpose of documentation of client care is the communication among healthcare professional to promote continuity of care among departments throughout 24 hours.
- **Quality assurance:** It provides substantiation of quality of care. An audit is a review of record.
- **Reimbursement:** Reimbursement for client care by insurance companies and other agencies are done after a review of client's records.
- **Legal accountability:** It serves as legal document. It may be used as evidences in court proceedings.
- **Research:** Nursing and healthcare research is often carried out by studying client records.
- **Diagnosis:** Documents are aids in diagnosis of patients' condition.
- **Evaluation:** Patient condition progress towards diseases condition will be evaluated based on his/her record.
- **Assessment:** The nurse and other healthcare members gather assessment data from the client records.

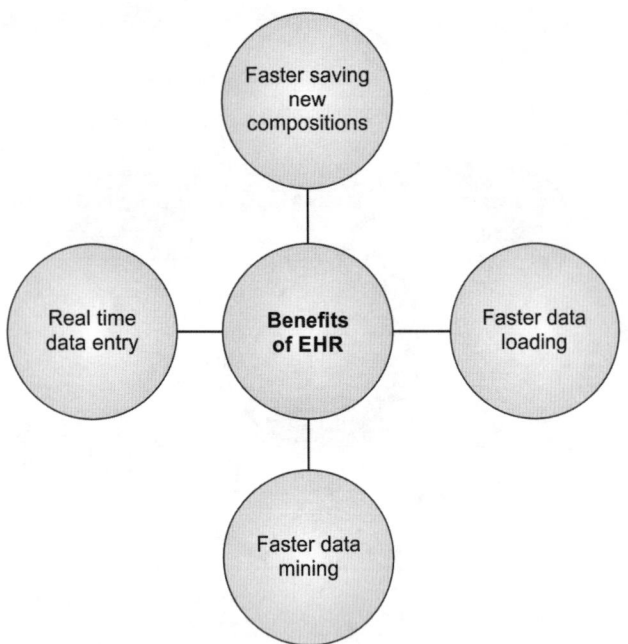

Fig. 18.11: Benefits of electronic health record (EHR).

- **Education:** Members of the health team including students utilize these records as an educational tool.
- **Vital statistics:** Client records, registers and reports furnish the vital statistics.
- **Health service planning:** Client record points out the health problems of the country and provides a baseline for local, state, national and international health service planning. **Figure 18.11** shows benefits of electronic health record.

Purpose of Documentation

- **Communication:** The primary purpose of documentation of client care is the communication among healthcare professional to promote continuity of care among departments throughout 24 hours.
- **Quality assurance:** It provides substantiation of quality of care. An audit is a review of record.
- **Reimbursement:** Reimbursement for client care by insurance companies and other agencies are done after a review of client's records.
- **Legal accountability:** It serves as legal document. It may be used as evidences in court proceedings.
- **Research:** Nursing and healthcare research is often carried out by studying client records.
- **Diagnosis:** Documents are aids in diagnosis of patients' condition
- **Evaluation:** Patient condition progress towards diseases condition will be evaluated based on his/her record.
- **Assessment:** The nurse and other healthcare members gather assessment data from the client records.
- **Education:** Members of the health team including students utilize these records as an educational tool.
- **Vital statistics:** Client records, registers and reports furnish the vital statistics.
- **Health service planning:** Client record points out the health problems of the country and provides a baseline for local, state, national and international health service planning.

Uses

- The information contained in the medical record allows healthcare providers to determine the patient's medical history and provide informed care.
- The medical record serves as the central repository for planning patient care and documenting communication among patient and healthcare provider and professionals contributing to the patient's care.
- An increasing purpose of the medical record is to ensure documentation of compliance with institutional, professional or governmental regulation.
- The traditional medical record for inpatient care can include admission notes, on-service notes, progress notes (SOAP notes), preoperative notes, operative notes, postoperative notes, procedure notes, delivery notes, postpartum notes, and discharge notes.
- Personal health records combine many of the above features with portability, thus allowing a patient to share medical records across providers and healthcare systems.

Contents

- A patient's individual medical record identifies the patient and contains information regarding the patient's case history at a particular provider.
- The health record as well as any electronically stored variant of the traditional paper files contains proper identification of the patient. Further information varies with the individual medical history of the patient.

Types of Patient Records

- **Medical history:** The medical history is a longitudinal record of what has happened to the patient since birth. It chronicles diseases, major and minor illnesses, as well as growth landmarks. It gives the clinician a feel for what has happened before to the patient. As a result, it may often give clues to current disease state. It includes several subsets detailed below.
- **Surgical history:** The surgical history is a chronicle of surgery performed for the patient. It may have dates of operations, operative reports, and/or the detailed narrative of what the surgeon did.
- **Obstetric history:** The obstetric history lists prior pregnancies and their outcomes. It also includes any complications of these pregnancies.
- **Medications and medical allergies:** The medical record may contain a summary of the patient's current and previous medications as well as any medical allergies.
- **Family history:** The family history lists the health status of immediate family members as well as their causes of death (if known). It may also list diseases common in the family or found only in one sex or the other. It may also include a pedigree chart. It is a valuable asset in predicting some outcomes for the patient.

- **Social history:**
  - The social history is a chronicle of human interactions. It tells of the relationships of the patient, his/her careers and trainings, and religious training.
  - It is helpful for the physician to know what sorts of community support the patient might expect during a major illness.
  - It may explain the behavior of the patient in relation to illness or loss. It may also give clues as to the cause of an illness (e.g., occupational exposure to asbestos).

Habits

- Various habits which impact health, such as tobacco use, alcohol intake, exercise, and diet are chronicled, often as part of the social history.
- This section may also include more intimate details, such as sexual habits and sexual orientation.

Immunization history: The history of vaccination is included. Any blood tests proving immunity will also be included in this section.

Growth Chart and Developmental History

- For children and teenagers, charts documenting growth as it compares to other children of the same age is included, so that healthcare providers can follow the child's growth over time.
- Many diseases and social stresses can affect growth, and longitudinal charting can thus provide a clue to underlying illness.
- Additionally, a child's behavior (such as timing of talking, walking, etc.) as it compares to other children of the same age is documented within the medical record for much the same reasons as growth.

Medical Encounters

- Within the medical record, individual medical encounters are marked by discrete summations of a patient's medical history by a physician, nurse practitioner, or physician assistant and can take several forms.
- Hospital admission documentation (i.e., when a patient requires hospitalization) or consultation by a specialist often take an exhaustive form, detailing the entirety of prior health and healthcare.
- Routine visits by a provider familiar to the patient, however, may take a shorter form, such as the problem-oriented medical record (POMR), which includes a problem list of diagnoses or a "SOAP" method of documentation for each visit. Each encounter will generally contain the aspects below:
  - **Chief complaint:** This is the main problem (traditionally called a complaint) that has brought the patient to see the doctor or other clinician. Information on the nature and duration of the problem will be explored.
  - **History of the present illness:** A detailed exploration of the symptoms the patient is experiencing that have caused the patient to seek medical attention.

Physical Examination

- The physical examination is the recording of observations of the patient.
- This includes the vital signs, muscle power and examination of the different organ systems, especially ones that might directly be responsible for the symptoms the patient is experiencing.

Assessment and Plan

- The assessment is a written summation of what are the most likely causes of the patient's current set of symptoms.
- The plan documents the expected course of action to address the symptoms (diagnosis, treatment, etc.).

Orders and prescriptions: Written orders by medical providers are included in the medical record. These detail the instructions given to other members of the healthcare team by the primary providers.

Progress notes:

- When a patient is hospitalized, daily updates are entered into the medical record documenting clinical changes, new information, etc.
- These often take the form of a SOAP note and are entered by all members of the healthcare team (doctors, nurses, physical therapists, dietitians, clinical pharmacists, respiratory therapists, etc.).
- They are kept in chronological order and document the sequence of events leading to the current state of health.

Test results: The results of testing, such as blood tests (e.g., complete blood count) radiology examinations (e.g., X-rays), pathology (e.g., biopsy results), or specialized testing (e.g., pulmonary function testing) are included. Often, as in the case of X-rays, a written report of the findings is included in lieu of the actual film.

Records Maintained by the Nurses

Vitals sign chart on this the temperature, pulse and respiration are written in a graphic form so that a slight deviation from the normal can be noted at a glance:

- **Intake and output chart:** Intake and output chart to be maintained for the critically-ill client those who received intravenous fluids, postoperative clients, clients with edema, and client suffering with vomiting and diarrhea,
- **Nurses notes:** Nurses notes are a record of treatments and nursing measures carried out by the nurse which reflects the observation of the client.
- **Other information:** Many other items are variably kept within the medical record. Digital images of the patient, flow sheets from operations/intensive care units, informed consent forms, EKG tracings, outputs from medical devices (such as pacemakers), chemotherapy protocols, and numerous other important pieces of information form part of the record depending on the patient and his or her set of illnesses/treatments.

NURSING RECORDS

Records are an account of something, written to perpetuate knowledge of events. Records and reports and indispensable aids to all who are responsible for giving best possible service to individuals, families and community. Good reports are time savers. They prevent duplication of work, decrease errors and show efficiency level of the staff. Records and reports hold an important place in the process of educational administration. The teacher should prepare records and reports after implementation of a plan over project and the educational administrator himself is expected to prepare a report about the organization and its function periodically (Figs. 18.12 to 18.14).

Characteristics of Good Recording and Reporting

- **Accuracy:** Information should be correct to prevent serious mistakes. Use of correct spelling and the institutions accepted abbreviation and symbols ensure accurate interpretation of information. It should be always complete with accurate signature. Do not use nick names.
- **Conciseness:** Use a few words as possible to give the necessary information.
- **Thoroughness:** Even a concise record or report must contain complete information.
- **Up to date:** Recording should be done on time. A definite time and routine for the reporting make more time and routine for the reporting makes more efficient management. Delay in recording can result in serious omissions and delay the work.
- **Organization:** Communicate all the information in a logical format or order.
- **Confidentiality:** The information should be confidential.
- **Objectivity:** Presentation of facts not personal feelings, to give true picture.

Types of Records (Fig. 18.15)

- **Patients clinical records:** It is the record of events in the patient illness, progress in his or her recovery and the type of care given by the hospital personnel.

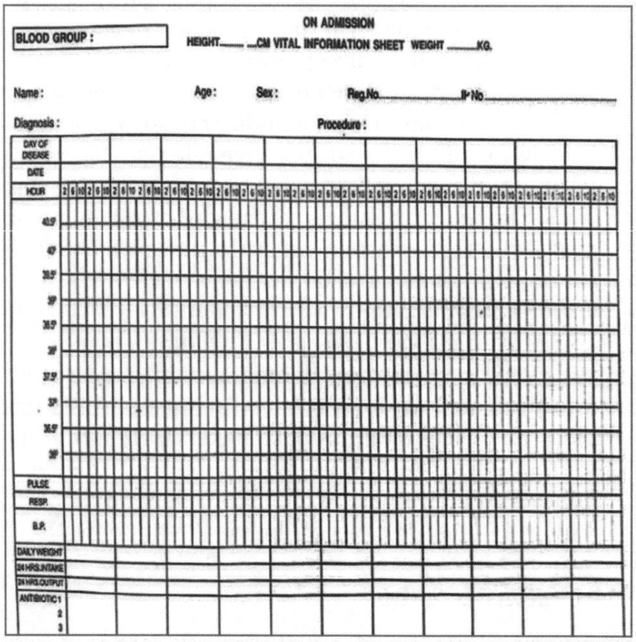

- **Individual staff records:** A separate set of record is needed for staff, giving details of their absences, their carrier development activities and a personnel note.

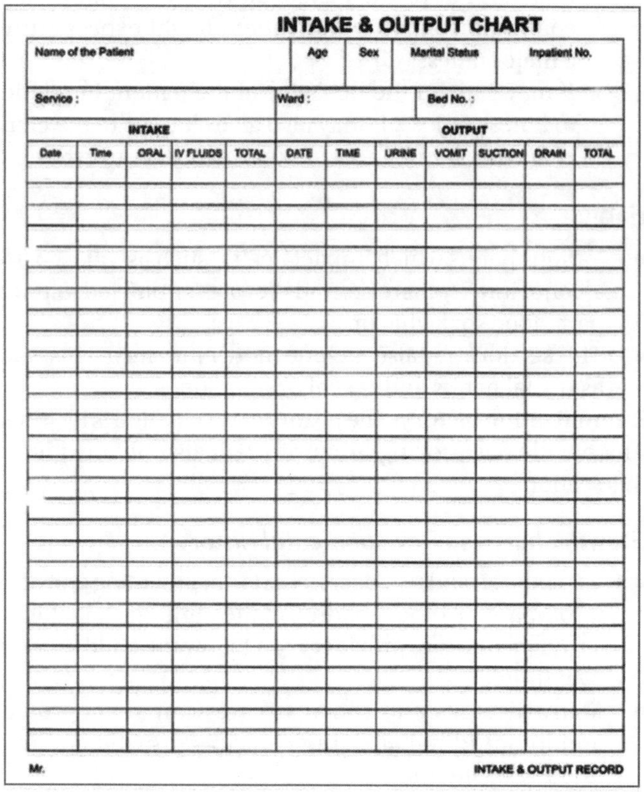

Fig. 18.13: Intake and output chart.

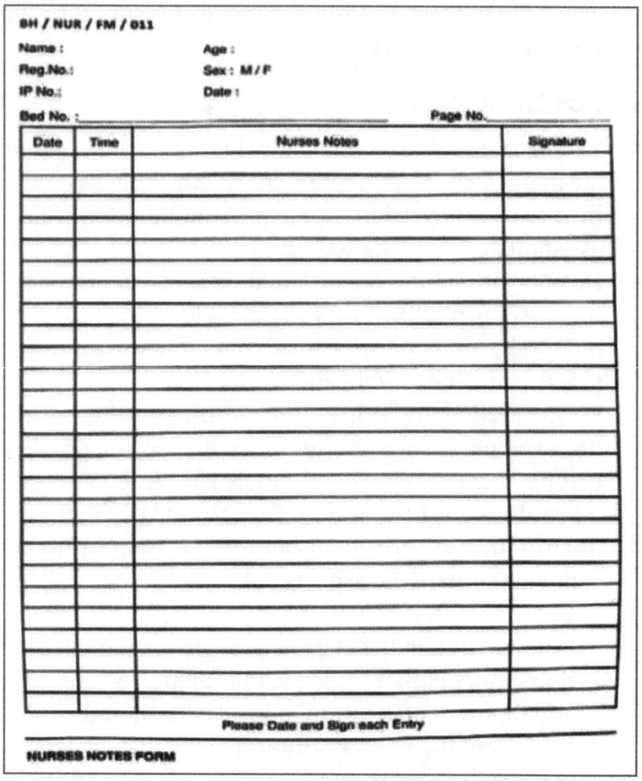

Fig. 18.12: TPR recording chart.

Fig. 18.14: Nurses notes form.

Chapter 18: Nursing Informatics/Information Management

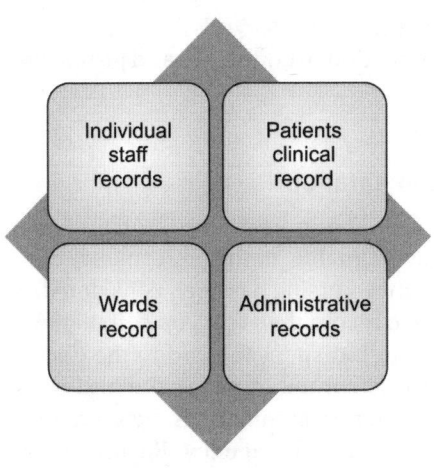

Fig. 18.15: Types of nursing records.

- **Ward records:** These records are maintained in the each ward, such as:
  - Census records.
  - Change in medical staff and non-nursing personnel for the ward. (Duty roaster)
  - Inventory and stock records
  - Staffs leave records
  - Admission records
  - Transfer records
  - Discharge records
  - Medicine records, etc.
- **Administrative records:** These records are maintained purely for administrative purpose of the hospital or unit
  - Legal documents: For the patients with poisoning, assault, rape, burns, etc.
  - Research or statistics data records
  - Audit and nursing audit records
  - Quality of care records
  - Personnel performance records
  - Other administrative records

Figure 18.16 shows nursing process recording system.

Principles of Documentation

- **Accuracy in charting**
  - Be specific and definite in using words or phrases that convey the meaning you wish expressed
  - Words that have ambiguous meanings and slang should not be used in charting
  - Chart objective facts, not your interpretations or opinions
- **Date and time:** Document the date and time of each recording.
- **Correct spelling:** It is essential for accuracy in recording.
- **Appropriateness:** Record only information that pertains to the client's health problems and care.
- **Legal protection:** Accurate complete documentation will give legal protection to the nurse other healthcare professional of the institution and the client.
- **Accuracy:** Client's name and identification data must be written on each page of the client's records and entries must be accurate.
- **Completeness:** Document all information necessary to explain the events in a shift. Anyone reading the document should have a clear picture of what took place.
- **Brief:** Only standard medical and nursing terminology and community recognized abbreviations and symbols should be used.
- **Organizations:** Recording of information on the clients must follow a chronological order charting statements must be logically organized according to time and content.
- **Omissions:** Blank spaces are not to be left on the chart and avoid writing outside the lines of the charting format.

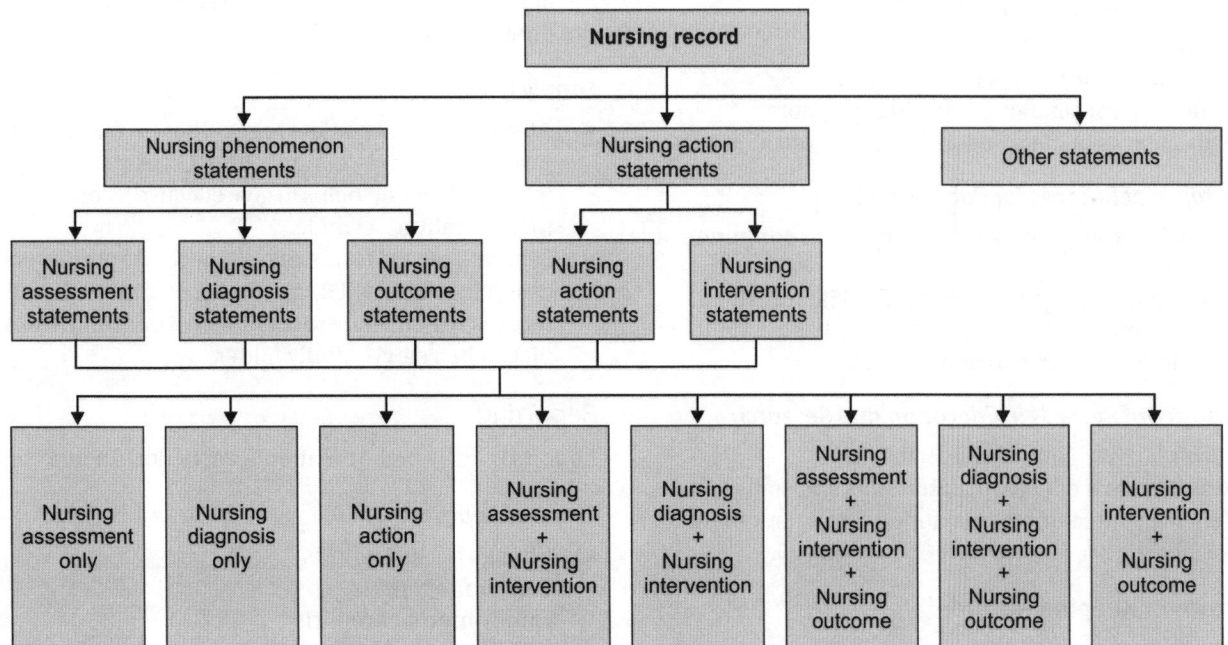

Fig. 18.16: Nursing process recording system.

- **Confidentiality:** Information within the chart is often of a personal matter as well as legal evidence of the care provided and should be available for the necessary health team members only.
- **Standard:** Spell correctly
  - Use proper grammar
  - Put signature
    - Affix signature, place at the end of charting at the right hand margin of the nurses notes.
    - Sign each entry with your full name and status, e.g., SN for student nurse, RN for registered nurse.
  - In case of error.
    - Correct errors by drawing a single horizontal line through the error
    - Write the word error above the line, and then sign your signature
    - No ink eradication, erasers or use of occlusive materials

Importance of Records and Reports

The importance of records can be described under following heads:

Importance of Records for Patients

- Legal evidence
- It avoids duplication of treatment measures.
- It avoids duplication of diagnostic and procedural measures.
- It will assist in continuity of patient care.
- It helps in health insurance of the patient.

Importance of Records for Doctor

- Assure quality of care
- It will help in evaluation of medical care given by doctors
- It protects the doctor from legal activities

Importance of Records for Hospital

- Legal protection of hospital
- Evaluate medical care given by doctor
- Evaluate performance of individual doctors
- It also assists in planning and justification of resources

Importance of Records for Public Health

- Helps in early warning of epidemic and communicable disease
- Assist in planning preventive and social measures
- Provide information of vital statistics like mortality rate, morbidity rate, infant death rate etc.

Importance of Records in Education and Research

- Forms basis of clinical research
- Aids in formal education of students and staff
- Reliable source of material for advancement in medical science.

Purposes of Keeping Records

- Communication
- Education
- Assessment
- Documentation of continuity and justification of case
- Research
- Auditing

Legal Documentation

Types and uses of nursing records: All professional persons need to be accountable for the performance of their duties to the public. Since nursing has been considered as profession, nurses need to record their work on completion. Records are a practical and indispensable aid to the doctor, nurse and paramedical personnel in giving the best possible service to the clients. Report summarizes the services of the person or personnel and of the agency. Records may be used for teaching and research.

For the Nurse

- Provide with documentation of services rendered, i.e., shows health condition of the client.
- Provide data essential for planning and evaluation of services for further improvement.
- Serve as a guide for professional growth.
- Enable to judge the quality and quantity of work done.
- Serve as communication tool between staff and other members involved in care.
- Indicate plans for the future.

For Authorities

- Provide the management with statistical information necessary for decision in regard to utilization of resources, planning for administrative control and future references.
- Help the supervisor evaluate the services rendered, teaching done and a person's action and reactions.

Cumulative or Continuing Records

This is found to be time saving, economical and also it is helpful to review the total history of an individual and evaluate the progress of a long period.

Family Records

- All records, which relate to members of family, should be placed in a single family folder. Gives the picture of the total services and helps to give effective, economic service to the family as a whole.
- Separate record forms may be needed for different types of service, such as TB, maternity, etc., all such individual records which relate to members of one family should be placed in a single family folder.

Reporting

Reports may be oral or written form of documentation

Types of Reports

- Change of shift reports
- Telephone reports
- Family member reports
- Incident reports
- Legal reports

Change of Shift Reports

- A change of shift reports is given by a primary nurse to the nurse who assumes responsibility for continuing care of the patient. The change of shift report might be given in written form or orally.
- It provides basic identifying information, such as patient condition, current appraisal of each patient's health status, current order by the physician, changes of medication, intravenous fluids, diet, and activity level.
- Summary of each newly admitted patient.
- Report on patients who have been transferred or discharged.

Telephone Reports

- Telephones and telemedicine equipment can link healthcare professionals immediately and enable nurses to receive and give critical information about patients in a timely fashion.
- Report the patients' current vital signs and clinical manifestation investigation, etc.

Family Member Reports

Nurses play a crucial role in keeping the patient family and updated about the patient's condition nurses should clarify their doubts and record their patient condition.

Incident Reports

It is a tool used by heath agencies to document the occurrence of anything out of the ordinary that results in harm to a patient, employee or visitor these reports are used for quality improvement.

Nursing Documentation Format

SOAPIER Format

S—SUBJECTIVE = What patient tells you. (e.g., I have leg pain).

O—OBJECTIVE = What you observe (observe the leg for swelling/injury and facial expressions).

A—ASSESSMENT = The critical analysis and evaluation or judgement of the patient condition

P—PLAN = What you are going to do. (plan for any nursing intervention to reduce pain, informing physician, giving medication and comfort position).

I—IMPLEMENTATION = Specific interventions implemented like hot or cold fomentation, administration of medication, etc.

E—EVALUATION = Patient response towards nursing care (patient may say, I am feeling better, my leg pain is reduced).

R—REVISION = Changes the treatment. (If the pain is not reduced modify the intervention).

APIE Charting

It is Similar to SOAP

A—Assessment

P—Problem Identification

I—Intervention

E—Evaluation

Focus charting: Focused only on nursing diagnosis, patient problem, signs and symptoms. It has three components (DAR)

- DATA—subjective or objective data that supports the focus
- ACTION—nursing intervention
- RESPONSE—patient response to intervention

Example:

- D—complaining of pain at incision site, pain score: 7/10
- A—repositioned for comfort—analgesics injection given.
- R—patient states pain reduced, "Feels Much Better."

Computer-assisted Charting

- Notes always legible and easy to read
- Quick communication among departments about patient needs
- Many providers have access to patient's information at one time
- Can reduce documentation time.
- Reimbursement for services rendered is faster and complete

Nurses Responsibility for Record Keeping and Reporting

- Keep under safe custody of nurses.
- No individual sheet should be separated.
- Not accessible to patients and visitors.
- Strangers are not permitted to read records.
- Records are not handed over to the legal advisors without written permission of the administration.
- Handed carefully, not destroyed.
- Identified with bio-data of the patients, such as name, age, admission number, diagnosis, etc.

USE OF COMPUTERS IN HOSPITAL, COLLEGE AND COMMUNITY (BOXES 18.4 AND 18.5)

The word computer comes from the word "compute", which means to calculate. Computer can be defined as an electronic device that is designed to automatically accept data, store and process then producing output results. Computers are used to store and process large amount of data and provide information to the user and to perform large number of calculations rapidly and accurately. Charles Babbage is

---

Box 18.4: Uses of computers in clinical nursing practice.

- **Admission, discharge and transfer (ADT)**
  - ADT system allows nurses to obtain basic biographical information on clients before they arrive to the unit.
  - When a discharge or transfer is entered in the computer, all the appropriate departments are automatically notified, thus saves many phone calls, information about beds and clients location on the unit is also readily available.
- **Nursing documentation**
  - Nursing assessments, clients care plan, medication administration records, nursing notes and discharge plans are some of the forms of nursing administration that are computerized.
  - Advantage of this documentation is legible and it can store standard nursing care plans in a format determined by the institutions, to be used by the nurses as the basis for developing individualized client care plan.

> **Box 18.5:** Use of computers in hospital and community.
>
> **Clinical implication**
> - Assessment
> - Patient monitoring
> - Documentation
> - Nursing minimum data sheet
> - Telemedicine
> - **Electronic medical records (EMR):**
>   - Increased efficiency
>   - Improved documentation
>   - Improved quality of care
>   - Improved security
>   - Reduced documentation expenses

considered to be father of modern computer

Computers are being increasingly used in medical profession. There are different levels of interface of medicine and computer technology.

Uses for Computers in Healthcare

- **Computers for medication and treatment:** Computers have revolutionized the way medication is administered and diagnosing medical treatment required. With access to accurate patient records, doctors and nurses can review an individual's full medical history in detail, enabling them to diagnose, treat, and administer medications in a timely manner.
- **Computers for security and organized record keeping:** A computer network is a far more secure way to store and organize patient records. Filing patient records in cabinets or on shelving is quickly being phased out, with computer systems offering a more efficient solution. A computer keeps patient records secure, organized, and easily accessible. A mobile computer cart gives doctors and nurses access to records anywhere in the hospital. There's no need for medical personnel to waste time running back and forth to retrieve patient files when they easily transport a laptop computer with network access.
- **Computers for every room:** Medical computer carts can serve as standing workstations in every room of a hospital or healthcare facility. If a rolling stand proves to be impractical to wheel around a medical facility constantly, one can be designated to each room. This still gives doctors and nurses access to a portable solution that's equipped with everything they need.

    Medical staff can quickly access patient records, or hook up other equipment to a computer, to perform their duties and still have full mobility around a room.
- **Computers for offsite care:** Not all patients can access a hospital due to their health condition, which means sometimes doctors and nurses have to go offsite to treat people. Laptop computers are portable so can accompany doctors and nurses on home visits, allowing them to access the hospital network even when not on site. Having access to patient information, especially when not in the hospital is crucial for ensuring there are no errors when treating a patient in their home.
- **Computers for surgical procedures:** The use of computers in operating theaters is helping save lives. Surgeons rely on computer systems for performing intricate procedures and monitoring the wellbeing of their patients. Mobile computer stands play a key role in the success of surgical procedures. Height adjustable industrial computer carts that are mobile are extremely useful for surgeons who need a clear line of sight to a computer screen that is being used as part of a surgical procedure. A laptop cart is widely used in surgical theaters as a solution for medical imaging, allowing surgeons to monitor a procedure closely.
- **Computers for communication and inventory management:** Computers enable better communication across different hospital departments, allowing them to quickly share updates or medical research. Doctors and nurses can also access the internet for information shared by their peers on conditions they are perhaps unfamiliar with, but others in their profession have treated.

USE OF COMPUTERS IN HOSPITAL

Computers are the excellent means for storage of patient related data. Big hospitals employ computer systems to maintain patient records. It is often necessary to maintain detailed records of the medical history of patients. Computers can keep track of prescriptions and billing information

Uses of Computers

- Computers can be used for storing data and using it while it is required.
- Mathematical calculations and other calculations can be done using computers.
- Computers can be also used for communicating through internet.
- Any kind of information can be achieved from the computers.
- We can share our views with people using internet from computers.
- At higher level, computers are used for weather predictions, medical science, space research, AI development and many more other things.
- Companies provide the employment in the field of computer jobs.

Ways Computers are Used in Medicine

Medical Imaging

- Medical imaging is a broad term that covers technology used to create images of the human body for study and diagnosis.
- It includes magnetic resonance imaging (MRI), ultrasound, CT scans and X-rays.
- All of these devices are controlled by computers. Even X-ray imaging, which has been used in medicine since the early 20th century, now uses computers for image adjustment and transfer.

Patient Monitoring

- Modern computer-based patient monitoring machines allow heart rate, respiratory activity, blood pressure and other critical vital signs to be collected automatically in digital form.
- Computer monitoring machines cut down on the time spent on routine tests in doctors' offices.
- In hospitals, they have the ability to automatically update a patient's chart and notify hospital staff of changes to a patient's vitals.

Computer-assisted Surgery

- Computers are used to assist in planning, teaching and performing many surgical procedures.
- One of the biggest recent developments in this area is robotically-assisted surgery (RAS), which allows surgeons to use robotic devices and computer software to complete minimally-invasive procedures.
- The surgeon remains in control and guides the robot device to complete complex operations in confined parts of the body.

Networks and Digital Communication

- Computer networks and the internet have increased the means of communication between medical professionals with email, instant messaging, video chats and webinars.
- Being able to connect digitally helps healthcare professionals stay current with the latest medical developments.
- They can also consult with colleagues in real-time and receive second opinions for diagnoses and treatment options.

Telemedicine

- The concept of a house visit is returning to healthcare in the form of telemedicine. Thanks to computers and smartphones, some medical professionals use video chats to visit with patients remotely.
- Besides benefitting patients who live in rural areas with limited healthcare options, telemedicine has proved useful following natural disasters and in war zones.

Electronic Health Records

- Perhaps one of the newest major developments in healthcare, the electronic health record (EHR) is also one of the most far-reaching.
- An EHR is a digital version of a patient's paper chart that is instantly available to authorized health providers.

Medical Databases

- Computers have brought the development of many useful software solutions in the medical field. Large public health organizations, such as the World Health Organization and the Centers for Disease Control have amassed huge databases of information related to diseases and health statistics.
- There are also public databases available with information about toxic substances, clinical research results and drug coverage.

Medical Research

- Much of the current research being done into incurable diseases, such as AIDS and cancer involves the creation of complex computer simulations.
- Supercomputers and distributed computer systems are able to handle massive amounts of research data and analyze millions of possible outcomes.
- The mapping of the human genome is one example of how computers are advancing medical research.

Computers and Hospital Administration

- Most hospitals depend heavily on computers and specialized software that handles patient records, supply inventory, personnel scheduling and all the other details required to care for patients.
- The use of a computer in a hospital extends to every department, from the surgical center to the cafeteria.
- Larger hospitals may have their own private computer servers and network and a team of IT specialists who maintain them.

Uses of Computer in Offices

- The typical doctor's office relies heavily on computer technology for day-to-day operations.
- Everything from patient scheduling to billing to filing insurance claims takes place through a computer.
- Many doctors no longer write prescriptions, but instead send a digital prescription from their office computer directly to the patient's pharmacy.
- During diagnosis, many doctors consult online databases of medical conditions using a computer instead of looking at a medical book.

COMPUTERS IN NURSING

Computers influence every sphere of human activity and bring in many changes in industry, education, healthcare, scientific research, social service, law and even in arts, music and painting. The computer revolutionized the nursing profession. Clinical and technological advancements led to a nursing specialty called nursing informatics the application of computer and information science to promote and support the practice of nursing and the delivery of nursing care (**Fig. 18.17**).

Box 18.6: Community setting.

The main uses of computers in community are:
- Gathering of epidemiological and administrative statistics
- Patient appointments—identification system
- Patient assessment and data gathering
- Monitoring
- Documentation
- Special need application

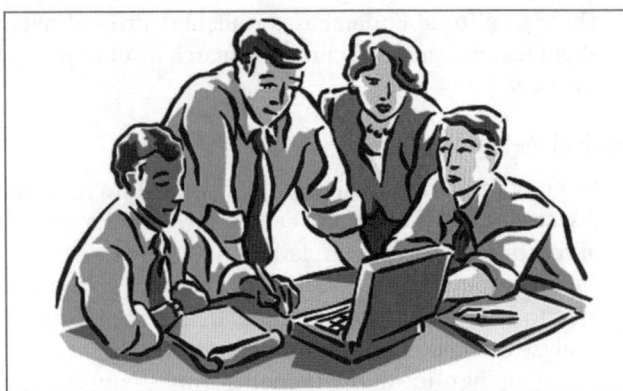

Fig. 18.17: Computer in nursing.

Historical Perspectives of Computers and Nursing

- In 1960's, use of computers in healthcare is questioned, but studies on computers in nursing are started.
- 1970's, nurses assisted in the design of HIS. Computers are used in financial and management functions, and several communities developed management information system.
- In 1980's, nursing Informatics is formally accepted as new nursing specialty
- In 1990's, computer technology became an integral part of the healthcare setting.
- In the year 2000, Clinical Information System became individualized in the electronic patient record, mobile computing device were introduced.

Uses of Computers in Clinical Nursing Practice

- Admission, Discharge and Transfer (ADT) ADT system allows nurses to obtain basic biographical information on clients before they arrive to the unit. When a discharge or transfer is entered in the computer, all the appropriate departments are automatically notified, thus saves many phone calls, information about beds and clients location on the unit is also readily available.
- Nursing documentation nursing assessments, clients care plan, medication administration records, nursing notes and discharge plans are some of the forms of nursing administration that are computerized. Advantage of this documentation is legible and it can store standard nursing care plans in a format determined by the institutions, to be used by the nurses as the basis for developing individualized client care plan.

Teaching Learning Process (Box 18.7)

- Instructing the students using PowerPoint slides, word documents or web pages and using hyperlinks for better concept daily.
- Readymade software could give practice material to students.
- Collecting notes from web pages for detailed information and projects/assignments.
- Saving the documents as soft copy for future use.

> **Box 18.7:** Teaching–learning process.
>
> - Instructing the students using PowerPoint slides, word documents or web pages and using hyperlinks for better concept daily.
> - Readymade software could give practice material to students.
> - Collecting notes from web pages for detailed information and projects/assignments.
> - Saving the documents as soft copy for future use.
> - Learning through animations, as they are much near to the students.
> - E-books/online libraries/online encyclopedia helps to guide in minutes and saves precious time and resources.
> - Publications of pamphlets brochures for awareness with institutions and among community members.

- Learning through animations, as they are much near to the students.
- E-books/online libraries/online encyclopedia helps to guide in minutes and saves precious time and resources.
- Publications of pamphlets brochures for awareness with institutions and among community members.

Computer in Education

Testing and Evaluation Process

- Keeping records of students for their academic scores
- Keeping records in relation to personal history
- Creating question bank for students
- Online testing and evaluation
- Analysis and interpretation of the data

Guidance Purposes

Testing for aptitude, interest, psychology using computers data bases and interest. Library:

- Documents stored as soft copy for students/faculty members use.
- Online magazines, journals, brochures, research articles.
- Records of the books, record of the books maintained using special library software.
- Records of the issues and returns of the books.

School Administration

- Records of students (personal/academic)
- Records of employee of school
- Accounts of the institutions
- Aid to memory with minimum paper work
- Circulation of instructions/notices and getting it in printed form

Nursing Software's

- Probably the most overlooked and underappreciated resource in the operating room which nursing professionals require is nursing that performs multiple services.
- It minimizes non-clinical time, improves time management and facilitates access to information allowing them to do the job they were trained to do that is deliver patient care.
- SIS nursing software includes a series of modules that address each nursing related phases of the surgery case and more.

It includes:
- Preadmission testing
- Preoperative
- Intraoperative
- Postoperative

Tech breakthroughs that will make you a better nurse:
- Better communication systems—some hospitals are incorporating advanced communication systems, in which nurses and other members of the healthcare team can text message, speak, and receive patient alarms through their smart phone devices using specialized apps.
- This concept replaces antiquated paging systems, and helps the whole nursing unit stay in touch and work more efficiently with each other.

Electronic healthcare records (EHR): The days of endless paperwork, filling out patient charts, and having doctors fax over medical records will be gone for good as more and more hospitals and facilities convert to EHR, which allows healthcare providers to access patient information with a few keystrokes. With an extensive patient history easily accessible and all in one place, it cuts down on human error, alerts nursing staff to possible drug interactions, and keeps track of diagnostic test results.

■ COMPUTERS APPLICATION IN HEALTHCARE

Medical laboratory: Computers used to analyze DNA, blood, urine, used to test for disease and genetic.

Electrocardiogram (EKG or ECG)
- Computer provides a printout of electrical activity of patient's heart.
- Computer can also "read" the EKG—tell the reader what the EKG means. This used to be done by the doctor.
- An EKG can be done at a remote location and sent to a doctor thousands of miles away.

Echocardiogram
- Computer directs sound waves into the heart, and then converts the reflection of the waves into an image of the heart.
- Used to reveal heart problems—valve problems, defects in the heart wall, etc.

Computerized Tomography (CT)
- It is a computerized body scanner.
- Shows cross-section views
- Allows us to see bone and body tissues
- Helps us find tumors

Magnetic Resonance Imaging (MRI)
- It is a body scanner that uses nuclear magnets instead of X-rays.
- Patient is placed in a large, circular magnet that measures the activity of hydrogen ions and converts it to a picture.
- Can see tumors, blood moving through veins

Ultrasonography
- Uses high frequency sound waves
- Body parts are viewed on a computer screen and printed on photo paper
- Used during pregnancy

Telemedicine
- Includes remote monitoring devices and videoconferencing
- Used to connect specialists to patients in remote locations
- Can transmit information from prisons, an ambulance, and other challenging locations
- Families can watch the care of high-risk newborns who are still in the hospital

Bioinformatics
- The use of computers to store retrieves, analyze or predict the composition or the structure of biomolecules.
- "Biomolecules" include your genetic material—nucleic acids—and the products of your genes: proteins.

Human Genome Project
- Computers play an important role in the Human Genome Project.
- The goals of the Human Genome Project are:
  - Identify all the approximate 30,000 genes in human DNA
  - Determine the sequences of the 3 billion chemical base pairs that make up human DNA
  - Store this information in databases and improve tools for data analysis.

Computers in Biotech
- IBM is working on a supercomputer called Blue Gene which may decipher some of the mystery behind how proteins work.
- "Computational biology," or "bioinformatics," can collect information "without having to do the experiment" This could make it easier to design drugs because we can make a reasonable prediction of the structure with a computer.

Bioinformatics: Bioinformatics is the term coined for the new field that merges biology, computer science, and information technology to manage and analyze data, with the ultimate goal of understanding and modeling living systems.

■ TELEMEDICINE

Telemedicine refers to the practice of caring for patients remotely when the provider and patient are not physically present with each other. Modern technology has enabled doctors to consult patients by using HIPAA compliant video-conferencing tools **(Fig. 18.18)**.

Definition by WHO Delivery of healthcare services, where distance is a critical factor, by all healthcare professionals using information and communication technology for exchange of valid information for diagnosis, treatment and

Chapter 18: Nursing Informatics/Information Management

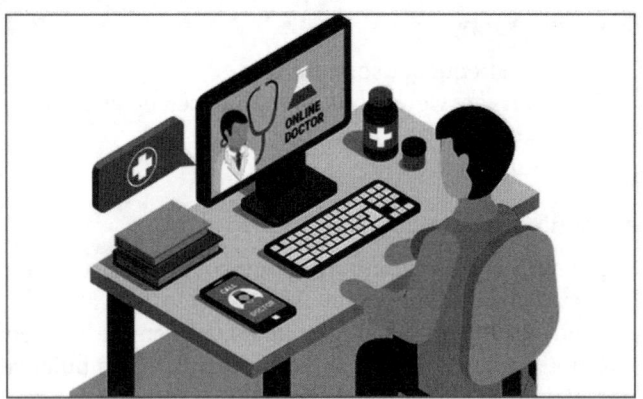

Fig. 18.18: Telemedicine.

prevention of diseases and injuries, research and evaluation, and for continuing education of healthcare providers, all in the interests of advancing the health of individuals and their communities.

Definition

- Telemedicine can be defined as the use of technology (computers, video, phone, messaging) by a medical professional to diagnose and treat patients in a remote location.
- Telemedicine is the exchange of medical information from one location to another using electronic communication, which improves patient health status.
- Telemedicine has multiple applications and can be used for different services, which includes wireless tools, email, two-way video, smartphone, and other methods of telecommunications technology.
- Tele-health is defined as "the use of electronic information and telecommunication technologies to support long-distance clinical healthcare, patient and professional health related education, public health and health administration"

Meaning of Telehealth

Tele" is a Greek word meaning "distance" and medicine derived from "mederi" is a Latin word meaning "to heal". Time magazine called telemedicine "healing by wire". Telemedicine is the use of electronic information to communicate technologies to provide and support healthcare when distance separates the participants.

"The delivery of healthcare services, where distance is a critical factor, by all healthcare professionals using information and communication technologies for the exchange of valid information for diagnosis, treatment and prevention of disease and injuries, research and evaluation and for the continuing education of healthcare providers, all in the interests of advancing the health of individuals and their communities." —By WHO

Objectives

- To provide specialized medical advice
- To monitor patient condition
- To guide other medical staff about treatment procedure

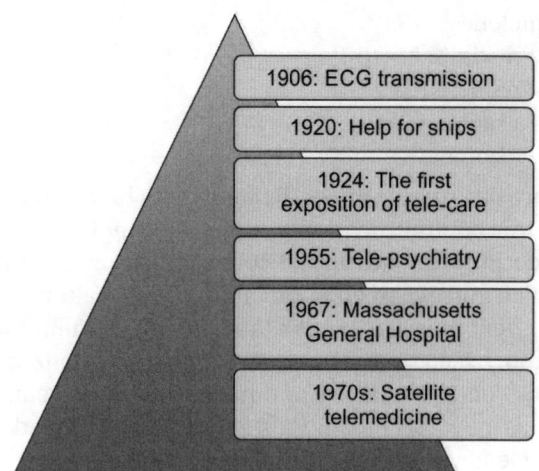

Fig. 18.19: History of telemedicine.

- Share patient data among institutions for research purpose. **Figure 18.19** shows history of telemedicine.

Functions

- Video conferencing between patient and specialist doctors
- Video conferencing between different specialist and other healthcare professionals
- Monitoring patient vitals and statistics in ICU's
- Security in data connection
- Transfer of patient's medical data among hospitals
- Storage of information

Uses of Telemedicine

- Interactive telemedicine services
- Specialist and primary care consultations
- Store-and-forward telemedicine
- Remote monitoring
- Imaging services

Telemedicine Benefits (Fig. 18.20)

Using telemedicine as an alternative to in-person visits has a host of benefits for patients and providers alike.

Benefits for Patients

Telemedicine can help treat a range of medical conditions. It is most successful when a person seeks care from a qualified physician and provides clear details about their symptoms. Some other benefits of telemedicine include:

- **Lower costs:** Some research suggests that people who use telemedicine spend less time in the hospital, providing cost savings. Also, less commuting time may mean fewer secondary expenses, such as childcare and gas.
- **Improved access to care:** Telemedicine makes it easier for people with disabilities to access care. It can also improve access for other populations, including older adults, people who are geographically isolated, and those who are incarcerated.
- **Preventive care:** Telemedicine may make it easier for people to access preventive care that improves their

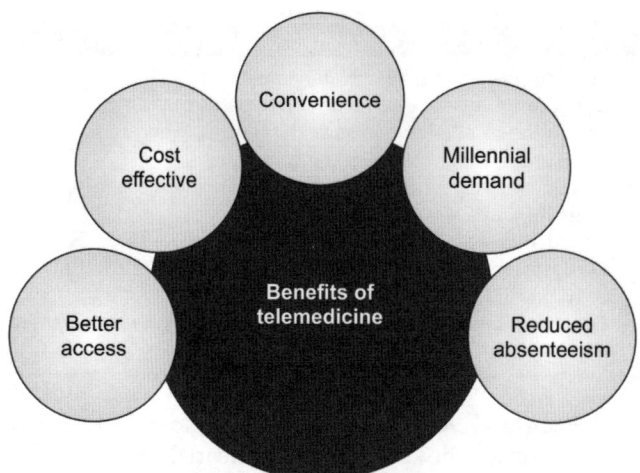

Fig. 18.20: Benefits of telemedicine.

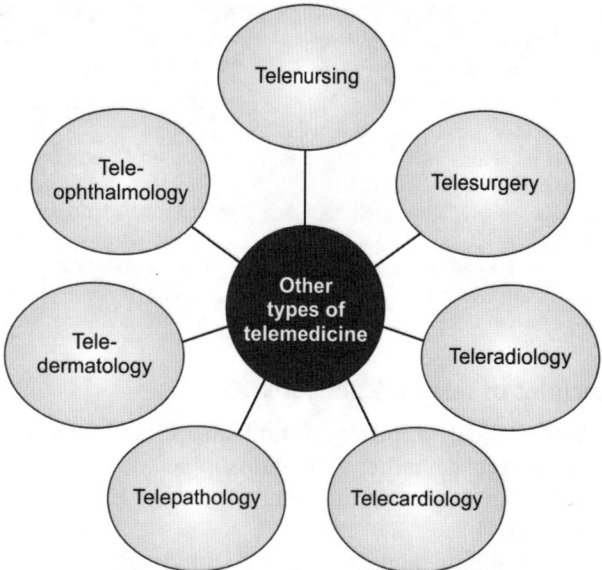

Fig. 18.21: Other types of telemedicine.

long-term health. This is especially true for people with financial or geographic barriers to quality care.

- **Convenience:** Telemedicine allows people to access care in the comfort and privacy of their own home. This may mean that a person does not have to take time off of work or arrange childcare.
- **Slowing the spread of infection:** Going to the doctor's office means being around people who may be sick, often in close quarters. This can be particularly dangerous for people with underlying conditions or weak immune systems.

Types of Telemedicine

There are three main types of telemedicine, which include store-and-forward, remote monitoring and real-time interactive services. Each of these has a beneficial role to play in overall healthcare and, when utilized properly, can offer tangible benefits for both healthcare workers and patients.

I. Store-and-Forward

- Store-and-forward telemedicine surpasses the need for the medical practitioner to meet in person with a patient.
- Instead, data, such as medical images or biosignals can be sent to the specialist as needed when it has been acquired from the patient.
- This practice is common in the medical fields of dermatology, radiology and pathology.
- With proper structure and care, this technique can save time and allow medical practitioners to serve the public with their services more fully.
- However, it relies on a history report and documented information or images, rather than a physical examination, which has the potential to cause complications, such as misdiagnosis.

II. Remote Monitoring

- Also known as self-monitoring or self-testing, remote monitoring uses a range of technological devices to monitor health and clinical signs of a patient remotely.
- This is extensively used in the management of chronic diseases, such as cardiovascular disease, diabetes mellitus and asthma.
- Benefits of remote monitoring include cost effectiveness, more frequent monitoring and greater patient satisfaction.
- There is some risk that tests conducted by the patients themselves may be inaccurate, but the outcomes are generally thought to be similar to professional-patient tests.

III. Real-time Interactive Services

- Interactive services can provide immediate advice to patients who require medical attention.
- There are several different mediums utilized for this purpose, including phone, online and home visits.
- A medical history and consultation about presenting symptoms can be undertaken, followed by assessment similar to those usually conducted in face-to-face appointments. **Figure 18.21** shows other types of telemedicine.

Benefits for Healthcare Providers

Healthcare providers who offer telemedicine services may gain several benefits, including:

- **Reduced overhead expenses:** Providers who offer telemedicine services may incur fewer overhead costs. For example, they may pay less for front desk support or be able to invest in an office space with fewer exam rooms.
- **Additional revenue stream:** Clinicians may find that telemedicine supplements their income because it allows them to provide care to more patients.
- **Less exposure to illness and infections:** When providers see patients remotely, they do not have to worry about exposure to any pathogens the patient may carry.
- **Patient satisfaction:** When a patient does not have to travel to the office or wait for care, they may be happier with their provider. **Table 18.2** describes benefits and challenges of telemedicine.

Table 18.2: Benefits and challenges of telemedicine.	
Pros	Cons
• You can take it anywhere • You can save patients a visit to the office • You can bill for a visit that might not have occurred • You can expand your catchment area of patients • You can alleviate some time constraints associated with an in-person visit	• Physical examination limited • Potential loss of personal connection with patient • Potential reimbursement challenges • State credentials (required in every state in which you see patients)

> **Box 18.9:** Telemedicine: Areas of challenge.
> - **Confidence**—to share when vulnerable
> - **Confidentiality**—to discuss person to person
> - **Candour**—to admit when something went wrong to patient or loved ones—either failure or complication
> - **Courage**—to face 'fud' together/to act in an emergency/to act when the stakes are life
> - **Collegiality**—to give team members support
> - **Compassion**—to see the bigger picture and when struggle is not the right choice
> - **Complications**—to hold the relationship in the face of unwanted events

Principles of Telemedicine (Box 18.8)

- Telemedicine applications and sites should be selected pragmatically, rather than philosophically
- Clinician drivers and telemedicine users must own the systems
- Telemedicine management and support should be from the 'bottom up', rather than from the 'top down'
- The technology should be as user-friendly as possible
- Telemedicine users must be well trained and supported, both technically and professionally
- Telemedicine applications should be evaluated in a clinically appropriate and user-friendly manner
- Information about the development of telemedicine must be shared

Applications

There are few limitations to how telemedicine can be applied. Here are a few examples of how it is being used today.

- **Follow-up visits:** Using health software for routine follow-up visits is not only more efficient for providers and patients, but it also increases the likelihood of follow-up, reducing missed appointments and improving patient outcomes.
- **Remote chronic disease management:** The increasing rate of chronic disease is a major challenge for our health system. It is a prime candidate for the use of telemedicine software because it makes it easier and less expensive for patients to maintain control over their health.
- **Remote post-hospitalization care:** One telehealth program for patients with congestive heart failure reduced 30-day hospital readmissions by 73% and six-month readmissions by 50%.
- **Preventative care support:** Weight loss and smoking cessation are the keys to reducing heart disease and a host of other conditions. Telemedicine can be a valuable tool in connecting providers with patients to make sure they get the support they need to be successful.
- **School-based telehealth:** When children become ill at school, they might visit a school nurse or be picked up by their parents and taken to an urgent care center. Some innovative districts have teamed up with doctors to conduct remote visits from the school. The provider can assess the urgency of the case and provide instructions or reassurance to parents.
- **Assisted living center support:** Telemedicine software has already proven to be useful in keeping residence of assisted living facilities out of the hospital. Problems often occur at night or on weekends, making hospitalization the only option even for less urgent problems. With telemedicine, on-call doctors can conduct a remote visit to determine if hospitalization is necessary. **Box 18.9** describes area of challenge of telemedicine.

Advantage of Telemedicine System

- Easy access to remote areas
- Using telemedicine in peripheral health set-ups can significantly reduce the time and costs of patient transportation
- Monitoring home care and ambulatory monitoring
- Improves communications between health providers separated by distance
- Critical care monitoring where it is not possible to transfer the patient
- Continuing medical education and clinical research
- A tool for public awareness
- A tool for disaster management
- Second opinion and complex interpretations
- Bring the expertise to medical practices
- Tele-mentored procedures-surgery using hand robots
- Disease surveillance and program tracking
- It provides an opportunity for standardization and equity in provision of healthcare, both within individual countries and across regions and continents.
- The center for International Rehabilitation recognizes that telecommunication and telemedicine are important technologies to improve and provide rehabilitation services in remote areas.

> **Box 18.8:** Principles of telemedicine.
> - Telemedicine applications and sites should be selected pragmatically, rather than philosophically
> - Clinician divers and telemedicine users must own the systems
> - Telemedicine management and support should be from the 'bottom up', rather than from the 'top down'
> - The technology should be as user-friendly as possible
> - Telemedicine users must be well trained and supported, both technically and professionally
> - Telemedicine applications should be evaluated in a clinically appropriate and user-friendly manner
> - Information about the development of telemedicine must be shared

- Telemedicine cannot be substitutes for physicians in rural areas especially in developing countries where resources are scarce and public health problems are in plenty.

Barriers in Telehealth (Fig. 18.22)

- **Perspective of medical practitioners:** Doctors are not fully convinced and familiar with e-medicine.
- **Patients' fear and unfamiliarity:** There is a lack of confidence in patients about the outcome of e-medicine.
- **Financial unavailability:** The technology and communication costs being too high sometimes make Telemedicine financially unfeasible.
- **Lack of basic amenities:** In India, nearly 40% of population lives below the poverty level. Basic amenities like transportation, electricity, telecommunication, safe drinking water, primary health services, etc., are missing. No technological advancement can change anything when a person has nothing to change.
- **Literacy rate and diversity in languages:** Only 65.38% of India's population is literate with only 2% being well-versed in English.
- **Technical constraints:** e-medicine supported by various types of software and hardware still needs to mature. For correct diagnosis and pacing of data, we require advanced biological sensors and more bandwidth support.
- **Quality aspect:** "Quality is the essence" and every one wants it but this can sometimes create problems. In case of healthcare, there is no proper governing body to form guidelines in this respect and motivate the organizations to follow—it is solely left to organizations on how they take it.
- **Government support:** The government has limitations and so do private enterprises. Any technology in its primary stage needs care and support. Only the government has the resources and the power to help it survive and grow. There is no such initiative taken by the government to develop it.

Disadvantages for Patients

Telemedicine is not a good fit for all patients. Some drawbacks of this type of care include:

- **Insurance coverage:** Not all insurers cover telemedicine. Currently require insurers to cover or reimburse the costs of telemedicine. However, these laws are constantly changing.

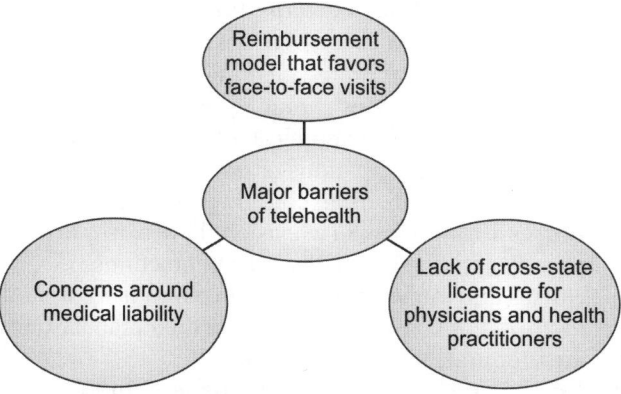

Fig. 18.22: Major barriers of telehealth.

- **Protecting medical data:** Hackers and other criminals may be able to access a patient's medical data, especially if the patient accesses telemedicine on a public network or via an unencrypted channel.
- **Care delays:** When a person needs emergency care, accessing telemedicine first may delay treatment, particularly since a doctor cannot provide life saving care or laboratory tests digitally.

Disadvantages for Healthcare Providers

Healthcare providers may also face some drawbacks associated with telemedicine, including:

- **Licensing issues:** State laws vary, and clinicians may not be able to practice medicine across state lines, depending on the state in which they hold their license and the state in which the patient lives.
- **Technological concerns:** Finding the right digital platform to use can be challenging. Also, a weak connection can make it difficult to offer quality care. Clinicians must also ensure that the telemedicine program they use is secure and fully compliant with privacy laws.
- **An inability to examine patients:** Providers must rely on patient self-reports during telemedicine sessions. This may require clinicians to ask more questions to ensure that they get a comprehensive health history.

Challenges of Telemedicine in India

Implementing telemedicine needs good infrastructure and faces issues, such as:

- Ignorance and lack of awareness
- Rural India lacks basic infrastructure
- Language and communication issues
- Acceptance for both doctors and patients will be a challenge
- Lack of regulations by the government

TELENURSING

Tele is a prefix meaning "at a distance," and it is used in terms, such as telescope, or telemetry. The prefix tele, when combined with the term scope, has the single clear following meaning: an instrument to view phenomena at a distance. Telenursing refers to the use of information technology in the provision of nursing services whenever physical distance exists between patient and nurse, or between any numbers of nurses. As a field, it is part of telemedicine, and has many points of contacts with other medical and non-medical applications, such as telediagnosis, teleconsultation, and telemonitoring.

Definition of Telenursing

- Telenursing is a subset of tele health in which the focus is an nursing practice via telecommunication.
  —*By American Nurses Association*
- Tele nursing is defined as the practice of nursing using protocols through telecommunication technology.
  —*Arkansas Staff Board of Nursing*

Concept of Telenursing

- Telehealth is the use of electronic information and telecommunications technologies to support long distance clinical healthcare, patient and professional health related education, public health and health administration.
- Telenursing is a subset of telehealth in which technology is used to deliver nursing care and conduct nursing practice. It is specific to nursing as a profession.
- Telenursing is not a new mode of healthcare delivery rather it is an evolving mode of healthcare delivery that begun from the advent of telephone use in 1876.

Technologies used

Technologies used in telenursing may include, but are not limited to:
1. Telephones (land lines and cell phones)
2. Personal digital assistants (PDAs)
3. Facsimile machines (faxes)
4. Internet
5. Video and audio conferencing
6. Teleradiology
7. Computer information systems
8. Telerobotics

Figure 18.23 shows needs of telenursing.

Types of Telenursing

1. **Remote monitoring:**
   - The nurse monitors the patient remotely from his/her house.
   - Patient collects and transmits data to nurses; the nurse plans the intervention.
   - Used for handling chronic diseases, such as heart disease, diabetes, asthma, etc.
2. **Interactive telenursing services:** It involves series of interactive sessions with client via phone conversations and online communication. Used to obtain history, physical tests, psychiatric assessments, ophthalmology evaluation.
3. **Store and forward telenursing:** Used to obtain medical images, audio or video data that can be forwarded to a nurse at a suitable time for evaluation offline. Areas utilized are dermatology, radiology and pathology
4. **Specialist and primary care consultations:** Patient sees a nurse over a live video connection or using diagnostic images/video along with patient data to a specialist for viewing later
5. Imaging services used in radiology, pathology and in cardiology

Principles of Telenursing

These guidelines are based on the principles of telenursing, which state that effective telenursing should:

- Augment existing healthcare services
- Enhance optimum access where appropriate and necessary
- Provide immediate access to healthcare services
- Follow position descriptions that clearly define comprehensive, yet flexible roles and responsibilities
- Improve and/or enhance the quality of care
- Reduce the delivery of unnecessary health services
- Protect the confidentiality/privacy and security of information related to nurse-client

Guidelines for Telenursing

- Nurses and midwives practicing in telenursing shall be registered nurses or midwives. Enrolled nurses involved by telenursing need to be under the supervision of registered nurse or midwife.
- Nurses and midwives practicing telenursing are personally responsible for ensuring that their nursing and or midwifery skills and expertise remain current for their practice.
- Nurses and midwives who are practices telenursing in Australia are effected to practice with is the framework of the ANMC National Competences standards of the midwife the ANMC code of professional conducts for nurses in Australia, code of ethics for nurses in Australia and other relevant professional standards.
- Nurses and midwives should inform consumers of the telehealth process including other persons/professionals who may be participations or presence is the telehealth consultations and urban consent before proceeding.
- Nurses are midwives in televisions have a duty to provide privacy and confidentiality in all interactions.
- Nurses and midwives practices in telenursing should be aware of both the evidence base for their practice and the areas or practice is need or research.
- Nurses and midwives practicing telenursing should engage in evaluation of their practice in relations to issue

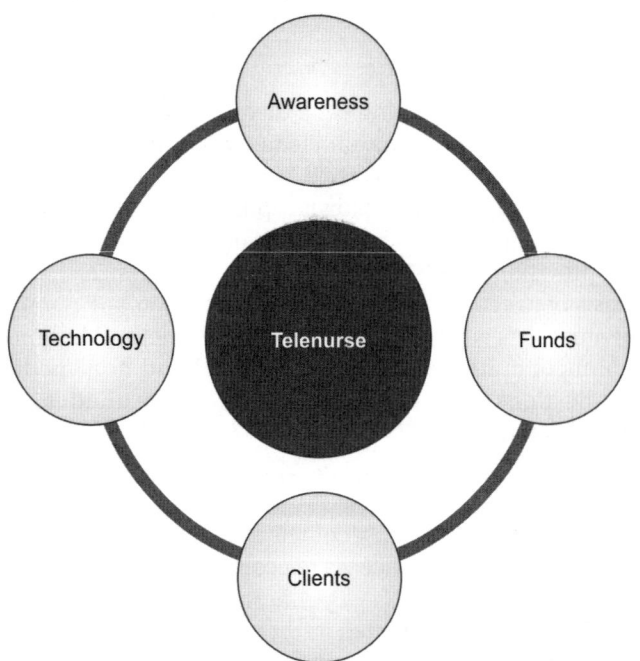

Fig. 18.23: Needs of telenursing.

Chapter 18: Nursing Informatics/Information Management

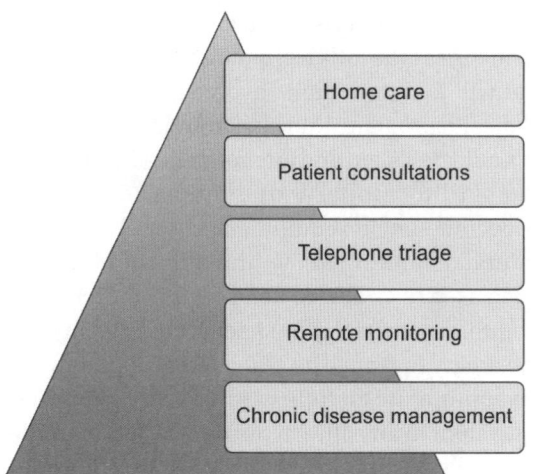

Fig. 18.24: Application of telenursing.

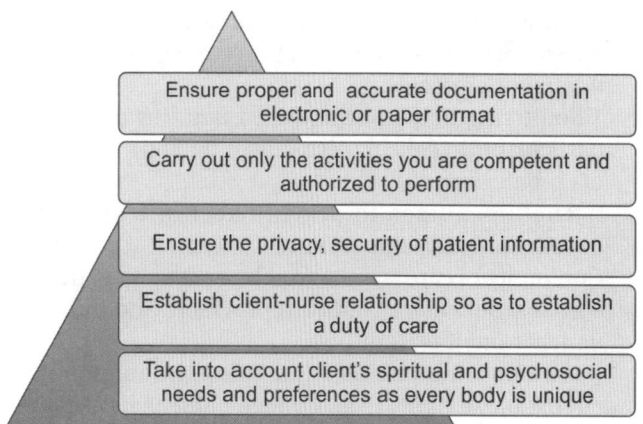

Fig. 18.25: Role of nurses in telenursing.

of quality safety and patient outcomes. **Figure 18.24** shows application of telenursing.

Benefits of Telenursing (Table 18.3)

- When patient stand seeing of their own day, they stand connecting the data above their processes.
- Managing their disease better reduce their utilization of acute case services, such as emergency department visits and hospitalization.
- Saving time achievable because driving time to reach patient residence by significantly reduced.
- Nurses are able to spend more time on direct patient care.

Telehealth Nurses Provide Nursing Care by

- Using Clinical Algorithms, Protocols, or Guidelines to Systematically Assess Patient Needs and Symptoms.
- Prioritizing the urgency of patients needs.
- Collaborating and developing a plan or care with the patient and supportive, disciplines which may include recommendation for cure, call back educations.
- Evaluation outcomes

Role of Nurses in Telenursing (Fig. 18.25)

- Ensure proper and accurate documentation in electronic or paper format
- Carry out only the activities you are competent and authorized to perform
- Ensure the privacy, security of patient information
- Establish client-nurse relationship so as to establish a duty of care
- Take into account client's spiritual and psychosocial needs and preferences as everybody is unique

Recommendations

- Nurses should support the expanded role of telenursing.
- Seminars and workshops should be put in place so as to increase the level of awareness among nurses.
- Government should support the establishment of telenursing services in the country.

Uses of Telenursing

- One of the most distinctive telenursing applications is home care. For example, patients who are immobilized, or live in remote or difficult to reach places, citizens who have chronic ailments, such as chronic obstructive pulmonary disease, diabetes, congestive heart disease, or disabilitating diseases, such as neural degenerative diseases (Parkinson's disease, Alzheimer's disease, ALS), etc., may stay at home and be "visited" and assisted regularly by a nurse via videoconferencing, internet, videophone, etc. Still other applications of home care are the care of patients in immediate post-surgical situations, the care of wounds, ostomies, handicapped individuals, etc.
- In normal home healthcare, one nurse is able to visit up to 5–7 patients per day. Using telenursing, one nurse can "visit" 12–16 patients in the same amount of time.
- Telephone nursing is the use of the nursing process to provide care to patients over the telephone.
- Telephone triage is the largest and most recognized component of telephone nursing.
- Telephone nursing services include advice and information, appointments and referrals, symptom management and disease management.
- A common application of telenursing is also used by call centers operated by managed care organizations, which are staffed by registered nurses who act as case managers or perform patient triage, information and counseling as a means of regulating patient access and low and decrease the use of emergency rooms.
- Telenursing can also involve other activities, such as patient education, nursing teleconsultations, and

Table 18.3: Benefits of telenursing.

Patient benefits	Nurses' benefits	Hospital benefit
• Increase access to healthcare • Economical • Saves time	• Saves time • More seeing distant patients • Rural providers can receive continuing education • Available as a specialty as a specialty program	• Administrators save travel time and funds by attending meetings via telenursing • Addresses shortage of nurses • Service available to more clients

examination of results of medical tests and exams, and assistance to physicians in the implementation of medical treatment protocols.
- Telenursing helps patients and families to be active participants in care, particularly in the self management of chronic illness.
- It enables nurses to provide accurate and timely information and support line.
- Continuity of care is enhanced by encouraging frequent contacts between healthcare providers and individual patients and their families.
- Use videoconferencing to provide continuing nursing education sessions (e.g., College's Telehealth sessions, CNA's Nurse ONE).
- Assist with client surgeries from a distant site.

Application of Telenursing

Telenursing applications are available in the home, hospital through telenursing centers and through mobile units. Telephone triage and home care are the fastest growing applications today. In home care, nurses use systems that allow home monitoring of physiologic parameters, such as blood pressure, respiratory peak flow and weight measurements, via the internet.
- Collecting data from patient
- Assessing data using knowledge
- Document all retrieved data
- Utilize critical thinking skills
- Provide nursing interventions
- Continue to monitor and utilize available technology

Advantages
- Increase public access to healthcare
- Provide access in rural areas
- Decrease wait times
- Decrease unnecessary hospital visits
- Decrease healthcare costs
- Increase continuity of care
- Increase patient compliance with aftercare
- Transcending miles and borders

Disadvantages
- Decreased face-to-face interaction
- Dehumanizing effects
- Risk of decreasing quality of care
- Equipment malfunction
- Concerns with security
- Concerns with maintaining confidentiality
- Knowledge base of the nurse

Competency, Qualifications and Skills

In general, the competencies required in telenursing practice mirror the competencies required of all registered nurses (e.g., clinical competence and assessment skills in the nurses' area of practice; an understanding of the scope of service being provided). However, registered nurses practicing telenursing should also possess:

- Personal characteristics (e.g., positive attitude, open-mindedness towards technology and good people skills) that will facilitate their involvement and advance the telehealth program. Knowledge and ability to navigate the technology system and environment (e.g., the knowledge and skill to properly operate hand-held cameras, videoconferencing equipment, computers, etc.)
- An understanding of the limitations of the technology being used (e.g., able to determine if vital signs are being monitored accurately by specific equipment)
- The ability to recognize when telehealth approaches are not appropriate for a client's needs (i.e., not 'reasonably' equivalent to any other type of care that can be delivered to the client, considering the specific context, location and timing, and relative availability of traditional care), includes assessment of a client's level of comfort with telehealth.
- Ability to modify clients' care plans based on above noted assessments.
- Awareness of client risks associated with telehealth and willingness to develop back-up plans and safeguards.
- Knowledge, understanding and application of telehealth operational protocols and procedures
- Competent enhanced communication skills
- Appropriate video/telephone behaviors.
- Awareness of the evidence base for their practice and areas of practice in need of research
- The ability to deliver competent nursing services by regularly assessing their own competence, identifying areas for learning, and addressing knowledge gaps in relation to the area of practice and relevant decision-based software and technology.
- Requisite clinical knowledge for competent telenursing.
- Registered nurses employed in a call-center responsible for triaging health concerns should possess clinical competencies in emergency and/or critical care nursing practice.
- Assessment of the needs of seniors, through the use of in-home video monitoring systems, should be conducted by nurses with expertise in home care and gerontological nursing.

■ ELECTRONIC MEDICAL RECORDS

An electronic medical record (EMR) includes information about a patient's health history, such as diagnoses, medicines, tests, allergies, immunizations, and treatment plans. Electronic medical records can be seen by all healthcare providers who are taking care of a patient and can be used by them to help make recommendations about the patient's care. Also called EHR and electronic health record. They have the potential to provide substantial benefits to physicians, clinic practices, and healthcare organizations. These systems can facilitate workflow and improve the quality of patient care and patient safety.

Definition

Electronic medical record (EMR) systems, defined as "an electronic record of health-related information on an individual that can be created, gathered, managed, and consulted by authorized clinicians and staff within one healthcare organization".

Functions

Eight key functions for safety, quality, and care efficiency that EMRs should support:
1. Physician access to patient information, such as diagnoses, allergies, lab results, and medications.
2. Access to new and past test results among providers in multiple care settings.
3. Computerized provider order entry.
4. Computerized decision-support systems to prevent drug interactions and improve compliance with best practices.
5. Secure electronic communication among providers and patients.
6. Patient access to health records, disease management tools, and health information resources.
7. Computerized administration processes, such as scheduling systems.
8. Standards-based electronic data storage and reporting for patient safety and disease surveillance efforts.

Benefits of EMR (Figs. 18.11 and 18.26)

There are many benefits of implementing the use of an EMR System. The overall improvement of workflow and reimbursement assure that the initial expense is recuperated quickly and the office runs efficiently.

- **Realize space savings:** Paper charts take up space and as they grow they it becomes necessary to find alternate storage facilities for older chart volumes. EHR software replaces paper charts completely.
- **No more misfiled or lost charts:** EMR system eliminates the chance of a misfiled or lost chart, while also increasing office operations by making one chart available electronically to multiple employees at the same time.
- **Legible chart notes:** EMR software eliminates the legibility issue because notes are no longer written, but typed or picked from multiple choices in a predefined system.
- **Reduced need for transcription staff:** EMR Software is able to eliminate most filing tasks or at least reduce them to a point where staff hours can be reduced.
- **Ability to recruit young physicians:** New doctors are looking for a practice to grow with, and the technology offered in an EMR is not only something they have grown accustomed to in residency, but shows them that a practice is progressive and keeping up with industry changes.
- **Lab interface fast tracks availability of results:** Through an interface between external systems and EMR software, the return time on these reports will be reduced and reduce employee hours by placing the report in the respective chart for the physician to review.
- **Pharmacy interface improves prescription process:** EMR software can communicate directly to the pharmacy eliminating the need for a nurse or medical assistant to cal the pharmacy with the prescription, but also reduce call backs from the pharmacy for clarification of quantities or dosage on prescription that are written out quickly or are less than legible.

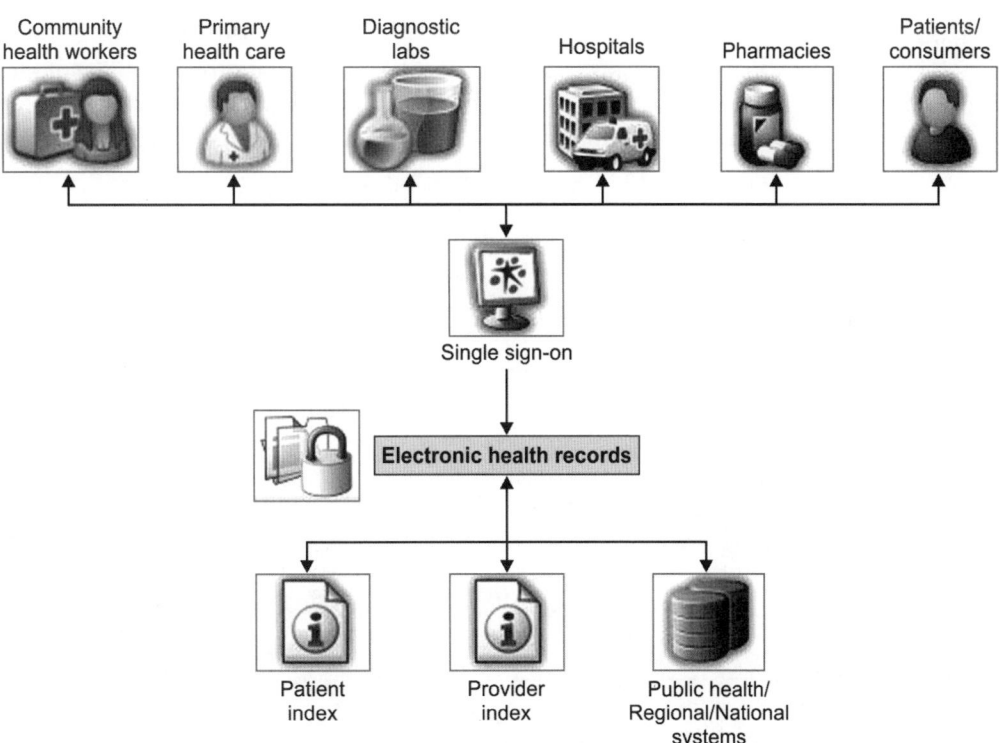

Fig. 18.26: Benefits of EMR.

Table 18.4: Differences between EHR and EMR.

EHR (electronic health records)	EMR (electronic medical records)
A digital record of health information	A digital version of a chart
Streamlined sharing of updated, real-time information	Not designed to be shared outside the individual practice
Allows a patient's medical information to move with them	Patient record does not easily travel outside the practice
Access to tools that providers can use for decision making	Mainly used by providers for diagnosis and treatment

- **Faster identification of interactions and allergies:** Accidents can happen, and sometimes patients may be prescribed medication that is either contraindicated because of an allergy or because they are on another medication that should not be taken with the new choice.
- **Improves ability to handle unforeseen disasters:** EMR software can be set to back up data daily or weekly to a location onsite or offsite thereby creating a safe duplicate of information.
- **Improves coding and enhances compliance:** Proper coding speeds up reimbursement, frees the physicians time up to see more patients and also allows the office to properly bill for procedures without duplication. **Table 18.4** shows difference between EHR and EMR.

Advantages

Electronic medical records (EMRs) are a digital version of the paper charts in the clinician's office. An EMR contains the medical and treatment history of the patients in one practice. EMRs have advantages over paper records. For example, EMRs allow clinicians to:

- Track data over time
- Easily identify which patients are due for preventive screenings or checkups
- Check how their patients are doing on certain parameters, such as blood pressure readings or vaccinations
- Monitor and improve overall quality of care within the practice

Barriers

Among the most significant barriers to adoption are:
- High capital cost and insufficient return on investment for small practices and safety net providers.
- Underestimation of the organizational capabilities and change management required.
- Failure to redesign clinical process and workflow to incorporate the technology systems.
- Concern that systems will become obsolete.
- Lack of skilled resources for implementation and support.
- Concern that current market systems are potentially not meeting the needs of rural health centers or federally qualified health centers (FQHC).
- Concern regarding negative unintended consequences of technology.

ELECTRONIC HEALTH RECORDS

Electronic health records (EHRs) focus on the total health of the patient—going beyond standard clinical data collected in the provider's office and inclusive of a broader view on a patient's care. EHRs are designed to reach out beyond the health organization that originally collects and compiles the information. They are built to share information with other healthcare providers, such as laboratories and specialists, so they contain information from all the clinicians involved in the patient's care.

Definition

Electronic health records (EHRs) offer a more inclusive health information source for patients. The government has mandated that health records should all be transferred over to EHRs for several reasons, including reducing errors and harm, cutting costs, improving the decision-making process, and making access to patient information by providers and quality personnel easier.

Elements of EHRs

Compared to paper records, electronic health records contain more information about the patient and their care. Most EHRs contain the following information:
- Patient's demographic, billing, and insurance information
- Physical history and physicians orders
- Medication allergy lists
- Nursing assessments, notes, and graphics of vital signs
- Laboratory and radiology results
- Trending labs, vital signs, results, and activities pages for easy reference
- Links to important clinical information and support
- Reports for quality and safety personnel

Benefits of EHRs (Figs. 18.27 and 18.28)

Examples of the numerous benefits of electronic medical records in hospitals and other healthcare facilities include:

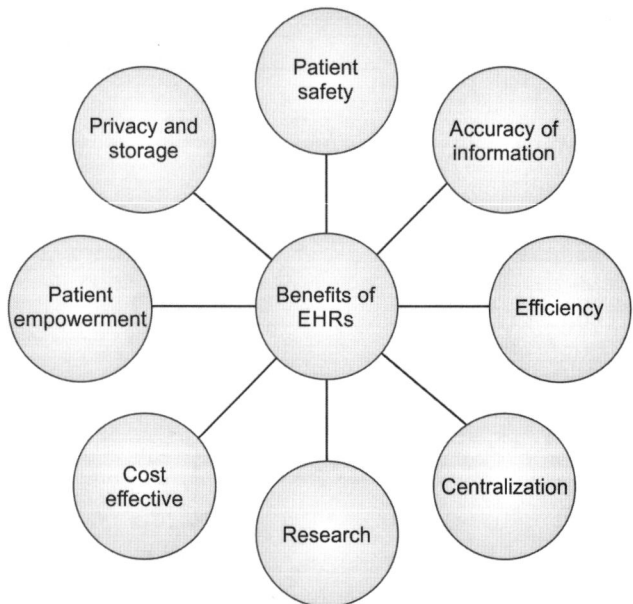

Fig. 18.27: Benefits of EHRs.

Chapter 18: Nursing Informatics/Information Management

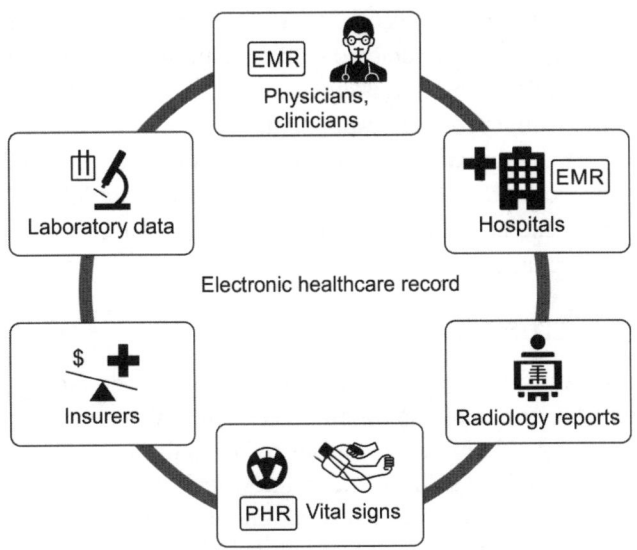

Fig. 18.28: Electronic healthcare record.

- **Improved quality of care:** Computerized notes are often easier to read than a physician's handwriting. This reduces the risk of errors and misinterpretations that can negatively impact the quality of patient care.
- **Convenience and efficiency:** Medical and office staff no longer have to waste time sorting through cumbersome paper records. Users can access electronic health records quickly and efficiently with just a few strokes on a keyboard.
- **Saving space:** Electronic health records eliminate the need to store documents in bulky file cabinets, which frees up more space in the office for medical supplies and equipment and other essentials.
- **Patient access:** Many EHR systems include a patient portal that allows patients to view their medical history and information whenever they wish.
- **Financial incentives:** Installing a certified EHR can help you fulfill the meaningful use requirements for medicaid and medicare, making you eligible for various incentives from the federal government. **Figure 18.29** shows patient's EHR.

EHRs May Improve Risk Management By

- Providing clinical alerts and reminders
- Improving aggregation, analysis, and communication of patient information
- Making it easier to consider all aspects of a patient's condition
- Supporting diagnostic and therapeutic decision making
- Gathering all relevant information (lab results, etc.) in one place
- Support for therapeutic decisions
- Enabling evidence-based decisions at point of care
- Preventing adverse events
- Providing built-in safeguards against prescribing treatments that would result in adverse events
- Enhancing research and monitoring for improvements in clinical quality. **Figure 18.30** shows essential elements.

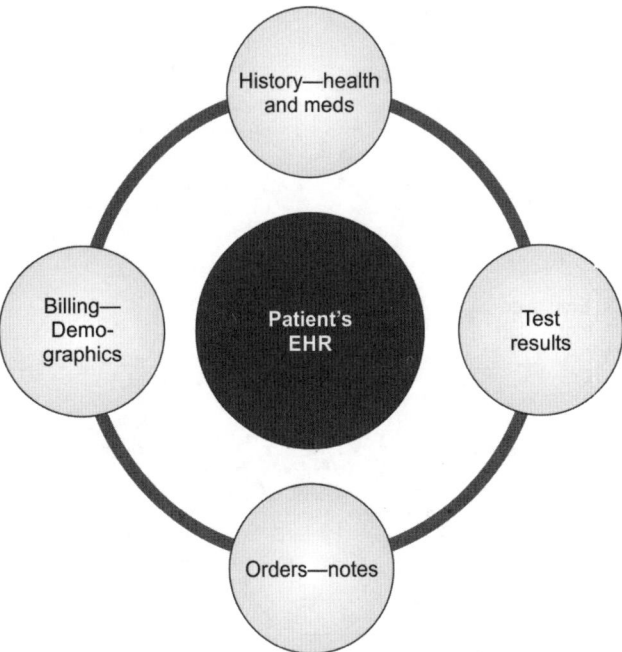

Fig. 18.29: Patient's EHR.

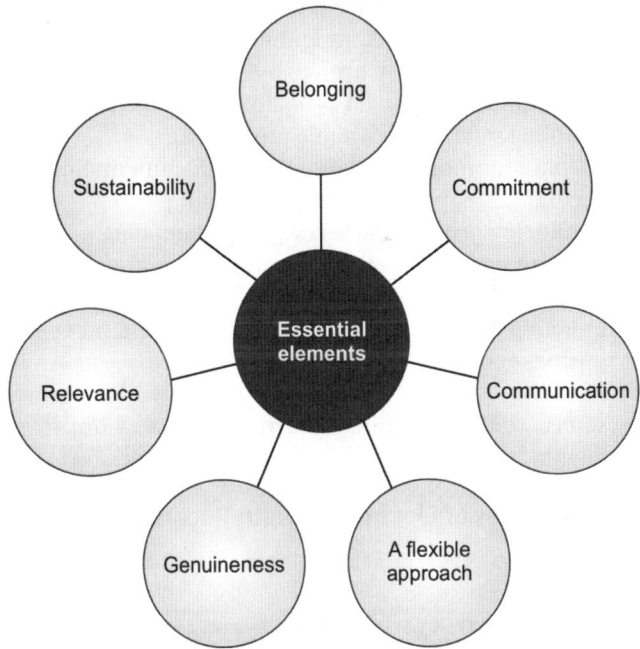

Fig. 18.30: Essential elements.

Advantages of Electronic Health Records (Fig. 18.31)

EHRs and the ability to exchange health information electronically can help you provide higher quality and safer care for patients while creating tangible enhancements for your organization. EHRs help providers better manage care for patients and provide better healthcare by:

- Providing accurate, up-to-date, and complete information about patients at the point of care
- Enabling quick access to patient records for more coordinated, efficient care
- Securely sharing electronic information with patients and other clinicians

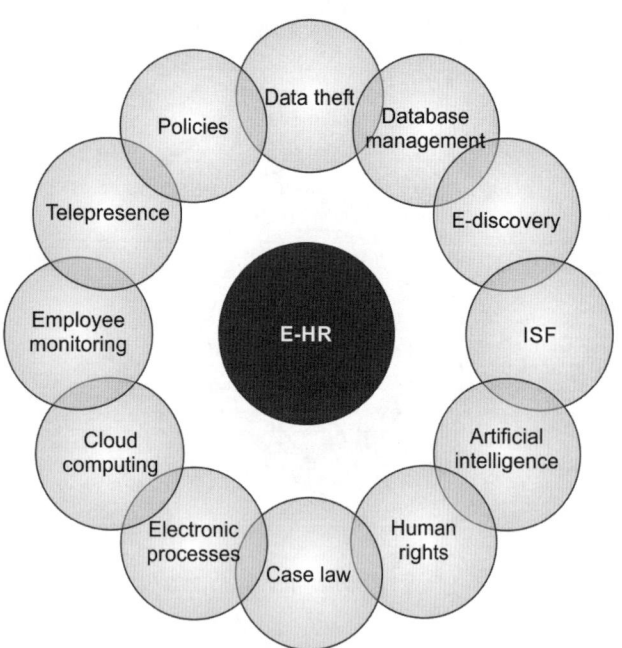

Fig. 18.31: Advantages of electronic health records.

- Helping providers more effectively diagnose patients, reduce medical errors, and provide safer care
- Improving patient and provider interaction and communication, as well as healthcare convenience
- Enabling safer, more reliable prescribing
- Helping promote legible, complete documentation and accurate, streamlined coding and billing
- Enhancing privacy and security of patient data
- Helping providers improve productivity and work-life balance
- Enabling providers to improve efficiency and meet their business goals
- Reducing costs through decreased paperwork, improved safety, reduced duplication of testing, and improved health.

Disadvantages of Electronic Health Records

There are also several disadvantages of electronic medical records, such as:

- **Potential privacy and security issues:** As with just about every computer network these days, EHR systems are vulnerable to hacking, which means sensitive patient data could fall into the wrong hands.
- **Inaccurate information:** Because of the instantaneous nature of electronic health records, they must be updated immediately after each patient visit—or whenever there is a change to the information. The failure to do so could mean other healthcare providers will rely on inaccurate data when determining appropriate treatment protocols.
- **Frightening patients needlessly:** Because an electronic health record system enables patients to access their medical data, it can create a situation where they misinterpret a file entry. This can cause undue alarm, or even panic.
- **Malpractice liability concerns:** There are several potential liability issues associated with EHR implementation. For example, medical data could get lost or destroyed during the transition from a paper-based to a computerized EHR system, which could lead to treatment errors. Since doctors have greater access to medical data via EHR, they can be held responsible if they do not access all the information at their disposal.

CONCLUSION

Nursing informatics is a growing field. As nurses, we face ever changing and challenging practice situations; competency in nursing informatics promises to strengthen our clinical decision-making skills. Although new technology may be a challenge for some, informatics will enhance nursing practice. We will have quicker access to patient information, improve overall efficiency, and see a reduction in potential errors.

REVIEW QUESTIONS

Long Essays

1. Define nursing informatics; explain the purposes and scope of nursing informatics.
2. Describe the competencies of nursing informatics.
3. Define telemedicine; explain the objectives and uses.
4. Define telenursing; explain the uses, principles and types.
5. Define electronics medical records; explain the functions and benefits.

Short Essays

1. Application of nursing informatics.
2. Nursing informatics areas.
3. Importance of nursing informatics.
4. Nursing informatics inpatient care.
5. Nursing informatics model.
6. Duties of nurse in informatics.
7. Legal issues in nursing informatics.
8. Benefits of computer automation in healthcare.
9. Current trends and issues in nursing informatics.
10. Nursing career in informatics.
11. Uses for computers in healthcare.
12. Electronic health records.

Short Answers

1. Telehealth.
2. Purpose of documentation.
3. Types of patient records.
4. Characteristics of good recording and reporting.
5. Principles of documentation.
6. Computer-assisted charting.
7. Use of computers in hospital.
8. Uses of computers in clinical nursing practice.
9. Principles of telemedicine.
10. Advantage of telemedicine system.
11. Barriers in telehealth.
12. Uses of telenursing.
13. Benefits of EMR.

BIBLIOGRAPHY

1. Ainsley B, Brown A. The impact of informatics on nursing education: a review of the literature. Journal of Continuing Education in Nursing. 2009;40:228.
2. Arnaert A, Delesie L. Telenursing for the elderly. The case for care via video telephone. Journal of Telemedicine and Telecare. 2001;7(6):311-6.
3. Bakken S. An informatics infrastructure is essential for evidence-based practice. J Am Med Inform Assoc. 2001;8(3):199-201.
4. Ball M, Hannah K (Eds). Nursing Informatics: Where Caring and Technology Meet. New York: Springer-Verlag; 2000.
5. Bohnenkamp SK, McDonald P, Lopez AM, et al. Traditional versus telenursing outpatient management of patients with cancer with new ostomies. Oncology Nursing Forum. 2004;31(5);1005-10.
6. Button D, Harrington A, Belan I. E-learning and information communication technology (ICT) in nursing education: A review of the literature. Nurse Educ Today. 2013;13:162-5.
7. Gassert C. The Challenge of Meeting Patients' Needs with a National Nursing Informatics Agenda. J Am Med Inform Assoc. 1998;5:263-8.
8. Grady JL, Fairchild L. Report of International Telenursing Survey. Computer-information-nursing. 2007;25:18-67.
9. Hersh W. Who are the informaticians? What we know and should know. J Am Inform Assoc. 2006;13:166-70.
10. Kierkegaard P. "Electronic health record: Wiring Europe's healthcare". Computer Law and Security Review. 2011;27(5):503-15.
11. Lee TT. Nurses' experiences using a nursing information system: early stage of technology implementation. Computers Informatics Nursing. 2007;25(5):294-300.
12. Little BB, Passmore D, Schullo S. Using synchronous software in Web-based nursing courses. Comput Inform Nurs. 2006;24(6):317-25.
13. Thede LQ. Summer Institute in Nursing Informatics 2008. CIN: Computers, Informatics, Nursing. 2008(a);26(6):307-8,310.
14. Tilley DS, Boswell C, Cannon S. Developing and establishing online student learning communities. Comput Inform Nurs. 2006;24(3):144-9.

CHAPTER 19

Personnel Management—Review

LEARNING OBJECTIVES

- Emotional Intelligence
- Resilience Building
- Stress and Time Management—Destressing
- Career Planning

INTRODUCTION

Personnel management deals with the managerial function of estimating and classifying human resources requirements for meeting organizational goals through people at work and their relationships with each other. It involves strategies that ensure right number of staff, a right combination of talent, training, and performance in jobs. Personnel management is defined as an administrative specialization that focuses on hiring and developing employees to become more valuable to the company. It is sometimes considered to be a sub-category of human resources that only focuses on administration.

DEFINITION

Personnel management can be defined as obtaining, using and maintaining a satisfied workforce. It is a significant part of management concerned with employees at work and with their relationship within the organization **(Fig. 19.1)**.

- "Personnel management is the planning, organizing, compensation, integration and maintenance of people for the purpose of contributing to organizational, individual and societal goals." —*Flippo*
- "Personnel management is that part which is primarily concerned with human resource of organization." —*Brech*
- "Personnel management is concerned with the obtaining and maintaining of a satisfactory and a satisfied work force." —*George R Terry*
- "Personnel management is an extension of general management that of promoting and stimulating every employee to make fullest contribution to the purpose of the business." —*HN North Scott*
- 'Personnel management is that aspect of management having as its goal the effective utilization of the labour resources of an organization". —*Paul G Hastings*

Box 19.1 describes principles of personnel management.

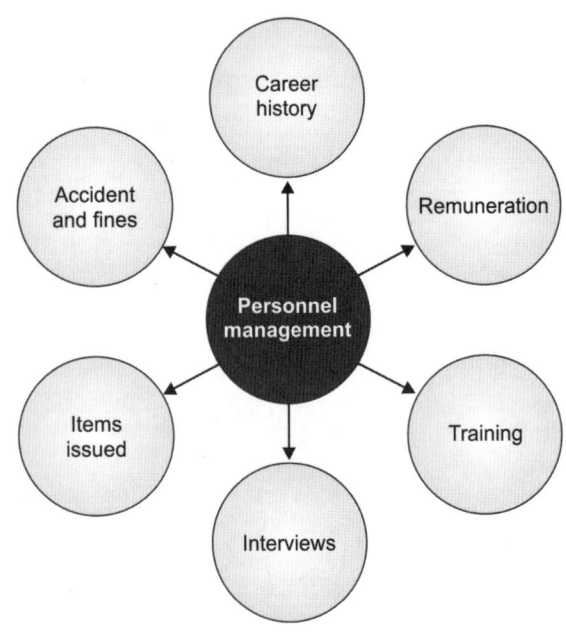

Fig. 19.1: Personnel management.

Box 19.1: Principles of personnel management.

Principles of personnel management are the rules which help the personnel managers to conduct and direct the policies in a proper way.
- Principle of maximum industrial development.
- Principle of scientific selection.
- Principle of high morale.
- Principle of dignity of labor.
- Principle of team spirit.
- Principle of effective communication.
- Principle of joint management.
- Principle of fair award.
- Principle of effective utilization.
- Principle of contribution of national prosperity.

MEANING OF PERSONAL MANAGEMENT

- Men, material and money are regarded as the three important factors of production. Human beings constitute

the organization at all levels and are regarded as the only dynamic factor of production.
- A business unit comes into existence with certain well defined objectives. An effort is made by the management to coordinate human and material resources in such a way that the objectives of the business are achieved.
- In order to get the best results from the people, management must be aware of as to what the employees expect from a business enterprise. The needs of human beings may be classified as physical, social and egoistic.
- Physical needs refer to basic necessities of life without which an individual can not live, such as food, shelter and clothing.
- Social needs, on the other hand, refer to an environment on the job where he is recognized as an individual. His morale increases if the individual is identified with a small group or a team.
- Man is a social animal and feels unhappy if his companions treat him unfairly. Egoistic needs include praise for work, recognition and importance of work, etc.
- It is for the management to ensure that all the employees get economic, social and individual satisfaction.

OBJECTIVES OF PERSONNEL MANAGEMENT

- To attract and secure appropriate hands, capable of performing effectively the organizations specific task.
- To utilize the manpower effectively.
- To generate maximum individual development of the people working within the organization.
- To establish and maintain an adequate organizational structure and a desirable working relationship.
- To secure the integration of the individuals and groups within an organization.
- To recognize and satisfy individual needs and group goals by offering an adequate and equitable remuneration, economic and social security.
- To maintain a high morale and better human relations inside an organization.

NATURE OF PERSONNEL MANAGEMENT

- Personnel management includes the function of employment, development and compensation—these functions are performed primarily by the personnel management in consultation with other departments.
- Personnel management is an extension to general management. It is concerned with promoting and stimulating competent work force to make their fullest contribution to the concern.
- Personnel management exists to advice and assists the line managers in personnel matters. Therefore, personnel department is a staff department of an organization.
- Personnel management lays emphasize on action rather than making lengthy schedules, plans and work methods. The problems and grievances of people at work can be solved more effectively through rationale personnel policies.
- It is based on human orientation. It tries to help the workers to develop their potential fully to the concern.

Table 19.1: Personnel vs human resource management.

	Personnel management	Human resource management
Time and planning perspective	Short-term, reactive, "ad hoc", marginal	Long-term, proactive, strategic, integrated
Psychological contract	Compliance	Commitment
Control system	External controls	Self-control
Employee relations perspective	Pluralist, collective, low trust	Unitarist, individual, high trust
Preferred structures	Bureaucratic/mechanistic, centralized, formal roles	Organic, devolved, flexible roles
Roles	Specialist/professional	Integrated into line m
Evaluation criteria	Cost minimization	Maximum utilization

- It also motivates the employees through its effective incentive plans so that the employees provide fullest co-operation.
- Personnel management deals with human resources of a concern. In context to human resources, it manages both individual as well as blue-collar workers. **Table 19.1** shows relationship between personnel and human resource management

CHARACTERISTICS OF PERSONNEL MANAGEMENT

From the various definitions given above, the following important characteristics emerge, which also explains its nature:

- **It is concerned with employees:** Personnel management is a management of human resources. It is primarily concerned with the efficient utilization and conservation of these resources. It considers employees as individuals and also as a member of a group.
- **It is concerned with personnel policies:** Personnel management is concerned with formulation of personnel policies with regard to recruitment, selection, training, promotion, transfer, job evaluation, merit rating, working conditions, etc.
- **Creation of cordial environment:** A cordial environment is created in the enterprise where each employee contributes his maximum for the achievement of organization's goals. It becomes possible because each employee is treated on equitable basis and is given humane treatment.
- **It is of a continuous nature:** The personnel function is of a continuous nature "It cannot be turned on and off like water from a faucet; it cannot be practiced only one hour each day or one day a week. Personnel management requires a constant alertness and awareness of human relations and their importance in every day operations".
  —*George R Terry*
- **It ensures economic, social and individual satisfaction:** Personnel management is mainly concerned with the satisfaction of physical, social and egoistic need of the employees at all levels covering both 'blue-collar' and 'white-collar employees.

ELEMENTS OF PERSONNEL MANAGEMENT

- **Organization:** Organization is said to be the framework of many activities taking place in view of goals available in a concern. An organization can be called as a physical framework of various interrelated activities.
- **Job:** The second element, i.e., jobs tells us the activities to be performed in the organization. It is said that the goals of an enterprise can be achieved only through the functional department in it.
- **People:** The last and foremost element in personnel management is people. In a organizational structure, where the main aim is to achieve the goals, the presence of manpower becomes vital.
- **Personnel manager:**
  - Personnel manager is the head of personnel department.
  - He performs both managerial and operative functions of management.

SCOPE OF PERSONNEL MANAGEMENT (BOX 19.2)

The scope of personnel management is very wide and it is as follows:
- Organizational planning and development
- Staffing and employment
- Training and development
- Compensation, wage and salary administration
- Employee services and benefits
- Employee records
- Labor relations, and
- Personnel research and personnel audit

Box 19.2: Scope of personnel management.

Personnel management covers four types of functions:
1. **Advisory function: Establish good relations** between management and employees.
2. **Management function:** Recruitment, training, education, etc., of personnel.
3. **Administrative function:** Covers major administrative matters.
4. **Workers welfare:** Pay attention to workers' physical and mental health, and their social and economic conditions.

ROLE OF PERSONNEL MANAGER (FIG. 19.2)

Personnel manager is the head of personnel department. He performs both managerial and operative functions of management. His role can be summarized as:

1. **Personnel manager provides assistance to top management:** The top management are the people who decide and frame the primary policies of the concern. All kinds of policies related to personnel or workforce can be framed out effectively by the personnel manager.
2. **He advices the line manager as a staff specialist:** Personnel manager acts, such as a staff advisor and assists the line managers in dealing with various personnel matters.
3. **As a counselor:** As a counselor, personnel manager attends problems and grievances of employees and guides them. He tries to solve them in best of his capacity.
4. **Personnel manager acts as a mediator:** He is a linking pin between management and workers.
5. **He acts as a spokesman:** Since, he is in direct contact with the employees, he is required to act as representative of organization in committees appointed by government. He represents company in training programs. **Figure 19.3** shows roles of personnel management.

FUNCTIONS OF PERSONNEL MANAGEMENT

Following are the four functions of personnel management:
1. Manpower planning
2. Recruitment
3. Selection
4. Training and development

Manpower Planning

Manpower planning which is also called as Human Resource Planning consists of putting right number of people, right kind of people at the right place, right time, doing the right things for which they are suited for the achievement of goals of the organization. Human Resource Planning has got an important place in the arena of industrialization. Human Resource Planning has to be a systems approach and is carried out in a set procedure. The procedure is as follows:
- Analyzing the current manpower inventory
- Making future manpower forecasts

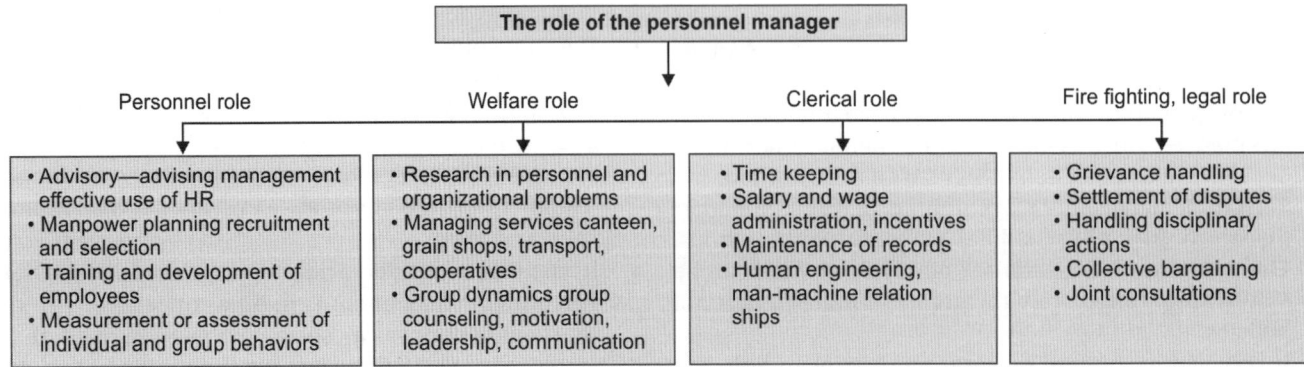

Fig. 19.2: The role of the personnel manager.

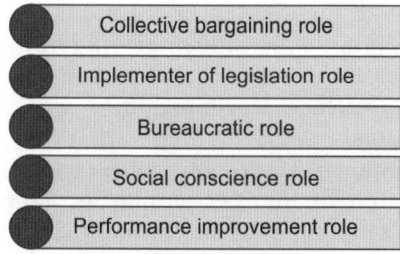

Fig. 19.3: Roles of personnel management.

> **Box 19.3:** Steps of manpower planning.
> - **Analyzing organizational objectives:** The objective to be achieved in future in various fields, such as production, marketing, finance, expansion and sales gives the idea about the work to be done in the organization.
> - **Inventory of present human resources:** From the updated human resource information storage system, the current number of employees, their capacity, performance and potential can be analyzed. To fill the various job requirements, the internal sources (i.e., employees from within the organization) and external sources (i.e., candidates from various placement agencies) can be estimated.

- Developing employment programs
- Design training programs

Steps in manpower planning (Box 19.3): Analyzing the current manpower inventory: Before a manager makes forecast of future manpower, the current manpower status has to be analyzed. For this the following things have to be noted:
- Type of organization
- Number of departments
- Number and quantity of such departments
- Employees in these work units

Once these factors are registered by a manager, he goes for the future forecasting.
- **Making future manpower forecasts:** Once the factors affecting the future manpower forecasts are known, planning can be done for the future manpower requirements in several work units.

  The manpower forecasting techniques commonly employed by the organizations are as follows:
  - **Expert forecasts:** This includes informal decisions, formal expert surveys and Delphi technique.
  - **Trend analysis:** Manpower needs can be projected through extrapolation (projecting past trends), indexation (using base year as basis), and statistical analysis (central tendency measure).
  - **Work load analysis:** It is dependent upon the nature of work load in a department, in a branch or in a division.
  - **Work force analysis:** Whenever production and time period has to be analyzed, due allowances have to be made for getting net manpower requirements.
- **Other methods:** Several mathematical models, with the aid of computers are used to forecast manpower needs, such as budget and planning analysis, regression, new venture analysis.
- **Developing employment programs:** Once the current inventory is compared with future forecasts, the employment programs can be framed and developed accordingly, which will include recruitment, selection procedures and placement plans.
- **Design training programs:** These will be based upon extent of diversification, expansion plans, development programs, etc. Training programs depend upon the extent of improvement in technology and advancement to take place. It is also done to improve upon the skills, capabilities, knowledge of the workers. **Figure 19.4** shows steps in human resources planning.

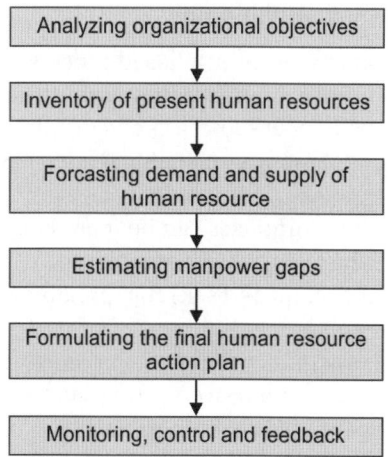

Fig. 19.4: Steps in human resources planning.

Importance of Manpower Planning

- **Key to managerial functions:** The four managerial functions, i.e., planning, organizing, directing and controlling are based upon the manpower. Human resources help in the implementation of all these managerial activities. Therefore, staffing becomes a key to all managerial functions.
- **Efficient utilization:** Efficient management of personnel's becomes an important function in the industrialization world of today. Setting of large scale enterprises requires management of large scale manpower. It can be effectively done through staffing function.
- **Motivation:** Staffing function not only includes putting right men on right job, but it also comprises of motivational programs, i.e., incentive plans to be framed for further participation and employment of employees in a concern. Therefore, all types of incentive plans become an integral part of staffing function.
- **Better human relations:** A concern can stabilize itself if human relations develop and are strong. Human relations become strong trough effective control, clear communication, effective supervision and leadership in a concern. Staffing function also looks after training and development of the work force which leads to co-operation and better human relations.
- **Higher productivity:** Productivity level increases when resources are utilized in best possible manner. Higher productivity is a result of minimum wastage of time, money, efforts and energies. This is possible through the staffing and its related activities (Performance appraisal, training and development, remuneration).

Need of Manpower Planning

Manpower planning is a two-phased process because manpower planning not only analyses the current human resources but also makes manpower forecasts and thereby draw employment programs. Manpower planning is advantageous to firm in following manner:

- Shortages and surpluses can be identified so that quick action can be taken wherever required.
- All the recruitment and selection programs are based on manpower planning.
- It also helps to reduce the labor cost as excess staff can be identified and thereby overstaffing can be avoided.
- It also helps to identify the available talents in a concern and accordingly training programs can be chalked out to develop those talents.
- It helps in growth and diversification of business. Through manpower planning, human resources can be readily available and they can be utilized in best manner.
- It helps the organization to realize the importance of manpower management which ultimately helps in the stability of a concern.

Recruitment (Fig. 19.5)

Types of recruitment: Recruitment is of two types:

1. Internal Recruitment

- It is a recruitment which takes place within the concern or organization.
- Internal sources of recruitment are readily available to an organization.
- Internal sources are primarily three: Transfers, promotions and re-employment of ex-employees.
- Internal recruitment may lead to increase in employee's productivity as their motivation level increases.
- It also saves time, money and efforts. But a drawback of internal recruitment is that it refrains the organization from new blood.
- Also, not all the manpower requirements can be met through internal recruitment. Hiring from outside has to be done.

Internal sources are primarily 3:
1. Transfers
2. Promotions (through internal job postings) and
3. **Re-employment of ex-employees:** Re-employment of ex-employees is one of the internal sources of recruitment in which employees can be invited and appointed to fill vacancies in the concern. There are situations when ex-employees provide unsolicited applications also.

2. External Recruitment

- External sources of recruitment have to be solicited from outside the organization.
- External sources are external to a concern. But it involves lot of time and money.
- The external sources of recruitment include—employment at factory gate, advertisements, employment exchanges, employment agencies, educational institutes, labor contractors, recommendations, etc.

Employment at Factory Level

- This a source of external recruitment in which the applications for vacancies are presented on bulletin boards outside the factory or at the gate.
- This kind of recruitment is applicable generally where factory workers are to be appointed.
- There are people who keep on soliciting jobs from one place to another.
- These applicants are called as unsolicited applicants. These types of workers apply on their own for their job.
- For this kind of recruitment workers have a tendency to shift from one factory to another and therefore they are called as "badli" workers.

Advertisement

- It is an external source which has got an important place in recruitment procedure.

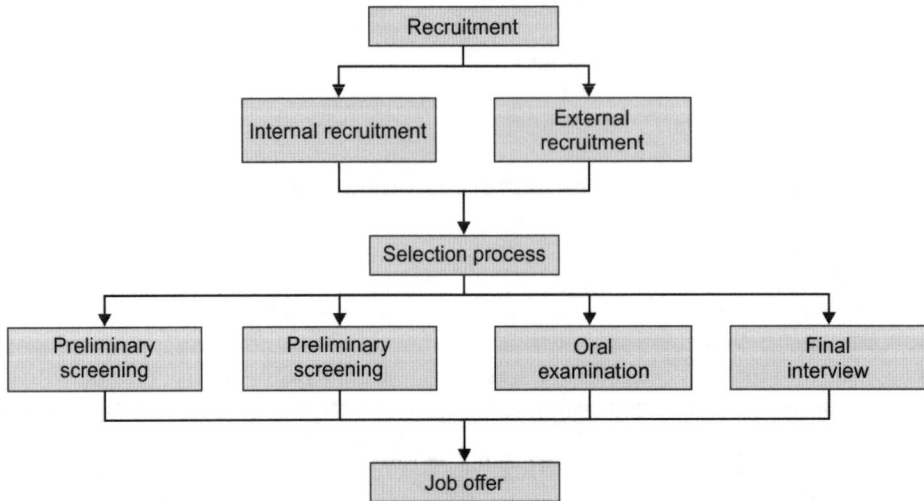

Fig. 19.5: Recruitment and selection.

- The biggest advantage of advertisement is that it covers a wide area of market and scattered applicants can get information from advertisements. Medium used is newspapers and television.

Employment Exchanges

- There are certain employment exchanges which are run by government. Most of the government undertakings and concerns employ people through such exchanges.
- Nowadays recruitment in government agencies has become compulsory through employment exchange.

Employment Agencies

There are certain professional organizations which look towards recruitment and employment of people, i.e., these private agencies run by private individuals supply required manpower to needy concerns.

Educational Institutions

- There are certain professional institutions which serve as an external source for recruiting fresh graduates from these institutes.
- This kind of recruitment done through such educational institutions is called as Campus Recruitment.
- They have a special recruitment cell which helps in providing jobs to fresh candidates.

Recommendations

- There are certain people who have experience in a particular area. They enjoy goodwill and a stand in the company.
- There are certain vacancies which are filled by recommendations of such people.
- The biggest drawback of this source is that the company has to rely totally on such people which can later on prove to be inefficient.

Labor Contractors

- These are the specialist people who supply manpower to the factory or manufacturing plants.
- Through these contractors, workers are appointed on contract basis, i.e., for a particular time period.
- Under conditions when these contractors leave the organization, such people who are appointed have to also leave the concern.

Selection Process

Employee selection is the process of putting right men on right job. It is a procedure of matching organizational requirements with the skills and qualifications of people. Effective selection can be done only when there is effective matching. By selecting best candidate for the required job, the organization will get quality performance of employees. Moreover, organization will face less of absenteeism and employee turnover problems. By selecting right candidate for the required job, organization will also save time and money. Proper screening of candidates takes place during selection procedure. All the potential candidates who apply for the given job are tested. **Table 19.2** shows differences between personnel management and human resource management.

Employee selection process takes place in following order:

- **Preliminary interviews:**
  - It is used to eliminate those candidates who do not meet the minimum eligibility criteria laid down by the organization.
  - The skills, academic and family background, competencies and interests of the candidate are examined during preliminary interview.
  - Preliminary interviews are less formalized and planned than the final interviews.
  - The candidates are given a brief up about the company and the job profile; and it is also examined how much the candidate knows about the company.
  - Preliminary interviews are also called screening interviews.
- **Application blanks:** The candidates who clear the preliminary interview are required to fill application blank. It contains data record of the candidates, such as details about age, qualifications, reason for leaving previous job, experience, etc.
- **Written tests:** Various written tests conducted during selection procedure are aptitude test, intelligence test, reasoning test, personality test, etc. These tests are used to objectively assess the potential candidate. They should not be biased.
- **Employment interviews:**
  - It is a one-to-one interaction between the interviewer and the potential candidate.
  - It is used to find whether the candidate is best suited for the required job or not. But such interviews consume time and money both. Moreover the competencies of the candidate cannot be judged.
  - Such interviews may be biased at times. Such interviews should be conducted properly. No distractions should be there in room.

Table 19.2: Differences between personnel management and human resource management.

Personnel management	Human resource management
Careful delineation of written contracts (employment contract)	Aim to beyond contract (employment contract)
Pay after job evaluation (fixed grades)	Performance-related pay system
Collective bargaining is a means of labor management	Individual contracts are the basis for labor management
Labor is treated as a tool which is expendable and replaceable	People are treated as assets to be used for the benefit of an organization, its employees and the society as a whole
Interests of the organization are uppermost	Mutuality of interests
Indirect communication	Direct communication
Job design is division of labor oriented	Job design is teamwork oriented

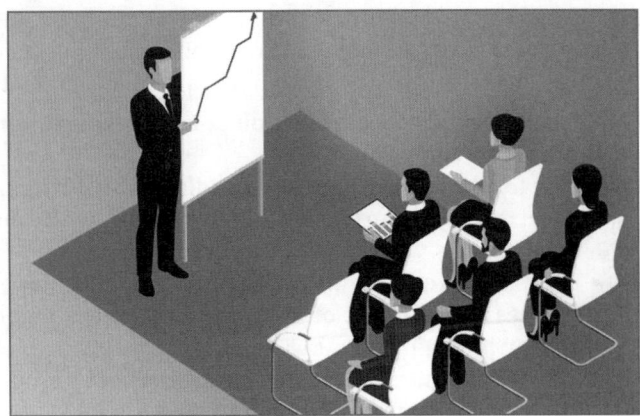

Fig. 19.6: Training of employees.

- There should be an honest communication between candidate and interviewer.
- **Medical examination:** Medical tests are conducted to ensure physical fitness of the potential employee. It will decrease chances of employee absenteeism.
- **Appointment letter:** A reference check is made about the candidate selected and then finally he is appointed by giving a formal appointment letter.

Training of Employees (Fig. 19.6)

Training of employees takes place after orientation takes place. Training is the process of enhancing the skills, capabilities and knowledge of employees for doing a particular job. Training process moulds the thinking of employees and leads to quality performance of employees. It is continuous and never ending in nature.

Importance of Training

Training is crucial for organizational development and success. It is fruitful to both employers and employees of an organization. An employee will become more efficient and productive if he is trained well.

Training is given on four basic grounds:
1. New candidates who join an organization are given training. This training familiarizes them with the organizational mission, vision, rules and regulations and the working conditions.
2. The existing employees are trained to refresh and enhance their knowledge.
3. If any updations and amendments take place in technology, training is given to cope up with those changes. For instance, purchasing new equipment, changes in technique of production, computer implantment. The employees are trained about use of new equipments and work methods.
4. When promotion and career growth becomes important. Training is given so that employees are prepared to share the responsibilities of the higher level job.

Benefits of Training

- **Improves morale of employees:** Training helps the employee to get job security and job satisfaction. The more satisfied the employee is and the greater is his morale, the more he will contribute to organizational success and the lesser will be employee absenteeism and turnover.
- **Less supervision:** A well-trained employee will be well acquainted with the job and will need less of supervision. Thus, there will be less wastage of time and efforts.
- **Fewer accidents:** Errors are likely to occur if the employees lack knowledge and skills required for doing a particular job. The more trained an employee is, the less are the chances of committing accidents in job and the more proficient the employee becomes.
- **Chances of promotion:** Employees acquire skills and efficiency during training. They become more eligible for promotion. They become an asset for the organization.
- **Increased productivity:** Training improves efficiency and productivity of employees. Well trained employees show both quantity and quality performance. There is less wastage of time, money and resources if employees are properly trained.

Ways/Methods of Training

Training is generally imparted in two ways:
1. **On the job training:**
   - On the job training methods are those which are given to the employees within the everyday working of a concern.
   - It is a simple and cost-effective training method. The in proficient as well as semi- proficient employees can be well trained by using such training method. The employees are trained in actual working scenario.
   - The motto of such training is "learning by doing." Instances of such on-job training methods are job-rotation, coaching, temporary promotions, etc.
2. **Off the job training:**
   - Off the job training methods are those in which training is provided away from the actual working condition.
   - It is generally used in case of new employees. Instances of off the job training methods are workshops, seminars, conferences, etc. Such method is costly and is effective if and only if large number of employees have to be trained within a short time period.
   - Off the job training is also called as vestibule training, i.e., the employees are trained in a separate area (may be a hall, entrance, reception area, etc., known as a vestibule) where the actual working conditions are duplicated.

ROLES OF A PERSONNEL MANAGER

- Personnel manager provides assistance to top management
- The top management is the people who decide and frame the primary policies of the concern. All kinds of policies related to personnel or workforce can be framed out effectively by the personnel manager.

- He advices the line manager as a staff specialist
- Personnel manager acts, such as a staff advisor and assists the line managers in dealing with various personnel matters.
- **As a counselor:** Personnel manager attends problems and grievances of employees and guides them. He tries to solve them in best of his capacity.
- **As a mediator:** He is a linking pin between management and workers.
- **As a spokesman:** Since, he is in direct contact with the employees, he is required to act as representative of organization in committees appointed by government. He represents company in training programs.

EMOTIONAL INTELLIGENCE (FIG. 19.7)

Emotional intelligence or EQ is one's ability to be aware of their own emotions as well as the emotions of others and to use that knowledge to help manage the expression of emotions. It is also the capacity to handle interpersonal relationships judiciously and empathetically. Emotional intelligence is the capacity to understand and manage the emotions. The skills involved in emotional intelligence are self-awareness, self-regulation, motivation, empathy, and social skills.

Definition

- **Salovey and Mayer, 1990:** Emotional intelligence is a set of skills associated with monitoring one's own and others' emotions, and the ability to use emotions to guide one's thinking and actions.
- **Salovey and Mayer:** "Emotional intelligence is the ability to perceive emotions, to access and generate emotions so as to assist thought, to understand emotions and emotional knowledge, and to reflectively regulate emotions so as to promote emotional and intellectual growth."
- **Goleman:** "Emotional intelligence is the capacity for recognizing our own feelings and those of others, for motivating ourselves, and for managing emotions effectively in ourselves and others. An emotional competence is a learned capacity based on emotional intelligence that contributes to effective performance at work."
- **Reuven bar-on:** "Emotional Intelligence is an array of non-cognitive capabilities, competencies, and skills that influence one's ability to succeed in coping with environmental demands and pressures."

Components of Emotional Intelligence

- **Self-awareness:** When we are self-aware, we know our strengths and weaknesses, as well as how we react to situations and people.
- **Self-regulation:** Because they are self-aware, emotionally intelligent people can regulate their emotions and keep them in check as necessary.
- **Motivation:** People with high emotional intelligence tend to be highly motivated as well, which makes them more resilient and optimistic.
- **Empathy:** People with empathy and compassion are simply better at connecting with other people.
- **Social skills:** The social skills of emotionally intelligent people show they genuinely care for and respect others and they get along well with them. **Table 19.3** shows emotional intelligence domains and competencies.

Emotional Intelligence Skills

- **Reflect on your emotions:** This is where self-awareness begins. To grow in emotional intelligence, think about your own emotions and how you typically react to negative situations, whether they involve a co-worker, family member or stranger. When you're more aware of your emotions and typical reactions, you can start to control them.
- **Ask for perspective:** What we perceive to be reality is often quite different from what those around us are seeing. Start getting input from others to understand how you come across in emotionally charged situations.
- **Observe:** Once you have increased your self-awareness and you understand how you are coming across, pay more attention to your emotions.
- **Pause for a moment:** Stop and think before you act or speak. It is hard to do, but keep working at it and it will become a habit.
- Become more empathetic by understanding the "why" Try to understand the "why" behind another person's feelings or emotions.

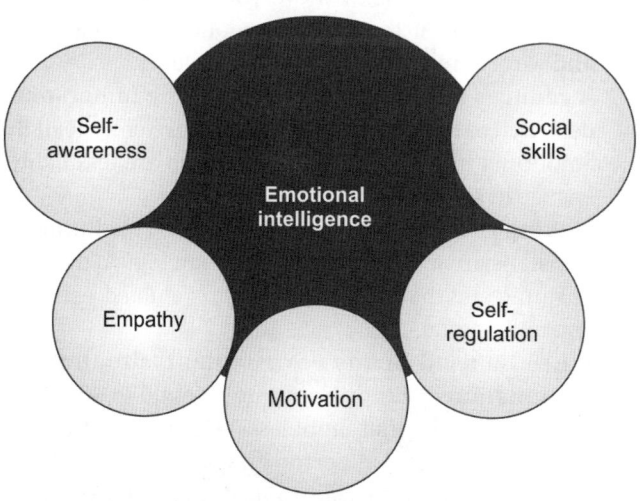

Fig. 19.7: Emotional intelligence.

Table 19.3: Emotional intelligence domains and competencies.

Self-awareness	Self-management	Social awareness	Relationship management
Emotional self-awarenesss	Emotional self-control	Empathy	Influence
	Adaptability		Coach and mentor
	Achievement orientation	Organizational awareness	Conflict management
	Positive outlook		Teamwork
			Inspirational leadership

- Choose to learn from criticism. Who likes criticism? Possibly no one. But it is inevitable. When we choose to learn from criticism rather than simply defend our behaviors, we can grow in emotional intelligence.
- Practice, practice, practice. Becoming more emotionally intelligent would not happen overnight, but it can happen-with effort, patience, and a lot of practice.

Importance of Emotional Intelligence
- Psychological health
- Work performance
- Teamwork
- Conflict management
- Patient satisfaction
- Coaching skills
- Employability and re-employment
- Workplace incivility
- Institutional climate
- Job satisfaction

Benefits of Emotional Intelligence in the Workplace
- Providing effective communication
- Predicting staff reactions to negative news and aptly preparing for this
- Effectively listening
- Successfully managing difficult situations
- Recognizing potential mental health risks to staff
- Making employees feel comfortable in sharing ideas and concerns with you
- Remaining optimistic and having a positive attitude
- Gaining trust and loyalty quickly which subsequently increases staff performance
- Being empathetic and compassionate towards staff and clients
- Remaining calm and handling pressure effectively
- Being open to positive and negative feedback
- Influencing and inspiring staff which helps when trying to gain support for future projects
- Motivating yourself and your staff
- Resolving conflict fairly

Types of Emotional Intelligences
There are four types of emotional intelligences:
1. **Perceiving emotions:** This involves understanding nonverbal signals, such as body language and facial expressions and perceiving them accurately.
2. **Reasoning with emotions:** This involves using emotions to promote thinking and cognitive activity. Emotions help prioritize what we pay attention and react to; we respond emotionally to things that grab our attention.
3. **Understanding emotions:** This is the ability to determine if regarding another person, their emotions are about themselves or directed to you or in response to particular occurrence. Also means you have the ability to be aware that you are upset at someone.
4. **Reflective regulation of emotions:** Ability to analyze and manage emotions. **Figure 19.8** shows Academic success (CGPA).

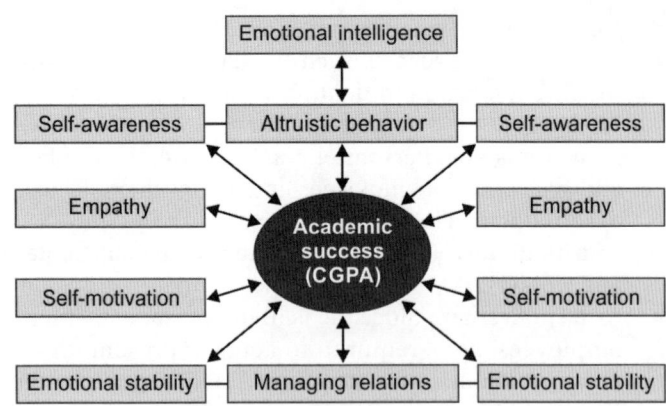

Fig. 19.8: Academic success (CGPA).

Developing or Improving Emotional Intelligence
Emotional intelligence comes more naturally to some than others. Unlike IQ, which remains fairly constant throughout life, emotional intelligence develops with age. This shows us that it is something that can be learnt. There are many different types of interventions aimed at developing emotional intelligence. The following key components are essential to provide successful interventions aimed at improving Emotional Intelligence
- They need to be specifically emotional intelligence based
- They need to be constructed using a specific, clear and well documented conceptual framework (such as the Bar-On Emotional-Social Intelligence Model).
- They need to use exercises that are based on scientific evidence.

Pros of Emotional Intelligence (Fig. 19.9)
- **It is something that anyone can learn:** Emotional intelligence is not a genetic trait or a natural talent. It is a skill that anyone can learn.
- **It can help to reduce bullying:** When we understand our emotions and can tap into the emotions of others, then we get to feel a little bit of what others are feeling around us.
- **It improves a person's social effectiveness:** By understanding the emotions of everyone else around them, a person exercising their skills of emotional intelligence can find ways to relate to others at a core level.
- **It reduces the likelihood of engaging in personally destructive behaviors:** People who have enhanced their emotional intelligence skills over time are less likely to engage in self-destructive behaviors.
- **Making decisions becomes a lot faster:** Emotional decisions are a lot easier to make than logical decisions. Logic dictates that every scenario be evaluated, estimated, and anticipated.
- **It can be used in any environment, situation, and circumstance:** Emotional intelligence is a skill that transcends industries, hobbies, and situations because it is always applicable. A person exercising their skills in this area can find a way to relate to anyone in any circumstance or situation.

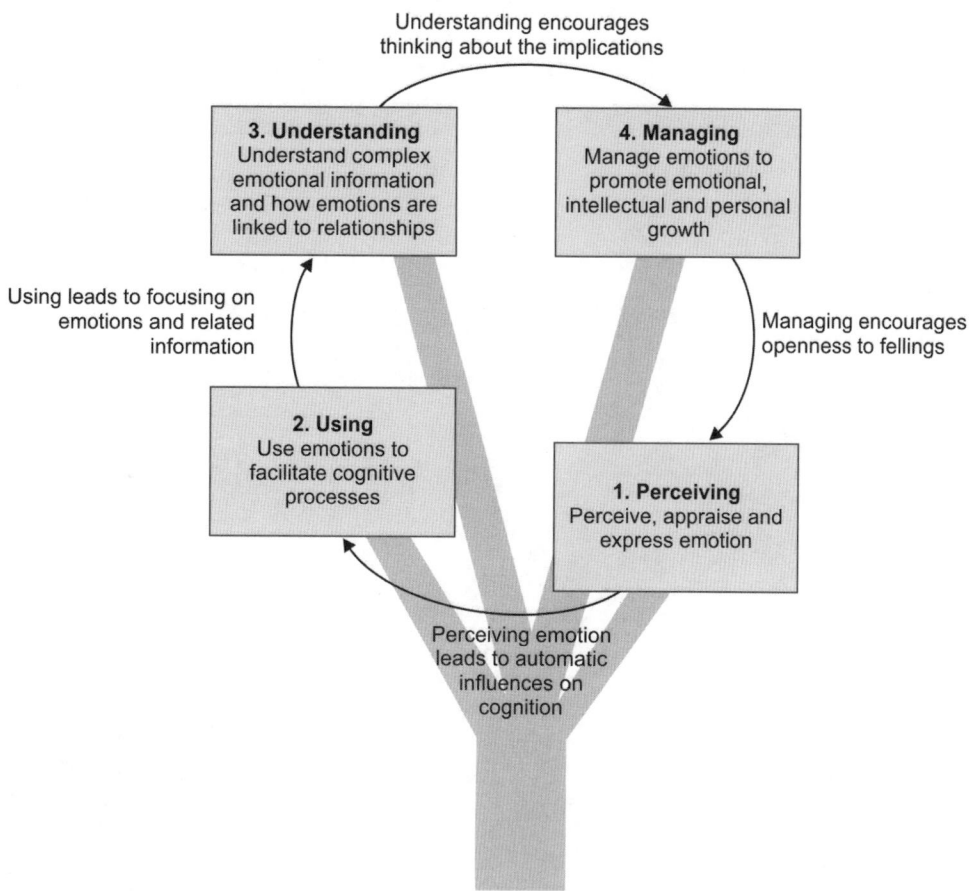

Fig. 19.9: Pros of emotional intelligence.

Cons of Emotional Intelligence

- **It can be used to manipulate people:** Emotions are one of the core components of our being. We experience emotions in virtually every moment of every day.
- **It prevents others from using their critical thinking skills:** When someone knows how to "put their emotion on a plate," then that emotional exposure can help others relate through that contact.
- **It can be used for personal gain:** Emotional intelligence can also be used to manipulate others for personal gain.
- **It can make a person more open and agreeable:** Social factors are very important within the scope of human existence. Rare is the individual who can live on their own without any personal contact of any kind for an extended period of time.
- **It takes time to develop this skill:** Although everyone can develop emotional intelligence skills, this is a time investment that can be quite extensive and personal.
- **Emotional intelligence is a skill that not everyone takes seriously:** Information is the primary currency today and society often separates emotions from words.

RESILIENCE BUILDING (FIGS. 19.10 AND 19.11)

Resilience is the ability to withstand adversity and bounce back from difficult life events. Being resilient does not mean that people do not experience stress, emotional upheaval, and suffering. Some people equate resilience with mental toughness, but demonstrating resilience includes working through emotional pain and suffering.

Meaning

Resilience is the process of being able to adapt well and bounce back quickly in times of stress. This stress may manifest as family or relationship problems, serious health problems, problems in the workplace or even financial problems to name a few.

Characteristics

In general, resilient people have many of the following characteristics:

- **Locus of control:** Focus on how you, as opposed to external forces, can control the outcome of events.
- **Social support:** Rely on family, friends, and colleagues when needed.
- **Problem-solving:** Skills Identify ways within your control to work and resolve a problem.
- **Optimism:** When the going gets tough, believe in your ability to handle it.
- **Coping skills:** Find techniques to reduce stress and anxiety.
- **Self-care:** Make your mental, emotional, and physical health top priorities.
- **Self-awareness:** Know your strengths and weaknesses and how to put internal resources to work.

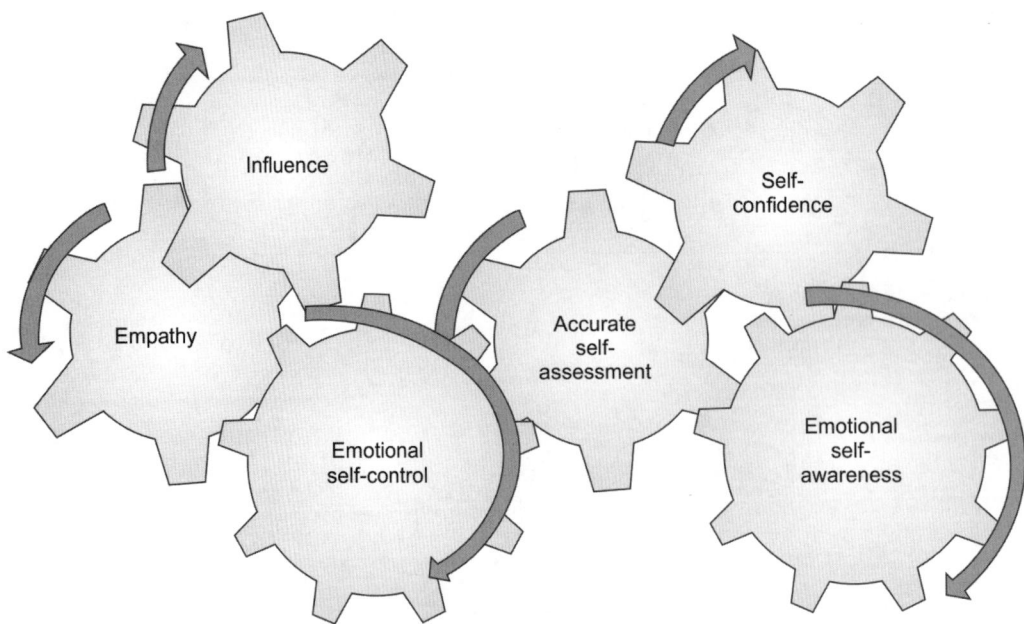

Fig. 19.10: Resilience characteristics.

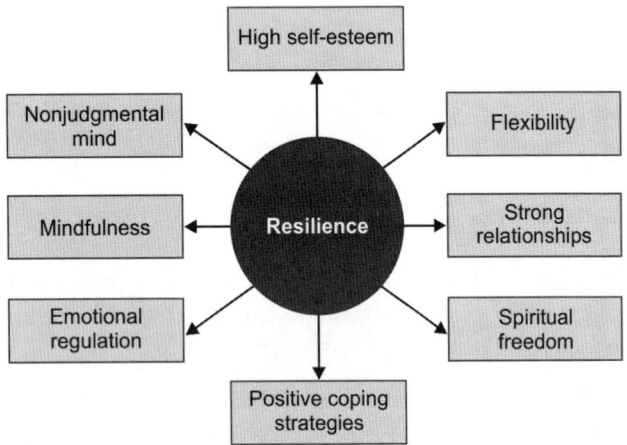

Fig. 19.11: Resilience.

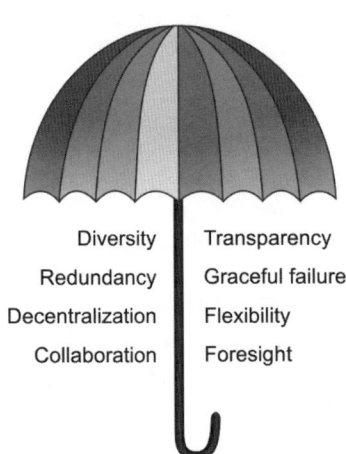

Fig. 19.12: Eight principles of resiliency.

Traits, Qualities, and Characteristics of the Resilient Person

According to Conner and Davidson (2003), resilient people have certain characteristics. These characteristics may include:
- Viewing change as a challenge or opportunity
- Commitment
- Recognition of limits to control
- Engaging the support of others
- Close, secure attachment to others
- Personal or collective goals
- Self-efficacy
- Strengthening effect of stress
- Past successes
- Realistic sense of control/having choices
- Sense of humor
- Action-oriented approach
- Patience
- Tolerance of negative affect
- Adaptability to change
- Optimism
- Faith

Figure 19.12 shows eight principles of resiliency.

Principles of Resilience

Resilience measures should be discussed and incorporated during the predevelopment and planning stages:
- Identifying hazards
- Assessing vulnerabilities
- Analyzing scenarios and impacts
- Establishing performance targets
- Assessing how resilient interventions can create value in terms of underwriting building operations and mitigating harm.
- Balancing costs and long-term value over the intended service life.
- Developing lines of communication about potential hazards to build resilience between owners, operators and users.

Factors of Resilience

These factors include:
- **Social support:** Social systems that provide support in times of crisis or trauma support resilience in the individual. Social support can include immediate or extended family, community, friends, and organizations.
- **Realistic planning:** The ability to make and carry out realistic plans helps individuals play to their strengths and focus on achievable goals.
- **Self-esteem:** A positive sense of self and confidence in one's strengths can stave off feelings of helplessness when confronted with adversity.
- **Coping skills:** Coping and problem-solving skills help empower a person who has to work through adversity and overcome hardship.
- **Communication skills:** Being able to communicate clearly and effectively helps people seek support, mobilize resources, and take action.
- **Emotional regulation:** The capacity to manage potentially overwhelming emotions (or seek assistance to work through them) helps people maintain focus when overcoming a challenge.

7 Cs of Resilience (Fig. 19.13)

The 7 Cs model is centered on two key points:
1. **Competence:** This is the ability to know how to handle situations effectively. To build competence, individuals develop a set of skills to help them trust their judgments and make responsible choices.
2. **Confidence:** True self-confidence is rooted in competence. Individuals gain confidence by demonstrating competence in real-life situations.
3. **Connection:** Close ties to family, friends, and community provide a sense of security and belonging.
4. **Character:** Individuals need a fundamental sense of right and wrong to make responsible choices, contribute to society, and experience self-worth.
5. **Contribution:** Ginsburg says that having a sense of purpose is a powerful motivator. Contributing to one's community reinforces positive reciprocal relationships.
6. **Coping:** When people learn to cope with stress effectively, they are better prepared to handle adversity and setbacks.
7. **Control:** Developing an understanding of internal control helps individuals act as problem-solvers instead of victims of circumstance. When individuals learn that they can control the outcomes of their decisions, they are more likely to view themselves as capable and confident.

Types of Resilience

The word resilience is often used on its own to represent overall adaptability and coping, but it can be broken down into categories or types:
1. **Psychological resilience:** Psychological resilience refers to the ability to mentally withstand or adapt to uncertainty, challenges, and adversity. It is sometimes referred to as "mental fortitude."
2. **Emotional resilience:** There are varying degrees of how well a person copes emotionally with stress and adversity. Some people are, by nature, more or less sensitive to change. How a person responds to a situation can trigger a flood of emotions.
3. **Physical resilience:** Physical resilience refers to the body's ability to adapt to challenges, maintain stamina and strength, and recover quickly and efficiently. It's a person's ability to function and recover when faced with illness, accidents, or other physical demands.
4. **Community resilience:** Community resilience refers to the ability of groups of people to respond to and recover from adverse situations, such as natural disasters, acts of violence, economic hardship, and other challenges to their community.

Building and Cultivate Resilience (Fig. 19.14)

Components of Building Resilience

The 4-Rs: The NIAC (2009) determined that resilience can be characterized by four key features:
1. **Robustness:** The ability to maintain critical operations and functions in the face of crisis. This includes the building itself, the design of the infrastructure (office buildings, power generation, distribution structures, bridges, dams, levees), or in system redundancy and substitution (transportation, power grid, communications networks).
2. **Resourcefulness:** The ability to skillfully prepare for, respond to and manage a crisis or disruption as it unfolds. This includes identifying courses of action and business continuity planning; training; supply chain management; prioritizing actions to control and mitigate damage; and effectively communicating decisions.
3. **Rapid recovery:** The ability to return to and/or reconstitute normal operations as quickly and efficiently as possible after a disruption. Components of rapid recovery include carefully drafted contingency plans, competent emergency operations, and the means to get the right people and resources to the right places.
4. **Redundancy:** It is proposed as another key feature, which mean that there are back-up resources to support the originals in case of failure that should also be considered when planning for resilience.

Steps that can help build resilience: It is helpful to think of resilience as a process. The following are steps that can help build resilience over time:

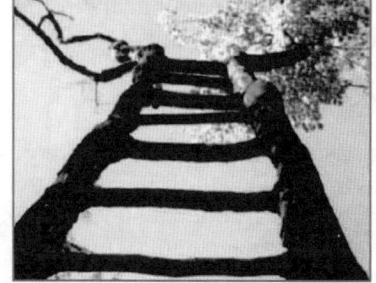

Fig. 19.13: Seven Cs of resilience.

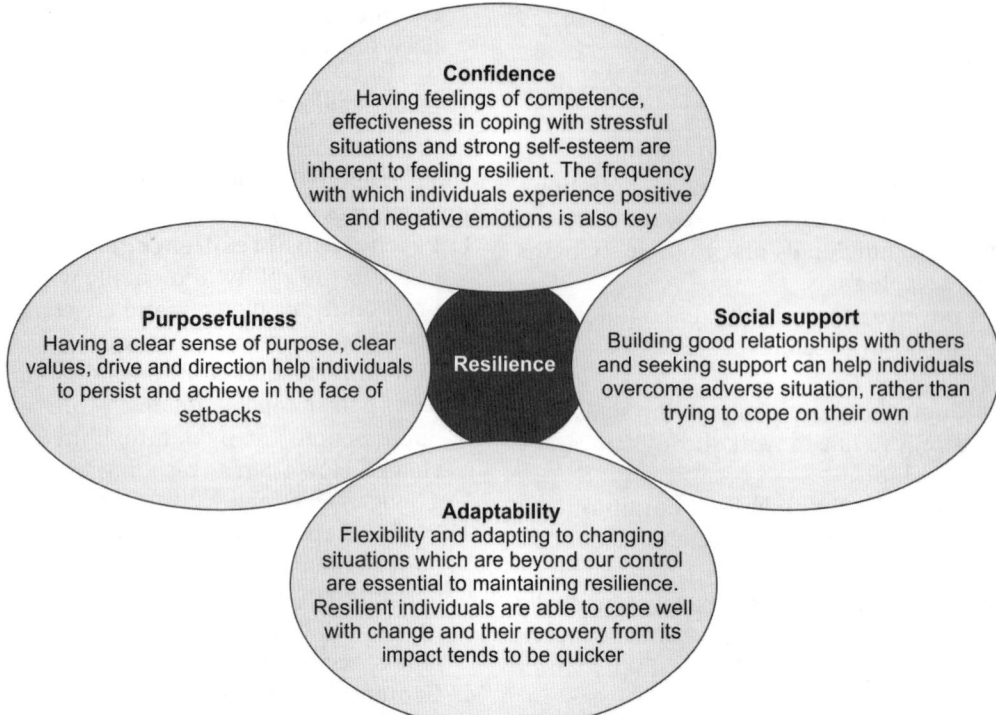

Fig. 19.14: Building and cultivate resilience.

- **Develop self-awareness:** Understanding how you typically respond to stress and adversity is the first step toward learning more adaptive strategies. Self-awareness also includes understanding your strengths and knowing your weaknesses.
- **Build self-regulation skills:** Remaining focused in the face of stress and adversity is important, but not easy. Stress-reduction techniques, such as guided imagery, breathing exercise, and mindfulness training, can help individuals regulate their emotions, thoughts, and behaviors.
- **Learn coping skills:** There are many coping skills that can help in dealing with stressful and challenging situations. They include journaling, reframing thoughts, exercising, spending time outdoors, socializing, improving sleep hygiene, and tapping into creative outlets.
- **Increase optimism:** People who are more optimistic tend to feel more in control of their outcomes. To build optimism, focus on what you *can* do when faced with a challenge, and identify positive, problem-solving steps that you can take.
- **Strengthen connections:** Support systems can play a vital role in resilience. Bolster your existing social connections and find opportunities to build new ones.
- **Know your strengths:** People feel more capable and confident when they can identify and draw on their talents and strengths.

Resilience Scale

Conner-Davidson resilience scale
- Able to adapt to change
- Close and secure relationships
- Sometimes fate or God can help
- Can deal with whatever comes
- Past success gives confidence for new challenge
- See the humorous side of things
- Coping with stress strengthens
- Tend to bounce back after illness or hardship
- Things happen for a reason
- Best effort no matter what
- You can achieve your goals
- When things look hopeless, you do not give up
- Know where to turn for help
- Under pressure, focus and think clearly
- Prefer to take the lead in problem-solving
- Not easily discouraged by failure
- Think of self as a strong person
- Make unpopular or difficult decisions
- Can handle unpleasant feelings
- Have to act on a hunch
- Strong sense of purpose
- In control of your life
- You like challenges
- You work to attain your goals
- Pride in your achievements

STRESS MANAGEMENT

Stress is basically the tension or anxiety caused by any sort of pressure in everyday life. The ability to handle or minimize the physical and emotional effects of such anxiety is known as one's stress management skills.

The importance given to stress management skills in workplace can be guessed from the fact that employers, in many countries, have been burdened with a legal responsibility of recognizing as well as coping with the workplace stress in order to ensure good mental and physical health of employees in organization.

Symptoms of Stress (Fig. 19.15)

Although we all experience stress differently, some common symptoms include:

- Difficulty sleeping
- Weight gain or weight loss
- Stomach pain
- Irritability
- Teeth grinding
- Panic attacks
- Headaches
- Difficulty concentrating
- Sweaty hands or feet
- Heartburn
- Excessive sleeping
- Social isolation
- Fatigue
- Nausea
- Feeling overwhelmed
- Obsessive or compulsive behaviors

14 Facts about Stress and Burnout

If you are not yet convinced about the need to prioritize stress management, these 14 facts might help:

1. Stress has been referred to as the "silent killer" as it can cause heart disease, high blood pressure, chest pain, and an irregular heartbeat.
2. Telogen effluvium is the result of hair loss caused by stress that can happen up to three months after a stressful event.
3. Stress accounts for 30% of all infertility problems. In women, stress can cause spasms in the fallopian tubes and uterus. In men, it can reduce sperm count and cause erectile dysfunction.
4. Researchers have found that stress worsens acne, more so than the prevalence of oily skin.
5. Stress can cause weight gain too. The stress hormone cortisol has been found to cause both the accumulation of abdominal fat and the enlargement of fat cells, causing "diseased" fat.
6. Correlations have been found between stress and the top six causes of death: cancer, lung ailments, heart disease, liver cirrhosis, accidents, and suicide.
7. In children, chronic stress has been found to negatively impact their developmental growth due to a reduction of the growth hormone in the pituitary gland.
8. The word itself, "stress" stems from the Latin word stringere, meaning "to draw tight".
9. In the event of chronic stress, dominant hormones are released into our brain. These hormones are intended for short-term emergencies and in the event where they exist for extended periods they can shrink, impair and kill brain cells.
10. Stress can increase the likelihood of developing blood clots since the blood prepares itself for injuries and becomes "stickier".
11. Chronic stress can place pressure on, and cause damage to arteries and organs. This occurs due to inflation in our bodies caused by cytokines (a result of stress).
12. Stress is also responsible for altering our blood sugar levels, which can lead to fatigue, hyperglycemia, mood swings, and metabolic syndrome.
13. On a positive note, we can reduce our stress levels by laughing. Having a chuckle, lowers the stress hormones, including cortisol, epinephrine, and adrenaline. Laughing also strengthens our immune system by releasing positive hormones.
14. More good news, especially for chocolate lovers-dark chocolate has been found to reduce stress hormones.

Prevention of Workplace Stress

The prevention of workplace stress is most successful when a combination of both organizational change and individual stress management is used. That is, like any healthy relationship, both parties—the employee and the employer make an effort.

- Promote leave, rest and breaks
- Encourage exercise and meditation, both within and outside of work hours
- Ensure the workload is in line with workers' abilities and resources
- Provide stimulation and opportunities for workers to use skills
- Boost workplace morale by creating opportunities for social interactions
- Clearly set out workers' roles and responsibilities
- Encourage participation in decision making that affects individuals roles
- Encourage open communication
- Establish no tolerance policy for workplace discrimination
- Engage an external consultant to suggest a fresh approach to any existing issues
- Create family-friendly policies to encourage work-life balance
- Provide training for workplace stress management. **Figure 19.16** shows preventing and managing stress.

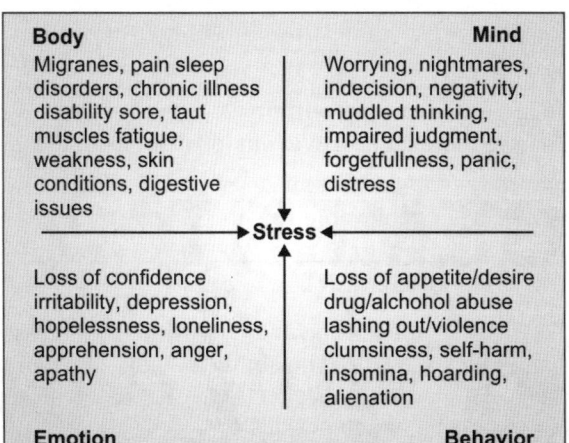

Fig. 19.15: Stress.

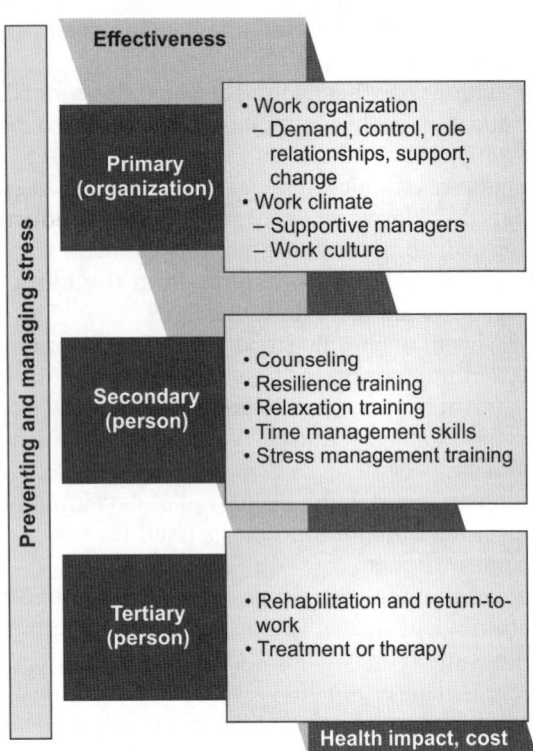

Fig. 19.16: Preventing and managing stress.

Stress Management Tips

People can learn to manage stress and lead happier, healthier lives. Here are some tips to help you keep stress at bay.
- Keep a positive attitude
- Accept that there are events that you cannot control.
- Be assertive instead of aggressive. Assert your feelings, opinions, or beliefs instead of becoming angry, defensive, or passive.
- Learn and practice relaxation techniques; try meditation, yoga, or tai-chi for stress management.
- Exercise regularly. Your body can fight stress better when it is fit.
- Eat healthy, well-balanced meals
- Learn to manage your time more effectively
- Set limits appropriately and learn to say no to requests that would create excessive stress in your life.
- Make time for hobbies, interests, and relaxation.
- Get enough rest and sleep. Your body needs time to recover from stressful events.
- Do not rely on alcohol, drugs, or compulsive behaviors to reduce stress.
- Seek out social support. Spend enough time with those you enjoy.
- Seek treatment with a psychologist or other mental health professional trained in stress management or biofeedback techniques to learn healthy ways of dealing with the stress in your life.

TIME MANAGEMENT (FIG. 19.17)

Time management is the process of planning and exercising conscious control of time spent on specific activities, especially to increase effectiveness, efficiency, and productivity. It involves a juggling act of various demands upon a person relating to work, social life, family, hobbies, personal interests and commitments with the finiteness of time.

Definition

Time management is the process of planning and controlling how much time to spend on specific activities. Good time management enables an individual to complete more in a shorter period of time, lowers stress, and leads to career success.

Meaning

- Time management refers to managing time effectively so that the right time is allocated to the right activity.
- Effective time management allows individuals to assign specific time slots to activities as per their importance.
- Time management refers to making the best use of time as time is always limited.

Objectives of Time Management

- Understand the concept of time management
- Implement such concept in an activity
- Recognize some facts and principles of time management
- Overcome challenges to time management.
- Develop effective time management skills

Need of Time Management

- To save time
- To reduce stress
- To function effectively
- To increase our work output
- To have more control over our job responsibilities

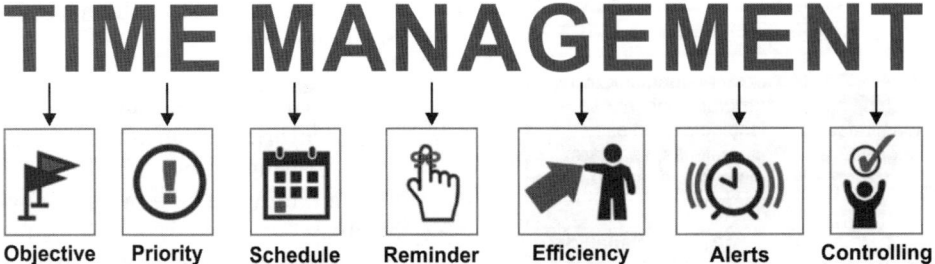

Fig. 19.17: Time management.

Important of Time Management

- Bad time management = stress
- Time is a special resource that you cannot store or save for later use.
- Wise time management can help you find the time for what you desire to do or need to do.
- Time management will help you set up your priorities.
- Time management helps you make conscious choices, so you can spend more of your time doing things that are important and valuable to you.
- To avoid damage to our personal life
- It keeps you healthy and stress free.

Benefits of Time Management

The ability to manage your time effectively is important. Good time management leads to improved efficiency and productivity, less stress, and more success in life. Here are some benefits of managing time effectively:

- **Stress relief:** Making and following a task schedule reduces anxiety. As you check off items on your "to-do" list, you can see that you are making tangible progress. This helps you avoid feeling stressed out with worry about whether you're getting things done.
- **More time:** Good time management gives you extra time to spend in your daily life. People who can time-manage effectively enjoy having more time to spend on hobbies or other personal pursuits.
- **More opportunities**: Managing time well leads to more opportunities and less time wasted on trivial activities. Good time management skills are key qualities that employers look for. The ability to prioritize and schedule work is extremely desirable for any organization.
- **Ability to realize goals**: Individuals who practice good time management are able to better achieve goals and objectives, and do so in a shorter length of time.

Time Management Skills (Fig. 19.18)

Stay Organized

- The workstation must be kept clean and organized.
- Keeping important files organized helps you retrieve them immediately and thus saves time which goes on unnecessary searching. Staple important documents together.
- Do not keep stacks of files and heaps of paper on your desk. Throw whatever you do not need.

- Keep stationery items and your personal belongings like cell phone, car keys, wallet at their proper places.
- Develop the habit of using an organizer. Plan your day well in advance.
- Never write on loose papers. Keep a notepad and pen handy.

Learn to Prioritize

- Set your priorities. Do not work just for the sake of working.
- Prepare a "Task Plan" or a "To Do" List the moment you settle down for work. Jot down all the activities you wish to do in a single day as per importance and urgency.
- High priority tasks must be attended to immediately. Do not start your day with something which does not require your immediate attention.
- Tick off completed tasks. It gives you a sense of relief and satisfaction.
- An employee must understand the difference between high and low priority tasks and also between important and urgent work.
- Do not indulge in irrelevant activities. You will waste your entire day and the output would be zero.
- Be clear about your roles and responsibilities at the workplace.

Be Punctual and Disciplined

- Being punctual helps you complete tasks way ahead of deadline.
- Avoid taking too many leaves from work. Such an attitude is completely unprofessional.
- Make sure you are there at your desk five minutes before your actual time.
- Strive hard to complete tasks on time. Do not keep assignments pending and wait for the last minute.

Take Ownership of Work

- Do not work only when your boss is around. Work for yourself. The dedication has to come from within.
- Be responsible for your work and learn to accept your mistakes.
- If you have accepted something, then it becomes your responsibility to complete it within the allotted time slot.

Be a Little Diplomatic

- Do not accept everything which comes your way. A polite "NO" in the beginning will save your reputation later.
- The employees must be delegated responsibilities as per their specialization and background. This way they take more interest and eventually finish work on time.

More Focused

- Be a little focused and concentrate on work. Do not waste time by loitering and gossiping around.
- Do not take long personal calls at work. Finish off work and leave for the day on time. You will have ample time to catch up with your friends or log on to social networking sites. Playing games while you are at work is something which is not expected out of a professional.

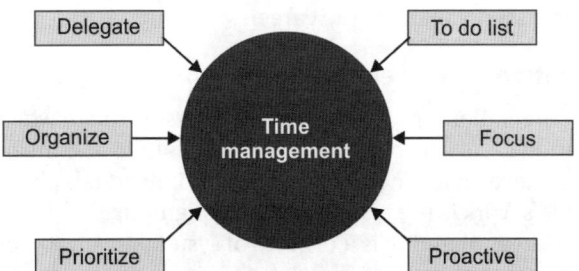

Fig. 19.18: Time management skills.

Be Reasonable

- No individual can work for the whole day. Do include some time in your daily schedule to speak to your team member sitting next to you.
- Do not over burden yourself.

Tips for Effective Time Management (Fig. 19.19)

After considering the benefits of time management, let us look at some ways to manage time effectively:

- **Set goals correctly:** Set goals that are achievable and measurable. Use the SMART method when setting goals. In essence, make sure the goals you set are **S**pecific, **M**easurable, **A**ttainable, **R**elevant, and **T**imely.
- **Prioritize wisely:** Prioritize tasks based on importance and urgency. For example, look at your daily tasks and determine which are:
  - Important and urgent: Do these tasks right away.
  - Important but not urgent: Decide when to do these tasks.
  - Urgent but not important: Delegate these tasks if possible.
  - Not urgent and not important: Set these aside to do later.
- **Set a time limit to complete a task:** Setting time constraints for completing tasks helps you be more focused and efficient. Making the small extra effort to decide on how much time you need to allot for each task can also help you recognize potential problems before they arise. That way you can make plans for dealing with them.
- **Take a break between tasks:** When doing a lot of tasks without a break, it is harder to stay focused and motivated. Allow some downtime between tasks to clear your head and refresh yourself. Consider grabbing a brief nap, going for a short walk, or meditating.
- **Organize yourself:** Utilize your calendar for more long-term time management. Write down the deadlines for projects, or for tasks that are part of completing the overall project. Think about which days might be best to dedicate to specific tasks.
- **Remove nonessential tasks/activities:** It is important to remove excess activities or tasks. Determine what is significant and what deserves your time. Removing non-essential tasks/activities frees up more of your time to be spent on genuinely important things.
- **Plan ahead**: Make sure you start every day with a clear idea of what you need to do-what needs to get done THAT DAY. Consider making it a habit to, at the end of each workday, go ahead and write out your "to-do" list for the next workday.

Implications of Poor Time Management

- **Poor workflow**: The inability to plan ahead and stick to goals means poor efficiency. For example, if there are several important tasks to complete, an effective plan would be to complete related tasks together or sequentially.
- **Wasted time:** Poor time management results in wasted time. For example, by talking to friends on social media while doing an assignment, you are distracting yourself and wasting time.
- **Loss of control**: By not knowing what the next task is, you suffer from loss of control of your life. That can contribute to higher stress levels and anxiety.
- **Poor quality of work:** Poor time management typically makes the quality of your work suffer. For example, having to rush to complete tasks at the last minute usually compromises quality.
- **Poor reputation:** If clients or your employer cannot rely on you to complete tasks in a timely manner, their expectations and perceptions of you are adversely affected. If a client cannot rely on you to get something done on time, they will likely take their business elsewhere.

CAREER PLANNING

Career planning is an individual's lifelong process of establishing personal career objectives and acting in a manner intended to bring them about. Career planning is a continuous process of setting individual professional goals and exploring ways to achieve them through self-evaluation, market research, and continuous learning. It is an important exercise to successfully manage the career.

Definitions of Career Planning

- Career planning is an ongoing process through which an individual sets career goals and identifies the means to achieve them. The process by which individuals plan their life's work is referred to as career planning.
- "Career planning is a process of systematically matching career goals and individual capabilities with opportunities for their fulfillment."

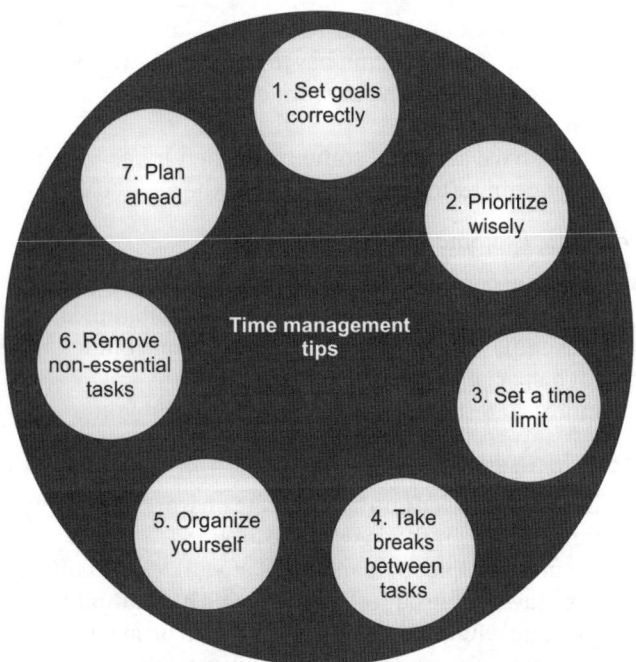

Fig. 19.19: Time management tips.

- A career may be defined as 'a sequence of jobs that constitute what a person does for a living'.
- According to Schermerborn, Hunt, and Osborn, 'Career planning is a process of systematically matching career goals and individual capabilities with opportunities for their fulfillment'.

Objectives of Career Planning

Career planning seeks to meet the following objectives:
- To provide and maintain appropriate manpower resources in the organization by offering careers, not jobs.
- To provide environment for the effectiveness, efficiency and growth of its employees and motivating them to contribute effectively towards achieving the objectives of the organization.
- To map out careers of various categories of employees suitable to their ability, and their willingness to be 'trained and developed for higher positions.
- To have a stable workforce by reducing absenteeism and employee turnover.
- To cater to the immediate and future human resources need of the organization on a timely basis.
- To increase the utilization of managerial reserves within organization.

Features of Career Planning and Career Development

- It is an ongoing process.
- It helps individuals develop skills required to fulfill different career roles.
- It strengthens work-related activities in the organization.
- It defines life, career, abilities, and interests of the employees.
- It can also give professional directions, as they relate to career goals.

Nature of Career planning

The following are the salient features of career planning:
- **A process:** Career planning is a process of developing human resources rather than an event.
- **Upward movement:** It involve upward movement in the organisational hierarchy, or special assignments, project work which require abilities to handle recurring problems, human relations issued and so on.
- **Mutuality of interest:** The individual's interest is served as his needs and aspirations are met to a great extent and the organization's interest is served as each of its human resources is provided an opportunity to develop and contribute to the organizational goals and objectives to the optimum of its ability and confidence.
- **Dynamic:** Career planning is dynamic in nature due to an ever changing environment.

Important Elements of Career

Analyzing definitional context, it is clear that career has following important elements—
- It is a proper sequence of job-related activities. Such job related activities vis-a-vis experience include role experiences at different hierarchical levels of an individual, which lead to an increasing level of responsibilities, status, power, achievements and rewards.
- It may be individual-centered or organizational-centered, individual-centered career is an individually perceived sequence of career progression within an occupation.
- It is better defined as an integrated pace of internal movement in an occupation of an individual over his employment span.

Career Anchors

Career anchors denote the basic drives that create the urge to take up a certain type of a career. These drives are as follows:
- **Managerial competence:** Person having this drive seek managerial positions that provide opportunities for higher responsibility, decision making, control and influence over others.
- **Technical competence:** People having this anchor seek to make career choices based on the technical or functional content of the work. It provide continuous learning and updating one's expertise in a technical or specialized area, such as quality control, engineering, accounting, advertising, public relations, etc.
- **Security:** If one's career anchor is security than he is willing to do what is required to maintain job security (through compliance with organisational prescriptions), a decent income and a stable future.
- **Creativity:** This drive provides entrepreneurial and innovative opportunities to the people. People are driven by an overwhelming desire to do something new that is totally of their own making.
- **Autonomy:** These people seek a career that provides freedom of action and independence.

Importance of Career Planning

- Career planning ensures a constant supply of promotable employees
- It helps in improving the loyalty of employees.
- Career planning encourages an employee's growth and development.
- It discourages the negative attitude of superiors who are interested in suppressing the growth of the subordinates.
- It ensures that senior management knows about the calibre and capacity of the employees who can move upwards.
- It can always create a team of employees prepared enough to meet any contingency.
- Career planning reduces labor turnover.
- Every organization prepares succession planning towards which career planning is the first step.

Steps in Career Planning Process (Fig. 19.20)

1. **Step 1:** Self-assessment—the first and foremost step in career planning is to know and assess yourself. You need to collect information about yourself while deciding about a particular career option. You must analyze the interests,

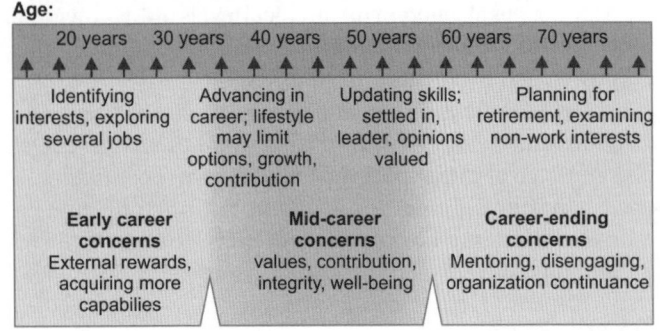

Fig. 19.20: Steps in career planning process.

abilities, aptitudes, desired lifestyle, and personal traits and then study the relationship between the career opted for and self.
2. **Step 2:** Goal setting—set the goals according to the academic qualification, work experience, priorities and expectations in life. Once the goal is identified, then you determine the feasible ways and objectives how to realize it.
3. **Step 3:** Academic/career options—narrow your general occupational direction to a particular one by an informatory decision making process. Analyze the career option by keeping in mind your present educational qualification and what more academic degrees you need to acquire for it.
4. **Step 4:** Plan of action—recognize those industries and particular companies where you want to get into. Make the plan a detailed one so that you can determine for how many years you are going to work in a company in order to achieve maximum success, and then switch to another. Decide where you would like to see yourself after five years and in which position.
5. **Step 5:** Catch hold of opportunities—opportunity comes but once. So, whenever you get any opportunity to prove yourself and get into your desired career, try to convert it in every way for suiting your purpose. Remember, a successful professional is also quite opportunistic in his moves, examining every opening to turn to his favor.

Different Phases in the Career of an Employee

Most working people go through career stages and it has been found that individual's needs and expectations change as the individual moves through these stages.

- **Exploration stage:** This is the stage where an individual builds expectations about his career. Some of them are realistic and some are not. But the fact is that these could be a result of the individual's ambitions.
- **Establishment stage:** This could be at the stage where the individual gets his first job, gets accepted by his peers, learns in this job, and also gains the first tangible evidence of success or failure. The establishment/advancement stage tends to occur between ages 25 and 44. In this stage, the individual has made his or her career choice and is concerned with achievement, performance, and advancement. This stage is marked by high employee productivity and career growth, as the individual is motivated to succeed in the organization and in his or her chosen occupation. Opportunities for job challenge and use of special competencies are desired in this stage. The employee strives for creativity and innovation through new job assignments. Employees also need a certain degree of autonomy in this stage so that they can experience feelings of individual achievement and personal success.
- **Mid-career stage:** The individual's performance levels either continue to improve, or levels, or even deteriorates.
- **Late career:** This is regarded as a pleasant phase, where one is allowed to relax and play the role of an elderly statesman in the organization.
- **Decline:** The stage, where the individual is heading towards retirement.

Benefits of Career Planning

- Career planning helps to develop internal supplies of promotable talent. If vacancies occur, it is easy to locate a good successor.
- The increased attention and concern for individual careers generate more organizational loyalty, and therefore, lower employee turnover. Career planning improves the organization's ability to attract and retain high talent personnel.
- Career planning encourages employees to tap more of their potential abilities because they have specific career goals.
- Career plans and goals motivate employees to grow and develop, without career planning; it is easier for managers to hoard key subordinates. Career planning causes employees, managers, and the HR department to become aware of employee qualifications. Key subordinates can be placed in different departments.
- It reduces employee frustration as the employee knows what he should do to the career goal. Assists affirmative action plans. Career planning can help members of protected groups prepare for more important jobs. This preparation can contribute to meeting affirmative action timetables.
- It-ensures needed talents and promotes organizational goodwill.
- Career planning helps the individual have the knowledge of various career opportunities, his priorities, etc.
- It helps him select the career which is suitable to his lifestyle, preference, family environment, the scope for self-development, etc.
- It helps the organization identify talented employees who can be promoted.
- Internal promotions, up gradation and transfers motivate the employees, boost their morale and also result in increased job satisfaction.

- Each employee will await his turn of promotion rather than changing to another organization. This would lower employee turnover.
- It improves employee's performance on the job by tapping their potential abilities and stimulating their personal growth.
- Increased job satisfaction due to career planning enhances employee commitment and creates a sense of belongingness and loyalty to the organization.
- Being an integral part of the manpower planning and corporate planning, career planning contributes towards individual development and organizational development and effective achievement of corporate goals.
- An organization with well-designed career plans is able to have a better image in the employment market, and it will attract and retain competent people.

Limitations of Career Planning

Though career planning helps an organization in numerous ways, it has a few limitations that undermine the importance and relevance of career planning. These are:
- Time factor
- Unsuitable for a large workforce
- Lack of objectivity
- External interventions
- Lack of knowledge and awareness
- Lack of flexibility
- Difficulty in measuring career success

CONCLUSION

Personnel management is one of the cornerstones of a human resource department. It comprises all administrative and routine tasks in a human resources department. Planning and development are other central responsibilities. Personnel management is also referred to as personnel administration or transactional personnel work. This kind of administration deals intensively with the relationship between employees and the company. In the course of transactional tasks, data is also transferred to third parties. For example, payroll accounting is forwarded to the responsible authorities.

REVIEW QUESTIONS

Long Essays

1. Define personnel management; explain nature, objectives and characteristics.
2. Explain the differences between personnel management and human resource management.
3. Define emotional intelligence; explain the components and skills.
4. Define resilience building; explain the characteristics, factors and principles.
5. Define stress; explain the symptoms and prevention of workplace stress.
6. Define time management; explain the needs, objectives and importance of time management.
7. Define career planning; explain the objectives, nature and benefits.

Short Essays

1. Elements of personnel management.
2. Functions of personnel management.
3. Importance of manpower planning.
4. Training of employees.
5. Types of recruitment.
6. Benefits of emotional intelligence in the workplace.
7. Types of resilience.
8. Time management skills.
9. Steps in career planning process.

Short Answers

1. Scope of personnel management.
2. Manpower planning.
3. Need of manpower planning.
4. Methods of training.
5. Roles of a personnel manager.
6. Importance of emotional intelligence.
7. Types of emotional intelligences.
8. Pros of emotional intelligence.
9. Benefits of time management.

CHAPTER 20

Establishment of Nursing Educational Institutions

LEARNING OBJECTIVES

- Indian Nursing Council Norms and Guidelines: Faculty Norms, Physical Facilities, Clinical Facilities, Curriculum Implementation, and Evaluation/Examination Guidelines
- Coordination with Regulatory Bodies: INC and State Nursing Council
- Accreditation—Inspections
- Affiliation with University/State Council/Board of Examinations

INTRODUCTION

Modern nursing is a dynamic, therapeutic and educative process in meeting the health needs of the individuals, the family and the community. Nursing is one of the health professions which functions in conjunction with other healthcare agencies in assisting individuals, families and communities to achieve and maintain desirable standards and maintain desirable standards of health. A nursing education at a technical college aims to fulfill two primary goals. The first goal is to prepare nursing students to become registered nurses by taking and passing the National Council Licensure Examination. The other goal is to prepare students to become dedicated and competent professional nurses. These nurses will have the capability to administer effective healthcare to a diverse population, including the poor and underserved. To graduate from nursing programs at technical colleges, a nursing student must meet and maintain a number of requirements. Students must also meet grade standards and consistently operate according to high technical standards.

AIMS OF NURSING EDUCATION

The ultimate purpose of nursing education is to produce well qualified and competent professional nurses.
Specific aims of nursing education:
- Knowledge aim
- Leadership aim
- Professional development aim
- Personality development aim
- Nursing research
- Democratic citizenship

Knowledge Aim

- Nursing education aims at imparting scientific and up-to-date knowledge in the area of biological, behavioral, social and medical science.
- Nursing education's primary focus is to inculcate the appropriate nursing skills and the right attitude among the student nurses.
- Theoretical and practical knowledge is essential for rendering intelligent and efficient nursing services.
- Nursing education curriculum should have sufficient theory content and practical experience.

Leadership Aim

- Nursing education aims at the preparation of nurses as good leaders. Nurses are in a pivotal position not only to render quality care but also to assess and monitor the quality of care.
- Nursing education prepares nurses to participate in decision making and policy making with respect to health matters. Nurses are educated to plan, organize and manage the healthcare programs of the country.
- Nurses are educated to suitably evaluate the quality and structure of the healthcare services.
- Nurses are prepared to collaborate and coordinate the healthcare functions of the members of the healthcare team.
- The nurse leaders are responsible for effective nursing education and hence aim at identifying potential nursing leaders and facilitate their development.

Professional Development Aim

- Nursing education aims at the professional development of each individual nurse.
- A nurse should be trained to keep up the ethics and standards in the profession.
- The nursing education system aims at educating a nurse in a manner so as to enable the nurse to develop appropriate skills and attitudes required for the practice of the profession.
- The nurse in turn should aim to contribute for the growth and development of her profession.

Personality Development Aim

- Nursing education also aims at contributing to the all round development of the individual.
- The focus of nursing education system is to help a nurse in developing positive personal attributes, such as self-awareness, self-direction and self-motivation.

Nursing Research

Research opens the horizons for the growth of a profession and nursing education aims at preparing nurses to carry out research so as to add to the body of knowledge by means of scientific investigations.

Democratic Citizenship

Nursing education includes values, such as respect to individuality, equality, toleration, cooperative living and faith in change through persuasion.

NURSING PROGRAMS IN INDIA

Most students are enrolled in different nursing programs, such as Auxiliary Nurse and Midwife, GNM (General Nursing and Midwifery), BSc, (Bachelor Basic), BSc, (Post Basic), MSc, (Master), MPhil and PhD programs. After school, students can enroll in BSc Basic program, Auxiliary Nurse and Midwife and GNM, if students need specialization, they can do BSc Basic or if they interested diploma course, they can join in ANM or GNM. Duration of these programs is different, for example, BSc Basic is 4 years, GNM is 3 years and ANM is 2 years.

Aims of Nursing Programs

Nursing education focuses on educating healthcare people about effective ways to deliver the healthcare to patients. It educates nurses about how to administer different medicines, to examine patient and to deliver best services to patients. The aims of nursing program are to:

- Produce knowledgeable competent nurses with clear critical thinking skills who are caring, motivated, assertive and well-disciplined responding to the changing needs of profession, healthcare delivery system and society.
- Prepare graduates to assume responsibilities as professional, competent nurses and midwives in providing promotive, preventive, curative and rehabilitative healthcare services in hospital or public health settings.
- Prepare nurses who can make independent decisions in nursing situations within the scope of practice, protect the rights of individuals and groups and conduct research in the areas of nursing practice and apply evidence-based practice.
- Prepare nurses to assume role of practitioner, teacher, supervisor and manager in clinical or public health settings.

Types of Nursing Education Programs in India

Nursing programs	Training duration	Examination	Registration
Auxiliary nurse and midwife	2 years	Nursing Examination Board	R ANM
General nursing and midwifery	3 and 1/2 years 3 years from 2015–2016	Nursing Examination Board	RN and RM
BSc (Basic)	4 years	University	RN and RM
BSc (Post Basic)	Regular: 2 years Distance: 3 years	University	Additional qualification
MSc	2 years	University	Additional qualification
MPhil	1 year (full time) 2 years (part time)	University	Additional qualification
PhD	3–5 years	University	

Goals and Objectives of Nursing Education

Nursing goals are as individualized as you are and go way beyond merely the desire to become a nurse. Some nurses want to specialize, while others intend to attend a number of graduate nursing programs to achieve their career and preferred nursing position goals. A number of options are available to nurses, so breaking down your ultimate objective will help you decide on the correct path of education and skills necessary to achieve those goals.

Communication

Nursing education objectives differ depending on the topic under study. For example, you can have nursing objectives for nutrition, communication and pharmacology studies, as well as a greater understanding of patient-centered care in different healthcare and delivery scenarios. For example, one goal of adequate nursing education is to teach nursing students the importance of communication through verbal, written and visual skills.

- **Critical thinking:** A very important skill, the mastering of which is the goal of most nurses, is the ability to use critical thinking methods in order to make effective and correct decisions. Critical thinking is essential in problem-solving that requires immediate attention in many medical care scenarios. Teaching students to gather data, analyze that data and evaluate a problem or potential solution is the goal of instructors in nursing schools.
- **Ethics:** The ethical responsibilities and obligations of nurses are at the foundation of structure for nursing instruction and education in a wide range of fields like pediatrics, oncology and geriatric care. Questions of ethics and potential "what-if" scenarios offered by nursing instructors may help nursing students evaluate legal, regulatory and ethical or moral issues and beliefs.
- **Skills:** Attention to detail and competency in basic nursing skills are important aspects of the overall nursing education curriculum. Student nurses must be able to provide basic hands-on skills, such as taking vital signs, wound care and dressing, range of motion and knowledge regarding proper ambulation and transfer techniques to ensure and support patient safety. While a nurse should have empathy and compassion for others, professionalism and the proper attitude are also desired.

- **Stress:** A nurse must be able to think, analyze and make decisions under stress and time constraints. As such, it's important to teach nurses how they can function under pressure, manage and deal with constant change, communicate and make effective decisions.

Competencies for Nursing Programs

- **Patient-centered care:** Provide holistic care recognizing individual patient's preferences, values and needs, that is compassionate, coordinated, age and culturally appropriate safe and effective care.
- **Professionalism:** Demonstrate accountability for the delivery of standard-based nursing care as per INC standards that are consistent with moral, altruistic, legal, ethical, regulatory and humanistic principles.
- **Leadership:** Influence the behavior of individuals and groups within their environment and facilitate establishment of shared goals.
- **System-based practice:** Demonstrate awareness and responsiveness to the context of healthcare system and ability to manage resources essential to provide optimal quality of care.
- **Health informatics and technology:** Use technology and synthesize information and collaborate to make critical decisions that optimize patient outcomes.
- **Communication:** Interact effectively with patients, families and colleagues fostering mutual respect and shared decision making to enhance patient satisfaction and health outcomes.
- **Teamwork and collaboration:** Function effectively within nursing and interdisciplinary teams, fostering open communication, mutual respect, shared decision making, team learning and development.
- **Safety:** Minimize risk of harm to patients and providers through both system effectiveness and individual performance.
- **Quality improvement:** Use data to monitor the outcomes of care processes and utilize improvement methods to design and test changes to continuously improve the quality and safety of healthcare system.
- **Evidence-based practice:** Identify, evaluate and use the best current evidence coupled with clinical expertise and consideration of patient's preferences, experience and values to make practical decisions.

Basic Bachelor of Nursing (BSc Nursing)

Graduate nursing education started in India in the year 1946 in CMC, Vellore and in the RAK College of nursing at Delhi University.

At present 1373 colleges have been recognized by INC to conduct the course under several universities in India.

Eligibility for Admission

A candidate seeking admission should have:
- Pass the 2 years of pre-university exam or equivalent as recognized by concerned university with science subjects, i.e., physics, biology and chemistry.
- Students of vocational courses
- Obtained at least 45% of total marks in science subjects in the qualifying exam, if belongs to a scheduled caste or tribe, should have obtained not less than 40% of total marks in science subjects.
- Completed 17 years of age at the time of admission or will complete this age on or before 31st December of the year of admission
- Is medically fit

Objectives of study: The program is designed:
- To provide a balance of professional and general education
- To enable a student to become a professional nurse practitioner who has self direction and is a responsible citizen. Through planned guided experiences students are provided with opportunities to develop:
- A broad concept of the fundamental principles of nursing care based on sound knowledge and satisfactory levels of skill in providing care to people of all ages in community or institutional setting.
- Understanding of the application of principles from the physical biological and social sciences for assessing the health status
- Ability to investigate healthcare problems systematically
- Ability to work collaboratively with members of allied disciplines towards attaining optimum health for all members of the society
- Understanding of fundamental principles of administration and organization of nursing service
- Understanding of human behavior and appreciation of effective interpersonal relationship with individuals families and groups
- Ability to assume responsibility for continuing learning
- Appreciation of professional attitudes necessary for leadership roles in nursing appreciation of social and ethical obligations to society.

Course of study: The course of study leading to bachelor of nursing degree comprises four academic years.

Post Basic-Bachelor of Nursing Course (Post Certificate) for Qualified Nurses

INC has recognized two modes of programs at this level.
1. **Regular** BSc (Post Basic) course for those who have 10+2 + GNM (General Nursing and Midwifery) which has a duration of 2 years.
2. **Distance** BSc (Post Basic) course for those who have 10+2 GNM + 2 years experience which has duration of 3 years.

Philosophy and Aims of the Program

- Nursing is an integral part of the healthcare delivery system and shire responsibility in collaboration with other allied health professions for the attainment of optimal health for all members of the society.
- Education as a lifelong learning process. It seeks to render appropriate behavioral changes in students in order to facilitate their development, which assists them to live personally satisfied and socially useful lives.

- The goal of post certificate degree program leading to Bachelor of Science in nursing is the preparation of the trained nurse as a generalist who accept responsibility for enhancing the effectiveness of nursing care.

Eligibility for admission: The candidate seeking admission must:
- Hold a certificate in general nursing.
- Be a registered nurse
- Have minimum of two years of experience. Now it is relaxed that no experience after GNM is required for admission to this course.
- Have passed pre-university exam in the arts/science/commerce or its equivalent which is recognized the university
- Be medically fit
- Have a good personal and professional record
- Have working knowledge of English

Program of Study

Duration: the program of the study is two academic years from the date of commencement of program. Terms and vacations shall be as notified by the university from time to time.

Objectives: The goal of the post certificate program leading to the bachelor of nursing is the preparation of the trained nurses as a generalist who accept responsibility for enhancing the effectiveness of nursing care.
- Administer high quality nursing care to all people of all ages in homes, hospitals and other community agencies in urban and rural areas.
- Apply knowledge from the physical, social and behavioral sciences in assessing the health status of individuals and make critical judgment in assessing the health status of the individuals and make critical judgment in planning, directing and evaluating primary, acute and long-term care given by themselves and others working with them.
- Investigate healthcare problems systematically
- Work collaboratively with members of other health disciplines
- Teach and counsel individuals, families and other groups about health and illness
- Understand human behavior and establish effective interpersonal relationships
- Teach in clinical nursing situations
- Identify underlying principles from the social and natural sciences and utilize them in adapting to, or initiating changes in relation to those factors
- Acquire professional knowledge and attitude in adapting for leadership role.

Degree of Master Nursing (MSc Nursing)

- First two years course in masters of nursing was started at RAK College of Nursing in 1959 and in 1969 in CMC Vellore.
- At present, there are 401 colleges imparting MSc Nursing degree course in different specialties.
- INC recognized List of Colleges of Nursing for MSc(N) course (2010–2011)

Philosophy

- The master of nursing program is offered by institution of higher education and is built up on a recognized bachelor's curriculum in nursing (in India—by Indian Nursing Council).
- The program prepares nurses for leadership position in nursing and other health fields who can function as specialist's nurse practitioners, consultants, educators, administrators and investigators in a wide variety of professional setting in meeting the national priorities and the changing needs of the society.
- The program prepares nursing graduates who are professionally equipped, creative and self-directed and socially motivated to effectively meet with the needs of the social change.
- The program encourages accountability and commitment to lifelong learning which fosters improvement of quality care.

Objectives: Graduates of master of nursing program demonstrate:
- Increased cognitive, affective and psychomotor competencies and the ability to utilize the potentials for effective nursing performance.
- Expertise in the utilization of concepts and theories for the assessment, planning and intervention in meeting the self-care needs of an individual for the attainment of fullest potentials in the field of specialty.
- Ability to practice independently as a nurse specialist
- Ability to function effectively as nurse educators and administrators
- Ability to interpret the health-related research
- Ability to plan and initiate change in the healthcare system
- Leadership qualities for the advancement of practice of professional nursing
- Interest in lifelong learning for personal and professional learning advancement

Eligibility: The candidate seeking admission must:
- Have passed BSc Nursing/post certificate BSc, or nursing degree of any university
- Have a minimum of one year of experience after obtaining BSc, in hospitals or nursing educational institutions or community health setting
- For BSc, nursing post certificate, no such experience is needed after graduation the candidate shall be—a registered nurse or registered midwife for admission to medical surgical nursing, community health nursing, pediatric nursing obstetric and gynecological nursing.
- A registered nurse for admission to psychiatric nursing
- The candidate shall be selected on merit judged on the basis of academic performances in BSc nursing, post certificate BSc, or nursing and selection tests.

Specialties: Candidate will be examined in any of the following branches:
1. Medical surgical nursing—cardiovascular and thoracic nursing
   - Medical surgical nursing—critical care nursing
   - Medical surgical nursing—oncology nursing

- Medical surgical nursing—neurosciences nursing
- Medical surgical nursing—nephrourology nursing
- Medical surgical nursing—orthopedic nursing
- Medical surgical nursing—gastroenterology nursing
- Obstetric and gynecological nursing
- Pediatric (child health) nursing
- Psychiatric (mental health) nursing
- Community health nursing

Four common papers are there included in the syllabus. They are:
1. Advanced concepts of health and nursing
2. Education and nursing education
3. Biostatistics, research methodology and nursing research
4. Administration and nursing administration

Master of Philosophy Program in Nursing (MPhil)

In 1980 RAK college of nursing started an MPhil program as a regular and part time course. Since then several universities started taking students for the MPhil course in nursing. Prominent among these are: MGR Medical University, Rajiv Gandhi University of Health Sciences, SNDT University and Delhi University and Manipal Academy of Higher Education.

- **Philosophy:** Nursing shares with the whole university a main focus of preparing its students for service and assisting them to achieve a meaningful philosophy of life. The student is encouraged to develop judgment and wisdom in handling knowledge and skills and achieve mastery of problem-solving and creative skills. Commitment to lifelong learning is the mark of truly professional person. In order to maintain clinical competencies and enhance professional practice, the student must stay abrupt of the new developments and contribute to the advancement of nursing knowledge.
- **Objectives:** The objectives of MPhil degree course in nursing are:
  - To strengthen the research foundations of nurses for encouraging research attitudes and problem solving capacities
  - To provide basic training required for research in undertaking doctoral work
- **Duration:** Duration of the full term MPhil course will be one year and part time course will be two year.
- **Course of study:** At the time of admission, each candidate will be required to indicate her priorities in regard to the optional courses a candidate may offer one course from MPhil program from the department of anthropology, education, sociology and physiology or any suitable department. The MPhil studies will be into two distinct parts, part 1 and part 2.
  - **Part 1:** It consist of 3 courses, i.e., research methods in nursing, major aspects of nursing, allied disciplines
  - **Part 2:** After passing the part 1 examination, a student shall be required to write a dissertation. The topic and the nature of the dissertation of each candidate will be determined by the advisory committee consist of 3 members. The dissertation may include results of original research, a fresh interpretation of existing facts, and date or a review article of critical nature of may take.

Doctorate of Philosophy in Nursing (PhD in Nursing)

1. Ealier Indian nurses were sent abroad for PhD program.
2. PhD programs in nursing was first started in India in 1992
3. Universities where PhD programs are conducted in India include.

Philosophy: A candidate for admission to the course for the degree of doctor of philosophy in the faculties of medical science must have obtained an MPhil degree of a university or have a good academic record with first or second class master's degree of an Indian or a foreign university in the concerned subject.

The candidate shall apply to the university for the admission stating his qualifications and the subjects he proposes to investigate enclosing a statement on any work he may have done in the subject. Every application for the admission of the course must be analyzed by the board of research studies.

Board of research studies (medical sciences)—members
- Dean and the head of the departments concerned
- Principals/head of institutions recognized for postgraduate medical studies.
- Two members nominated by the medical academic council.
- Three persons nominated by the medical faculty (for their special knowledge in the medical science.

Eligibility Criteria

- The candidate should be post graduate in nursing with more than 55% of aggregates of marks.
- Should have research background
- May/may not published articles in journals
- The course duration is for regular PhD course is 3 years and for part time is 4 years.

COORDINATION WITH REGULATORY AND AFFILIATING BODIES

Many professional bodies perform professional certification to indicate a person possesses qualifications in the subject area, and sometimes membership in a professional body is synonymous with certification, but not always. Sometimes, membership in a professional body is required for one to be legally able to practice the profession. Many professional bodies also act as learned societies for the academic disciplines underlying their professions.

Definition

Regulatory bodies is a public authority or government agency responsible for exercising autonomous authority over some area of human activity in a regulatory or supervisory capacity.

Meaning of Regulatory Bodies

Regulatory agencies are usually a part of the executive branch of the government, or they have statutory authority to perform

> **Box 20.1:** Major types of regulating bodies.
> - International Council for Nurses.
> - Indian Nursing Council.
> - State Nursing Council.
> - Trained Nurses Association of India
> - Student Nursing Association.
> - Maharashtra University of Health Sciences.
> - National League for Nursing.

their functions with oversight from the legislative branch. Their actions are generally open to legal review. Regulatory authorities are commonly set up to enforce standards and safety

- Professional body or professional organization, also known as a professional association or professional society, is an organization, usually nonprofit, that exists to further a particular profession, to protect both the public interest and the interests of professionals.
- Associations is organizations of persons with common interests. Merton defined a professional association as, "an organization of practitioners, who judge one another as professionally competent and have united together to perform social functions, which they cannot perform in their separate capacity as individuals".
- Associations exist in all profession and in all parts of the world. Associations serve their individual members through a variety of services.
- Professional associations provide a vehicle for nurses to meet present and future challenges and work toward positive profession wide changes that keep pace with societal changes.
- As for as the educational institution is concerned the employee associations are formed among the teachers and office staff to promote their own welfare.

Box 20.1 describes major types of regulating bodies.

Role, Characteristics and Principles

Role of Regulatory Bodies
- To ensure the public's light to quality healthcare service
- To support and assist professional members
- Set and enforce standards of nursing practice
- Monitor and enforce standards for nursing education
- Set the requirements for monitor and enforce standards of nursing practice
- Set the requirements for registration of nursing professionals

Characteristics
- It is relatively permanent.
- It is voluntary in nature.
- It is an instrument of defense against exploitation.
- It is an association of educated persons.
- It is for the common purpose.

Principles of Regulatory Bodies
- Unity is strength
- Collective bargaining
- Promotion of common interest
- Career advancement
- Opportunity for the self career development
- Economic security
- Security of service

Benefits of Professional Bodies
- Developing leadership skills
- Recognition through certification. Certification is a formal but voluntary process of demonstrating expertise in particular areas of nursing.
- Legislative lobbying power. Association lobbies the government to influence the laws affecting nursing.
- Other benefits—publications, continuing nursing education, discounts in train, eyeglasses goods and services.
- To negotiate collective bargaining to get the dues in terms of finance and nonfinance
- To get along with their fellow-workers in a better way and to gain respect in the eyes of their peers
- To safe guard the common interest of the professionals
- To promote public relations

Importance of Professional Bodies

The Public
Serve public by establishing codes of ethics and standards of practice, socializing new members to these codes and standards and enforcing codes and standards in practice.

The Profession
- Serve by being the mechanism through which the collective interests of its members are pressed collectively and focused politically.
- Collective action means the activities are undertaken on behalf of a group of people, who have common interests.
- Professional association help nurses use collective action to push for political responses to benefit consumers of healthcare and members of the profession.

Individual Members
- Serve by providing continuing education and ensuring mechanisms for a professional work place.
- They work by forming relationships with the public and other professions and by ensuring that the professions work is properly understood and supported by the public, government officials and other healthcare professionals.

University
A university is an institution of higher (or tertiary) education and research which awards academic degrees in various academic disciplines. Universities typically provide undergraduate education and postgraduate education.

Permanent Affiliation Guidelines
- Conditions laid down for granting of permanent affiliation to colleges/institutions:

Chapter 20: Establishment of Nursing Educational Institutions

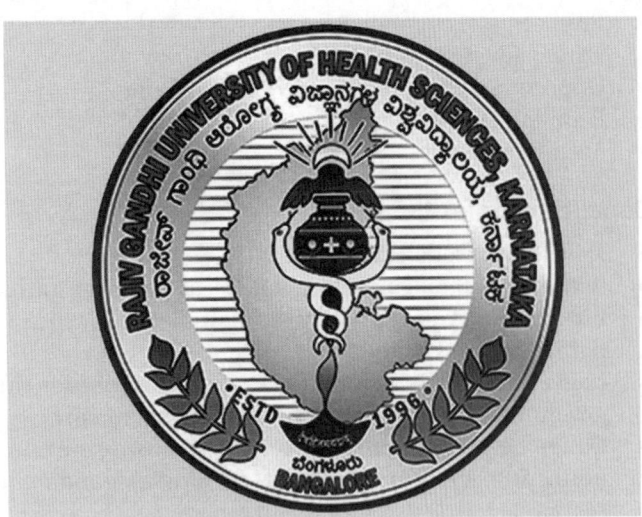

Fig. 20.1: Rajiv Gandhi University of Health Sciences, Karnataka.

- Permanent affiliation to college will be granted after standing of five years and has fulfilled and complied with all the conditions of affiliation as given below and also the recommendations of various LICs that have been visiting the Institutions from time to time.

Document require for affiliation following document submitted in two copy files:

- An affidavit prescribed format
- Copy of land document
- Building plan approved by authority
- Land use certificate by authority
- No objection certificate of Gujarat government
- Original Khatauni of land
- Trust deed and trust registration certificate
- Certificate of verification of land from competent authority or Tehsildar.
- Affidavit regarding acceptance of norms and guidelines of the university.
- Application fee demand draft in favor of university.

Figure 20.1 shows logo of Rajiv Gandhi University of Health Sciences, Karnataka.

Functions of the University

- Provide education at university standard
- Provide facilities for, and encourage, study and research
- Encourage the advancement and development of knowledge, and its application to government, industry, commerce and the community.
- Provide courses of study or instruction, at levels of achievement the council considers appropriate, to meet the needs of the community.
- Confer higher education awards
- Disseminate knowledge and promote scholarship
- Provide facilities and resources for the wellbeing of the University's staff, students and other persons undertaking courses at the university
- Perform other functions given to the university under the Act or another Act
- Conduct examination

Indian Nursing Council/Apex Body (Fig. 20.2)

The Indian Nursing Council, which was authorized by the Indian Nursing Council Act of 1947, was established in 1949 for the purpose providing uniform standards in nursing education and reciprocity in nursing registration throughout the country.

The only national legislation directly related to nursing practice, also provides a basis from which rules for nursing practice can be developed. Among other responsibilities, this Act gives authority to the Indian Nursing Council for prescribing curricula for nursing education and recognizing qualifications of institutions with teaching programs for nursing.

- **Definition:** Indian Nursing Council (INC) is a statutory body that regulates nursing education in the country through prescription, inspection, examination, certification and maintaining its stands for a uniform syllabus at each level of nursing education.
- **Aim:** To establish a uniform standard of training for nurses midwives and health visitors INC is a regulatory body for nurses and nursing education in India It is an autonomous body under the Government of India, Ministry of Health and Family Affairs.

Functions of INC

- To establish and monitor uniform standards of nursing for nurse midwives, auxiliary nurse midwives and health visitors' education by doing inspection of the institutions.
- To recognize the qualification(s) under section 10(2)(4) of the Indian Nursing Council Act, 1947 for the purpose of registration and employment in India and abroad.
- To prescribe minimum standards of education and training in various nursing programs and prescribe the syllabus and regulations for nursing programs under section 16 of the Indian Nursing Council Act, 1947.

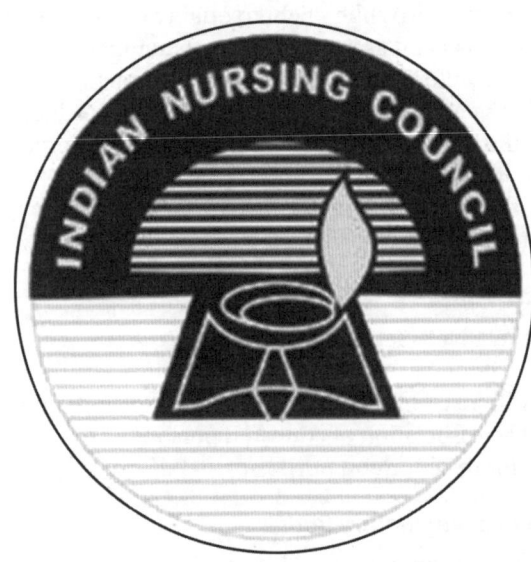

Fig. 20.2: Indian Nursing Council.

Chapter 20: Establishment of Nursing Educational Institutions

- Power to withdraw the recognition of qualification under Section 14 of the Indian Nursing Council Act, 1947 in case the institution fails to maintain its standards under Section 14(1)(b) of the Act when an institution recognized by a State Council for the training of nurses midwives, Auxiliary Nurse Midwives or health visitors does not satisfy the requirements of the Council.
- To recognize Degree/Diploma/Certificate awarded by Foreign Universities.
- To give approval for registration of Indian and Foreign Nurses possessing foreign qualification under Section 11(2)(a) of the Indian Nursing Council Act, 1947.
- To maintain Indian Nurses Register for registration of nursing personnel.
- To advise the State Nursing Councils, Examining Boards, State Governments and Central Government in various important items regarding nursing education in the country.
- To promote research in nursing.
- To prescribe code of ethics and professional conduct.
- To regulate the policies of training of nursing programs in the field of nursing to improve the quality of nursing education.

Objectives and Roles of (INC)

- Recognizing the qualification/s of the INC Act, 1947 under section 10(2)(4) for the purpose of employment and registration in India, as well as abroad.
- Monitoring and establishing uniform standards of nursing education for auxiliary nurse midwives, health visitors, nurse midwives by conducting inspections of different institutions.
- Prescribing minimum education and training standards in different nursing programs along with regulations and syllabus under section 19 of the INC Act, 1947.
- Indian Nursing Council holds the power of withdrawing the recognition of an institution under Section 14 of the INC Act, 1947. This happens if a State Council recognized institute fails to meet or maintain its standards as prescribed under Section 14(1) (b) of the INC Act.
- The council is responsible to provide recognition to a Degree/Certificate/Diploma awarded by Foreign Universities.
- Under Section 11(2)(a) of the INC Act, 1947, the council gives approval for registration of Foreign and Indian Nurses possessing qualifications from a foreign country.
- For the registration of nursing personnel, it maintains the Indian Nurses Register.
- Advising different State Nursing Councils, State Governments, Central Governments and Examining Boards in different crucial items regarding nursing education in India.
- Promoting research in nursing.
- Regulating policies for nursing training programs for the improvement of the quality of nursing education.
- Prescribing professional conduct and code of ethics.

Types of Inspection

1. **First inspection:** The first inspection is conducted on the receipt of proposal.
2. **Re-inspections:** Re-inspections are conducted for those institutions, which are found unsuitable by INC.
3. **Periodic inspection:** INC conducts the periodical inspections once the institution is found suitable by INC.

Guidelines for Establishment of New Nursing Schools/Colleges

- Any organization under the central, state government, local body or a private trust should obtain the no objection certificate from the state government.
- The INC on the receipt of the proposal from the institution to start nursing program, will undertake the first inspection to assess the suitability.
- After the approval from INC, the institution shall obtain the approval from state nursing council and examination board.

The INC conducts the inspection every year till the first batch completes the program.

- Apply in state government for the essentiality certificate
- After essentiality inspection government issued the certificate
- Then apply for state nursing council and university affiliation
- LIC inspection from affiliation department of university
- Then after university syndicate meting diced for the course permission
- University gives affiliation certificate
- Then GNC inspection carried out
- After GNC meeting give consent letter of the permission
- Then apply in INC for the permission
- INC inspection is carried out after inspection report and INC meting
- Give the permission letter for starting the program.

State Registration Council

In India, there are 29 State Nursing Councils that carry out the functions of a Nursing Council for its state. The work of these bodies is to provide recognition to its nursing colleges/universities, withdrawing recognition (if needed), conducting state-level nursing exams and admissions, maintaining the standards of nursing education in that state and many more.

The functions of the councils are to:

- Inspect and accredit schools of nursing in their State.
- Conduct examinations
- Prescribe rules of conduct, take disciplinary actions, etc.
- Maintain register of nurses, midwives, ANMs and health visitors in the State.

The State Registration councils are autonomous to a great extent except that they do not have powers to prescribe syllabi for the various training courses, recognize examining bodies and to negotiate reciprocity. These powers are vested with the INC and State Councils ensure that the prescribed syllabi are followed and standards are maintained.

Figure 20.3 shows The Karnataka State Nursing Council.

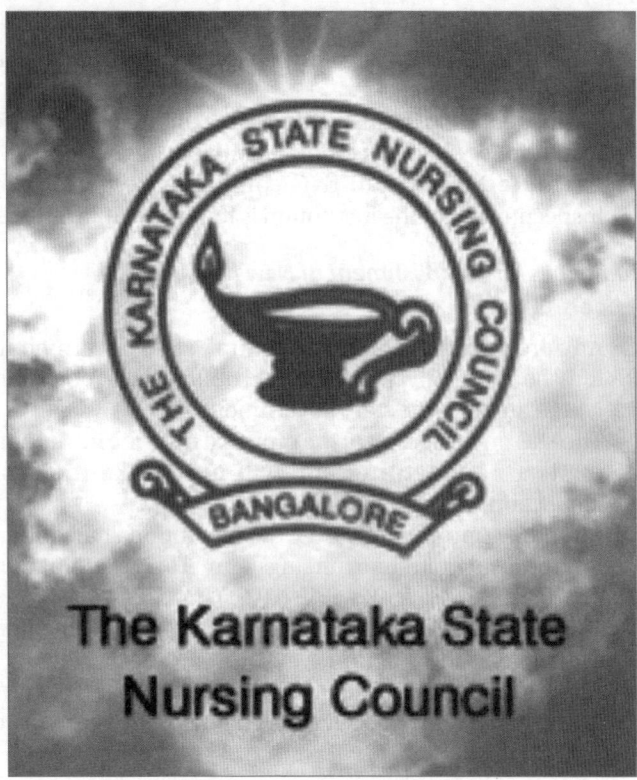

Fig. 20.3: The Karnataka State Nursing Council.

Mission and Vision of the Council

- To bring a quality in healthcare system through proper A practices of nurses in the state.
- To improve the quality of nursing education and healthcare.
- To enable the nurses, ANM/FHW, midwives, female health assistants to provide care to the patients by safe practices

Objectives

- Maintenance of database of the persons practicing as nurse, auxiliary nurse midwives, female health workers lady health visitors.
- Restriction for enrollment in the registered list
- Publication of notification for the registers and lists
- Monitoring of issues and appeals of aggrieved persons related to recognition, affiliation and registration.
- To conduct inspection and licensing of nursing institution in the state.

Function

- Registration
- Conduct of examinations
- Changing surname
- Inspection of training institutions and granting recognition.
- Maintenance of registers related to different category of nurses.
- Change of address for trained nurses
- Issue of duplicate certificates if original is lost
- Additional qualification registration for up-to-date statistics for higher qualifications
- Renewal of registration
- Reciprocal registration
- Abroad verification
- Publication
- Construction of syllabus
- In-service education program.
- Research

State Government

The state government controls nursing practice throughout the state Nurses Registration Acts. The state Nurses Registration Councils have authority to prescribe rules of conduct, to take disciplinary action and to maintain registers of nurses. Except for the uniform standards given by the INC, the state nurse practice act is the important law affecting nursing practice act that protects the public by broadly defining the legal scope of nursing practice.

Functions

- It registers nurse/midwives.
- It serves as legal protections to the nurse.
- It protects the public from incompetent nursing practice or poor nursing care.
- It accredits and inspects schools of nursing and college of nursing.
- It prescribes the rules of conduct, table disciplinary action.

International Council of Nurses (ICN)

The International Council of Nurses, founded in 1899 by Mrs Bedford Fenwick, is a federation of nonpolitical and self-governing national nurses association. The headquarters are in Geneva, Switzerland. The main purpose of the ICN is to provide a mean through which the national associations can share their interest in the promotion of health and care of the sick.

Functions

- To promote the development of strong national nurses associations.
- To assist national nurses association to improve the standards of nursing and the competencies of nurses.
- To assist national nurses associations to improve the status of nurses within their countries.
- To serve as the authoritative voice for nurse and nursing internationally.

The International Council of Nurses is the global voice of nursing. The governing body of the ICN is the council of national representative which is made up of the ICN Honorary officers and the presidents of the national members associations.

Trained Nurses' Association of India (TNAI) (Fig. 20.4)

In 1937, the TNAI adopted the Nurses' Charter, which formed the basis for TNAI'S representations to government and other

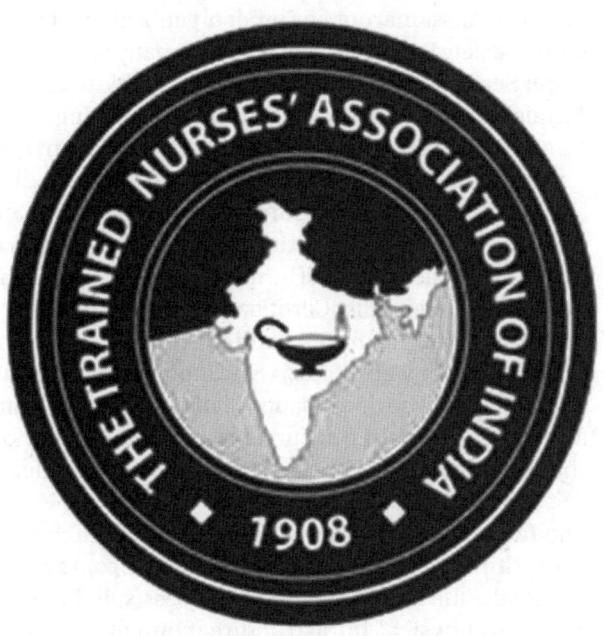

Fig. 20.4: Trained Nurses' Association of India.

employing authorities on vital matters, such as upgrading, development and standardization of nursing education (Basic and Post basic), improvement of living and service conditions for nurses throughout India and registration of qualified nurses.

Sustained efforts of the TNAI also brought about the constitution of the Indian Nursing Council and also State Nursing Councils, which established a uniform system of nursing education in the country and nurses qualified from recognized institutions could practice in any part of the country. The Indian Nursing Council Act was passed by an ordinance on December 31, 1947. The council was established in 1949.

Objectives

Upholding every way the:
- Dignity and honor of the nursing profession
- Promoting a sense of esprit de corps among all nurses
- To advance professional, educational, economic and general welfare of nurses

Functions

- To enunciate standards of nursing education and implement these through appropriate channels.
- To establish standards and qualifications for nursing practice.
- To enunciate standards of nursing service and implement these through appropriate channels.
- To establish a code of ethical conduct for practitioners.
- To stimulate and promote research designed to enhance the knowledge for evidence-based nursing practice.
- To promote legislation and to speak for nurses in regard to legislative action.
- To promote and protect the economic welfare of nurses.
- To provide professional counseling and placement service for nurses.
- To provide for the continuing professional development of practitioners.
- To represent nurses and serve as their spoke person with allied national and international organizations, governmental and other bodies and the public.
- To serve as the official representative of the Nurses of India as a member of the International Council of Nurses.
- To promote the general health and welfare of the public through the association programs, relationships and activities, e.g., Disaster Management.
- To render care as per the changing needs of the society.

Standardization of Nursing Education

- In the early days, TNAI assisted in the formulation of basic nursing curricula and, in later years, the association was instrumental in promoting the establishment of degree courses and post-certificate programmers in teaching and administration. As early is 1933, an Education Committee was appointed.
- The Committee of Nurses appointed through the TNAI to advise the Bhore Committee (The Health Survey and Planning Committee, 1941–1944) took up again the question of establishing degree courses which were accepted by the government.
- The colleges of nursing were established in Delhi and Vellore (Tamil Nadu) in 1946.
- The recent educational activities of the association are conducting educational conferences and workshops.
- Various conferences and workshops were organized on various nursing topics from time to time by TNAI.

Service Condition for Nurses

- The association is officially recognized by the government of India as a service organization.
- The voice of the association is accepted as the voice of nurses in India, and the resolutions adopted by it and presented to the various authorities, are well received and generally accepted for implementation, sooner or later.

ORGANIZATION OF ANM PROGRAM

Auxiliary Nurse Midwife (ANM) is one and a half years (18 months) of certificate level course offered by various prominent institutions in India. The course makes aspirants familiar with the ways through which they can take care of the health-related problems of sick, injured, recovering mothers, newborn mentally challenged and old people. The course also provide knowledge regarding setting up the equipment of an operation theater, providing medication, maintaining health records of patients and other routine jobs. The selection is done on the basis of merit in qualifying examination. After an Auxiliary Nurse Midwife (ANM) certificate, one can always opt for higher studies or can consider pursuing career in related field. Check out the list of colleges offering ANM.

Aim of the Program

- Prepare nurses with a sound educational program in nursing to enable them to function as efficient members of the health team.
- Help nurses develop an ability to cooperate and coordinate with members of the health team in the prevention of disease, promotion of health and rehabilitation of the sick.
- Serve as a base for further professional education and specialization in nursing.
- Understanding healthcare.
- Understanding the basic symptoms of ailments
- Understanding the preventive measures to be taken
- Tackle emergency situation and handle the patients effectively
- Assist the doctors and nurses in emergency
- Prepare the patients to undergo necessary treatments
- Be selfless for the cause of medical care and attention
- Educate common people about misconceptions and approach then with proven facts and figures.

Objectives of the Program

- To help in understanding the principles of healthful living related to all age groups in the community.
- To help society deal in basic healthcare activities in community and institutional settings.
- Importance of nutrition and health education activities in the home, clinic and community.
- Explain and understand basic material and child healthcare including immunization services, family healthcare, and family planning services.
- Develop skills in first-aid and emergency nursing care, elementary medical care including treatment of minor ailments.
- Lead and motivate as a responsible member of the health team.
- To understand and develop community resources which could be utilized for health promotion, health maintenance, and prevention of disease.
- Develop training module for the training of community/village level health worker.
- Promote community development activities
- Education people and self and environmental sanitation
- To perform basic healthcare activities in assigned role.
- Planning and also to carry them out about health and nutrition for mother and child
- Provide immunization services, family healthcare and family planning services
- Work towards societal development, prevent communicable diseases and keep a health environment.

Guidelines Establishing New School

Guidelines for establishment of new auxiliary nurse and midwives.

School of Nursing

- Any organization under: (i) Central Government/State Government/Local body (ii) Registered Private or Public Trust (iii) Missionary or any other organization registered under Society Registration Act (iv) Company incorporated under Section 25 of company's act are eligible to establish Auxiliary Nurse and Midwives School of Nursing.
- Above organization shall obtain the Essentiality Certificate/No Objection Certificate for the Auxiliary Nurse and Midwives Program from the respective State Government. The institution name along with Trust Deed/Society address shall be mentioned in No Objection Certificate/Essentiality Certificate.
- An application form to establish Nursing Program is available on the website viz., www.indiannursingcouncil.org, which shall be downloaded. Duly filled in application form with the requisite documents mentioned in the form shall be submitted before the last date as per the calendar of events of that year.
- The Indian Nursing Council on receipt of the proposal from the Institution to start nursing program, will undertake the **first inspection** to assess suitability with regard to physical infrastructure, clinical facility and teaching faculty in order to give permission to start the program.
- After the receipt of the permission to start, the nursing program from Indian Nursing Council, the institution shall obtain the approval from the State Nursing Council and Examination Board.
- Institution will admit the students only after taking approval of State Nursing Council and Examination Board.

Minimum requirement to establish auxiliary nurse and midwives Program for 40–60 students

Physical Facilities

Sl. No.	Teaching block	Area: Sq/ft
1.	Staff room	500
2.	Faculty room	1200
3.	Classroom	2 × 1080 = 2160
4.	Nursing laboratory	1500
5.	Nutrition laboratory	900
6.	Library cum study	1200
7.	Audio-visual aids	600
8.	Provision for toilets	500
9.	Multipurpose hall	1500
	Total	10060 sq/ft

Hostel Block

Sl. No.	Hostel block	Area: Sq/ft
1.	Double room	12000
2.	Sanitary	One bathroom and one latrine (for 5 students—500
3.	Visitor room	250
4.	Reading room	125
5.	Store	250

Sl. No.	Hostel block	Area: Sq/ft
6.	Recreation room	250
7.	Dining hall	1500
8.	Kitchen and store	750
9.	Total	15625 sq/ft

Grand total: 10060 + 15625 = 25685 sq/ft

Note:
1. Nursing educational institution should be in institutional area only and not in residential area.
2. If the institute has non-nursing program in the same building, nursing program should have separate teaching block.
3. Shift-wise management with other educational institutions will not be accepted.
4. Separate teaching block shall be available if it is in hospital premises.
5. School and college of nursing can share laboratories, if they are in same campus under same name and under same trust, that is the institution is one but offering different nursing programs. However, they should have equipment and articles proportionate to the strength of admission. And the class rooms should be available as per the requirement stipulated by Indian Nursing Council of each program.

- **School building:** There should be separate building/block for the school and hostel. It should have an open space to facilitate outdoor games for the students.
- **Office:** There should be individual furnished office rooms for—Principal, Teachers, and Clerical Staff. A separate telephone connection for the school is necessary.
- **Class-room:** There should be two adequately large classrooms, accommodating required number of students (i.e., for 20-40 students size of the room should be 720 sq ft). Rooms should be well ventilated and properly lighted. There should be chairs with arms or desks according to the number required. Suitably placed black/green or white board should be available in the classrooms.
- **Nursing laboratory:** There should be a demonstration room with at least two to four beds and adequate number of cupboards with necessary articles for demonstration. Provision should be made for community, midwifery and first aid demonstration and practice.
- **Nutrition laboratory:** There should be provision for nutrition practical. Cooking gas, stove and wash basin with tap connections, suitable working tables and sufficient number of necessary utensils for conducting cooking classes should be available.
- **Library-cum-study:** There should be a room of adequate size in order to accommodate 40 students at a time, with sufficient number of cupboards, library books and adequate number of chairs and tables for the students. Library should have updated edition of textbooks, referral books, few professional journals and general knowledge magazines as well as storybooks, etc., in sufficient numbers.
- **Audio-visual aid:** School must have a TV, DVD player, an overhead projector, LCD projector, laptop for projection computer facility, models, charts, skeleton and manikin/simulators, neonatal resuscitation equipment, home visiting bags, delivery kits, etc.
- **Toilets:** There should be adequate toilets facility in the school building for the students and teachers at least in the ratio 1:10.
- **Garage:** There should be a garage for the mini bus.

Nursing Teaching Faculty

Teaching faculty for 20-40 annual admission:

Sl. No.	Teaching faculty	Qualifications and experience
1.	Principal	MSc Nursing with 3 years of teaching experience or BSc Nursing with 5 years of teaching experience.
2.	Nursing tutor	BSc Nursing/Diploma in Nursing Education and Administration/Diploma in Public Health Nursing with 2 years of Clinical experience.

Note: Teacher student ratio should be 1:10 on sanctioned strength of students (excluding tutor for interns).

Clinical Facilities

- A Rural Hospital (RH) having minimum bed strength of 30 and maximum 50 and serving an area with community health programs.
- Affiliated to district hospital or a secondary care hospital with minimum 150 beds, in order to provide adequate maternity, childcare and basic medical surgical experiences. The hospital to have adequate number of trained nursing staff round the clock. Bed occupancy on the average to be between 60-70%.
- An organization having a hospital with 150 beds with minimum 30-50 obstetrics and gynecology beds, and 100 delivery cases monthly can also open Auxiliary Nurse and Midwives school. They should also have an affiliation of PHC/CHC for the community health nursing field experience.

Note: Pollution control Board certification wherein beds of the hospital are mentioned for both affiliated and parent hospital to be submitted.

Roles and Responsibilities

Box 20.2 describes role of auxiliary nurse midwife.
- Health is a fundamental human right. Maintenance of optimum level of health entails individual as well as social responsibility. However, health can never be adequately protected by health services without active involvement of the community.
- Indian Nursing Council (INC) believes that ANM plays a vital role in the rural healthcare delivery system. She should be sensitive and accountable to meet the health needs of the community. She should be able to provide accessible, equitable, affordable and quality healthcare. ANM can act as a catalyst for promoting intersectoral convergence in promotive and preventive healthcare.
- ANM curriculum intends to prepare skilled and effective female health workers to achieve the goals of National Rural Health Mission which aims at bringing about dramatic improvement in the health system and health status of the country.

Box 20.2: Roles of ANM.
- Education about prevailing health problems and method of preventing and controlling
- Promotion of food supply and proper nutrition
- An adequate supply of safe water and basic sanitation
- Maternal and child healthcare, including family **planning**
- Immunization against infectious diseases
- Prevention and control of endemic diseases
- Appropriate treatment of common diseases and injuries
- Provision of essential drugs

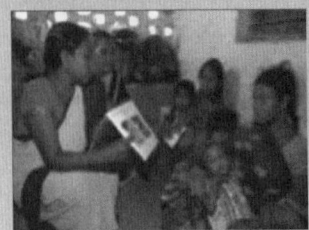
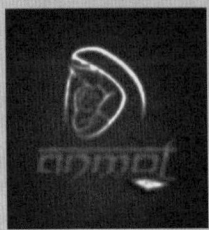

- ANM in community health skills to practice healthcare at a defined level of proficiency in accordance with local conditions and to meet local needs. Further, the program fits into the general educational pattern as well as nursing education system.

ORGANIZATION OF GNM PROGRAM

General nursing and midwifery, popularly known as GNM, is a diploma course offered in many nursing colleges across India. The course is aimed at producing competent nurses. It is a divine service to humanity and is considered one of the prestigious courses. After pursuing GNM course, one can work as nurse in private/government hospitals, nursing homes, clinics or serve in community health services, especially in rural areas. Working as home nurse is also a bright option, after doing GNM. The course is taught to develop an aptitude for nursing and to provide the required knowledge and skills, to make the nurses capable of providing proper medical care to patients suffering from any type of illness.

Philosophy

The Indian Nursing Council believes that the basic course in nursing is a formal educational preparation which should be based on sound education principles. The council recognizes that the program as the foundation on which the practice of nursing is built and on which depends further professional education. It also recognizes its responsibility to the society for the continued development of student as individual nurse and citizens.

Purpose

- The purpose of general nursing program is to prepare general nurse who will function as member of the health team beginning with competence for first level position in both hospital and community.
- The program is generated to the health needs of the society, the community and the individual and will assist nurses in their personal and professional development so that they may take their maximum contribution to the society as individual citizens and nurses.

Aims of GNM Program

The aims of the Diploma in General Nursing and Midwifery Program are:
- To prepare nurses with a sound educational program in nursing to enable them to function as efficient members of the health team, beginning with the competencies for first level positions in all kinds of healthcare settings.
- To help nurses develop and ability to cooperate and coordinate with member of the health team in the prevention of disease, promotion of health and rehabilitation of the sick.
- To help nurses in their personal and professional development, so that they are able to make maximum contribution to the society as useful and productive individuals, citizens as well as efficient nurses.
- To serve as a base for further professional education and specialization in nursing.
- To prepare nurses to keep pace with latest professional and technological developments and use these for providing nursing care services.

Objectives of GNM Program

The nurse on completion of this course will be able to:
- Demonstrate competency in providing healthcare to individual, sick or well, using nursing process.
- Assess the nursing need of clients from birth to death.
- Plan and carry out appropriate action to meet nursing needs.
- Provide effective nursing care for maintaining best possible level of health in all aspects.
- Promote self-care in people under their care.
- Apply problem solving techniques in nursing practice.
- Evaluate effectiveness of nursing care.
- Apply knowledge from the humanities, biological and behavioral sciences in functioning as a nurse.
- Function effectively with members of the health team and community applying the knowledge of human relations and communication skills in her work.
- Participate as member of the health team in delivery of curative preventive, promotive and rehabilitative healthcare services.
- Mobilize community resources and their involvement in working with the communities.
- Demonstrate use of ethical values in their personal and professional life.
- Demonstrate interest in activities of professional organizations.
- Recognize the need of continuing education for professional development.
- Demonstrate basic skills in teaching patients and giving nursing care to them.
- Demonstrate basic skills in administration and leadership while working with other members of health team and community.
- Assist in research activities

Student's Admission

- Age for the entrance shall be 17–35 years, provided they meet the minimum educational requirement ie 12 years of schooling.
- Minimum education all students should pass 12 classes or its equivalent, preferably with science subjects
- Admission of students shall be once a year.
- Students should be medically fit.

The selection committee should comprise tutors, nurse administrators, and educationalist/psychologist. The principal of the school shall be the chairperson.

Guidelines and Minimum Requirements to Establish School of Nursing

Guidelines for establishment of New General Nursing and Midwifery:

School of Nursing

- Any organization under: (i) Central Government/State Government/Local body, (ii) Registered Private or Public Trust, (iii) Missionary or any other organization registered under Society Registration Act, (iv) Company incorporated under Section 25 of company's act are eligible to establish General Nursing and Midwifery School of Nursing.
- Any organization having 100-bedded Parent (Own) hospital is eligible to establish General Nursing Course.
- Above organization shall obtain the Essentiality Certificate/No Objection Certificate for the General Nursing and Midwifery Program from the respective State Government. The institution name along with Trust Deed/Society address shall be mentioned in No Objection Certificate/Essentiality Certificate.
- An application form to establish nursing program is available on the website viz., www.indiannursingcouncil.org, which shall be downloaded. Duly filled in application form with the requisite documents mentioned in the form shall be submitted before the last date as per the calendar of events of that year.
- The Indian Nursing Council on receipt of the proposal from the Institution to start nursing program, will undertake the first inspection to assess suitability with regard to physical infrastructure, clinical facility and teaching faculty in order to give permission to start the program.
- After the receipt of the permission to start the nursing program from Indian Nursing Council, the institution shall obtain the approval from the State Nursing Council and Examination Board.
- Institution will admit the students only after taking approval of State Nursing Council and Examination Board.

Minimum requirement to establish General Nursing and Midwifery Program.

Physical Facilities

- The School of Nursing has a separate building. If the school is situated in hospital premises, the area marked for the building of the school should be at a suitable distance from hospital which enables a calm environment ideally required for a school.
- Minimum land area recommended by INC for a school of nursing is four acres of land owned and possessed by the applicant to set up the proposed nursing school. For a school with an annual admission capacity of 20 students, the constructed area of the school should be 4000 square feet.
- For every additional 10 seats, an additional constructed area can be increased.
- Constructed area is increased in a phased manner between first and second year.

Teaching Block

- The School of Nursing should have a separate building/teaching block. For a school with an annual admission capacity of 40–60 students, the constructed area of the School should be 23720 square feet.
- The School of Nursing can be in a rented/leased building for first two years.
- After two years, institute shall have own building in an institutional area.
- Otherwise ₹ 3 lakh penalty has to be paid for every year for 3 years. During the penalty period if the institute is not able to construct own building the permission/suitability will be withdrawn and will be taken as a fresh proposal.
- Adequate hostel/residential accommodation for students and staff should be available in addition to the above mentioned built up area of the Nursing School respectively.

The details of the constructed area are given below for admission capacity of 40–60 students:

Sl. No.	Teaching block	Area: Sq/ft
1.	Lecture hall	4 × 1080 = 4320
2.	Nursing foundation	1500
	CHN	900
	Nutrition	900
	OBG and pediatrics	900
	Preclinical science laboratory	900
	Computer laboratory	1500
3.	Multipurpose hall	3,000
4.	Common room (male and female)	1100
5.	Staff room	1000
6.	Principal room	300
7.	Vice principal	200
8.	Library	2400
9.	AV aids room	600
10.	One room for each head of the departments	800

Sl. No.	Teaching block	Area: Sq/ft
11.	Faculty room	2400
12.	Provisions for toilets	1000
	Total	23720 sq/ft

Note:
1. Nursing educational institution should be in Institutional area only and not in residential area.
2. If the institute has non-nursing program in the same building, Nursing program should have separate teaching block.
3. Shift-wise management with other educational institutions will not be accepted.
4. Separate teaching block shall be available if it is in hospital premises.
5. Proportionately, the size of the built-up area will increase according to the number of students admitted.
6. School and College of Nursing can share laboratories, if they are in same campus under same name and under same trust, i.e., the institution is one but offering different nursing programs. However, they should have equipment and articles proportionate to the strength of admission. And the classrooms should be available as per the requirement stipulated by Indian Nursing Council of each program.

- **Classrooms:** There should be at least four classrooms with the capacity of accommodating the number of students admitted in each class. The rooms should be well ventilated with proper lighting system. There should be built in black/green/white boards. Also there should be a desk/dais/a big table and a chair for the teacher and racks/cupboards for keeping teaching aids or any other equipment needed for the conduct of classes also should be there.
- **Laboratories:** There should be at least six laboratories as listed below:

Sl. No.	Laboratories
1.	Nursing foundation laboratory
2.	Community health nursing practice laboratory
3.	Nutrition laboratory
4.	Computer laboratory
5.	OBG and pediatric laboratory
6.	Preclinical sciences laboratory

- **Auditorium:** Auditorium should be spacious enough to accommodate at least double the sanctioned/actual strength of students, so that it can be utilized for hosting functions of the college, educational conferences/workshops, examinations, etc. It should have proper stage with green room facilities. It should be well-ventilated and have proper lighting system. There should be arrangements for the use of all kinds of basic and advanced audio-visual aids.
- **Multipurpose hall:** It should have multipurpose hall, if there is no auditorium in the school.
- **Library:** There should be a separate library in the school. It should be easily accessible to the teaching faculty and the students. It should have comfortable seating arrangements for half of the total strength of the students and teachers in the school. There should be separate budget for the library. The library committee should med regularly for keeping the library updated with current books, journals and other literature.
  - The library should have proper lighting facilities and it should be well-ventilated. It should have a cabin for librarian with intercom phone facility.
  - There should be sufficient number of cupboards, books shelves and racks with glass doors for proper and safe storage of books, magazines, journals, newspapers and other literature.
  - There should be provision for catalogue-cabinets, book display racks, bulletin boards and stationery items, such as index cards, borrower's cards, labels and registers.
  - Current books, magazines, journals, newspaper and other literature should be available in the library.
  - A minimum of 500 single titled nursing books (all new editions), in the multiple of floor, 3 kinds of nursing journals, 3 kinds of magazines, 2 kinds of newspapers and other kinds of current health-related literature should be available in the library.
- **Offices requirements**
  - **Principal's office:** There should be a separate office for the Principal with attached toilet and provision for visitor's room. Independent telephone facility is a must for the Principal's office with intercom facility connected/linked to the hospital and hostel.
  - **Office for Vice-principal:** There should be a separate office for the Vice-principal with attached toilet and provision for visitor's room. Independent telephone facility is a must for Vice-principal's office with intercom facility connected/linked to the hospital and hostel.
  - **Office for faculty members:** There should be adequate number of office rooms in proportion to the number of teaching faculty. One office room should accommodate **two** teachers only. Separate toilet facility should be provided for the teaching faculty with hand washing facility. There should be a separate toilet for male teachers.
  - One separate office room for the office staff should be provided with adequate toilet facility. This office should be spacious enough to accommodate the entire office staff with separate cabin for each official.
    Each office room should be adequately furnished with items, such as tables, chairs, cupboards, built-in racks and shelves, filing cabinets and book cases. Also there should be provision for typewriters, computers and telephone.
- **Common rooms:** A minimum of **three** common rooms should be provided. One for the teaching faculty, one for the student and one for the office staff.
  Sufficient space with adequate seating arrangements, cupboards, lockers, cabinets, built-in-shelves and racks should be provided in all the common rooms. Toilet and hand washing facilities should be made available in each room.
- **Record room:** There should be a separate record room with steel racks, built-in shelves and racks, cupboards

and filing cabinets for proper storage of records and other important papers/documents belonging to the college.

- **Store room:** A separate store room should be provided to accommodate the equipment and other inventory articles which are required in the laboratories of the college. This room should have the facilities for proper and safe storage of these articles and equipment like cupboards, built-in-shelves, racks, cabinets, furniture items like tables and chairs. This room should be properly lighted and well-ventilated.
- **Room for audio-visual aids:** This room should be provided for the proper and safe storage of all the audio-visual aids. The school should possess all kind of basic as well as advanced training aids, such as chalk boards, overhead projectors, slide and film-strip projector, models specimen, charts and posters, TV and VCR, photostat machine, tape recorder and computers.
- **Other facilities:** Safe drinking water and adequate sanitary/toilet facilities should be available for both men and women separately in the school. Toilet facility to the students should be in the ratio of 1:25 students is to be made available for students along with hand washing facility. There should be a separate toilet for men.
- **Garage:** Garage should accommodate a 50 seater vehicle.
- **Fire extinguisher:** Adequate provision for extinguishing fire should be available as per the local bye-laws.
- **Playground:** Playground should be spacious for outdoor sports, such as volleyball, football, badminton and for athletics.

Hostel Block

Hostel provision is mandatory and shall also be owned by the institute within the period of two years.

Sl. No.	Hostel block	Area: Sq/ft
1.	Single room/double room	24,000
2.	Sanitary	One bathroom and one latrine (for 5 students—500
3.	Visitor room	500
4.	Reading room	250
5.	Store	500
6.	Recreation room	500
7.	Dining hall	3000
8.	Kitchen and store	1500
9.	Total	30750 sq/ft

Grand total (total requirement for the nursing program): –23720 (Teaching block) + 30750 (Hostel block) = 54470 sq/ft

Hostel facilities: There should be a separate hostel for the male and female students. It should have the following facilities:

- **Hostel room:** It should be ideal for two students. The furniture provided should include a cot, a table, a chair, a book rack, a cupboard and a cloth rack for each student.
- **Toilet and bathroom:** Toilet and bathroom facilities should be provided on each floor of the student's hostel at the rate of one toilet and one bathroom for 2-6 students. Geysers in bathroom and wash basins should also be provided.
- **Recreation:** There should be facilities for indoor and outdoor games. There should be provision for TV, radio and video cassette player.
- **Visitor's room:** There should be a visitor room in the hostel with comfortable seating, lighting and toilet facilities.
- **Kitchen and dining hall:** There should be a hygienic kitchen and dining hall to seat at least 80% of the total students strength at one time with adequate tables, chairs, water coolers, refrigerators and heating facilities. Hand washing facilities must be provided.
- **Pantry:** One pantry on each floor should be provided. It should have water cooler and heating arrangements.
- **Washing and ironing room:** Facility for drying and ironing clothes should be provided in each floor.
- **Sick room:** A sick room should have a comfortable bed, linen, furniture and attached toilet. Minimum of five beds should be provided.
- **Room for night duty nurses:** Should be in a quiet area.
- **Guest room:** A guest room should be made available.
- **Warden's room:** Warden should be provided with a separate office room besides her residential accommodation.
- **Canteen:** There should be provision for a canteen for the students, their guests, and all other staff members.
- **Transport:** School should have separate transport facility under the control of the Principal. 25 and 50 seats bus is preferable.
- **Residential accommodation:** Residential family accommodation for faculty, should be provided, according to their marital status. Telephone facility for the Principal at her residence must be provided. Residential accommodation with all facilities is to be provided to the Hostel Warden.
- **Crèche:** There should be a crèche in the college campus.
- **Staff for the hostel:**
  - Warden (Female)—3: Qualification—BSc Home Science or Diploma in Housekeeping/Catering. Minimum three wardens must be there in every hostel for morning, evening and night shifts. If number of students are more than 150, one more warden/Asst. Warden/House keeper for every additional 50 students.
  - Cook—1: For every 20 students for each shift.
  - Kitchen and dining room helper—1—for every 20 students for each shift.
  - Sweeper—3
  - Gardener—2
  - Security Guard/Chowkidar—3

Nursing Teaching Faculty

Qualification of teaching staff for General Nursing and Midwifery Program with 40 students intake:

Sl. No.	Teaching faculty	Qualifications and experience	No required
1.	Principal	MSc Nursing with 3 years of teaching experience or BSc Nursing with 5 years of teaching experience	1
2.	Vice-Principal	MSc Nursing or BSc Nursing (Basic)/Post Basic with 3 years of teaching experience	1
3.	Nursing tutor	MSc Nursing or BSc Nursing (Basic/Post Basic) or Diploma in Nursing Education and Administration with 2 years of professional experience	10
4.	Additional tutors for interns	MSc Nursing or BSc Nursing (Basic/Post Basic) or Diploma in Nursing Education and Administration with 2 years of professional experience	2
		Total	14

Note: Teacher student ratio should be 1:10 on sanctioned strength of students (excluding tutor for interns).

External Lecturers

- Besides the regular teaching faculty in the school of nursing, there should be provision for external lecturers for teaching the students.
- They should possess the desired qualifications in the respective subjects which are to be taught.
- Remuneration of these external lecturers may comprise of nursing experts, Medical Faculty and Scientists, General Educationists including teaching experts in English, Computer Education.
- Physical examination/Yoga, psychologists, sociologists, Hospital Dieticians, Nursing Service personnel, such as Nursing Superintendent, Ward-In-Charge or Ward Sister, Health Economists/Statistician, etc., working in or outside the institution.

Clinical Facilities

- There must be a parent hospital for providing practical experience to the students
- The parent hospital should have a minimum of 250 functional beds with daily of not less than 75% occupancy for an admission of 20 students per year. There should be out patient department, casualty department, operating rooms, central sterile supply department and incinerator in the hospital
- The parent hospital should provide the clinical learning experience required for the students in the areas of medical, surgical, pediatrics, eye, ENT, maternity, gynecology and orthopedic nursing.

There should be a variety of patients of age groups in all the clinical areas where the students are posted for obtaining the request the learning experience.

School of nursing should have a 100 bedded parent (own hospital) for 40-60 annual intakes in each program:

- **Distribution of beds in different areas:** Medical—30, surgical—30, obstetrics and gynecology—30, pediatrics 20, ortho—10

- **The size of the hospital/nursing home for affiliation:**
  - Should not be less than 100 beds apart from having own hospital.
  - Maximum three Hospital can be attached.
- **Bed occupancy** of the Hospital should be minimum 75%.
- **Other specialties**/Facilities for clinical experience required are as follows:
  - Major OT, Minor OT, Dental, Eye/ENT, Burns and Plastic, Neonatology with Nursery, Communicable disease, Community Health Nursing, Cardiology, Oncology, Neurology/Neuro-surgery, Nephrology, etc., ICU/ICCU
- Affiliation of psychiatric hospital should be of minimum 30–50 beds.
- The nursing staffing norms in the affiliated hospital should be as per the INC norms.
- The affiliated hospital should give student status to the candidates of the nursing program.
- Affiliated hospitals should be in the radius of 15–30 km.
- 1:3 student patient ratio to be maintained.

If the institution is having both General Nursing and Midwifery and BSc(N) Program, it would require affiliated hospital for 40-60 annual intake in each program to maintain 1:3 student patient ratio.

Note: *Parent Hospital*—The same trust which has established nursing institution and has also established the hospital will be considered as "Parent Hospital" of that institute.

Affiliation

If all the required learning experience is not available in the parent hospital, the students should be sent to affiliated hospitals/agencies/institutions where it is available.

Criteria for affiliation: The types of experiences for which a nursing school can affiliate are:

- Community health nursing
- Communicable diseases
- Mental health (Psychiatric) nursing
- Specialties, such as cardiology, neurology oncology, nephrology, etc.

The physical facilities, staffing and equipment of the affiliated hospitals should be of the same standard as required in the parent hospitals.

The staff of the selected hospitals should be prepared to recognize student status and their educational program.

Distribution of beds: At least one third of the total no of beds should be for medical patients and one third for surgical patients. The number of beds for male patients should be less than 1/6th of the total number of beds, i.e., at least 40 beds. There should be minimum of 750 deliveries per year (for annual admission capacity of 20 students). Provision should be made for maternity clinics, child health and family welfare services and for preventive social medicine.

Internal Assessment

- There shall be 25% internal assessment for all the theory papers and 50% internal assessment for all the practicals.

- A regular and periodic assessment for each subject and clinical/field experiences is to be carried out.
- For the purpose of internal assessment there shall be written test in each subject taken by the respective teacher each month.

    The student shall be required to maintain the practical record book and report of observation visits and diary for assessment by the teachers concerned, various other techniques for assessment must be also used. Marks shall be allotted for each of the following: (a) Case study, (b) Case presentation, (c) Nursing care plan, (d) Maintenance of record books (procedure book and midwifery record book), (e) Daily diary, (f) Area wise clinical assessment is to be carried out. Minimum two assessments are required in each clinical area.
- Regular record of theory and practical is to be maintained. Task-oriented assessment is to be undertaken. Assessment shall be maintained by teacher for each student each month. This can be checked by the council/board principal shall sign all the records of examination of the students.
- A candidate must secure 50% marks in internal assessment separately in each theory and practical. To be successful a student must get 50% marks in the internal as well as council or board examination of each year.
- For each student who appears for much supplementary examination her/his fresh internal assessment in the failed subject (s) practical (s) is to be sent to the council/board.
- State nursing council/board should prepare a model perform for performance evaluation for each of the clinical area and circulate to all; schools of nursing for maintaining uniformity.

Examinations for ANMs/LHVs/FHWs

These candidates will appear for all the examination in theory and practical's as per the scheme of examination for other candidates.

I. Eligibility for Admission to Examination

A candidate shall be eligible for the admission to the state council/board examination if the principal of the school certifies that:
- She/he has completed not less than eleven month of the course
- She/he has attended 75% of the formal instructions given on each subject and 75% of the clinical field experience in each area/subject separately during the academic year. However, the total clinical/field experience prescribed must be completed before the final council/board examinations and before the issue of diploma. (The diploma shall not be awarded to the student till she/he has completed the clinical field requirements).
- The overall performance of the student and her/his conduct during the entire academic year has been satisfactory.
- The student has passed in the internal assessment in each subject, i.e., both in the teaching and practical (5) by securing 50% marks separate in each theory and practical (s).
- The record of practical experience is complete (the principal shall send to the council/board the internal assessment for each subject, i.e., both theory and practical (s) before the start of the examination along with the examination form).
- ANM/LHV/FHW who have been exempted for six months during third year will be eligible for third year examination after completion of six months training.

II. Supplementary Examination

The council shall conduct supplementary examination within six months of the annual examination:
- If a student fails in one theory paper/practical. She/he may be allowed to proceed to the next year of study. She/he will sit for a supplementary examination held subsequently in the failed subject/practical. If she/he fails to clear supplementary examination she/he shall be allowed to sit again along with her next year annual examination.
- If a student fails in two or more papers or practical she/he will not be allowed to proceed to the next year. She/he shall sit for supplementary examination in the failed subjects/practicals only but shall be eligible for the next year's examination after one academic year from the date of passing the last examination.
- No candidate for category (a) shall be allowed to proceed to third year (higher class), unless she/he has passed in the subjects of the previous year (backlog to the second year).
- If a student fails in one theory paper/practical examination of the third year, she/he may be allowed to proceed for internship. She/he will sit for supplementary examination held subsequently in the failed subject/practical.
- If a student fails in two or more papers/practical's she/he will not be allowed to proceed for internship. She/he shall sit for supplementary examination in the failed subjects/practical's only. A student shall not be allowed to proceed for internship till he/she clears third year examination.

III. Grading of Examination

Examination shall be graded on aggregate marks of the entire three and a half years of the training program, as follows:
- Distinction 80% and above
- First division 70–79%
- Second division 60–69%
- Pass 50–59%.

IV. Theory Examination

- Nursing teacher with minimum of 5 years of teaching experience (recent) in a particular subject may be appointed as paper setters and examiners for that particular subject only.
- Question papers should have a combination of essay, short answer and objective type question (situation-based questions)

- All units of a subject and sub subject should be given due weight age in accordance with the instructional hours prescribed.

V. Practical Examination

- Practical examination is to be conducted in the respective clinical area.
- Nursing teacher with minimum of five years of teaching/clinical teaching experience (recent) in a particular subject/clinical area may be appointed as practical examiner.
- Not more than 10 to 15 students are to be examined in a day.
- Internal and external examiner shall jointly evaluate each candidate for practical examination.

Internship Period

General Objectives

Upon completion of the internship period the period shall be able to:
- Demonstrate skills in the discharge of professional responsibilities independently and effectively.
- Demonstrate beginning skills in teaching patients/client in healthcare setting and nursing student in clinical setting in an effective manner.
- Demonstrate beginning skills in administration and management of nursing units, health clinics and health centers
- Assist/participate in research activities of the institution/organization in various healthcare settings.
- Identify and participate the needs for continuing and in service education in practice of nursing.
  Details of internship period:
  - Total duration—26 weeks/6 months
  - Vacation—1 week
  - Examination—1 week
  - For the remaining 24 weeks students will be posted in different clinical areas and also undergo formal class room instruction
  - Total working hours of each day—8
  - Hours per week—8 × 6 = 48
  - Total hours of internship period—48 × 24 = 1152
  - Total hours of theory instruction—190
  - Total hours of clinical posting—1152 – 190 = 962
  - Student shall attend one hour class daily and 7 hours for clinical experience or one day for theory and five days for clinical experience shall be planned by institutes as per their suitability which shall come to 40 hours per week clinical and 8 hours for theory.

Breakup of Clinical Experience

- Medical nursing—3 weeks
- Surgical nursing—3 weeks
- Pediatric nursing—3 weeks
- Psychiatric nursing—3 weeks
- Community health nursing—4 weeks
- Midwifery—4 weeks
- Student's area of interest—2 weeks
- Two weeks of night clinical experience is to be given during this period with night supervisor

ORGANIZATION OF BASIC-BACHELOR OF SCIENCE IN NURSING PROGRAM

The Bachelor of Science (BSc) degree in nursing is one of the career pathways to becoming a registered nurse, the largest healthcare occupation Bachelor of Science programs are offered in universities and colleges and generally take four years to complete. Students usually take general education courses in the first two years and concentrate exclusively on the science and principles of nursing in the last two years. Nursing education programs include both classroom instruction and supervised clinical experience. The BSN degree provides a strong platform for career advancement and higher-level degrees, such as a Master of Science in nursing. BSN provides more training in communication, leadership and critical thinking and offer more clinical experience in nonhospital settings than diploma or associate degree in nursing programs, and a BSN or higher degree is often necessary for administrative positions, research, consulting and teaching.

Philosophy

The philosophical foundations of the BN course is based on the values and beliefs that underpin nursing, education, primary healthcare, Indigenous health and social justice.

Objectives of BSc Nursing Program

A nurse successfully completing the undergraduate training program should be able to:
- Describe the structure and function of the human body so as to permit her to appreciate aberrations from normal and their consequences. She should be able to observe and record vital functions of the body while nursing the sick and report the effects of therapeutic measures instituted. She should also be able to assist in common investigative procedures and recognize the deviations in the results from normal.
- Function effectively as part of the team in the delivery of comprehensive healthcare in a community, hospital in urban as well as rural location. She should demonstrate competence not only in curative aspects of nursing but also in its preventive and promotive aspects for individual as well as community level.
- Administer comprehensive as well as specialized nursing care to the sick in the hospital or home environments.
- Explain the actions, side effects and indications for use of common drugs administered to the sick. She should be able to administer them in the correct dosage and by the correct method and recognize and report any toxic effects thereof.
- Provide first aid to the injured or the sick in emergency independently in the absence of a doctor. She should be able to demonstrate skill in cardiopulmonary resuscitations in hospital or home environment.

- Explain the local patterns of diseases in the country and common diseases in the country. She should be able to administer special nursing care required for the management of these diseases. She should be able to recognize the symptoms of common diseases and suggest suitable therapeutic measures for diseases, such as malaria, cholera, gastroenteritis, etc., in the absence of the availability of a doctor. She should at the same time be able to recognize her limitations and be able to decide the
- Explain the national health problems and appreciate the role of social, cultural, economic, psychological and environmental factors in the causation and control of diseases. Thus, she should be able to describe the social and environmental factors necessary to function as a public health nurse.
- Provide antenatal supervision and conduct normal deliveries at home or in the hospital. She should be able to recognize the complications during antenatal, natal or postnatal period and seek help in time from a doctor. She should be able to suggest methods for the care of the newborn infant and to the mother. She should be able to suggest and implement various measures for fertility control necessary for the family welfare and planning program and render service in this aspect at the individual as well as the community level.
- Demonstrate adequate management and supervisory skill to coordinate the proper functioning of various personnel in the ward, outpatient department, rural health centers or the community. She should be able to teach both formally and informally in clinical nursing situations and in nursing education programs.
- Assist in common operative procedure and describe the surgical aspects, techniques and be skilled in its applications. She will be able to provide high quality team support to surgeons during operative procedures by cooperative planning and coordination of functions between nursing staff, surgical staff and anesthesia staff in an effort to improve the overall care of patient in the operating room.

Eligibility for Admission

A candidate seeking admission should have:
- Pass the 2 years of pre-university exam or equivalent as recognized by concerned university with science subjects, i.e., physics, biology and chemistry.
- Students of vocational courses
- Obtained at least 45% of total marks in science subjects in the qualifying exam, if belongs to a scheduled caste or tribe, should have obtained not less than 40% of total marks in science subjects.
- Completed 17 years of age at the time of admission or will complete this age on or before 31st December of the year of admission
- Is medically fit

Guidelines and Minimum Requirements to Establish BSc(N) College of Nursing

Guidelines for establishment of New BSc(N) College of Nursing
- Any organization under: (i) Central Government/State Government/Local body, (ii) Registered Private or Public Trust, (iii) Missionary or any other organization registered under Society Registration Act, (iv) Company incorporated under Section 25 of company's Act are eligible to establish BSc(N) College of Nursing.
- Any organization having 100-bedded parent (Own) hospital is eligible to establish BSc(N) Course.
- Above organization shall obtain the Essentiality Certificate/No Objection Certificate for the BSc(N) program from the respective State Government. The institution name along with Trust Deed/Society address shall be mentioned in No Objection Certificate/Essentiality Certificate.
- An application form to establish nursing program is available on the website viz., w.w.w.indiannursingcouncil.org, which shall be downloaded. Duly filled in application form with the requisite documents mentioned in the form shall be submitted before the last date as per the calendar of events of that year.
- The Indian Nursing Council on receipt of the proposal from the Institution to start nursing program, will undertake the first inspection to assess suitability with regard to physical infrastructure, clinical facility and teaching faculty in order to give permission to start the program.
- After the receipt of the permission to start the nursing Program from Indian Nursing Council, the institution shall obtain the approval from the State Nursing Council and University.
- Institution will admit the students only after taking approval of State Nursing Council and University.
- Upgradation is not a additional BSc(N) Program, but is the convert from School of Nursing into College of Nursing.

Note: If any School of Nursing wants to upgrade to College of Nursing, essentiality Certificate for BSc(N) course is not essential, as they already possess essentiality certificate for School of Nursing. However, the private institutions have to produce document with regard to resolution of the management for upgrading the School of Nursing into College of Nursing and INC norms will be followed. The School of Nursing should have been recognized by Indian Nursing Council. Minimum requirement to establish BSc(N) Program.

Physical Facilities

Building: The College of Nursing should have a separate building. The College of Nursing should be near to its parent hospital having space for expansion in an institutional area. For a college with an annual admission capacity of 40–60 students, the constructed area of the college should be 23720 square feet.

Adequate hostel/residential accommodation for students and staff should be available in addition to the above mentioned built up area of the nursing college respectively. The details of the constructed area are given below for admission capacity of 40–60 students:

- **Classrooms:** There should be at least four classrooms with the capacity of accommodating the number of students admitted in each class.

  The rooms should be well ventilated with proper lighting system.

  There should be built in black/green/white boards. Also there should be a desk/dais/a big table and a chair for the teacher and racks/cupboards for keeping teaching aids or any other equipment needed for the conduct of classes also should be there.

  Table 20.1 describes teaching block and their area in sq/ft.

  Departments: College should have following departments:
  - Fundamentals of Nursing including Nutrition
  - Medical Surgical Nursing
  - Community Health Nursing
  - Obstetric and Gynecological Nursing
  - Child Health Nursing
  - Psychiatry and Mental Health Nursing

- **Laboratories:** There should be at least seven laboratories as listed below:

Sl. No.	Laboratories
1.	Nursing Foundation Laboratory
2.	Community Health Nursing Practice Laboratory
3.	Nutrition Laboratory
4.	Computer Laboratory
5.	OBG and Pediatric Laboratory
6.	Preclinical Sciences Laboratory (Biochemistry, Microbiology, Biophysics, Anatomy and Physiology)

- **Auditorium:** Auditorium should be spacious enough to accommodate at least double the sanctioned/actual strength of students, so that it can be utilized for hosting functions of the college, educational conferences/workshops, examinations, etc. It should have proper stage with green room facilities. It should be well-ventilated and have proper lighting system. There should be arrangements for the use of all kinds of basic and advanced audio-visual aids.

- **Multipurpose hall:** College of Nursing should have multipurpose hall, if there is no auditorium.

- **Library:** There should be a separate library for the college. The size of the Library should be of minimum 2,400 sq ft. It should be easily accessible to the teaching faculty and the students. Library should have seating arrangements for at least 60 students for reading and having good lighting and ventilation and space for stocking and displaying of books and journals. The library should have at least 3000 books. In a new College of Nursing the total number of books should be proportionately divided on yearly basis in four years. At least 10 set of books in each subject to facilitate for the students to refer the books. The number of journals should 15 out of which one-third shall be foreign journals and subscribed on continuous basis. There should be sufficient number of cupboards, book shelves and racks with glass doors for proper and safe storage of books, magazines, journals, newspapers and other literature.

Table 20.1: Teaching block.

Sl. No.	Teaching block	Area: Sq/ft
1.	Lecture hall	4 × 1080 = 4320
2.	Nursing foundation	1500
	CHN	900
	Nutrition	900
	OBG and pediatrics	900
	Preclinical science laboratory	900
	Computer laboratory	1500
3.	Multipurpose hall	3000
4.	Common room (male and female)	1100
5.	Staff room	1000
6.	Principal room	300
7.	Vice-Principal	200
8.	Library	2400
9.	AV aids room	600
10.	One room for each head of the departments	800
11.	Faculty room	2400
12.	Provisions for toilets	1000
	Total	23720 sq/ft

Note:
1. Nursing educational institution should be in institutional area only and not in residential area.
2. If the institute has non-nursing program in the same building, nursing program should have separate teaching block.
3. Shift-wise management with other educational institutions will not be accepted.
4. Separate teaching block shall be available if it is in hospital premises.
5. Proportionately, the size of the built-up area will increase according to the number of students admitted.
6. School and college of nursing can share laboratories, if they are in same campus under same name and under same trust, that is the institution is one but offering different nursing programs. However, they should have equipment and articles proportionate to the strength of admission. And the classrooms should be available as per the requirement stipulated by Indian Nursing Council of each program.

In the library, there should be provision for:
- Staff reading room for six persons.
- Rooms for librarian and other staff with intercom phone facility
- Video and cassette/CD room (desirable)
- Internet facility.

- **Offices requirements**
  - **Principal's office:** There should be a separate office for the Principal with attached toilet and provision for visitor's room. Independent telephone facility is a must for the Principal's office with intercom facility connected/linked to the hospital and hostel and a computer with internet facility. The size of the office should be 300 sq ft.

- **Office for Vice-Principal:** There should be a separate office for the Vice-Principal with attached toilet and provision for visitor's room. Independent telephone facility is a must for Vice Principal's office with intercom facility connected/linked to the hospital and hostel and a computer with internet facility. The size of the office should be 200 sq ft.
- **Office for faculty members:** There should be adequate number of office rooms in proportion to the number of teaching faculty. One office room should accommodate two teachers only. Separate toilet facility should be provided for the teaching faculty with hand washing facility. There should be a separate toilet for male teachers. The size of the room should be 200 sq ft. Separate chambers for heads of the department should be there.
- One separate office room for the office staff should be provided with adequate toilet facility. This office should be spacious enough to accommodate the entire office staff with separate cabin for each official. Each office room should be adequately furnished with items, such as tables, chairs, cupboards, built-in racks and shelves, filing cabinets and book cases. Also there should be provision for typewriters, computers and telephone.
- **Common rooms:** A minimum of three common rooms should be provided. One for the teaching faculty, one for the student and one for the office staff.

  Sufficient space with adequate seating arrangements, cupboards, lockers, cabinets, built-in-shelves and racks should be provided in all the common rooms. Toilet and hand washing facilities should be made available in each room.
- **Record room:** There should be a separate record room with steel racks, built-in shelves and racks, cupboards and filing cabinets for proper storage of records and other important papers/documents belonging to the college.
- **Store room:** A separate store room should be provided to accommodate the equipment and other inventory articles which are required in the laboratories of the college. This room should have the facilities for proper and safe storage of these articles and equipment like cupboards, built-in-shelves, racks, cabinets, furniture items like tables and chairs. This room should be properly lighted and well-ventilated.
- **Room for audio-visual aids:** This room should be provided for the proper and safe storage of size 600 sq ft for all the audio-visual aids.
- **Other facilities:** Students' welfare hall of size 400 sq ft. Indoor games hall of size 4000 ft. Safe drinking water and adequate sanitary/toilet facilities should be available for both men and women separately in the college in each floor common toilets for teachers (separate for male and female), i.e., four toilets with wash basins. Common toilets for students (separate for male and female) 12 with wash basins for 60 students.
- **Garage:** Garage should accommodate a 60 seated vehicle.
- **Fire extinguisher:** Adequate provision for extinguishing fire should be available as per the local bye-laws.
- **Playground:** Playground should be spacious for outdoor sports, such as volleyball, football, badminton and for athletics.

Hostel Block

Hostel provision is mandatory and shall also be owned by the institute within the period of two years.

Sl. No.	Hostel block	Area: Sq/ft
1.	Single room/double room	24000
2.	Sanitary	One bathroom and one latrine (for 5 students—500
3.	Visitor room	500
4.	Reading room	250
5.	Store	500
6.	Recreation room	500
7.	Dining hall	3000
8.	Kitchen and store	1500
9.	Total	30750 sq/ft

Grand Total: 23720 + 30750 = 54470 sq/ft

Note: Proportionately, the size of the built-up area will increase according to the number of students admitted.

Hostel facilities: There should be a separate hostel for the male and female students. It should have the following facilities:
- **Hostel room:** It should be ideal for 2 students with the minimum 100 sq ft carpet area. The furniture provided should include a cot, a table, a chair, a book rack, a cupboard and a cloth rack for each student.
- **Toilet and bathroom:** Toilet and bathroom facilities should be provided on each floor of the student's hostel at the rate of one toilet and one bathroom for 2–6 students. Geysers in bathroom and wash basins should also be provided.
- **Recreation:** There should be facilities for indoor and outdoor games. There should be provision for TV, radio and video cassette player.
- **Visitor's room:** There should be a visitor room in the hostel with comfortable seating, lighting and toilet facilities.
- **Kitchen and dining hall:** There should be a hygienic kitchen and dining hall to seat at least 80% of the total students strength at one time with adequate tables, chairs, water coolers, refrigerators and heating facilities. Hand washing facilities must be provided.
- **Pantry:** One pantry on each floor should be provided. It should have water cooler and heating arrangements.
- **Washing and ironing room:** Facility for drying and ironing clothes should be provided in each floor.
- **Sick room:** A sick room should have a comfortable bed, linen, furniture and attached toilet. Minimum of 5 beds should be provided.

- **Room for night duty nurses:** Should be in a quiet area.
- **Guest room:** A guest room should be made available.
- **Warden's room:** Warden should be provided with a separate office room besides her residential accommodation.
- **Canteen:** There should be provision for a canteen for the students, their guests, and all other staff members.
- **Transport:** College should have separate transport facility under the control of the Principal. 50 seated bus is preferable.

Residential accommodation: Residential family accommodation for faculty, should be provided, according to their marital status. Telephone facility for the Principal at her residence must be provided. Residential accommodation with all facilities is to be provided to the Hostel Warden.

Crèche: There should be a crèche in the college campus.

Staff for the hostel:
- Warden (Female)—3: Qualification—BSc Home Science or Diploma in Housekeeping/Catering. Minimum three wardens must be there in every hostel for morning, evening and night shifts. If number of students s more than 150, one more warden/Assistant warden/house keeper for every additional 50 students.
- Cook—1: For every 20 students for each shift.
- Kitchen and dining room helper—1: For every 20 students for each shift.
- Sweeper—3
- Gardener—2
- Security guard/chowkidar—3

Nursing Teacher Faculty

Qualifications and experience of teachers of college of nursing

Sl. No.	Post, qualifications and experiences
1.	**Principal-cum-Professor:** 15 years experience with MSc(N) out of which 12 years should be teaching experience with minimum of 5 years in collegiate program. PhD(N) is desirable
2.	**Vice-Principal-cum-Professor:** 12 years experience with MSc(N) out of which 10 years should be teaching experience with minimum of 5 years in collegiate program. PhD(N) is desirable
3.	**Professor:** 10 years experience with MSc(N) out of which 7 years should be teaching experience. PhD(N) is desirable
4.	**Associate Professor:** MSc(N) with 8 years experience including 5 years teaching experience PhD(N) desirable
5.	**Assistant Professor:** MSc(N) with 3 years teaching experience PhD(N) desirable
6.	**Tutor:** MSc(N) or BSc(N)/PBBSc(N) with 1 year experience

Sl. No.	Designation	BSc(N) 40–60 (students intake)	BSc(N) 61–100 (students intake)
1.	Principal	1	1
2.	Vice-Principal	1	1
3.	Professor	0	1
4.	Associate Professor	2	4
5.	Assistant Professor	3	6
6.	Tutor	10–18	19–28

- Principal is excluded for 1:10 teacher student ratio norms (Teacher)
- Tutor student ratio will be 1:10 (For example, for 40 students intake minimum number of teacher required is 17 including Principal. The strength of tutors will be 10, and 6 will be as per Sl. No. 2 to 5)

Sl. No.	Designation	BSc(N) 40–60 (students intake)	PBBSc(N) 20–60 (students intake)
1.	Principal	1	
2.	Vice-Principal	1	
3.	Professor	0	
4.	Associate Professor	2	
5.	Assistant Professor	3	2
6.	Tutor	10–18	2–10

Sl. No.	Designation	BSc(N) 40–60 (students intake)	PBBSc(N) 20–60 (students intake)	MSc(N) 10–25 (students intake)
1.	Principal	1		
2.	Vice-Principal	1		
3.	Professor	0		1
4.	Associate Professor	2		1
5.	Assistant Professor	3	2	3
6.	Tutor	10–18	2–10	

- 1:10 teacher student ratio for MSc(N) if BSc(N) is also offered by the institution.
- Candidates having 3 years experience after MSc(N) only will be considered for MSc(N) Program.

Sl. No.	Designation	GNM 20–60	BSc(N) 40–60 (students intake)	PBBSc(N) 20–60 (students intake)	MSc(N) 10–25 (students intake)
1.	Principal		1		
2.	Vice-Principal		1		
3.	Professor		0		1
4.	Associate Professor		2		1
5.	Assistant Professor		3	2	3
6.	Tutor	6–18	10–18	2–10	

- 1:10 teacher student ratio for MSc(N) if BSc(N) is also offered by the institution.
- Candidates having 3 years experience after MSc(N) only will be considered for MSc(N) program.

Sl. No.	Designation	ANM 20–60	GNM 20–60	BSc(N) 40–60 (students intake)	PBBSc(N) 20–60 (students intake)	MSc(N) 10–25 (students intake)
1.	Principal			1		
2.	Vice-Principal			1		
3.	Professor			0		1
4.	Associate Professor			2		1
5.	Assistant Professor			3	2	3
6.	Tutor	4–12	6–18	10–18	2–10	

- 1:10 teacher student ratio for MSc(N) if BSc(N) is also offered by the institution.
- Candidates having 3 years experience after MSc(N) only will be considered for MSc(N) Program.
- Part time Teachers/External Teachers**

Sl. No.	Part-time teachers
1.	Microbiology
2.	Biochemistry
3.	Sociology
4.	Biophysics
5.	Psychology
6.	Nutrition
7.	English
8.	Computer
9.	Regicidal language
10.	Pharmacology
11.	Physical education
12.	Genetics
13.	Pathology
14.	Statistics
15.	Physical education

- The above teachers should have postgraduate qualification with teaching experience in respective area

Note:
1. No part time nursing faculty will be counted for calculating total no. of faculty required for a college.
2. Irrespective of number of admissions, all faculty positions (Professor to Lecturer) must be filled.
3. For MSc(N) Program appropriate number of MSc faculty in each specialty be appointed subject to the condition that total number of teaching faculty ceiling is maintained.
4. All nursing teachers must possess a basic university or equivalent qualification as laid down in the schedules of the Indian Nursing Council Act, 1947. They shall be registered under the State Nursing Registration Act.
5. Nursing faculty in nursing college except tutor/clinical instructors must possess the requisite recognized postgraduate qualification in nursing subjects.
6. All teachers of nursing other than Principal and Vice-Principal should spend at least 4 hours in the clinical area for clinical teaching and/or supervision of care every day.

Other Staff (Minimum Requirements)

(To be reviewed and revised and rationalized keeping in mind the mechanization and contract service)

Ministerial

- Administrative Officer 1
- Office Superintendent 1
- PA to Principal 1
- Accountant/Cashier 1
  - Upper Division Clerk 2
  - Lower Division Clerk 2
- Store Keeper 1
  - Maintenance of stores 1
  - Classroom attendants 2
  - Sanitary staff as per the physical space
- Security staff as per the requirement
- Peons/Office attendants 4

Library

- Librarian 2
- Library attendants as per the requirement

Hostel

- Wardens 2
- Cooks, Bearers, as per the requirement
- Sanitary Staff
- Ayas/Peons as per the requirement
- Security staff as per the requirement
- Gardeners and Dhobi depends on structural facilities (desirable)

College management committee: Following members should constitute the Board of Management of the College.
- Principal Chairperson
- Vice-Principal Member
- Professor/Reader/Senior Lecturer Member
- Chief Nursing Officer/Nursing Superintendent Member
- Representative of Medical Superintendent Member

Admission/Selection Committee

This committee should comprise of:
- Principal Chairperson
- Vice-Principal
- Professor
- Chief Nursing Officer or Nursing superintendent

CLINICAL FACILITIES

College of nursing should have a 100-bedded parent hospital.
- Distribution of beds in different areas/for 40 annual intakes is: Medical 30, surgical 30 and obstetrics and gynecology 30, pediatrics 20, ortho 10
- Bed occupancy of the hospital should be minimum 75%.
- The size of the hospital/nursing home for affiliation should not be less than 100 beds
- Other specialities/facilities for clinical experience required are as follows:

- Major OT, Minor OT, Dental, Eye/ENT, Burns and Plastic, Neonatology with Nursery, Communicable disease, Community Health Nursing, Cardiology
- Oncology, Neurology/Neurosurgery, Nephrology, etc., ICU/ICCU
• Affiliation of psychiatric hospital should be of minimum 50 beds.
• The nursing staffing norms in the affiliated hospital should be as per the INC norms.
• The affiliated hospital should give student status to the candidates of the nursing program.
• Affiliated hospitals should be in the radius of 15–30 km.
• 1:3 student patient ratio to be maintained.

If the institution is having both GNM and BSc(N) Program, it would require 240-bedded parent/affiliated hospital for 40 annual intake in each program to maintain 1:3 student patient ratio.

Parent hospital: The same trust which has established nursing institutions and has also established the hospital, then only it will be considered as "Parent Hospital" of that institute.

ORGANIZATION OF PBBSc(N) PROGRAM

The post basic BSc Nursing is a three year degree program for in-service nurses. The program was launched in July 1994 and is recognized by the Indian Nursing Council (INC). There are Program Study Centers, which are existing Colleges of Nursing, already conduction Post Basic BSc Nursing Program or BSc Nursing Program. These Colleges of Nursing are recognized by the Indian Nursing Council. One program Study Center at Seychelles was also established in 2001–02. The program has been revised based on the revised syllabus of INC (2001). The post basic BSc Nursing Program comprises 108 credits (40 credits in theory and 68 credits in practical).

Philosophy and Aims of the Program

- Nursing is an integral part of the healthcare delivery system and shire responsibility in collaboration with other allied health professions for the attainment of optimal health for all members of the society.
- Education as a lifelong learning process. It seeks to render appropriate behavioral changes in students in order to facilitate their development, which assists them to live personally satisfied and socially useful lives.
- The goal of post certificate degree program leading to Bachelor of Science in nursing is the preparation of the trained nurse as a generalist who accept responsibility for enhancing the effectiveness of nursing care.

Eligibility for Admission

The candidate seeking admission must:
- Hold a certificate in general nursing.
- Be a registered nurse
- Have minimum of two years of experience. Now, it is relaxed that no experience after GNM is required for admission to this course.
- Have passed pre-university exam in the arts/science/commerce or its equivalent which is recognized the university
- Be medically fit
- Have a good personal and professional record
- Have working knowledge of English

Objectives

The goal of the post certificate program leading to the bachelor of nursing is the preparation of the trained nurses as a generaralist who accept responsibility for enhancing the effectiveness of nursing care.

- Administer high quality nursing care to all people of all ages in homes, hospitals and other community agencies in urban and rural areas.
- Apply knowledge from the physical, social and behavioral sciences in assessing the health status of individuals and make critical judgment in assessing the health status of the individuals and make critical judgment in planning, directing and evaluating primary, acute and long-term care given by themselves and others working with them.
- Investigate healthcare problems systematically
- Work collaboratively with members of other health disciplines
- Teach and counsel individuals, families and other groups about health and illness
- Understand human behavior and establish effective interpersonal relationships
- Teach in clinical nursing situations
- Identify underlying principles from the social and natural sciences and utilize them in adapting to, or initiating changes in relation to those factors
- Acquire professional knowledge and attitude in adapting for leadership role

Guidelines and Minimum Requirements to Establish Post Basic BSc(N) College of Nursing

Guidelines for additional PBBSc(N) Program in the recognized College of Nursing

- Any organization under: (i) Central Government/State Government/Local body, (ii) Registered Private or Public Trust, (iii) Missionary or any other organization registered under Society Registration Act, (iv) Company incorporated under section 25 of company's act are eligible to establish PBBSc(N) College of Nursing.
- Indian Nursing Council recognized BSc(N) College of Nursing is eligible to establish PBBSc(N) Course.
- Above organization shall obtain the Essentiality Certificate/No Objection Certificate for the PBBSc(N) Program from the respective State Government. The institution name along with Trust Deed/Society address shall be mentioned in No Objection Certificate/Essentiality Certificate.
- An application form to establish nursing program is available on the website viz., www.indiannursingcouncil.org, which shall be downloaded. Duly filled in application form with the requisite documents mentioned in the form shall be submitted before the last date as per the calendar of events of that year.

- The Indian Nursing Council on receipt of the proposal from the institution to start nursing program, will undertake the **first inspection** to assess suitability with regard to physical infrastructure, clinical facility and teaching faculty in order to give permission to start the program.
- After the receipt of the permission to start the nursing program from Indian Nursing Council, the institution shall obtain the approval from the State Nursing Council and University.
- Institution will admit the students only after taking approval of State Nursing Council and University. Minimum Requirement to establish PBBSc(N) Program.

Physical Facilities

Additional 2 (Two) Lecture Halls: 2 × 1080 = 2160 sq ft for PBBSc(N) Program for 40–60 Students intake

Note: Proportionately, the rooms and other facilities will increase according to the number of students admitted.

Nursing Teacher Faculty

Qualifications and experience of teachers of college of nursing:

Sl. No.	Post, qualifications and experiences
1.	**Principal cum Professor:** 15 years experience with MSc(N) out of which 12 years should be teaching experience with minimum of 5 years in collegiate program. PhD(N) is desirable
2.	**Vice-Principal cum Professor:** 12 years experience with MSc(N) out of which 10 years should be teaching experience with minimum of 5 years in collegiate program. PhD(N) is desirable
3.	**Professor:** 10 years experience with MSc(N) out of which 7 years should be teaching experience. PhD(N) is desirable
4.	**Associate Professor:** MSc(N) with 8 years experience including 5 years teaching experience PhD(N) desirable
5.	**Assistant Professor:** MSc(N) with 3 years teaching experience PhD(N) desirable
6.	**Tutor:** MSc(N) or BSc(N)/PBBSc(N) with 1 year experience

Sl. No.	Designation	BSc(N) 40–60 (students intake)	PBBSc(N) 20–60 (students intake)
1.	Principal	1	
2.	Vice-Principal	1	
3.	Professor	0	
4.	Associate Professor	2	
5.	Assistant Professor	3	2
6.	Tutor	10–18	2–10

Sl. No.	Designation	BSc(N) 40–60 (students intake)	BSc(N) 61–100 (students intake)
1.	Principal	1	1
2.	Vice-Principal	1	1
3.	Professor	0	1
4.	Associate Professor	2	4
5.	Assistant Professor	3	6
6.	Tutor	10–18	19–28

BSc(N) + PBBSc(N) Teacher Student Ratio = 1:10

ORGANIZATION OF MSc(N) PROGRAM

National Health Policy (NHP) 2002 emphasizes the need to prepare nurses to function in superspecialty areas who are required in tertiary care institutions, entrusting some limited public health functions to nurses after providing adequate training, and increase the ratio of degree holding vis a vis diploma holding nurses. It is observed that there is an acute shortage of nursing faculty in undergraduate and post-graduate nursing program in India.

Philosophy of MSc(N) Program

Postgraduate program is essential to prepare nurses to improve the quality of nursing education and practice in India. Postgraduate program in nursing builds upon and extends competence acquired at the graduate levels, emphasizes application of relevant theories into nursing practice, education, administration and development of research skills. The program prepares nurses for leadership position in nursing and health fields who can function as nurse specialists, consultants, educators, administrators and researchers in a wide variety of professional settings in meeting the national priorities and the changing needs of the society. This program provides the basis for the post masteral program in nursing. Further the program encourages accountability and commitment to lifelong learning which fosters improvement of quality care.

Objectives MSc(N) Program

On completion of the two year MSc Nursing Program, the graduate will be able to:
- Utilize/apply the concepts, theories and principles of nursing science
- Demonstrate advance competence in practice of nursing
- Practice as a nurse specialist
- Demonstrate leadership qualities and function effectively as nurse educator and manager.
- Demonstrate skill in conducting nursing research, interpreting and utilizing the findings from health-related research.
- Demonstrate the ability to plan and effect change in nursing practice and in the healthcare delivery system.
- Establish collaborative relationship with members of other disciplines
- Demonstrate interest in continued learning for personal and professional advancement.

Eligibility

The candidate seeking admission must:
- Have passed BSc Nursing/post certificate BSc, or nursing degree of any university
- Have a minimum of one year of experience after obtaining BSc, in hospitals or nursing educational institutions or community health setting
- For BSc, nursing post certificate, no such experience is needed after graduation the candidate shall be—a registered nurse or registered midwife for admission to medical surgical nursing, community health nursing, pediatric nursing obstetric and gynecological nursing.
- A registered nurse for admission to psychiatric nursing
- The candidate shall be selected on merit judged on the basis of academic performances in BSc nursing, post certificate BSc, or nursing and selection tests.

Specialties

Candidate will be examined in any of the following branches:
- Medical surgical nursing—cardiovascular and thoracic nursing
- Medical surgical nursing—critical care nursing
- Medical surgical nursing—oncology nursing
- Medical surgical nursing—neurosciences nursing
- Medical surgical nursing—nephrourology nursing
- Medical surgical nursing—orthopedic nursing
- Medical surgical nursing—gastroenterology nursing
- Obstetric and gynecological nursing
- Pediatric (child health) nursing
- Psychiatric (mental health) nursing
- Community health nursing

Guidelines and Minimum Requirements to Establish MSc(N) College of Nursing

Guidelines for establishment of MSc Nursing Program
- **Guidelines and minimum requirements** for establishment of a MSc Nursing Program having recognized BSc(N) College.
  - Any organization under: (i) Central Government/State Government/Local body, (ii) Registered Private or Public Trust, (iii) Missionary or any other organization registered under Society Registration Act, (iv) Company incorporated under Section 25 of company's act are eligible to establish MSc(N) College of Nursing.
  - Indian Nursing Council recognized BSc(N) College of Nursing wherein one batch has passed out is eligible to establish MSc(N) Program.
  - Above organization shall obtain the Essentiality Certificate/No Objection Certificate for the MSc(N) Program from the respective State Government. The institution name along with Trust Deed/Society address shall be mentioned in No Objection Certificate/ Essentiality Certificate.
  - An application form to establish nursing program is available on the website viz., which shall be downloaded. Duly filled in application form with the requisite documents mentioned in the form shall be submitted before the last date as per the calendar of events of that year.
  - The Indian Nursing Council on receipt of the proposal from the institution to start nursing program, will undertake the **first inspection** to assess suitability with regard to physical infrastructure, clinical facility and teaching faculty in order to give permission to start the program.
  - After the receipt of the permission to start the nursing program from Indian Nursing Council, the institution shall obtain the approval from the State Nursing Council and University.
  - Institution will admit the students only after taking approval of State Nursing Council and University.
II. **Guidelines for super speciality hospital for establishment of a MSc Nursing Program**
  - Any organization under: (i) Central Government/State Government/Local body, (ii) Registered Private or Public Trust, (iii) Missionary or any other organization registered under Society Registration Act, (iv) Company incorporated under section 25 of company's act are eligible to establish MSc(N) College of Nursing.
  - Above organization shall obtain the Essentiality Certificate/No Objection Certificate for the MSc(N) Program from the respective State Government. The institution name along with Trust Deed/Society address shall be mentioned in No Objection Certificate/ Essentiality Certificate.
  - An application form to establish Nursing Program is available on the website viz., which shall be downloaded. Duly filled in application form with the requisite documents mentioned in the form shall be submitted before the last date as per the calendar of events of that year.
  - The Indian Nursing Council on receipt of the proposal from the institution to start nursing program, will undertake the **first inspection** to assess suitability with regard to physical infrastructure, clinical facility and teaching faculty in order to give permission to start the program.
  - After the receipt of the permission to start the nursing program from Indian Nursing Council, the institution shall obtain the approval from the State Nursing Council and University.
  - Institution will admit the students only after taking approval of State Nursing Council and University.
- **Cardiothoracic beds:** 50–100-bedded cardiac hospital, which has CCU, ICCU and ICU units with own thoracic unit or affiliated thoracic unit.
- **Critical care beds:** 250–500-bedded hospital, which has a 8–10 beds critical care beds and ICUs
- **OBG speciality beds:** 50-bedded parent hospital having:
  - Mother and neonatal units
  - Case load of minimum 500 deliveries per year
  - 8–10 level II neonatal beds.
  - Affiliation with level III neonatal beds

- **Neuro-speciality beds:** Minimum of 50 bedded Neuro care institution with advanced diagnostic, therapeutic and state of the art clinical facilities
- **Oncology specialty beds:** Regional Cancer centers/Cancer Hospitals having minimum 100 beds, with medical and surgical oncology units with chemotherapy, radiotherapy, palliative care, other diagnostic and supportive facilities.
- **Specialty beds:** 250–500 bedded Hospital, which has a 50 orthopedic beds and rehabilitation units.
- **Psychiatric beds:** Minimum of 50 bedded institutes of psychiatry and mental health having all types of patients (acute, chronic, adult psychiatric beds, child psychiatric beds and de-addiction facilities), with advanced diagnostic, therapeutic and state of the art clinical facilities.
- **Pediatrics beds:** 50–100 bedded pediatric Hospital/unit with pediatric surgery and level II or III neonatal units
- **Gastroenterology beds:** 50–100 bedded gastroenterology beds
- **Nephrourology specialty beds:** 50–100 bedded nephrourology hospital with dialysis and kidney transplants, urosurgery

Minimum requirement to establish MSc(N) Program Minimum 2 additional classrooms and one classroom as per the number of electives.

Note: Proportionately the rooms and other facilities will increase/decrease according to the number of students admitted.

Nursing Teaching Faculty MSc(N)

If parent hospital is super-specialty hospital like cardiothoracic hospital/cancer with annual intake 10 MSc(N) in cardio thoracic/cancer

- Professor cum coordinator 1
- Reader/Associate Professor 1

Lecturer 2: The above faculty shall perform dual role **BSc(N) and MSc(N)**

Sl. No.	Designation	BSc(N) 40–60 (students intake)	MSc(N) 10–25 (students intake)
1.	Professor cum Principal	1	
2.	Vice-Principal	1	
3.	Professor cum Professor	0	1
4.	Associate Professor	2	1
5.	Assistant Professor	3	3
6.	Tutor	10–18	

- 1:10 student patient ratio for MSc(N)
- One in each specialty and the entire MSc(N) qualified teaching faculty will participate in all collegiate programs. Teacher student ratio = 1:10 for MSc(N) Program.

Qualifications and experience of teachers of college of nursing:

Sl. No.	Post, qualifications and experiences
1.	**Principal cum Professor:** 15 years experience with MSc(N) out of which 12 years should be teaching experience with minimum of 5 years in collegiate program. PhD(N) is desirable
2.	**Vice-Principal cum Professor:** 12 years experience with MSc(N) out of which 10 years should be teaching experience with minimum of 5 years in collegiate program. PhD(N) is desirable
3.	**Professor:** 10 years experience with MSc(N) out of which 7 years should be teaching experience. PhD(N) is desirable
4.	**Associate Professor:** MSc(N) with 8 years experience including 5 years teaching experience PhD(N) desirable
5.	**Assistant Professor:** MSc(N) with 3 years teaching experience PhD(N) desirable
6.	**Tutor:** MSc(N) or BSc(N)/PBBSc(N) with 1 year experience

Note:
1. No part time nursing faculty will be counted for calculating total no. of faculty required for a college.
2. Irrespective of number of admissions, all faculty positions (Professor to Lecturer) must be filled.
3. For MSc(N) Program appropriate number of MSc faculty in each speciality be appointed subject to the condition that total number of teaching faculty ceiling is maintained.
4. All nursing teachers must possess a basic university or equivalent qualification as laid down in the schedules of the Indian Nursing Council Act, 1947. They shall be registered under the State Nursing Registration Act.
5. Nursing faculty in nursing college except tutor/clinical instructors must possess the requisite recognized postgraduate qualification in nursing subjects.
6. Holders of equivalent postgraduate qualifications, which may be approved by the Indian Nursing Council from time to time, may be considered to have the requisite recognized postgraduate qualification in the subject concerned.
7. All teachers of nursing other than Principal and Vice-Principal should spend at least 4 hours in the clinical area for clinical teaching and/or supervision of care every day.

Regulations for Examinations

Eligibility for appearing for the examination: About 75% of the attendance for theory and practical's. However, 100% of attendance for practical before the award of degree.

Classification of results:
- 50% pass in each of the theory and practical separately
- 50–59% Second division
- 60–74% first division
- 75% and above is distinction
- For declaring the rank aggregate of 2 years marks to be considered

If the candidate fails in either practical's or theory paper he/she has to reappear for both the papers (theory and practical) Maximum no. of attempts per subject is three (3) inclusive of first attempt. The maximum period to complete the course successfully should not exceed 4 years Candidate who fails in any subject, shall be permitted to continue the studies into the second year. However the candidate shall not be allowed to appear for the second year examination till such time that he/she passes all subjects of the first year MSc nursing examination.

Practicals:
- Four hours of practical examination per student.
- Maximum number of 10 students per day per specialty.
- The examination should be held in clinical area only for clinical specialties.
- One internal and external should jointly conduct practical examination.
- **Examiner:** Nursing faculty teaching respective specialty area in MSc Nursing Program with minimum 3 years experience after MSc Nursing.

Dissertation: Evaluation of the dissertation should be done by the examiner prior to viva duration: Viva-voce—minimum 30 minutes per student.

MASTER OF PHILOSOPHY PROGRAM IN NURSING

In 1980, RAK College of Nursing started an MPhil Program as a regular and part time course. Since then several universities started taking students for the MPhil course in nursing. Prominent among these are: MGR Medical University, Rajiv Gandhi University of Health Sciences, SNDT University and Delhi University and Manipal Academy of Higher Education.

Philosophy

- Nursing shares with the whole university a main focus of preparing its students for service and assisting them to achieve a meaningful philosophy of life.
- The student is encouraged to develop judgment and wisdom in handling knowledge and skills and achieve mastery of problem-solving and creative skills.
- Commitment to lifelong learning is the mark of truly professional person. In order to maintain clinical competencies and enhance professional practice, the student must stay abrupt of the new developments and contribute to the advancement of nursing knowledge.

Objectives

The objectives of MPhil degree course in nursing are:
- To strengthen the research foundations of nurses for encouraging research attitudes and problem-solving capacities
- To provide basic training required for research in undertaking doctoral work

Duration

Duration of the full term MPhil course will be one year and part time course will be two year.

Course of Study

At the time of admission, each candidate will be required to indicate her priorities in regard to the optional courses. A candidate may offer one course from MPhil Program from the department of anthropology, education, sociology and physiology or any suitable department. The MPhil studies will be into two distinct parts, part 1 and part 2.
- **Part-1:** It consist of 3 courses, i.e., research methods in nursing, major aspects of nursing, allied disciplines.
- **Part-2:** After passing the part 1 examination, a student shall be required to write a dissertation. The topic and the nature of the dissertation of each candidate will be determined by the advisory committee consist of three members. The dissertation may include results of original research, a fresh interpretation of existing facts, and date or a review article of critical nature of may take.

DOCTORATE OF PHILOSOPHY IN NURSING (PhD IN NURSING)

- Earlier Indian nurses were sent abroad for PhD Program.
- PhD Programs in nursing was first started in India in 1992
- Universities where PhD Programs are conducted in India include:
  - PhD Consortium by Indian Nursing Council, RUGHS and WHO
  - RAK College of Nursing
  - NIMHANS, Bengaluru
  - Manipal University

Philosophy

A candidate for admission to the course for the degree of doctor of philosophy in the faculties of medical science must have obtained an MPhil degree of a university or have a good academic record with first or second class master's degree of an Indian or a foreign university in the concerned subject.

The candidate shall apply to the university for the admission stating his qualifications and the subjects he proposes to investigate enclosing a statement on any work he may have done in the subject. Every application for the admission of the course must be analyzed by the board of research studies.

Board of research studies (medical sciences) members:
- Dean and the head of the departments concerned
- Principals/head of institutions recognized for post graduate medical studies.
- Two members nominated by the medical academic council.
- Three persons nominated by the medical faculty(for their special knowledge in the medical science.

Eligibility Criteria

- The candidate should be postgraduate in nursing with more than 55% of aggregates of marks.
- Should have research background
- May/may not published articles in journals
- The course duration is for regular PhD course is 3 years and for part time is 4 years.

ACCREDITATION OF NURSING EDUCATIONAL INSTITUTIONS

When selecting a college or university and before committing any money to a postsecondary educational institution, it is important to determine whether or not the institution is "accredited." This is even more important when considering a non-traditional form of instruction, such as distance learning. With an accredited institution, a student has some assurance of receiving a quality education and gaining recognition by other colleges and by employers of the course credits and degrees earned. Accreditation is an affirmation that a college provides a quality of education that the general public has the right to expect and that the educational community recognizes.

According to Selden "Accrediting is the process whereby an organization agency recognizes a college or university or a program of study as having met certain predetermined qualifications and standard".

Definition

Accreditation ensures a basic level of quality in the education you receive from an institution. It also ensures your degrees will be recognized for the true achievements they are.

- 'Accrediting' is the process whereby an organizations or agency recognizes a college or university or a program of study as having met certain predetermined qualifications and standard.
- 'Accreditation' refers to a voluntary review process of educational programs by a professional organization. The organization is called an 'accrediting agency', and is invited to compare the educational quality of the program with established standard and criteria.

Concept of Accreditation

- The concept of accreditation of educational programs in nursing is very important. Prospective nursing students should inquire about the accreditation status of any nursing program they are considering.
- Employers of nurses are usually only interested in hiring or employing nurses who are graduates of accredited programs. And acceptance into graduate program, in nursing is usually dependent on graduation from an accredited baccalaureate program.
- Accreditation is vital of the welfare of institution of higher education. Those institutions that fail to attain accreditation or removed from the list of accrediting agency may be handicapped in a number of ways.
- For example, an institution of higher learning that is not accredited by an accrediting agency may find the difficulty in getting grants from the foundation in government sector.
- Graduates from unaccredited professional programs in medicine, nursing, dentistry, pharmacy, veterinary medicine, law, engineering and certain other professional programs find it difficult to obtain state licensure to practice that profession.
- Thus, it becomes of vital importance to the institutions and to society that colleges and universities attain and maintain standards that will make institutions of higher learning eligible for accreditation.

Purpose of Accreditation

Accreditation refers to a voluntary review process of educational programs by a professional organization. At the end of seminar student will be able to understand the knowledge about accreditation and use it in hospital and college settings. The purpose of accreditation is to:

- Administration requirements
- Uniform standards of nursing education
- Institutional self-improvement by evaluation and inspection.
- Safeguard the institution from social, educational and political pressure.
  - Prescribe syllabus
  - Grant recognition
  - Inspection
  - Improve the quality of nursing education
- Protect the autonomy of health service program
- Preserves the quality of nursing education
- Protects the public from ill-prepared nurses
- Protects the institution from political pressure
- Helps the practitioner for the ever expanding or the broad scope of nursing practices

Principles of Accreditation

Accreditation is a voluntary process of self-regulation and peer review adopted by the educational community. Institutions of higher education have voluntarily entered into associations to evaluate each other in accord with an institution's stated goals. Non-accredited institutions must be able to demonstrate that they possess certain "characteristics of quality" before they are allowed to become members of the association of accredited institutions.

- To provide programs of study that is educationally sound, up-to-date, of high quality and is demonstrably effective.
- To maintain fair, ethical, and clearly stated advertising, admission, and enrollment practices by accurately and fairly representing the accredited institution and its service to its constituency.
- To provide effective student counseling and motivational programs that recognize individual differences and ensure successful student retention, graduation and, where applicable, employability.
- To demonstrate the ultimate benefit of private educational training programs through satisfied participants.
- To maintain an effective peer review system that ensures proper and ethical administration of all financial operations of the institution.
- To promote the concept of voluntary self-regulation inherent in the accreditation process.
- To demonstrate a commitment to educational services through community involvement and participation.

- To demonstrate the effectiveness of private education and training, thereby providing essential skills to support a productive American work force.
- To promote continuing education and training programs of the highest quality and integrity.

Objectives of Accreditation

Accrediting is carried on mainly by voluntary organization. Although these organizations are advisory in nature and do not have legal power to control institutions of higher education, they do exert influence. Accreditations have had extensive influence on the development of higher education. It has also been the focus of controversy. Accrediting agencies have been largely responsible for the development and maintenance of minimum academic standards and quality of instructions of higher learning. Accreditation safeguard to society. Accreditations have four major purposes which include the following:

- Maintenance of adequate admission requirements
- Maintenance of minimum academic standards
- Stimulation of institutional self improvements, and
- Protection of institutions of higher education against educationally and socially harmful pressures.

Accreditating Organizations in India

Accrediting organizations in higher education are generally classed into three types: 1. National accrediting agency, 2. National professional accrediting agency, 3. State accrediting bodies.

National Agencies

National accrediting agencies are concerned with appraising the total activities of the institutions of higher learning, and with safeguarding the quality of liberal education, the foundation of professional programs in colleges and universities. Each agency establishes criteria for the evaluation of institutions in its region and it reviews those institutions periodically, and it publishes from time to time a list of those agencies which it has accredited.

India has following all India educational councils:
- Central Advisory Board of Education
- All India Council for Elementary Education
- All India Council for Secondary Education
- University Grants Commission
- All India Council for Technical Education
- National Assessment and Accreditation Council.

National Professional Accrediting Agency

Professional accrediting is supported by State licensure laws. Individuals who hold a common body of knowledge and who have a desire to attain high vocational status tends to form professional organizations. This professional group aim to foster research, to improve service to the public and the number of individuals admitted to the profession. Controlling admissions is vital to a professional group particularly in the early stages when the professional is struggling for status.

These professional groups that tend to restrict admission through the state licensure laws and through the accreditation of colleges and universities which offer the program. In India, particularly in the field of health, national professional accrediting agencies have existed.

- Medical Council of India
- Indian Nursing Council
- Dental Council of India
- Pharmacy Council of India
- Central Council of Indian System of Medicine

Accridating Bodies in Nursing

- Indian Nursing Council (INC) is the official accrediting agency for all programs of nursing, which include Diploma (GNM), BSc, Nursing (both basic and post basic, Buccalaur, etc.), NM/MSc N/MPhil (Masters) and PhD (Doctoral programs in Nursing).
- Accreditation of nursing schools and colleges grew out of concern repeatedly expressed by the members of profession about the quality and standards for nursing education.
- An accredited program voluntarily adhere, to standards thus protect, the quality of education, public safety, and the profession itself.
- Accreditation provides both a mechanism and a stimulus for programs to initiate periodic self-examination and self-improvement.
- It assures students that their educational program is accountable for offering quality education for future practice.
- Areas generally scrutinized in accreditation review one administration and governance, finances and budget, faculty, students, curriculum and resources.
- Criteria or standards are established in each area, programs under review prepare reports, than show how school or college meets each criticism.
- Once accredited and in good standing, continuing accreditation review take place in every 8 years or 5 years.
- Programs that do not meet standards may be placed on warning and given a specific time period to correct deficiencies.
- Accreditation can be withdrawn if deficiencies are not corrected within the specified time.

Benefits of Accrediting Nursing Institutions

There are many benefits to attending an accredited nursing school. These benefits start helping you advance your healthcare education almost immediately. Some of the most important benefits are:

- For students to qualify for financial aid on a federal level and other federal programs, the institution to which they have been accepted must be accredited by an accrediting agency that is recognized by the federal government.
- Accreditation ensures that the level of education you receive meets certain criteria and standards.
- Attending an accredited school makes transferring to a different school more acceptable as it ensures the

accepting school that the credits you have are of a certain level of quality.
- As a graduate of an accredited nursing school, you have the opportunity to attend other schools offering advanced studies, including MSN and Doctorate programs.
- Present yourself to a prospective employer as a professional with impeccable academic preparation and credentials.

INSPECTIONS OF NURSING COLLEGES

The policy laid down by the Indian Nursing Council in respect of inspection of the existing nursing colleges/institutions is at Annexure. The policy as laid down by Indian Nursing Council (INC) is as follows:
- The School/College of Nursing desiring to open new nursing course are first required to obtain a No Objection Certificate/Essentiality Certificate from the concerned State governments; thereafter, the concerned institutions are to apply to the INC in the proforma prescribed indicating the teaching, clinical and infrastructural facilities available in the institution.
- After receipt of the complete proposal, the council conducts inspections through independent inspectors appointed under the provisions of section 13 of INC Act, 1947.
- The report of the independent inspector is placed before the Executive Committee of the INC which after evaluating the inspection report decides as to whether the institution has to be granted suitability/recognition or not.
- Two Ad-hoc inspectors are selected under the panel as per eligibility criteria.
- The ad-hoc inspectors are deputed to conduct inspection by Indian Nursing Council in the Country. Indian Nursing Council officials are not eligible to conduct inspection.

Objectives

- To establish and maintain a uniform standard of nursing education for nurses, auxiliary nurse midwives and health visitors by doing periodical inspection of the institution.
- To give registration to nurses and midwives who had undergone their training from recognized institutions.
- To conduct undergraduate courses and to issue diploma and registration certificate.
- To conduct examinations for GNM, ANM, Post Basic Diploma Courses and Health Supervisor Courses.
- Power to withdraw the recognition of qualification in case the institution fails to maintain its standards.

Periodic Inspection

- Indian Nursing Council conducts periodical inspection of the institution. Once the institution is found suitable by Indian Nursing Council, to monitor the standard of nursing education and the adherence of the norms prescribed by INC periodic inspection is conducted.
- Institutions are required to pay annual affiliation fee every year. However, if the institution does not comply with the norms prescribed by Indian Nursing Council for teaching, clinical and physical facilities, the institution will be declared unsuitable.

Renewal/Validity for Existing Institution

- Institution shall submit renewal/validity application form through respective State Nursing Council along with the affidavit. Then only the institutions are issued validity.
- This information was given by the Union Minister of Health and Family Welfare Shri Ghulam Nabi Azad in written reply to a question in the Lok Sabha today.

STAFFING IN COLLEGE OF NURSING

Staffing is a selection, training, motivating and retaining of a personnel in the organization. Nurse staffing is a constant challenge for healthcare facilities. Before the selection of the employees, one has to make analysis of the particular job, which is required in the organization, then comes the selection of personnel.

Principal Job Description

The school principal serves as the educational leader, responsible for managing the policies, regulations, and procedures to ensure that all students are supervised in a safe traditional Catholic learning environment that meets the approved curricula and mission of the school. Achieving academic excellence requires that the school Principal work collaboratively to direct and nurture all members of the school staff hired by the Board of Directors and to communicate effectively with parents. Inherent in the position are the responsibilities for scheduling, curriculum development, extracurricular activities, personnel management, emergency procedures, and facility operations.

Job Functions and Responsibilities

- Establish and promote high standards and expectations for all students and staff for academic performance and responsibility for behavior.
- Manage, evaluate and supervise effective and clear procedures for the operation and functioning of the school consistent with the philosophy, mission, values and goals of the school including instructional programs, extracurricular activities, and discipline systems to ensure a safe and orderly climate, building maintenance, program evaluation, personnel management, office operations, and emergency procedures. Ensure compliance with all laws, board policies and civil regulations.
- Establish the annual master schedule for instructional programs, ensuring sequential learning experiences for students consistent with the school's philosophy, mission statement and instructional goals.
- Supervise the instructional programs of the school, evaluating lesson plans and observing classes (teaching, as duties allow) on a regular basis to encourage the use of a variety of instructional strategies and materials consistent with research on learning and child growth and development.

- Establish procedures for evaluation and selection of instructional materials and equipment, approving all recommendations.
- Supervise in a fair and consistent manner effective discipline and attendance systems with high standards, consistent with the philosophy, values, and mission of the school. Ensure a safe, orderly environment that encourages students to take responsibility for behavior and creates high morale among staff and students. File all required reports regarding violence, vandalism, attendance and discipline matters.
- Establish a professional rapport with students and with staff that has their respect. Display the highest ethical and professional behavior and standards when working with students, parents and school personnel. Serve as a role model for students, dressing professionally, demonstrating the importance and relevance of learning, accepting responsibility, and demonstrating pride in the education profession. Encourage all teachers to do the same.
- Notify immediately the Board, and appropriate personnel and agencies when there is evidence of substance abuse, child abuse, child neglect, severe medical or social conditions, potential suicide or students appearing to be under the influence of alcohol or controlled substances.
- Keep the Board advised of employees not meeting their contractual agreement.
- Research and collect data regarding the needs of students, and other pertinent information including the collection of detail regarding the sacraments students have received or are preparing for. Keep the chaplain informed of this information.
- Keep the staff informed and seek ideas for the improvement of the school. Conduct meetings, as necessary, for the proper functioning of the school: weekly meetings for full-time staff; monthly staff meetings.
- Establish and maintain an effective inventory system for all school supplies, materials and equipment.
- Establish procedures that create and maintain attractive, organized, functional, healthy, clean, and safe facilities, with proper attention to the visual, acoustic and temperature.
- Assume responsibility for the health, safety, and welfare of students, employees and visitors.
- Develop clearly understood procedures and provide regular drills for emergencies and disasters.
- Maintain a master schedule to be posted for all teachers.
- Establish schedules and procedures for the supervision of students in non-classroom areas (including before and after school).
- Maintain visibility with students, teachers, parents and the Board.
- Communicate regularly with parents, seeking their support and advice, so as to create a cooperative relationship to support the student in the school. The Principal may not interfere with anyone's freedom to speak directly to the chaplain.
- Use effective presentation skills when addressing students, staff, parents, and the community including appropriate vocabulary and examples, clear and legible visuals, and articulate and audible speech.
- Use excellent written and oral English skills when communicating with students, parents and teachers.
- Complete in a timely fashion all records and reports as requested by the Board. Maintain accurate attendance records.
- Maintain and account for all student activity funds and money collected from students.
- Communicate with the Board regularly about the needs, successes and general operation of the school.
- Establish procedures for safe storing and integrity of all public and confidential school records. Ensure that student records are complete and current.
- Protect confidentiality of records and information gained as part of exercising professional duties and use discretion in sharing such information within legal confines.
- Organize and supervise procedures for identifying and addressing special needs of students including health-related concerns, and physical, emotional and spiritual needs (keeping the Chaplain informed of these).
- Supervise the exclusion from school of any pupil who shows departure from normal health, who has been exposed to a communicable disease, or whose presence may be detrimental to the health and cleanliness of other pupils. Assure that excluded pupil's parents or guardian are apprised of the reasons for exclusion.
- Maintain positive, cooperative and mutually supportive relationships with staff, parents and Chaplain.
- Attend required committee meetings (e.g., fund-raising, curriculum, etc.) and extra school sponsored functions and religious events, e.g., first communion, confirmation, graduation, etc.).
- Perform any duties that are within the scope of employment and certifications, as assigned by the Board and not otherwise prohibited by law or in conflict with contract.
- Ensure that schedule allows for regular mass and confessions.
- Oversee the development of Curriculum Committee and keep the Board apprised.
- Provide quarterly student grade and behavior reports to parents. Post honor roll lists each quarter.
- Work with the chaplain to guide and instruct the teachers to provide the spiritual atmosphere inherent in a traditional Catholic educational environment.
- Nurture both students and teachers to achieve their greatest potential academically, instructionally and spiritually.
- Maintain in the school a spirit conducive to prayer and study.
- Provide an atmosphere of piety, obedience and charity throughout the school day.
- Ensure that students and teachers attend scheduled prayers and mass throughout the school day.

- Enforce uniform policy and appearance policy so as to assure a school environment that is focused on group spiritual and academic achievement rather than on individuals.
- Provide and supervise a safe recreation and play period for the students.

Vice-Principal

Vice-Principals, more commonly known as assistant principals, work for both public and private school systems. The job of the vice principal is to assist the principal with the school's everyday administrative tasks. Vice principals are often in charge of scheduling, hiring, organizing clinical experiences and supplies, and dealing with behavioral issues.

Educational
- Assists Principal in planning, implementation and evaluation of the programs.
- Assists Principal in identifying needs for professional development of faculty and conducting staff development program.
- Supervises postgraduate students in conducting research.
- Participates in teaching of various educational programs.
- In the absence of Principal, chairs the assigned committee meetings.
- Supervises all educational programs in coordination with the coordinators.
- Guides faculty in day-to-day academic activities

Supervisory
- Shares responsibility with Principal and Professor in supervision of teaching and nonteaching staff.
- Plans academic staff assignments in consultation with Principal.
- Participates in conduct of orientation program
- Supervises and guides staff in conducting their activities.
- Writes staff performance report and reviews evaluation report of assigned staff.
- Assists Principal in monitoring students welfare activities, e.g., mess, hostel, health, sports, Student Nurses Association (SNA), etc.
- Assists Principal in administration and supervision of library.

Financial
- Assists Principal in carrying out financial activities
- Planning and revising budget
- Monitoring college expenditure
- In the absence of Principal, performs all the functions

Establishment
- Assists Principal in maintaining rules and regulations in college campus
- Supervizes overall functioning of staff and students' hostel.
- Assists Principal in maintaining discipline in the college.
- Assists Principal in reviewing recruitment and promotion policies of teaching and non-teaching staff.

Interpersonal
- Assists Principal in maintaining human relation and communication
- Identifies conflict among staff members, initiates solution and reports to Principal when necessary.
- Communicates with staff in explaining administrative constraints.
- Facilitates guidance and counseling students and staff as per need.
- Any other responsibility assigned by the Principal.

Professor: Job Description

Nursing professors are registered nurses (RNs) who also hold PhD's. They are at the forefront of every nursing student's education, teaching nursing in colleges, universities and hospital-based nursing schools. There is a high demand for nursing professors due to the increasing number of applicants to nursing schools.

- **Job description:** Nursing professors develop and implement curricula in order to prepare students adequately for the challenges presented within all aspects of the nursing field. In order to keep up with the current needs of nursing, professors revise their programs where and when necessary. Like nurses, professors often specialize, teaching the areas in which they have the most experience, such as pediatrics, mental health or acute care.
- **Duties:** The duties of a nursing professor are many and varied. In addition to classroom teaching, they supervise and advise students, conduct clinical research and present scholarly work at nursing conferences. They may be asked to chair committees or even become deans of the colleges of nursing where they teach.
- **Job requirements:** Excellent leadership, public speaking and oral communication skills are required of nursing professors in order to convey their knowledge face-to-face with students and graduate staff. In addition, they must think, such as instructors versus nurses and resist the urge to carry out nursing assignments and duties for students in the classroom. They keep current in their areas of expertise by reading professional journals, and some work as part-time clinicians in order to maintain clinical competence.

Associate Professor: Job Description

The responsibilities of the faculty are to develop a healthy and caring environment that offers a variety of opportunities for active participation by the students in the learning process. Major responsibilities of faculty include teaching, tutoring, and professional development.

Education

Master's degree preferred or Bachelor's degree with appropriate experience. Degrees must be within nursing or a related

subject. An Associate degree is acceptable with one of the following:
- In the processes of obtaining a bachelor's degree
- Have at least five years of full-time experience in a clinical setting in the role of a registered nurse.
- Have at least two years of full-time experience as an educator.

Qualification
- Must have an active registered nurses license or eligible to be licensed in the state of Florida.
- Demonstrated the ability to achieve goals, influence others, and meet deadlines.
- Proficient in computers (Word, Excel, Access, Outlook, PowerPoint and Adobe).
- Must be able to multitask.
- Experience with presenting information to both small and large groups.
- Proven strong communication skills and the ability to work with people from diverse backgrounds and experiences.

Experience
Five years of experience in academic, clinical or administrative nursing of any combination thereof.

Responsibilities
The following are the responsibilities of the Faculty, but not limited to the following:
- Ability to plan and prepare course content and curriculum, utilizing assessment and effective methodologies of instruction for the enhancement of learning.
- Maintain expertise in field of study and teaching pedagogy by attending seminars, workshops and classes for self improvement and/or professional enhancement.
- Maintain active participation in professional organizations as appropriate.
- Participate in enrollment management activities and sharing of professional expertise with colleagues and students beyond the classroom.
- Provide support and in some cases provide the leadership for student recruitment, marketing, and in general activities that "build" a program within the clinical setting.
- Support student activities, include course and career guidance to students, mentor, graduation, and foster a love of learning.
- Assist in the development of the departmental course schedule.
- Giving required forms and papers to Registrar's Office within the specified timeframe.
- Maintain appropriate records of student performance.
- Demonstrate procedures in nursing skills laboratory, supervise student demonstrations and evaluate student performances.
- Integrate theory with planned clinical performance.
- Orientate students to the clinical site and communicate clinical objectives to the student and the staff.

Duties and Responsibilities
- Teach courses as assigned (lecture, lab and clinical) in accordance with the established syllabi of the nursing program.
- Advise and register assigned students; participates in retention, placement and cooperative educational experiences. Make counseling services referrals as appropriate.
- Prepare and/or maintain current course syllabi, course outlines and develops classroom expectations for each assigned course.
- Maintain accurate academic records.
- Research and recommend adequate instructional materials for the assigned courses.
- Provide, prepare and maintain adequate classroom and lab facilities and equipment for assigned courses.
- Participate in the development of departmental budgets, reports and objectives.
- Participate in the development of course schedules.
- Serve on instructional committees
- Represent the nursing department, the Health Science Division and the college by participating in community and professional meetings.

Essential Physical Skills
- Acceptable eyesight (with or without correction).
- Acceptable hearing (with or without hearing aid).
- Ability to communicate both orally and in writing.
- Ability to access files cabinets for filing and retrieval of data.
- Ability to sit at a desk and view a display screen for extended periods of time.
- Ability to access input and retrieves information from a computer.
- Able to actively demonstrate and participate in the skills laboratory and clinical without physical limitations.

Environmental Conditions
- Works inside a classroom/laboratory environment.
- Clinical sites at various locations

Assistant Professor: Job Description
The job of an assistant clinical nursing professor is a vital role performed at colleges and universities. The nursing shortage has created healthcare gaps in patient care and clinical nursing professors Helps bridge this gap by teaching and guiding nursing students for direct patient care.
- **Function:** The assistant nursing clinical professor performs varied functions, including a combination of teaching and administrative duties. The assistant professor may work under the basic supervision of the director of nursing at a school or university.
- **Assistant nursing professor duties:** Assistant clinical nursing duties may range from teaching upper level nursing courses to performing nurse student advising, such as career direction. Some assistant nursing professors analyze and coordinate nursing educational programs.

- **Qualifications:** A Master of Science (MS) degree from an accredited college or university is a minimum requirement for most clinical nursing educational positions. Nursing master's program coursework may include health policies and nursing leadership skills. Current nursing licensure and certification may also be needed.
- **Work environment:** Assistant nursing professors enjoy flexible work schedules, including evenings. Some nursing professors may complete researching and writing nursing programs at home and perform clinical nursing classes on campus.

Clinical Instructor: Job Description

Nursing instructors, who are also referred to as nurse educators, play a vital role in the field of nursing. They teach students essential skills and knowledge which is required for nursing. According to the National League of Nursing, there is a current shortage of nursing instructors. Many schools are turning away students for this reason. Nursing educators must maintain an RN license at all times.

- Demonstrates and teaches patient care in classroom and clinical units to nursing students and instructs students in principles and application of physical, biological, and psychological subjects related to nursing: Lectures to students, conducts and supervises laboratory work, issues assignments, and directs seminars and panels.
- Supervises student nurses and demonstrates patient care in clinical units of hospital.
- Prepares and administers examinations, evaluates student progress, and maintains records of student classroom and clinical experience.
- Participates in planning curriculum, teaching schedule, and course outline.
- Cooperates with medical and nursing personnel in evaluating and improving teaching and nursing practices.
- May specialize in specific subject, such as anatomy, chemistry, psychology, or nutrition, or in type of nursing activity, such as nursing of medical or surgical patients.
- Collaborate with colleagues to address teaching and research issues.
- Plan, evaluate, and revise curricula, course content, and course materials and methods of instruction.
- Assess clinical education needs, and patient and client teaching needs, utilizing a variety of methods.
- Compile, administer, and grade examinations, or assign this work to others.
- Advise students on academic and vocational curricula, and on career issues.
- Maintain student attendance records, grades, and other required records.
- Maintain regularly scheduled office hours in order to advise and assist students.
- Supervise undergraduate and/or graduate teaching, internship, and research work.
- Conduct research in a particular field of knowledge, and publish findings in professional journals, books, and/or electronic media.
- Participate in student recruitment, registration, and placement activities.
- Serve on academic or administrative committees that deal with institutional policies, departmental matters, and academic issues.
- Coordinate training programs with area universities, clinics, hospitals, health agencies, and/or vocational schools.
- Compile bibliographies of specialized materials for outside reading assignments.
- Select and obtain materials and supplies, such as textbooks and laboratory equipment.
- Participate in campus and community events.
- Write grant proposals to procure external research funding.
- Act as advisers to student organizations.
- Demonstrate patient care in clinical units of hospitals.
- Perform administrative duties, such as serving as department head.
- Provide professional consulting services to government and/or industry.

CONCLUSION

Nursing profession has seen tremendous improvement over these years of its journey in practice as well as in education aspects. Still the main part of the regulatory bodies and institutions is not pertaining to merely increase the production of nursing professionals but to make them competent in their profession so as to make them visionary leaders lifting the banner of nursing—the Noble Profession. There are different courses offered in nursing, such as ANM, DGNM, BSc(N), PB BSc(N), MSc(N), MPhil, and PhD(N). The INC, SNC and the University with which an institution is affiliated plays a vital role in establishing and maintenance of standards in nursing education.

REVIEW QUESTIONS

Long Essays

1. Explain the aims of education; discuss about goals and objectives of nursing education.
2. Explain about nursing programs in India; discuss in detail about the types of Nursing Education Programs in India.
3. Define accreditation; explain the purposes, objective and principles.
4. Describe briefly about inspections of nursing colleges.

Short Essays

1. Competencies for nursing programs.
2. Define regulatory bodies; explain role, characteristics and principles.

3. Indian Nursing Council/Apex body: Objectives and roles.
4. Guidelines for establishment of new nursing schools/colleges.
5. State Registration Council: Objectives and functions.
6. Guidelines and minimum requirements to establish school of nursing.
7. Accrediting bodies in nursing.
8. Staffing in college of nursing.

Short Answers

1. Principles of regulatory.
2. Bodies importance of professional bodies.
3. Aims of GNM Program.
4. Objectives of BSc Nursing Program.
5. Accreditation Organizations in India.
6. Benefits of Accrediting Nursing Institutions.

BIBLIOGRAPHY

1. Basavanthappa BT. Nursing Administration, second edition, India: Jaypee Brothers; 2009. pp. 119-28, 145-52.
2. Harold K. Essentials of management, 6th edition. India: Tata McGraw-Hill publishing company limited; 2005. pp. 64-9, 127-9.
3. Sakharkar BM. Principles of hospital administration and planning. second edition, India. Jaypee Brothers; 2009. pp.120-5, 129-34.

CHAPTER 21

Planning and Organizing Educational Institutions

LEARNING OBJECTIVES

- Philosophy, Objectives and Mission of the College
- Organization Structure of School/College
- Review: Curriculum Planning
- Planning Teaching and Learning Experiences, Clinical Facilities—Master Plan, Time Table and Clinical Rotation
- Budget Planning—Faculty, Staff, Equipment and Supplies, AV Aids, Lab Equipment, Library Books, Journals, Computers and Maintenance
- Infrastructure Facilities—College, Classrooms, Hostel, Library, Labs, Computer Lab, Transport Facilities
- Records and Reports for Students, Staff, Faculty and Administrative
- Committees and Functioning
- Clinical Experiences

PHILOSOPHY, OBJECTIVES AND MISSION OF THE NURSING COLLEGE

A philosophy of nursing is a statement that outlines a nurse's values, ethics, and beliefs, as well as their motivation for being part of the profession. It covers a nurse's perspective regarding their education, practice, and patient care ethics.

A philosophy of care is a framework of care goals and values to help you make the best choices for your child and family. A spectrum of "philosophies of care" occurs along a spectrum from less intervention to more technical approaches. Perform a comprehensive assessment of individuals, families and aggregates utilizing current technologies when needed. Practice safe evidence based nursing care. Promote health through education, risk reduction, and disease prevention. Appreciate human diversity and the implications of a global healthcare environment.

Philosophy

The guiding philosophy of Nurse-Midwifery Program is based on the College/School of Nursing values: collaboration, social responsibility, integrity, respect, accountability, diversity, and excellence.

- **Collaboration:** Care of women occurs within a healthcare system that provides for consultation, collaborative management, and referral between nurse-midwives and other healthcare providers. This care enhances continuity in the best interests of the women and their families.
- **Social responsibility:** Social and reproductive justice are essential values of nurse-midwifery practice. There is a need to develop innovative systems to increase access to healthcare for all women and their families.
- **Integrity:** Nurse-midwives respect their own self-worth, dignity, and professional integrity. They provide an environment that promotes privacy and safety for women and their families, and protects them from harmful and unethical practices.

Mission	Vision
• A mission statement talks about HOW you will get to where you want to be	• A vision statement outlines WHERE you want to be
• It answers the question, "what do we do? What makes us different?"	• It answers the question, "where do we aim to be?"
• A mission statement talks about the present leading to its future	• A vision statement talks about the future
• It lists the broad goals for which the organization is formed	• It lists where you see yourself some years from now it inspires the organization to give its best

- **Respect:** Nurse-midwives respect the individuality, dignity, and basic human rights of all persons. They support the self-determination of women and their families through a partnership and empowerment. Nurse-midwifery recognizes the normalcy of women's life cycle events, including menarche, preconception, pregnancy, birth, newborn care, postpartum, miscarriage and abortion, well-woman care, and menopause. A central goal of care is to promote, maintain, and restore the well-being and health of women, families, and communities.
- **Accountability:** Nurse-midwives maintain a commitment to professionalism through reflective and systematic evaluation of practice and ongoing professional growth.
- **Diversity:** Nurse-midwives approach the care of women and their families from a position of cultural humility

and inquiry and provide care without discrimination or prejudice.
- **Excellence:** Nurse-midwives apply the scientific evidence from nursing science, midwifery, and related sciences to the care of women and their families. Nurse-Midwives educated at the graduate level are prepared to safely and competently practice the core competencies. Doctoral level practitioners are further prepared with skills in leadership, practice inquiry, and evaluation.

Mission
- Provide high-quality undergraduate education in nursing
- Maintain and develop superior graduate programs in nursing that respond to the needs of healthcare in general and nursing in particular within Pennsylvania, the nation, and the world
- Engage in research and other scholarly activities that advance learning through the extension of the frontiers of knowledge in healthcare
- Cooperate with healthcare, governmental, and related institutions to transfer knowledge in health sciences and healthcare
- Offer continuing education programs adapted to the professional upgrading and career advancement interests and needs of nurses in Pennsylvania
- Make available to local communities and public agencies the expertise of the School of Nursing in ways that are consistent with the primary teaching and research functions and contribute to the intellectual and economic development in healthcare within the commonwealth, the nation, and the world.

Objectives
The specific objectives of the Nurse-Midwifery track are to prepare graduate who:
- Provide competent, safe, high-quality and culturally sensitive nurse-midwifery care to address the health needs of diverse women, families, and communities.
- Critically evaluate theories, concepts, and research findings from nursing, midwifery, and related sciences for translation into clinical practice.
- Use effective communication and leadership skills in interprofessional teams to promote positive change in the healthcare of women, newborns and families.
- Use information systems and other technologies to improve the quality and safety of healthcare for women and newborns.
- Apply principles of distributive justice and the social determinants of health in the evaluation of health policies and advocacy for the health of women and newborns in local, national, and international contexts.
- Evaluate care systems by analyzing the needs of consumers, healthcare policies, service delivery and finance models, political contexts, and health indicators to increase access to healthcare for all women and their families in a variety of communities.

Goals
The College/School of Nursing's Goals are to:
- Prepare highly educated and competent nurses ready to enter the workforce;
- Contribute to and disseminate the scholarly evidence-base in nursing and healthcare
- Foster excellence in teaching
- Provide service to the profession and other communities of interest

CURRICULUM PLANNING

Curriculum is an important element of education. Aims of education are reflected in the curriculum. In other words, the curriculum is determined by the aims of life and society. Aims of life and society are subject to constant change. Hence, the aims of education are also subject to change and dynamic. The aims of education are attained by the school programs, concerning knowledge, experiences, activities, skills and values. The different school programs are jointly known as curriculum.

Meaning of Curriculum
The term curriculum has been derived from a Latin word 'Currere' which means a 'race course' or a runway on which one runs to reach a goal. Accordingly, a curriculum is the instructional and the educative program by following which the pupils achieve their goals, ideals and aspirations of life. It is curriculum through which the general aims of a school education receive concrete expression. Traditional concept- The traditional curriculum was subject-centered while the modern curriculum is child and life-centered.

Purpose of Curriculum
The systematic arrangement of certain courses designed with certain objectives for the pupil. Curriculum refers to the totality of activity and experiences planned by the school with a view to achieve the objectives of education.
1. Is based on the social aspirations of society,
2. Outlines the goals and aims of the program, and
3. Is expressed as goals and objectives.

There are three categories of goals and objectives:
1. Cognitive, referring to intellectual tasks,
2. Psychomotor, referring to muscular skills, and
3. Affective, referring to feeling and emotions

Concept of Curriculum
A curriculum is a "plan or program of all experiences which the learner encounters under the direction of a school". According to Gatawa, it is "the totality of the experiences of children for which schools are responsible". All this is in agreement with Sergiovanni and Starrat (1983), who argue that curriculum is "that which a student is supposed to encounter, study, practice and master... what the student learns". For others, such as Beach and Reinhatz (1989: 97), a curriculum outlines a "prescribed series of courses to take"

Modern concept of curriculum: Modern education is the combination of two dynamic processes. The one is the process of individual development and the other is the process of socialization, which is commonly known as adjustment with the social environment.

The four C's of curriculum planning
1. **Cooperative:** A program prepared jointly by group of persons.
2. **Continuous:** Preparation of program and its revision should be continuous.
3. **Comprehensive:** All the components of the program should be included.
4. **Concrete:** Concrete professional tasks must constitute the essential structure of a relevant program.

Definitions

The term curriculum has been defined by different writers in different ways:

- **Cunningham:** "Curriculum is a tool in the hands of the artist (teacher) to mould his material (pupils) according to his ideas (aims and objectives) in his studio (school)".
- **Morroe:** "Curriculum includes all those activities which are utilized by the school to attain the aims of education."
- **Froebel:** "Curriculum should be conceived as an epitome of the rounded whole of the knowledge and experience of the human race."
- **Crow and crow:** The curriculum includes all the learners' experience in or outside school that are included in a program which has been devised to help him developmentally, emotionally, socially, spiritually and morally".
- **TP Nunn:** "The curriculum should be viewed as various forms of activities that are grand expressions of human spirit and that are of the greatest and most permanent significance to the wide world".

Components of Curriculum

- Philosophy
- Objectives
- Total duration
- Detailed course plan
- Program evaluation
- The statement of philosophy of the educational program.
- The statement of the objectives of educational program.
- Total duration of the educational program. (Theortical, practical, clinical components)
- Detailed course plan for each course. (Placement, sequences and learning situations, instructional methods)
- Program evaluation (evaluation methods, plan and schedule of evaluation, results of evaluation).

Levels of Curriculum Planning

Goodland names curriculum in three levels.
1. Societal
2. Institutional
3. Instructional

Societal Curriculum

This curriculum which is planned for a large group or classes of students, e.g., BSc(N), it is planned by groups outside of an educational institution, e.g., National League for nursing. According to the needs of the society curriculum will be changed.

The institutional curriculum
- It is planned by faculty or teacher for a clearly identified group of students who will spend a specified period in a particular institution.
- Cooperative planning through curriculum committee of the particular institution.
- More active participation of each teacher generally brings about change and improvement.

The instructional curriculum: It consists of the content (subject matter and learning activities) planned day by day and week by week by a particular teacher for a particular group of students.

Principles of Curriculum Development

The conservative principles: This means that the present, the past, and the future needs of the community should be taken into considerations.

- **The forward-looking principles:** Children of today are the citizens of tomorrow.
- **The creative principle:** Curriculum should enable the child to exercise his creative and constructive powers.
- **Principle of totality form:** The curriculum should be total learning experience and total learning opportunity.
- **The activity principles:** The curriculum should be developed in terms of activity and experience.
- **Principle of preparation of life:** Enable the child to fulfill his responsibilities when he becomes an adult.

Principle of connecting to life: Curriculum should provide worthwhile life experiences.

- **Child-centered curriculum:** Consideration should be given to the student's age, their educational level, needs and individual differences.
- **Principle of integration and correlation:** While developing curriculum, each year's course should be built on what has been done in previous years and at the same time should serve as basis for subsequent learning.
- **Principle of comprehensiveness and balance:** The curriculum should be framed in such a way as every aspect of life, such as economic relationships, social activities and occupations.
- **Principle of loyalties:** Curriculum should be planned in such a manner that it teaches a true sense of loyalty to the family, the school, the country and the international community at large.
- **Principle of variety and flexibility:** Variety should be provided in terms of learning and teaching activities. It's not so rigid.
- **Principle of connecting to community needs:** Curriculum should address the community needs.

Principle of connecting with social life: Curriculum has to maintain to relation with social life.

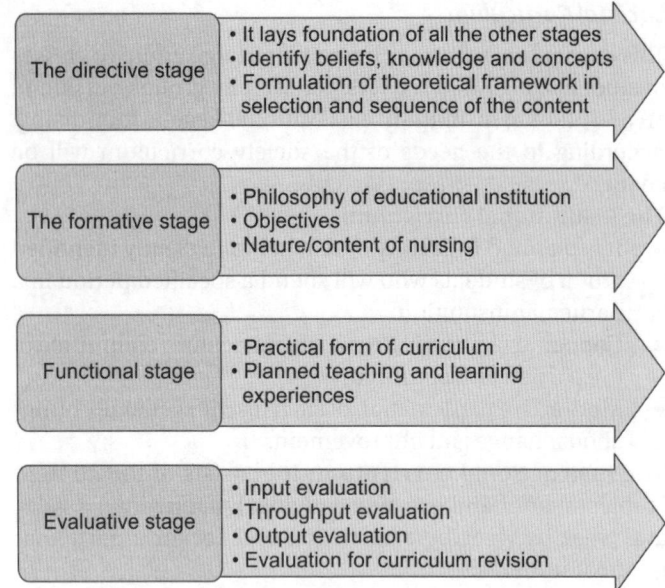

Fig. 21.1: Stages of curriculum development.

Box 21.1: Principles of curriculum development.
- The conservative principle
- The forward looking principle
- The creative principle
- Principle of totality form
- Activity principle
- Preparation for life
- Principle of connecting to life
- Child centered
- Integration and correlation

- **Training for leisure:** The curriculum should have some provision for the co-curricular activities, relaxation, and library utilization according to choice.
- **Principle of core or common subjects:** Broad areas of knowledge, skills and appreciation should be included. Cosubjects, such as maths, science, etc.
- **Principle of all round development of body, mind and spirit:** All kinds of experiences should be provided.
- **Principles of dignity of labor:** Curriculum should help students to develop a positive attitude towards all kinds of jobs.
- **Principle of character building:** Curriculum should promote human and social values.
- **Principle of democracy, secularism and socialism:** Curriculum should train the child to imbibe ideals and values of a democratic, secular and socialist state. Principle of connecting with social life: curriculum has to maintain relations with social life. **Figure 21.1** shows stages of curriculum development.

Principles Related to the Development of Nursing Curriculum (Box 21.1)

- Nursing curriculum should equip the students with the essential knowledge, skills and attitude.
- Curriculum should be clear to the students as well as to the teacher.
- Consider the community needs
- Curriculum should inculcate right attitude to students.
- Frame adequate teaching-learning activities in the classroom, clinical area and community settings.
- Consider the guidelines lay down by the statutory bodies line INC, universities, examination boards.
- High-Tech-High-Touch approach in the nursing care.
- Participatory approach in the teaching-learning process.
- The learning environment should resemble the life situation.

FACTORS AFFECTING CURRICULUM DEVELOPMENT

Several factors affect all curriculum development in meeting the needs of 21st century learners in both organized academic settings and corporation learning centers. Blueprinting curriculum development requires selecting learning goals, designing knowledge delivery models while creating assessment methods for individual and group progress. Factors affecting curriculum development include government norms, which in turn brings other factors into the process. Valid curriculum development requires awareness of the diversity of the target community socially, financially and psychologically.

- **Political factors:** How politics influences curriculum design and development starts with funding. Both private and public educational institutions rely on funding for hiring personnel, building and maintaining facilities and equipment. All aspects of curriculum depend on local, state and national political standards. From defining goals, interpreting curricular materials to approving examination systems, politics affects curriculum development.
- **Economical factors:** Curriculum developed for in house training in corporations focuses on educating employees for promotions that bring better returns in profits. Nations financing education expect an economic return from educated students contributing to the country's economy with global competition abilities in technical fields. Curriculum content influences learner goals, standards for academic achievement with an underlying influence of the nation's economy.
- **Technological factors:** The computer technology of the 21st century influences curriculum development at every level of learning. Learning centers and classrooms increasingly provide computers as requisite interaction for studies among students. Technological multimedia use influences educational goals and learning experiences among students. Undergraduate and graduate degrees in computer technology increases in popularity.
- **Social diversity:** Social diversity including religion, culture and social groupings affects curriculum development because these characteristics influence the types of topics and methods for teaching information. Developing relevant curriculum takes into account society's expectations, accommodating group traditions and promoting equality.

> **Box 21.2:** Major factors which influence curriculum development in nursing education.
> - Philosophy of nursing education
> - Educational psychology
> - Society
> - Student
> - Knowledge explosion and scientific advancements
> - Technological advancements in patient care
> - Educational technology
> - Transnational career opportunities
> - Resources

- **Learning theories:** Both child and adult learning theories within the psychology field influence curriculum development. Understanding the psychology behind learning theories implemented in curriculum development maximizes learning with content, delivery, interactive activities and experiences initiated at the most opportune teaching moment.
- **Environmental factors:** World awareness and action toward reversing and ending pollution continues affecting curriculum development. Typical elementary classrooms teach recycling and healthy environmental practices. Higher education in the sciences offer environmentally-focused degrees. **Box 21.2** shows major factors which influence curriculum development in nursing education.

Types of Curriculum

- **Formal curriculum:** According to Urevbu, formal curriculum refers to—what is laid down as the syllabus or that which is to be learnt by students. It is the officially selected body of knowledge which government, through the Ministry of Education or anybody offering education, wants students to learn.
- **Informal curriculum:** Urevbu refers to informal curriculum as the curriculum in use. Teachers or instructors may not adhere to the presented formal curriculum but can include other aspects of knowledge derived from other sources. This additional material is called the 'informal curriculum'.
- **Actual curriculum:** This refers to both written and unwritten syllabuses from which students encounter learning experiences (Tanner and Tanner 1975). Learning experiences can be selected from other sources rather than the prescribed, official and formal syllabuses. The actual curriculum is the total sum of what students learn and teachers teach from both formal and informal curricula.
- **Hidden curriculum:** Urevbu describes the hidden curriculum as the nonacademic but educationally significant component of schooling. Tanner and Tanner (1995) prefer to call it the 'collateral curriculum'. They argue that the word 'hidden' implies deliberately concealing some learning experiences from students. Since, this is not written or officially recognized, its influence on learning can manifest itself in students' attitudes and behavior, both during and after completing their studies. What is acquired or learned from hidden curriculum is usually remembered longer than information learned at school. Tanner and Tanner (1975) recommend that positive learning from the hidden curriculum should be acknowledged and treated as an integral part of the planned and guided learning experiences. As already implied, the hidden or collateral curriculum is often responsible for the values students may exhibit later in life.

Models of Curriculum Design (Fig. 21.2)

Curriculum design is a complex but systematic process. This unit describes a variety of models of curriculum design in order to make this complex activity understandable and manageable. The curriculum design models discussed show that curriculum designing is conducted stage by stage. Some of the models discussed consider the process to be more important than the objectives. Other models take objectives to be the most important feature of curriculum design. Generally, all models stress the importance of considering a variety of factors that influence curriculum.

- **The objectives model:** The objectives model of curriculum design contains content that is based on specific objectives. These objectives should specify expected learning outcomes in terms of specific measurable behaviors. This model comprises four main steps:
  1. Agreeing on broad aims which are analyzed into objectives,
  2. Constructing a curriculum to achieve these objectives,
  3. Refining the curriculum in practice by testing its capacity to achieve its objectives, and
  4. Communicating the curriculum to the teachers through the conceptual framework of the objectives. (Gatawa, 1990: 30)
- **The process model:** Unlike the objectives model, this model does not consider objectives to be important. Using this model presupposes that:
  1. Content has its own value. Therefore, it should not be selected on the basis of the achievement of objectives.

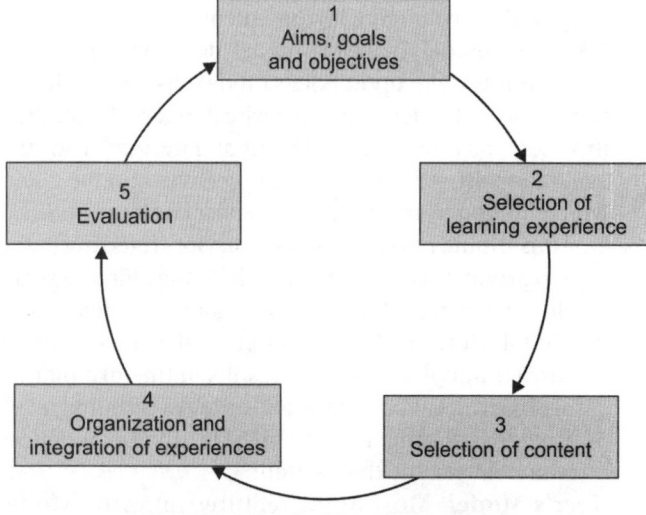

Fig. 21.2: Models of Curriculum Design.

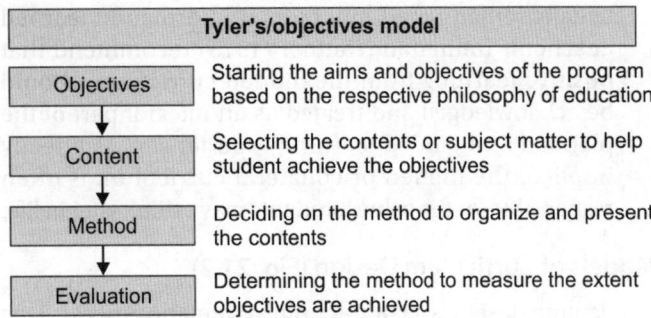

Fig. 21.3: Tyler's/objectives model.

2. Content involves procedures, concepts and criteria that can be used to appraise the curriculum.
3. Translating content into objectives may result in knowledge being distorted.
4. Learning activities have their own value and can be measured in terms of their own standard. For this reason, learning activities can stand on their own. (Gatawa, 1990: 31)

- **Tyler's Model (Fig. 21.3):** Tyler's model for curriculum designing is based on the following questions:
  1. What educational purposes should the school seek to attain?
  2. What educational experiences can be provided that are likely to attain these purposes?
  3. How can these educational experiences be effectively organized?
  4. How can we determine whether these purposes are being attained?

  The model is linear in nature, starting from objectives and ending with evaluation. In this model, evaluation is terminal. It is important to note that:
  1. Objectives form the basis for the selection and organization of learning experiences.
  2. Objectives form the basis for assessing the curriculum.
  3. Objectives are derived from the learner, contemporary life and subject specialist.

  To Tyler, evaluation is a process by which one matches the initial expectation with the outcomes.

- **Wheeler's model:** Wheeler's model for curriculum design is an improvement upon Tyler's model. Instead of a linear model, Wheeler developed a cyclical model. Evaluation in Wheeler's model is not terminal. Findings from the evaluation are fed back into the objectives and the goals, which influence other stages. Wheeler contends that:
  1. Aims should be discussed as behaviors referring to the end product of learning which yields the ultimate goals. One can think of these ultimate goals as outcomes.
  2. Aims are formulated from the general to the specific in curriculum planning. This results in the formulation of objectives at both an enabling and a terminal level.
  3. Content is distinguished from the learning experiences which determine that content.

- **Kerr's Model:** Most of the features in Kerr's Model resemble those in Wheeler's and Tyler's Models. However, Kerr divided the domains into four areas (Urevbu, 1985: 23):
  1. Objectives,
  2. Knowledge,
  3. Evaluation, and
  4. School learning experiences

A simplified version of Kerr's model of curriculum design is shown below.
What you should note about the model is that:
1. The four domains are interrelated directly or indirectly, and
2. Objectives are derived from school learning experiences and knowledge.

In Kerr's Model, objectives are divided into three groups:
1. Affective
2. Cognitive
3. Psychomotor

The model further indicates that knowledge should be (Urevbu, 1985):
1. Organized
2. Integrated
3. Sequenced
4. Reinforced

Evaluation in Kerr's Model is the collection of information for use in making decisions about the curriculum. School learning experiences are influenced by societal opportunities, the school community, pupil and teacher relationships, individual differences, teaching methods, content and the maturity of the learners. These experiences are evaluated through tests, interviews, assessments and other reasonable methods.

Curriculum Implementation

Curriculum implementation entails putting into practice the officially prescribed courses of study, syllabuses and subjects. The process involves helping the learner acquire knowledge or experience. It is important to note that curriculum implementation cannot take place without the learner. The learner is therefore the central figure in the curriculum implementation process. Implementation takes place as the learner acquires the planned or intended experiences, knowledge, skills, ideas and attitudes that are aimed at enabling the same learner to function effectively in a society.

Curriculum Evaluation

According to Gatawa, the term curriculum evaluation has three major meanings:
1. The process of describing and judging an educational program or subject.
2. The process of comparing a student's performance with behaviorally stated objectives.
3. The process of defining, obtaining and using relevant information for decision-making purposes.

What you need to understand about these definitions is that each does not exist in isolation from the others although each can be an activity on its own.

The first activity involves the collection of descriptive and judgmental information for the purpose of establishing whether an educational program or project is doing what it is expected to do. The evaluator pronounces judgment at the end of the exercise.

The second activity involves comparing the performance of one or more students with set standards. Such an evaluation determines the extent to which the objectives of a learning activity are being realized. This is the kind of evaluation teacher's conduct on a daily basis.

The third activity is concerned with the identification of deficiencies in an educational program or syllabus for the purpose of effecting revision and improvement.

Curriculum Evaluation Approaches

Gatawa (1990:60) has identified five curriculum evaluation approaches:
1. **Bureaucratic evaluation:** This evaluation is usually initiated by the government or the Ministry of Education. In your circumstances, the Ministry of Education could evaluate a course of study or subjects taught in schools to find out whether they need improvement or modifications. The results of the evaluation are used by the Ministry of Education or the government.
2. **Autocratic evaluation:** This evaluation focuses on what is considered to be the educational needs of a curriculum. Governments or ministries usually ask independent evaluators, such as consultants to conduct this evaluation. The government or ministry is not obliged to accept the results of the evaluation.
3. **Democratic evaluation:** This focuses on the experiences and reactions the curriculum initiators have had with the programs or project being evaluated. In this approach, the evaluation does not lead to firm recommendations to be considered by the initiators or program implementers.
4. **Norm-referenced evaluation:** This evaluates students' performance relative to other students' performance. The performance of current students or of previous students can be compared.
5. **Criterion-referenced evaluation:** Criterion referencing measures students' actual performance and compares it with the objectives of instruction identified in the syllabus.

Functions of Curriculum Evaluation

Urevbu (1985:64–70) has also identified some functions of curriculum evaluation:
1. Informing decision-makers on the state of affairs of certain curriculum programs or syllabuses, and
2. Enabling teachers to evaluate themselves.
- **Decision making:** With respect to the first function, Partlett and Hamilton, in Urevbu, argue that the principal purpose of evaluation is to contribute to decision making. In our circumstances, curriculum evaluations are conducted in order to correct deficiencies make improvements and establish new priorities. For meaningful decisions to be made, they must be supported by evidence from evaluation exercises.
- **Self-evaluation:** This puts you, the teacher, at the center of the evaluation exercise. You are a curriculum developer indulging in research based teaching. The advantage of self-evaluation is that it allows you to change the curriculum or instructional strategies if evaluations show that they could be more effective.
- **Forms of evaluation:** In the context of curriculum evaluation, there are formative and summative evaluations. Both can be conducted to provide information necessary for effective decision making.

Formative Evaluation

- The term 'formative evaluation' was originally coined by Scriven (1973) to classify evaluation that gathered information for the purpose of improving instruction as the instruction was being given.
- The performance of the learner was the primary focus in Scriven's version of formative evaluation.
- Information about the learner's immediate retention of skills and knowledge, retention over time and attitudes were used to shape instruction as it proceeded.
- Formative evaluation was considered to be an integral part of instructional design and delivery.
- In our curriculum context, formative evaluation can be considered to be the process that looks for evidence of success or failure of a curriculum program, a syllabus or a subject taught during implementation.

Summative Evaluation

- This type of evaluation assesses whether or not the project or program can perform as the originators and designers intended.
- It considers cost effectiveness in terms of money, time and personnel. It also assesses the training that teachers might need in order to implement a program successfully.
- It determines whether a new curriculum program, syllabus or subject is better than the one it is intended to replace or other alternatives. It is usually conducted at the end of the program cycle.
- Formative and summative evaluations can take place wherever an evaluation exercise is conducted. They can be conducted on educational projects and programs existing in the curriculum or on the teaching of individual subjects in the school systems.

Curriculum Change and Innovations

- **Curriculum change:** Hoyle defines change as embracing the concepts of innovation, development, renewal and improvement of a curriculum. Curriculum change is dictated by the changes in the economic, social and technological aspects of a society. Change has magnitude and direction and occurs within a definite time frame
- **Curriculum innovation:** Harris et al. describe innovation as "an intentional and deliberate process to bring out desired effects and change". Curriculum innovation refers to ideas or practices that are new and different from those that exist in the formal prescribed curriculum.

Types of Change

Change can be categorized into two types. Perhaps you are familiar with the types described below:
1. **Hardware types:** These changes are introduced by additions to facilities, such as new classrooms, equipment, books and play grounds.
2. **Software types:** These affect the content and range of the curriculum itself. They may be related to the methods of delivery recommended by curriculum initiators, designers and developers.

Forms of Change

Change can occur in the following forms (University of Zimbabwe, 1985:69):
- **Substitution:** In this change, one element replaces another previously in use. Examples are new textbooks, new equipment or the replacement of teachers and administrators.
- **Alteration:** This involves change in existing structures rather than a complete replacement of the whole curriculum, syllabus or course of study.
- **Addition:** This is the introduction of a new component without changing old elements or patterns. New elements are added to the existing program without seriously disturbing the main structure and content of the prescribed curriculum. These could be support inputs, such as audio-visual aids, workshops and equipment.
- **Restructuring:** This involves the rearrangement of the curriculum in order to implement desired changes. It may also involve the sharing of resources among a group of schools or institutions.

Strategies

- **Participative problem-solving:** This strategy focuses on the users, their needs and how they satisfy these needs. The system identifies and diagnoses its own needs, finds its own solution, tries out and evaluates the solution and implements the solution if it is satisfactory. The emphasis is on local initiative.
- **Planned linkage:** In this model, the intermediate agencies, such as schools, bring together the users of the innovation.
- **Coercive strategies:** These strategies operate on the basis of power and coercion by those in authority, using laws, directories, circulars and so forth. Ministries of Education usually use these strategies.
- **Open input strategies:** These are open, flexible, pragmatic approaches that make use of external ideas and resources.

The innovation process: Innovation and change generally follow several logical steps:
1. Identify a problem, dissatisfaction or need that requires attention.
2. Generate possible solutions to the identified problem or need.
3. Select a particular solution or innovation that has been identified as the most appropriate.
4. Conduct a trial
5. Evaluate the proposed solution
6. Review the evaluation
7. If the innovation has solved the identified problem, implement it on a wide scale.
8. Adopt and institutionalize the innovation or search for another solution.

Innovation planning: Effective planning for innovation cannot take place unless the following elements are considered in the process (University of Zimbabwe, 1995:83):
- The personnel to be employed
- The specification of the actual task
- The strategy or procedure to be used to undertake the task
- The equipment needed
- The buildings and conducive environment
- The costs involved
- Social contexts
- Time involved
- Sequencing of activities
- Rationale for undertaking the innovation
- Evaluation of the consequences or effects of the innovation.

Curriculum Development in Nursing

Curriculum development in nursing education is a means to arrange, employ and assess learning opportunities. Nursing curriculum is built on philosophical foundations and is generally structured to incorporate that philosophy by considering the nature of knowledge, how students learn it and what teaching approach will best impart it.

- **Linear development:** Linear nursing education models are objectives—driven, emphasizing desired student-nurse outcomes. Objectives or specific behaviors are established and a step-by-step program is developed to teach students and achieve desired outcomes. As an educational blueprint, linear models can be assessed to determine if the stated objectives have been reached.
- **Cyclic development:** Cyclic models portray nursing curriculum development as a coherent and logical procedure involving five specific mechanisms including situational analysis, choice of objectives, content selection and arrangement, methods selection and arrangement and learning assessment. This model assumes that what is being taught is circular with no specific starting or ending point.
- **Dynamic models:** A third nursing education curriculum model is the dynamic model. Complex, flexible, interactive and dynamic, this model encourages curriculum development participants to debate, argue and discuss the curriculum approach until arriving at an agreed-upon result. The model urges nursing educators, nurses, doctors, students and healthcare community leaders to have involvement and input in the curriculum design and development.

Chapter 21: Planning and Organizing Educational Institutions

■ PLANNING TEACHING AND LEARNING EXPERIENCES

Organizing and planning of teaching-learning is the framework on which effective teaching is based. Careful and thoughtful planning allows instructional time to be maximized, standards to be addressed, prior knowledge to be activated, misconceptions to be confronted and the diverse characteristics and learning needs of students to be considered.

Classroom management issues are resolved and the focus can be on instruction and increasing student achievement. In addition, instruction can be scaffolded more effectively and assessments of learning goals and content can be aligned to maximize understanding. For curricular planning, it should be done before the academic year. In this case, selection of textbooks, their distribution, conduct of exams, preparation of time-table, allotment of staff for each subject in different classes, monitoring of each class by teachers, etc., are very important. All these activities highlight the importance of annual planning, unit planning and lesson planning which are presented in details in the subsequent paragraphs. **Table 21.1** describes principles to be followed while providing learning experience.

Objectives

- Examine the importance of planning in teaching-learning process in social sciences
- Identify the various areas of planning in social sciences
- Implement various learning experiences in a classroom
- Describe the planning of Annual Plan, Unit Plan and Lesson Plan
- Differentiate between behaviorist and constructivist classroom
- Organize constructivist classroom activities
- Prepare lesson plan based on the principles of constructivism.

The Six Aspects

There are six aspects of planning learning experiences and instruction:
1. Check students' prior knowledge, skill levels and potential misconceptions
2. Identify a series of specific learning goals/intentions
3. Organize and sequence the specific learning goals/intentions
4. Use WHERETO to inform learning events/experiences
5. Code learning events/experiences
6. Decide how progress will be monitored during learning events. How will students get feedback?

I. Check Students' Prior Learning

Understanding students' prior knowledge and skills will guide any differentiated instruction/assessment that may be needed, but do not grade pre-assessments. To check prior learning: **Know, Want to know, Learnings (K-W-L)**.

- **Know:** Prior to the introduction of a new topic or skill, ask students what they already know, or think they know, about the topic or skill, and record them on a whiteboard or chart paper under a 'K' column (sometimes, students make statements that are incorrect or reveal misconceptions).
- **Want to know:** Secondly, ask them what they want to know (or what questions they have) about the topic/skill. These are recorded under the 'W' column (their questions often reveal interests or 'hooks' to the topic and their questions may reveal misconceptions that will need to be addressed).
- **Learnings:** As the lesson or unit proceeds, learning's are summarized and recorded in the 'L' column as they occur (this provides an opportunity to go back and correct any misconceptions that may have been initially recorded in the 'K' column).

Pre-Test

Give students a pre-test to check their prior knowledge of key facts and concepts. Use the results to plan instruction and selection of resources. Ensure students know that the results will not count toward final grades.

Skills Check

Have students demonstrate their proficiency with a targeted skill or process. It is helpful to have a proficiency checklist or developmental rubric to use in assessing the degree of skill competence. Students can then use the checklist or rubric for on-going self-assessment.

Web/Concept Map

Ask students to create a web or concept map to show the elements or components of a topic or process. This technique is especially effective in revealing whether students have gaps

Table 21.1: Principles to be followed while providing learning experience.

• Proceed	• Principle of diagnostic and remedial teaching
• Principle of aim	• Principle of looking ahead
• Learning by doing	• Principle of creativity
• Principle of linking	• Systematic exposition
• Principle of planning	• Clear understanding
• Principle of interest and motivation	• Principle of revision and fixation
• Principle of sympathy and kind atmosphere	• Area to be selected for learning experience
• Principle of flexibility and cooperation	

Box 21.3: Criteria for selection of learning experiences.

- Should be consistent with the philosophy and objectives
- Should be varied and flexible
- Opportunity for self-activity
- Opportunity for development of independent thinking and decision making
- Should be adapted to the needs of the students
- Continuity, correlation and integration of theory and practice
- Planned and evaluated cooperatively by the teacher and the student
- Select according to relative importance

in their knowledge and the extent to which they understand relationships among the elements.

Misconception

Check present students with common errors or predictable misconceptions regarding a designated topic, concept, skill or process. See if they are able to identify the error or misconception and explain why it is erroneous or flawed. The misconception check can also be presented in the form of a true-false quiz, where students must agree or disagree with statements or examples.

II. Identify Specific Learning Goals/Intentions

Identify a series of specific learning goals/intentions by considering the acquisition, meaning and transfer learning goals and breaking them down into specific learning intentions (these could be for a week, a few days or a lesson). Share and discuss these with students and display prominently.

III. Organize and Sequence

- Organize the specific learning intentions/goals into a sequence and decide on learning events/experiences.
- Consider the sequence of learning intentions that best suits the desired results.
- Decide on the learning events/experiences that are most appropriate for the desired results.
- How will you support students to understand important ideas and processes?
- How will you prepare them to autonomously transfer their learning?
- What enabling knowledge and skills will students need in order to perform effectively and achieve desired results?
- Which activities, sequence, and resources are best suited to accomplish the learning intentions/goals?

IV. Use WHERETO (Fig. 21.4)

Use WHERETO to inform learning events and experiences.

W = Where and Why

- Where are the students coming from? Where are they headed? How will I help learners know what they will be learning? Why is this worth learning? What evidence will show their learning? How will their performance be evaluated?
- Learners of all ages are more likely to put forth effort and meet with success when they understand the learning goals and see them as meaningful and personally relevant.
- The 'W' in WHERETO reminds teachers to clearly communicate the goals and help students see their relevance.
- Also, learners need to know the performance expectations and assessments through which they will demonstrate their learning, so that they have clear learning targets and the basis for monitoring their progress toward them.

H = Hook and Hold

- How will I hook and engage the learners? How will I keep them engaged?
- The best teachers have always recognized the value of 'hooking' learners through introductory activities that tease the mind and engage the heart in the learning process.

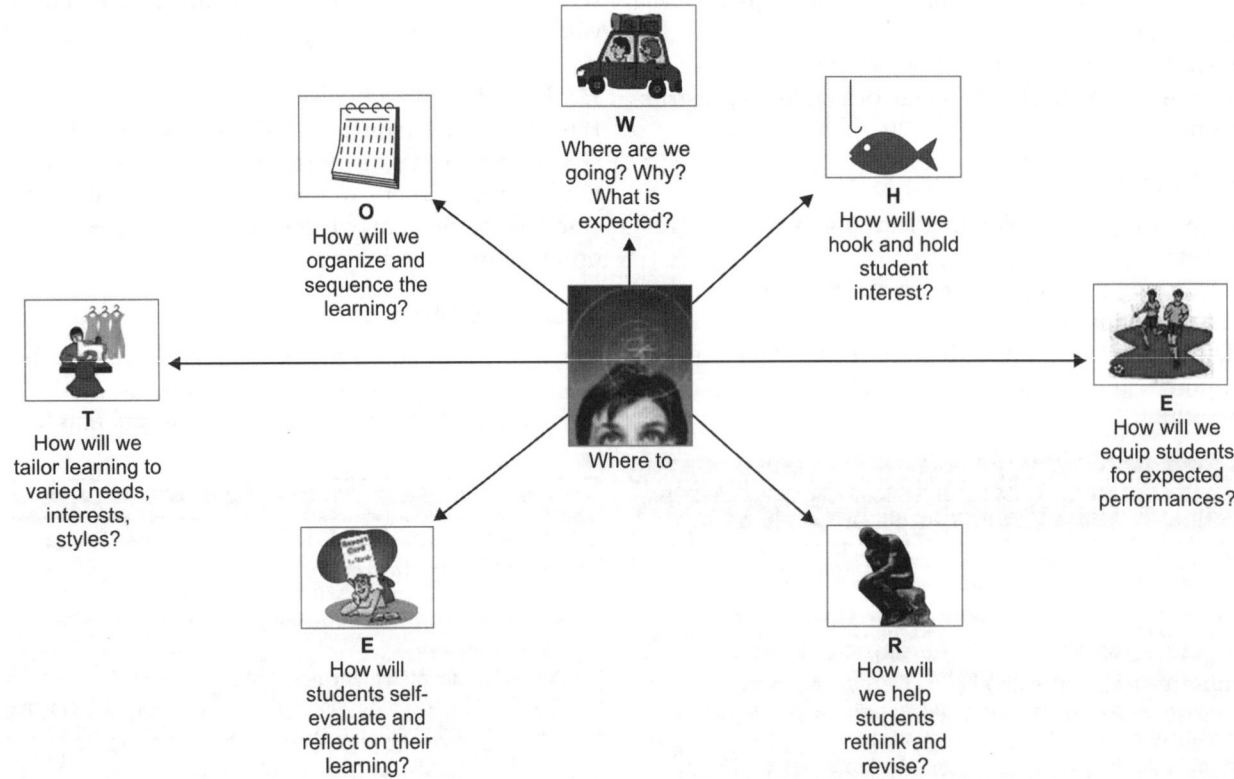

Fig. 21.4: Planning teaching and learning experiences.

- Teachers are encouraged to deliberately plan ways of hooking their learners to the topics they teach.
- The intent is to match the hook with the content and the experiences of the learner—by design—as a means of drawing them into a productive learning experience.
- Examples of effective hooks include provocative essential questions, counter-intuitive phenomena, controversial issues, authentic problems and challenges, emotional encounters, and humor.
- One must be mindful, of course, of not just coming up with interesting introductory activities that have no carry-over value.

E = Explore and Experience, Enable and Equip

- **Consider:** How will I equip students to master identified standards and succeed with the transfer performances? What learning experiences will help develop and deepen understanding of important ideas?
- Understanding cannot be simply transferred, such as a load of freight from one mind to another.
- Coming to understand requires active intellectual engagement on the part of the learner. Therefore, instead of merely covering the content, effective educators 'uncover' the most enduring ideas and processes in ways that engage students in constructing meaning for themselves.
- To this end, teachers select an appropriate balance of constructivist learning experiences, structured activities, and direct instruction for helping students acquire the desired knowledge, skill, and understanding.
- There is a place for direct instruction and modeling, teaching for understanding asks teachers to also adopt a facilitative role—to engage learners in making meaning through active inquiry and diverse experience with the content.

R = Reflect, Rethink, Revises

- How will I encourage the learners to rethink previous learning? How will I encourage on-going revision and refinement?
- Few learners develop a complete understanding of abstract ideas on the first encounter. Indeed, the phrase 'coming to understand' is suggestive of a process.
- Over time, learners develop and deepen their understanding by thinking and re-thinking, by examining ideas from different points of view, from examining underlying assumptions, and by receiving feedback and revising.
- Just as the quality of a piece of writing benefits from the iterative process of drafting and revising, so to do understandings become more mature. The 'R' in WHERETO encourages teachers to explicitly include such opportunities.

E = Evaluate Work and Progress

- How will I promote students' self-evaluation and reflection?
- Capable and independent learners are distinguished by their capacity to set goals, self-assess their progress, and adjust as needed.
- Yet one of the most frequently overlooked aspects of the instructional process involves helping students to develop the meta-cognitive skills of self evaluation, self-regulation, and reflection.
- The second 'E' of WHERETO remind teachers to build in time and expectations for students to regularly self assess, reflect on the meaning of their learning, and set goals for future performance.

T = Tailor and Personalize the Work

- How will I tailor the learning experiences to the nature of the learners I serve?
- How might I differentiate instruction to respond to the varied needs of students?
- 'One size fits all' teaching is rarely optimal. Learners differ significantly in terms of prior knowledge, skill levels, interests, talents, and preferred ways of learning.
- Accordingly, the most effective teachers get to know their students and tailor their teaching and learning experiences so as to connect the material with the kids.
- A variety of strategies may be employed to differentiate content (how subject matter is presented), process (how students work), and product (how learners demonstrate their learning).
- The logic of backward design offers a cautionary note here: the content standards and understandings should not be differentiated (except for students with Individual Education Plans). In other words, we differentiate means while keeping the ends in mind for all.

O = Organize for Optimal Effectiveness

- How will I organize the learning experiences for maximum engagement and effectiveness? What sequence will be optimal given the understanding and transfer goals?
- When the primary educational goals involve helping students acquire basic knowledge and skills, teachers may be comfortable 'covering' the content by telling and modeling. However, when we include understanding and transfer as desired results, educators are encouraged to give careful attention to how the content is organized and sequenced.

V. Code Learning Events/Experiences

Code learning experiences to ensure all three types of goals (acquisition, meaning and transfer) are addressed in the plan. Beside each learning event/experience record A T or M (or a combination) to check that all 3 areas are being covered in the learning plan.

VI. Monitor Progress and Feedback

Decide how progress will be monitored during learning events, and how students will get feedback. The following on-going assessment techniques can be used to obtain a quick 'pulse check' of a whole class or group of students.

Hand Signals

Ask students to display a designated hand signal to indicate their understanding of a designated concept, principle, or process. For example,
- I understand [X] and can explain it (for example, thumbs up)
- I do not yet understand [X] (for example, thumbs down)
- I am not completely sure about [X] (for example, wave hand)
  - **Mini white boards:** Have students record a response on a mini white board and hold it up. For example,
    a. Prediction—what number should appear next in the sequence?
    b. Agree/disagree—is this an example of adaptation
  - **Student response systems:** Use student response systems (SRS) 'clickers' to have students record a response to a question or a prompt. The results can be tabulated on the teacher's computer to provide immediate feedback.
  - **Misconception check:** Present students with common or predictable misconceptions about a designated concept, principle, or process. Ask them to agree or disagree.
  - **Observations:** Carefully observe students as they work or respond to questions. Observe the work they produce. What areas of strength and weakness do you notice?

ORGANIZING CLINICAL FACILITIES FOR NURSING STUDENTS

One of the main features of nursing both as a science and a profession is integration of theory and practice. Clinical training is an important component of nursing education. Clinical learning takes place in a complex social context of the clinical environment. Learning in a clinical setting creates challenges that are absent in a classroom setting. Facilitators have control of the environmental conditions in the classroom whereas in the clinical setting, the teaching and learning are modified according to the situation of the real environment. The safety of patients that the students are assigned to care for must be maintained. Clinical experience prepares student nurses to be capable of knowing as well as doing the clinical principles in practice. Moreover, the clinical practices stimulate students to use their critical thinking skills in problem solving
- Most of the time, the clinical learning is based on the dyadic approach consisting of clinical environment and supervisory relationship between students and the teachers.
- This approach warrants a lot of commitment from both the lecturers and students to foster effective learning. Sometimes the student and lecturer ratio ranges from 1:6 to 1:12 in the clinical area.
- The high acuity and increased number of the patients in the clinical area creates challenges and influences the clinical teaching and learning.
- The nursing students prepared at a higher diploma level are expected to be evaluated on more than twenty clinical procedures during their practicum according to their level in nursing program.

INC Requirements

- College of nursing should have a 100-bedded parent hospital.
- Distribution of beds in different areas/for 40 annual intakes is
  - Medical 30
  - Surgical 30
  - Obst and Gynecology 30
  - Pediatrics 20
  - Ortho 10
- Bed occupancy of the hospital should be minimum 75%.
- The size of the hospital/nursing home for affiliation should not be less than 100-beds.
- Other specialties/facilities for clinical experience required are as follows:
  - Major OT
  - Minor OT
  - Dental
  - Eye/ENT
  - Burns and plastic
  - Neonatology with nursery
  - Communicable disease
  - Community health nursing
  - Cardiology
  - Oncology
  - Neurology/neurosurgery
  - Nephrology, etc.
  - ICU/ICCU
- Affiliation of psychiatric hospital should be of minimum 50 beds.
- The nursing staffing norms in the affiliated hospital should be as per the INC norms.
- The affiliated hospital should give student status to the candidates of the nursing program.
- Maximum distance between affiliated hospitals and institutions: (a) Institutions generally can be in the radius of 15–30 km. from the affiliated hospital, (b) Hilly and Tribal area, it can be in the radius of 30–50 km from the affiliated hospital.
- 1:3 student patient ratio to be maintained.
- For the grant of 100 students minimum 300-bedded parent hospital is mandatory.

Parent hospital for a nursing institution having the same trust which has established nursing institutions and has also established the hospital.

OR

For a nursing institution (managed by trust) a "Parent Hospital" would be a hospital either owned and controlled by the trust or managed and controlled by a member of the trust. In case, the owner of the hospital is a member of the Trust that the hospital would continue to function as a "Parent Hospital" till the life of the nursing institution. The undertaking would also be to the effect that the Member of the Trust would not allow the hospital to be treated" Parent/Affiliated Hospital" to any other nursing institution and will be for minimum 30 years [i.e., signed by all members of trust] to the undertaking to be submitted from the Members of the Trust.

Types of Clinical Areas

- **Hospitals:** Hospitals are the ultimate "catch-all" healthcare facility. Their services can vary greatly depending on their size and location, but a hospital's goal is to save lives. Hospitals typically have a wide range of units that can be loosely broken into intensive care and non-intensive care units. Intensive care units deal with emergencies and the most serious illnesses and injuries. Patients with imminently life-threatening problems go here. Non-intensive care units include things like childbirth, surgeries, rehabilitation, step-down units for patients
- **Orthopedic and other rehabilitation centers:** Orthopedic medicine deals with muscles and bones. Physical therapists are typically the practitioner patients see for problems in these areas of the body. If you are experiencing chronic lower back pain, for example, you might see a physical therapist at an orthopedic center or clinic to get a diagnosis and a plan of treatment.

  Orthopedic centers deal in everything from athletic injuries to therapy for patients with disabilities. They typically offer evaluation and diagnosis of the problem, as well as prevention, treatment and rehabilitation work involving bone, tendon, ligament, muscle and joint conditions.
- **Mental health and addiction treatment centers:** This type of healthcare facility is a grouping for many different types of facilities. Specialty treatment centers exist all across America for specified mental health issues and addictions. Mental health treatment facilities sometimes exist as a general institution for any mental health issue and are sometimes specialized. Examples of these kinds of facilities are suicidal thoughts (or suicidal ideation) treatment, depression treatment, trauma and post-traumatic stress disorder (PTSD) treatment, treatment for anxiety disorders, behavioral disorders and more.
- **Community clinical facilities:** College of Nursing students are given opportunity to participate in immunization programs, school health programs, MCH programs, home visit, street play, puppet show, role play, projects, health talk, mass health programs, Nutritional assessment and cooking demonstration are carried out in areas attached to both rural and urban health centers. Apart from home visit students participate in the programs and activities of the health centers.

MASTER ROTATION PLAN (FIG. 21.5)

- Master rotation plan is an overall plan which shows rotation of all the students in a particular educational institution.
- It shows the placement of the students belonging to various groups/classes in a clinical nursing as well as community.
- It denotes duration of the placement that includes theoretical (teaching) block, partial block (half clinical and half theory) block and clinical block.

Definition

- Master rotation plan is an overall plan which shows rotation of all the students in a particular educational institution.

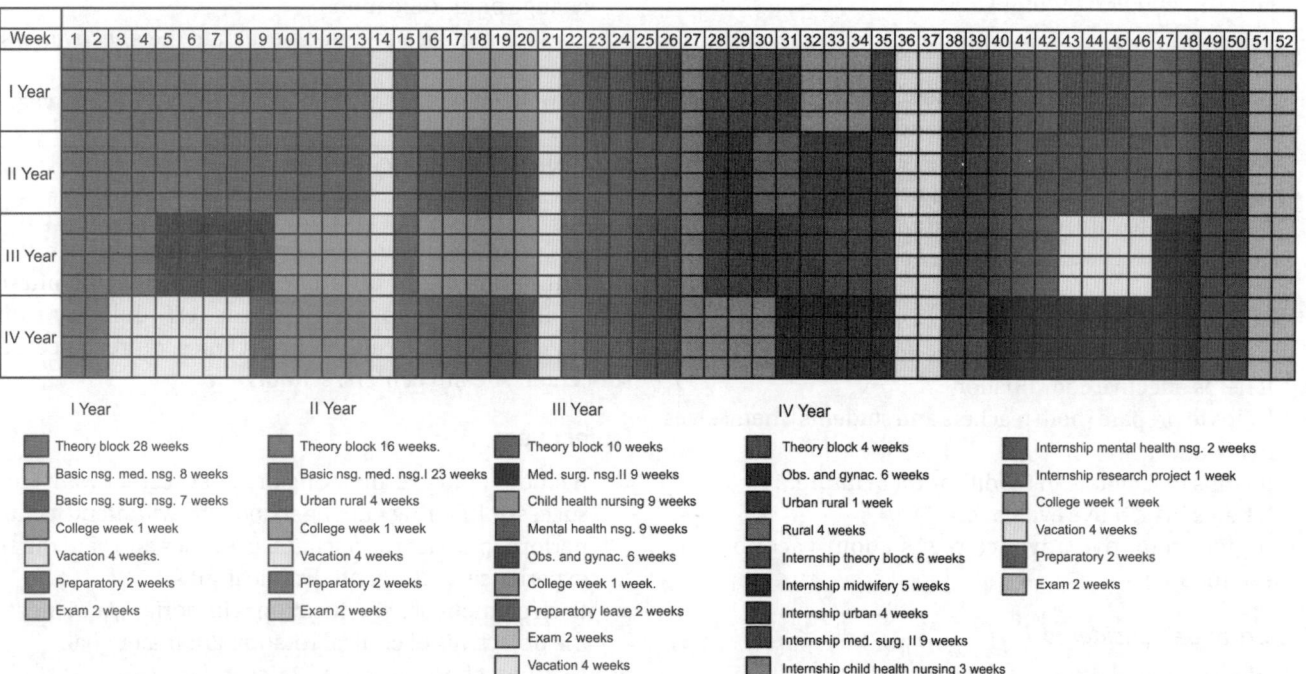

Fig. 21.5: Master rotation plan BSc Nursing (4 Years).

- Master rotation plan denotes duration of the placement that includes theoretical block, partial block (Half clinical, half theory block) and clinical block.

Purposes

- Availability of an advance plan before implementation of curricular activities during an academic year for the entire program.
- All concerned are aware of the placement of students in clinical fields.
- Coordination becomes more effective when theory, practice correlates, and integrity exist.
- Helps the students and teachers to prepare themselves for working in the areas.
- Any modifications are required based on situations concerned, collaborations between the faculty and service staff can be made for smooth running of organizational activities, and meeting the objectives of educational program.
- Assessment of the curricular program is more effective.

Nature of Plan

- It is prepared in advance for the whole year.
- It gives complete and clear picture about the students
- It must include period of vacation, teaching block, preparation time, examination and vacation.
- Master rotation plan for each year can be prepared separately than putting up combined chart.
- The teacher should be aware of the student's placement.
- Overlapping particular area or shortage in particular area can be noted
- The teacher should follow Indian Nursing Council and University syllabus.
- The teacher should consider all three domains (cognitive, affective and psychomotor).

Domains used in Planning

- **Cognitive domain:** It includes knowledge, comprehension, application, analysis, synthesis and evolution.
- **Affective domains:** It includes receiving, responding, valuing, organization and characterization.
- **Psychomotor domain:** It includes imitation, manipulation, precision, articulation and naturalism.

Purpose of Master Rotation Plan

- It gives information about entire course plan
- It helps effective coordination
- Helps to prepare (both teachers and students) themselves in advance.
- It helps to facilitate in modification in future.
- It helps in effective evaluation.
- It gives tentative advance plans about vacation and examination.

Factors to be Considered

- Objectives of the courses
- Number of students in the class
- Number of departments/areas
- Size of the department, e.g., surgical ward, MSW, FSW and POP (postoperative ward)
- Duration of experience
- Number of persons available for supervision
- Indian Nursing Council/University requirements.

Principles of Master Rotation Plan

- Theoretical instruction should proceed as closely as possible the clinical experience, ward classes, clinical care presentations should be held simultaneously.
- There should be at least one instructor (in clinical area) who is well prepared in her field—available to students at least 1:4 or prescribed by the INC and/or according to the type of patient nursed.
- Selection of areas of experience should proceed from simple to complex.
- The teaching staff should be involved whenever feasible and must be familiar with the rotation plan.
- Each student must be provided experience in each block - no block should be missed.
- The rotation plan must be made in advance
- Continuity of experience, which is considered essential, must be maintained.
- Overlapping should be avoided.

Responsibility of Teaching Staff

- Correlate theory and practice
- Participate in teaching, supervision and evaluation.
- Prepare the student in theory block before they enter the clinical block
- Maintain adequate and regular attendance at both the class room and clinical areas.
- Report to the principal or concerned person for any change or modification.
- Plan for regular meeting to evaluate the effectiveness of a plan
- Domain of educational objective should be followed.

■ CLINICAL ROTATION PLAN (FIG. 21.6)

In nursing education clinical rotation refers to "regular, successive and recurrent posting of various groups of nursing student belonging to different classes in specific nursing fields, i.e., OPD's, specialty, wards, OT, delivery room, clinics, community health fields—clinics, outreach centers, subcenters, health centers, schools, etc.

Objectives

- A student nurse embarking on a new career wants to be successful. During nursing school, she will attend lectures, perform practical application exercises and gain nursing experience at designated clinical sites.
- Each element of her education is important, and meeting the objectives of clinical rotation is a major goal.
- Nursing schools provide clinical rotations to give student nurses an opportunity to care for actual patients.

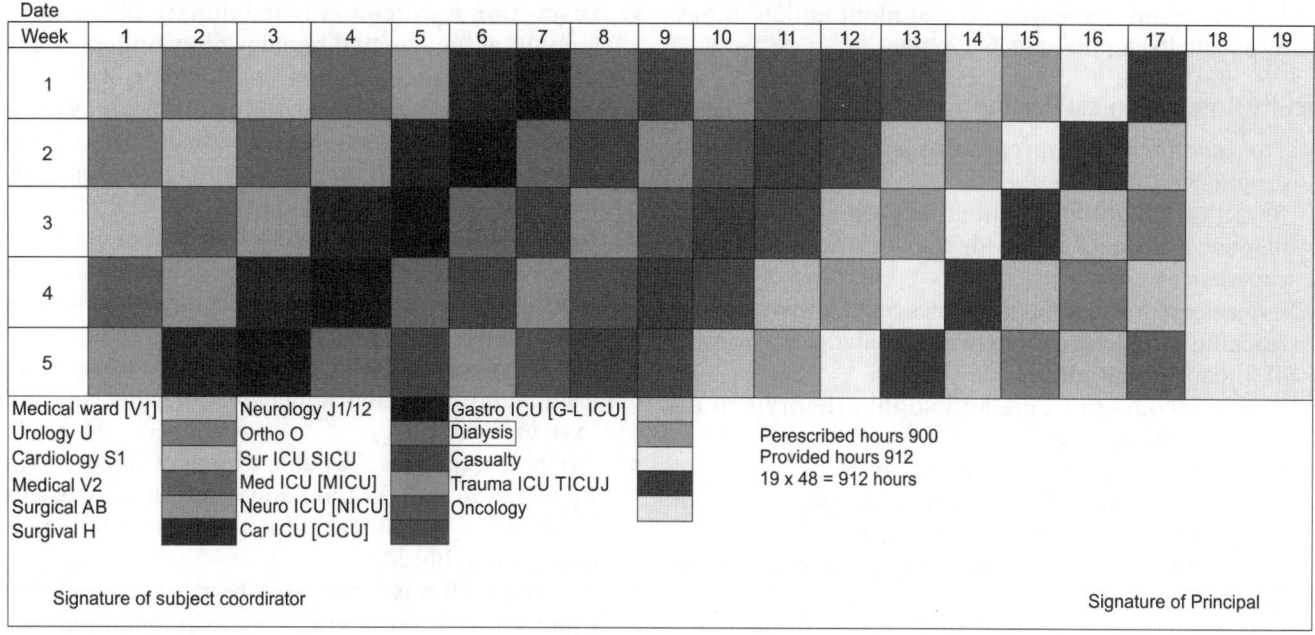

Fig. 21.6: Clinical rotation plan.

- Clinical rotations are required periods of practical application and training conducted in a medical facility.
- The nursing school, in accordance with accrediting institutions, design coursework and mandate hours of clinical care.
- The clinical rotations will complement the nursing coursework. The nursing lessons are generally divided into foundations of nursing, adult care, childcare, maternal health and childbearing, mental health, critical care, pharmacology, and medical-surgical care.
- The nursing school designates an instructor to accompany and train the nursing student at the clinical rotation site.

Basic Principles

- Select the type of learning experience from simple to complex.
- Clinical supervisor must be familiar with the rotation plan.
- Each student should get all the experience on rotation wise.
- All students should enter and leave the clinical area at the same time and they should complete the assignment in time.

Factors Considered

- The objectives of the course have to be clearly stated.
- Number of students in each class.
- Number and size of department teaching units, or wards where student should be given opportunity for practicing clinical skills/clinical experience.
- The duration of clinical experience in each area as per INC and university/Board norms.
- The number of teaching faculty available for clinical supervision. Adhere to rotation plan.
- The clinical rotation plan must be in accordance with the total curriculum plan.
- It has to be prepared in advance.
- Theoretical instructions should proceed as closely as possible with clinical experience.
- The teacher and student ratio will be 1:4 or as prescribed by INC.

Responsibilities of clinical instructor:

- The instructor coordinates with the nursing course lecturer to devise practical application exercises that reinforce/re-emphasize the classroom lecture.
- The instructor fosters a relationship with the staff who work at the hospital or medical facility where the nursing students practice.
- The students impose on time and resources of the medical facilities where they train, so forming a good working relationship benefits the nursing school and prolongs the association between the school and clinical site.
- Additionally, the instructor encourages learning, questioning, self-development and critical thinking in her students.
- She evaluates students and ensures the safety of patients assigned to her students.

Responsibilities of nursing student:

- The student nurse has the responsibility of observing procedures, documenting procedures that she performs and practicing her nursing skills.
- Prior to meeting a patient, she reviews the patient's medical record and familiarizes herself with the patient's condition and treatment.
- The student also follows the rules and regulations of medical facility.
- In meeting the clinical rotation objectives the student assesses the patients mental and physical condition defines the patient's health problem then makes and implements a plan of care.

- The instructor supervises the student and assumes responsibility for the student's actions.

Faculty Role in Clinical Posting

- The teacher has to prepare objectives for clinical experience.
- Based on objectives, clinical experience has to be planned in advance to provide specific planned learning experiences.
- If necessary for some of the topics provide spot clinical teaching and such topic has to be repeated to each group of student as they rotate.
- Plan the course outline and so that theory can be correlated to practice.
- Get permission from clinical authority.
- Ensure that each student is aware of the objectives and assignments and criteria for evaluation.
- Place and guide the student to get required clinical experience.
- Orient the student to the clinical area, ward staff, etc., where they are posted.
- Participate in teaching, supervision, and evaluation of students in the ward.
- Arrange ward teaching, ward discussions and case presentation.
- Help the students for effective charting of records and reports.

BUDGET PLANNING FOR COLLEGE OF NURSING

Budgeting in nursing school can present several unique challenges. In addition to paying normal living expenses and school costs, nursing students also must save up money for certifications, clinical, and uniforms. Students with full-time employment or dependents may face additional strains on their time and resources. However, taking the time to develop and maintain a financial plan can help manage these obstacles.

- School/college of nursing should have a separate budget; principal in charge of the school of nursing should be drawing the budget. (As per government rules regulations and as seemed necessary for running an educational institutions.)
- Both the school/college and hospital should have separate budget. The budget for the school or college is annually planned by the nursing director, principal and general manager and approved by the managing director.

Budgeting Terminology

- **Total income:** Total income refers to the total amount of funding students have when they enter school. Students should include financial aid, outside assistance, and paychecks.
- **Monthly income:** Monthly income refers to the specific amount of income students receive every month. Most often, monthly income comes from a job. This amount can vary depending on the number of hours students work.
- **Discretionary income:** Discretionary income is the amount of income that remains after students pay for necessary expenses, such as food and rent. Students can use discretionary income for savings or spending money.
- **Essentials:** Students absolutely need essentials to live and succeed in school. Common essential expenses include rent, food, fees, books, and utilities.
- **Nonessentials:** Nonessentials may still be important. However, a student's survival likely does not hinge on whether or not they have them. Examples include gym membership, coffee shops, dining out, and entertainment.
- **Fixed expenses:** Fixed expenses cost the same amount each month. Rent and student loan payments count as fixed expenses.
- **Variable expenses:** Variable expenses fluctuate from month to month. While many variable expenses are nonessential, essential expenses, such as utilities can also change monthly.
- **Emergency funds:** Emergency funds cover unexpected expenses, such as car repairs, vet visits, or hospital stays.

Types

Classification of budget is classified into two heads:
1. **Revenue:** It includes assets, fixed deposits, investments, loan and income.
2. **Expenditure:** It includes all expenses.

Revenue Expenditure

- College fees (from students)
- Fixed deposits
- Government salary (for employees)
- Donation (trustees)
- Guest lecturers
- Staff salary
- University payment
- Workshop or conferences
- Maintenance

Objectives in Budgeting

The main objective of a firm is to make an excess of revenue over expenses to maximize profit. But it is not a matter of a dream or chance. There is no magic formula for boosting the figure of profit overnight. Budgeting can increase the chances of making profits within the given environment. The main objectives of budgets are as follows:

- To provide a realistic estimate of income and expenses for a period and of the financial position at the close of the period.
- To provide a coordinated plan of action which is design to achieve the estimates reflected in the budget.
- To provide a comparison of actual results with those budgeted and an analysis and interpretation of deviations by areas of responsibility to indicate courses of corrective actions and to lead to improvement in future plans.
- To provide a guide for management decisions in adjusting plans and objectives if there is an uncontrollable change in conditions.

- To provide a ready basis for making forecasts during the budget period to guide management in making day to day decisions.

Purpose of Budget

- Budget supplies the mechanism for translating fiscal objective into projected monthly spending pattern.
- Budget enhances fiscal planning and decision-making.
- Budget clearly recognizes controllable and uncontrollable cost areas.
- Budget offers a useful format for communicating fiscal objectives.
- Budget allows feedback of utilization of budget.
- Budget helps to identify problem areas and facilitates effective solution.
- Budget provides means for measuring and recording financial success with the objectives of the organizations.

Characteristics of Budget

A budget is a financial document or an action plan which is prepared and used to project future income and expenses. It outlines an organization's financial and operational goals. It can also include non-monetary information with the monetary information. They need to be made and approved in advance of the year in which they are to be used or implemented.

Following are the characteristics of a good budget:

- It is expressed in quantitative or monetary terms.
- It is prepared for a fixed period of time It is prepared before the period in which it commences.
- Practical to implement
- It spells out the objects and the policies to be pursued in order to achieve the objective of the organization.
- Many people are involved in drawing up a budget.
- Flexible enough to allow changes in the changing environment.
- Prepared on the basis of established standards of performance.
- Analysis of cost and revenues
- On the basis of budget report performance of the organization is constantly monitored.

Classifications of Budget

- **Master budgets:** This is a comprehensive summary budget, incorporating all the functional and operational budgets, generally including sales, production, material and labor costs, any overhead costs, profit, etc.
- **Materials and utilities budget:** This budget also known as operations budget includes budgeting for raw materials required for production, spare parts for maintenance, labor time, machine time, energy consumption, etc. Labor time and machine time is the output per unit of time.
- **Control of liquidity:** This involves cash flow and is very important in controlling and meeting current financial obligations. This budget forecasts cash receipts and outlays in a set time basis and is necessary to control the income and expenses, so that there is no shortage of cash to pay bills, and also no excessive unused cash which may be unproductive.
- **Revenue and expenses budgets:** The revenue budgets should show anticipated sales by product or by geographical area or department, etc. The expense budgets should cover all necessary and relevant areas, such as rent, utilities, supplies, security, etc.
- **Capital expenditure budgets:** These budgets plan for long-term investments and include expenditures for new plant and equipment, major installations, replacement of existing equipment, building, etc.
- **Sales budget:** The sales budget is the direct outcome of sales forecast and is based on the consideration of the following factors: demand and supply, competition, past sale trends, future prediction of sales, seasonal changes that affect sales, etc. The sales forecasting is based on such factors as population trends, consumer's purchasing power, disposable income, price trends of the products, inflation rate and the general business economy, etc.
- **Production budget:** The production budget contains manufacturing program for future operations and is based upon the sales forecasts and sales budgets. It aims at obtaining maximum utilization of manufacturing methods and facilities.
- **Balance sheet:** It is a composite budget and reflects anticipated assets, liabilities and owner's equity or net worth at the end of a given period in the future. It provides a forecast of the anticipated financial status of the company at a future date.
- **Flexible budget:** Flexible or variable budget reflects and combats the changes in expenditure as a result of changes in volume of production and revenues. These expenditures are primarily variable costs since the fixed costs are not generally affected by changes in revenues.

Importance of Budget

Budget is a numerical description of expected income and planned expenditure for an organization for a specified period of time. It is a concrete, precise, picture of the total operation of an enterprise/organization/institution in monetary term, i.e., finance.

The following point serves the importance of budget:

- Budget is needed for planning for future course of action and to have a control over all activities in the organization.
- Budget facilitates co-coordinating operation of various departments and sections for realizing organizational objectives.
- Budget serves as a guide for action in the organization.
- Budget helps one to weigh the values and to make decision when necessary on whether one is of a greater value in the program than the other.

Benefits of Budget

Budgets are produced in all organizations, whether they are small, large, private or public sector. They are important and are produced for the following reasons:

- To compel planning—by having a formal budgeting procedure, managers are forced to consider business objectives and ways in which those objectives can be achieved
- To coordinate the activities of the various parts of the business and to ensure that the parts are working together
- To communicate plans to the various responsibility managers within the enterprise
- To motivate managers to work towards the business objectives
- To control activities—the budget provides a yardstick against which the performance of the business can be compared
- To evaluate the performance of the managers
- The budgeting process helps management learn from past experience. Management can critically look at the success or failure of the past budgets and isolate errors and analyze their causes and establish steps to avoid repetition of the same errors.
- Budgets help in the just measurement of performance. Due to quantification of budgets, the measurement is more objective, thus eliminating biases that might be introduced due to subjective evaluations.
- The budgeting process induces the management to shift attention to the future operations. It forces managers to anticipate and forecast the trends and changes in the external environment.

Limitations of Budget

Some of the problems associated with budgeting are:
- Budgets are often too rigid and restrictive and supervisors are given little free hand in managing their resources. The budgets may either be changed too often or not at all, making it difficult for employees to meet performance levels.
- Budgets are used to evaluate the performance and results, but the causes of failures and successes are not thoroughly investigated.
- Budgets may be used punitively. The employees may regard budgets simply as rating tools or as a device for catching their mistakes. This will lower their morale and dilute their sense of dedication.
- Budget goals may be conceived as too high. A high production level or sales level may be presented as unrealistic and may create tension and pressures which could very well result in worker inefficiency and create conflict between workers and the management.

Essential Requisition for Budget

- **Forecasting:** Sound forecasting may be related to making decisions on purchases, expansion, advertising, services, working capital needs, etc.
- **Accounting** well conceived accounting system must be needed to compare the budget information with actual accomplishment. The cost information tells as to how much it will cost to produce or give service.
- **Lines of authority:** Budget preparation, operation and supervision need/require clearly defined lines of authority.
- **Budget committee:** Budget needs budget committee in an organization (i) to receive and approve all forecasts, departmental budgets, periodic reports showing comparison of actual and budgeted income and expenditure and (ii) to request for special studies of deviations from the budget and consider revision of budget to meet changed conditions.
- Business policies clearly defined business policies serve as basis for budget preparations.
- Statistical information In the form of figures, i.e., estimates regarding the budget terms are essential for budget.
- Top level management support is essential to ensure successful installation of the budget program.
- **Period of budget:** Length of budget period (usually a year) should be specified.

Steps in Budgeting

While designing and implementing a planning program, the nurse administrator/manager should follow steps as given below:

1. Review the goals of the agency or hospital to identify activities of highest priority, because these are most likely to receive funding.
2. Review the objectives of the existing programs and written for proposed programs to ensure that achievement of these objectives will support agency.
3. Existing programs are revised and proposed programs designed to maximum goal accomplishment.
4. Manpower, capital and operating expenses are computed for each program, old and new.
5. Alternative methods are identified for realizing designated objectives and price of each alternative is determined.
6. Comparisons are made to determine which alternative is most cost-effective.
7. A budget request is developed which details a fiscal plan for the preferred program indicates alternative methods for meeting the same objective, and explains why the recommended program is preferred.
8. Request the assistant nursing officers and supervisors to present their needs for the coming year by a specified date, and confer with those who have presented such need.
9. Review the budget appropriation and actual expenditure for the current year in conjunction with statistical data as to the numbers and distribution of patient, nursing hours, per patient by services, operations and others.
10. Ascertain whether any changes are contemplated, such as opening new facilities for patients or changes in other departments, which affect the nursing services required.
11. Prepare the program which the new budget is to cover in terms of the nursing hours to be given to patients, the distribution of the hours among the various groups of personnel, the ratio of supervisors and head nurses to patients' care and the provision for the administration of nursing unit.

12. Determine the percentage of salaries of personnel who have both educational and nursing service function to be allocated to each function on the basis of time devoted to each.
13. Estimate the requirement for the coming year from the information supplied as the expenditure for supplies, equipments and repairs to date.
14. Prepare a summary of new needs, both personnel and material with data to support the request.

The budget report submitted to the head of the nursing department after carefully reviewed by her/his associates.

BUDGET AUDIT

It developed in 19th century; the nursing audit is similar to an audit performed by accounting departments. It is a process that offers the nursing personnel in a health agency the opportunity to create and enforce standards of nursing care and to examine their own practice in systematic manner.

Meaning of auditing: Auditing is broadly defined as a systematic process of objectively obtaining and evaluating evidence in respect of certain assertions about economic actions and events, to ascertain the degree of correspondence between those assertions and established criteria and reporting the results to interested parties. Auditing usually covers a particular period of time. Auditing may be narrowly defined as a written report on the examination of financial statements for a particular period of time.

Types of Auditing

- **Nursing management audit:** This type is more structure oriented focusing on administrative aspects of the nurse's responsibilities and nurses that the health facilities are suitably equipped to provide care.
- **Retrospective audit:** This is the evaluation of nursing care by examining the records and charts of discharged patients.
- **Concurrent audit:** It is the evaluation of the nursing care by the observation and retrospective method during the delivery of care. The best method of audit depends on the objective of audit.

Characteristics of Audit

- Audit looks at the entire process of care including administration and not just at clinical management.
- Compares the care which actually is given. Standard procedures are agreed to decide which care should be given.
- Concentrates on finding solutions for the problems identified.

Principles of auditing: Fundamental principles are those according to which the books of business accounts are audited. These principles can be changed according the desire of the auditor. We discuss the main principles of auditing under these headings:

- **Planning:** It is the basic principle of auditing. The auditor should plan before starting the work. In planning auditor decides accounting about the system and internal control procedure.
- **Honesty:** Honesty and sincerity is the second important principle of auditing. The loyalty of auditor to work and profession must be beyond the doubt.
- **Impartiality:** In case of audit, the attitude of the auditor must be impartial. Keeping in view this principle his personal views may not be included in the audit report.
- **Secrecy:** Secrecy must be maintained by the auditor during the process of audit. He cannot disclose any information to the third party.
- **Evidence:** During the audit, the auditor can collect the evidence. He can frame his opinion on the audit evidence. The nature and source of evidence must be kept in view by the auditor.
- **Consistency:** It is an important principle of auditing. In case of selecting the rates of depreciation and valuation of stock the accountant must follow the rates of the coming years. In this regard, there should be consistency and changes are not acceptable.
- **Legal framework:** The business activities may run within the rules and legal formalities. To protect the rights of the interested parties rules must be applied.
- **Working paper preparation:** The auditor collects documents providing evidence that audit was carried out according the principles. The auditor prepares the working paper and kept in this custody as a proof.
- **Internal control:** The auditor will examine the accounting system and inter control. To frame his opinion, he keeps in view the evidence obtained from the books.
- **Report:** According the principle of auditing, a report will be prepared by the auditor at the end. It may be conditional or unconditional. The auditor can draw conclusion and disclose the facts and figures about the business for general information.

RECORDS AND REPORTS FOR STUDENTS, STAFF, FACULTY AND ADMINISTRATIVE

Documentation is process of communicating in written form about essential facts for the maintenance of continuous history of events over a period of time. Recording and reporting are the other ways of documentation. Record is the permanent written communication that document information relevant to a client's healthcare management. Record means all documents facilities evaluation of the program and provides continuity from the time the institution is established.

Definition of Records

- A record is a clinical, scientific, administrative and legal document relating to the nursing care given to individual family or community.
- Reports are oral or written exchanges of information shared between caregivers or workers in a number of ways.

Purposes

- Provides staff member, administrator, or any other members and not only members of the health team with

documentation of the services that have been rendered and supply data that are essential for program planning and evaluation.
- To provide the practitioner with data required for the application of professional services for the improvement of family's health.
- Records are tools of communication between health workers, the family, and other development personnel.
- Effective health records show the health problem in the family and other factors that affect health. Thus, it is more than a standardized sheet or a form.
- A record indicates plans for future.
- It provides baseline data to estimate the long-term changes related to services.

Important of Records and Reports

- **Decision making:** Records play an important role for making decision. Based upon the previous data, future planning, even decisions can be made.
- **Planning client care:** Records are very helpful for planning nursing care to the patients.
- **Communication:** Records and reports are very important for conveying the information to the employees, employer as well as to the public.
- **Legal documentation:** Records are helpful for the legal purposes especially in medicolegal cases.
- **Education:** Records are helpful for teaching the nursing as well as medical students. Medical students learn from the previous records of the patients.
- **Research:** Records are the secondary source for data collection while conducting research; investigator did the recording of all the activities he/she performed during data collection.
- **Vital statistics:** Records are used especially for assessing mortality and morbidity rate.

Principles of Maintaining Records

- There must be standards framed for record keeping that focuses on content quality.
- Record should be for a specific purpose which should be clearly understood.
- Records should contain only relevant information and records should not be duplicated.
- Records which are required by the teaching staff should be easily accessible to them.
- Persons responsible for maintaining records should be aware for their particular responsibility and every effort should be made to keep records up to date and accurate.
- There should be sufficient number of filing cabinets and appropriate equipments to operate a filing system which is simple and safe and requires the minimum possible time.
- There should be provision for periodic review of all records.
- There should be adequate, safe and fire proof storage arrangements.
- Records should be audited by trained peer auditors at regular interval.

Characteristics of Good Recording and Reporting

- **Accuracy:** Information should be correct to prevent serious mistakes. Use of correct spelling and the institutions accepted abbreviation and symbols ensure accurate interpretation of information. It should be always complete with accurate signature. Do not use nick names.
- **Conciseness:** Use a few words as possible to give the necessary information.
- **Thoroughness:** Even a concise record or report must contain complete information.
- **Up-to-date:** Recording should be done on time. A definite time and routine for the reporting make more time and routine for the reporting makes more efficient management. Delay in recording can result in serious omissions and delay the work.
- **Organization:** Communicate all the information in a logical format or order.
- **Confidentiality:** The information should be confidential.
- **Objectivity:** Presentation of facts not personal feelings, to give true picture.

General School Records

These consist of:
- The philosophy, objectives and curriculum of the school
- Written policies of the school
- Statement of budget proposals and allotments
- Letters of agreement with affiliating agencies
- Minutes of staff meetings
- Copy of school brochure (or prospectus)
- Inventories of stocks
- Admission

Students Records

The list of records is:
- Application forms and other reports—concerning selection and admission, such as references, medical reports, including mark lists, certificates and results of written test and interview at the time of selection.
- Admission register
- A cumulative health record
- Class attendance and leave record
- Clinical and field experience, student rotation
- Internal assessment register—both theory and practical
- Mark list (state council/board results)
- Records of extracurricular activities
- Practical record book
- Permanent cumulative student record, student details, examination and results, theory hours, practical experience, marks, rank class for each student.
- Student evaluation internal practical and theory

Records and Reports for INC

- Admission register
- Students attendance register
- Clinical experience records
- Students health records

- Staff attendance records
- Acquittance register
- Internal assessment register
- External marks register
- Report of various committee

Staff Records

- Application form
- Copy of letter of appointment and any subsequent letter showing change in status
- Job description/functions
- Record of the staff members
  a. Educational qualification
  b. Previous experience
  c. Any short-term educational course attended
  d. Membership in professional societies and activities
  e. Contribution of articles to journals
  f. Holding office in organization
  g. Participation in seminars, conferences etc updated every year
- Periodic evaluation or progress report
- Leave record
- Health record
- Anecdotal record

Administrative Records

- Philosophy, purposes and curriculum
- Course content and course plan record for each subject
- Record of academic requirements
- Rotation plans for each academic year
- Record of committees
- Record of the stocks
- Application records
- Records of educational programs organized for teaching faculty and students
- Annual reports
- Written policies
- Statement of budget proposals and allotments
- Copy of brochure
- Inspection/accreditation record
- Minutes of committee meeting
- Photograph/video/paper cuttings of important events
- Computerized records (Floppy, CD)

Records Used in Hospitals

A medical record contains information about a patient and the healthcare he has received. Hospital medical records can be electronic or paper-based, and include documentation that describes patient encounters and procedures. Medical records are also known as legal medical records, or LMR, as the information contained within them is required by federal and state law.

Each medical record must contain the patient's name, address, and hospital identification number. The patient's age, sex, marital status, legal status for admission, emergency contact information, and religious preference should be included, as well as date and time of admission and discharge, the name of the attending physician and any advanced medical directives on file.

- **Medical history:** Required medical history includes immunizations, allergies, nutritional and psychiatric evaluations as necessary, past medical and surgical history, social and family history, and any screening tests that have been performed.
- **Physical examination:** A thorough physical evaluation should be performed and documented in the chart record. This includes the patient's vital signs, general appearance, HEENT, neck, chest, cardiovascular system, abdomen, extremities and neurological evaluation.
- **Laboratory and radiology:** Results of all laboratory tests and radiological assessments are required in hospital documentation. Pathology reports of any tissue or body fluid also should be contained within the record.
- **Patient orders:** Any order given to the patient must be documented in the chart. This includes orders for medication, treatment, prescriptions, nutritional orders as well as screening tests, laboratory work, physical or occupational therapy or radiological imaging that the patient is advised to have performed.
- **Impression and diagnosis:** The patient's initial impression is documented on the history and physical performed as the patient enters the hospital. Final diagnosis is required on the discharge summary performed when the patient is discharged from the hospital.
- **Operative procedures:** Documentation for both minor and major procedures is required. This includes preoperative and postoperative diagnosis, techniques and instruments used, anesthesia administered and operative findings. Consent forms for all procedures need to be included in the record. Any preoperative or postoperative instructions should be written and given to the patient, with a copy stored in the medical record.
- **Nursing notes:** Documentation for encounters by the nursing staff is required, including nutritional, psychosocial and functional evaluation, patient care administered, medication administration including amount and method of dosage and any restraint or isolation that was deemed to be necessary.
- **Consultations:** Any consulting physician must document the patient visit. This includes all documented information required for a typical patient encounter, such as medical history, physical examination, laboratory and radiological evaluation, orders, impression and diagnosis.
- **Discharge information:** The discharge summary is prepared as the patient is leaving the hospital. This record includes findings and events during hospitalization, final diagnosis, the condition of the patient and recommendations for future care, as well as any discharge instructions to the patient.
- **Records used in the community:** Nurses are the backbone of the medical community. A nurse cares for the patient when the doctor is not there and is required to create an informative history of injury and care via her

nursing reports. Every nurse needs to know how to write a nursing report. Doctors use nursing reports to follow the patient's progress once treatment has been prescribed. More than that, nurses need to learn how to write nursing reports that accurately reflect every action taken on the patient's behalf.
- **Records and reports used in PHC and subcenters:** There is considerable uniformity in records being used and yet there are differences in forms used by municipalities' states and private agencies. Nurse should study the record forms and systems b and make recommendations for changes that will help meet the needs of the organization and community in the most effective manner.

I. Cumulative or Continuing Records

- This is found to be time saving, economical and also it is helpful to review the total history of an individual and evaluate the progress of a long period. For example, child's record should provide space for newborn, infant and preschool data.
- The system of using one record for home and clinic services in which home visits are recorded in blue and clinic visit in red ink helps coordinate the services and saves the time.

II. Family Records

The basic unit of service is the family and so the central record unit should be family unit. In practice because of difficulty in defining "family" The unit is the "household" meaning the group of people who live together and share a cooking facility?. Separate records forms may be needed for different types of services, such as TB maternity infant and preschool, school and industrial are family may be making use of any are or all of these services. All records which relate to members of one family should be placed in a single family folder. The family folder which contains all the individual records of one family has all the identifying data observations about the general social and environmental factors that at least health in the family on it.

III. Registers

The registers usually provide only an indication of the total volume of service and of the types of cases seen. It gives no idea of the quality of services on the results achieved.

Filing Records

Different systems may be adopted depending on the purposes of the records and on the merits of a system. The records could be arranged: Alphabetically, numerically, geographically and with index cards.

Role of Administrator

The nurse administrator should see that everybody is following common guidelines for recording information:
- Information recorded is true and complete.
- Entries should be legible and written in link.
- Only facts should be recorded.
- Entries should be brief, accurate, legible and correctly spelt.
- If item error is made while written, the nurse should not erase or overwrite, instead draw a single line over it and sign it. Then note it down correctly.
- Do not leave blank space in a note.
- Always make chart for yourself and never for someone else.
- Should write in chronological order of date and time.
- Each page of record should be properly identified with identification data.

Keeping records and reports is an important responsibility of the nurse administrator. The main points include:
- The records and reports should be kept under safe custody.
- No individual sheet is separated from the complete record.
- Records must place confidentially.
- No stranger is permitted to read the record.
- All records to be handled carefully.
- Protection from loss
- Filling should be done alphabetically, numerically with cards and geographically.
- Assess periodically to determine the use of record and reexamine for means of simplification.

Keeping records and reports is necessary activities in every administrative and educational program. Reports also serve as a source of reference and it has legal value too. The nurse administrator should see her role in maintaining records and reports in nursing education in order to save time. The form of record should be simple and easy to fill.

COMMITTEES AND FUNCTIONING

Committees are essential for good organization and management. The committee is a group of persons to whom as a group, some matter is entrusted. Committees can also be defined as a group of employees engaged in some aspect of the management function. A committee may have coordinating, informational or advisory responsibility. Sometimes committees are referred to as boards, task forces, commissions or teams.

A committee can facilitate coordination of activities throughout an institution. To handle1 solve intradepartmental problems, a committee can be formed having members representing from different departments. These committees can help to obtain the information from various departments and they can also disseminate the information to 4 their departments. In order to plan and execute a complex organizational project, the top-level executive may need continuous advice from the various subject specialists, who must contribute towards progress of the project. Regular meetings can be scheduled to ensure the availability of the required advice.

Need of Committees

The use of committees is increasing. They are highly effective tools'for accomplishing certain objectives. Some of the important reasons for using committees are as follows:

- **Group deliberation and judgment:** Group deliberation can bring people together with wider range of experience and a greater variety of opinion to solve the problems. Thorough probing leads to clarification of problems and generation of new ideas.
- **Representation of varied interests:** When there is a difficult problem involving aspects of different departments, the administrator can choose committee members so as to get representation of the interested partners. This helps to ensure that the group develops a sense of loyalty and commitment to the decision reached.
- **Coordination of departmental policies and plans:** Committees promote coordination among departments. It is useful for coordinating policies and plans. The concerned members obtain a picture of overall plans and their place in them. The members also contribute suggestions for improvement of plans. A committee brings managers together and helps them gain a better understanding of their role.
- **Sharing of information:** All the group members affected by a problem can transmit and share information so as to crystallize the problem.
- **Motivation:** If the committees work skillfully and effectively, they motivate the subordinates to take part in making a decision, accept and execute it with enthusiasm and commitment.
- **To diffuse resentment and responsibility:** When a decision is almost certain to be highly unpopular in the organization, a committee can be used to diffuse resentment and responsibility.

I. Governing Council/Advisory Committee

Objectives: To obtain approval of updated policies and procedures of the institution based on revision of syllabus.
- To obtain permission to modify and renew infrastructure, staffing, teaching and learning resources, new facilities and achievements to sustain the quality teaching process and to meet norms as per apex body.
- To conduct meeting once in a year
- Plan and obtain approval for institutional budget
- To review and recruit teaching and non-teaching staff based on requirement.
- To update regarding admission and the results of the academic year.

II. General Faculty Committee

All faculties are involved in this meeting.
Objectives: To implement curricular, co-curricular and extracurricular activities
Activities:
- To analyze the implementation of each month classroom and clinical hours
- To provide general academic/professional/any other related information to the other staff members

Students through faculty:
- To suggest and guide the faculty regarding activities carried out
- To know the attendance shortage of students in order to take appropriate action
- To analyze student performance regarding IA test and take appropriate action for needful improvement
- To review the class meeting and other activities of the class as per the calendar of events
- Conduct meeting once in a month

III. Curriculum and Evaluation Committee

Objectives:
- To ensure that UG and PG curriculum is designed, implemented and evaluated as per apex body.
- To ensure that the design and structure of a curriculum meets the established curricular goals and objectives
- To monitor all aspects of the curriculum.
- To evaluate all aspects of the curriculum periodically

Activities:
- Plans calendar of events for all the courses
- Selection of class coordinators and course coordinators
- Prepare course wise master rotation plan for the academic year
- Designing the course developments in accord with the overall academic objectives.
- Supervise the instructional plans for each class/course.
- Ensure on provision of adequate instructional resources
- Conduct periodic committee meetings once a year.
- Investigate specific curriculum problems present and discuss them, find solutions and take corrective measures.
- Plan and organize staff development activities relating to curriculum needs in coordination with staff welfare committee.
- Obtain and review feedback from various sources of the curriculum and instructional programs, such as students, alumni and stakeholders.
- Define student evaluation procedures.
- Plan and conduct evaluation of particular instructional program and also the entire curriculum plan of each program.
- Plant and obtain objective specific curriculum evaluation.

IV. Library Committee

Objectives:
- To promote the smooth access and utilization of books, journals video caste, computer and digital facilities to staff and students.
- Conduct meeting every six months once to discuss about the development of the library.
- Prepares library schedule batch wise and displays in the notice board/informs to the concerned class-coordinators
- Prepare a library budget based on admission rate and files
- Provides a proposal to the principal to purchase department/subject wise text books and Journals to purchase to the library.
- Monitors students and staffs utilization of library
- Collect the important articles specific to nursing profession and display on the notice board

- Promotes and maintains a conducive environment in the library
- Conducts stock verification once in a year

V. Student Welfare Committee
Objectives:
- Review the conditions that contribute to the academic success, personal development and well-being of students.
- Collect and share information relating to student welfare matters.
- Coordinate and communicate with teachers and students on matters concerning to the welfare of the students.
- Invite guest speakers on aspects of student welfare.
- Conducting meetings three times in a year.
- Arranging for physical examination and vaccination.
- Preparing health in-charges rotation plan for students.
- Arranging recreational and cultural activities in coordination with SNA

VI. Disciplinary Committee (Staff and Students)
Objectives:
- Maintain professional behavior/etiquettes among students
- Plan, develop and display the rules and regulations at college, clinical and hostel
- Reporting incident within 24 hours to principal's office
- Verify and analyze the issues
- Classify minor or major incidents
- Notifying to the parents or guardian
- Taking necessary action

VII. Students Counseling Cell
Objectives:
- To provide counseling services to the students
- To provide appropriate services to the students for their emotional, psychological and personal development in order to enhance their academic and overall performance
- To reduce stress among students and thereby improving their performance
- To inculcate good lifestyle pattern among students.
- To provide sustainable psychosocial support in order to gain control over all the circumstances.

Activities:
- Providing guidance and counseling to the students wherever it is required.
- Planning and conducting seminars and other programs to improve over all development of the students in co-ordination with student welfare committee.
- Conducting one to one sessions with students to find out problems and helping them to cope with the demanding situation.
- To provide information and literature about stress management and personality development.
  To guide the students for good lifestyle pattern by conducting regular group discussions.

Parent Teacher Association
Objectives:
- To foster better relationships between parents and their children's college.
- To promote open communication and cooperation between teaching staff and parents.

Activities:
- Plan and organize meetings with teaching staff and parents twice a year (after 1st and 3rd IA test) and when ever required.
- To update parents regarding their children performance in the classes, clinical and on overall development in the college and to get feedback for the same.

Placement Cell
Objectives:
- To provide a platform of support service for the students in developing their clinical skills, communication ability, personal development and confidence to perform better.
- To provide support services to the students to face the challenges with regard to competitive examinations without any stress.
- Provide guidance and counseling to the students regarding various traditional and Job oriented courses.
- To provide or display the information related to vacant jobs

Activities:
- To provide carrier guidance twice in a year
- To provide information and literature about the various possible careers available in India and abroad.
- To help students to resolve career problems.
- To equip them career related information to cope with the career challenges.
- To provide information further academic courses and scholarship, etc.

National Service Scheme
Objectives:
- Understand the community in which they work.
- Understand themselves in relation to their community.
- Identify the needs and problems of the community and involve them in problem-solving process.
- Develop among themselves a sense of social and civic responsibility.
- Utilize their knowledge in finding practical solution to individual and community problems.
- Develop competence required for group-living and sharing of responsibilities.
- Gain skills in mobilizing community participation.
- Acquire leadership qualities and democratic attitude.
- Develop capacity to meet emergencies and natural disasters.
- Practice national integration and social harmony

Activities:
- General orientation of NSS volunteers
- Skill development (first aid, disaster management, public speaking, leadership motivation, HIV/AIDS awareness, etc.).

- Community development activities (in the adopted village)—survey in the village, green plantation, health, cleanliness, road safety, visits to homes, technical training for rural youth and SHG, sanitation, women development programs, consumer awareness, etc.
- Conduct blood donation camp
- Conduct Swachh Bharat Campaign at urban slums and rural area.

Alumni Association

Objectives:
- To create a forum to promote and foster relationship among the alumni and institution.
- To actively and constructively participate in the well being of Institution by utilizing the good will, rich experience and services of the alumni.
- To initiate scholarships, prizes/medals for the deserving students of college of nursing.
- To provide and disseminate information regarding the institution, its graduates, facilities and students to alumni.
- To arrange lecture by eminent alumni and other eminent personality for the benefit of students and alumni.
- To organize career guidance program for outgoing UG and PG students.

Activities:
- To enroll and maintain membership of the association.
- Conduct meeting twice in a year
- To establish and maintain a link with all the students and with the community at large.
- To maintain a close relationship between the ex-students and the present students of the college.

Continuing Nursing Education

Objectives:
- Update the knowledge with current trend, information and technology in nursing.
- Maintain standards of healthcare at acceptable level, and setting standard of performance.
- Develop/built a healthy working environment and faster good relationship among the faculty.
- Provide the faculty with personal and professional enrichment.
- Provides a platform to exercise their professional capabilities.
- Encourage to conduct EB a research activities.

Activities:
- Conducts or organizes in-service education programs
- Encourages the faculty to attend seminars/workshops/conferences
- Maintains documents of the program conducted.

Student's Nurses Association

Objectives:
- To help students to uphold the dignity and ideals of profession for which they are qualifying.
- To promote a corporate spirit among students for common goal.
- To furnish nurse in training with advice in their courses of study leading up to professional qualifications.
- To encourage leadership abilities and help students to gain a wide knowledge of the nursing profession in all its different branches and aspects.
- To increase the students social contacts and general knowledge in order to help them take their place in the community when they have finished their training.
- To encourage both professional and recreational meetings, games and sports.
- To encourage students to compete for prizes in the student nurses exhibition and to attend national and regional conferences.

Activities:
- Plans calendar of events every year.
- Conducts general body meetings once in a year and executive meeting as and when required.
- Elects SNA office bearers once in a year.
- Celebrates various national days, such as Independence Day, Republic day and Kannada Rajyostava day.
- Organizes significant days, such as Nurses Day, Teachers day and New Year.
- Celebrates various festivals, such as Onam and Christmas.
- Plans and conducts college events, such as Freshers Day, Graduation and lamp lighting ceremony and farewell of students and staff.
- Arranges picnic for students and staff.
- Arranges guest lecturers for enhancement of knowledge for students and staff.
- Maintain documents and registers of meetings and financial expenditure.

VIII. Research Committee

Objectives:
- Promote nursing research activities by facilitating the development and maintenance of research interest among students and staff.
- Provide a forum for discussion of research study/research project, conducted by students.
- Support the need for evidence-based practice and activities that facilitate the appropriate transfer of best evidence into practice.
- Promote collaboration among members in their research related activities.
- Conducting regular UG/PG research/project presentation
- Assist and review in refining the research proposals.
- Provide research consultation when appropriate.
- Appraise the research activities of the students periodically.

IX. Institutional Ethics Committee

Institutional Ethics Committee of College of nursing was constituted for discussion and approval of institution/collaborative research projects with respect to safeguard dignity, right, safety and well being of all research participants and to ensure that the research is carried under prescribed guidelines.

Objectives:
- To ensure the competent review and evaluation of all ethical aspects of research projects received in an objective manner.
- To protect the safety, right and well being of the potential research participants.
- To conduct scientific evaluation and to ensure technical appropriateness of the proposed study.
- To ensure that universal ethical values and international scientific standards are expressed in terms of local community values/customs.
- To assist in the development and education of a research community responsive to local healthcare requirement.
- Creation, developing, revising and implementing ethical guidelines (SOPs)
- Academic assistant who will help the IEC member Secretary in executing functions of the IEC, documentation and archiving documents.
- All documents, communication of IEC will be dated, filed and preserved in a secure place.
- Only person who are authorized by chairman of IEC will have access t to various documents.
- All documents related to research project will be archived for a minimum period of three years in the institute following completion or termination of project.
- All the agenda and minutes of meeting will be filed and archived the records shall be made available to relevant statutory authorities upon request.
- Once in a year General Body Meeting will be conducted.
- Executive meeting will be conducted as and when required.

X. Staff Welfare Committee

Objectives:
- Uphold the staff code of ethics, rules and regulation framed by the institution.
- Built a healthy working environment and faster good relationships among staff (create work friendly environment).
- To coordinate for benevolent facilities for staff members.
- Identifies communication and coordinate matters concern to welfare and development of staff.
- Equity of work issues, reinforcement for the good work done.
- Motivates and improved the sense f security among staff.
- Provide a platform to exercise their professional capabilities.
- Establish a formal means to identify specific issues relevant to staff welfare at the college.
- Advise the management on work matters of interest and concern to staff.
- Share with management the staff ideas and suggestions for improvement to achieve the institution objectives.
- Facilitate effective communication between staff and the various management structures within the college.

XI. Anti-Ragging Committee

Objectives:
- To prevent ragging occurrence by using regulations.
- To punish those who indulge in ragging in spite of prohibition and prevention.
- To keep a continuous monitory and vigilance over ragging, to prevent its occurrence and recurrence.
- To promptly deal with the incidents of ragging brought to the notice.
- Punish the guilty either by itself or by putting-forth its finding/recommendation/suggestion before the competent authority for decision.

XII. Staff and Students Recruitment and Selection Committee

Objectives:
- To recruit the right student to the right program and right person to right job
- Selection of teaching and non-teaching staff and students as per the criteria given by apex bodies and institutional policy.
- Planning orientation to the selected staffs and students on rules and regulations of the college.
- Explaining the rules, regulations of the institution and responsibilities of particular post.
- The meeting is conducted as and when required.

XIII. Grievance Redressal Committee

Objectives:
- Reviewing and resolving staff/students grievances.
- Complaints and grievances are handled according to regular requirements of institutional policy.
- Maintain compliance with regulatory requirements.
- Provide a forum to ensure appropriate and timely review and resolution of staff grievances.

Activities:
- The grievance committee meeting will be conducted as and when the complaints are received.
- To provide an opportunity in the institution that may provide easy access for ventilating personal grievances.
- Impart a degree of objectively and fair play in the whole process.
- Establish good communication between the employee and management.
- Make every effort to remove misunderstanding and to develop congenial atmosphere in the institution.

Youth Red Cross Unit/National Service Scheme

Objectives: The Youth Red Cross Unit of College of Nursing is organized for the purpose of inculcating in Indian Youth the ideal and practice of service especially in relation to:
- Taking care of their own health and that of others
- Understanding and accepting of civic responsibility.

- Maintaining a spirit of friendliness and helpfulness towards other youth in India and all over the world.
- Dissemination of the Red Cross movement.

Activities of Youth Red Cross Unit

Preparing year action plan. Celebrating of:
- World Health Day—7th April
- World Red Cross Day—8th May
- World Environment—5th June
- World Blood Donor's Day—14th June
- World AIDS Day—1st December
- Relief Work during Emergencies.

Alumni Association

Objectives:
- To create a forum to promote and foster relationship among the alumni and institution.
- To actively and constructively participate in the well being of Institution by utilizing the good will, rich experience and services of the alumni.
- To initiate scholarships, prizes/medals for the deserving students of college of nursing.
- To provide and disseminate information regarding the institution, its graduates, facilities and students to alumni.
- To arrange lecture by eminent alumni and other eminent personality for the benefit of students and alumni.
- To organize career guidance program for outgoing UG and PG students.

Activities:
- To enroll and maintain membership of the association.
- Conduct meeting twice in a year
- To establish and maintain a link with all the students and with the community at large.
- To maintain a close relationship between the ex-students and the present students of the college.

XIV. Hostel Committee

Objectives:
- To maintain friendly and homely atmosphere to the students.
- To develop social integrity among students.
- To provide general comfort and welfare to the students.
- To maintain discipline in the hostel.

Activities:
- Periodic review of cleanliness of hostel and mess.
- Periodic review of matters related to mess and hostel.
- Periodic review of policies related to hostel and mess
- Conducting hostel meetings once in 6 months/whenever required.
- Conducting social nights and encouraging group prayers
- Arranging for recreational activities.
- Monitoring of quality and preparation of food.
- Monitoring maintenance work.
- Reviewing mess menu based on student's feedback.

CONCLUSION

Planning is an important attribute of management in achieving the aims and objectives required of education. The plan being a policy statement and is equally required helps in to policy making. Planning is a process that determines the future course of action and is undertaken at all levels of management. It is continuous and includes the process of perception, analysis and conceptual issue. Organization is a means to bring the plan into existence. It is a media through which goals and the objectives of administration are achieved. Management is an art and a science. It is the process of decision making and a control over the action. Management is a social process, involves group effort; aims at achieving pre-determined goals, a distinct entity and is required at all levels of organization.

REVIEW QUESTIONS

Long Essays
1. Discuss about nursing philosophy of nursing colleges.
2. Define curriculum planning; explain the purposes and principles.
3. Describe organizing, clinical facilities for nursing students.

Short Essays
1. Objectives of nursing colleges.
2. Factors affecting curriculum development.
3. Types of curriculum.
4. Models of curriculum design.
5. Curriculum evaluation approaches.
6. Formative evaluation.
7. Curriculum change and innovations.
8. Curriculum development in nursing.
9. Planning teaching and learning experiences.
10. Master rotation plan.
11. Clinical rotation plan
12. Budget planning for college of nursing.

Short Answers
1. Components of curriculum.
2. Levels of curriculum planning.
3. Stages of curriculum development.
4. Formal curriculum.
5. Curriculum implementation.
6. Curriculum evaluation.
7. Wheeler's model.
8. Self-evaluation.
9. Curriculum change.
10. Curriculum innovation.
11. Participative problem-solving.
12. Linear development.
13. Cyclic development.
14. Principles of master rotation plan.

CHAPTER 22

Staffing and Student Selection

LEARNING OBJECTIVES

- Faculty/Staff Selection, Recruitment and Placement, Job Description
- Performance Appraisal
- Faculty Development
- Faculty/Staff Welfare
- Student Recruitment, Admission, Clinical Placement

■ PERFORMANCE APPRAISAL

Performance appraisal or merit rating is one of the oldest and most universal practices of management. The approach resulted in an appraisal system in which the employee's merits like initiative, dependability, and personality were compared with others and ranked or rated. The trend now a day is in the direction of attempting to measure what man does (performance appraisal) rather than what he is (merit rating). Appraisal can be made by one or more supervisors or by subordinate or by peers. There can be even be a system of self-appraisal in which an employee evaluate his own performance and potentials **(Fig. 22.1)**.

Definition

- Performance appraisal refers to all the formal procedures used in the working organizations to evaluate the personalities and contribution of group members.
- Performance appraisal is a periodic formal evaluation of how well personnel have performed their duties during specific period.
- Performance appraisal (also called merit rating or efficiency or service rating) is the process of reviewing an individual's performance and progress in job and assessing his/her potentials. **Figure 22.2** shows components of performance appraisal

Meaning of Performance Appraisal

Performance appraisal is the systematic evaluation of the performance of employees and to understand the abilities of a person for further growth and development. Performance appraisal is generally done in systematic ways which are as follows:

- The supervisors measure the pay of employees and compare it with targets and plans.
- The supervisor analyzes the factors behind work performances of employees.

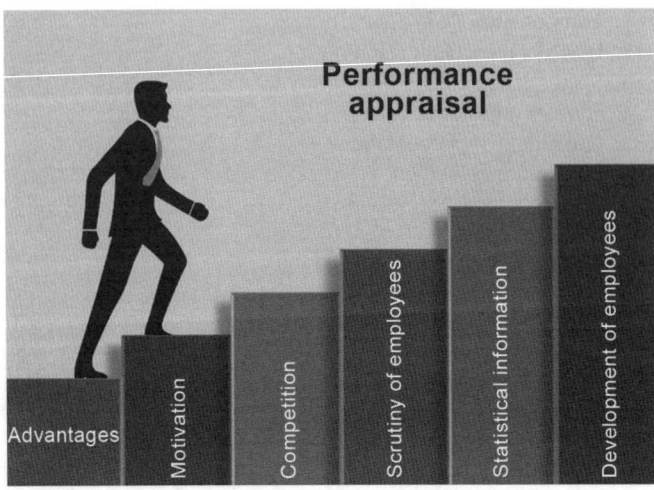

Fig. 22.1: Performance appraisal.

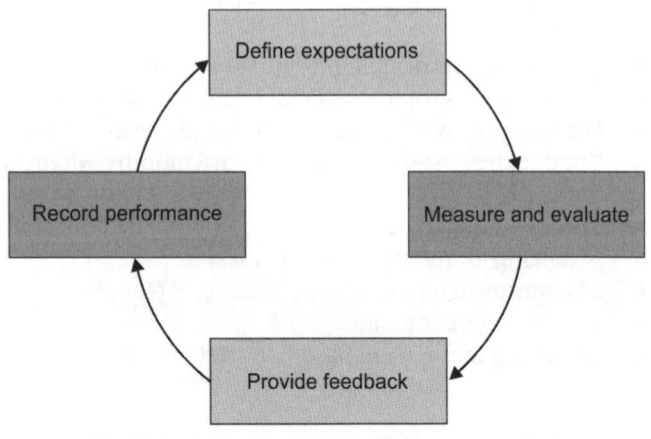

Fig. 22.2: Components of performance appraisal.

- The employers are in position to guide the employees for a better performance.

Objectives of Performance Appraisal

Performance appraisal can be done with following objectives in mind:
- To maintain records in order to determine compensation packages, wage structure, salaries raises, etc.
- To identify the strengths and weaknesses of employees to place right men on right job.
- To maintain and assess the potential present in a person for further growth and development.
- To provide a feedback to employees regarding their performance and related status.
- To provide a feedback to employees regarding their performance and related status.
- It serves as a basis for influencing working habits of the employees.
- To review and retain the promotional and other training programs.

Purpose of Performance Appraisal

- It can serve as a basis for job change or promotion. By establishing whether the nurse can contribute still more in a different or higher job, it helps in his suitable promotion and placement.
- By identifying the strengths and weakness of an employee, it serves as a guide for formulating a suitable training and development program to improve his quality of performance in his present work.
- It serves as a feedback to the employee. By letting the employee know how well he is doing or where he stands with his superior, it tells him what he can do to improve his present performance and go up in the management hierarchy.
- It serves as an important incentive to all the employees who are by the existence of an appraisal system assured of the management's continued interest in them and of their continuous possibility to develop. The employees realize that not only are they being continuously observed but that they have not been forgotten.
- The existence of regular appraisal system tends to make the supervisors and executive more observant of their subordinates because they will be expected periodically to fill out rating forms and would be called upon to justify their estimates. Their knowledge results in improved supervision.
- Performance appraisal often provides the rational foundation for payment of piecework, wages, bonuses, etc., the estimates of the relative contributions of employees of their characteristics help to determine the rewards and privileges.
- Performance appraisal serves as a mean for evaluation the effectiveness of devices for the selection and classification of workers. Alternatively, knowledge of the characteristics of supervisor and inferior workers can be helpful in selection and placement of workers.
- Permanent performance appraisal records of employees help the management to give up sole reliance upon personal knowledge of supervisors who may be shifted. **Figure 22.3** shows performance Appraisal steps.

Need of Performance Appraisal

Performance appraisal is needed in order to:
- Provide information about the performance ranks basing on which decision regarding salary fixation, confirmation, promotion, transfer and demotion are taken.
- Provide feedback information about the level of achievement and behavior of subordinate. This information helps to review the performance of the subordinate, rectifying performance deficiencies and to set new standards of work, if necessary.
- Provide information which helps to counsel the subordinate.
- Provide information to diagnose deficiency in employee regarding skill, knowledge, determine training and development needs and to prescribe the means for employee growth provides information for correcting placement.
- To prevent grievances and in disciplinary activities.

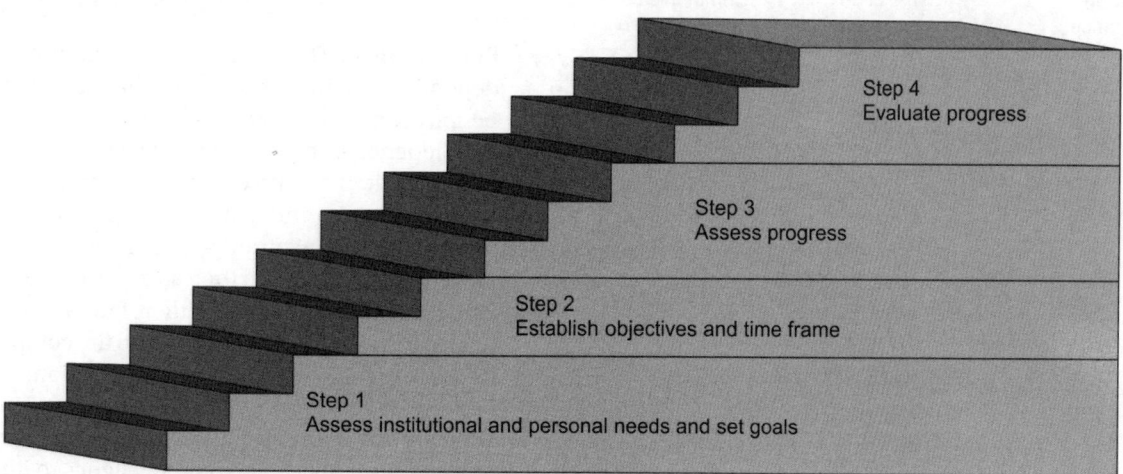

Fig. 22.3: Performance appraisal steps.

Characteristis of Performance Appraisal

The performance appraisal system must have the following characteristics:
- It must be bias free the evaluator must be objective and the methods of appraisal must be fair and equitable. The atmosphere must be that of confidence and trust.
- It must be relevant, it should only measure behaviors that are relevant to the successful job performance and not any other personal traits.
- It should be acceptable to all the performance standards as well as the appraisal methods should be developed by joint participation and joint collaboration.
- It should be reliable, dependable, stable and consistent. High reality is essential for correct decision making and valid action studies: It should be sufficiently scientific so that if an employee is evaluated by two different evaluators, then the result should be significantly the same.
- It must be able to objectively differentiate between a good employee and an ineffective employee. Rating an employee "average" does not adequately the degree of effectiveness. Hence, the technique must be sufficiently sensitive to pick up the differences between an effective and an ineffective employee.
- It must be practical, sound, clear and unambiguous, so that all parties 'concerned understand its implications.

Principles of Performance Evaluation (Fig. 22.4)

- Evaluation must contain content this is relevant to individuals being evaluated in a particular setting.
- Criteria that are used to evaluate performance should be stated and standards should be specified whenever possible.
- Performance evaluation should be able discriminate between excellent, good and poor performance.
- Any performance evaluation must be practical or in measurement terminology. It must have utility.

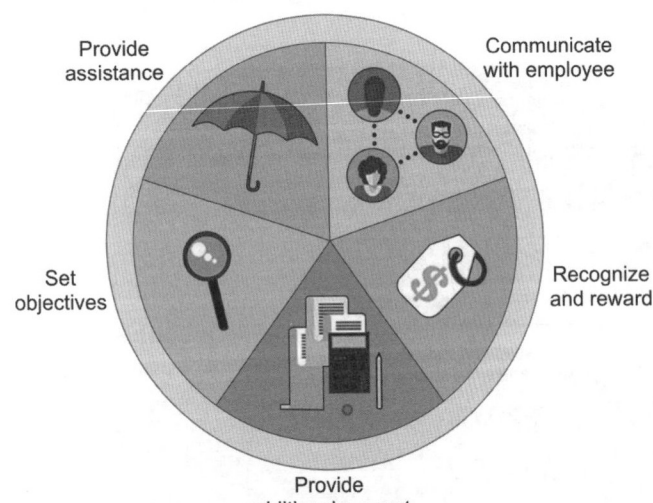

Fig. 22.4: Principles of performance evaluation.

Factors Affecting Performance Appraisal (Fig. 22.5)

Performance appraisal is one business activity that most of employees look forward to. After all, this is one of the most important factors that drives employees to put in that extra effort in their jobs day-in and day-out. Performance appraisals are conducted to review the performance of the employee, and decide his/her compensation package according to his/her achievements. Performance appraisal may not be a very exciting proposition for those employees who have not performed as per the expectations, but it is nevertheless important as apart from revising the salary; performance appraisals also help in setting core competencies and future goals for the employees.

Factors	Description	Factors
1.	Job knowledge	5 factors, such as responsibilities, duties, understanding of job, requirements, etc.
2.	Skill level	5 factors skill to perform the assigned job, acumen, basic knowledge, new ideas, computers, etc.
3.	Job execution	5 factors executes the job with perfection, use of resources, effective use of time, handling of unusual situation, etc.
4.	Initiative	5 factors develops new avenues skills, works independently with minimum supervision, demonstrates interest, follows instructions.
5.	Client orientation	5 Handling of colleagues, understands the instruction well, implementation of project, etc.
6.	Cooperation and ability work in teams	5 factors, can work with the team, rapport with co-workers, interpersonal relations, behavior with colleagues
7.	Compliance to policies and practices	5 factors understanding of internal procedures, practices, responsibilities, loyalty, etc.
8.	Overall rating	10 overall performance: leadership, communication skills, execution of job, effective use of available resources, wastage management, time management, reporting, etc.

- **Performance:** The appraisal of an employee is directly dependent on the performance that he has shown over a period of time. Every business wants to maximize its profits and depends upon the collective effort of its employees to achieve it. If certain employees perform up and above the expectations and help the company to achieve better results, the organization would appreciate their efforts and give them a raise in their salary. However, employees who have not performed to their full potential and have not led to any major contribution to the company may not find any such favors from the organization.
- **Teamwork:** The way you behave in your office also has a huge impact on the appraisal process. If you are known as a team player and help your colleagues to improve their performance, it is highly likely that the organization would

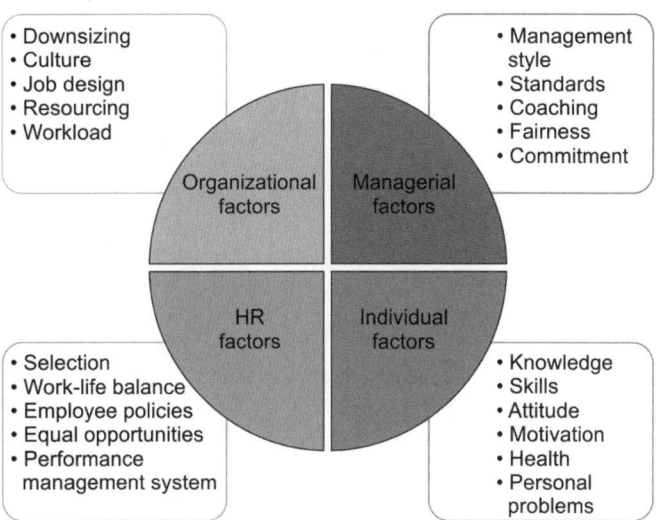

Fig. 22.5: Factors affecting performance appraisal.

recognize your efforts and reward you handsomely. This is one of the prime reasons that some employees whose performance has not been exceptional still manage to have a healthy raise in their appraisals. On the other hand, if you are someone who spreads rumors and negativity in the workplace, there is a possibility that you would have a tough time during your appraisals.

- **Attendance and punctuality:** While it is OK to take a day off once in a while, but frequent absenteeism can hamper your appraisal. Once you start calling in sick, your managers develop a negative perception which is hard to shed. Tardiness on your part can also affect your appraisal as organizations put this to intense scrutiny. Various surveys have found that 'average' employees who have lesser absenteeism and are punctual get more favors from the managers, and this is one of the important factors that plays a part during your appraisal.
- **Assertiveness/motivation:** Assertiveness and motivation are important characteristics that every organization looks forward to in their employees. Employees who go about their jobs with vigor and excitement, take initiatives and show a desire to perform exceptionally are looked upon highly by the managers. Employees with a positive attitude and self-belief are respected by the organization and are likely to be rewarded for their efforts.
- **Process knowledge:** A friend of mine was disappointed when she came to know that her colleague had been awarded a higher rating than her, even though she had generated more sales. She was in a dilemma for a few days before her manager sensed the situation and decided to have a word with her so that there is no ambiguity. He told her that, the reason she was not able to get a very good rating was because she lacked process knowledge. Ignorance about your products can hamper your customer experience besides marring the reputation of your company. When you do not know enough about your products, it is difficult to convince the customers about the benefits that they will derive from it.

- **Organizational skills:** A well-organized employee is always ready for any additional responsibilities and the managers can trust him for his ability to get something done. Organizational skill is an important attribute and plays an important part in the appraisal process.
- **Customer service:** If you are someone who has generated a lot of revenue for your company at the cost of your customer service, then there is a likelihood that your managers would not be able to rely on you, and your relationship with them would be marked by a trust-deficit. Customer complaints are crucial for an organization and can also result in a possible disciplinary action being taken against you.
- **Appearance:** The way you dress up to office also plays an important part in determining the course of your appraisal process. Employees who are presentable are more likely to create a positive image in the minds of managers than employees who are disheveled and do not dress up poorly to office.
- **Biased managers:** These factors are disadvantageous for an organization and promote ill-will and negativity in an organization. Managers sometimes show bias towards employees with whom they have a friendly relationship as compared to those who are just acquaintances. This creates nepotism and negativity in the workplace and hampers the morale of hard-working employees.

Essentials of Good Appraisal System (Box 22.1)

- **It must be easily understandable:** If the system is too complex or too time consuming, it may be anchored to the ground by its own dead weight of complicated from which nobody but the experts understands.
- **It must have the support of all line people who administer it:** If the line people think it is too theoretical, too ambitious, too unrealistic, or that it has been foisted on them by ivory-towered, staff-consultant who have no comprehension of the demands on the time of line operators, they will resent it. A similar goodwill and understanding must exist between the rater and the rates.
- **The system should fit the organization's operations and structure:** A system that may work extremely well at a company those activities are compact. Similarly, where the operations are interdependent and interlinked,

---

Box 22.1: Essentials of good performance appraisal.

- Standardized performance appraisal system
- Uniformity of appraisals
- Defined performance standards
- Trained raters
- Use of relevant rating tools or methods
- Should be based on job analysis
- Use of objectively verifiable data
- Avoid rating problems, such as halo effect, central tendency, leniency, severity, etc.
- Consistent documentations maintained
- No opportunity for discrimination based on cast, creed, race, religion, region

performance data pertaining to any one individual cannot be regard as sufficiently discrete or reliable for appraising his performance.
- **The system should be both valid and reliable:** The validity of rating is the degree to which they are truly indicative of the intrinsic merit of employees. The reliability of rating is the consistency with which the ratings are made, either by different raters, or by on rater at different times.
- The system should have built in incentives, that is awarded should follow satisfactory performance.
- **The system should be periodically evaluated to be sure that is continuing to meet its goals:** Not only is there the danger that subjective criteria may become more salient than the objective standards originally established, there is the further danger that the system may become rigid in a tangle of rules and procedure many of which are no longer useful.

Criteria of Performance Appraisal

Criteria may be classified into two main categories: Objective criteria and subjective criteria. Amount of quality of production, work sample tests, length of service, amount of training necessary, absenteeism, accidents, etc., are all examples of objective criteria. Rating of employee's job proficiency by their supervisors, peers and subordinates, extent of upward communication of ideas, degree of knowledge about corporate goals, contribution to sociocultural values, etc., are all examples of subjective criteria. Since all subjective criteria depend upon human judgment and opinion, they are subject to certain kinds of errors likely to be found in the rating process.

Performance Appraisal Methods (Fig. 22.6)

- **Rating method:** Rating means the judgment of one person by another. Rating is, in essence, direct observation. Rating is a team applied to expression of opinion or judgment regarding some situation, object or character. Opinions are usually expressed on a scale or values. Rating techniques are devices by which such judgments may be quantified. The oldest and simplest method of performance appraisal is to compare one man with all other men band place him in a simple rank order. In this way, ordering is done from best to worst of all individuals comprising the group.
- **Rating-scale method:** As the very name implies, these methods provide some kind of a scale for measuring absolute differences between individuals. The scales used are generally of two types:
    1. **Discrete:** Where two or more categories are provided, representing discrete amounts of ability or degrees of the characteristics, the rater can tick mark the category which he feels best describes the person being rated. Thus, for example, the characteristic job knowledge may be divided into five categories on a discrete scale. Exceptionally good, above average, average, below average and poor.

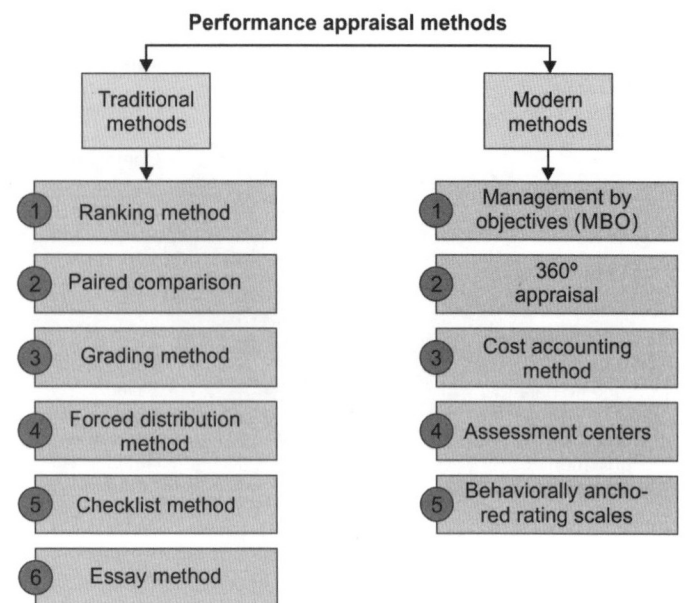

Fig. 22.6: Performance appraisal methods.

2. **Continuous (or graphic):** Where just above the category notation as uninterrupted line is provided. There are four kinds of standards used in rating scale, namely, numerical or alphabetical, descriptive-adjective, man to man and behavior sample.
- **Checklist method:** Sometimes, the method used for performance appraisal is a list consisting of a number of statements about the worker and his behavior. Each statement on this list is assigned a value depending upon its importance. The method has advantages of requiring only a reporting of facts from the rater. Since, the values assigned to different statements do not appear on list, the rater does not know how highly he has rated a given individual. He also does not have to distinguish among various categories for each of the several traits considered for each of the several employees working under him.
- **Forced-choice method:** A forced-choice rating form consists of a number of statements which desired an individual being rated. These statements are grouped in twos, threes, or fours. Sometimes, the groups on the rating form are made of favorable statements only, sometimes all above unfavorable statements only and sometimes they have both favorable and unfavorable statements in equal number. When all groups on the rating form contain favorable statements only, the rater must check one statement in each group which he believes best characterizes the individual being rated. When all group are made of unfavorable statements, the rater must check one statement in each group which he believes is the least descriptive of the individual being rated. When each group has two favorable and two unfavorable statements, the rater makes two checks in each group, one for the statements which best describes the individual and one for the statement which is least descriptive.
- **Field review:** Under this method, appraisal of worker is done by the personal officer by collecting oral rating

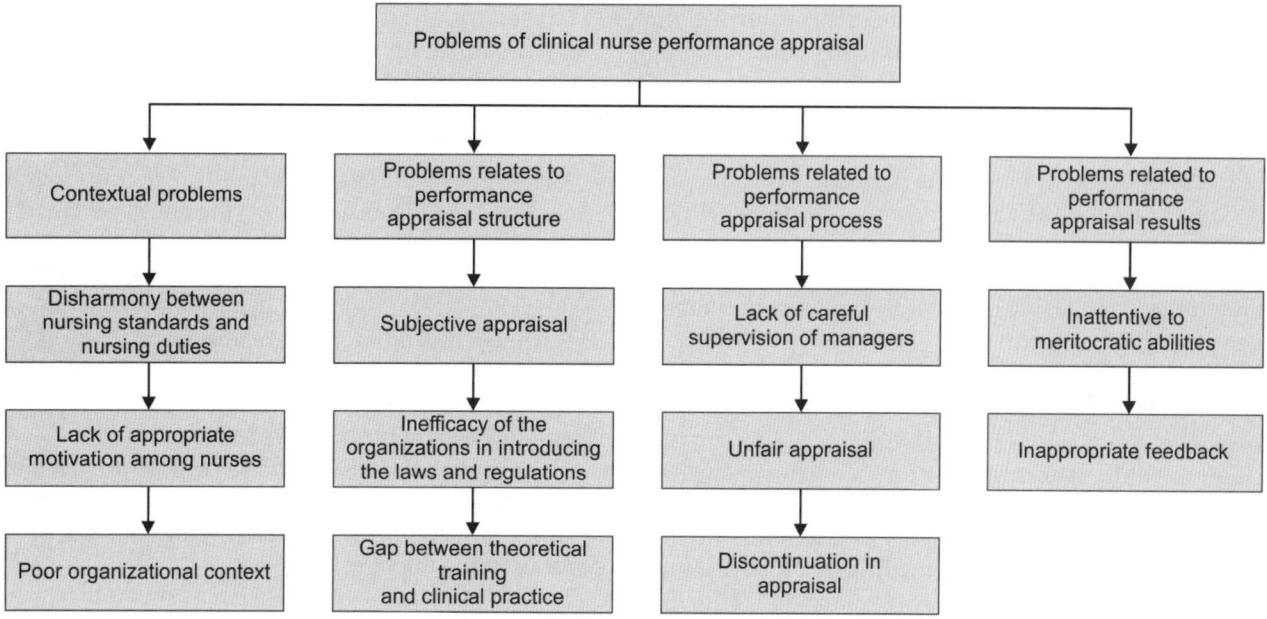

Fig. 22.7: Problems of clinical nurse performance appraisal.

about them from the supervisor at the place of work. The personnel officer later writes his notes and initiates the supervisor to make additions or corrections. This method is not widely used because supervisors generally resent what they consider the staff interference.

- **Critical incident technique:** In this method, the first step is to draw-up for each job a list of critical job requirements, that is, those requirements which are vital for success for failure on the job. The concept of a critical incident differs from that off an anecdote. Fivers and Gosnell define a critical incident as one that makes a significant difference in the outcome of an activity. It may be the positive factors that contribute towards the cusses of the behavior or it may be the negative factors that interfere with the completion of the assignment.
- **Confidential report:** A confidential report by the immediate supervisor is still a major determinant of the subordinate promotion or transfer. The format and pattern of this varies with each organization.

Performance Appraisal Tool

The type of appraisal tool used is not so important as how it is utilized. A formal written tool may have specific guidelines or a more open-ended format. General topics may be addressed in an anecdotal or incident-type format. The tool or evaluation form should facilitate accurate appraisal of the individual's performance as well as provide an opportunity to stimulate personals goals of the individual and goals of the organization. They are primary two categories of performance appraisal tools: structured and fixed.

1. **Structured (traditional) method:** The forced distribution scale is a norm-referenced tool that prevents the evaluator from rating all individuals in the same manner. The evaluator is provided a schematic diagram and asked to rate the individual according to all individuals the manager evaluates. The evaluator has indicated that the individuals rated are in the top 10% of employee, but is not the best employee. This scale also provides the employee with a brief visual picture of how this evaluator has ranked performance in reference to others. This type of scale can undetermined group cohesion and communication effectiveness by its very nature of rank ordering individual performance.
2. **Flexible (collaborative) method:** The evaluation focus can also be conducted with a collaborative approach. One method that has been used for many years is management by objectives (MBO). The MBO method is similar but more rigid in structure. An MBO approach requires that the employee establish clear and measurable objectives at the beginning of each rating period. These objectives are then addressed individually and in writing by both the employee and the employee and the manager during the performance appraisal interview. The approach can be simplified if it is performance based and outcome or results oriented. Then, in effect, the employee has created a performance contact as well having defined goals for future professional performance. **Figure 22.7** shows problems of clinical nurse performance appraisal.

Performance Appraisal in Clinical Practice

- The term clinical practice is familiar to individuals involved in nursing, but perception of this term varies considerably. To some it implies a series or an aggregate of tasks and to others the term implies a process.
- Clinical practice may be viewed as the way or the medium through which a professional practitioner ministers to his/her client.
- The clinical practice may be conceptualized as the way the nurse utilizes a particular consultation of abilities to meet the health needs of the client.
- Performance appraisal implies systematic or formal evaluation of the individual with respect to his performance on the job and his potential for development.

- It is the rational and continuous process of evaluating the performance of employees on a particular job in terms of the job required.
- Performance appraisal should be differentiated from job evaluation. Job evaluation involves the determination of worth of different jobs while performance appraisal is concerned with the measurement of the worth of individuals to the organization.
- In job evaluation, the focus is on the job while under performance appraisal the emphasis is on the performance and potentials of an employee.

Benefits of Performance Appraisal (Fig. 22.8)

Performance appraisal, in simple words, is the process of deciding the worth of an employee for an organization. The supervisor who conducts performance checks compares the employee performance with the set standards by the organization, and rate him accordingly. Performance appraisals are a part of any corporate organization. They are essential for organizational management and for handling the workforce effectively. Let us see the advantages that these appraisals have for the different parties involved in it.

Benefits for Employees

- One of the most important benefits for an employee is that he clearly understands his role in the organization, and what is exactly expected from him.
- When a person knows this, he can focus on his work better and deliver quality work which will match the standards set by the management. Moreover, they get to know the way the performance appraisal process is conducted by their supervisors.
- Performance appraisals are mainly conducted for employees to help them understand their strengths and weaknesses and improve themselves accordingly.
- The management also suggests some ways through which the employees can improve their performance.
- In the appraisal session, the employee can discuss the areas where he needs more training and support with the management so that he does not lag behind in the work allotted to him.
- Benefits of performance appraisals also include recognition for good work done and getting opportunities for further career development.
- They can be very useful in providing employees with much-needed motivation, satisfaction and support.

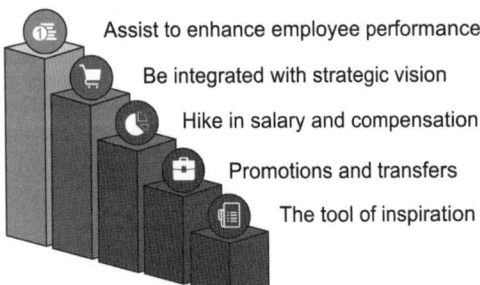

Fig. 22.8: Benefits of performance appraisal.

- These appraisals help an individual understand that the organization is taking keen interest in their career development and performance.

Benefits for Supervisors

- As said above, the benefits of performance appraisals are also for supervisors who direct the entire process.
- During the appraisal process, the supervisors get the time to interact with the employees and understand their difficulties. From the way an employee talks, they can judge his confidence levels and spot his weaknesses.
- The appraisals give them knowledge of the available human resources and a chance of motivating the employees to achieve better results.
- In the appraisals, the supervisors reward ace performers, develop a rapport with all employees, uplift the morale of teams and identify employees needing special attention for uplifting their performance.
- Supervisors/seniors can also get a lot of job satisfaction and understand the importance of their job through the appraisal process.
- A supervisor gets to know of the training and development needs of an employee through appraisal sessions. Once this happens, they can arrange for special sessions in the areas of concern to increase the efficiency of employees in performing their job.

Benefits for the Organization

- For all kinds of organizations, performance appraisals are very important to identify candidates with high potential.
- The company can get to know about the expectations of the employees from the company, and what is their view about the promotion and pay policies of the management.
- Employee training plans can be chalked out after considering the areas where maximum employees need improvement.
- Performance appraisals help organizations improve the overall workforce efficiency, skills and productivity and build good relationships with each employee.
- The database which is prepared after the performance appraisal can help to decide how successful the company's induction and recruitment policies are.
- The company management, with the help of appraisals know whether the quality of their workforce has improved or declined.
- Keeping the employees motivated and rewarding the top performers is vital to boost their morale, as this has a direct effect on the overall performance of the company. So, it is the duty of the management to make this process more transparent and efficient to see better results going ahead.

Importance of Performance Appraisal (Fig. 22.9)

- **Performance feedback:** Most employees are very interested in knowing how well they are doing at present and how they can do better in a future. They want this information to improve their performance in order to get

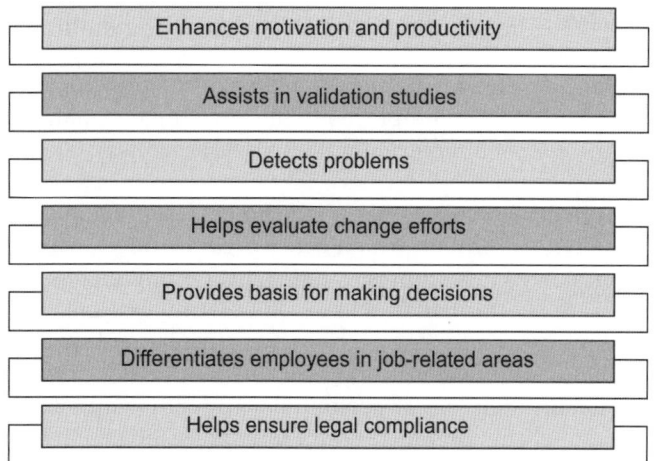

Fig. 22.9: Importance of performance appraisal.

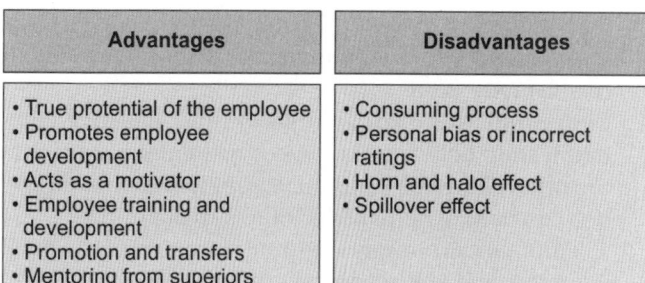

Fig. 22.10: Performance appraisal.

promotions and merit pay. Proper performance feedback can improve the employee's future performance. It also gives him satisfaction and motivation.

- **Employee training and development decisions:** Performance appraisal information is used to find out whether an employee requires additional training and development. Deficiencies in performance may be due to inadequate knowledge or skills. For example, a professor may improve his efficiency by attending workshops or seminars about his subject. Performance appraisal helps a manager to find out whether he needs additional training for improving his current job performance. Similarly, if the performance appraisal results show that he can perform well in a higher position, then he is given training for the higher level position.
- **Validation of selection process:** Performance appraisal is a means of validating both internal (promotions and transfers) and external (hiring new employees from outside) sources. Organizations spend a lot of time and money for recruiting and selecting employees. Various tools used in the selection process are application blanks, interviews, psychological tests, etc. These tools are used to predict (guess) the candidate's performance on the job. A proper performance appraisal finds out the validity of the various selection tools and so the company can follow suitable steps for selecting employees in future.
- **Promotions:** Performance appraisal is a way of finding out which employee should be given a promotion. Past appraisals, together with other background data, will enable management to select proper persons for promotion.
- **Transfers:** Performance appraisal is also useful for taking transfer decisions. Transfers often involve changes in job responsibilities, and it is important to find out the employees who can take these responsibilities. Such identification of employees who can be transferred is possible through the performance appraisal.
- **Layoff decisions:** Performance appraisal is a good way of taking layoff decisions. Employees may be asked to lay off, if the need arises. The weakest performers are the first to be laid off. If there is no performance appraisal, then there are chances that the best men in the department may be laid off.
- **Compensation decisions:** Performance appraisal can be used to compensate the employees by increasing their pay and other incentives. This is truer in the case of managerial jobs and also in the case of employees in non-unionized organizations. The better performances are rewarded with merit pay.
- **Human resource planning (HRP):** The appraisal process helps in human resource planning (HRP). Accurate and current appraisal data regarding certain employees helps the management in talking decisions for future employment. Without the knowledge of who is capable of being promoted, demoted, transferred, laid off or terminated, management cannot make employment plans for the future.
- **Career development:** Performance appraisal also enables managers to coach and counsel employees in their career development. **Figure 22.10** shows performance appraisal.

Advantages of Performance Appraisal

It is said that performance appraisal is an investment for the company which can be justified by following advantages:
- **Promotion:** Performance appraisal helps the supervisors to chalk out the promotion programs for efficient employees. In this regards, inefficient workers can be dismissed or demoted in case.
- **Compensation:** Performance appraisal helps in chalking out compensation packages for employees. Merit rating is possible through performance appraisal. Performance sppraisal tries to give worth to a performance. Compensation packages which include bonus, high salary rates, extra benefits, allowances and pre-requisites are dependent on performance appraisal. The criteria should be merit rather than seniority.
- **Employees development:** The systematic procedure of performance appraisal helps the supervisors to frame training policies and programs. It helps to analyse strengths and weaknesses of employees so that new jobs can be designed for efficient employees. It also helps in framing future development programs.
- **Selection validation:** Performance appraisal helps the supervisors to understand the validity and importance of the selection procedure. The supervisors come to know

the validity and thereby the strengths and weaknesses of selection procedure. Future changes in selection methods can be made in this regard.
- **Communication:** For an organization, effective communication between employees and employers is very important. Through performance appraisal, communication can be sought for in the following ways:
  - Through performance appraisal, the employers can understand and accept skills of subordinates.
  - The subordinates can also understand and create a trust and confidence in superiors.
  - It also helps in maintaining cordial and congenial labor management relationship.
  - It develops the spirit of work and boosts the morale of employees.

  All the above factors ensure effective communication.
- **Motivation:** Performance appraisal serves as a motivation tool. Through evaluating performance of employees, a person's efficiency can be determined if the targets are achieved. This very well motivates a person for better job and helps him to improve his performance.

Staff Development Program (Fig. 22.11)

Staff development activities consist of the training and education provided by an employer to improve employee's occupational knowledge, skills and attitudes and to provide the employee with the opportunity to grow professionally. Professional nurses one education in a variety of ways staff development program have greater responsibility to develop characteristics, abolition work assignments and uptake knowledge among staff. Nursing managers are challenged to provide creative and consistent high guilty education to learner she frequently perform the staff development role, sometimes a director of nursing in a health care organizations as nurse manger or from other management positions.

Definition
- Staff development program are designed to motivate learner in the way of the train and education to improve their knowledge, skills and attitudes.
- Staff development is the process directed towards the personal and professional growth of nurses and other personnel while they are employed by a health care agency.
- Staff development refers to all training and education provided by an employee to improve the occupational and personal knowledge, skills and attitudes of vested employees.
- Staff development refers to the processes, programs and activities through which every organization develops, enhances and improves the skills, competencies and overall performance of its employees and workers.
- A process consisting of orientation, in-service education and continuing education for the people of promoting the development of personnel within any employment setting, consistent with the goals and responsibilities of the employment (ANA).

Meaning of Staff Development
Staff development refers to the continuing improvement of the nursing personnel. It also includes setting standards for jobs, providing on the—job growth experiences, considering potential growth opportunities in all assignment planning, supervising and appraising performance proficiencies and assuming responsibility for reparative or corrective training measures. Staff development program are designed to motivate learner in the way of the train and education to improve their knowledge, skills and attitudes.

Objectives of Staff Development
- To assist each employee to improve performance in present position.
- To keep in pace with medical sciences.
- New development in medical science and technology.
- New diagnostic and treatment techniques.
- To motivate each staff member and create a sense of security and loyalty.
- To improve work productivity and for promotion.
- To reduce staff turnover, absenteeism and tardiness.
- To acquire personal and professional abilities that maximizes the possibility of career advancement.

Need for Staff Development (Box 22.2)
- Social change and scientific advancement
- Advancement in the field of science, such as medical science and technology.
- To provide the opportunity for nurses to continually acquire and implement the knowledge, skills, attitudes, ideals and valued essentials for the maintenance of high quality of nursing care:
  - As part of an individual's long-term career growth.
  - To add or improve skills needed in the short term
  - Being necessary to fill gap in the past performance
  - To change or correct long-held attitudes of employee
  - Need to increase the productivity and quality of the work.
  - To motivate employees and to promote employee loyalty
  - Fast growing organizations.

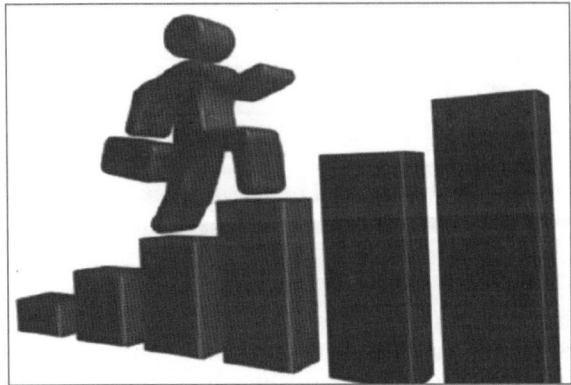

Fig. 22.11: Staff development.

> **Box 22.2:** Need for staff development.
> - Social change and scientific advancement
> - Advancement in the field of science, such as medical science and technology
> - To provide the opportunity for nurses to continually acquire and implement the knowledge, skills, attitudes, ideals and valued essentials for the maintenance of high quality of nursing care:
>   - As part of an individuals long-term career growth.
>   - To add or improve skills needed in the short term

Staff Development Process (Fig. 22.12)

The major processes involved in the staff development programs are presented graphically in the following chart prepared by Silver (1981): The goals and objectives of the training program must first of all be defined. This will give focus and guidance to the entire program. Then, the strengths and weaknesses of staff must be identified. This will be useful in developing long-term plans and specific training programs which will involve specific outlines of major annual training goals, the number of individuals who will benefit from such training and the cost implication of the plan.

The next stage involves detailed training programs which will be undertaken. The acquisition of text and training materials, the preparation of teaching or instructional aides, the selection and appointment of instructors and their remunerations are determined. This stage is followed by the implementation of the program which will involve the use of consultants and resource persons. Meeting places are provided. The trainees are released from their regular duties for the training programs. The last stage is the evaluation of the efforts and performance of the training programs with a view to detecting the need for improvement in certain areas of the program.

Functions of Staff Development (Fig. 22.13)

Personnel assigned to staff development should provide the following consultative functions for health care agency:

- Determination of the administrative structure of the staff development program.
- Determination and establishment of organizational methods, policies and procedures for a staff development program.
- Determination and establishment of lines of communication for the utilization of facilities and resources personnel for a staff development program.
- Determination of organizational and individual staff development needs and priority.
- Development of measurable short- and long-term objectives for staff development programs.
- Promotion, development, implementation and evaluation of programs to meet these objectives.
- Planning, coordination, and utilization of community resources to assist in meeting these objectives.
- Provision of a consultative service and a resource for information relative to staff development.

Staff Development Activities

Staff development includes formal and informal, group or individual training and education. Staff development activities include (**Fig. 22.13**): 1. Induction training, 2. Orientation, 3. In-service education, 4. Continuing education, and 5. Training for special functions, such as management, team building, and budgeting method.

- **Induction training (3 days):** It is a brief introduction to agency philosophy, purpose, administrators, programs, policies and regulations that is given to new employee during the first three days of employment.
- **Orientation (2–24 weeks):** It is individualized training given each employee during the first period of his job to familiarize him with his job's duties, work place, clients and co-worker.
- **In-service education (2–8 hours):** It includes all on-the-job instruction and training that is given to enhance employee's present job performance.
- **Continuing education (1–5 days):** It includes all planned learning that is intended to increase employee's knowledge or skills beyond that needed for satisfactory performance in the present job.

Importance of Staff Development

- It is focus on developing nursing skills and knowledge.
- Introduce the employees to new situations and orientated to philosophy, soils, politics, and physical sanities.
- It provider job-relate counseling, which involves promoting the professional growth of employees.
- It provider learning experiences in the work setting for the purpose of refining and developing new skills and knowledge related to job performance.

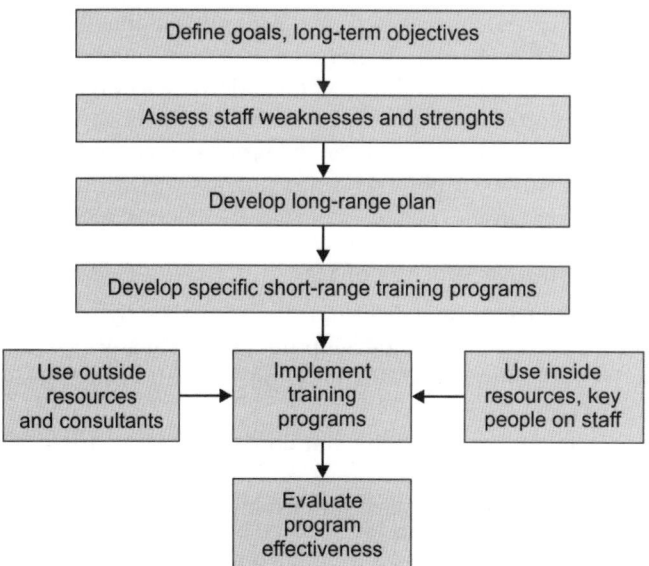

Fig. 22.12: Staff development process.

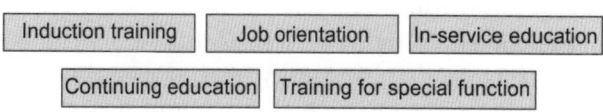

Fig. 22.13: Types of staff development.

- It is planned and organized around learning experiences in variety of setting.
- To reduce staff turnover and absenteeism.

Staff Development Organization

The staff development program philosophy based on nursing organization. It includes: 1. How learning takes place, 2. Various teaching methods, 3. Responsibility for their learning, 4. Rights of the clients

1. **Organization:** There are two methods of organization.
   a. Centralized model here, all department collaborating determining and planning the job needs of their staff
   b. Decentralized model: Each department its own organized staff development programs.
2. **Committees:** Committees identifying needs and resources for program committees member maintain relationship and communicable between each one to accomplish the god.
3. **Budgets:** Budgets based on staff size, no of new employees and resource person, program manager is responsible for budget preparation.
4. **Personnel:** Staff development manager to work on planning, implementing and evaluating staff development programs. The size of staff depends on the size it the agency.

Staff Development Assessment Methods

Staff development planning, organizers to assessment needs of participants. Following faction should be considered to assess needs of the program
- Population
- Time
- Cost/financial
- Analysis time
- Objectivity

Various methods of needs assessment
- Questionnaire method
- Survey
- Interview
- Observation
- Group meeting
- Performance appraisal
- Individual need assessment method.

Goals of Staff Development (Fig. 22.14)

Staff development includes formal and informal group and individual training and education. The goals of staff development programs are to assist each employee to improve performance in her or his present position and to acquire personal and professional abilities that maximize the possibility of career advancement. Staff development activities include the following:

1. **Induction training** is a brief, standardized indoctrination to an agency's philosophy, purpose, policies and regulations given to each worker during her or his first two or three days of employment in order to ensure his

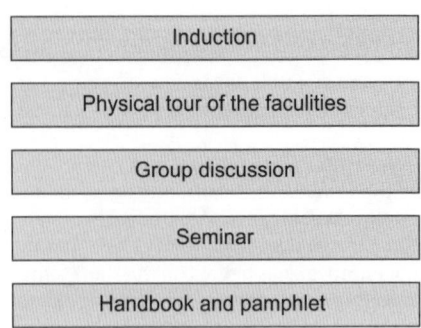

Fig. 22.14: Methods of delivering staff development program.

or her identification with agency's philosophy, goals and norms.

2. **Job orientation** is an individualized training program intended to acquaint a newly hired employee with job responsibilities work place, clients and co-workers.
3. **In-service education** refers to an ongoing-on-the-job instruction that is given to enhance, the workers' performance in their present job.

   In-service education is a planned educational experience provided in the job setting and closely identified with service in order to help the person to perform more effectively as a person and as a worker (NLN). In-service education is defined as a continued program of education provided by the employing authority, with the purpose of developing the competence of personnel in their functions appropriate to the position they hold, or to which they will be appointed in the service.
4. **Continuing education** is "any extension of opportunities for reading, study and training to any person and adult following their completion of or withdrawal from full time school and/or college programs". It is there education for adults provided by specific schools, centers, colleges or institutions that emphasize flexible rather than traditional or academic programs. Adult education is a formal and informal instruction and aids to study for mature persons; all activities with educational purposes carried on by mature persons on a part time basis; any voluntary, purposeful effort towards the self development of adults conducted by public or private agencies, for informational, cultural, remedial, vocational, recreational, and professional and other purposes (Dictionary of Education).

Administrative Structure of SDP

The major factors that determine the administrative structure of an agency-wide staff development program are:
- Administrative philosophy, policies and practices of health care agency.
- Policies, practices and standards of nursing and other health professions.
- Human and material resources within a healthcare agency and the community.
- Physical facilities within a healthcare agency and the community.

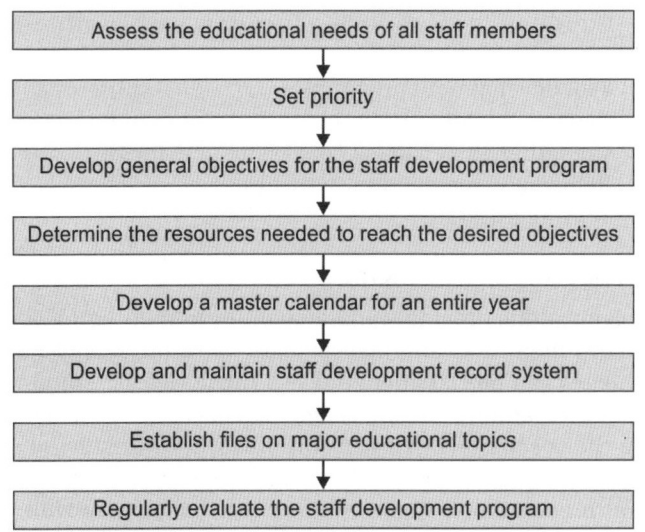

Fig. 22.15: Step of staff development program.

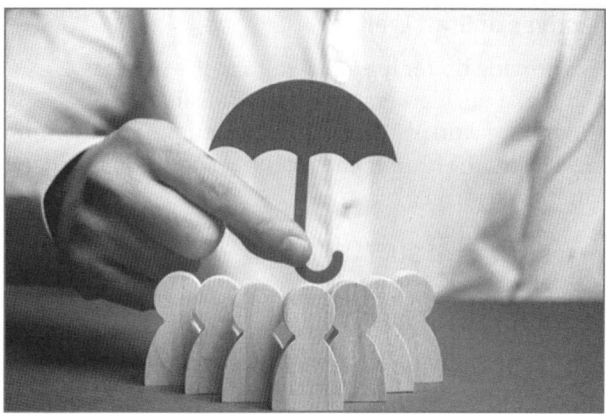

Fig. 22.16: Staff welfare.

- Financial resources within a healthcare agency and the community. **Figure 22.15** shows step of staff development program.

Centralization vs decentralization: In some cases, a centralized structure will be more effective than a decentralized structure. There are advantages and disadvantages to both types of structure. Usually, the coordination of staff development is more readily facilitated in a centralized structure. However, in a decentralized structure, it is possible to involve a larger number of personnel in planning and implementing programs. One alternative is a centralized structure for an agency-wide staff development program and decentralized structure for programs related to learning a specific job skill. Whatever be the administrative structure, it is vital to circumvent redundancy, repetition and ineffective utilization of personnel and facilities,

Role of Head Nurse in SD

- Involves staff members in developing high standards of patient care and in establishing objectives and criteria for their attainment.
- Discover leadership's skills and creative abilities among staff and arrange for their development.
- Encourage staff to participate in planning for the improvement of nursing care and to apply findings of nursing practice research.
- Provide learning opportunities for professional advancement of staff in order to develop to their highest potential.
- Share in planning and participate in staff educational programs of professional and non-professional personnel.
- Allot time for discussions, observations and questions.
- Set a good example in everyday practice.

STAFF WELFARE (FIG. 22.16)

The institution should serve various facilities for the staff members to enable them to function effectively at their work. The institution expects from its staff a commitment to serve, in the spirit of god, the patients and others who come in search of the services. Some of the provisions provided are unique to the institution and we believe will faster a fellowship and friendship amongst the staff to develop a team spirit which is critical for successful medical services.

Definition

Staff welfare is an all-encompassing term covering a wide range of facilities that are essential for the well-being of your employees.

Meaning of Staff Welfare

- Welfare includes anything that is done for the comfort and improvement of employees and is provided over and above the wages.
- Welfare helps in keeping the morale and motivation of the employees high so as to retain the employees for longer duration.
- The welfare measures need not be in monetary terms only but in any kind/forms.
- Employee welfare includes monitoring of working conditions, creation of industrial harmony through infrastructure for health, industrial relations and insurance against disease, accident and unemployment for the workers and their families.

Vision and Mission

- **Vision:** Creation of competitive, amicable and healthy atmosphere within the campus.
- **Mission:** Overall development of staff members by applying different welfare scheme

Purposes of Staff Welfare

- It motivates the staff to work effectively.
- It improves interest to serve to the particular institution.
- It facilitates the staff member to participate with full involvement.
- It improves the team work in the institution.
- It helps to meet the psychological, social and educational need of the employee.
- It helps to meet the psychological, social and educational and of the employee.

Objectives of Staff Welfare

- To provide better life and health to the workers
- To make the workers happy and satisfied.
- To relieve workers from industrial fatigue and to improve intellectual, cultural and material conditions of living of the workers.

Characteristics of Staff Welfare

The basic features of labor welfare measures are as follows:
- Labor welfare includes various facilities, services and amenities provided to workers for improving their health, efficiency, economic betterment and social status.
- Welfare measures are in addition to regular wages and other economic benefits available to workers due to legal provisions and collective bargaining.
- Labor welfare schemes are flexible and ever-changing. New welfare measures are added to the existing ones from time to time.
- Welfare measures may be introduced by the employers, government, employees or by any social or **charitable** agency.
- The purpose of labor welfare is to bring about the development of the whole personality of the workers to make a better workforce.

Goals

- To provide platform to the staff for expressing their ideas.
- To felicitate outstanding achievements of staff members in various fields
- To develop cooperation and coordination among the staff
- To create opportunities for exchange of inter disciplinary knowledge
- To provide opportunities for updating their knowledge

Staff Welfare Activities (Fig. 22.17)

- Conducting journal club meetings based on innovative themes.
- Deputing the staff to attend conferences to update their knowledge
- Conducting in-service education and continuing education programs
- Staff development programs
- Capacity building training for all the staff to realize and strengthen their capacity in various activities
- Retreat and recreational activities
- TNAI registration

Employee Welfare Schemes

Organizations provide welfare facilities to their employees to keep their motivation levels high. The employee welfare schemes can be classified into two categories viz. statutory and non-statutory welfare schemes. The statutory schemes are those schemes that are compulsory to provide by an organization as compliance to the laws governing employee health and safety. These include provisions provided in industrial Acts, such as Factories Act 1948, Dock Workers Act (safety, health and welfare) 1986, Mines Act 1962. The non-statutory schemes differ from organization to organization and from industry to industry.

Statutory Welfare Schemes

The statutory welfare schemes include the following provisions:

- **Drinking water:** At all the working places safe hygienic **drinking water** should be provided.
- **Facilities for sitting:** In every organization, especially factories, suitable seating arrangements are to be provided.
- **First aid appliances:** First aid appliances are to be provided and should be readily assessable so that in case of any minor accident initial medication can be provided to the needed employee.
- **Latrines and urinals:** A sufficient number of latrines and urinals are to be provided in the office and factory premises and are also to be maintained in a neat and clean condition. **Figure 22.18** shows pride approaches of staff welfare.

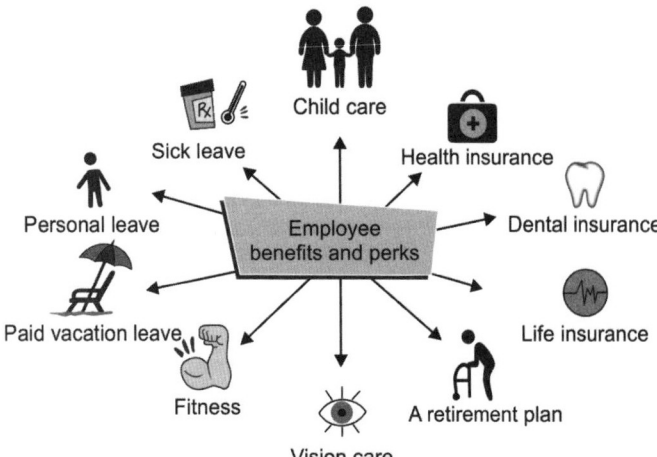

Fig. 22.17: Employee benefits and perks.

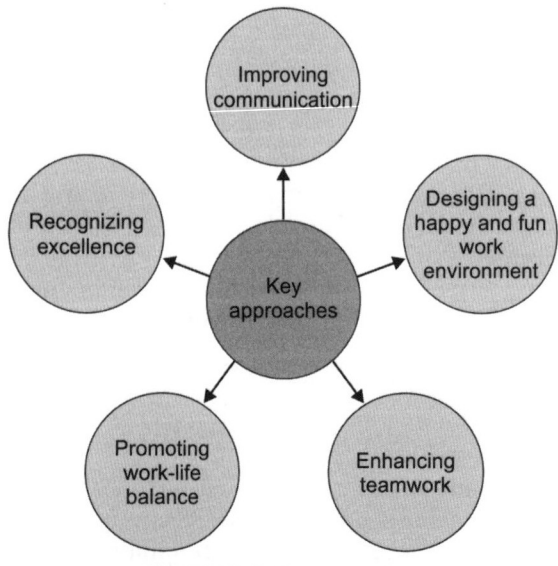

Fig. 22.18: Pride approaches.

- **Canteen facilities:** Cafeteria or canteens are to be provided by the employer so as to provide hygienic and nutritious food to the employees.
- **Spittoons:** In every work place, such as ware houses, store places, in the dock area and office premises spittoons are to be provided in convenient places and some are to be maintained in a hygienic condition.
- **Lighting:** Proper and sufficient lights are to be provided for employees, so that they can work safely during the night shifts.
- **Washing places:** Adequate washing places, such as bathrooms wash basins with tap and tap on the stand pipe are provided in the port area in the vicinity of the work places.
- **Changing rooms:** Adequate changing rooms are to be provided for workers to change their cloth in the factory area and office premises. Adequate lockers are also provided to the workers to keep their clothes and belongings.
- **Restrooms:** Adequate numbers of restrooms are provided to the workers with provisions of water supply, wash basins, toilets, bathrooms, etc.

Nonstatutory Schemes

- **Personal health care (regular medical check-ups):** Some of the companies provide the facility for extensive health check-up.
- **Flexi-time:** The main objective of the flextime policy is to provide opportunity to employees to work with flexible working schedules. Flexible work schedules are initiated by employees and approved by management to meet business commitments while supporting employee personal life needs.
- **Employee assistance programs:** Various assistant programs are arranged, such as external counseling service so that employees or members of their immediate family can get counseling on various matters.
- **Harassment policy:** To protect an employee from harassments of any kind, guidelines are provided for proper action and also for protecting the aggrieved employee.
- **Maternity and adoption leave:** Employees can avail maternity or adoption leaves. Paternity leave policies have also been introduced by various companies.
- **Medi-claim insurance scheme:** This insurance scheme provides adequate insurance coverage of employees for expenses related to hospitalization due to illness, disease or injury or pregnancy.
- **Employee referral scheme:** In several companies employee referral scheme is implemented to encourage employees to refer friends and relatives for employment in the organization.

Faculty Improvement Techniques

- Encourage and stimulate faculty
- Take positive attitude towards problems of teachers
- Provide resources and facilities for the implementation of instructions.
- Give recognition to abilities

- Create a climate which stimulates creative participation by faculty members.
- While making changes in the curriculum, invite suggestions from the faculty.
- Given opportunity to plan, experiment and explore
- Assist in developing teaching techniques
- Maintain good relation with faculty members.

Staff Welfare Activities

The conditions under which the teaching staff have an effect on the implementation of the program besides contributing towards the stability of the staff. Frustrations, conflicts, resignations and frequent requests for transfer can often be reduced when there are clearly defined policies related to hours of work, teaching load, welfare of the staff and other matters. The policies should be written down known to everyone. The following are some of these matters employee welfare activities are social security measures provided by the institution for the welfare of the employees. Some of them are:

- Employees provident fund
- Gratuity benefit
- Maternity benefit
- Risk allowances
- Compensations for work injuries
- Family pension schemes
- Employee state insurance

Box 22.3 describes types of employee welfare.

Types of faculty welfare include:

- Opportunity for leave on the basis of leave rules by the institution policies These leave rules incorporate existing annual leave, maternity leave, sabbatical leave, study leave, leave on loss of pay, official leave.
- Gratuity-cum-retirement benefit scheme
- Hospital concessions
- Staff special superannuation benefit scheme for long-term service.
- Provident fund
- Death benefit schemes
- Providing opportunity to develop cognitive skills by staff development programs, in-service program and continuing education programs.

Box 22.3: Types of employee welfare.

- **Statutory welfare work:** Comprising the legal provisions in various pieces of labor legislation.
- **Voluntary welfare work:** Includes those activities which are undertaken by employers for their voluntary work. Different ways of Social Security Provision in India
    1. **Social insurance:** Common fund is established with periodical contribution from workers out of which all benefits in terms of cash or kind are paid. The employers and state prove major portion of finances. Benefits, such as PF, Group Insurance, etc., are offered.
    2. **Social assistance:** Benefits are offered to persons of small means by government out of its general revenues, e.g., old age pension

Formulation of Policies

Condition under which the teaching staff work, has an effect on the implementation on the program besides contributing towards the stability of the staff trust rations, conflicts, resignations and frequent requests for transfer, can often be reduced when there are clearly defined policies relating to hour of work, teaching load, welfare of staff and other matters. Such policies are particularly effective when the staff have been involved in formulating them, when they are known to everyone. The following are some of the matters in which it would be helpful to have stated policies and some of the factors to be considered in formulating them are.

- **Hours of work:** The policy should given direction on
  - The maximum number of working hours per week.
  - The number of days off per month, to which the staff is entitled.
  - The procedure to be followed regarding public holidays.
- **Teaching work load:** The policy regarding the maximum teaching work load to be carried by each tutor should allow time for preparation for classes and laboratory sessions, student guidance and counseling, evaluation of student assignments, committee work, record keeping and all other functions expected of a tutor. A teaching load of 14-16 hours per week will permit attention to these functions. In cases, where this in not possible, 20 hours of formal teaching per week should not be exceeded.
- **Residence:** There should be policy regarding the residence of staff quarters facilities. Residence for some staff is essential if student's curricular and extracurricular activities are implemented satisfactorily. The accommodation for married and unmarried staff including family quarters depends on institution's policy.
- **Leave:** The college should have clear policy about leaves.
  - Time of year during which annual leave may normally be taken.
  - How many leaves may be taken at one time.
  - The purpose for which casual or special leave may be granted.
  - The provision for maternity leave.
- **Sickness:** In regard to the care which will be given to staff members who are sick the college policy should state clearly about sick leave, medical expenses, reimbursement facility, etc.
- **Attendance at conference and study care:** The college should state policies regarding the selection and deputation of the staff for further education, including attendance at formal courses, refresher courses, work shop and conferences.
- **Promotion and transfer:** Promotion is the transfer of an employee to a job that pays more money or one that enjoys some preferred status. A promotion is the advancement of an employee to a better job better in terms of greater responsibilities.

Leave Facilities

- Leave shall be granted in accordance with the leave rules of institution.
- Leave cannot be claimed by any employee as right.
- The administrative officer concerned shall be the competent authority to sanction by the administrative officer concerned depending up on the necessities.
- Ordinarily no employee shall absent himself or herself from work unless leave is sanctioned. Employees remaining absent unauthorized shall be subjected to disciplinary action.
- Normally, leave application shall be made in prescribed forms.
- All leave applications forwarded to the administrative officer concerted for sanctioning shall contain the recommendation of the head of the department.
- The administrative officer concerned shall arrange to intimate the unvoiled leave to the credit of the employees of each department.

I. **Annual leave:** The quantum of annual leave shall be on the following scale.
   Council appointees—35 days, non-council appointees—25 days
   Annual leave for unconfirmed employees shall be calculated on priority basis on the number of days spent on duty by on employee in the leave year. For arriving at the number of days spent on duty the days availed on annual leave, casual leave, and sick leave, maternity leave will be taken into account.
   Annual leave cannot follow casual leave. However, casual leave up to a maximum of five days can be added on to the annul leave by prior permission of administrative officer concerned. Annual leave shall not be granted in more than three installments in a leave year.

II. **Casual leave:** Casual leave may be granted to a employees for a total of 10 days in each year subject to the necessities and exigencies of work. Casual leave may be either prefixed or suffixed to Sundays or holidays. Casual leave may be availed for half a day. Unexpected casual leave up to 2 day may be carried over to the following year to be used within the first six months.

III. **Compensatory and institutional holidays:** If any member of staff is on any leave other than official leave on a declared holiday of the institution, no compensatory leave shall be given to him/her. However, if the day off given to a staff member falls on a declared. If Christmas, New Year's Day, Republic Day, Good Friday and Independence day, which are National and Institutional holidays falls on a Sunday, compensatory leave will be given which may be taken within 6 months.

IV. **Sick leave:** Sick leave with full pay for a total of 15 days may be granted in a leave year. In addition to 15 days sick leave full pay as above, sick leave with half pay for a further period up to 18 days may be granted in a leave year. However, this cannot be converted to 9 days sick leave with full pay.

Sick leave normally is granted only on production of a sick leave recommendation slip issued by the medical officer, staff student health service. Sick leave shall be sanctioned according to the number of days indicated in the sick leave slip issued by the staff student health service.

V. **Maternity leave:** Women employees in the institution shall be granted maternity leave for 8 weeks with full pay. Part of the maternity leave may be availed just prior to delivery.

Incentives

Incentives are provided by some organization in order to attract and retain good employees. Incentives may be monetary and non-monetary. The monetary incentives may be the form of payment of bonuses, merit increments, housing facilities, medical care, loans, provision of transportation, education of children, etc. The non-monetary incentives are also used to motivate the employees for higher education. They are in the form of status and recognition, job security, responsibility; participation is decision making, training facilities, promotion, discipline, team spirit, etc., negative incentives are in the form of fine, demotion, suspension.

■ CONCLUSION

Employee welfare means anything done for the comfort and (intellectual or social) improvement of the employees, over and above the wages paid. In simple words, it means "the efforts to make life worth living for workmen." It includes various services, facilities and amenities provided to employees for their betterment. These facilities may be provided voluntarily by progressive entrepreneurs, or statutory provisions may compel them to provide these amenities; or these may be undertaken by the government or trade unions, if they have the required funds.

■ REVIEW QUESTIONS

Long Essays

1. Define performance appraisal; explain the objectives, purposes and need.
2. Define staff development program; explain the objectives, purposes and process.
3. Define staff welfare; explain the purpose, objectives, goals and characteristics.

Short Essays

1. Characteristic of performance appraisal.
2. Factors affecting performance appraisal.
3. Principles of performance evaluation.
4. Criteria of performance appraisal.
5. Performance appraisal methods.
6. Performance appraisal tool.
7. Performance appraisal in clinical practice.
8. Benefits of performance appraisal.
9. Importance of performance appraisal.
10. Staff development activities
11. Goals of staff development.

Short Answers

1. Teamwork.
2. Organizational skills.
3. Assertiveness.
4. Essentials of good performance appraisal.
5. Rating method.
6. Checklist method.
7. Advantages of performance appraisal.
8. Importance of staff development.
9. Staff development organization.
10. Job orientation.
11. In-service education.
12. Continuing education.
13. Role of head nurse in staff development.
14. Staff welfare activities.

CHAPTER 23

Directing and Controlling

Learning Objectives

- Review: Curriculum Implementation and Evaluation
- Leadership and Motivation, Supervision—Review
- Guidance and Counseling
- Quality Management—Educational Audit
- Program Evaluation, Evaluation of Performance
- Maintaining Discipline
- Institutional Records and Reports—Administrative, Faculty, Staff and Students

GUIDANCE AND COUNSELING

Guidance counseling, by name counseling and guidance, the process of helping individuals discover and develop their educational, vocational, and psychological potentialities and thereby to achieve an optimal level of personal happiness and social usefulness. The concept of counseling is essentially democratic in that the assumptions underlying its theory and practice are, first, that each individual has the right to shape his own destiny and, second, that the relatively mature and experienced members of the community are responsible for ensuring that each person's choice shall serve both his own interests and those of society. It is implicit in the philosophy of counseling that these objectives are complementary rather than conflicting.

Definition

Definition of Guidance

- Guidance is an assistance made available by a competent counselor to an individual of any age to help him direct his own life, develop his own point of view, make his own decision and carry his own burden.
  —*Hamrin and Erikson*
- Guidance is a process of helping every individual, through his own effort to discover and develop his potentialities for his personal happiness and social usefulness.
  —*Ruth Strang*

Definition of Counseling

- Counseling is essentially a process in which the counselor assists the counselee to make interpretations of facts relating to a choice, plan or adjustment which he needs to make. —*Glenn F Smith*
- Counseling is a series of direct contacts with the individual which aims to offer him assistance in changing his attitude and behaviors. —*Carl Rogers*

Concept of Guidance

Guidance is broad term. Counseling is only a part of guidance which deals pupils at problem points. Counseling refers to a process in which the individual is helped to make a decision, to make a choice or to find a direction about all the important matter like a program in the school, getting employment, planning for life, etc. Counseling is considered as one of the techniques in guidance program.

Definition: Fundamental of all guidance is the help or assistance given by a competent person to an individual so that the latter may direct his life by developing his point of view, make his own decision and carry-out these decisions."

Elements of Guidance

- Guidance focuses our attention on the individual and not the problem.
- Guidance helps the discovery of abilities of an individual.
- Guidance is based on the interest, abilities, assets, needs and limitations of the individual.
- Guidance gives rise to self—development and self-direction.
- Guidance makes the individual to plan wisely for present and the future.
- Guidance makes the individual to become adjusted to the new environment.
- Guidance is helpful in achieving success and happiness.

Principles of Guidance

- The basis of guidance is individual differences.
- Guidance is the basis of rigid code of ethics.
- The basis of guidance is an educational and vocational objective.
- Guidance is able to develop the insight of an individual
- Guidance regards most of the individuals as average normal person.
- Guidance is slow but a continuous process.

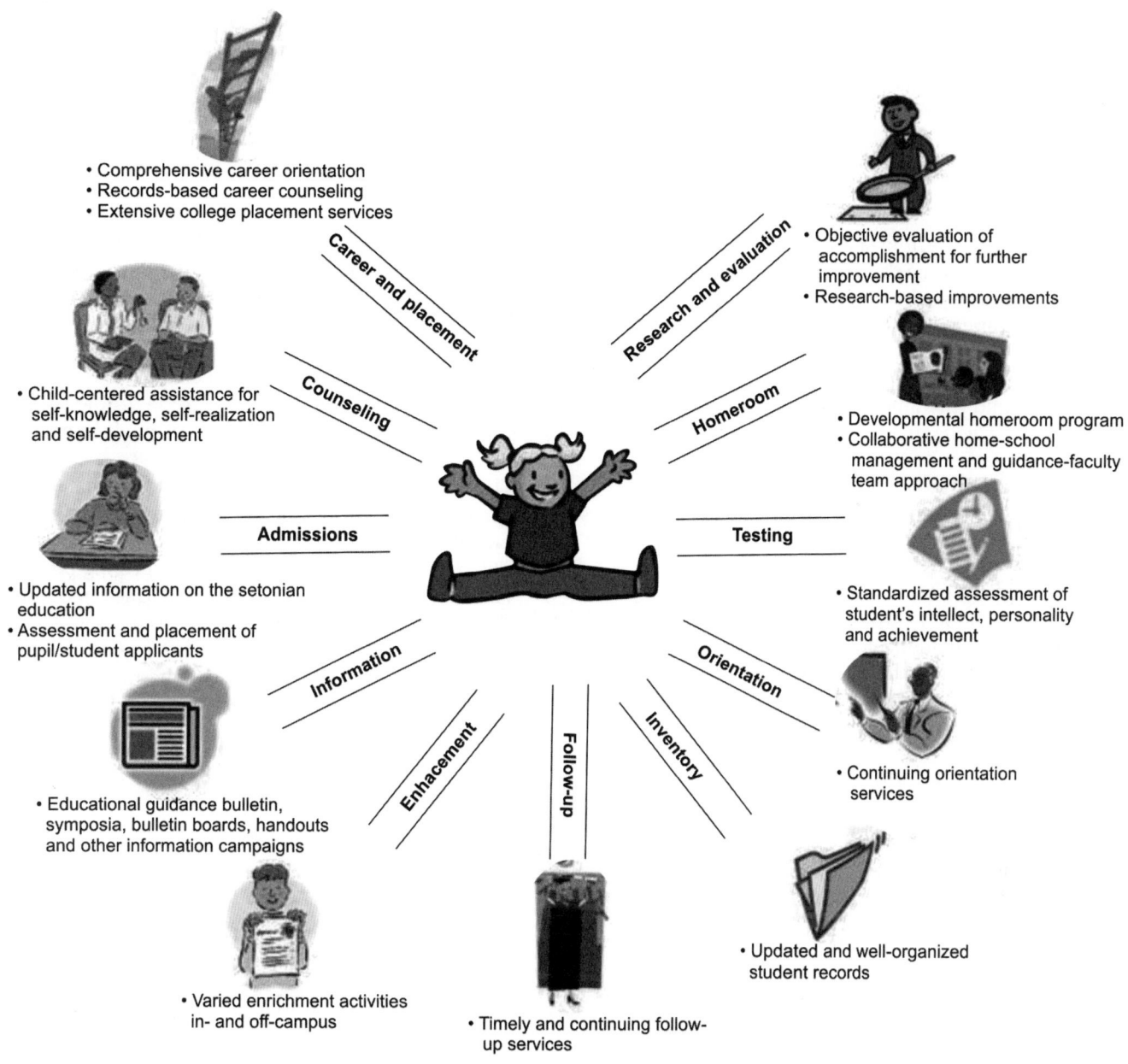

Fig. 23.1: Guidance services.

- Guidance is developed as well as comprehensive.
- Guidance is practical side of education.
- Guidance is mainly child centered.
- Guidance is specialized and generalized service (**Fig. 23.1**).

Purposes of Guidance

- **Understand the individual:** The main purpose of guidance is to discover and understand capacities, potentialities, abilities, aptitudes, interests, weak and strong points of the individual and to make evaluation of the self in relation to personal and social experience and to use the self more efficiently in every day of living.
- **Help the individual in making adjustment:** Another aim of guidance is to assist the individual so as to be making satisfactory and maximum adjustments at home, school, to teacher, to pupils and to society by giving him informational services, such as individual inventory service and occupational information's services, counseling service, placement and follow-up services.
- **Develop personal abilities and potentialities:** Another purpose of guidance is to help the individuals to develop their abilities, potentialities and points of view, to develop their body, mind, personality and character, to utilize their efforts, to make their own decisions and choices; to direct their lives; to develop their points of view and to solve their problems independently in an efficient manner.
- **Improve school activities:** The guidance program helps the school staff to solve various problems and improve all the activities of the school.
- **Coordinating home, school, and society:** Erickson has correctly said that one of the important purposes of guidance has been coordinating home, school, and community influence on the child.

Erickson has given the following purposes of guidance:

- **Careful study of individual:** In order to make the guidance program effective, an attempt is made to study the individual thoroughly. Guidance helps in doing so with the help of tests and techniques at its disposal.
- **Informational services:** By guidance, it means help given to pupils, so that they may be able to solve their problems. Now in order to solve these problems, they require information in various aspects of life. The guidance programme is to see that this information comes from either various information services, such as individual inventory service, occupational information services or by many other agencies of the school.
- **Counseling:** By counseling, it means the help of a personal kind when individual is faced with adjustment problems. In general, there a provision of counseling for pupils requesting special and personal help.
- **Placement and follow up:** Guidance program is quite helpful in placing pupils in various jobs. Later, it also studies as to how far they have been a success. It makes them to succeed also.
- **Assisting the school staff:** The guidance program serves the entire school by providing available information to others. In fact guidance program aims at improving all the activities of the school.
- **Coordination:** Finally, guidance makes various effects to coordinate home, school and community influences on the child.

Basis for comparison	Guidance	Counseling
Meaning	Guidance refers to an advice or a relevant piece of information provided by a superior, to resolve a problem or overcome from difficulty	Counseling refers to a professional advice given by a counselor to an individual to help him in overcoming from personal or psychological problems
Nature	Preventive	Remedial and curative
Approach	Comprehensive and extroverted	In-depth and introverted
What it does?	It assists the person in choosing the best alternative	It tends to change the perspective, to help him get the solution by himself or herself
Deals with	Education and career related issues	Personal and socio-psychological issues
Provided by	Any person superior or expert	A person who possesses high level of skill and professional training
Privacy	Open and less private	Confidential
Mode	One to one or one to many	One to one
Decision making	By guide	By the client

Concept of Counseling

Counseling is a personal and dynamic relationship between the individuals an older nurse experienced and wiser (counselor) and a younger less experienced and less wise (counselee). The later has problem for which he seeks the help of the former. The two work together so that the problem may be more clearly defined and the counselee may be helped to a self-determined solution.

Counseling is assisting an individual in the solution of his problem. The interview has an important place in guidance, but only one stage in the whole process of counseling.

Characteristics of Counseling

- Counseling is based on a person-to-person relationship.
- It involves two individuals, one seeking help and the other, a professionally trained person who can help the first.
- The main aim is to help and assist properly. The counselor must establish a relationship of mutual respect, co-operation and friendliness between the two individuals.
- The counselor will try to discover the problems of the client and helps him to set up goals and guide him through difficulties and problems.
- The counselor will try to discover the problems of the client and helps him to set up goals and guide him through difficulties and problems.
- The main emphasis in the role of counseling process is laid on the counselor's self-direction and self-acceptance.
- Counseling is democratic and the counselor sets up a democratic pattern and allows the counselee to do freely whatever he likes while with consultant and not under the consultant.

Objectives of Counseling

- Achievement of positive mental health
- Resolutions of problems
- Improving personal effectiveness
- Maximizing change of behavior
- Decision making as a goal of nursing
- Modification of behavior as a goal

Principles for Counseling

Siddiqui (2013) has listed 10 principles of counseling which are the following:

1. Communicate personal warmth and make the client feel welcome and valued as individuals.
2. Act with care and respect considering the individual and cultural differences and diversity of human experience.
3. Be honest and trustworthy in all of the individual's professional relationships, being open, friendly and not defensive.
4. Respect the confidence with which the individual is entrusted.
5. Be empathetic and sense the feelings and experience of another person.
6. Promote the safety and wellbeing of individuals, families, and communities.
7. Seek to increase the range of choices and opportunities for the clients.
8. Practice within the scope of the individual competence.
9. Treat colleagues and other professionals with respect.
10. Focus on finding solutions to the existing problems and future decisions of the individual.

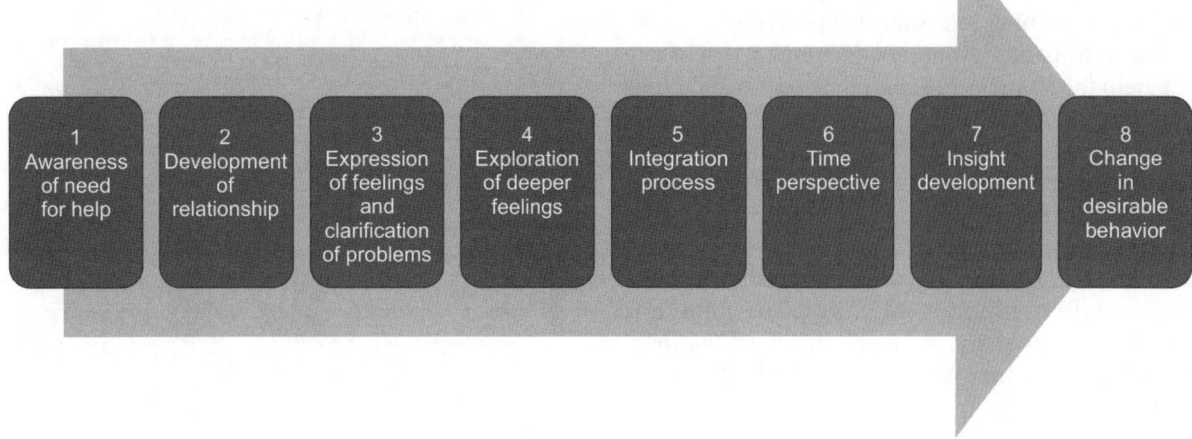

Fig. 23.2: Steps in counseling.

Counseling Skills

- Attending
- Observing
- Active listening
- Reflecting
- Questioning
- Summarizing
- Silence
- Independence
- Concreting
- Empathy and acceptance
- Cultural sensitivity

Steps of Counseling (Fig. 23.2)

1. **Analysis:** Collection of data is carried out from a variety of sources by using a variety of tools and techniques. The data is essential for an adequate understanding of the client.
2. **Synthesis:** Summarizing and organizing the data are to be carried out so as to reveal the client's assets, liabilities, adjustments and maladjustments.
3. **Diagnosis:** At this stage, an attempt should be made to find out the root cause of the problem exhibited by the client.
4. **Prognosis:** At this stage, the future development of the client's programs should be predicted.
4. **Treatments or counseling:** It may include some or all of the following procedures:
   - To establish rapport with the client
   - To interpret the collected data to the student
   - To advise or plan a program of action with the student
   - To assist the student in carrying out the plan of action
   - To refer to other counselors for getting assistance in diagnosing or counseling.
6. **Follow up**—here the counselor makes an attempt to help the client with new problems or with recurrences of the original problem and ascertain the effectiveness of counseling provided to them.

Advantages

- It is more economical in time.
- Emphasis is mainly laid on the problem but not on the individual the counselor can examine the client more objectively then the client himself.
- Directive counseling lays more emphasis on the intellectual rather than the emotional aspect of personality of the individual.
- In directive counseling methods used to have been direct persuasive and explanatory.

Scope of Counseling Services

- The scope of guidance and counseling is extremely comprehensive **(Fig. 23.3)**. As the life is getting complex day by day, the problems in which expert help is required are increasing proportionately.

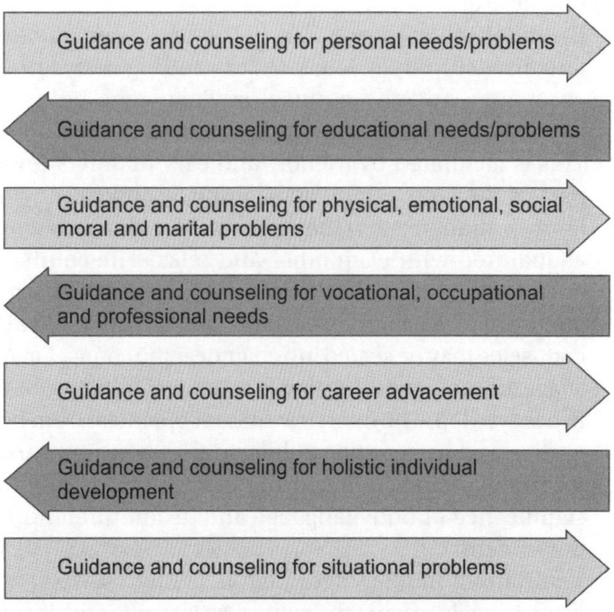

Guidance and counseling for personal needs/problems

Guidance and counseling for educational needs/problems

Guidance and counseling for physical, emotional, social moral and marital problems

Guidance and counseling for vocational, occupational and professional needs

Guidance and counseling for career advacement

Guidance and counseling for holistic individual development

Guidance and counseling for situational problems

Fig. 23.3: Scope of guidance and counseling.

- It helps the students in the selection of educational courses, profitable occupations, job placement, higher education and training, selection of improvement of study skills and study habits formation, maintenance of mental health, help the students to achieve maximum efficiency in meeting their needs.
- Individual services will be provided, granting loans, and scholarships, handling discipline cases, selection of roommates, advice on students activities and programs, helping the students to choose vocational objectives, selecting optional courses to the study, concerns about educational progress, course program planning, financial and health matters, problems of family, social, educational, vocational, a vocational, personal, moral, marital are the context of counseling.

Levels of Counseling

It is a face-to-face interview in which the counselor attempts non-coercively to help the client or counselee to make personal decisions. There are three levels of activity related to training.

- **In formal counseling:** Any helping relationship by a responsible person who may have little or no training for the work.
- **Non-specialist counseling by professionals:** It is help provided by professional who do a great deal of face-to-face work with psychological problems in the course of their work.
- **Professional counseling:** It is helping another person with decision and life-plans whether personal or educational or vocational by a person specially trained for this work.

Counseling Process (Fig. 23.4)

Several models have been proposed for the process of counseling. Basic counseling model. This model has five stages. These are:

1. **Establishing rapport:** This is the first stage, creating a relationship by mutual understanding between the counselee and the counselor. This stage helps the counselee to relax and openly discuss her problems. This is facilitated by friendly and easy manners on the part of the counselor. Establishing a rapport may not happen suddenly, but may take time for both to become acquainted with each other and relax. The counselor attempts to relate to the counselee and establish a friendly atmosphere in which conversation will flow naturally. The counselee may be seated in a chair near the counselor. Any suggestion of an authoritative relationship between the two is avoided. The interview calls for openness from both parties and uses a style of language that is appropriate for the occasion. The counselor must understand the significance of body language and its interpretation by the student.
2. **Ventilation:** In this stage, the role of the counselor is to listen actively to what the counselee is saying and observe nonverbal cues, such as posture, gesture, eye contact, etc.

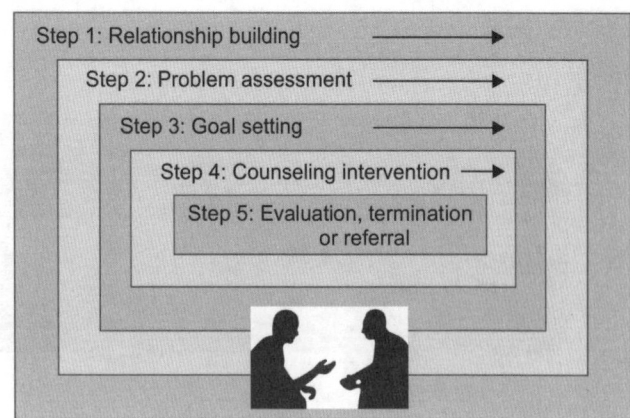

Fig. 23.4: Counseling process.

He may encourage the counselee by saying 'yes 'go on, etc., to continue the conversation.

3. **Understanding the problem:** This involves assisting the counselee to gain the fullest awareness of her problem. As the counseling progresses, the counselee begins to feel less fearful and gains an insight into her problem.
4. **Decision-making:** This stage consists of an examination of the various possible solutions to a problem and choosing the best one and also the method of implementing this solution. The counselor does not make the decision for the counselee; rather he guides the decision-making process.
5. **Terminating the interview:** This is a summary stage, which reviews the progress made and consolidates the solution which has been decided. It must be remembered that an interview cannot be terminated during the process of counseling by the end of a single session. A counseling process may take many months to reach its final stage. However, this model explains the process of counseling and the course of action to follow.

Thorne's model: Brian J Thorne proposed this model which has nine stages.

1. Counselee approaching for help
2. Counselor attempting to relate to the counselee
3. Defining a helping situation
4. Encouraging the counselee to express
5. Counselor agreeing to help
6. Developing an insight into the problem
7. Establishing new goals
8. Decision-making
9. Terminating the counseling process

Qualities of a Counselor

The qualities and skills required of a counselor can be summarized as follows:
- A good and active listener
- A good observer—watching the counselee's nonverbal behavior for its meaning and stress if any.
- Attentiveness—showing complete attention to the counselee by her posture, non-verbal signals, eye contact, etc.
- A warm, approachable and genuine personality
- Maintaining confidentiality

- Reflective, creative and imaginative—paraphrasing the counselees' words or saying what he thinks about what the counselee feels
- Using good techniques of questioning—using open questions rather than closed, to allow expansion by the counselee
- Maintaining silence when necessary—effective use of silence can encourage the counselee to talk
- Not getting impatient over long gaps of silence on the part of the counselee, but interrupting if necessary
- Giving independence to the counselee for solving her own problems by appropriate questioning

A counselor-counselee relationship is very fruitful but very demanding. A counselor/tutor can get help from co-counselors/co-tutors whenever necessary to discuss problems related to counseling. For example, when teachers take up the role of student counseling, they may feel inadequate in certain aspects of counseling. To tackle such inadequacies, co-counselors/co-tutors can be of immense help. The principle of confidentiality must be maintained when a counselor needs such help. Guidance and counseling services must be arranged in all colleges. It is important to have guidance and counseling departments in Institutions where the services of trained counselors are available.

Functions of Guidance and Counseling (Fig. 23.5)

Guidance and counseling have three-folded functions, namely—adjust mental, orientation and developmental. They also assist the their students, especially in identifying the gifted and backward children. This will help the teachers to recognize the individual difference among students.

Adjustmental

- Guidance and counseling are adjustmental in the sense that they help the students in making the best possible adjustment to the current situations in the educational institution, in the home and the community.
- Professional and individual aid is given in making immediate and suitable adjustment at problem points.
- In accordance with the words of Reniold, guidance and counseling should enable the students to accept the things which they cannot change in life, to modify or change the things which they can in order to achieve success in life and to differentiate between what they can change and cannot change in life.
- For instance, a student cannot change his short stature but he can change, i.e., get rid of the inferiority complex that has arisen out of the short stature by giving more importance to his good character and academic achievements.
- In fact, the ability to differentiate between the things which we can change and cannot will help us a lot in leading a happy life.

Orientation

- Guidance and counseling have orientation function also. They orient the students in the problems of career planning, educational programming and direction towards long-term personal aims and values.
- This orientation will serve as a foundation for formulating realistic plans regarding future education and after education career.

Developmental

- Guidance is developmental in that it is concerned with helping the pupils to achieve self-development and self-realization.
- Through assisting in the achievement of self-development and self-realization, they can prevent problems and maladjustments rather than curing the damage occurred as a result of problems.

Need of Guidance and Counseling (Box 23.1)

The problems of students must be properly tackled with an intention to solve them. Unresolved problems may affect not only the academic performance of students but also their personality development. Guidance and counseling help teachers to solve the student's problems with their active involvement. They also assist the teacher in creating a healthy climate in the institution by ensuring harmonious and integrated personality development of students.

The need for counseling and guidance can be summarized as follows:
- To help in the total development of students.
- To assist students in leading a healthy life by abstaining from whatever is deleterious to health.

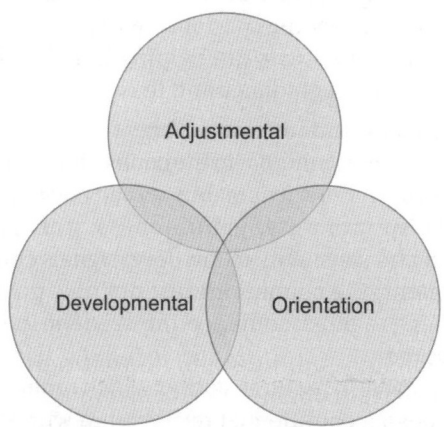

Fig. 23.5: Functions of guidance and counseling.

> **Box 23.1:** Need of guidance and counseling in nursing education.
> - To help nursing students in establishing proper identity.
> - To help them to develop a positive attitude towards life.
> - To help to overcome periods of turmoil and confusion.
> - To help students in developing their leadership qualities.
> - To motivate them for taking membership in professional organizations after competing their studies.
> - Helps them to make advantages of technological advancement in a patient care.
> - Helps them to readiness for changes and face challenges
> - To carryout responsibilities as a health team member
> - Helps them to proper selection of career
> - Motivate them for higher studies

- To help in the proper selection of educational programs.
- To help in the selection of careers according to their interests and abilities.
- To help the students in vocational development.
- To develop readiness for changes and to face challenges.
- To minimize the mismatching between education and employment and help in the efficient use of man power.
- To help fresher's establish proper identity.
- To identify and motivate the students from weaker sections of society.
- To help students to overcome the period of turmoil and confusion.
- To identify and render help to students who are in need of special help.
- To ensure proper utilization of time spent outside the classrooms.
- To help in tackling problems arising out of student explosion and co-education. To make up the deficiencies at home.
- To minimize the incidence of indiscipline.
- To motivate the youth for self-employment.
- To assist the needy students in availing financial assistance from appropriate organizations.

Puposes of Student Nurse Counseling

Dunsmoor and miller are of the view that the core of student counseling is to help the student to help himself. From this point of view they describe the following purposes of student counseling:

- To give the student information on matters important to success.
- To get information about student which will be of help in solving his problems?
- To establish a feeling of mutual understanding between student and teacher.
- To help the student work out a plan for solving his difficulties.
- To help the student know himself better-his interests, abilities, aptitudes and opportunities.
- To encourage and develop special abilities and right attitudes.
- To inspire successful endeavor toward attainment.
- To assist the student in planning for educational and vocational choices.

It is obvious that goal of counseling is problem clarification and self-directed needs. The counselor helps the student to understand the problems and helps the student to help himself. In this process, the role of the student is objective self-assessment of the situation and the role of counselor is to formulate the decision making process and to act as a stimulator of insights and sensitivities of the student. Counseling does not solve the problems but helps in solving and if solution is not possible, to help face challenges and to live with them. In short, counseling aims at developing student's self-understanding, self-acceptance and self-confidence.

Planning for Comprehensive Guidance and Counseling

Annual school division and school plans should include the components of guidance and counseling. An effective guidance/counseling program includes planned programs and activities, based on the needs of students that result in student outcomes in terms of knowledge, skills, and attitudes in areas of personal/social, educational and career development. Planning should include all four components of the comprehensive guidance and counseling model.

Plans should address issues of diversity and inclusion and should identify the range of programs and services to address diverse needs of all students.

The process of planning should involve key stakeholders, including students, school staff, families, and the community in a meaningful way.

Planning for comprehensive guidance and counseling programs and services should include:

- Statement of vision and mission
- Identification of priorities or key target areas
- Statements of expected outcomes
- Strategies and activities to achieve the outcomes
- Measurable indicators of success (strategies for evaluating the effectiveness of activities).

Special consideration in planning should be given to the role of guidance and counseling in supporting and contributing to the six priorities of Manitoba Education and Youth:

- Improving outcomes especially for less successful learners
- Strengthening links among schools, families and communities
- Strengthening school planning and reporting
- Improving professional learning opportunities for educators
- Strengthening pathways among secondary schools, post-secondary education and work
- Linking policy and practice to research and evidence.

Guidance and Counseling for Nursing Personnel

- To help adolescents with normal developmental problems.
- To help individual through temporary crisis.
- To identify signs of disturbed behavior at the earliest,
- To refer cases needing specialist treatment.
- To support tutors who are helping individual but who themselves want guidance and reassurance.

The problems in student counseling:

- major problems inherent in the counseling process derive from its very nature. It demands certain personal qualities, such as spontaneity, genuineness, non-possessive warmth and sensitivity to low-level signals coming from the student; the counselor must not only possess these qualities, he must convince the student that he does possess them.
- Counseling also requires skills of a high order—an ability to establish a confidential relationship with students of all types, a knowledge of the techniques of eliciting and

analyzing information, an understanding of the prevalent, so called, 'youth culture' and acquaintance with a variety of social environments.

- Its success involves patience and persistence. In Roger's words, it requires the creation of a non-threatening, non-judgmental environment, characterized by an attitude of empathy and respect for the student.
- Above all, perhaps, it requires more than a superficial acquaintance with the principles of psychotherapy.
- The formidable list of desirable qualities in the student counselor is a pointer to and a warning against, the morass in which the well-intentioned, but ill-equipped, amateur may find himself.
- Further problems may arise from the possible clash of goals and beliefs in the interviewing process which is inseparable from counseling. How is the strong minded counselor, possessed of a morality founded on deeply-held ethical principles, to react when faced with 'values of nihilism'? How does the professional teacher respond to the expressions of an 'anti-culture' which denies the validity of that in which he believes? In short, how does the counselor achieve the 'understanding neutrality' said to be required in the counseling process?
- The complexities of the counseling relationship are outlined by Munro in the enumeration of essential conditions of such a relationship. These conditions are described as 'of an ethical nature' and include a higher degree of confidentiality than is normally expected from a teacher, an insistence on the essentially voluntary nature of the relationship; insistence on the client's responsibility for his or her own behavior.
- Some teachers who have practiced as counselors have reported their feelings of inadequacy when the complex reality of problems of a classroom deviance is uncovered. Family backgrounds, financial difficulties, health concerns and emotional entanglements may have woven a web, from which the student cannot be extricated, save by a long term process of adjustment, requiring assistance which is totally beyond the counselor's power and resources. Frustration on both sides is deepened when. The counselor's diagnosis reveals a situation from which escape seems quite impossible.
- The problem of confidentiality often emerges at an early stage in student counseling, sometimes in the first meeting where the interviews produce criticisms of a counselor's teaching colleagues, is it to be

Conveyed to them? Where an interview reveals activities of a criminal nature, are the police to be informed? What is the legal situation of a counselor who, aware of such activities fails to inform the authorities?

Role of Nurse Manager in Guidance and Counseling

The modern nursing managers are facing many problems in today's competitive environment, but the basic management challenge is the management to work. No matter how good the plans, how flexible the policies and procedure of lab organization. Despite all "getting work done through people" is a major task for the nurse managers. Human resources are considered the single most important organizational asset. Managing the people of the organization is two tasks in one: The task of dealing with each employee as an individual with a uniquely different set of needs and behaviors.

While dealing with each employee or each work group, all managers experience interruption, but lower—level managers experience the most frequent work interruptions result in situational stress and lowered job satisfaction many of the times, it is due to scarce resources [organizational resources] like

- Money
- Information
- Materials
- Human resources, etc., lead to conflict developments.

Causes of Conflicts

- Unclear job boundaries and responsibilities
- Communication breakdown may be defective causes misunderstanding and conflict among people and groups.
- Personality clashes
- Power and status differences
- Goal differences

To avoid unpleasantness, to make people happy in good working environment and to maintain good moral among employees. Counseling (may be individual or group) and Guidance are provided whenever and wherever required. In organizations, giving guidance and counseling to individuals working must be continuous to help the individual develop in the maximum of their capacity in the direction most beneficial to him and to the organization.

On part of a nurse manager, the following steps may be taken to improve morale among employees while giving counseling and guidance.

Evolving good effective system of two way communication.
Keeping the employees informed about the organizational policies.

- To provide suitable job incentives relating to job, security, working conditions, opportunity for promotion, benefits and social status.
- Making provision of welfare amenities, such as recreation, housing and medical facilities.
- Encouraging staff participation in management.
- Analyzing and removing the causes of workers dissatisfaction in the organization.
- Encouraging group activities by the employees, such as social get together picnics, etc.

QUALITY MANAGEMENT IN NURSING INSTITUTIONS

Nursing and midwifery schools were urged to develop viable quality assurance systems and to regularly monitor evaluate and strengthen them in order to continuously improve the quality of education. Quality of education can be measured with many indicators, including the number of students that pass the national examination, the number of those securing jobs in the nursing and midwifery sector in recognized health facilities immediately after they graduate, the level of satisfaction of employers, supervisors and clients of the care providers, and the percentage of students who further their education at the graduate level.

Objectives

- To review the strategies used for quality improvement in nursing and midwifery education.
- To agree upon guidelines on quality assurance and accreditation.
- To provide recommendations on the roles and function of nursing and midwifery educational institutions, nursing and midwifery councils or regulatory bodies and national authorities on the quality of education.

Strategies

Strategies or methods used for quality improvement in their educational institutions. These were:
- Standards for curriculum and educational institution
- Upgrading of student admission criteria,
- Recruitment of students by central examination
- Curriculum revision upgrading of level of nursing education, i.e., from diploma to degree program
- External committee to review the test or sit in on the final examination
- Formal study for higher degree of teachers
- Refresher courses for teachers
- Nursing council offering comprehensive examination to all schools.

Role of Indian Nursing Council

- The Indian Nursing Council prescribes the syllabus, including unit plan and hours of each subject, scheme of examination and admission criteria.
- This ensures that the education offered in all nursing institutions is uniform.
- Minimum standards are also set for the physical facility, teaching facility and clinical facility to start a nursing program.
- The Indian Nursing Council conducts yearly or periodic inspections of the institutions in order to ensure that the set standards are being implemented.

Quality Assurance

- The goal of education is to prepare people to function properly in society according to societal needs.
- Quality assurance (QA) is one of the mechanisms developed by educational institutions to ensure that graduates attain adequate standards of education and training. It may consist of internal and external QA.
- Internal QA refers to the audit and assessment done by a team from within the organization.
- External QA refers to the audit and assessment done by a team from outside the organization, with the purpose of making the evaluation more objective. There should be tools for audit and assessment.
- The audit examines whether the school has performed the activities described in the checklist.
- The auditor simply checks a "yes" or "no" column. The assessment aims to judge the level of quality.
- On the assessment form, criteria and a score for achievement are given for each item. The assessor selects the column that reflects the level of achievement.
- The total score indicates the readiness or level of quality. The school must review the results and improve the quality in areas that are not yet at the highest level, while maintaining the quality of those that already meet the standards.
- The scope of assessment includes curriculum; student guidance, teaching and assessment; teaching and learning environment; available resources; and standards, quality control and procedures.
- The assessment results range from "excellent", "highly satisfactory" and "satisfactory" to "improvement required".
- In case of a grade of "improvement required", a repeat visit after one year is planned to assess the status of recommendations for improvement.

EDUCATIONAL AUDIT IN NURSING EDUCATION

The Academic Audit, such as more traditional program reviews, is a peer review process including a self-study and a site visit by peers from outside the institution. However, the similarities end there. Unlike the traditional approach to program evaluation, this process emphasizes self-reflection and self-improvement rather than compliance with predetermined standards.

Purposes

- Enabling students to have appropriate educational opportunities
- Maintaining/improving the students practice placement experience
- Giving recognition to the staff working in areas of excellence
- Improving the quality of the practice learning environment
- Identifying those areas in which staff needs help and support to maintain, improve and develop the quality of the learning environment.

Principles of the Academic Audit

- **Define quality in terms of outcomes**
  - Learning outcomes should pertain to what is or will become important for the department's students.
  - Learning, not teaching per se, is what ultimately matters.
- **Focus on process**
  - Departments should analyze how teachers teach, how students learn, and how to best approach learning assessment.

- Departments should study their discipline's literature and collect data on what works well and what does not.
- Experimentation with active learning should be encouraged.
- Faculty should be encouraged to share and adopt their colleague's successful teaching innovations.

- **Work collaboratively**
  - Teamwork and consensus lead to total faculty ownership of and responsibility for all aspects of the curriculum and make everyone accountable for the success of students.
  - Dialogue and collaboration should be encouraged over territoriality and the "lone wolf" approach.

- **Base decisions on evidence**
  - Departments should collect data to find out what students need.
  - Data should be analyzed and findings incorporated in the design of curricula, learning processes, and assessment methods.

- **Strive for coherence**
  - Courses should build upon one another to provide necessary breadth and depth.
  - Assessment should be aligned with learning objectives.

- **Learn from best practice**
  - Faculty should seek out good practices in comparable departments and institutions and adapt the best to their own circumstances.
  - Faculty should share best practices and help "raise the bar" for their department.

- **Make continuous improvement a priority:** Departments should continually and consciously strive to improve teaching and learning.

Steps for audit of educational institutions are as follows:
1. Study of the trust deed or regulations
2. Examine the previous financial statements
3. Noting of provisions applicable
4. Evaluation of internal control system
5. Examine the minute of the meeting and resolution
6. Verification of students fee register
7. Authorization for fee concessions
8. Verification of cashbook with respect of counterfoils of receipts and payments
9. Examination of capital fund regarding admission fees
10. Verify free studentship and concessions
11. Confirmation of fines for late payment or absence
12. Check hostel dues recovery
13. Verification of rental income or expenses
14. Examine the bank pass book of different nature
15. Verification of investment register and also ask about any interest and dividend from investment if any
16. Verify grants from any local bodies or Government with reference to memo or sanction letter
17. Reporting of any arrears
18. Vouch counterfoils of receipts taken from donors
19. Confirmation of any deposits and caution money and its treatment
20. Examination of expenses for library books and sports equipment
21. Checking of acknowledgement letter if any with regards to scholarship
22. Examination of payments with respect to prizes, if any
23. Examine the salary register
24. Verify the Provident Fund Register
25. Check annual report with accurate supporting documents
26. Vouching of all establishment expenses
27. Vouch payment for electricity and water bill
28. Examination of payment for hostel maintenance and any other miscellaneous expenses
29. Inspection of facilities given to students under any schemes associated with government
30. Verification of Fixed Assets Register
31. Verify ownership and existence of Fixed Assets
32. Confirmation of statutory compliance, i.e., PF, income tax, etc.
33. Verification of separate statements of accounts for different funds.
34. Checking of calculation of salary payable and deductions. At last, cross check all procedure.

Audit of Educational Institutions

The auditor may thoroughly study the trust deed of the trust to which the school or the college belongs and in the case of the audit of a university, he may study the Act of Legislature and the rules that are applicable to that university.

The institution may receive the following:
- Grant from government, local authority or governing bodies
- Legacies
- Donation in cash and in kind
- Income from Investments
- Admission fees, tuition fees, hostel fees, etc.
- Fines and penalties
- Contribution towards specific fund
- Rental income, etc.

Records to be Verified by Auditor in Educational Institutions

To verify the above, the auditor may examine the following books and records:
- Minutes of the managing committee.
- Students' fees Register.
- Cash book and counterfoils of receipts for fees, caution deposit, fine, etc.
- Rental and lease agreements.
- Correspondence and other documents relating to legacies, grants, etc.

Role of an Auditor in Audit of Educational Institutions

- He shall evaluate and confirm the effectiveness of internal check system of accounting of the receipts.
- He should verify that the fees are collected from all the students and if there is any concession, the same is granted by a person who is so authorized.

- He should also ensure that the fees received in advance and fees receivable are properly accounted and irrecoverable fees are written off under the authorization of the appropriate person.

An auditor may ensure the following while verifying records of educational institutions:
- That the admission fees are credited to capital fund account
- That the fines and penalties are collected after due authorization and accounted properly.
- That a separate register is maintained for caution deposit received from students and the refund due out of caution deposit is refunded to the students.
- That long outstanding tuition fees, hostel fees, etc., are periodically reviewed and reported to the management for further action.
- That the funds created for specific purpose are maintained separately, the investments representing such funds are kept separately and the surplus income from such funds are accumulated and invested along with the capital fund maintained for the purpose.
- That the amounts that are refundable to the students are shown as liability in the Balance sheet.
- That all the capital expenditure is approved by the managing committee.
- That the internal control procedure relating to purchase of stationery, provisions, clothing and other items are effective and chances of pilferage and fraud are minimum.

The auditor may verify all the expenditure in the usual manner and examine the payment out of funds created for specific purpose thoroughly and ensure that the receipts and payments out of these funds are accounted and presented separately in the Balance Sheet.

PROGRAM EVALUATION IN NURSING COURSE

Program evaluation is a common practice in nursing education programs; however, evidence indicates that many schools only focus on program evaluation around the scheduled accreditation period, thus reducing the potential value of the evaluation.

BSc Nursing Program
- **Nursing knowledge:** Apply knowledge from physical, biological and behavioral sciences, medicine including alternative systems and nursing in providing care to individuals, families and communities.
- **Nurse and the community:** Demonstrate understanding of lifestyle and other factors, which affect health of individuals and groups.
- **Care giver:** Provide nursing care based on steps of nursing process in collaboration with the individuals and groups.
- **Problem analysis/Decision making:** Demonstrate critical thinking skill in making decisions in all situations in order to provide quality care.
- **Technology update:** Utilize the latest trends and technology in providing healthcare.
- **Nurse and the healthcare system:** Provide promotive, preventive and restorative health services in line with the national health policies and programs.
- **Nurse and the profession:** Practice within the framework of code of ethics and professional conduct, and acceptable standards of practice within the legal boundaries.
- **Communication:** Communicate effectively with individuals and groups and members of the health team in order to promote effective interpersonal relationships and teamwork.
- **Information education and counseling:** Demonstrate skills in teaching to individuals and groups in clinical/community health settings.
- **Nurse as a collaborative care giver:** Participate effectively as members of the health team in healthcare delivery system.
- **Nursing administration and management:** Demonstrate leadership and managerial skills in clinical/community health settings.
- **Nursing research:** Conduct need based research studies in various settings and utilize the research findings to improve the quality of care.
- **Life-long learning:** Demonstrate awareness, interest and contribute towards advancement of self and of the profession.

Examinations and Assessment

Evaluation for a course shall be done on a continuous basis. The uniform procedures to be adopted shall be to conduct at least three theory assessments and if practical has been prescribed two practical continuous internal assessments (CIA) followed by one end year university examination (EY) for each course.
- For the category of Core Theory courses offered the assessment will comprise of Continuous Internal Assessment (CIA) and the end-year (EY) examination. For each course, the total of 100% per course is determined from the CIA evaluation weighted at 30% and the EYT weighted at 70%.
- For the category of core clinical rotation/ skills lab (CR/CL) and dissertation (RP) courses offered the assessment will comprise of Continuous Internal Assessment (CIA) for 50% and the end-year (EYP) examination for 50%. Or it can be evaluated internally as CIA for 100% as defined in the scheme of examinations table
- Courses (with separate course codes) wherein theory and clinical rotation/skills/lab are assessed jointly (results in group, RG), the passing minimum 60% for the theory exams and CR/CL, exams have to be obtained separately, in order to be declared passed in the individual courses. Reappearance in any one of the components is treated as reappear in both these components.
- Courses wherein curriculum includes both theory and lab hours, the CIA shall include evaluations for both components.
- Candidates having 100% attendance and obtaining 60% in the theory and practical internal assessments in each

of the courses can alone qualify to appear for the end year examinations.
- Candidate is declared passing a course if he/she has obtained 60% minimum in CIA and 60% minimum in end year examinations and in aggregate.

Continuous Internal Assessment

- There will be internal assessment (CIA) of students' performances in terms of theory and practical as given in the scheme 13.2 below.
- There will be internal assessment of students' performances in terms of theory and practical as given in the scheme of examination.
- To qualify for appearing for the university examination, a candidate should secure a minimum of 60% of marks in theory/practical separately in each subject.
- At least, three theory examinations and if practical has been prescribed two practical examinations, will be conducted in the subject concerned and marks as per the weightage will be taken into consideration for award of internal assessment marks.
- The written theory examination should be similar to the pattern of university examination.
- If a candidate fails in internal assessment in any subject(s) he/she will be given an opportunity to improve the internal assessment marks by conducting a minimum of two examinations in theory and in practical if prescribed, in the subject concerned.
- The details of internal marks awarded to the candidates should be submitted to the university by the Head of the Institution at least 15 days prior to the commencement of the university examinations.

EVALUATION OF PERFORMANCE IN NURSING EDUCATION

Performance evaluation is defined as a formal and productive procedure to measure an employee's work and results based on their job responsibilities. It is used to gauge the amount of value added by an employee in terms of increased business revenue, in comparison to industry standards and overall employee return on investment (ROI).

Aims

The aim of the undergraduate nursing program is to:
- Produce knowledgeable competent nurses with clear critical thinking skills who are caring, motivated, assertive and well-disciplined responding to the changing needs of profession, healthcare delivery system and society.
- Prepare graduates to assume responsibilities as professional, competent nurses and midwives in providing promotive, preventive, curative and rehabilitative healthcare services in hospital or public health settings.
- Prepare nurses who can make independent decisions in nursing situations within the scope of practice, protect the rights of individuals and groups and conduct research in the areas of nursing practice and apply evidence-based practice.
- Prepare nurses to assume role of practitioner, teacher, supervisor and manager in clinical or public health settings.

Practical Examination

Practical exams will be conducted for the following courses: Advanced Health/Physical Assessment in Critical Care Nursing, Foundations of Critical Care Nursing Practice, Critical Care Nursing I, Critical Care Nursing II. Examination will be conducted in the clinical area for duration of six hours

Practical examination includes OSCE and viva voce:
- Theory and practical examinations shall be conducted at the end of first year and second year respectively in the subjects as per the syllabus. If the candidate fails, he/she will be allowed to appear in supplementary examinations (February/August) in failed subjects.
- A candidate can take a maximum of TWO attempts within the maximum prescribed period of 4 (four) years.
- A candidate registered for the Nurse Practitioner in Critical Care Postgraduate Residency Program must pass the first year and second year examinations within four years from the date of his/her admission otherwise he/she shall be discharged from the course.
- The candidate who fails in any subject shall be permitted to continue the studies into the second year. However, the candidates shall not be allowed to appear for the second year examination till such time that he/she passes all subjects of the first year MSc (Nurse Practitioner in Critical Care) examination.
- For the courses offered, three examiners shall be appointed from the list provided by the Head/approved by BoS consisting of external/internal/interdepartmental examiners. Of the three examiners for practical examination, two will be internal examiners appointed by the office of the controller of examinations.
- The team of practical examiners will include one internal examiner [MSc faculty with minimum two years of experience in teaching the NPCC program/MSc faculty (Medical Surgical Nursing preferable) with five years of Post PG experience], one external examiner and one medical internal examiner who should be the preceptor for NPCC program.

Maintenance and Submission of Log Book

- Every candidate shall maintain a record of skills he/she has acquired during the two years of study period, duly certified by various Heads of Departments under whom he/she has undergone training.
- At the end of each clinical posting, log book (Specific procedural competencies/Clinical skills and clinical requirements) has to be signed by the preceptor every fortnight
- The Head of the Department shall scrutinize the log book once every three months.

- At the end of the program, the candidate should summarize the contents and get the log book certified by the Head of the Department.
- At the time of practical examination, each candidate shall submit the log book duly certified by the Principal as a bonafide record work done by the candidate for the scrutiny by the Board of Examiners.
- In addition to the above, the preceptors shall involve the candidates in seminars, journal club, group discussions, nursing conferences and in the teaching and training program of undergraduate students.
- Every candidate should be encouraged to present short title papers in conferences and to make improvements in it and submit them for publication in reputed Nursing journals.

Dissertation

- Every candidate shall be required to submit the research proposal by six months in first year.
- Every candidate shall be required to submit three copies of dissertation with attached CD, six months before the commencement of the Nurse Practitioner in Critical Care Postgraduate Residency Program II year final examination to the Controller of Examinations through the Head of the Department/Institution.
- The dissertation should be neatly typed on one side only in double line spacing on A4 size paper and it should not exceed 80 pages excluding certifications, acknowledgements and annexures
- The dissertation shall be evaluated by two examiners prior to the commencement of the second year university theory examinations.
- When certain corrections are suggested in relation to the dissertation, the Chairman, Board of Examiners would furnish a detailed report to the Controller of Examinations about the corrections that the candidate has to carry out. In such case, the candidate should resubmit the dissertation carrying out the corrections suggested, within one month from the date of receipt of communication from the Controller of Examinations to the effect, and till the dissertation is approved on such resubmission, the issue of mark statement to the candidate will be withheld.
- If the dissertation of a candidate is approved, but he/she fails in the University theory/practical examination, the marks awarded for his/her dissertation shall be carried over for the subsequent examination(s).
- When the dissertation of a candidate is rejected, the candidate shall submit a fresh dissertation two months prior to the commencement of the subsequent University examination(s).
- Administrative approval and ethical clearance should be obtained.

MAINTAINING DISCIPLINE IN NURSING COLLEGES

Every student shall conduct herself in accordance with and for the fulfillment of her declaration in her application for admission in the School of Nursing to the effect that she sincerely believes in the basic principles of the institution, that care for services of humanity at large, without any distinction of religion, race, color, caste, or creed, with complete dedication, love and as much renunciation and sacrifice as possible, as worship of God and advancement of her spiritual powers, and in furtherance of this objective she:

- Shall abide by and obediently maintain discipline in the school, hostel, and hospital as well as outside when permitted to go out.
- Shall be strictly punctual in studies, recreation and work and shall pass her life in purity in the hostel, the hospital and the outside world.
- Shall pursue her studies, theoretical and practical, faithfully and obediently with interest, and diligence, both in the classrooms as well as in the hospital.
- Shall abstain from anything deleterious or mischievous.
- Shall not take herself or administer to anyone else any drug which may be harmful.
- Shall learn and acquire patients' bedside manners and ethics and shall never lose temper and shall do everything in her power to observe, follow and maintain the standards of the profession of nursing.
- Shall keep secret and confidential all personal matters or affairs of patients and his/her family matters which may be confided to her or may come to her knowledge in, or in connection with the practice of nursing.
- Shall loyally render all possible help and assist the doctor.
- Shall devote herself faithfully with love, tenderness and sympathy to the welfare of patients committed to her care as nurse.
- Shall see to it that the patients committed to her care, their relatives or visitors are not made to incur and do not on their own accord incur any expense or service, or obtain service or concession, in connection with the college, the hostel, or the hospital, which is not legal or ethical.
- Shall honor faithfully and shall try to fulfill all the aims and objectives enumerated.
- Shall learn to be courteous to the patients and their visitors.
- Shall not organize unauthorized meetings or assemblies within the hostel premises or undertake collection of Union Subscription. Collection of any money for any other purpose also cannot be done without prior permission from the Principal in writing.
- Shall refrain from unruly behavior, defiance, and/or disobedience of lawful instructions and/or order of the superiors. Such behavior will expose a boarder for disciplinary action which includes removal from the School. Decision of the Secretary will be final and binding in all cases.
- Shall refrain from damaging hostel or hospital properties, misuse of water and electricity causing wasteful expenditure. In the event of any breach thereof, the cost will be recovered from the erring student

Breach of any of the foregoing shall attract disciplinary action: The candidates as well as their parents, at the time of admission of the students to the school will be required to furnish an undertaking in the form of an affidavit that the student shall not participate in any form of ragging, strike, etc. If found guilty, the school may take appropriate action against the erring students.

Rules and Regulations

- Every student admitted to the nursing course shall have to follow rules and regulations of the nursing college.
- It is compulsory for all students to attend the general assembly in the morning.
- All decisions taken by the management are final and binding on the students.
- Students should maintain silence in the classes, library, reading room and in the corridors. Students should make every effort to take care of the college and hospital property and help in maintaining the same. They should not write on the black board, scribble on tables, chairs, walls, etc.
- Students are not allowed to come directly in the Principal's office. They can come only with the permission of the class in charge.
- Boys MUST have a short hair cut always. Long hair will NOT be allowed.
- If the students have any problem, they should inform the class representative and the class representative will intimate it to the class coordinators. If the problem is not solved at the class coordinator's level, then the class coordinator will present it to the principal. No students should by-pass the above mentioned channels. Exceptions are allowed only if the problem is utmost urgent/serious.
- A student nurse is not allowed to receive gift or gratuity of any sort at any time from the patients of the hospital or their relatives.
- If a student is in need to get leave from the college or hospital in the middle of a day, for any emergency, he/she should get sanction from the class coordinator and a letter to that effect must be produced from the parent or guardian.
- Regular and punctual attendance in all class activities, such as lectures, demonstrations, practical's, clinical teaching, tutorials, tests, etc., is a must. Usual college time is 9 AM–4.30 PM and in clinics 8 AM–4 PM. Students must have to participate in all college activities, such as clinical meetings, conferences, guest lectures, seminars as well as sports, cultural activities, etc.
- No student shall be allowed to appear in the annual examination of the concerned subject if his/her practical, hospital posting and bedside clinical areas, etc., the attendance should not fall short of 100% of the total sessions.
- Use of cell phone by students is strictly prohibited in class rooms, hospital and community health postings.
- In case of illness, permission shall have to be obtained from the principal to remain absent from studies.
- The student must clear all the dues of the college and hostel before the commencement of exam; otherwise she/he will not be allowed to attend the exams.
- Any student who damages the reputation of the college in any way is liable to be expelled. If any student discontinues the course, he/she shall clear all dues for the remaining duration of the course. If he/she fails to pay, his/her original certificates will not be returned. Original certificates will be returned at the time of leaving the college when students clear the dues.
- Students are required to maintain ethical and professional standards in behavior both inside and outside the college, hospital, hostel and community premises.
- Each student is responsible for the proper handling and safe custody of any apparatus or equipment that he/she may be using in different nursing labs. Misuse or negligence will result in replacement of the particular by the candidate. Any willful damage done to the property of the college and hospital will be treated as breach of discipline.
- All books are to be used with care. If a book while under issue to anyone be damaged or lost, the person in whose name the book is issued, will be held responsible for the cost of repair to the satisfaction of the Library Committee or replacement if the damage cannot be satisfactorily made good or if the book is lost. In case of irreparable damage to or loss of a book which cannot be replaced, to Dean and the Chairman, Library Committee will decide the amount of compensation to be paid. The term "Book" also includes Pamphlet, Magazine, Journal, etc.
- Students are forbidden to communicate with any outside authority directly. All such communications must be submitted through the office of the principal. Any student infringing this rule is liable to be suspended.
- For any kind of misbehavior with staff or creating disturbances in classroom and in the college premises by a student or group of students, a full range of disciplinary action will be taken, i.e., student will be expelled from the institute and depending upon his/her fault can be under legal action. A student expelled on disciplinary grounds will never be readmitted to this college.
- If any student found in use of liquor or narcotics on hospital duty or in institute premises, he/she will be suspended from the institute for a specific period or be expelled from the institution.
- Possession of weapons, explosive and other objectionable material in institute/hostel will result in being expelled from the institution.
- Taking active part in politics will result in being expelled from the institution. Coming on hospital duty or entering the institute premises in a UN presentable appearance will be liable to punishment.
- Ragging is an offense. Ragging is strictly prohibited in the college campus as well as in the hostel. Any student/students involved in such activities will be immediately expelled from the institution. Both junior and senior

students are required to maintain cordial relationship with each other and a disciplined atmosphere in the college campus.

- Students are required to wear full uniform during college and hospital. Jewellery, ear rings, painted fingernails, threads and bracelets on hands, etc., are not allowed. Students must wear white apron in college laboratories. Students must be neat and tidy in their dress, avoiding expensive clothes and exaggerated fashions.
- Students are required to carry their identity cards during college hours, clinical and whenever they are going out and must be produced whenever it is asked by the concerned authority.
- Membership in the recognized Student Nurses' Association is compulsory.
- The hostellers who desire to go home during the working days will take written permission from the Principal on the recommendation of HOD of the respective department and approval from the hostel warden before leaving the hostel.
- All lights and fans must be switched off before leaving the room, failing which a fine will be imposed for each item found to be on when the room is locked.
- Student will cooperate to keep campus neat, clean and green.

CONCLUSION

Controlling is one of the important functions of a manager. In order to seek planned results from the subordinates, a manager needs to exercise effective control over the activities of the subordinates. In other words, controlling means ensuring that activities in an organization are performed as per the plans. Controlling also ensures that an organization's resources are being used effectively and efficiently for the achievement of predetermined goals. Controlling is, thus, a goal-oriented function.

REVIEW QUESTIONS

Long Essays

1. Define guidance; explain the elements and principles.
2. Define counseling; explain the characteristics, objective, principles and stages of counseling.
3. Discuss the program evaluation in nursing course.

Short Essays

1. Scope of guidance and counseling.
2. Counseling process.
3. Functions of guidance and counseling.
4. Quality management in nursing institutions.
5. Educational audit in nursing education.
6. Evaluation of performance in nursing education.
7. Maintaining discipline in nursing colleges.

Short Answers

1. Levels of counseling.
2. Thorne's model.
3. Qualities of a counselor.
4. Student nurse counseling.
5. Causes of conflicts.
6. Principles of the academic audit.
7. Continuous internal assessment.
8. Practical examination.

CHAPTER 24: Professional Considerations

LEARNING OBJECTIVES

Review: Legal and Ethical Issues
- Nursing as a Profession: Characteristics of a Professional Nurse
- Nursing Practice: Philosophy, Aim and Objectives
- Regulatory Bodies: INC and SNC Constitution and Functions

Review: Professional Ethics
- Code of Ethics and Professional Conduct—INC and ICN
- Practice Standards for Nursing—INC
- International Council for Nurses (ICN)

Legal Aspects in Nursing
- Consumer Protection Act, Patient Rights
- Legal Terms Related to Practice, Legal System—Types of Law, Tort Law and Liabilities
- Laws Related to Nursing Practice—Negligence, Malpractice, Breach, Penalties
- Invasion of Privacy, Defamation of Character
- Nursing Regulatory Mechanisms—Registration, Licensure, Renewal, Accreditation, Nurse Practice Act, Regulation for Nurse Practitioner/Specialist Nursing Practice

NURSING AS A PROFESSION (FIG. 24.1)

Nursing has been called the oldest of the arts and the youngest of the profession. The word nurse evolved from the Latin word nutritious, which means nourishing. The roots of medicine and nursing are intertwining and found in mythology, ancient eastern and Western cultures and religion. Nursing is defined by various authors at various times.

Hansderson says "nursing is primarily assisting the individuals (sick or well) in the performances of those activities, contributing or its recovery (or to a peaceful death) that he would perform unaided, if he had the necessary strength, will or knowledge. The unique contribution of nursing is to help the individual to be independent or, such assistance as soon as possible.

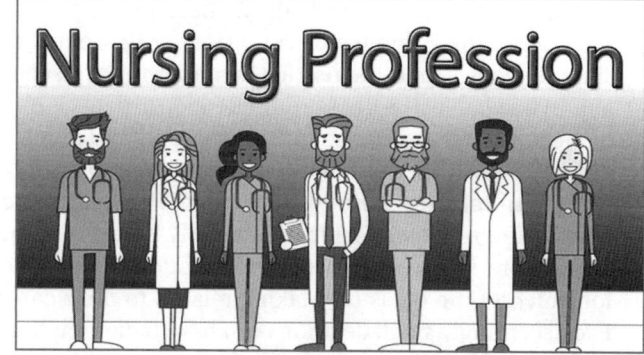

Fig. 24.1: Nursing profession.

Definition

- The International Council of Nurses defines "Nursing is to assist the individual, sick or well in the performance of those activities contributing to health or to its recovery (or to peaceful death) that he would perform unaided if he had the necessary strength, will or knowledge."
- **Florence Nightingale:** Nursing defined as the act of utilizing the environment of the patient to assist him in his recovery.
- **Canadian Nurses Association-1987:** Nursing practice as a dynamic, caring and helping relationship in which the nurse assists the client to achieve and obtain optimal health.
- **American Nurses Association:** Nursing practice as direct goal oriented and adaptable to service the needs of the individual, the family and community during health and illness.

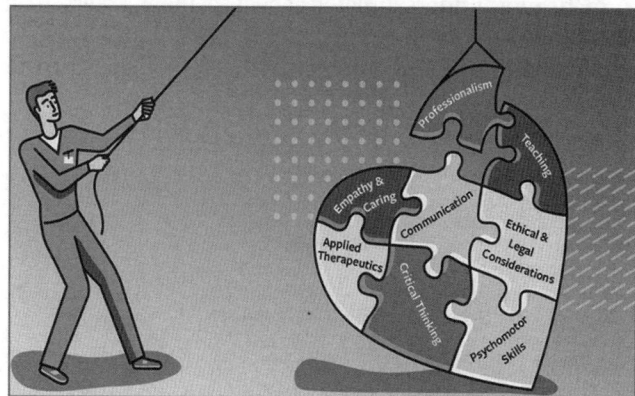

Fig. 24.2: Professional responsibilities of a nurse.

Qualities of Professional Nurse (Fig. 24.3)

- **Caring:** Many nurses who choose the nursing career path prioritize job security, are interested in using it as a starting point for another career, or have a lack of alternative ideas/options. A nurse showing a natural tendency to truly care about how their patients feel (and in turn, how well they perform their job) will have a significant impact on their success in the nursing field, which makes caring a key indicator of a nurse's success.
- **Communication skills:** Strong communication skills are critical characteristics of a nurse. A nurse's role relies on the ability to effectively communicate with other nurses, physicians, disciplines across other units, patients, and their families. By prioritizing and practicing communication skills, nurses will provide safer care and benefit their patients, their unit, and the entire hospital/health system—not to mention, their long-term career.
- **Empathy:** A characteristic of a good nurse is one that shows empathy to each patient, making a true effort to put themselves in their patients' shoes. By practicing empathy, nurses are more likely to treat their patients as "people" and focus on a person-centered care approach, rather than strictly following routine guidelines.
- **Attention to detail:** Nurses are undoubtedly under immense pressure as they balance receiving orders from physicians with using their own knowledge skills and critical judgement to provide the highest quality patient care. Add to this combination caring for multiple patients simultaneously, and the risk for human error can seem almost inevitable. Having a strong attention to detail is one of the nurse personality traits that can easily and quickly determine how successful they will be in their role.
- **Problem-solving skills:** Problem-solving skills are essential to nursing, as nurses generally have the most one-on-one time with patients and are often responsible for much of the decision-making related to their care. Even seemingly small decisions can have major impacts and cause adverse patient outcomes if incorrectly made.
- **Stamina:** The physical demand on nurses is perhaps one of the most underestimated aspects of their careers. In an average 12-hour shift, nurses exercise a unique balance of physical and emotional stamina that few other industries encounter. Effectively managing this skill is what makes a great nurse. This extremely important skill impacts nurses, their coworkers, and of course, the patients. Having sufficient stamina is one of the most important qualities of a great nurse.
- **Sense of humor:** Having a good sense of humor also helps spread positivity to other nurses, patients, and their families. A good sense of humor is not only a characteristic of a nurse leader, but reminds patients and their families that "nurses are people, too" and ultimately increases their trust and openness with sharing feedback and concerns. In especially stressful times, patients and their family members are appreciative of any efforts (no matter how small) to help bring a bit of cheer.
- **Commitment to patient advocacy:** This concept is the foundational core tenet of healthcare from the Hippocratic Oath to nearly every hospital's mission statement in one phrase or another: keep patients safe, deliver the highest quality of care. In other words, be an advocate for patients, with special attention on their overall safety. As one of the leading qualities of a nurse leader, a great nurse understands that patient advocacy is a mindset that must be practiced every day, with every patient, throughout every stage of the care continuum.
- **Willingness to learn:** Nurses spend more bedside time with patients than any other role in healthcare and their willingness to learn and put new knowledge into practice is one of the leading traits of a good nurse. Improvements in education approaches (e.g., multidisciplinary training, personalized learning, etc.) can help foster successful learning environments, but a good nurse must possess a natural willingness to learn for them to be truly beneficial. This important skill applies to nurses of all ages, throughout every stage of their career, from recent graduates to the highly experienced.
- **Critical thinking:** A nurse with highly functioning critical thinking skills is one of the most important characteristics of a professional nurse. After years of education and training, the ability to apply clinical guidelines and best practices on the floor depends on a nurse's ability to think critically, which is quickly noticed (either positively or negatively) by leadership, other nurses, and ultimately, patients.
- **Time management:** Balancing multiple patients, stressful care settings, and competing priorities is no small feat during a 12-hour shift. Having the ability to implement effective time management is a key personality trait for nursing, as is being able to concentrate on the most critical issues first, which is not necessarily the patient/family that is demanding the most.
- **Leadership:** A quality of a good nurse that will become more and more valuable in the growing nursing field is the ability to successfully lead. However, if a nurse manager recognizes that their role is not perhaps the right fit, knowing when/how to voice that concern is equally as admirable as thriving in the role. Exercising leadership skills in any role/level of the organization

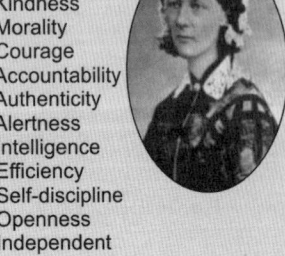

- Truthfulness, loyalty and honesty
- Love for the fellowmen
- Caring
- Commitment
- Compassion, generosity
- Acceptance, assertiveness
- Punctuality
- Fairness
- Self-esteem and tolerance
- Appreciation
- Creativity
- Imagination
- Confidence
- Empathy
- Humor
- Kindness
- Morality
- Courage
- Accountability
- Authenticity
- Alertness
- Intelligence
- Efficiency
- Self-discipline
- Openness
- Independent

Fig. 24.3: Qualities of professional nurse.

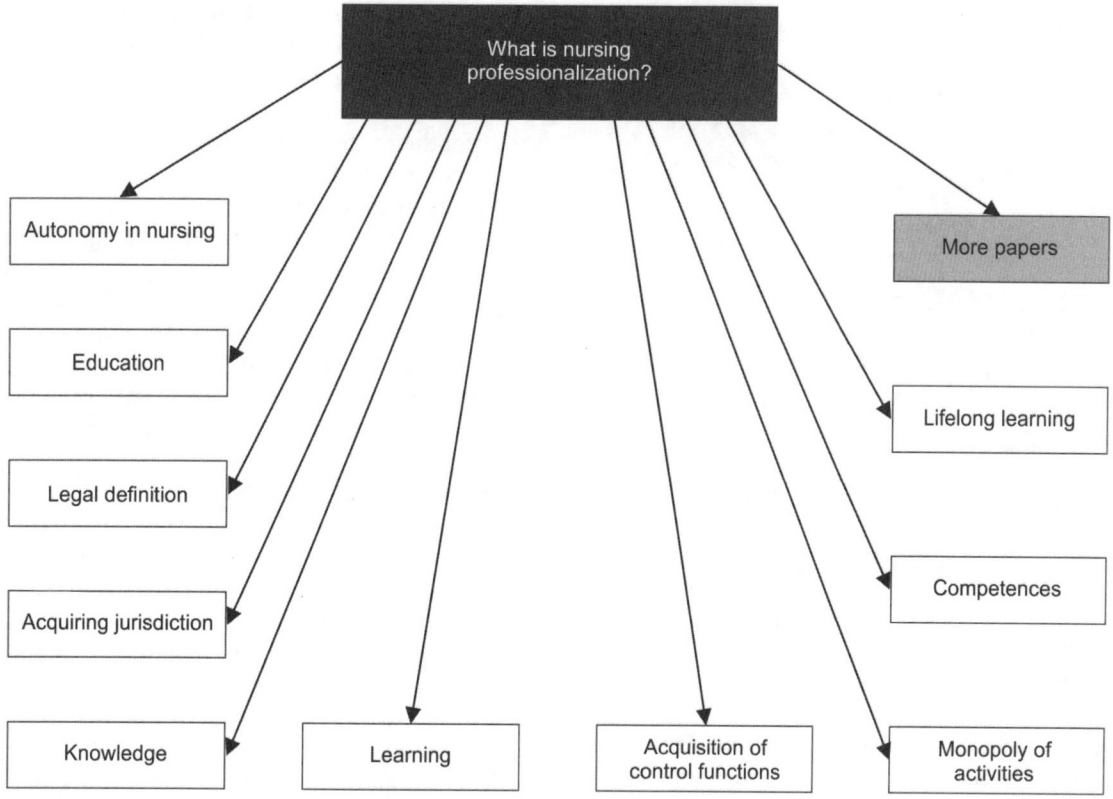

Fig. 24.4: Characteristics of professionalism.

shows a willingness to grow and adapt at one's own pace. Mentorships from nursing leaders can also teach invaluable lessons on how to become a great nurse.
- **Experience:** It is important to note that as veteran nurses leave the healthcare industry and begin retirement, they are taking with them years of experience and knowledge that cannot be quickly replaced. As nursing leaders work to bring new nurses in the door, most available candidates are predominantly new graduate nurses—a stark contrast to their predecessors in terms of experience and the many patient care skills and knowledge that can only come with time and practice.

Scope of Nursing

There was a time when professional nurses had very little choice of service because nursing was centered in the hospital and bedside nursing. Career opportunities are more varied now for a numbers of reasons. The list of opportunities available is given under:
1. **Staff nurse:** Provides direct patient care to one patient or a group of patients. Assists ward management and supervision. She is directly responsible to the ward supervisor.
2. **Ward sister or nursing supervisor:** She is responsible to the nursing superintendent for the nursing care management of a ward or unit. Takes full charge of the ward. Assigns work to nursing and non-nursing personnel working in the ward. Responsible for safety and comfort of patients in the ward. Provides teaching sessions if it is a teaching hospital.
3. **Department supervisor/assistant nursing superintendent:** She is responsible to the nursing superintendent and deputy nursing superintendent for the nursing care and management of more than one ward or unit. Example —surgical department, out-patient department.
4. **Deputy nursing superintendent.** She is responsible to the nursing superintendent and assists in the nursing administration of the hospital.
5. **Nursing superintendent:** She is responsible to the medical superintendent for safe and efficient management of hospital nursing services.
6. **Director of nursing:** She is responsible for both nursing service and nursing educations within a teaching hospital.
7. **Community health nurse (CHN):** Services rendered mainly focusing Reproductive Child Health Programme.
8. **Teaching in nursing:** The functions and responsibilities of the teacher in nursing are planning, teaching and supervising the learning experiences for the students. Positions in nursing education are clinical instructor, tutor, senior tutor, lecturer, and associate professor, Reader in nursing and Professor in nursing.
9. **Industrial nurses** are providing first aid, care during illness, health educations about industrial hazards and prevention of accidents.
10. **Military nurse:** Military nursing service became a part of the Indian Army by which means nurses became commissioned officers who are given rank from lieutenant to major general.
11. **Nursing service abroad:** Attractive salaries and promising professional opportunities, which cause a major increase for nursing service in abroad.

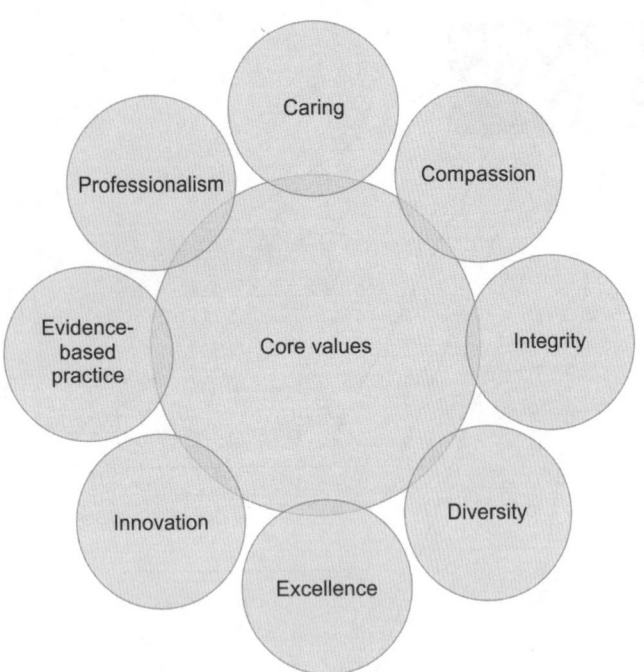

Fig. 24.5: Core values of professional nursing.

12. **Nursing service administrative positions**: At the state level, the Deputy Director of Nursing at the State Health Directorate. The highest administrative position on a national level is the Nursing Advisor to the Government of India. **Figure 24.5** shows core values of professional nursing.

New Perspectives of Nursing Profession

Historically, only medicine, law and the ministry were accepted as profession.

Criteria of a profession: Genevieve and Roy Bixler first wrote about the status of nursing as a profession in 1945. These criteria include the following.

- The services provided are vital to humanity and the welfare of the society. Nursing is the service that is essential to the wellbeing of the people and to the society. Nursing promotes, maintains and restores the health of individuals, groups and communities. Assisting others to attain the highest level of wellness is the goal of nursing. Caring, meaning nurturing and helping others are the basic components of professional nursing.
- There is a special body of knowledge that is continually enlarged through research. In the past, nursing was based on principles borrowed from the physical and social sciences and other disciplines. Today there is a unique body of knowledge to nursing.
- The services involve intellectual activities. Individual responsibilities (accountability) are a strong feature. Nursing has developed and refined its own unique approach to practice.
  - Nursing process is a cognitive activity that requires both critical and creative thinking and serves as the basis of providing nursing care.
  - Individual accountability in nursing has become the hallmark of practice.
- Accountability is 'is being answerable to someone for something one has done'.
- Through legal opinion and court cases, society has demonstrated that nurses are individually responsible for their actions as well as for those of personnel under their supervision.
- Practitioners are educated in institution of higher learning. There are basic nursing program, baccalaureate program, masters and doctoral program in nursing
- Practitioners are relatively independent and control their own policies and activities. Autonomy or control over one's practice is another controversial area for nursing. Although many nursing actions are independent, most nurses are employed in hospitals where authority resides in one's position.
- Practitioners are motivated by service (altruism) and considered their work an important component of their lives. Nurses are dedicated to the ideal of service to others, which is known as altruism
- There is a Code of Ethics to guide the decisions and conduct of practitioners. The International Council of Nurses (ICN) has established Code of Nursing Ethics through which standards of practice are established, promoted and refined.
- There is an organization (Association) that encourages and supports high standards of practice. Nursing has a number of professional associations that were formed to promote the improvement of the profession. Foremost among these, is the Trained Nurses Association of India (TNAI). The purposes of TNAI are to foster high standards of nursing practice, promote professional and educational advancement of nurses and promote the welfare of the nurses.

Concept of Professionalism in Nursing

Nursing, besides being an honorable profession, is one of the oldest arts and an essential modern occupation. Nursing is one of the greatest of humanitarian services and all people whether ill or well, rich or poor, literate or illiterate, young or old, at work or at play, in or out of hospital, are in some way or other, directly or indirectly closely associated with it. Nursing has its own body of knowledge scientifically based and humanitarianism that promises expanded benefits to people and society. It assists the individual or family to achieve their potential for self-direction for health.

Art of nursing: Professional nursing practice is grounded in the art of nursing, described as taking a holistic, client-centered focus; being caring and ethical in interactions with patients, families and colleagues; having above-average interpersonal skills; and making sound judgments based on experience and knowledge, thus averting potential problems.

Competence: Professional practice demands competence in relation to knowledge and technical skills. This requires not only a broad base of knowledge, but also depth of knowledge in a chosen area of practice, a desire and ability to continue developing that knowledge base and to share it with others and critical thinking in decision-making.

 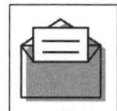 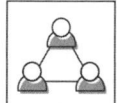
Advocate for patients | Communicate effectively | Work as a team

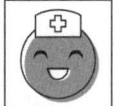 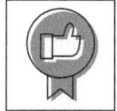 
Keep a positive attitude | Deliver top-quality care | Maintain your integrity

Fig. 24.6: Professionalism in nursing.

Attributes of practice: Professional practice reflects a particular approach to one's work, with collaboration by far most salient characteristic. Professional nursing practice means working in partnership with other nurses and health professionals in providing client care, being highly organized in managing activities and time, having the ability to manage many complex tasks simultaneously, working autonomously as appropriate and having an open mind and nonjudgmental manner.

Personal commitment: In describing this element of professional practice, respondents referred to the importance of having confidence in one's abilities and taking responsibility for one's actions, including having a sound understanding of the boundaries and limitations of nursing practice. Having a balanced lifestyle and supporting the advancement of the profession were also considered important characteristics of a professional nurse. **Figure 24.6** shows professionalism in nursing.

Values of a Professional Nurse

To be successful, nurses must be equipped with certain tools and abilities. These skills are developed over time as a nurse gains experience and confidence (**Fig. 24.6 and Table 24.1**).

- **Confidentiality and autonomy:** Nurses have to have an awareness of legislation on patient confidentiality and the policies of their own organization. Nurses should not breach confidentiality, unless the circumstances are exceptional—for instance, if the patient is threatening harm to himself or others. Nurses must not discuss patients' details outside of the care setting, and must take care of notes, paper and computer files. Nurses should make all efforts to promote the patient's rights to make her own decision whenever possible.
- **Protection from harm:** The nurse's conduct must protect the patient from harm. He must not undertake something he thinks might cause harm to the patient even if he has been told or asked to do so by another person. The nurse is accountable for her own actions, and might be asked' to explain these in later proceedings. If the nurse sees anything she fears may endanger the patient, she must immediately report this to management.
- **Professional development:** The nurse has a duty to keep up-to-date with all developments that may have an impact on his job. He must attend professional development and training activities. Part of his duty may involve training and mentoring new and junior staff. Nurses must meet training requirements and pay any fees needed to maintain licensing.
- **Dedication:** Professional nursing is a difficult profession with many stressful scenarios. Nurses must work long shifts and deal with many vastly different issues on a daily basis. The combination of long work hours, constant Care of patients, and the stress of seeing death can cause nurses to unravel. Thus, professional nurses need to be Calm and overlook, able to quickly handle a multitude of problems effectively. Nurses are responsible for patient quality of care and the execution of the healthcare plan. A dedication to the job is essential for a nurse to fulfill her nursing duties.
- **Systems thinking:** A nurse is faced with a plenty of situations throughout each workday. Each patient has individual problems and requires a different approach. Nurses are expected to develop individualized decisions of care depending on the patient and the specific circumstances.
- **Caring:** Nurses are required to take care of the patient throughout the entire healthcare process. Their goal is to make the healing process and painless and comfortable as possible, without inflicting any unnecessary grief for the patient. Nurses must console the patients and the families in order to ease the transition. According to the American Association of Critical Care Nurses, these duties of care

Table 24.1: Essential nursing values and behaviors.

Values	Professional behaviors
Altruism Nurse's concern for the welfare of patients, other nurses, and other healthcare providers	• Understands cultures, beliefs, and perspectives of others • Advocates for patients • Take risks on behalf of patients and colleagues
Autonomy Nurses respects patient's right to make decisions about their healthcare	Plans care in partnership with patients
Human dignity Nurses values and respects the inherent worth and uniqueness of all patients and colleagues	• Provides culturally competent and sensitive care • Protects patient's privacy • Designs care to individual patient needs
Integrity Nurses acts honestly and provides care based on an ethical framework	• Provides honest information to patients and the public • Document care honestly and accurately • Seeks to remedy errors made by self or others • Demonstrates accountability of own actions
Social justice Nurse upholds moral, legal, and humanistic principles by ensuring equal treatment under the law and equal access to quality healthcare	Supports fairness and nondiscrimination in the delivery of care

include "vigilance, engagement, and responsiveness of caregivers, including family and healthcare personnel."
- **Ethnic and religious sensitivity:** Nurses take care of patients from a variety of ethnic and religious backgrounds. Professional nurses must be sensitive to the specific requirements of various cultures and religions in order to facilitate the patient's healthcare. Nurses must demonstrate a desire to respect various practices while continuing to adhere to professional standards.

Roles and Responsibilities of Professional Nurse (Figs. 24.7 and 24.8)

The professional nurse occupying a position of a professional nurse accepts responsibility and accountability in:
- Provide quality nursing to the clients in their care, placing emphasis on the medical psychosocial, spiritual needs of the clients and be mindful of the needs of the relatives or attendants.
- Cooperating with the nursing units and all other departments within the hospital
- Understanding all activities in relaxation to patient care and other assigned duties
- Actively participating in the nursing team.
- Actively pursuing continuing self-education.
- Actively providing appropriate health education to the individuals, families and groups and community at large in various settings.

Nursing Practice

Nursing practice is underpinned by values that guide the way in which nursing care is provided. The Nursing and Midwifery Board of Ireland considers that the following values should underpin nursing practice and provide the basis for the formulation of a philosophy of nursing:

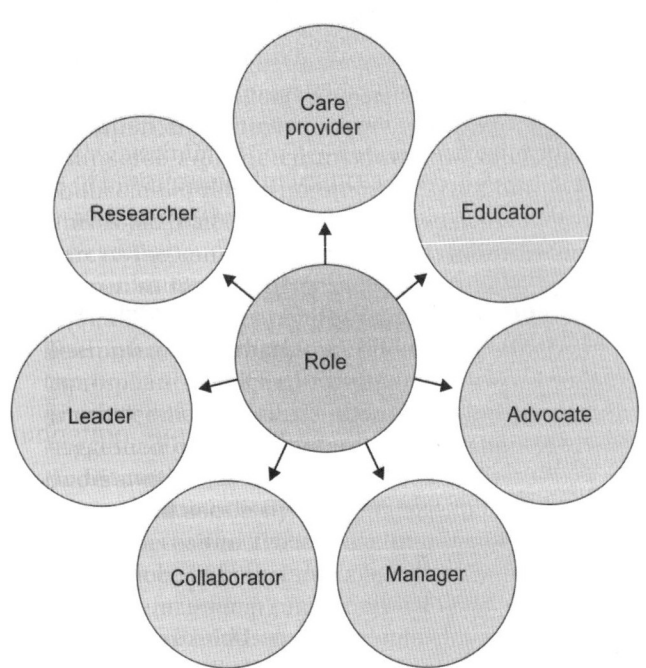

Fig. 24.7: Role of professional nurse.

- In making decisions about their individual scope of practice; nurses should keep to the fore the rights, needs and overall benefit to the patient and the importance of promoting and maintaining the highest standards of quality in the health services.
- Nurses respect all people equally without discriminating on the grounds of age, gender, race, ethnicity, religion, civil status, family status, sexual orientation, disability (physical, mental or intellectual), or membership of the Traveller community.
- Fundamental to nursing practice is the therapeutic relationship between the nurse and the patient that is based on open communication, trust, understanding, compassion and kindness, and serves to empower the patient to make life choices.
- Nursing practice involves advocacy for the rights of the individual patient and for their family. It also involves advocacy on behalf of nursing practice in organizational and management structures within nursing.
- Nurses recognize their role in delegating care appropriately and providing supervision to junior colleagues and other healthcare workers, where required.
- Nursing care combines art and science. Nursing care is holistic in nature, grounded in an understanding of the social, emotional, cultural, spiritual, psychological and physical experiences of patients, and is based upon the best available research and experiential evidence.
- Nursing practice must always be based on the principles of professional conduct stated in the latest edition of the Code of Professional Conduct and Ethics for Registered Nurses and Registered Midwives (2014).

Professional Practice Model: The Professional Practice Model incorporates our organization's mission and values, which are key to the caring relationships developed between our providers, families and staff members. Our professional nurses focus on high-quality, safe patient care incorporating the entire seven puzzle pieces of our model. Our nursing practice is based on scientific evidence, and we are committed to providing the excellent care needed in today's complex healthcare environment.

Functions and Responsibilities

- **Client care:** Providing safe and effective nursing care within a healthcare set up or community. It includes participating in the delivery of nursing care based on the best practice principles stated by statutory body, maintaining nursing standards, observing and participating in quality improvement programs, fostering congeniality between all members of the healthcare team, assisting with cost containment by utilizing resources effectively, participating in appropriate meetings, workshops or committees related to improving nursing care.
- **Professional practice:** In professional practice, the aspects included are maintaining confidentiality, taking reasonable care in health and safety of persons on the unit, being familiar with the resources to be used in case of any

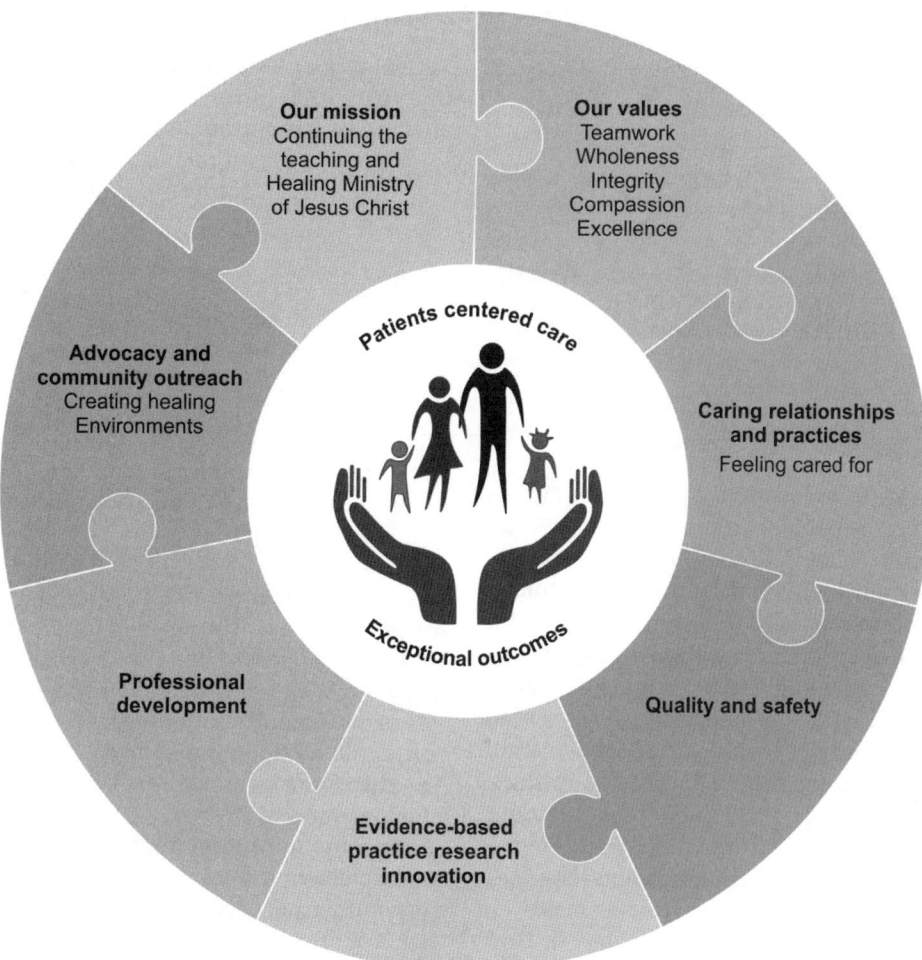

Fig. 24.8: Responsibilities of professional nurse.

emergency or disaster, adhering to all infection control policies and safety rules, cooperating with management for health, safety and welfare provisions, actively seeking knowledge of the diagnosis and treatment given, actively participating with a zeal as a member of multidisciplinary team, complying with the professional code of ethics, demonstrating accountability and responsibility for the professional conduct, practicing with limits of own abilities and qualification, initiating and maintaining effective communication with others.

- **Management:** There are three kinds of management roles, i.e., in planning, in organizing, and in implementation and in evaluation.
  - In planning, the management roles are to describe the planning process in the assigned clinical area, to assess client's needs, work environment and available resources, to set appropriate priorities for day's work, to anticipate and plan for potential problems or unpredictable events.
  - In organizing, the management roles are to organize work activities, to delegate tasks and share responsibilities, to adhere to organizational policies and procedures, to describe instances of the incorporation of risk management concepts in the assigned clinical setting.
  - In implementation, the management roles are to perform nursing procedures safely, accurately and scientific knowledge based, to describe the decision making process, to assure continuity of care, to communicate effectively with patients, families and other health personnel, to show sensitivity to the patients' needs, to bring change in the status quo of the organization as required.
  - In evaluation, the management roles are to analyze the flow of communication in the unit and within the organization, to describe the nurse manager's role as evaluator of personnel performance, to assess patient care evaluation activities that are done in clinical setting.

ETHICAL ISSUES IN NURSING

Ethics are the rules or principles that govern right contact. Ethics are designed to protect the rights of human being. Ethics are characteristics of a healthy profession. The code of ethics will state what kind of conduct is expected from the members of a profession, what are the responsibilities of its members towards those whom they serve, their coworker, the profession and the society as a whole.

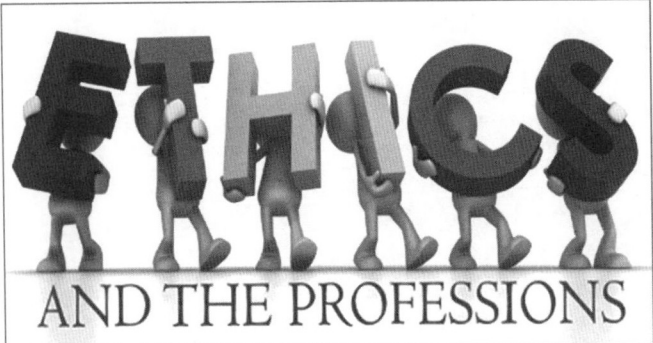

Fig. 24.9: Nursing ethics.

Nursing Ethics (Fig. 24.9)

The nursing ethics provide professional standards for nursing activities which protect the nurse and the patient. In 1973, the International Council for Nurses (ICN) adopted code of ethics. The fundamental responsibility of the nurse is fourfold-to promote health, to prevent illness, to restore health and to alleviate suffering. The need for nursing is universal. Inherent in nursing is respect for life dignity, and rights of men. It unrestricted by considerations of nationality, race, creed, color, age, sex, politics or social status. Nurses render health services to the individual, the family and the community and coordinate their services with those of related groups. Examples of duties are: (WD Ross's Seven Prima Facie Duties):

- Beneficence—the duty to do good and promote happiness
- Nonmaleficence—the duty to do no harm and to prevent harm
- Fidelity—duties arising from past commitments and promises
- Reparation—duties that stem from past harms
- Gratitude—duties based upon past favors and unearned services
- Self-improvement—the duty to improve our knowledge and virtue
- Justice—the duty to give each person equal consideration
- Retributive justice—punishment for wrongdoing
- Distributive justice—fair distribution of benefits and burdens. **Figure 24.10** shows concept of ethics.

Ethical Principles

Ethical principles actually control professionalism nursing practice much more than to ethical theories. Principles encompass basic promises from which rules are developed. Principles are the moral norms that nursing, as a profession, both demands and strives to implement to every day clinical practice. Ethical principle that the nurse should consider when making decisions are as follows **(Fig. 24.11)**:

- Respect for persons
- Respect for autonomy
- Respect for freedom
- Respect for beneficence (doing good)
- Respect for nonmaleficence (avoiding harm to others)
- Respect for veracity (truth telling)
- Respect for persons
- Respect for justice (fair and equal treatment)
- Respect for rights
- Respect for fidelity (fulfilling promises)
- Confidentiality (protecting privileged information)

Respect for persons: Respect for persons not only applies to clinical situations, but also to all life's situations. It directs individuals to treat themselves and other, with a respect inherent to man's humanness. It requires recognition on a sense that all mankind shared a common human destiny. The respect to persons needs to be simplified as it affects nursing practice.

Autonomy: Autonomy that individuals are able to act for themselves to the level of their capacity. It is the right of individual to govern their actions according to their own purpose and reason. Respect for autonomy requires that persons honor another's right to govern him or her. The legal doctrine of informed consent is the direct reflection of autonomy.

Disclosure: Adequate presentation of relevant information about the proposed treatment or study.

Understanding: Adequate comprehension of the disclosed information.

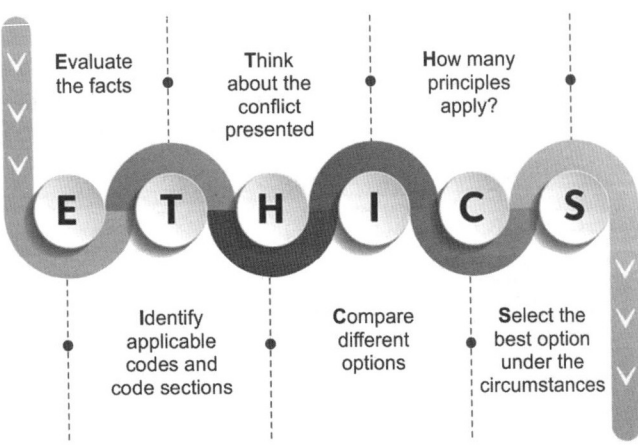

Fig. 24.10: Concept of ethics.

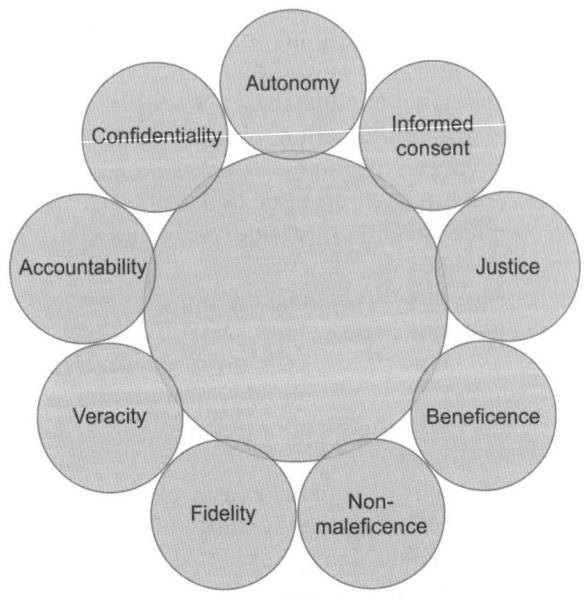

Fig. 24.11: Ethical principles.

Voluntary agreement: Free assent, influenced by external controlling factors.

Competence: Adequate decision making capacity. There are three type of autonomy, i.e., freedom of action, freedom of choice and effective deliberation.

Freedom: The principle of individual freedom decrease that patients be exempt from control by others to select and pursue personal health goals. Nurses as a group believe that patient should have greater freedom of choice within the nation's healthcare system. This principle should be observed by staff nurses when planning patient care; by nurse manager when leading subordinates.

Beneficence: The beneficence principle states that the actions one takes should promote good. It dictates that a person is obliged to help others to advance their legitimate and important interests; it requires the balancing of harms and benefits. Benefits promote the clients' welfare and health, whereas harms or risks detract from the client's health and welfare. In other words, providing benefits that enhance the others welfare.

Nonmaleficence: The corollary of beneficence, the principle of Nonmaleficence states that one should do no harm. The nurse should interpret the term 'harm' to mean emotional and social as well as physical injury. Harm is thwarting, defeating, or setting back one person's interest through invasive action by another. Many nurses find it difficult to follow the principle when performing treatment and procedures that bring discomfort and pain to patients.

Veracity: Veracity concerns truth telling an incorporates the concept that individuals should always tell the truth. It requires professional caregivers to provide with accurate, reality-based information about their health status and care or treatment prospect. Truth telling is an ethical concern for nurse, because truth is the basis for mutual trust between patient and nurse, and trust is the basis for patient's hope of benefit from nursing services.

Justice: Justice concerns the issue that persons should be treated equally and fairly. This principle of justice requires treating others fairly and giving persons their due. When there are resources to distribute in healthcare, nurses should allocate them in such a way that equal shares go to equal recipients. The following problems complicate the application of justice:

- Not everyone is equal in every way; sometimes, there are situations in which it seems that one person should receive a greater or lesser share than another.
- Resources are limited. There is not always enough for each person to receive an equal share.
- Questions of justice relate to the fairness with which benefits and burdens are distributed among people. Experience in turn found various principles have to be proposed to guide fair distribution of society's good are as follows:
  - Each person should receive an equal share.
  - The amount given to each person should be proportional to his/her need.
  - The amount given to each person should be proportional to the amount of his/her work effort,
  - The amount given to each person should reflect the value of his/her work product.
  - The amount given to each person should reflect his to her value to society.
  - The amount given to each person should be determined by free market exchange. These principles usually arise in times of short supplies or when there is competition for resources of benefits.

Rights: Right is an entitlement to behave in certain way under circumstances, such as nurse's entitlement to freely express personal beliefs and preferences by voting in a political election. Another right is the prerogative to define another's behavior in selected situations, such as manager's prerogative to give assignments to subordinates. A right is also a claim to a specific good, service or prerequisite, such as tea break time. Right is also used to mean agreement with justice, law and morality. So right may be mental rights or legal rights related to respective profession.

- The patient has the right to every consideration of his privacy concerning his own medical care program.
- The patient has the right to expect that all communications and records pertaining to his care should be treated as confidential.
- The patient has the right to expect that within its capacity a hospital must make reasonable response to the request of a patient for services.
- The patient has the right to obtain information as to any relationship of his hospital to other healthcare and educational institutions in so far as his care is concerned and any professional relationships among individuals, by name, who are treating him.
- The patient has the right to be advised if the hospital proposes to engage in or perform human experimentation affecting his care or treatment (and) has the right to refuse to participate.
- The patient has the right to expect reasonable continuity of care.
- The patient has the right to examine and receive an explanation of his bill regardless of source of payment.
- The patient has the right to know what hospital rules and regulations apply to his conduct as a patient.

Fidelity: Fidelity is keeping one's promises or commitments. The principle of fidelity holds that a person should faithfully fulfill his duties and obligations. Fidelity is important in a nurse because a patient's hope for relief and recovery rests on evidence of caregiver's conscientiousness. Nurse managers abide by this principle when they follow through on any promise they have previously made to employees, such as promised leave, a certain shift to be worked or a promotion to perception within the unit.

Confidentiality: Confidentiality is the duty to respect privileged information. The principle of confidentiality provides that caregivers should respect a patient need for privacy and use personal information about him or her only to improve care. Nurses should practice confidentiality to decrease patient vulnerability and share from widespread knowledge of personal information divulged during care.

Ethical Dilemmas

A dilemma is defined as situations requiring a choice between two equally desirable or undesirable alternatives. In ethical dilemma, each alternative course of action can be justified by two ways in which a person views the course of action based on his/her value system. Issues in healthcare delivery practices present different alternatives based on whether the issue or course of action is viewed by the patient, the healthcare agency, the legal system or the nurse. Increasingly, staff nurses and nurse managers face difficult decisions caused by tensions between technological capabilities, budgetary structures, and quality of life concerns. Nurses in all clinical and functional specialties face the following ethical dilemmas **(Boxes 24.1 and 24.2)**:

- Need to ration patient care to conserve scarce resources.
- Need to make treatment and care decisions for terminally-ill patients.
- Need to obtain patients informed consent for care and treatment orders and measures, such as:
  - Do not resuscitate order
  - Withholding/withdrawing nutrition and fluids
  - Starting/discontinuing life support system
- Response to patient request for assisted suicide
- Need to balance the patients need for confidentiality and privacy against society's needs for protection from unreasonable risk.
- Need to protect autonomy rights of children and incompetent adults concerning consent for research participation.
- Need to protect justice rights of patients who participate in random trials of experimental treatment.

Usually, the dilemma occurs when opposing views are seen for the solution of an issue and a decision must be made. There is no set of procedures or easy answers for how an ethical dilemma should be resolved. Ethical decision making is needed in all steps of the nursing process and all phases of the nursing management process. Ethical reasoning is similar to the nursing process in that it requires critical thinking skills. A nurse can best resolve ethical dilemma, by systematically considering all options for solving the dilemma. A ethical dilemma occurs as a result of conflict between moral principles that support different courses of action.

Ethical Decision Making (Fig. 24.12)

Nurse's decisions are increasingly constrained by ethical issues. Ethical decision making involves reflection on the following:

1. Who should make the choice?
2. Possible options or courses of action
3. Available options
4. Consequences, both good and bad, of all possible options
5. Rules, obligations and values that should direct choices, and
6. Desired outcomes

When making decisions, nurses need to combine all of these elements using an orderly, systematic, and objective method. There are various models for ethical decision making. Perhaps the easiest ethical decision making model to remember and to implement in practice is the "moral model" developed by Thirona and Halloraw as follows:

- **M—Massage the dilemma:** Identify and define the issues in the dilemma. Consider the opinions of all major players in the dilemma as well as their value system. This includes patient's family members, nurses, doctors, priest and any other interdisciplinary healthcare team member.
- **O—Outline the options:** Examine all options including those less realistic and conflicting, this stage is designed only for considering options and not for making final decision.

Box 24.1: Common ethical dilemmas.

- **Conflict of interest:** Examples include interviewing friends; only interviewing one grade or those with a specific point of view; covering clubs and teams that you are a member of, "getting even" with those who might have wronged you
- **Plagiarism:** Claiming others' work as one's own, essentially stealing from them. Students must credit other people's materials and ideas. This includes "borrowing" or downloading visuals from the Internet to use without permission with stories.
- **Anonymous/unnamed sources:** Although reporters sometimes use anonymous sources, most news organizations have strict guidelines about when to use them. A reporter has to determine the information's value and whether is it possible to get it any other way.

Box 24.2: Common ethical dilemmas in nursing.

- Euthanasia, assisted suicide, and aid in dying
- Nursing care and do not resuscitate (DNR) and allow natural death (AND) decisions
- Forgoing nutrition and hydration
- Registered nurses' roles and responsibilities in providing expert care and counseling at the end

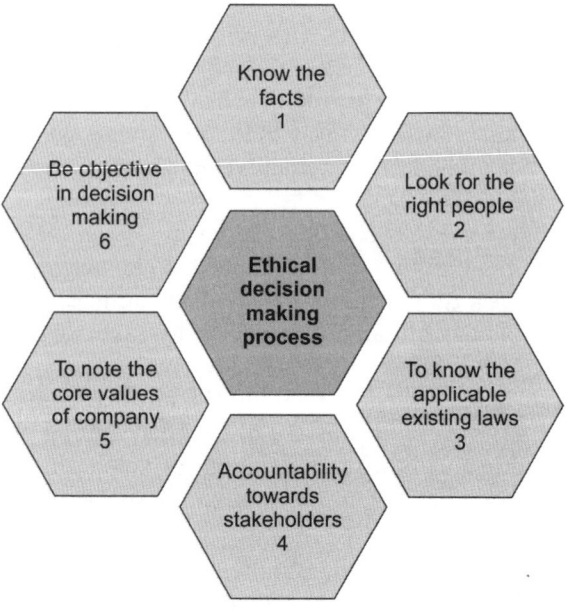

Fig. 24.12: Ethical decision making process.

- **R—Resolve the dilemma:** Review the issues and options, applying the basic principles of ethics to each option. Decide the best option based upon the views of all those concerned in the dilemma.
- **A—Act by applying chosen action:** This step is usually the most difficult as it requires actual implementation. While the previous steps had only allowed for dialogue or discussion.
- **L—Look back and evaluate the entire process including the implementation:** No process is complete without a thorough evaluation. Ensure that those involved are able to follow through on the final option. If not, a second decision may be required and process must start again at the initial step.

Another exchange of traditional model of ethical decision making is as follows:

- Identify the problem
- Gather data to analyze the causes and consequence of the problem
- Explore the optional solutions to the problem
- Evaluate the optional solution
- Select the appropriate solution from all the options
- Implement the selected solution
- Evaluate the result

Ethical Responsibility

- Caring demands the provision of helping services that are appropriate to the needs of the client and significant others.
- Caring recognizes the client's membership in a family and community and provides for the participation of significant others in his/her care.
- Caring acknowledges the reality of death in the life of every person, and demands that appropriate support the provided for the dying person and family to enable that to prepare for, and to cope with death when it is inevitable.
- Caring acknowledges that the human person has the capacity to fact up to health needs and problems in his/her own unique way, and directs nursing action in a manner that will assist the client to develop, maintain or gain personal autonomy, self-respect and self-determination.
- Caring, as a response to a health need, requires the consent and the participation of the person who is experiencing the need.
- Caring dictates that the client and significant others have the knowledge and information adequate for free and informed decisions concerning care requirements, alternative and preferences.
- Caring demands that the needs of the client supersede those of the nurse.
- Caring acknowledges the vulnerability of a client in certain situations, and dictates restraint in actions which might compromise the client's rights and privileges.
- Caring involving a relationship which is, in itself, therapeutic, demands mutual respect and trust.
- Caring acknowledges that information obtained in the course of the nursing relationship is privileged, and that

> **Box 24.3:** Need for nursing ethics.
> - Helps the students/RN to practice ethically
> - Helps the nurse to identify the ethical issues in her work place
> - Protecting patients right and dignity
> - Providing care with possible risk to the nurses health
> - Staffing patterns that limit the patients access to nursing care
> - Ethical reasoning helps the nurse to respond to ethical conflicts
> - Helps to differentiate right/wrong behavior
> - Guide for a professional behavior
> - Help teachers plan education
> - Prevent below standard practice

is requires the full protection of confidentiality unless such information provides evidence of serious impending harm to the client or to a third party, or is legally required by the courts.
- Caring requires that the nurse represents the needs of the client and that the nurse takes appropriate measures when fulfillment of these needs is jeopardized by the actions of other persons.
- Caring acknowledges the dignity of all persons in the practice of educational setting.
- Caring acknowledges, respects and draws upon the competencies of others.
- Caring establishes the conditions for the harmonization of efforts of different helping professionals in providing required services to clients.
- Caring seeks to establish and maintain a climate of respect for the honest dialogue needed for effective collaboration.
- Caring establishes the legitimacy of respectful challenge and! or confrontation when the service required by the client is compromised by incompetency, incapacity or negligence or when the competencies of the nurses are not acknowledged or appropriately utilized.
- Caring demands the provision of working conditions which enable nurses to carry out their legitimate and responsibilities.
- Caring demands resourcefulness and restraint-accountability for the use of time, resources, equipment, and funds, and requires accountability to appropriate individuals and/or bodies.
- Caring requires that the nurse bring to the work situation in education, practice, administration or research, the knowledge, affective and technical skills required, and that competency in these areas be maintained and updated.
- Caring commands fidelity oneself, and guards the right and privilege of the nurse to act in keeping with an informed moral conscience.

CODE OF ETHICS AND PROFESSIONAL CONDUCT

Ethics in nursing is a particular code of behaviors, characters, conducts and relationship unique only to the nursing personnel. Nursing ethics is "a system of principles governing the conduct of a nurse, her relationship to the patient and his family, her associates and society at large." As a guidelines to all those in the nursing profession, the Grand Council of the

International Council of Nurses held at Sao Paulo, Brazil on July 10, 1953, adopted, viewed and revised in the year 1964.

Definitions

- The Oxford dictionary defines ethics as "a science of human duty in its widest extent."
- The Chambers describes it as "the science of morals that branch of philosophy which is concerned with human character and conduct."
- Webster defines it as "the morals concerned with or relating to what is right and wrong in matters of human behavior."
- A code is needed to educate and orient members of the profession to distinguish desirable from the undesirable behaviors, to regulate relationships with coworkers and clients, and to guide the public in understanding professional conduct.
- A group of nurses stated, "Ethics is knowledge and attitudes that determine man's relationship to him, to others and to the society."
- Ethics is a science that endeavors to interpret the highest standards of written or unwritten principles or doctrines or morals of human duty, human character and conduct of human behavior and human relationships in day-to-day life.

Code of Ethics (ICN)

In accordance with these requests the Professional Service Committee of the ICN selected a sub-committee for the revision of the code. The final revised code was submitted to the ICN Council of National Representatives in Mexico in May 1973 at the 15th Quadrennial Congress. The sub-committee on the Code of Ethics tried to concentrate their attention on the most vital aspects of nursing and built their revised ethical code around five major headings **(Figs. 24.13 and 24.14)**.

- **Nurses and people:** The nurse's primary responsibility is to those people who require nursing care. The nurse holds in confidence personal information's and use judgment in sharing this information.
- **Nurses and practice:** The nurse maintains the highest standards of nursing care possible within the reality of a specific situation. The nurse when acting in a professional capacity should at all times maintain standards of personal conduct which credit upon the profession.
- **Nurses and society:** The nurse shares with other citizens the responsibility for initiating and supporting action to meet the health and social needs of the public.
- **Nurses and coworker:** The nurse maintains a co-operative relationship with coworkers in nursing and other fields. The nurse takes appropriate action to safeguard the individual when his care is endangered by a coworker or any other person.
- **Nurses and the profession:** The nurse acting through the professional organization participates in establishing and maintaining equitable social and economic working conditions in nursing.

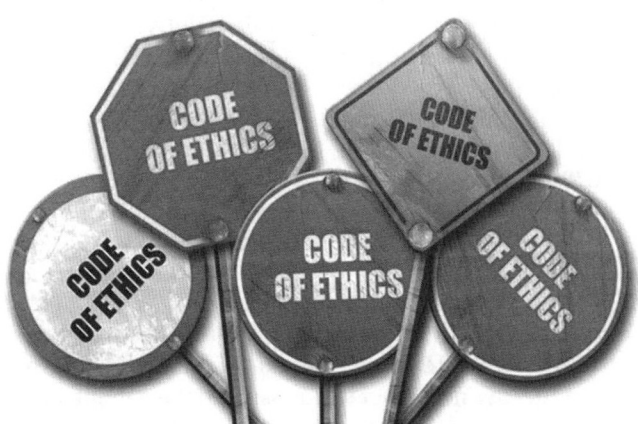

Fig. 24.13: Code of ethics in nursing.

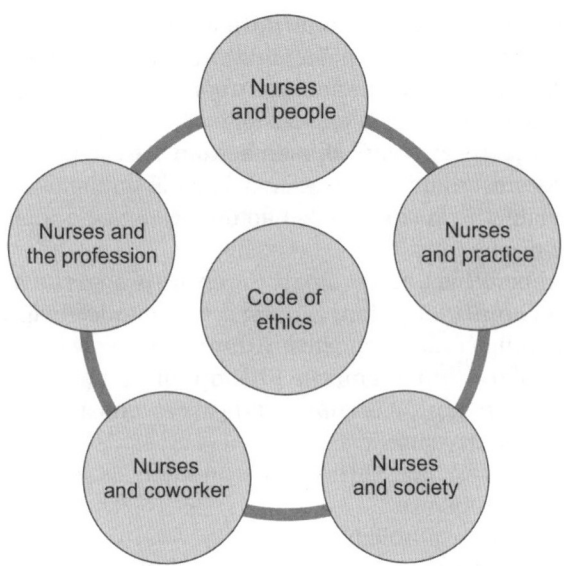

Fig. 24.14: Code of ethics by ICN.

Application of Code of Ethics in Nursing

Code of Ethics as applied to nursing, the codes of ethics is as follows:

- The nurse provides services with respect for human dignity irrespective of social or economic status, personal attributes, or the nature of health problems.
- The fundamental responsibility of the nurse is three-fold; to conserve life, to alleviate suffering and to promote health.
- The nurse shall maintain at all time the highest standards of nursing care and of professional conduct.
- The nurse must not only be well prepared to practice but shall maintain knowledge and skills at a consistently high level.
- The religious beliefs of a patient shall be respected.
- Nurses hold in confidence all personal information entrusted to them.
- Nurses recognize not only the responsibilities but the limitations of their professional functions not to recommend or give medical treatment without medical orders except in emergencies, and report such action to a physician as soon as possible.

- The nurse is under an obligation to carry out the physician's orders intelligently and loyally and to refuse to participate in unethical procedures.
- The nurse assumes responsibility and accountability for individual nursing judgments and actions.
- The nurse sustains confidence in the physician and other members of the health team; incompetence or unethical conduct of associates should be exposed but a only to the proper authority.
- The nurse safeguards the patients and the public when healthcare and safety are affected by the incompetent, unethical or illegal practice of any person.
- The nurse cooperates with the health team and maintains harmonious relationships with members of other professions and with nursing colleagues.
- The nurse adheres to standards of personal ethics, which reflect credit upon the profession.
- In personal conduct nurses should not knowingly disregard the accepted pattern of behaviors of the community in which they live and work.
- The nurse participates and shares responsibility with other citizens and other health professions in promoting forts to meet the health needs of the public—local, state, national and international.

Requests poured in from many quarters of the nursing world to review and revise this code against and representation for this purpose was made through several national councils.

INC Code of Ethics for Nurses in India

1. **The nurse respects the uniqueness of individual in provision of care**
   1.1. Provides care for individuals without consideration of caste, creed, religion, culture, ethnicity, gender, socioeconomic and political status, personal attributes, or any other grounds
   1.2. Individualizes the care considering the care considering the beliefs, values and cultural sensitivities.
   1.3. Appreciates the place of the individual in family and community and facilitates participation of significant others in the care.
   1.4. Develops and promotes trustful relationship with individual(s).
   1.5. Appreciates the place of the individual in family and community and facilitates participation of significant others in the care.
2. **The nurse respects the rights of individuals as partner in care and helps in making informed choices**
   2.1. Appreciates individual's right to make decisions about their care and therefore gives adequate and accurate information for enabling them to make informed choices.
   2.2. Respects the decisions made by individual(s) regarding their care.
   2.3. Protects public from misinformation and misinterpretations.
   2.4 Advocates special provisions to protect vulnerable individuals/groups.
3. **The nurse respects individual's right to privacy, maintains confidentiality, and shares information judiciously**
   3.1. Respects the individual's right to privacy of their personal information.
   3.2. Maintains confidentiality of privileged information except in life-threatening situations and uses discretion in sharing information.
4. **Nurse maintains competence in order to render quality nursing care**
   4.1. Nursing care must be provided only by registered nurse.
   4.2. Nurse strives to maintain quality nursing care and upholds the standards of care.
   4.3. Nurse values continuing education, initiates and utilizes all opportunities for self-development.
   4.4. Nurse values research as a means of development of nursing profession and participate in nursing research adhering to ethical principles.
5. **The nurse is obliged to practice within the framework of ethical, professional and legal boundaries**
   5.1. Adheres to code of ethics and code of professional conduct for nurses in India developed by Indian Nursing council.
   5.2. Familiarizes with relevant laws and practices in accordance with the law of the state.
6. **Nurse is obliged to work harmoniously with the members of the health team**
   6.1. Appreciates the team efforts in rendering care.
   6.2. Cooperates, coordinates and collaborates with the members of the health team to meet the needs of the people.
7. **Nurse commits to reciprocate the trust invested in nursing profession by society**
   7.1. Demonstrates personal etiquettes in all dealings.
   7.2. Demonstrates professional attributes in all dealings.

Code of Professional Conduct

Need of Professional Conduct

A profession conduct is needed for the following purposes:
- To promote and safeguard the interest and well-being of the patients.
- To improve and maintain professional knowledge and competence.
- To acknowledge any limitation in gained knowledge and competence and declaim any duties or responsibilities unless the nurse is not able to perform in a safe and skilled manner.
- To work in an open and a cooperative manner with the patients and their families in order to foster their independence and to recognize and respect their involvement in the planning and delivery of care.
- To recognize and respect the dignity of each patient as a client and respond to the needs of the patients with care, irrespective of their ethnic origin, religious beliefs, and personal attributes and the nature of their health problems.

- To report to the concerned authority at the earliest about any physical, psychological and social problems identified in the patients, which helps to start the treatment at the earliest and prevent the complications of the illness later.
- To work in a collaborative and cooperative manner with healthcare professionals and others involved in providing care and to recognize and respect their particular contribution within the care team.
- To avoid any abuse of the privileged relationship with patients in the workplace.

Code of Professional Conduct (for Nurses in India) (Box 24.4)

- **Professional responsibility and accountability:** To maintain professional responsibility and accountability the nurses:
  - Appreciate a sense of self- worth and nurtures it.
  - Maintains standards of personal conduct, reflecting credit upon the profession.
  - Carriers out responsibility within a framework of the professional boundaries.
  - In accountable for maintaining practice standards let by the Indian nursing council.
  - Is compassionate
  - Is responsible for the continuous improvement of current practices.
  - Provides adequate information to individuals these allows then to make informed choice
  - Practices healthful behavior
- **Nursing practice:** In the course of practice of nursing the nurse:
  - Provide care in accordance with set standards of practice.
  - Treats all individuals and families with human dignity in providing the physical, psychological emotional, social and spiritual and aspects of care.
  - Respects individuals and families, promoting healthy practices and discouraging harmful practices.
  - Presents realistic pictures truthful in all situations for facilitating autonomous decision making by individuals and families.
  - Endure is safe practice.
  - Consults coordinates, collaborates and follows up approximately when an individual's care needs exceed this/her competence.
- **Communication and interpersonal relationships:** This plays a key role in the interaction of the nurse with his/her client to effect optimal interaction nurses:

> **Box 24.4:** Codes of professional conduct for nurses.
> - Professional responsibility and accountability
> - Nursing practice
> - Communication and interpersonal relationship
> - Valuing human being
> - Management
> - Professional advancement

- Establishment and maintains effective interpersonal relationships with individuals families and communities.
- Upholds the dignity of team members and maintains effective interpersonal relationship with them.
- Appreciates and nurtures the professional role of team members.
- Cooperators with other health professionals to meet the needs of individual's families and communities.

- **Valuing human being:** The nurse values human life—he/she:
  - Takes appropriate action to protect individuals from harmful an ethical principles.
  - Considers relevant facts while taking particular decision in the best interest of individuals.
  - Encourages and supports individuals in there. Right to speak for themselves on issues affecting health and welfare.
  - Respects and supports choices made by individuals.
- **Management:** Proper management of resources and infrastructure is essential for improving the overall efficiency of the nurse. Hence, the nurse:
  - Ensures appropriate allocation and utilization of available response.
  - Participates in supervision and education of students and other formal provides.
  - Uses judgment in relation to individual competence. While accepting and delegating responsibility.
  - Facilities conducive work culture in order to achieve institutional objective.
  - Participates in performance appraisal.
  - Participates in evaluation of nursing services.
  - Work with individuals to identify the needs and sensitizes policy makers and funding agencies for resource allocation.
- **Professional advancement:** To escape that he/she is at part with contemporaries in the nursing field the nurse must:
  - Ensure the protection of human rights, while pursing the advancement of knowledge.
  - Participate in determining and implementing quality care.
  - Take responsibility for updating one's own knowledge and competencies. Contribute to the care of professional knowledge and conducting and participating in research.

Professional Etiquette for Nurses

Professional etiquette for nurses refers to the ethical manners and moral behavior that a nurse should follow throughout his/her life of nursing. Maintaining good etiquette reflects good morality in the nurse. The important qualities that make up good professional' etiquette are as follows:
- Being gentle and polite to all patients, seniors and other health workers in the hospital.
- Giving respect to the seniors, coworkers and clients.
- Addressing seniors with proper title, such as Sir/Madam.

- Answering politely and humbly to any questions asked or clarifications sought by the seniors.
- Giving way to the seniors and standing aside and allowing the senior nurse to pass.
- Maintaining discipline wherever needed, such as in the ward, conference meeting with seniors, classroom and library.
- Keeping the uniform neat and tidy.
- Not wearing any gold jewelry or applying make-up while on duty.
- Obeying the rules and regulations of the hospital at all times.
- Getting proper prior permission from colleagues and the sister-in-charge before taking any articles from the ward.

LEGAL ISSUES IN NURSING

The law constitutes body of principles recognized or enforced by public and regular tribunals have the administration of justice. The law is the body of principles recognized and applied by the state and the administrations of justice. Law is that portion of the established thought and habit which has gained district and formal recognition and the shape of uniform rules backed by the authority and power of the government **(Fig. 24.15)**.

Types of Laws (Table 24.2)

Civil law includes rules and regulations that specify the required course of action to be followed by an individual in business and social relationships with others. It is concerned with relationships among people and the protection of a person's rights.

Criminal law defines offences that affect public welfare and security and impose penalties. It includes rules forbidding conduct that is injurious to public order and specifying punishments to be administered to individual who exhibits injurious conduct.

The four legal elements are:
1. Duty (established relationship between the plaintiff and the defendant)

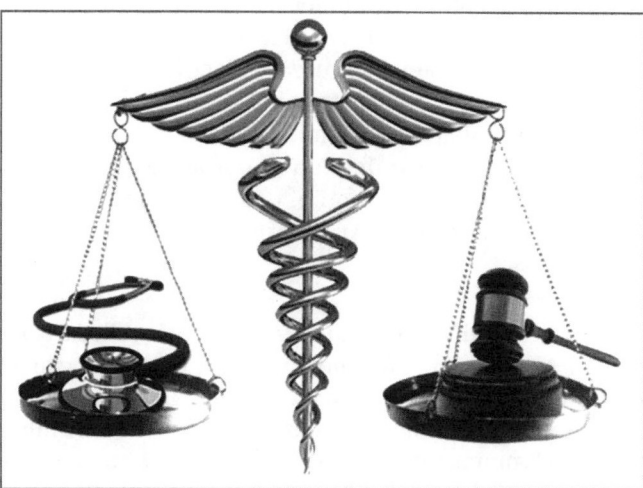

Fig. 24.15: Law in clinical practice.

Table 24.2: Types of law.

	Definition	Punishment	Burden of proof	Examples
Civil	Concerns private rights	Relief or remedy	Preponderance of the evidence	Divorce, law suit
Criminal	This type of case violates a specific penal law	Fine, imprisonment, or both	Beyond a reasonable doubt	Traffic violation, felony charge

2. Breach of Duty (failure to do what a reasonable and prudent professional would do under similar circumstances)
3. Damages (injuries)
4. Causation (An established correlation between the acts of negligence and the injuries)

Good Samaritan Act: The Good Samaritan Act in legal terms refers to someone who administers aid in an emergency situation to an injured person on a voluntary basis. Usually, if a volunteer comes to the aid of a person who is a stranger, the person giving the aid owes the stranger a responsibility of being reasonably careful. A person is not obligated by law to do first aid in most states, unless it is part of a job description.

Legal Terms

Legal terms that you must be familiar with include these:
- **Common law**: Common law is law that results from previous legal decisions. They are based on legal precedent.
- **Statutory law**: Statutory law is law that is passed by a legislative body, such as the state's legislature.
- **Constitutional law**: Constitutional law is law that is included in the Constitution of the United States of America and its amendments.
- **Administrative law**: Administrative law is rules and regulations that are legally enacted to support some statutory law. For example, nursing boards enact administrative rules and regulations relating to state enacted laws, such as the state's nurse practice act and legislated continuing education requirements for the relicensure of nurses.
- **Criminal law**: Criminal law, part of public law, covers acts that are illegal and against the law. Criminal law includes felony and misdemeanor infractions of the law.
- **Civil law**: Civil law, also part of public law, covers torts and contract laws.
- **Torts**: Torts are civil laws that address the legal rights of patients and the responsibilities of the nurse in the nurse patient relationship. Some torts specific to nursing and nursing practice include things like malpractice, negligence and violations relating to patient confidentiality.
- **Unintentional torts**: Unintentional torts include things like malpractice and negligence.
- **Intentional torts**: Intentional torts include things, such as false imprisonment, assault, battery, breaches of privacy and patient confidentiality, slander and libel.

- **Liability**: Liability is vulnerability and legal responsibility, simply stated. For example, nurses are liable when they fail to carry out doctor's orders.
- **Respondeat superior**: Respondeat superior is the legal doctrine or principle that states that employers are legally responsible for the acts and behaviors of its employees. Respondeat Superior does not, however, relieve the nurse of legally responsibility and accountability for their actions. They remain liable.
- **Negligence**: Negligence is a nonintentional tort. Negligence occurs when the nurse fails to follow established policies, procedures and standards of care in the same manner that another "reasonable" nurse would do in the same situation.
- **Malpractice**: Malpractice, also a nonintentional tort, has six elements. The elements of malpractice include a duty, a breach of duty as a nurse, reasonable foreseeability that the nurse's act has a connection with the patient injury that occurred, the patient was harmed, the link that act directly led to the harm and the patient has the right to financial compensation or damages.
- **Assault**: Assault, an intentional tort, is threatening to touch a person without their consent.
- **Battery**: Battery, another intentional tort, is touching a person without their consent.
- **False imprisonment**: False imprisonment is restraining, detaining and/or restricting a person's freedom of movement. Using a restraint without an order is considered false imprisonment.
- **Defamation**: Defamation is making false statements about a person in writing or orally that leads to the destruction of a person's reputation.
- **Slander**: Slander is oral defamation of character using false statements.
- **Libel**: Libel is written defamation of character using false statements.

Common Legal Issues

- Wrong medications, wrong dosage, wrong route of administration and wrong concentration.
- **Mistaken identity**: Prepare the wrong patient for an operation, to exchange babies in the labor room. To exchange dead bodies in the mortuary.
- Failure to communicate
- Maintenance of record
- Giving explanation and getting the concerned
- Bums and false
- Counting sponges and instruments during surgery
- Loss or damage to patient's property and fame
- **Euthanasia or mercy killing**: Taking positive step to kill a person in order to end his suffering is a murder. **Figure 24.16** shows role and functions of nurse manager in legal issues.

Law and Nurse

- **Responsibility of appointing and assigning**: The nurse administrators have responsibility for staffing

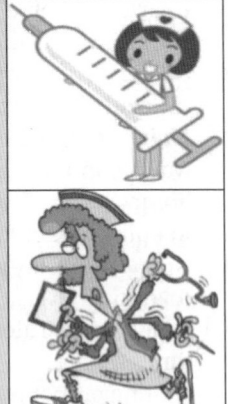

1. Services as a role model by providing nursing care that meets or exceeds accepted standards of care
2. Reports substandard nursing care to appropriate authorities
3. Practices nursing within the area of individual competence
4. Prioritizes patients right and welfare first in decision making
5. Delegates to subordinates wisely, looking at the managers scope of practice and that of those they supervice

Fig. 24.16: Role and functions of nurse manager in legal issues.

and supervising nursing units to ensure safe, effective patient care. Therefore, they have the authority to temporarily reassign a nursing employee to compensate for emergency staff shortages.
- **Responsibility in quality control:** A nurse manager's legal responsibility for quality control of nursing service imposes a duty to observe report and correct the incompetence of any patient care provider.
- **Responsibility for equipment:** To protect the patients and employees from injury, a nurse manager must ensure that all patient care equipment are fully functional and that defective equipment is promptly repaired or replaced.
- **Responsibility for observation and reporting:** Consequently nurses have a legal duty to observe patients frequently and report findings that have diagnostic or treatment value for the patient's physician and other members of the patient's treatment team.
- **Responsibility to protect public:** The nurse has a legal duty to protect the public from injury by dangerous patients. The manager must ensure that nursing personnel follow the procedures to alert community members to the presence of a potentially dangerous patient in their midst.
- **Responsibility for record keeping and reporting:** Nurses have legal responsibility for accurately reporting and recording patient's conditions, treatments and response to care. The medical record is an information source document that should be used to plan care, evaluate care, allocate costs, educate personnel, research care measure, and substantiate legal claim.
- **Responsibility for death and dying:** Nurses must be aware of legal definition of death because they must document all events that, when the patient is in their care.

Legal Issues in Nursing

- **Nurse Practice Act:** Each state has what is called a Nurse Practice Act. The Guidelines and laws outlined in the act pertain to all nurses who are licensed in that particular state. Nurse limitation is one of those laws. Each nurse has a limitation on what he is allowed and trained to do. He must follow the chain of command, especially with the care of a patient. If he does not have the authority or

knowledge to give a prescription, analyze a lab report, or advise the patient on treatment, he may not legally do so. Any wrong information or practice he commits is punishable by the law and the patient or family may file a suit against him and the health agency or hospital he works for.
- **Patients advocate:** A nurse has a legal obligation to act as the patients advocate in case of emergency. The nurse is to act as the liaison between the patient and the healthcare provider, such as a physician. The nurse will monitor the patient, ensuring that if any complications or abnormalities arise, a physician notified immediately. The nurse is legally obligated to keep the personal data and information of the patient confidential not doing so is a violation of the code of ethics for nurses.
- **Administering medication:** Nurses are responsible for administering the correct doses and medications to patients. If the nurse gives a fatal dosage amount, she may face legal malpractice suits. It is also the responsibility to research the patient's records, or ask the patient and family members if there are any allergies or complications that may pose a risk if a certain medication is administered.
- **Informed consent:** When a nurse is administering treatment, she must explain what the effects and outcomes could be, and any other important information. It is the responsibility of the nurse to confirm that the patient or family member who will sign the informed consent form is coherent, and understands all the negatives and aspects of the treatment. The nurse, patient, or patient family member will sign the informed consent form in front of a witness, a physician or another nurse. Not having this legal document signed and in front of a witness could be a legal issue for the nurse if complications arise during treatment.
- **Negligence:** It is the responsibility of the nurse to monitor the patient. If a patient calls for a nurse to come and assist him in going to the restroom for example, the nurse is to assist, or if the is busy with another patient, have another nurse assist the patient. Ignoring the patient or responding after a a lengthy delay could be considered negligence, and if the patient is hurt from trying to move himself, the nurse could face legal suits. Also, it could be considered negligence if a physician orders the nurse to administer a prescription, and the nurse did not do so.

Legal Aspects Related to Nursing Registration

A Registered Nurse (RN) is a nurse who has graduated from a college's nursing program or from a school of nursing and has passed a national licensing exam. A registered nurse helps individuals, families, and groups to achieve health and prevent disease.
- They care for the sick and injured in hospitals and other healthcare facilities, physicians' offices private homes, public health agencies, schools, camps, and industry.
- Some registered nurse, are employed in private practice. A registered nurses scope of practice is determined by each state's Nurse Practice Act.
- It outlines what is legal practice for registered nurses and what tasks they may or may not perform.
- Nurse Practice Acts also dictates the scope of practice for nurse practitioners (NP5). An example is prescriptive authority for NPs.
- In some states, NPs can practice completely autonomously and prescribe any category of medications in other states; NPs cannot prescribe controlled substances and may only practice with the collaboration of a physician.

Civil Law Penalties for Registered Nurses
- Registered nurses have penalties that are inflicted on them for transgressions, such as medical malpractice and breach of confidentiality.
- These civil law penalties can cause them to be suspended or banned from the nursing practice.

Patient's Bill of Right

In 1973, the American Hospital Association adopted Patient's Bill of Rights as national policy statement and distributed it to its members in the healthcare organizations throughout the nation. There are twelve rights summarized below:
1. The patient has a right to a considerate and respectful care.
2. The patient has a right to obtain complete and concerned information concerning the diagnosis, treatment and prognosis from his physician for the patient's expected understanding.
3. The patient has a right to receive the necessary information from his physician regarding the treatment and the procedures involved in it.
4. The patient has a right to refuse the treatment to the extent permitted by the law and to be informed about the medical consequences of his action.
5. The patient has a right to privacy concerning his own medical care program.
6. The patient has a right to expect all communications and records pertaining to his care should be treated as confidential.
7. The patient has a right to expect within the capacity a hospital must make reasonable response to the request made by the patient for services.
8. The patient has a right to obtain information as to any relationship of his hospital to other healthcare institution is concerned.
9. The patient has a right to be advised if the hospital proposes to engage him in or perform human experimentation affecting his treatment.
10. The patient has a right to expect reasonable continuity of care.
11. The patient has a right to examine and receive an explanation of his hospital bills regardless of the source of payment.
12. The patient has a right to know what hospital rules and regulations apply to his conduct as a patient.

Important Practice Standards for Breach Sanctions

The disparity in organizational response to employee malfeasance has a far-reaching impact on the healthcare industry. Consequences include the following:

Patients have the right to:

- Be treated for the life-threatening, chronic disease of addiction with honesty, respect and dignity
- Know what to expect from treatment, and the likelihood of success
- Be treated by licensed and certified professionals
- Evidence-based treatment
- Be treated for co-occurring behavioral health conditions simultaneously
- A individualized, outcomes-driven treatment plan
- Remain in treatment as long as necessary
- Support, education and treatment for their families and loved ones
- A treatment setting that is safe and ethical

Fig. 24.17: Patient's right.

- Licensure
- Good Samaritan Law
- Good rapport
- Standards of care
- Standing orders
- Informed consent
- Correct identity
- Documentation
- Reporting

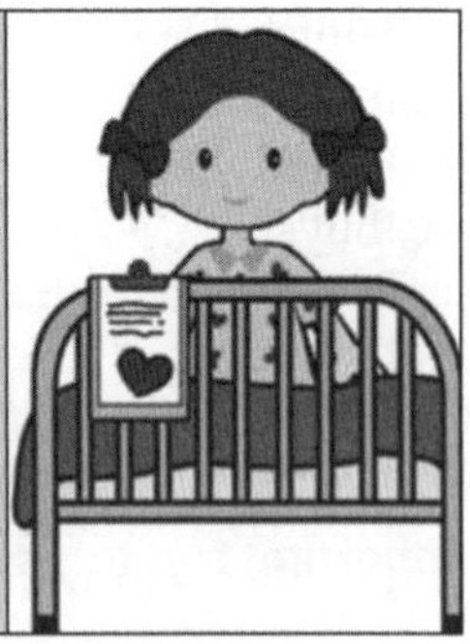

Fig. 24.18: Legal safeguards in nursing practice.

- **Confusing message:** An inconsistent organizational response to a breach sends a confusing message to both staff and the public. Healthcare workers moving from one organization to another find differing tolerance levels for enforcing the same directives.
- **Poor compliance:** Staff in organizations with less stringent enforcement may weigh the level of risk to themselves against the potential advantages. Inequity in sanction application encourages poor compliance by individuals who know they will escape any serious consequence for breaching privacy and security policies.
- **Erosion of public trust:** Public trust is eroded when significant variation is blatantly apparent in how healthcare organizations respond to a privacy or security breach both within and across entities and systems. The public must feel assured their personal health information has sufficient protections across the healthcare spectrum, particularly in this era of health information exchange.
- **Weakened position for dispute resolutions:** Inequitable application of sanctions can affect the outcome of personnel actions at arbitration and grievance proceedings. Unequal penalties for similar offenses undermine the organization's ability to prevail in dispute resolutions.
- **More regulation:** Poor and inconsistent implementation of privacy and security safeguards invites further state and federal intervention. Such laws place an additional administrative and financial burden on facilities. If the industry does not self-correct, then it leaves open the door to state and federal government intervention.
- **Questionable research:** The validity of research may be called into question when privacy or security breaches are not handled consistently and expeditiously patients

Safeguarding the Nurse (Fig. 24.18)

- **Licensure:** All nurses who are in nursing practice have to possess a valid licensure, issued by the respective state nursing council/Indian Nursing Council
- **Good Samaritan laws:** In response to health professionals, fear of malpractice claims, most states enacted Good Samaritan Laws that exempt doctors and nurses from liability when they render help during emergency. These laws limit liability and offer legal immunity for people helping in an emergency.
- **Good rapport:** Developing good rapport with the client is very important to prevent malpractice. The ability to develop good rapport with client is dependent on the nurse having good interpersonal communication skills, e.g., listening.
- **Standards of care:** All professional practicing in the medical field are held to certain standards when administering care. It is always better to follow standards of care to avoid malpractice and do not attempt anything beyond the level of competence.
- **Standing orders:** Although a nurse may not legally diagnose illness or prescribe treatment, she/he may after assessing patients condition apply standing orders or treatment guideline that have been established by the physician or doctor as appropriate for certain problems and conditions.
- **Consent for operation and other procedures:** A patient coming into hospital still retains his rights as a citizen and his entry only denotes his willingness to undergo an investigation or a course of treatment. Any investigation or treatment of a serious nature, or an operation in which an anesthetic is used, requires the written consent of the patient.
- **Correct identity:** The nurse or the midwife has the great responsibility to make sure that all babies born in the hospital are correctly labeled at birth and to ensure that at no time they are placed in the wrong cot or given to the wrong mother.
- **Counting of sponge instrument and needles:** Nurses advocate that sponge, instrument and needle counts be performed for all surgical procedures taking place in operation theatre. When an instrument left in a patient's body the nurse will probably be liable for any patient injury caused by the presence of foreign body.
- **Contracts:** A contract is a written or oral agreement between two people in which goods or services are exchanged.
- **Documentation:** Documentation is by far the best once a lawsuit field. The medical record is a legal document admissible in court as evidence.

Consumer Protection Act (Figs. 24.19 and 24.20)

Consumer protection act was passed by the parliament in the year 1986. This act considers patients as consumers, i.e., buyers of services and doctor as the provider of these services on payment. During last few years, due to increased availability of sophisticated investigative and therapeutic technology, modern practice of medicine is dehumanized. This fact is partly responsible for loss of mutual trust.

Important features of this Act are following:
- Services rendered by a doctor, hospital or any other healthcare organization for carrying out consultation, diagnosis, investigations and treatment fall within the purview of this Act.
- The services rendered may be free, on payment, in charitable hospital or in profit making paying hospital
- If the charges are reimbursible or there is third party payment, e.g., employer, insurance company, etc., and then also the act is applicable.
- If the services rendered are totally free, then the act is not applicable.
- The act is applicable to the patients who are treated free in paying hospitals.
- The act is applicable to all the patients free and paying in the free hospitals having paying beds, paying section or payment required for any service.
- Consumer does not have to pay court fees or process fees.
- Prescribed time limit for settling the dispute is three months. If expert examination is required, longer time is permitted.

The Act permits examination by the following bodies:
- **District forum:** The forum consists of three persons.
  - District judge as president
  - Two persons having knowledge of any of the following: (i) Law, (ii) Economics, (iii) Commerce, (iv) Accounting, (v) Administration, (vi) Industry.

  They should be having ability and integrity. At least one person should be a woman. Compensation not exceeding ₹ 5 lakhs is the limit of this body. Complaints demanding higher compensation are outside its purview.

  If the complainant is not satisfied with the decision he/she can appeal to state commission within 30 days.
- **State commission:** Consists of three members—
  - Sitting or past judge of high court as president

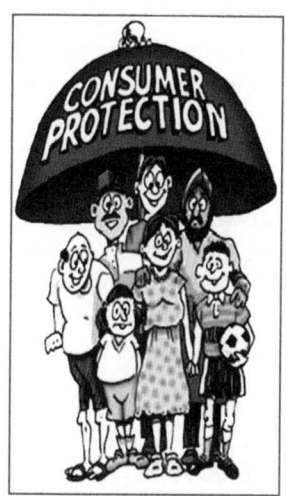

Fig. 24.19: Consumer protection.

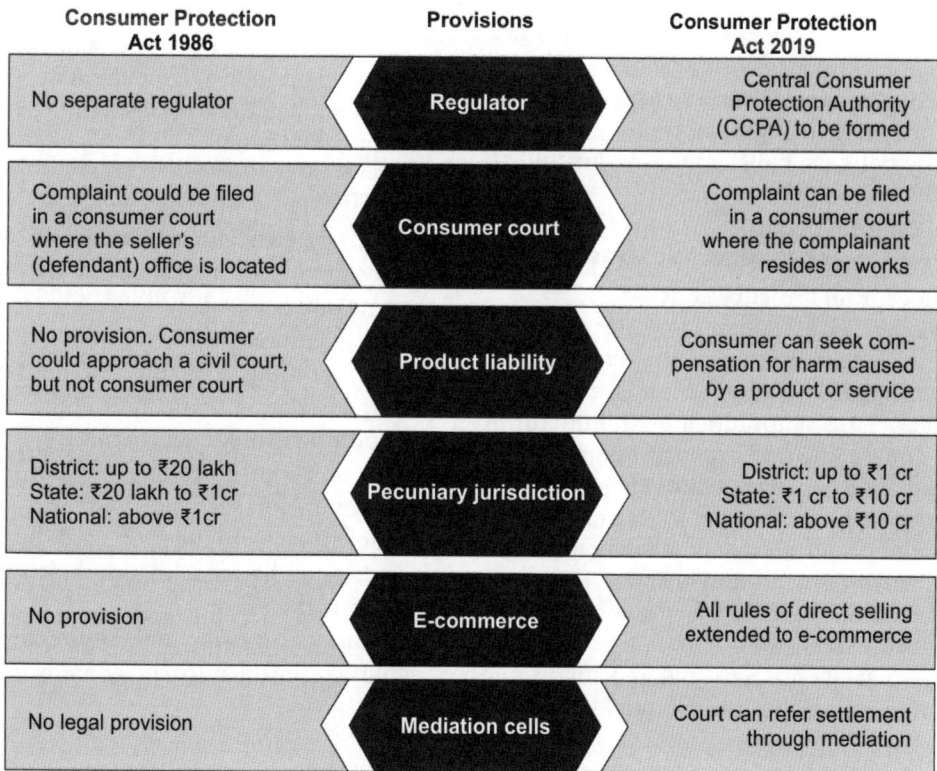

Fig. 24.20: Consumer Protection Act.

- Two persons as described in the composition of district forum.

This commission attends to the complaints asking for compensation (i) Which is more than ₹ 5 lakhs, (ii) Less than ₹ 20 lakhs.

If the complainant is not satisfied with the judgment, the appeal can be made to the National Commission within 30 days.

- **National commission:** Consists of five persons.
  - Sitting or past judge of Supreme Court
  - Four persons as described in the previous two committees.

This commission handles complaints demanding more than ₹ 20 lakhs as compensation.

Consumer Protection Act also provides for:
- State level consumer protection council
- Central consumer protection council for the purpose of: (i) Protecting rights of the consumers, (ii) Promoting rights of the consumer's, (iii) Educating consumers

Advantage of the Act:
- Doctors are accountable for their actions of:
  - Omission
  - Commission
- Speedy justice to consumers
- Decisions are made on the basis of law, faith and fairness.
- It encourages:
  - Proper communication with patient's
  - Proper documentation
  - Better performance
  - Reasonable charges

Disadvantages:
- Medical services are personalized and cannot be standardized. Hence, there may be unnecessary complaints.
- Doctors tend to practice defensive medicine by ordering more tests, ordering opinions, from other specialists and treating doubtful conditions vigorously
- Black mailing by patients, colleagues, lawyers and so called social workers
- Likely damage to the reputation
- Doctors may refuse to take up complicated cases.

Indemnity insurance for malpractice suits:
- In the event of dissatisfied consumer, i.e., patient claiming damages either through district forum, state commission, and National Commission or through court of law alleging medical negligence or malpractice by the doctor, it becomes time consuming and expensive issue for the doctor to prove that there had been no negligence.
- If the judgment goes against the doctor, than payment of a very large sum becomes necessary. As the number of such litigations against doctors and hospitals is steadily increasing. it has become necessary for the doctor to have medical indemnity insurance.
- At present, there are some nationalized insurance companies having scheme for professional indemnity insurance for:
  - Doctor as an individual
  - Shared practice i.e., partners
  - Diagnostic centers
  - Nursing homes
  - Laboratories
  - Hospitals
  - Blood banks, etc.
- In individual doctor's policy the policy holder can include the names of qualified assistants or qualifies employees mentioning their status.
- Hospitals can have comprehensive group policy which will cover all the staff employed by the hospital.
- If there are claims for compensation against an individual person or more persons of the hospital, the insurance company takes up the issue and if the act committed.

Laws Related to Nursing Practice

Some of the most commonly occurring legal issues that impact on nursing and nursing practice are those relating to informed consent and refusing treatment as previously detailed, licensure, the safeguarding of clients' personal possessions and valuables, malpractice, negligence, mandatory reporting relating to gunshot wounds, dog bites, abuse and unsafe practices, for example, informed consent, documentation, accepting an assignment, staff and client education relating to legal issues, and strict compliance with and adherence to all national, state, and local laws and regulations.

Liability

Liability is an obligation that can be enforced by law. In the nursing profession, it can be further broken down into subcategories:
1. Administrative liability—violation of regulation, such as failing to renew your license
2. Civil liability—imposing penalties in the form of payment or compensation to the patient who was harmed
3. Criminal liability—imposing fines or imprisonment for crimes committed

Malpractice

- Malpractice is an act of omission or commission that does not meet established standards of care and causes some injury.
- Nurses, therefore, must provide all aspects of nursing care according to established standards of care, in a safe and competent manner, and also done in a complete, appropriate and timely manner.
- The six essential components of malpractice include causation, foreseeability, damages to the patient, a duty that was owed to the client and this duty was breached, and, lastly, this breach of duty led to direct and/or indirect harm to the client.
- Actions of omission and commission that lead to client injury place the nurse in jeopardy for malpractice.

Negligence

- Negligence is also an act of omission or commission that does not meet established standards of care.

- It differs from malpractice because it lacks one or more of the six elements of malpractice that are essential to be considered malpractice.
- Actions of omission and commission that lead to client injury place the nurse in jeopardy for negligence.

Elements of Negligence
- Duty to act (Nurse—Patient relationship)
- Breach of duty (SOC not followed—reasonably prudent nurse)
- Damage (Physical and psychological) No damage no case!
- Causal connection (reasonably close connection between nurse's conduct and injury)

Professional Misconduct
- Violating any guidelines set forth by your state nursing board places you at risk of being charged with professional misconduct.
- Obtaining license fraudulently
- Practicing while impaired by ETOH, drugs, physical or mental disability.
- Habitual drunk or dependent on narcotics and other drugs with similar affects
- Refusing to provide professional service to a person based on race, creed, color, or national origin
- Practicing beyond authorized scope, with gross incompetence, with gross negligence on a particular occasion or negligence or incompetence on more than one occasion.

Documentation
- All documentation and all forms of documentation are considered legal documents.
- Some of the legal aspects of documentation, in addition to the legal mandates associated with confidentiality, include the strict legal prohibitions against altering a record, obliterating entries in the medical record, and falsifying documentation.
- Other guidelines for documentation include the use of permanent ink, the use of only accepted terms and abbreviations, legible writing, accurate spelling, proper grammar, accurate dating and time of the entry, the signature and title of the person who documented the entry, and a professional tone.
- If an error in documentation occurs, a thin line that does NOT obliterate the entry is drawn through the erroneous entry, the notation "Error" is written above the entry and the nurse signs this notation with their name and title.

Breach
- Failing to perform any term of a contract, written or oral, without a legitimate legal excuse.
- This may include not completing a job, not paying in full or on time, failure to deliver all the goods, substituting inferior or significantly different goods, not providing a bond when required, being late without excuse, or any act which shows the party will not complete the work ("anticipatory breach").
- Breach of contract is one of the most common causes of law suits for damages and/or court-ordered "specific performance" of the contract.

Penalties
A penalty is a punishment or consequence for doing something wrong, such as having to pay a fee for not bringing your library book back when it was due.

Invasion of Privacy
Invasion of privacy is the unjustifiable intrusion into the personal life of another without consent. However, invasion of privacy is not a tort on its own; rather it generally consists of four distinct causes of action. States vary on both whether they recognize these causes of action as well as what elements are necessary to prove them, so you should be sure to check your state's laws or consult with a lawyer before bringing legal action. The four most common types of invasion of privacy torts are as follows:

1. **Appropriation of name or likeness:** Appropriation of name or likeness laws protects the right to control the use of the own identity for a business or economic purpose. Typically, these claims involve the unauthorized use of a person's picture or name. While state laws vary, the elements necessary to prove appropriation are generally as follows:
   a. The defendant (the party being sued) used the plaintiff's (the party initiating the lawsuit) name, likeness or identity;
   b. The use was for the defendant's benefit, whether the benefit is economic or otherwise;
   c. The use was without the plaintiff's consent; and
   d. The use caused injury to the plaintiff.
2. **Intrusion upon seclusion:** Intrusion upon seclusion laws protects your right to privacy while you are in solitude or seclusion. This right extends to you or the private affairs. For example, it is an invasion of privacy for a neighbor to peek through the windows or take pictures of you in your home. Likewise, it is also an invasion of privacy to use electronic equipment to eavesdrop on a private conversation. The general elements of this tort are as follows:
   a. The defendant intruded into the plaintiff's private affairs, seclusion or solitude
   b. The intrusion would be objectionable to a reasonable person

   The defendant does not need to communicate the details of the intrusion to a third party; once the defendant has committed the intruding act (and the plaintiff proves the necessary elements), the defendant is liable for invasion of privacy.
3. **False light:** False light laws protect your right to not have potentially misleading or damaging information about yourself publicly disclosed. This includes the disclosure of information that may be true, but is nonetheless misleading or damaging. For example, it may be an invasion of privacy if a caption published with

a photograph in a news article about a protest describes a person as a participant, when in fact; the person was only observing the protest. Generally, the elements of false light are as follows:
   a. The defendant publicly disclosed information about the plaintiff;
   b. The information placed the plaintiff in a false light; and
   c. The false light would be highly offensive to a reasonable person.
4. **Public disclosure of private facts:** Public disclosure of private facts laws protect your right to keep the details of your private life from becoming public information. For example, publicizing facts about a person's health, sexual conduct, or financial troubles is likely an invasion of privacy. While state laws vary, the general elements of this tort are as follows:
   a. The defendant publicized a matter regarding the private life of the plaintiff;
   b. The publicized matter would be highly offensive to a reasonable person; and
   c. It is not of legitimate concern to the public.

To publicize a private matter, laws generally require that private information is disseminated in such a way that it is substantially certain to become public knowledge.

Defamation of Character

Defamation of character is an issue of importance in the legal realm. A person's livelihood can be severely hurt when they are defamed. Falsehood and intent to harm are important to consider when determining if defamation of character occurred.

- **Types:** The two types of defamation of character are libel and slander. Libel is the writing of false accusations against another person with intent to harm.
   1. Slander is saying false accusations against someone with intent to harm. Slander is what the parent told a reporter in the scenario with the principal.
   2. There are three areas that need to be proven to win a defamation of character.
- **Lawsuit:** False—first, what was said or written against a person must be proved false. Proving that an accusation is false can be challenging. Kevin the principal was told this by his lawyer friend. However, it can be done. In fact, in Kevin's case, it could be done quite easily. As we delve further into Kevin's situation, this will become clear. The accusation must indeed be proven false.
- **Intending harm:** Second, it must be proven that the one who said or wrote the falsehood intended harm. While proving that an accusation may be false is challenging, proving that the accuser intended harm can be even more challenging. Clear and convincing evidence is needed.

Nursing Regulatory Mechanisms

Regulatory body is the formal organization designated by a statute or an authorized governmental agency to implement the regulatory forms and process whereby order, consistency and control are brought to the profession and its practice

Main functions:
- To protect patient or society
- To define the scope of nursing practice
- To identify the minimum level of nursing care that must be provided to clients

Licensure:
- All registered and licensed practical, or vocational, nurses must be currently licensed to practice nursing in their state of practice.
- Licensure protects the consuming public and insures that the nurse has completed a state approved nursing school, has successfully passed their licensure examination and has also continuously met the requirement(s) for relicensure each biennium without any suspensions or revocations of their license.
- Practicing without a current and valid license is illegal and it amounts to practicing without a license.
- A license is a legal permit that a government agency grants to individual to engage in the practice of profession and to use a particular title.
- Each country has its own method to grant or maintain and revoke the licensure.
- However, a nurse can practice anywhere within the country with her state's licensure. This is known as mutual recognition model.

Certification: Certification is the voluntary practice of validating that an individual nurse has met minimum standards of nursing competence in specialty areas, such as maternal-child health nursing, pediatrics, school nursing, etc.,

Accreditation

It is the function of a state board of nursing is to ensure that schools preparing nurses maintain minimum standard of education.
- "Accreditation is the process whereby an organization or agency recognizes a college of university of program of study as having met certain predetermined qualifications of standards" — *Selden, 1962*
- A process of review and approval by which an institution, program or specific service is granted a time-limited recognition of having met certain established standards beyond those that are minimally acceptable. —*ICN*
- Organization or agency recognizes a college or university or a program of study as having met certain predetermined qualifications and standard' voluntary review process of educational programs by a professional organization

Purposes of Accreditation

- For the maintenance of adequate administration requirement.
- Maintaining a uniform standard for nursing education and nursing service.
- Stimulation of institutional self-improvement by evaluation and inspection.
- It safeguards the institution from social education and political pressures.
- It helps in the registration of nurses.

- It prescribes the syllabus.
- It grants recognition to school and colleges.
- It guides the school/college of nursing, according to recommendation and criteria.
- It also services to prepare the competent to serve the public.

Types of Accreditation Agencies
- National accrediting agency
- National professional accrediting agency
- State accrediting bodies

Functions of Accreditation
- It aims to protect the autonomy of various health service programs.
- It preserves the quality of nursing education.
- It protects the public from ill prepared nurses.
- It protects the institutions unsound and unsafe political pressure.
- It helps the practitioner for the broad scope of nursing practice.

National Agencies
- Concerned with appraising the total activities of the institutions of higher learning, and with safe guarding the quality of liberal education, the foundation of professional programs in colleges and universities.
- Each agency establishes criteria for the evaluation of institutions in its region it reviews those institutions periodically, and it publishes from time to time a list of those agencies which it has accredited.
- Central advisory board of education
- All India Council for elementary education
- All India Council for secondary education
- University Grants Commission
- All India Council for technical education
- National Assessment and Accreditation council

National Professional Accrediting Agency
- Aim to foster research, to improve service to the public and the number of individuals admitted to the profession.
- Medical Council of India
- Indian Nursing Council
- Dental Council of India' Pharmacy Council of India
- Central Council of Indian System of Medicine
- Indian Nursing Council, (INC) is the official accrediting agency for all programs of nursing, which include Diploma (GNM), BSc Nursing (both basic and post basic), MSc N/Mphil (Masters) and PhD (Doctoral programs in Nursing).

State Accrediting Bodies
- A state nursing councils, which is called reciprocity, was possible only if uniform standards of nursing education were maintained.
- Providing the registration to the nurses
- Maintains a register of names of professional nurses
- All degree holding nurses also have to get the registration in State Council.

Licensure/Registration
Licensure is defined as the "process by which an agency of State Government grant permission to an individual to engage in a given profession upon finding that the applicant has attained the essential degree of competency necessary to perform a unique scope of practice. A document issued by a body charged with the exclusive right to determine eligibility for practice in a specified profession, or field in the profession. It is generally used within a regulatory system that prohibits practice without a license. —*ICN*

Purpose:
- Licensure offers protection to the public
- It ensure minimum competency among professional.
- It ensures minimum standard among the professionals.
- It helps to prevent malpractice.
- It helps to regulate the professional conduct.

Licensing permits a person to offer special skills and knowledge to the public in a particular jurisdiction when such practice would otherwise be unlawful. A particular jurisdiction or area is covered by the license.

In India, all nurses are required to be licensed to work in any part of the country, for that they have to be registered in any of the State Nursing Council. All over India each state running their own nursing council. Registration councils are functioning in all states of India and they are affiliated to INC.

Renewal of Licensure
- The process for periodic reissuing of the legal authority to practice.
- Renewal system in a proper way it will help to improve the professional competencies in nursing.
- In TNMC instructed that all the nurses renew their registration every 5 years for that they need specific (150) credit hours.

Nurse Practice Act
- **Government service conduct rules:** The rule governs conduct of all government employees. This rule is basically applicable for nurse's practice employed by government.
- **Indian Nursing Council Act:** Indian Nursing Council, an autonomous body under Ministry of Health and Family Welfare (Government of India) was constituted under Section 3(1) of Indian Nursing Council Act, 1947 of parliament to establish a uniform standard of training for nurses, midwives and health visitors.
- **English laws:** This law generally hold care provider including nurses liable for negligence/answerable for act of carelessness. The Central Government is a source of legal authority.

Rights and Responsibilities of Nurses
Some of the rights and responsibilities applicable for nurses are:

- Right to refuse to treat patient except in case of an emergency. (Though it can be debatable as patient should not ideally be refused for treatment but in certain scenario nurses hold this right).
- Right to sue for fee
- The right to add a title or descriptions to one's name. Any title, description, abbreviation or letter which implies holding a degree, diploma, license or certificate showing particular qualification.
- The right to set standards for excellence in nursing.
- The right to participate in policy making affecting nursing.
- Rights to work and serve in a safe and health work environment.
- Right to refuse or protest formally a physician's order if a nurse believes it is harmful for the client.
- Right of appointing and assigning
- Right of quality control
- Right for record keeping
- Right to care public
- Right of using equipment's
- Right for observation and reporting

Duties of Nurses

Some of the fundamental duty of nurses includes:
- To exercise a reasonable degree of skill and knowledge in treating patients (the standard held is the one exercised by other reputable members of the same profession in similar circumstance).
- Once a relationship of a patient has been established there is an obligation to attend a patient as long as necessary unless the patient requests withdrawal of notice is given of intention to withdraw.

Regulation for Nurse Practitioner/Specialist Nursing Practice

The nurse practitioner (NP) is a registered nurse who possesses additional preparation and skills in physical diagnosis, psychosocial assessment, and management of health-illness needs in primary healthcare, who has been prepared in a program that conforms to Board standards

Primary Healthcare

- Primary healthcare is defined as, that which occurs when a consumer makes contact with a healthcare provider, who assumes responsibility and accountability for the continuity of healthcare regardless of the presence or absence of disease.
- This means that, in some cases, the NP will be the only health professional to see the patient and, in the process, will employ a combination of nursing and medical functions approved by standardized procedures.

Clinically Competent

Clinically competent means that one possesses and exercises the degree of learning, skill, care ordinarily possessed and exercised by a member of the appropriate discipline in clinical practice.

Child (Neonatal Specialty)

Neonatal nurse practitioners are registered in the child category and have specialized education relevant to neonatology which includes the complex management, resuscitation and stabilization of extremely premature and critically-ill neonates. Practice settings include high-risk newborn centers as well as Level 2 and 3 neonatal intensive care units. They are restricted to working with the neonate population

Treatment/Advanced Interventions

- Nurse practitioners are authorized to perform both invasive and non-invasive procedures integral to the clinical management of clients, determined by the competence of the individual nurse practitioner.
- These may include but are not limited to suturing, incision and drainage, excisions, intubation, limb immobilization and casting and reducing dislocation of joints.

Monitoring Client

Outcomes nurse practitioners collaborate with clients in monitoring their response to therapeutic interventions and adjusting interventions as needed to address healthcare needs in the provision of initial and ongoing care.

Consultation and Referral

- Nurse practitioners consult and refer to another healthcare provider when the client's condition warrants it.
- Referral to another healthcare provider (e.g., physiotherapist, another nurse practitioner, and physician) is required when the nurse practitioner approaches or reaches the limits of their competence beyond which they cannot provide care independently and additional information or assistance is required.
- Nurse practitioners are also consulted by other healthcare providers, including physicians, when the nurse practitioner is the most appropriate care provider.
- The nurse practitioner is accountable for identifying when collaboration, consultation, and referral are necessary for safe, competent, and comprehensive client care.

■ EXPANDED ROLE OF THE NURSE

Contemporary nursing requires that the nurse possess knowledge and skills in a variety of areas. In the past, the principal role of nurses was to provide care and comfort as they carried out specific nursing functions, but changes in nursing have expanded the role to include increased emphasis on health promotion and illness prevention, as well as concern for the client as a whole. The contemporary nurse functions in the interrelated roles of care giver, clinical and ethical decision maker, protector and client advocate, case manager, rehabilitator, comforter, communicator, and teacher.

Care Giver

- As care giver, the nurse helps the client regain health through the healing process.

- Healing is more than just curing a specific disease, although treatment skills that promote physical healing are important to care givers.
- The nurse addresses the holistic healthcare needs of the client, including measures to restore emotional, spiritual, and social well-being.
- The care giver helps the client and family set goals and meet those goals with a minimal cost of time and energy.

Clinical Decision Maker

- To provide effective care, the nurse uses critical thinking skills throughout the nursing process.
- Before undertaking any nursing action, whether it is assessing the client's condition, giving care, or evaluating the results of care, the nurse plans the action by deciding the best approach for each client.
- The nurse makes these decisions alone or in collaboration with the client and family. In each of these situations, the nurse collaborates and consults with other healthcare professionals.

Protector and Client Advocate

- As protector, the nurse helps maintain a safe environment for the client and takes steps to prevent injury and protect the client from possible adverse effects of diagnostic or treatment measures.
- Confirming that a client does not have an allergy to a medication and providing immunization against disease in a community-based practice are examples of the nurse's protective role.
- In the role of client advocate, the nurse protects the client's human and legal rights and provides assistance in asserting those rights if the need arises.
- For example, the nurse may provide additional information for a client who is trying to decide whether to accept treatment.
- The nurse may also defend clients' rights in a general way by speaking out against policies or actions that might endanger client's well-being or conflict with their rights.

Case Manager

- As case manager, the nurse coordinates the activities of other members of the healthcare team, such as nutritionists and physical therapists, when managing a group of clients' care.
- In addition, nurses must also manage the own time and the resources of the practice settings.
- Differentiated practice models offer nurses opportunities to ma decisions about their career paths.

Rehabilitator

- Rehabilitation is the process by which individual's maximal levels of functioning after illness, other disabling events.
- Frequently clients experience physical or emotional impairments that change their lives, and the nurse helps them adapt as fully as possible.
- Rehabilitative and restorative care activities range from teaching clients to walk with crutches to helping clients cope with lifestyle changes often associated with chronic illness.

Comforter

- The role of comforter, caring for the client as a person, is a traditional and historical one in nursing and has continued to be important as nurses have assumed new roles.
- Because nursing care must be directed to the whole person rather than simply the body, comfort and emotional support often help give the client strength to recover.
- While carrying out nursing activities, nurses can provide comfort by demonstrating care for the client as an individual with unique feelings and needs. As comforter, nurses should help the client reach therapeutic goals rather than encourage emotional or physical dependence.

Communicator

- The role of communicator is central to all oilier nursing roles. Nursing involves communication with clients and families, other nurses and healthcare professionals, resource persons, and the community.
- The quality of communication is a critical factor in meeting the needs of individuals, families, and communities.

Teacher

- As teacher, the nurse explains to clients concepts and facts about health, demonstrates procedures, such as self-care activities, determines that the client fully understands, reinforces learning or client behavior, anti-evaluates
- Progress in learning or client behavior, and evaluates progress in learning. Some teaching can be unplanned and informal, such as when a nurse responds to a question about a health issue in casual conversation.
- Other teaching activities may be planned and more formal, such as when the nurse teaches a client with diabetes to self-administer insulin injections.
- The nurse uses teaching methods that match the client's capabilities and needs and incorporates other resources, such as the family, in teaching plans.

Career Roles

- The proceeding roles and functions apply to all nurses in most practice settings.
- Career roles, on the other hand, are specific employment positions. Because of increasing educational opportunities for nurses, the growth of nursing as a profession, and greater concern for job enrichment, the nursing profession offers expanded roles and different kinds of career opportunities.
- Examples of career roles include nurse educators and advanced practice nurses, such as clinical nurse specialists, nurse practitioners, certified nurse midwives, anesthetists, administrators, and researchers. Additional no clinical roles include risk managers, quality improvement nurses, and product consultants.

Nurse Educator

- A nurse educator works primarily in schools of nursing, stall development departments (ii health re agencies, and client education departments.
- Nursing educators generally have a background in clinical nursing, which provides them with practical skills and theoretical knowledge. A faculty member in a school of nursing prepares students to function as nurses.
- Nursing faculty members are responsible for teaching current nursing practice theory and necessary skills in laboratories or clinical settings.
- Nurse educators in nursing schools are usually required to have graduate degrees in nursing education. In addition, they generally have a specific clinical specialty and advanced clinical experience.
- Nurse educators in staff development departments of healthcare institutions provide educational programs for nurses within their institution.
- These programs include orientation of new personnel, critical care nursing courses and instruction about new equipment or procedures.
- The primary focus of the nurse educator in an agency's department of client education is to teach or disabled clients and families to provide care in the home.

Advanced Practice Nurse

- The advanced practice nurse (APN) has a master's degree in nursing, advanced education in pharmacology and physical assessment, and certification and expertise in a specialized area of practice (ANA, 1995).
- An APN usually works in primary, acute, restorative, or community healthcare agency.
- In addition, arm APN may specialize in the management of a disease, such as cancer, diabetes, or cardiovascular or pulmonary disease or in a specific field, such as pediatrics or gerontology.

Clinical Nurse Specialist

- **Clinical nurse specialist:** The clinical nurse specialist (CNS) has a master's degree in nursing and expertise in a specialized area of practice.
- A CNS may work in primary care, acute care, restorative care, and community-based settings.
- In addition, the CNS may specialize in specific diseases, such as diabetes mellitus, cancer, or congestive heart failure or in a specific field, such as pediatrics or gerontology.
- The INS functions as an expert clinician, educator, case in manager, consultant, and researcher to plan or improve the quality of care provided to the client and family.

Nurse Practitioner

- The nurse practitioner provides healthcare to clients, usually in an outpatient, ambulatory care, or community-based setting and comprehensiveness of care.
- A significant percentage of primary care encounters extend beyond the boundaries of medicine and demand the expertise of the nurse.
- The nurse practitioner is able to establish a collaborative provider-client relationship.
- The major nurse practitioner categories are adult, family, pediatric, obstetrics-gynecology, and geriatric nurse practitioner.
- A nurse practitioner has the knowledge and skills necessary to detect and manage limited acute and chronic stable conditions.
- The nurse practitioner's educational preparation includes a practitioner program or a master's degree in nursing.

Adult Nurse Practitioner (ANP)

- ANP provides primary, ambulatory care to adults with a non emergency acute or chronic illness, and in some settings tertiary care.
- ANPs are usually employed in ambulatory care centers or outpatient clinics and work in collaboration with a primary physician.

Family Nurse Practitioner

- A family nurse practitioner (FNP) provides primary ambulatory care for families, usually in collaboration with a family care physician.
- The FNP meets the family's general healthcare needs, manages some illnesses by providing direct care, and guides or counsels the family as needed.

Pediatric Nurse Practitioner

- A pediatric nurse practitioner (PNP) provides healthcare to infants and children, An obstetrics-gynecology nurse practitioner (OB-GYN) provides primary ambulatory care to women seeking obstetrical or gynecological healthcare.
- The nurse practitioner who is also a certified nurse-midwife may independently deliver infants.
- Pediatric nurse practitioner (GNP) provides ambulatory or inpatient care to older adults.
- The GNP's activities include interventions for health maintenance, illness prevention, or health restoration.

Certified Nurse Midwife

- A certified nurse-midwife (CNM) is an RN who is also educated in midwifery and is certified by the American College of Nurse-Midwives.
- The practice of nurse-midwifery involves providing independent care for women during normal pregnancy, labor, and delivery, as well as care for the newborn; it may include some gynecological services, such as routine Papanicolaou (Pap) smears, family planning, and treatment for minor vaginal infections.
- A CNM practices with a healthcare agency that provides medical consultation, collaborative management and referral.

Nurse Anesthetist

- A nurse anesthetist is an RN who has received advanced training in an accredited program in anesthesiology.
- Nurse anesthetists provide surgical anesthesia under the guidance and supervision of an anesthesiologist,

who is a physician with advanced knowledge of surgical anesthesia.

Nurse Administrator

- A nurse administrator manages client care and the delivery of specific nursing services within a healthcare agency.
- This administrator may hold a middle-management position, such as head nurse or supervisor, or an upper-level management position, such as assistant or associate director or director of nursing services.
- Functions of administrators include budgeting, staffing, strategic planning of programs and services, employee evaluation, and employee development.
- Middle-management position usually requires at least a baccalaureate degree in nursing, and upper-level positions generally require a master's degree.

Nurse Researcher

- The nurse researcher investigates problems to improve nursing care and to further define and expand the scope of nursing practice.
- The nurse researcher may be employed in an academic setting, hospital, or independent professional or community-service agency.
- The minimum educational requirement is now a doctoral degree, with at least a master's degree in nursing.

■ CONCLUSION

The consumers are patients with complex needs. With increased awareness of healthcare, healthcare facilities and Consumer Protection Act, patients are getting aware about their rights. Nurses also have now the expanded role. Issues which seem not feasible, and ideal, may become practice with the change of time. These issues are base for the future trends in care. The legal implications of nursing practice are tied to licensure, state and federal laws, scope of practice and a public expectation that nurses practice at a high professional standard. The nurse's education, license and nursing standard provide the framework by which nurses are expected to practice. When a nurse's practice falls below acceptable standards of care and competence, this exposes the nurse to litigation.

■ REVIEW QUESTIONS

Long Essays

1. Define profession; explain the qualities of professional nurse and scope of profession.
2. Describe code of ethics and professional conduct.
3. Explain legal issues in nursing, discuss about types of laws.
4. Define accreditation; explain the purposes, types and functions.
5. Explain in detail about the expanded role of a nurse.

Short Essays

1. Concept of professionalism in nursing.
2. Values of a professional nurse.
3. Roles and responsibilities of professional nurse.
4. Ethical issues in nursing.
5. Ethical decision making in nursing.
6. Application of code of ethics in nursing.
7. INC code of ethics for nurses in India.
8. Professional etiquette for nurses.
9. Legal issues in nursing.
10. Legal aspects related to nursing registration.
11. Consumer Protection Act.
12. Nursing regulatory mechanisms.
13. Adult nurse practitioner.

Short Answers

1. Confidentiality.
2. Professional development.
3. Nursing practice.
4. Professional practice model.
5. Ethical principles.
6. Fidelity.
7. Ethical dilemmas.
8. Good Samaritan Act.
9. Patient's Bill of Right
10. Civil law penalties for registered nurses.
11. Laws related to nursing practice.
12. Malpractice.
13. Negligence.
14. Professional misconduct.
15. Invasion of privacy.
16. Breach.
17. Defamation of character.

CHAPTER 25

Professional Advancement

LEARNING OBJECTIVES

- Continuing Nursing Education
- Career Opportunities
- Membership with Professional Organizations—National and International
- Participation in Research Activities
- Publications—Journals, Newspaper

■ CONTINUING EDUCATION IN NURSING

Continuing education courses are sometimes grouped with adult education courses. Both types of courses usually have similar formats: they are offered at times, such as evenings and weekends when most adults are not working, and they are developed for those with an older-adult mindset. Adult education courses, however, often focus on remedial areas and helping a student to gain the equivalent of a high school education; continuing education courses, on the other hand, assume that the student already has a high level of understanding of the subject matter, and builds upon that.

Definition (Fig. 25.1)

- Continuing education is any extension of opportunities for reading, study and training to any person and adult following their completion of or withdrawal from full time school and/or college programs.
- Continuing education is an educational activity, primarily designed to keep the registered nurses abreast of their particular field of interest and do not lead to any formal advanced standing in the profession.

Purpose of Continuing Nursing Education (CNE)

The purpose of the approver unit is to provide for a system of peer review of continuing education events by applying the American Nurses Credentialing Center's Commission on Accreditation approved criteria for continuing education activities and providers and to provide for maintenance of records regarding the system of peer review.

- Nursing is a humanistic, socially essential service which is instrumental in providing quality healthcare to all people.
- The Association can contribute to the provision of quality nursing care by facilitating professional growth.
- Registered nurses benefit from an association which promotes the individual's social, educational, political, and economic development and/or advancement.
- The promotion of professional growth through a variety of association activities is important to facilitate the advancement of nursing as a profession.
- Nurse participation in ISNA approved continuing nursing education benefits the individual and the recipient of care.

Need for Continuing Education (Box 25.1 and Fig. 25.2)

- Respond effectively to the challenge of current social changes.
- To improve the healthcare, economic and educational opportunities.
- To improve the new health patterns of healthcare.
- Due to increasing trend towards specialization.
- Due to legislation and its impact on the education of health personnel.

Goals of CNE in Nursing (Box 25.2)

- Provide a system of approval of continuing nursing education in the State of Indiana for activities and for providers

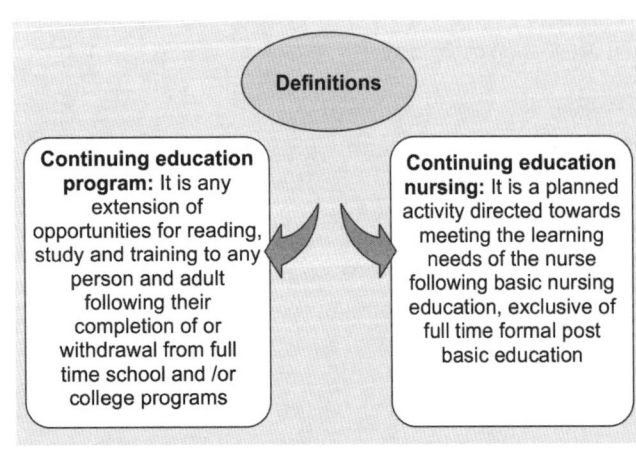

Fig. 25.1: Definitions of continuing education.

> **Box 25.1:** Need.
>
> - Rapid technological advances related to knowledge explosion have greatly altered the practice of nursing.
> - The gap between scientific knowledge and its application grows wider each year as a result of multiple influences.
> - Elimination of certain illnesses, particularly the communicable diseases.
> - New drugs to cure some illnesses and alter the course of many.
> - Surgeries are being performed successfully in areas that would not have been attempted 10–20 years ago.
> - Organ transplants are no more a novelty.
> - Complex and intricate machinery can extend lives.
> - All these advances require more highly skilled nursing care in a great variety of settings.
> - Continuing education is an accepted way of life.

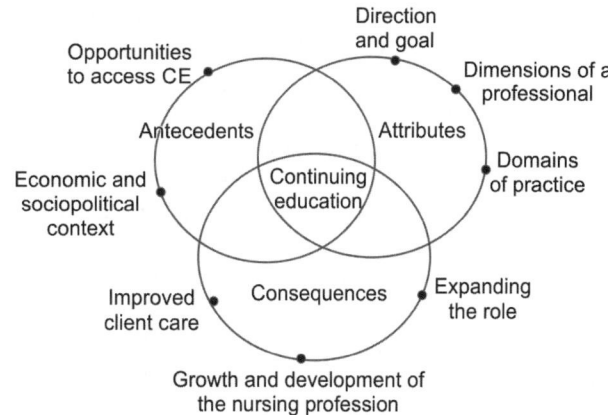

Fig. 25.3: Continuing education—a concept analysis.

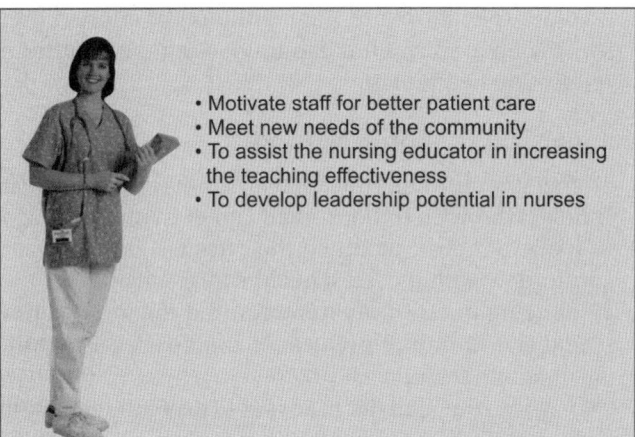

Fig. 25.2: Need of continuing education.

> **Box 25.2:** General goals of continuing education/staff development.
>
> - Rapidity of change in nursing care delivery systems necessities attendance of CE programs to ensure an updated knowledge.
> - Fostering innovative and creative approaches to the nursing care of patients for the purpose of achieving improved competence in nursing practice.
> - Assisting nursing personnel in becoming increasingly knowledgeable and competent in fulfilling role expectations.

- Maintain American Nurses Credentialing Center accreditation as an approver of continuing nursing education
- Publish a calendar of ISNA approved continuing education events.
- Evaluate the effectiveness of the approval unit's activities
- Assess the need, availability, and accessibility of quality continuing education opportunities for nurses
- Utilize the American nurses association's scope and standards of practice for nursing professional development as a means for assuring the quality of continuing nursing education.
- Maintain a mechanism for identification and resolution of problems and issues related to continuing education in nursing
- Maintain appropriate communication with membership of state regulatory agencies who have an impact on continuing education in nursing.
- Maintain contact with providers and inform them of ANCC updates.
- Conduct inter-rater reliability evaluation at least biennially.
- Utilize evaluation data to improve the approval process.
- Provide orientation session for new members of the ISNA Committee on Approval each year. **Figure 25.3** shows continuing education—a concept analysis.

Philosophy of Continuing Education

It has been believed that the system of higher education which provides the basic preparation or the members of a profession must also provide opportunities for practitioners to keep abreast of advances in their field. The Committee on Approval is an integral part of the State Nurses Association and, as such, adheres to the philosophy of the Nursing Association about the profession, the nature of nursing, and the importance of quality continuing education for nurses. In addition, the Committee adheres to the Nurses Association definition of nursing from the Nursing Policy Statement: "Nursing is the diagnosis and treatment of human responses to actual or potential health problems."

- Today's contemporary world is in an unrelenting, constant process of change.
- To respond effectively to the demands of change, the nursing profession believes that learning needs to be a continuous process throughout the lifespan.
- Learning is individual and diversified for each person. As such, the professional organization must recognize and respond to a commitment to registered nurses as unique persons, as individual learners, and as citizens.
- Individual nurses are responsible for their own learning and should participate in the identification of their own learning needs to meet these identified needs.
- Providers of continuing nursing education must have a commitment to involve learners in the learning process from the initial stages of planning through the evaluation of organized learning experiences.

- Continuing nursing education should be provided in a well-planned, organized educational environment. Strong support and leadership is expected from all groups providing continuing education.
- Continuing nursing education should assist individual practitioners in the continued acquisition of knowledge, the extension of professional responsibilities, the expansion of interpersonal skills, and the improvement of problem solving approaches to professional practice.
- Continuing nursing education should serve as a viable means of improving the professional competence of the practitioner with the outcome of improved healthcare.
- Continuing nursing education also should include such important concerns as—the realization of the health potential of each individual, the quality of life, and the understanding of the current health problems of modern society.
- Through its role as an approval body for continuing nursing education, the State Nurses Association should promote quality continuing nursing education for its membership as well as for the profession.
- This assurance of quality is needed to provide the citizens of Indiana with nursing practitioners who are accountable for developing, implementing and maintaining standards of nursing practice.

Principles of Continuing Education

The continuing education scheme is postulated on the principles of (**Box 25.3**):
- Treating basic literacy, post literacy and continuing education as one sustained, coherent learning process.
- Establishing a responsive and alternative structure for life-long learning.
- Responding to the needs of all sections of society.
- Learning not to be seen as a function of alphabets, but as all modes of human capacity building.
- Addressing the socioeconomic situations of the community to provide infrastructure for larger development initiatives.

Scope of Continuing Education

- A continuing education program is defined as "postsecondary instruction designed to meet the educational needs and interests of adults, including the expansion of available learning opportunities for adults who are not adequately served by current educational offerings in their communities".

Box 25.3: Principles of continuing nursing education.

- Provision for school and nursing faculty involvement in planning and teaching the continuing nursing education courses tend to maintain high educational standards for the program.
- An adequate staff is essential.
- Responsibility of the Director of Continuing Nursing Education are:
  - Determination of learning needs of the nurse population
  - Development and implementation of a program to meet these needs.

- The accreditation agency provides institutional accreditation for organizations whose primary function is for educational purposes and also for organizations offering continuing education as a clearly identified institutional objective within the operational entity, such as in-service corporate training.

Planning for Continuing Education

- Planning is the key stone for the administrative process. Without adequate planning, continuing education offerings are fragmented, haphazardly constructed, and often unrelated.
- A successful continuing education program is the result of careful and detailed planning.
- Effective planning is required at all levels, local, state, regional and national and eventually international—to avoid duplication and fragmentation of efforts and to help keep at minimum gap in meeting the continuing education needs of nurses.

Continuing Education in Nursing

- Nursing continuing education programs are designed for nurses who wish to boost their career by specializing in a particular area, maintain their license, or simply stay up-to-date with the latest healthcare trends.
- Practicing nurses are often required to earn a certain number of continuing education units each year in order to maintain their license.
- Nurses can even pursue an advanced degree by continuing education, which is ideal for people who are interested in moving to a management position.
- Practicing nurses that do not earn continuing education units often find it hard to stay abreast with the latest medical and technology developments.
- By continuing education, nurses can also select a field of specialization from a wide variety of branches ranging from psychiatric to palliative nursing.

Continuing Education Units (CEU) for Nurses

- Almost all practicing nurses are required to complete some continuing education units (CEU) each year.
- The number of continuing education units a nurse needs to complete varies institution to institution.
- Attending an approved nursing continuing education class or activity for 50 consecutive minutes' amounts to one contact hour.
- Each CEU comprises of 10 contact hours. Nursing Continuing Education Credits (CE) can be earned by participating in workshops, conferences, and nursing seminars.
- Nurses can even get CE credits for taking part in courses or activities that are related to nursing.

Importance CNE in Nursing

Nurses enter the field armed with the knowledge they need to excel at their jobs. However, healthcare is a changing field with constant new developments. Continuing education prepares nurses for these changes. When the H1N1 flu was spreading, most nurses received extra training, allowing them to spot and correctly care for patients with potential cases of this flu strain. Continuing education is also necessary for nurses who want to work as an advanced or specialized nurse.

Changing technology: Although nursing programs are designed to teach new nurses the very latest in healthcare technology, there are new products coming out each year that the nurses need to understand. For example, many medical facilities are in the process of switching to electronic health records. Nurses who have been in the field more than a few years may require training to learn how to use the new digital patient files and healthcare software.

Career advancement: The first stage in nursing is a licensed practical nurse (LPN). Training to become an LPN generally takes 12 months. To move past that and become a registered nurse (RN), nurses are required to take another two to four years of schooling. If an RN wants to continue his education, there are both master's and PhD nursing degrees available. Nurses can also pursue continuing education in specialties, such as pediatric or oncological nursing. Each additional certification or specialization can lead to an increase in pay and benefits. This type of continuing education can also open up new job opportunities, as certain types of nurses are frequently in demand.

Special situations: Nurses must continually educate themselves to keep up to date on arising situations in healthcare. As with the case of the H1N1 flu virus, sometimes there is a need for nurses to receive immediate additional training for a particular condition or medical development. Nurses must be prepared to implement changes in patient care as soon as changes become necessary.

State nursing requirement: Almost all nurses are required by state laws to meet a continuing education requirement. For example, nurses need 25 hours of continuing education from conferences, courses or seminars within two years of renewing their nursing licenses. Without taking the necessary courses, nurses cannot continue to work with patients. This ensures that medical patients get the very best care possible from nurses who are up to date on their training.

Consequences of not continuing education: If a nurse does not participate in continuing education opportunities, she will not be able to renew her license to practice medicine. On a larger scale, if continuing education were not mandatory for nursing, the quality of care the nursing community provided would diminish drastically. Each nurse would only have the formal education he received before graduation, whether that was 10 months or 10 years before. Care would be inconsistent and dangerous mistakes could easily become commonplace through lack of understanding. The need for continuing education reflects the constantly developing nature of the nursing field. **Figure 25.4** shows process for continuing nursing education (CNE) certification.

Types of Continuing Education (Fig. 25.5)

The dynamic and ever-evolving field of nursing requires medical professionals to stay current with developments

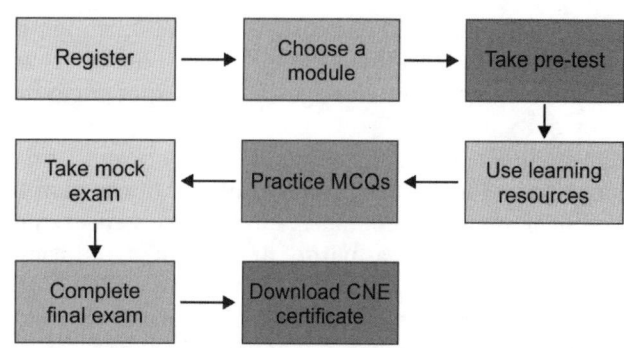

Fig. 25.4: Process for continuing nursing education (CNE) certification.

Types

- **Orientation** to introduce new recruits to the basic aspects of the job so that they can perform their job effectively
- **Continuing education** for the improvement of knowledge, skills and attitudes
- **Management skills and leadership training**
- **Staff development program** is directed toward expanding to the fullest all the potentials of an individual
- **Individual interest promotion programs**
- **Future oriented programs** to prepare learners for the future activities

Fig. 25.5: Types of continuing education.

as they happen. Technology that alters the way illnesses are diagnosed and treated, new medicines and alternative medicine options are becoming available on a regular basis. Because nurses need to know the most current trends, most states require nurses to take continuing education courses not just for their educational value, but also as a condition of maintaining a license to practice as nurses. The required courses vary and are available in different formats.

Seminars and Workshops

- Nurses who like the in-person approach to education can earn their continuing education credits by attending seminars and workshops.
- Seminars are available in different parts of the country in topics, such as career alternatives, case management, mediation, and also in specific skills that nurses must have to be successful.
- Seminars about developing nursing techniques and technology that is shaping the field are also available.

Online Courses

- Hundreds of online courses provide continuing education opportunities and credits for nurses. Courses are offered through organizations, such as NurseCEU.com, UniNursety, RnCeus.com and CE-Solutions.com.
- The courses cover topics that include neonatal care, pain management, treatment of older adults, sleeplessness, critical care, ambulatory nursing, emergency nursing, pediatrics and home health.

Chapter 25: Professional Advancement

- Nurses complete these courses entirely through the Internet, which allows them to work on their own schedule to gain continuing education experiences.

HIV/AIDS Training

- As a condition of license renewal and because of the critical nature of the information, many states require HIV/AIDS training as part of the continuing education process.
- A nurse needs these courses, which are available in both online and seminar form, fairly quickly after beginning practice

Domestic Violence Training

- The recognition and reporting of domestic violence is increasing in importance in the continuing education of nurses.
- As nurses are on the front lines of the medical treatment of young people, they are often in position to observe and help stop domestic violence.
- Courses in the recognizing domestic violence include specific training on what to do when it is suspected.

Benefits of Continuing Education (Fig. 25.6)

- One of the biggest benefits of continuing education is that it can improve one's skills in a current job or help gain new skills in preparation for a career change. Necessary skills in many job fields can change over time, so one must continue learning to be prepared for potential changes.
- This type of education also is critical for those who plan to switch careers or need cross-functional skills in a current job.
- Online learning and company training facilities have made it easier to further one's education without the need to quit working.
- Some employers require employees to learn new skills to maintain their current job or move to positions that require advanced skill levels.
- Companies that upgrade existing equipment or introduce a new computer program may ask employees to take a training course.
- Other employment fields may require continuing education to keep a license or to receive a salary increase.

- Many companies offer some kind of educational assistance program that can help cover a portion or all of one's educational expenses.
- Continuing education also does not have to take place in a classroom. One can choose to attend company workshops, take online courses or volunteer in a new field.
- Company workshops give one the opportunity to network with other business professionals and learn more about how the company functions.
- Online courses make it easy for working professionals to update current skills and do not require one to rearrange schedules or worry about travel costs.
- If one is considering changing careers, an internship can provide the chance to gain skills and try out the field before committing to a formal educational program.

CAREER OPPORTUNITIES IN NURSING

The term "nurse" is a generic label usually applied to all nurses working within the healthcare industry; however, there are four different groups of nurses, each of which has its own level of education, clinical experience and respective title.

- The specific career opportunities in nursing available to each group can vary greatly, and the choices often depend on the type of degree the nurse has earned. Within the general field of nursing, there are licensed practical nurses, registered nurses, advanced practice nurses and nurses with PhDs.
- Unlike many vocations, there is no direct career path in nursing. Because the field of nursing is so broad, there are many options to explore.
- A registered nurse might remain a registered nurse for his entire career, but he also has the option of working within many different departments or even specializing within a particular medical field.
- Likewise, the nurse who has worked in labor and delivery might decide to go back to school, earn her Master's degree and train as a nurse midwife, or even earn her PhD in order to teach other nurses.

Different Education Levels in Nursing (Fig. 25.7)

Licensed Practical Nurse

A licensed practical nurse (LPN), also known as a licensed vocational nurse (LVN), is one with the most limited career choices. The experience and duties associated to an LPN are somewhere in between that of a certified nurse's aide and a registered nurse (RN). Although an LPN may have similar responsibilities to that of a registered nurse, she is under the direct supervision of other RNs and physicians. The primary responsibility of an LPN is to provide bedside patient care, which might include assessing vitals, dressing wounds and administering medication. LPNs can work in a variety of clinical settings, including hospitals and office practices.

Registered Nurse

- According to the Bureau of Labor Statistics, three out of five registered nurses work in hospitals.

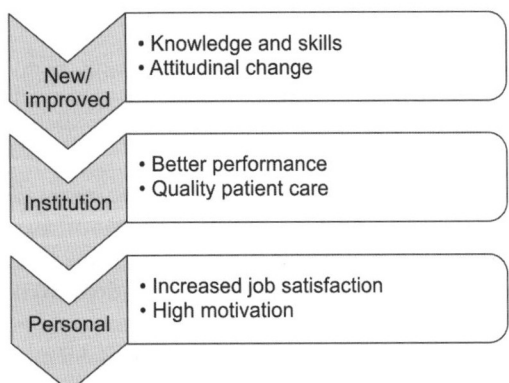

Fig. 25.6: Benefits of continuing nursing education.

Nurses can pursue a variety of educational paths to practice at different levels of nursing

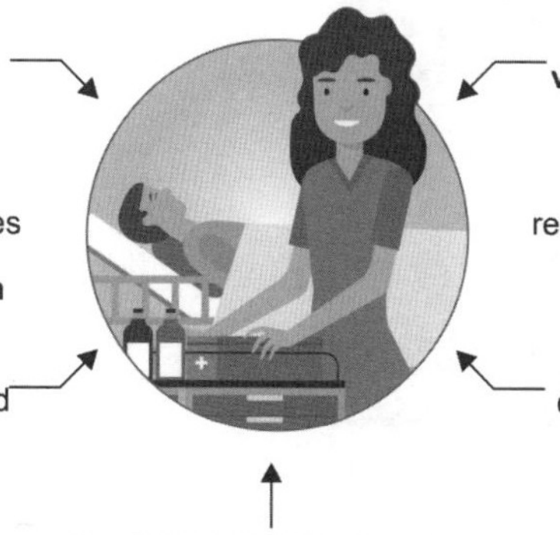

Certified nursing assistant: some CNA programs can be completed in as few as four weeks. CNAs are eligible to perform entry-level nursing duties

Bachelor of science in nursing (BSN): BSN holders have additional career opportunities and are eligible for more nursing jobs

Licensed practical nurse (LPN)/Licnsed vocational nurse (LVN): LPNs work under the supervision of MDs and RNs and have more responsibilities than CNAs

Master of science in nursing (MSN): MSN graduates often work in managerial positions

Doctor's of nursing practice (DNP): DNP holders have greater autonomy and responsibility and are eligible for high-level nursing positions

Fig. 25.7: Different education levels in nursing.

- A registered nurse enjoys the most flexibility within the healthcare industry
- Although RNs typically specialize in patient care according to the department for which they work, such as pediatrics, they can also sub-specialize.
- For example, a nurse trained in pediatrics might further specialize in the field of pediatric oncology.
- Registered nurses generally continue their education and broaden their experience through on-the-job training and classes relevant to their department or specialty

Advanced Practice Nurse

- An advanced practice nurse (APN) is a registered nurse who chooses to further her education and obtain a master's degree in nursing.
- Advanced practice nurses are considered expert clinicians, and they specialize in a particular field of nursing.
- Nurse anesthetists, nurse practitioners, nurse midwives and clinical nurse specialists are all APNs. These nurses are certified by the national organizations that govern each of their specialties.
- Advanced practice nurses can operate their own practice, although they generally work closely with other physicians. Such as registered nurses, advanced practice nurses work in various private and public settings.

PhD

- Nurses who earn a PhD in nursing have obtained the highest level of education in their field. PhD nursing programs prepare nurse researchers and scientists to better address the healthcare needs of individuals and their families, as well as the communities in which they live.
- These individuals are often more focused on academia and research rather than direct patient care, and they are usually affiliated with teaching hospitals, research facilities and universities.

Classification of Nurses by Nature of Work

Nurses generally fall into several main groups, depending on where they work—in hospitals, in private practice, in private homes, etc.

Hospital Nurses

- Hospital nurses, the largest group, are staff nurses who provide bedside nursing care and carry out the medical regimen prescribed by physicians.
- They also supervise licensed practical nurses and aides. Hospital nurses are typically assigned to one area, such as surgery, maternity, pediatrics, emergency, ICU, or oncology, but they sometimes rotate among departments.

Office Nurses

- **Office nurses care for outpatients in physicians' offices, clinics, and** emergency medical centers.
- They assist with examinations, administer injections and medications, dress wounds and incisions, assist with minor surgery, and maintain records. Some also perform routine laboratory and office work.

Nursing Home Nurses

- Nurses who work in nursing homes manages manage care for residents with conditions ranging from a fracture to Alzheimer's disease. Although they often spend much of their time on administrative and supervisory tasks, nursing home nurses also assess residents' health, develop treatment plans, supervise licensed practical nurses and nursing aides, and perform invasive procedures, such as starting intravenous fluids.
- They also work in specialty-care departments, such as long-term rehabilitation units for patients with strokes and head injuries.

Public Health Nurses

- Public health nurses work in government and private agencies, including clinics, schools, retirement communities, and other community settings.
- They focus on populations, working with individuals, groups, and families to improve the overall health of communities.
- Public health nurses work with communities to help plan and implement programs for immunizations, blood pressure testing, and other health screening.

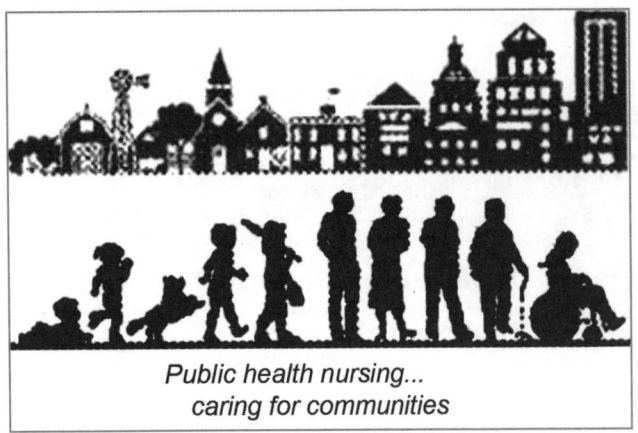

Fig. 25.8: Public Health Nursing.

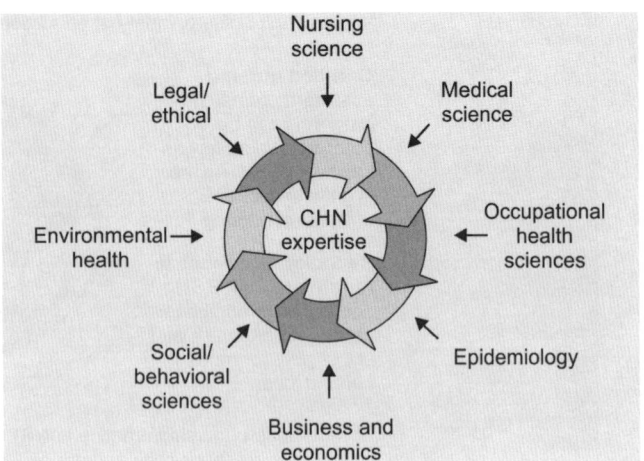

Fig. 25.9: CHN expertise.

- They instruct individuals, families, and other groups regarding health issues, such as preventive care, nutrition, and childcare. **Figure 25.8** shows public health nursing.

Nurse Practitioners

Nurse practitioners are the most advanced nurses, with the power to write prescriptions and independently diagnose and treat patients.

Registered Nurses

- Registered nurses (RNs) work to promote health, prevent disease, and help patients cope with illness. They are advocates and health educators for patients, families, and communities.
- When providing direct patient care, they observe, assess, and record symptoms, reactions, and progress in patients; assist physicians during surgeries, treatments, and examinations; administer medications; and assist in convalescence and rehabilitation.
- RNs also develop and manage nursing care plans, instruct patients and their families in proper care, and help individuals and groups take steps to improve or maintain their health.
- While State laws govern the tasks that RNs may perform, it is usually the work setting that determines their daily job duties.

Home Health Nurses

Home health nurses provide nursing services to patients at home. They assess patients' home environments and instruct patients and their families. Home health nurses care for a broad range of patients, such as those recovering from illnesses and accidents, cancer, and childbirth. They must be able to work independently and may supervise home health aides. Home health nurses provide periodic services, prescribed by a physician, to patients at home. They also provide support to patients and their families, and at times work independently.

Occupational Health Nurses (Industrial Nurses)

Occupational health nurses, also called industrial nurses, provide nursing care at worksites to employees, customers, and others with injuries and illnesses. They give emergency care, prepare accident reports, and arrange for further care if necessary. They also offer health counseling, conduct health examinations and inoculations, and assess work environments to identify potential or actual health problems. **Figure 25.9** shows CHN expertise.

Head Nurses or Nurse Supervisors

Head nurses or nurse supervisors direct nursing activities, primarily in hospitals. They plan work schedules and assign duties to nurses and aides, provide or arrange for training, and visit patients to observe nurses and to ensure that the patients receive proper care. They also may ensure that records are maintained and equipment and supplies are ordered.

Different Branches in Nursing Career

There are several paths for a nursing career, each differing in its educational requirements. When deciding to become a nurse it is wise to figure out where you would like to specialize. Knowing this information can help you streamline your training and start your nursing career as soon as possible. Four popular nursing careers include nurse practitioner, registered nurse, home health nurse and perinatal nurse.

Nurse Practitioner

- A career as a nurse practitioner requires the most advanced training and education.
- This type of nurse performs several functions that are similar to a physician, such as prescribing medicine and independently treating and diagnosing patients.
- Nurse practitioners are independent for the most part, reporting only to one medical doctor.
- A nurse practitioner career requires a master's degree and several years of nursing experience before the candidate will be accepted for training.

Registered Nurse (Fig. 25.10)

- Registered nurses provide education to patients, families and communities about disease prevention, health and illness. Furthermore, RNs are responsible for providing

Chapter 25: Professional Advancement

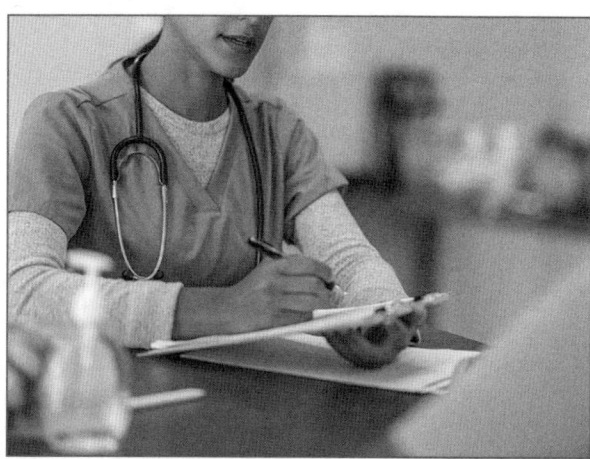

Fig. 25.10: Role of registered nurse.

direct patient care by observing, assessing and reporting a patient's symptoms, treatment reactions and progress.
- RNs also assist doctors during surgery and administer medicine. They play a major role in the patient's recovery, including instructing patients and family about out-of-hospital healthcare. Becoming an RN requires a bachelor's degree in nursing.

Home Health Nurse
- Home health nurses help and advise patients receiving home care. Their job is to analyze a patient's home environment, provide advice for improvement and instruct patients and family.
- Moreover, home health nurses work independently and care for a wide range of patients recovering from illness and injury.
- They also provide health aid to homebound patients under the instruction of a physician. A home health nursing career requires several years of experience as an RN.

Perinatal Nurse
- Perinatal nurses specialize in helping people with pregnancy and childbirth issues.
- Perinatal nurses are involved in helping pregnant women and couples prepare for childbirth and early infant care by offering health advice and instruction on watching for symptoms.
- Furthermore, perinatal nurses help doctors during delivery and are trained for independent delivery.
- A career in perinatal nursing training programs are often offered as continuing professional development for registered nurses.

Nursing Career Opportunities

Advanced Practice Registered Nurse
- The term Advanced Practice Registered Nurse is a general title granted to those registered nurses that have completed advanced educational and clinical requirements, usually a master's degree at the least.
- Advanced Practice Registered Nurses can be employed in a wide variety of positions and locations, from hospitals to community clinics and private practices.
- Nurse practitioners that are able to act independently of physicians, Certified Nurse Midwives that provide midwifery skills for pregnant women and newborns, Clinical Nurse Specialists who are experts in diagnosing and treating illnesses, and Certified Registered Nurse Anesthetists who are specialized in administering anesthesia

Ambulatory Care Nurses
- Ambulatory care nurses provide care to patients of all types outside of a traditional hospital environment.
- They primarily focus on pain management and general health education for those patients diagnosed with chronic injuries or illnesses on an episodic or outpatient basis.
- The type of care they provide includes screening, triage, case management, discharge planning, and other interventions to maintain or restore patients' health and ability to live independently.
- Ambulatory care nurses typically work in community clinics, schools, dialysis center, urgent care centers and pain management centers.

Camp Nurse
- Camp nurses provide healthcare and medical expertise to people of all ages attending camps and retreats.
- Their settings could range from a summer long camp of boy scouts in the forest, to a group of terminally ill cancer patients during a weekend retreat at a hotel.
- Because the campers could include youths and adults, chronically ill or perfectly healthy, camp nurses should possess a wide range of medical knowledge and skills.
- From treating poison ivy and mosquito bites to broken bones and camp fire burns, the list of conditions they could possibly be faced with is endless.

Cardiac Care Nurse (Fig. 25.11)
- Cardiac care nurses work primarily with patients that suffer from heart diseases and conditions.
- They can work in a wide variety of settings including coronary care units, intensive care units, operating theatres, cardiac rehabilitation centers, private clinics and ambulatory care facilities.
- **The conditions they treat can include:** Angina, cardiomyopathy, coronary artery disease, congestive heart failure, myocardial infarction, cardiac dysrhythmia and post-surgical care after bypasses, angioplasties and pacemaker implants.
- They also perform stress test evaluations, cardiac monitoring, vascular monitoring, and health assessments. Cardiac care nurses must also possess certification in Basic Life Support and Advanced Cardiac Life Support.
- Specialized skills include electrocardiogram monitoring, defibrillation and medical administration through

Chapter 25: Professional Advancement

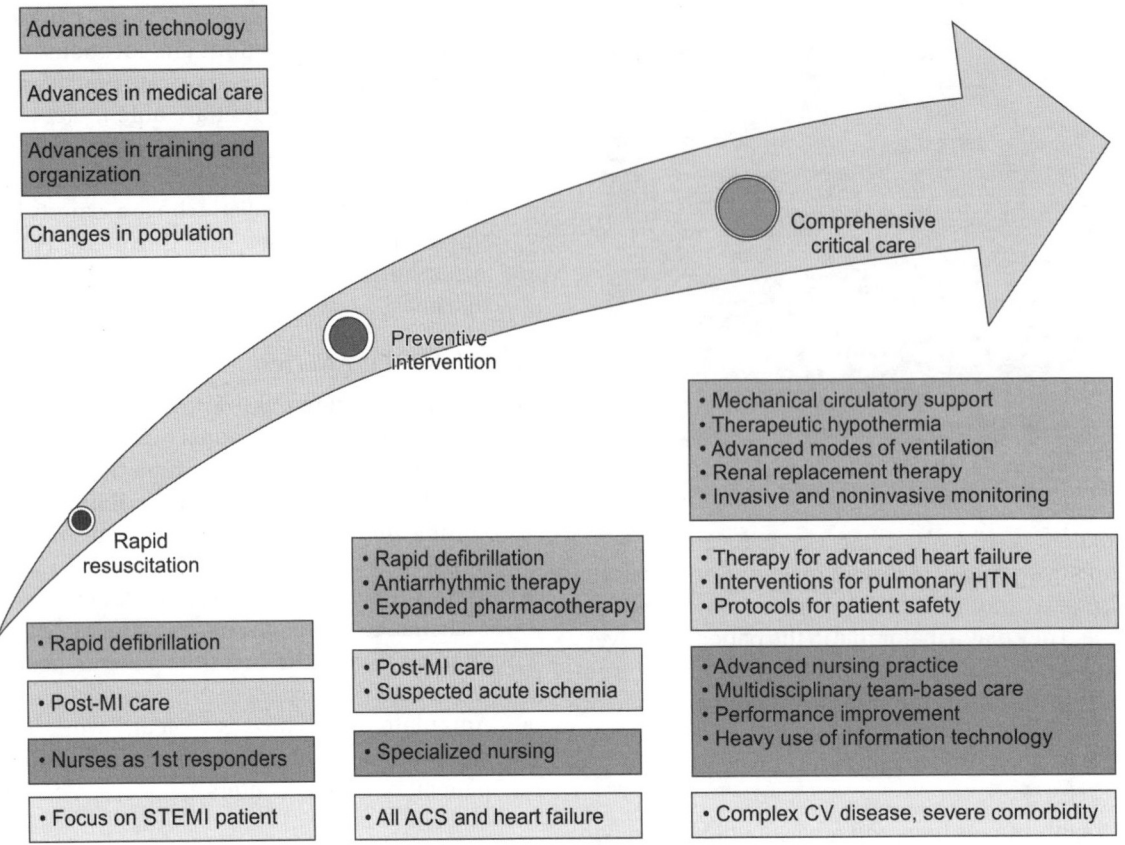

Fig. 25.11: Role of cardiac nurse.

intravenous drip. Cardiac care nurses have a wide variety of environments and conditions with which to specialize in. From pediatrics or geriatrics to post-surgical or ambulatory care, the possibilities are numerous.

Cardiac Cath Lab Nurse

- Cardiac catheterization, or heart cath, is the insertion of a catheter into a heart chamber or vessel.
- Cauterization can be used as a diagnostic tool to investigate possible cardiac conditions or used as a form of treatment.
- A specialized subset of cardiac catheterization is coronary catheterization, which involves catheterizing coronary arteries. From angioplasties, valvuloplasties, to stent placements, catheterization procedures take place in state of the art labs.
- During a catheterization procedure, the catheter, or thin, flexible tube, is inserted into a vein in the patient's leg or arm then moved into the arteries or heart.
- Cardiac cath lab nurses can also assist physicians in implanting pacemakers and implantable cardioverter-defibillators (ICDs).
- They must be good with technology and able to learn quickly. The majority of cardiac cath lab nurses work in hospitals and clinics, generally stationed in intensive care units and cardiovascular catheterization labs if they are available.

Case Management Nurse

- A case management nurse is responsible for providing and coordinating the long term care of patients.
- They aim to provide the proper treatments at the optimal times to maintain their patient's health and minimize the opportunity for hospitalization.
- Their duties can include coordinating primary care visits, surgery and other specialized treatments.
- They also assess and monitor their patients, determine their eligibility for treatments or procedures, and make use of all clinical pathways to achieve their desired outcomes.
- Case management nurses generally work with a specific group of patients and conditions, such as AIDS/HIV, cancer, geriatrics and pediatrics.

Certified Nurse Midwife

- Having a baby is an exciting time for any new parents, but ensuring the safe delivery of a healthy baby can be a tricky business.
- Certified nurse midwives are responsible for assisting women who have relatively low risk pregnancies.
- Patients who do not necessarily need the close supervision of a physician during pregnancy and delivery can instead be cared for by a certified nurse midwife.
- These nurses provide routine check-ups during the nine childbearing months, making certain that the baby is developing normally and that the mother's health is optimal.

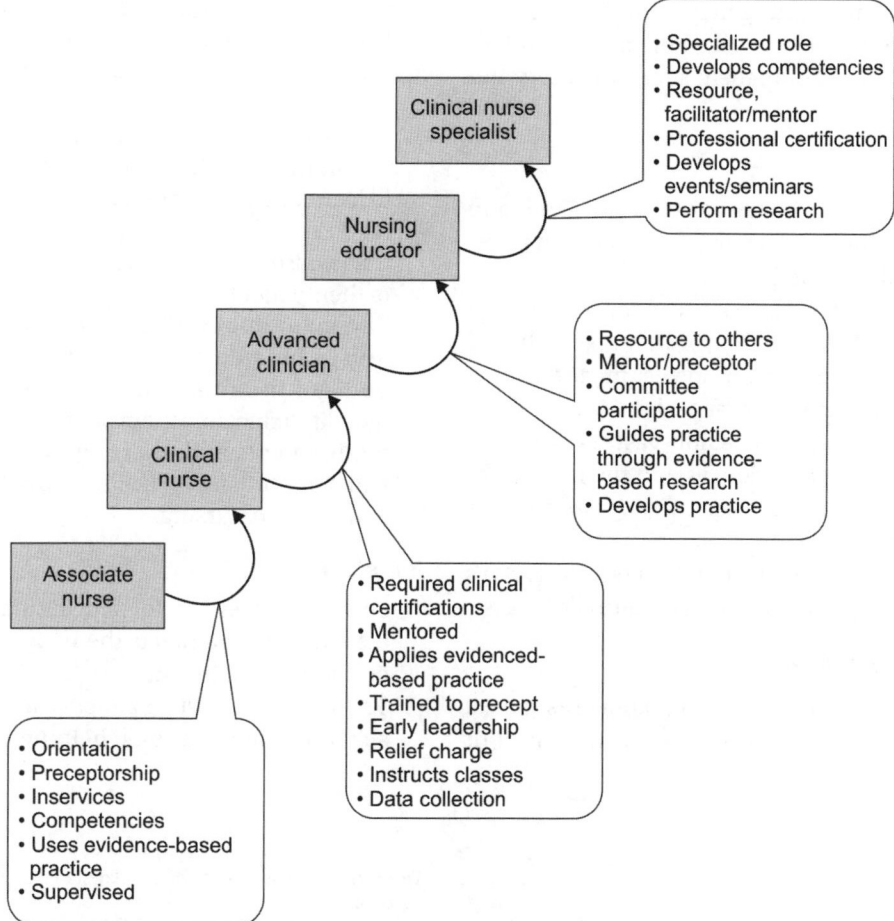

Fig. 25.12: Role of nurse in clinical areas.

Clinical Nurse Leader

- The clinical nurse leader is a new role and certification that has emerged in the healthcare industry.
- They are responsible for overseeing the lateral integration of care for a very specific set of patients and can also actively participate in the care of those patients.
- They also put the latest medical technologies and innovations into practice to provide their patients with the absolute best care possible.
- Clinical nurse leaders collect and evaluate patient outcomes, assess risk and have the decision making authority when it comes to patient care and treatments. **Figure 25.12** shows role of nurse in clinical areas.

Clinical Nurse Specialist

- A clinical nurse specialist (CNS) is an advanced practice nurse with an graduate or doctorate level education.
- They are traditionally found in acute care settings, but are working more and more today in non acute care environments.
- Clinical nurse specialists are experts at diagnosing and treating illnesses and they are responsible for providing evidence based treatments and interventions.
- They also work with other nurses and specialists to provide clinical expertise in an effort to bring about practical improvements to the overall health system.

Correlation Faculty Nurses

- Correctional facility nurses provide care and medical support for inmates of correctional facilities, such as prisons, juvenile homes, jails and penitentiaries.
- They specialize in acute care, such as trauma and influenza. They must also address and be prepared to treat chronic health problems, such as AIDS, substance abuse, mental illness, renal failure and dialysis, respiratory disease and terminal cancer, as well as other infectious diseases, such as TB and hepatitis.

Critical Care Nurse

- Critical care nurses are licensed professional nurses that ensure all critically-ill patients receive optimal care for the illnesses and injuries.
- They perform complex assessments, high intensity therapy and intervention, and advocate on behalf of the patients.
- They employ a specialized skill set and knowledge of the human body in order to care for their patients.
- The critical care nursing umbrella also includes subsets of adult, pediatric and neonatal care.
- The majority of these nurses work in hospital settings where critically-ill patients are present, including intensive care units, cardiac care units, telemetry units,

progressive care units, emergency departments, and recovery rooms. Some critical care nurses also work in nursing homes, schools, outpatient surgery centers and flight units.

Dermatology Nurse

- Nurses in dermatology provide patients with care and education concerning the treatment of wounds, injuries, diseases and conditions of the skin.
- These nurses can screen for skin cancer, assist with dermatological surgery, teach, conduct research and perform such procedures as biopsies, mesotherapy, microdermabrasion and chemical peels.
- The field of dermatology is incredibly vast, as skin is an organ, just like the heart or kidneys and the number of diseases and disorders are just as numerous as with other organs of the body.
- The majority of nurses in this field work for private doctor's offices, usually with plastic surgeons or dermatologists.

Developmental Disability Nurse

- Developmental disabilities nurses, also known as special needs nurses, provide care for those with mental or developmental disabilities, including mental retardation, Down's syndrome, pervasive developmental disorders, autism, Rett's syndrome, Asperger's syndrome and many more.
- These disorders are generally chronic, permanent conditions that develop at birth and affect one's ability to learn and perform basic life skills.
- Aside from working with their patients, these special nurses also provide education and support to the families of their patients.
- The main duties of these developmental disabilities nurses include—assisting patients with feeding and bodily functions, encouraging their independent mobility, educating them on the condition and its medical requirements and assisting the patient with language and communication skills. **Figure 25.13** shows levels of education in nursing.

Diabetes Nurse

- Diabetes nurses care for patients that suffer from diabetes, a condition that affects the body's ability to produce or absorb enough insulin.
- This includes assisting patients in monitoring their blood sugar and medications, helping to minimize diabetic

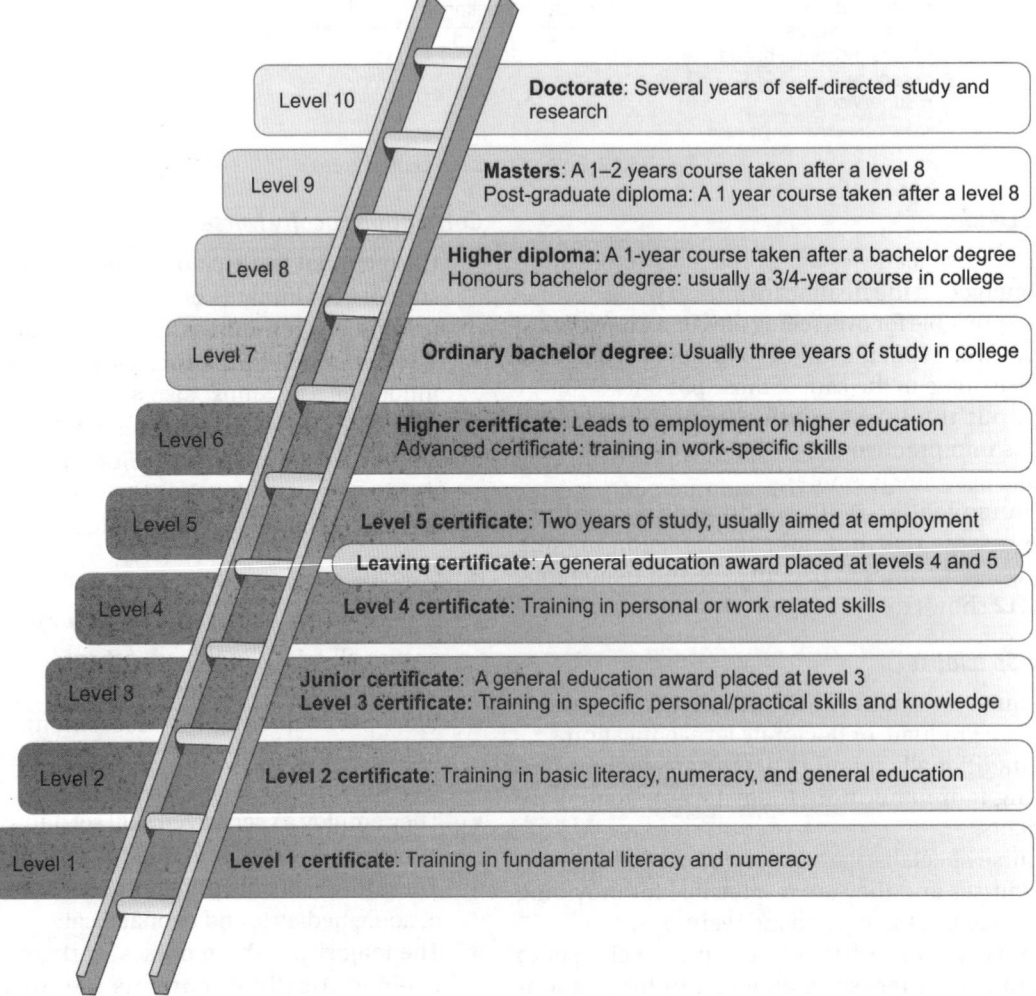

Fig. 25.13: Levels of education in nursing.

nerve damage, conducting nutritional therapy, dealing with psychosocial issues and behavioral management.
- They also spend a considerable amount of time educating patients and families on proper dietary, exercise and lifestyle habits to keep symptoms under control. These nurses also have a specialized knowledge of the endocrine system,

Domestic Violence Nurse

- Also known as violence nurses, violence prevention nurses, child abuse nurses and elder abuse nurses, these types of nursing professionals generally work with children, adults and the elderly to provide care, support and education concerning domestic violence.
- This position is considered a part of the relatively new field of forensic nursing, which links healthcare with the criminal justice system on behalf of the victims.
- These nurses must be incredibly compassionate, sensitive, supportive, and be a voice of advocacy for their victims and patients.
- Their utmost priorities are to keep them safe and care for their wounds physically, mentally and emotionally.

Emergency Nurse

- Emergency nurses provide medical care for patients in the critical or emergency phase of their illness, trauma or injury.
- They must work quickly and efficiently and be able to recognize life-threatening problems and subsequent solutions without hesitation.
- Emergency nurses must possess both general and specific medical expertise as they encounter a wide variety of conditions ranging from sore throats to broken bones to heart attacks for patients of all ages, races, genders and medical backgrounds.
- They can work in hospital emergency rooms, ambulances, helicopters, urgent care centers, sports arenas and any other place a person could encounter an emergency medical condition.

Family Nurse Practitioner

- A family nurse practitioner is a registered nurse that has completed the requirements to become a registered nurse, but also earned an advanced degree as well, either a Master's or Doctorate in Nursing and received training in more specific areas of medicine.
- They provide a broad range of services and can practice independently of a physician.
- Within their scope of duties, FNPs diagnose, treat and manage illnesses and diseases; order, perform and interpret diagnostic tests; prescribe and perform physical therapy and rehab; prescribe medication; assist in minor surgical procedures; and provide many other primary healthcare services.

Flight/Transport Nurse

- Flight nursing, or transport nursing, includes critical care, emergency medical services and disaster response services to patients prior to hospital admittance.
- They are highly trained medical professions that make life and death decisions very quickly.
- They must be able to work well in teams and react quickly to changes in patient and environmental conditions. These nurses can work with patients located in remote areas that cannot reach hospitals in time or disaster sites like car accidents and scenes of natural disasters.
- Flight nurses perform the necessary medical care while airlifting patients to safety and to the proper medical facilities.
- Some flight nurses can even travel with private patients that suffer from dangerous medical conditions during airline flights to ensure their safety

Forensic Nurse

- Forensic nurses are medical professionals trained in evidence collection, the criminal justice system and its procedures, and legal testimony expertise. They specialize in aiding the investigations of crimes like sexual assault, accidental deaths, abuse and physical assaults.
- Forensic nurses are the link between the medical profession and the criminal justice department.
- The majority of forensic nurses work in hospital emergency rooms, interpreting the first signs of wrong doing or foul play.
- Forensic nurses should be thorough, calculating and still sympathetic to their patients and victims.
- Their duties can include taking samples of blood and tissue, photographing and measuring wounds, testifying in court and collecting other vital evidence on the body.

Gastroenterology Nurse

- Gastroenterology nurses, also known as endoscopy nurses, work with physicians in treating and diagnosing patients with conditions affecting the digestive system and gastrointestinal (GI) tract, such as reflux, bleeding, cancer and abdominal pains.
- Other conditions they deal with regularly include carcinoma, ulcers, dysphagia, dyspepsia and the removal of foreign bodies.
- Gastroenterology nurses can work in a variety of setting including acute care hospitals, outpatient clinics, private medical offices and even manufacturing companies.
- A large part of the job of a gastroenterology nurse is also educating their patients on the conditions they have and various ways to manage their symptoms in daily life.

Geriatric Nurse

- Geriatric nurses are especially trained to work with elderly patients. They have experience meeting the healthcare needs of older adults, who are at greater risk of injuries and diseases, such as osteoporosis, Alzheimer's and cancer.

Chapter 25: Professional Advancement

- Geriatric nurses focus on preventing and treating diseases and disabilities in the elderly, and educate older adults and their families on how to cope with certain medical conditions that develop later in life.
- They help rehabilitate patients after injuries, and perform routine screenings, such as mammograms.
- Many times you can find geriatric nurses working in nursing homes, home healthcare services and in hospice facilities caring for bedridden patients, those with impaired mental faculties, and those experiencing severe pain.

Gynecology/Obstetrics Nurse

- Gynecology/obstetrics nurses are also known as OB/GYN nurses, and are especially trained to provide nursing care for women during pregnancy, labor and childbirth, as well as provide nursing care for women with health problems of or related to their reproductive system.
- OB/GYN nursing is a broad field, so nurses often further specialize in a specific area, such as perinatal nursing or labor and delivery nursing at hospitals and birthing centers or in gynecology nursing in a physician's office.
- OB/GYN nurses provide care and support for women from the moment they start their first period all the way through menopause.

Hematology Nurse

- Hematology nurses are especially trained to provide nursing care for patients with blood diseases or disorders. Some of the more commonly-known blood diseases and disorders a hematology nurse may encounter include— leukemia, lymphoma, sickle cell anemia and hemophilia.
- Hematology nurses initiate a plan of care to manage symptoms that result from such blood problems.
- Hematology nursing is often closely associated with oncology nursing, and some nurses will help patients with pain management if their cancer is particularly aggressive.
- Hematology nurses may work with adults only or specialize in working only with children.

HIV/AIDS Nurse

- HIV/AIDS nurses are especially trained to provide nursing care for patients with AIDS, a deadly, incurable disease that attacks a patient's immune system.
- AIDS is the disease that results from contracting the HIV virus. Because AIDS has such a social stigma attached to it, patients often struggle with both emotional and physical symptoms. Therefore, usually part of the role of the HIV/AIDS nurse is to connect AIDS patients to support groups and services.
- One of an HIV/AIDS nurse's biggest responsibilities is helping AIDS patients cope with and manage the disease.

Holistic Nurses

- Holistic nurses are especially trained to assist in providing complementary and alternative medicine (CAM) by itself or in combination with conventional Western medicine when treating patients.
- Holistic nursing is based on the premise that you cannot treat a patient's physical health without addressing the "whole" person—including a patient's mental, spiritual and emotional health and well-being. For this reason, holistic nurses are said to approach nursing in a different way than the average staff nurse.
- Some holistic nurses are certified to provide alternative medical treatments, such as acupuncture; others focus of stress management and incorporate aromatherapy and massage.

Home Healthcare Nurse

- Home healthcare nurses are especially trained to provide nursing care for patients from their homes. Most home healthcare nurses work with the elderly, but some work with younger populations with developmental disabilities and/or limited mobility.
- Home healthcare nurses may work on a long-term basis in end-of-life care; they may also work on a temporary basis, helping to rehabilitate patients so they can regain their physical independence after a serious or complex injury.
- Due to the nature of their work, home healthcare nurses may work with only one patient day after day for months and years at a time, while a staff nurse working in a hospital or clinic will see different patients every day.

Hospice Nurse

- Hospice nurses are especially trained to provide nursing care for dying patients.
- They help those with terminal illnesses to live as comfortably and independently as they can in the time they have left. Hospice patients are not expected to recover, so the primary focus of the hospice nurse is often pain management.
- Hospice patients often have serious terminal health problems due to end-stage cancer, heart disease, renal disease or COPD (a progressive lung disease).
- A hospice nurse closely monitors the patient to identify which stage of the disease the patient has entered, adjusting the pain management and treatment schedule accordingly.

Independent Nurse Contractor

- Independent nurse contractors perform the same duties as other nurses, only they work on a contractual basis rather than being directly employed by a healthcare provider.
- Travel nurses are typically independent nurse contractors as well. Because they work under contract, they are free to choose to work wherever they want for whichever client is in need of their services, including hospitals, outpatient clinics, physician's offices, nursing homes and home healthcare agencies.
- Since the US is currently in the midst of a nursing shortage, independent nurse contractors play a major role

in filling the gap in under-served areas and at medical facilities that are having difficulty hiring and retaining qualified nurses.

Infection Control Nurse

- Infection control nurses, also known as infection prevention nurses, are especially trained to help reduce the number of patient infections in hospitals and other healthcare facilities and to help prevent the spread of communicable diseases.
- To accomplish this, they instruct other nurses and healthcare staff in proper hand-washing and sanitation procedures, as well as study bacterial cultures taken from patients to identify any infections that resulted from the way a patient's healthcare was managed.
- In this way, the infection control nurse helps develop a plan to produce better patient outcomes in the future.

Labor and Delivery Nurse

- Labor and delivery nurses are especially trained to provide nursing care for women who are about to give birth to a baby and who are in labor.
- They monitor the fetal heart rate, the patient's blood pressure, time contractions and examine the mother-to-be to see how close she is to delivering the baby. Labor and delivery nurses also identify any complications.
- Before labor, they educate a woman and her family on the stages of giving birth, and what to expect.
- During labor, they may coach a woman to do breathing exercises and when to push.
- They assist other nurses and physicians in administering pain medications or performing epidurals, episiotomies and C-section deliveries.

Lactation Consultant

- Lactation consultants are especially trained to help new mothers breastfeed their newborn and to recommend solutions for women who are having difficulties breastfeeding their baby.
- They educate mothers on the importance of breastfeeding as well as give them informed advice on positioning and using a breast pump.
- Common problems mothers encounter during breastfeeding that a lactation consultant might address include: latching troubles, pain during nursing and not producing enough milk.
- A lactation consultant may recommend certain products or clothing especially designed for nursing mothers. While lactation consultants work in hospitals, clinics and doctor's offices, many are self-employed.

Legal Nurse Consultant

- A legal nurse consultant provides medical expertise in the proceedings of legal cases.
- They assist attorneys and other legal professions with interpreting complex medical records and charts, consulting on healthcare-related topics and generally understanding medical terminology.
- Their duties can also include medical record research, explaining complex medical information to clients, identifying medical standards of care, preparing reports, and testifying as an expert witness in court proceedings involving worker's compensation, malpractice, fraud, abuse and other medical matters.
- Aside from lawyers, legal nurse consultants can work with insurance companies, hospitals, pharmaceutical companies, clinics and government agencies.

Licensed Practical Nurse

- Licensed practical nurses (LPNs) are also known as licensed vocational nurses (LVNs) in Texas and California.
- They perform both simple and complex medical procedures and tasks under the supervision of a registered nurse or physician.
- They can administer medications and injections, perform measurements, such as taking vital signs, keep records including medical histories, perform CPR, administer basic care, educate patients and families about medical conditions and treatments, collect lab samples, and maintain sterile conditions. In private practices, LPNs can answer telephones, make appointments, keep records and other clerical tasks.

Long-term Care Nurse

- A long-term care nurse is especially trained to provide nursing care for patients of any age who have a chronic illness or disability and need long-term medical care. While the vast majority of long-term care patients are elderly, some are younger and have developmental disabilities or other physical and mental disabilities.
- A patient often moves into a long-term care facility when a stint in the hospital is not enough to rehabilitate them.
- A good many long-term care nurses work in nursing homes and assisted living facilities, but some work in home healthcare.
- Some long-term care nurses also assist patients with activities of daily living, such as dressing, bathing and using the bathroom, but their primary focus is on caring for their health.

Manage Care Nurse

- Managed care nurses are especially trained to evaluate the individual healthcare needs of patients, especially those using social services, and connect them to the most cost-effective healthcare providers who can meet those needs.
- They also educate patients on preventive healthcare and counsel them on getting regular check-ups and taking their children for regular check-ups and vaccinations.
- Managed care nurses emphasize prevention because they know that regular low-cost check-ups can head off higher medical costs later, especially if health problems are caught early.

- Managed care nurses need to have good communication skills and must be comfortable working with diverse populations.

Medical Assistants

- Medical assistants are especially trained to take care of certain administrative and/or clinical duties in doctor's offices, as well as the offices of various specialists, such as OB/GYNs, podiatrists, chiropractors, or optometrists.
- A medical assistant's responsibilities will vary depending on where they work, but many perform routine duties, such as taking a patient's blood pressure, height and weight and collecting lab specimens before a patient is seen by a physician, as well as recording medical histories.
- Medical assistants may report to an office manager or directly to a physician or other healthcare practitioner.

Military Nurse

- Military nurses are especially trained to provide nursing care to military personnel during war and peacetime, overseas and stateside.
- They are best known for setting up triage in warzones and treating soldiers who have been wounded in battle, but a large number of military nurses work in various military hospitals throughout the US Military nurses are also called upon to participate in providing humanitarian nursing care to innocent civilians who fall victim to war injuries or natural disasters.

Missionary Nurse

- Missionary nurses are especially trained to meet both the physical and spiritual needs of people in other nations who are in dire need of healthcare. Not only do missionary nurses treat illnesses and injuries, but they also share their faith with people from other cultures.
- In fact, they tend to believe faith and healing go hand-in-hand. Many missionary nurses also do humanitarian work in third-world countries, and view their work as a calling, rather than a profession. In addition to meeting healthcare needs.

Neonatal Intensive Care Nurse

- Neonatal intensive care nurses are especially trained to work with premature and critically-ill newborns in the neonatal intensive care unit (NICU) of a hospital. These newborns are often born needing immediate medical attention and must be connected to special technology that assists with their breathing and allows them to be fed intravenously to help them gain weight.
- Neonatal ICU nurses work under the direction of one or more physicians, and they are responsible for managing and carrying out an at-risk newborn's plan of care, monitoring the newborn's condition, administering any necessary medications and recording the progress of the newborn's development and recovery.

Nephrology Nurse

- Nephrology nurses are especially trained to provide nursing care for patients with kidney disease or abnormal kidney function.
- One of the most important duties of most nephrology nurses is to assist patients with getting dialysis treatments, the process by which toxins and excess water that would normally be filtered by healthy kidneys are removed artificially from the bloodstream.
- Nephrology nurses implement treatment plans for patients with kidney diseases and disorders, helping the patient to live a fuller and healthier life.
- They also play an important role in educating those who are at risk of developing kidney disease on how to prevent its onset.

Neuroscience Nurses

- Neuroscience nurses work with patients with brain and central and peripheral nervous system disorders, and care for their physical, behavioral, and cognitive needs.
- They provide specialized post-operative care for patients after neurosurgery and work with those that have experienced brain injury, neuro trauma, and spinal damage, as well as patients with conditions, such as multiple sclerosis, motor neurone disease, meningitis, encephalitis and Parkinson's disease.
- The nature of their work requires neuroscience nurses to be sensitive and remain calm as they treat patients who are often confused and restless, as well as those who have experienced severe trauma.
- Neuroscience nurses perform wide variety duties like monitoring neurological exams, administering medication, maintaining health records, and consulting physicians about patient progress.

Nurse Advocate

- A nurse advocate acts as a liaison between patients and their healthcare providers in order to improve or maintain the quality of care that patients receive.
- To help patients make the best decision regarding their health, these nurses educate them about illness, ensure that they understand their diagnosis and inform them about all of the possible treatment options.
- Although nurses take orders from doctors, they must be able to speak up for patients when those orders conflict with what the patients want. With each patient having different circumstances, beliefs, and preferences.

Nurse Anesthetists

- Nurse anesthetists are advanced practice nurses who are especially trained to provide anesthesia and anesthesia-related care to patients before, during and after surgical procedures.
- They also provide anesthesia during therapeutic, diagnostic and obstetrical procedures.
- A nurse anesthetist's patients may be coming in to a physician's office or hospital for a planned outpatient

diagnostic procedure, such as a colonoscopy, or be brought from the emergency room needing emergency surgery. Therefore, nurse anesthetists need to be prepared for a wide variety of situations.

Nurse Attorney

- By earning an education in both nursing and law, a nurse attorney is a professional expert on both legal and health issues. With such a set of unique qualifications, these types of nurses can choose to represent healthcare professionals in court or work to change healthcare policies.
- Nurse attorneys who choose a career in the courtroom work with doctors or nurses that have been wrongly accused of malpractice, as health consultants at law firms and on disputes with insurance companies.
- They analyze personal injury or insurance claims, and are expert witnesses in medical legal cases.
- Nurse attorneys who choose a career in healthcare are involved in advocating certain healthcare policies, lobbying for nursing associations or educating lawmakers about important issues and concerns within the healthcare industry.

Nurse Educator

- Nurse educators teach and mentor nursing students. They oversee instruction to ensure that the education students receive is of the highest quality in order to prepare them for a career in the healthcare field.
- Working in the classroom and practice settings, they design and teach academic curriculum, as well as evaluate curriculum and revise it as necessary.
- They instruct courses in formal academic programs for students working toward a bachelor's or associate degree in nursing, and also teach continuing education programs for nurses looking to advance their knowledge of nursing specialties.

Nurse Entrepreneurs

- Nurse entrepreneurs use their nursing education and business skills to employ themselves, and take on the responsibilities involved in creating a business, such as organization and management.
- They can work on business ventures within the healthcare industry, and even establish, promote and run their own companies.
- Using their creativity and knowledge, they carry out entrepreneurial efforts including the development of medical devices, computerized systems, and home health products.
- Not operating under a specific employer, they can also work independently and provide a variety of nursing services, such as patient care, nursing education, home health and consulting services.

Nurse Executives

- Nurse executives design, facilitate and manage patient care delivery. Mainly involved in management and administrative issues, they plan and develop patient procedures and institutional policies, as well as handle the budgets of healthcare facilities, such as hospitals, nursing homes and health clinics.
- Serving in a leadership position, nurse executives carry out the mission of their organization and are responsible for being effective communicators who value diversity, encourage creativity and demonstrate financial accountability.
- To foster a positive working environment, nurse executives establish and continuously develop professional relationships with staff and fellow colleagues.

Nurse Manager

- Nurse managers coordinate patient services by managing and communicating with all the nurses within their departments.
- These types of nurses supervise employees and evaluate their job performance, and are largely responsible for staff recruitment as well as retention. Along with consistently working with nurses, they also occasionally collaborate with physicians on patient care activities within specific units, and provide assistance to patients and their families.
- Nurse Managers conduct administrative work and handle paperwork pertaining to patients' medical records, department budgets and disciplinary actions against employees.

Nurse Practitioner

- Nurse practitioners are advanced practice nurses who are especially trained to serve as primary and specialty healthcare providers, under the authority of a physician.
- They are educated at the master's level or higher and offer a wide variety of nursing and healthcare services to a wide variety of patients.
- Nurse practitioners may specialize in a particular area, such as family practice, adult practice, women's health, pediatrics, acute care and geriatrics.
- Other specialties might include neonatology or mental health. In most states, nurse practitioners have some degree of prescriptive authority, meaning they can prescribe medications-even narcotics.

Nurse Researcher

- Nurse researchers conduct research on health-related issues in order to improve healthcare services and patient outcomes.
- They are scientists who design and implement scientific studies, and identify research questions, collect and analyze data, and report their findings. Those findings can be applied to practice innovations in patient care and be used to solve clinical problems.
- Through the hard work and dedication of nurse researchers, new and better ways are found to deliver healthcare services, improve the quality of life in chronically ill patients, provide care for patients at the end of life, prevent injury and illness, and inform patients about healthy nutrition, fitness and lifestyle choices.

- Nurse researchers work on individually funded projects, which can involve repetitive and detailed work like collecting and tabulating data, managing databases, reviewing documents, writing grants and recruiting subjects.

Nurse Informaticists

- Nurse informaticists, also known as nurse informatics specialists, are especially trained to help manage, interpret and communicate the vital medical data and information that flows into and out of doctor's offices, hospitals, clinics and other healthcare facility computer systems.
- Nurse informaticists usually work in the information systems department of a healthcare setting, and they are skilled in three primary areas: computer science, information technology and nursing science.
- Nurses are needed in this department to evaluate the computer systems, applications, tools and processes that nurses use to manage healthcare data.

Occupational Health Nurse

- An occupational health nurse provides monitoring and emergency care services in order to prevent job-related injuries and illnesses.
- Combining their healthcare expertise with their knowledge of business, occupational health nurses assist a wide range of work environments with prevention services.
- They help employers carry out health and safety standards, and observe and assess employees' health statuses relating to job duties and work environment hazards.
- Occupational health nurses work closely with employers in the development of health and safety programs and customize them according to each individual organization's type of work, workforce and community.

Oncology Nurse

- An oncology nurse provides care for patients who either have cancer or are at risk of developing it.
- For cancer patients who are critically and chronically ill, these types of nurses monitor their physical conditions and symptoms, create management strategies and prescribe medication, and administer treatments, such as chemotherapy.
- For patients at risk of developing cancer, they provide counseling services in cancer prevention, screening and detection.
- Advanced practice oncology nurses not only serve patients as caregivers but educators, consultants and researchers.

Operating Room Nurse

- Operating room nurses, more accurately referred to as perioperative nurses, provide care for patients before, during and after surgical procedures.
- Using a comprehensive and multidisciplinary approach, they work alongside surgical teams and ensure that patients are receiving the best possible care. Before surgery, operating room nurses interview and assess patients to identify potential problems and determine the proper care they should receive on the day of surgery.
- Working closely with patients and their families, they are able to serve as a liaison between them and the surgical team to provide efficient communication and support.
- During surgery, operating room nurses monitor patients, coordinate patient care, and make sure that the surgical team is providing the best possible patient care.
- They support the surgical team by maintaining a sterile environment and assist the surgeon by selecting and handing him or her instruments and supplies needed for surgery.

Ophthalmic Nurse

- Ophthalmic nurses care for patients who are diagnosed with disorders of the eyes. The eyes are indicators of a person's health, and keeping them in good shape is vital to one's wellness. Therefore, these types of nurses, who work under the supervision of an ophthalmologist, are an essential part of healthcare.
- As vision problems can be related to medical problems, such as hypertension and diabetes, when patients suffer from common eye disorders and diseases, such as glaucoma, cataracts, eye trauma, and partial or full blindness, ophthalmic nurses conduct tests that examine their health in other areas.

Orthopedic Nurse

- Orthopedic nurses care for patients with musculoskeletal diseases and disorders, such as arthritis, broken bones, joint replacements, fractures, diabetes, genetic malformations and osteoporosis.
- They evaluate how these types of problems will interfere with patients' daily lives, and assist in providing the proper treatment to help patients overcome or live with their conditions.
- This can include teaching patients new ways to conduct personal tasks, helping them redesign their personal space for better functionality, and providing them with information about resources, such as support groups or assistance programs.

Otorhinolaryngology Nurse

- Otorhinolaryngology nurses, also known as head and neck nurses, care for patients with head and neck disorders and diseases.
- These medical issues can be related to the throat, such as thyroid problems and tonsillitis, or the ears and nose, such as ruptured eardrums and allergies.
- Patients within the broad medical practice of otorhinolaryngology can also suffer from deformities, such as cleft palates or injuries that have resulted in maxillofacial trauma.
- Nurses in this specialized field perform a wide variety of duties.

Pain Management Nurse

- Pain management nurses care for patients experiencing acute or chronic pain by assessing, treating and monitoring their pain levels.
- They conduct pain assessments by observing patients' physiological signs and behavior as well as through patient self-reports.
- These assessments help to determine if the source of a patient's pain is neurological, muscular, skeletal or visceral, what medical condition is causing pain and what treatments will be the most effective in managing it.
- When it comes to treatment, pain management nurses work alongside other healthcare providers consulting with them about the patients' condition and coordinating their care.

Parish Nurse

- Parish nurses have essentially the same duties and responsibilities as any other nurse. The difference with general nursing and parish nursing is in the fact that parish nurses work within faith communities to provide healthcare services to those of the same religion.
- These nurses educate members of the same faith on health topics, provide counseling, and offer care to patients within the faith community from infancy to adulthood.
- Many parish nurses follow a holistic healing approach, meaning that their view on healthcare is that balance of the body and mind is essential in achieving good overall health.

Pediatric Endocrinology Nurses

- Pediatric endocrinology nurses care for children who have diseases of the endocrine system.
- These young patients, who range from infancy to adolescence, experience problems with physical growth and sexual development, such as constitutional growth delay and intersex disorders, endocrine diseases, such as diabetes and hypoglycemia, and endocrine gland disorders concerning adrenal, thyroid and pituitary problems.
- Nurses in this field work closely with pediatricians and help treat patients by administering medications and providing routine medical care.

Pediatric Nurse

- Pediatric nurses care for patients ranging from infancy to late adolescence.
- They work closely with other healthcare professionals, such as family doctors, pediatric physicians and other nurses, to provide preventative and acute care.
- Typical duties include conducting routine developmental screenings, "well child" examinations, administration of immunizations, and the diagnosis and treatment of common childhood illnesses, such as chickenpox, ear infections and tonsillitis.
- Pediatric nurses also work closely with patients' families, educating them about the role of health during child development and bringing awareness to issues that are vital during childhood, such as child disease prevention, proper nutrition, and growth and development.

Pediatric Nurse Practitioner

- Nurse practitioners are a type of advanced practice nurse. They are registered nurses who are also licensed to provide the same type of basic care that physicians provide, such as diagnosing illnesses and conditions, conducting health examinations, and even prescribing medication and therapy treatments.
- This is unlike lower level nursing where nurses are not allowed to make diagnoses or prescribe treatments without the supervision of a doctor. Those who specialize in pediatrics therefore perform essentially the same duties as a pediatrician

Perianesthesia Nurse

- When people think of the team involved in surgical procedures, they often only think of the work of surgeons, operating room nurses, and anesthesiologists.
- Though these are undoubtedly important figures in surgery, when it comes to patient recovery immediately after surgeries, the work of perianesthesia nurses is key.
- These nurses work with patients who are unconscious due to the use of anesthesia and care for them until after they regain consciousness.
- Though most patients who have undergone surgery with anesthesia wake up calm, perianesthesia nurses must still be prepared to handle the odd cases where patients react aversely to the anesthesia

Prenatal Nurse

- Pregnancy can be a complicated time for many women. Their bodies begin to change and those who are pregnant for the first time or have a history of prior health-related issues need to be constantly monitored to ensure that they and the baby are developing normally.
- Even healthy women pregnant for the second, third, or fourth time need specialized care throughout their pregnancy to make certain that everything is going along normally.
- That is where perinatal nurses come in. Perinatal nurses work with pregnant women to educate them about the things they will experience during the time they will be carrying the baby.

Plastic Surgery Nurse

- As the name suggests, plastic surgery nurses work in the field of plastic surgery. These nurses care for patients who are about to undergo plastic surgery as well as those who are recovering from the procedure.
- They even work in the surgery room alongside surgeons, acting as an extra pair of hands to help surgeons with

the procedure, so that it may be completed as quickly, efficiently, and safely as possible.
- Oftentimes, these nurses are also responsible for prepping the surgery room before the surgery team arrives with the patient.

Psychiatric Nurse
- A psychiatric nurse is, as the name implies, a nurse who specializes in treating patients with psychiatric disorders and conditions.
- Psychiatric nurses treat patients of all ages and commonly deal with those who have been diagnosed with conditions like schizophrenia, bipolar disorder, depression, and psychosis.
- Psychiatric nurses will often administer medication, teach patients and their loved ones how to deal with the behavioral challenges inherent in patients suffering from mental disturbance, and they also often deal with such behavioral challenges themselves.

Psychiatric Nurse Practitioner
- Nurse practitioners typically perform the same duties that physicians and other specialists perform, except that they are much more affordable to employ. Psychiatric nurse practitioners are no exception.
- These nurses perform much of the same duties as psychiatrists. They talk to patients and assess their mental health, diagnose mental illnesses, provide counseling to those who need it, and can even prescribe medications.
- Most psychiatric nurse practitioners act, such as therapists, participating in talk therapies for those whose mental conditions can be remedied with counseling, such as depressed or suicidal individuals, or those with anxiety disorders.
- Some also act as educators, talking over a patient's condition with the patient's family members and loved ones so that these people can better understand the patient's condition and know how to react in certain scenarios.

Public Health Nurse
- All nurses work with patients from the communities surrounding the healthcare facility. This means that in essence, all nurses deal with public health. However, public health nurses work more specifically in this area, striving to improve the health of the public and educate the community on health issues that are prevalent in the area.
- Many public health nurses work with specific populations, such as young children living in poverty. Their work is akin to social service work because they provide aid to that in need.
- These nurses identify populations that are at risk for health issues and work to remedy specific ones, such as the lack of clean water or malnutrition

Pulmonary Care Nurse
- The nursing field has many specialties related to different parts of the human body.
- This is because oftentimes, different organs come with their own set of delicate and complex characteristics and therefore demand specialized expertise and skills.
- Pulmonary care, which is the care of the lungs and respiratory system, is no exception.
- Pulmonary care nurses work with patients who have respiratory problems, such as tuberculosis, asthma, and cystic fibrosis.

Radiology Nurse
- Radiology nurses care for patients who are in the process of undergoing treatment involving various forms of radiation imaging. These include ultrasonography, magnetic resonance, or radiation oncology.
- Radiology nurses have to keep up to date on the latest in radiology technology, so that they can explain to their patients exactly how radiology procedures work.
- The radiology nurse assists the radiologist in preparing patients for procedures, such as CAT scans and MRIs. Nurses prepare patients by easing their worries, administering sedatives, inserting IVs, and monitoring patients while undergoing such procedures.

Registered Nurse
- Registered nursing is the general term for a large group of individuals in the nursing profession. Think of registered nursing as an umbrella term that covers a variety of more specific nursing occupations.
- For example, registered nurses can be surgical nurses, pediatric nurse practitioners, or pulmonary nurses. However, all registered nurses perform largely the same duties no matter what specific niche they work in.
- All registered nurses work to promote health, prevent disease, and help patients cope with illnesses, injuries, and disabilities.
- They also can assist physicians and other healthcare professionals in taking vital signs, recording symptoms, noting treatment progress, looking over health records, and conducting basic examinations and health screenings.

Rehabilitation Nurse
- Rehabilitation nurses aid patients with long-term physical disabilities or other chronic illnesses in learning how to cope with and deal with their limitations.
- A rehabilitation nurse is a rewarding career because it helps others reach their full potential in the face of medical illness.
- On a daily basis, rehabilitation nurses work with patients and their family members shortly after patients begin the recovery process that starts after having experienced a debilitating physical injury or long-term illness.
- Rehabilitation nurses work in a variety of settings that include hospitals, long-term care facilities, home healthcare agencies, or private practices.

Reproductive Nurse
- Reproductive nurses work with families, couples and individuals to provide educational information, treatment and support in the areas of fertility, conception and other matters concerning reproduction.
- They also work with women currently going through menopause, providing them with the necessary information about symptoms and treatment options.
- Reproductive nurses can work in a variety of settings from counseling programs, private reproductive clinics, obstetrics and gynecological practices, hospitals and even egg donor centers.
- These nurses should be especially sympathetic, compassionate and patient as they are dealing with people facing very sensitive life issues

Rheumatology Nurse
- Rheumatology nurses provide support and treatment for patients dealing with Rheumatic diseases including lupus, Lyme disease, Rheumatoid arthritis, fibromyalgia, myositis, and spondylitis.
- Working with these types of patients involves duties, such as monitoring blood work, patient counseling and managing pain and the effectiveness of their medication.
- They can work in a variety of settings from patient assessment clinics, drug surveillance and counseling clinics, private rheumatology practices and hospitals.

School Nurse
- Chances are that when you were a child, you made several trips to the school nurse due to stomach aches, headaches, or a bad cold.
- School nurses are an integral part of keeping school children healthy. They are responsible for caring for students who get sick or injured during school hours.
- School nurses who work at universities may even be available at all hours of the day just in case a student needs medical attention on campus.
- They perform the same duties as any other nurse, including taking vital signs, such as the patient's temperature, recording symptoms, and administering basic medical aid.

Substance Abuse Nurse
- Nurses that work in substance abuse are often specialized in pain management and help to regulate the treatment and administering of medication for patients addicted to drugs, alcohol and other substances.
- To work as a substance abuse nurse, one must have a thick skin, be compassionate and sympathetic. These nurses also spend a great deal of time educating their patients about the dangers of substance abuse and possible treatment options.
- They provide a great deal of support for people that have little else in their lives besides addiction.
- Substance abuse nurses can work in private facilities, mental health clinics, psychiatric wards, hospitals and inpatient or outpatient treatment center.

Surgical Nurse
- Surgical nurses, often called medical-surgical nurses, are especially trained to provide nursing care for patients before, during and after surgery.
- They are valued members of a medical facility's surgical team who assist surgeons, anesthesiologists, and other healthcare professionals during surgical procedures.

Toxicology Nurse
- Toxicology nurses are especially trained to work with patients who have ingested poisons or have otherwise come into contact with hazardous toxins.
- Some toxicology nurses even work with patients who have been bitten by venomous snakes or who are having a severe allergic reaction to a bee, wasp or scorpion sting.
- It all comes down to developing an individual plan of care for patients who have been exposed in one way or another to a poisonous or toxic substance.
- Toxicology nurses often work alongside pharmacists at poison control centers as telenurses, although they may work directly with patients in a variety of other healthcare facilities.

Transplant Nurse
- Transplant nurses are especially trained to provide nursing care and support for patients before, during and after they receive an organ transplant.
- They also work with living donors, educating them on their upcoming surgical procedure, how they should prepare, and any risks involved in donation.
- Living donors are those who voluntarily choose to donate organs and tissues, such as bone marrow, a kidney or even a portion of their liver.
- Other patients, however, receive essential organs, such as a heart or lungs, from donors who have already died.
- Transplant nurses take medical histories, ensure that the proper documentation is signed, order lab tests to confirm an organ match, and clear patients and donors for surgical procedures with the help of one or more physicians

Trauma Nurse
- A trauma nurse specializes in caring for patients who are in a state of emergency.
- This means that the trauma nurse is especially equipped to handle urgent medical situations in which a diagnosis has not been made and the causes of injury or disease are not yet known.
- Trauma nurses often work in emergency rooms and other chaotic environments.
- A typical task assigned to a trauma nurse is the processing of patients in an emergency room setting.
- They also run into a high degree of stressful situations and are often called upon to coordinate with doctors, family members, and other nurses.

Travel Nurse

- A travel nurse is in many ways, such as a Registered Nurse (RN). In fact, all travel nurses are registered; the only difference is that travel nurses work temporary shifts at hospitals around the country and in some cases, overseas.
- The typical domestic shift is 4–13 weeks, while an overseas stint can be for up to a year or two long.
- After receiving the required training, education, and initial experience, a travel nurse first applies through a nursing placement agency.

Urology Nurse

- A urologic nurse is a nurse who specializes in treating patients with diseases related to the kidney, bladder, urethra, and other parts of the human urinary system.
- In some cases, urologic nurses are also involved in the treatment of the male and female reproductive systems. Since urinary and reproductive health are part and parcel of achieving and maintaining a healthy body overall, the work of urologic nurses is both important and rewarding.
- Urologic nurses often deal with kidney or renal stones, which are solidified substances from crystallized urine which impair the proper functioning of the kidney.

Wound Care Nurse

- Wound care nurses, sometimes referred to as wound, ostomy, and continence (WOC) nurses, specialize in wound management, the monitoring and treatment of wounds due to injury, disease or medical treatments.
- Their work promotes the safe and rapid healing of a wide variety of wounds, from chronic bed sores or ulcers to abscesses, feeding tube sites and recent surgical openings.
- The majority of wound care nurses work in hospitals, nursing homes or travel to patients' homes as home health workers.
- Their main objectives are to assess the wounds, develop a treatment plan, clean wounds and monitor for signs of infection. If the wounds become worse, the nurses must be able to recognize symptoms that could require surgical debridement or surgical drains.

■ PROFESSIONAL ORGANIZATION MEMBERSHIP

Nurses in all stages of their professional practice must commit to ongoing career growth and development. Professional nurse organizations offer unique opportunities for networking, career advancement, and promotion of best practice guidelines. Professional nurse organizations may also offer access to mentoring and leadership development that may not be widely accessible to professionals in their employing organization.

Definition

- Professional associations have been defined as groups of people who share a set of professional values and who decide to join their colleagues to affect a change.

—*Poder-Wise (2007)*

- The Professional Organization is the one that provides a means through which efforts can be channeled with authority because of the number it represents. —*Hunt*

Meaning

- Organizations provide a means through which united efforts are made to elevate standards of nursing education and practice.
- It also offers a means of voicing and opinions, developing our abilities and keeping informed of new trends. Nursing regulatory bodies are also known as 'Professional Associations which are responsible for the licensing of nurses within their respective province or territory.
- These regulatory bodies set the enforced standards of nursing practice, Monitor and enforce standards for nursing education, Monitor and enforce standards for nursing practice and set the requirements for registration of nursing professionals.
- The professional nurse must be aware of these associations so as to participate in various nursing professional activities of these organizations.
- To be a part of these associations, the nurse must have life membership with these organizations through proper registration which is must.

Functions of Professional Bodies

- These associations provide a means through which the professional development of a nurse can be channeled with the authority because of its representative character.
- These associations also provide the nurses with the opportunities for expression a of their viewpoints, development of their leadership qualities and abilities
- These associations keep the nurses informed of professional news and trends throughout the country and worldwide.
- To advance excellence in nursing education to prepare nurses to meet the needs of a diverse population in a healthcare diverse population in a healthcare environment.
- To set standards for excellence and innovation of nursing education.
- To focus on specific areas.
- To help in presenting the educational program and publish journals.

Indian Nursing Council

The Indian Nursing Council was authorized by the Indian Nursing Council Act of 1947. It was established in 1949 to provide uniform standards in nursing education and reciprocity in nursing registration throughout the country.

Member Represents

The council is composed of:
- State registration councils
- Central and state health departments
- Military nursing service
- Indian Red Cross Society

important to renew the registration in order to upgrade the status of the nurse within the state register.

Student Nurse Association

The foundation of the National Student Nurses Association (NSNA) was created in 1969 to honor Frances Tompkins, the association's first executive director, organized exclusively for charitable and educational purposes." This association was organized twenty-four years ago, helps to bring students from all over India together for educational, professional, and recreational activities.

The student Nurses Association organized in 1929 is associated under the jurisdiction of the TNAI, in addition to providing a means of personnel and professional development for the nursing students. It serves as a source of membership for the parent organization. In addition, the TNAI serves as the advisor for the SNA.

Functions of SNA are:
- Project undertaking
- Socio cultural activities
- Exhibitions, public speaking and writing
- Organization of conferences
- Maintenance of SNA diary
- Propagation of profession
- Improvement of nursing education to improve healthcare
- Aid in the development of the nursing student
- Encourage optimal achievement in the professional role of the nurse.
- Fund Raising

Christian Medical Association of India

The Nurse's League of the Christian Medical Association (CMAI) was founded in 1930.

CMAI is a registered, non-profit, charitable organization. CMAI is the health arm of National Council of Churches in India (NCCI). They undertake programs in training, researcher community service, institutional consultancy, policy advocacy, interface of theology and medicine, information dissemination and others.

Objectives of CMAI
- Prevention and relief of human suffering irrespective of caste, creed, community, religion and economic status.
- Promotion of knowledge of the factors governing health.
- Coordination of activities for training doctors, nurses, allied health professionals and others involved in the ministry of healing.
- Implementation of schemes for comprehensive healthcare, family planning and community welfare.
- Rendering health in calamities and disasters of all kinds.

Functions of the Nursing Examination Board
- To coordinate and bring a uniform standard of nursing education, in accordance with the requirements of the Indian Nursing Council and State Nursing Council.
- To verify the eligibility requirements of the students before each examination.
- To arrange to conduct examination and issue diploma certificates to successful candidates.
- To maintain and enhance the educational standards of Schools of Nursing by arranging continuing education programs/workshops/exhibitions.
- To prepare the calendar of events at the beginning of each academic year.
- To decide the disciplinary action against students/concerned staff in case of malpractice in examinations.
- To nominate members for the panel of examiner's for 1st, 2nd and 3rd year of GNM nursing examinations.
- To appoint the examiners before annual and supplementary examination.
- To appoint an auditor to audit the board accounts.

The current objectives:
- To promote cooperation and encouragement among Christian nurse
- To promote efficiency in nursing education and services.
- To secure the highest standard possible in Christian Nursing Education through the Christian Schools of Nursing and
- To consider the special work and problems of Christian nurses working.

Nursing considered being an occupation now attains the status of profession.

International Professional Organizations in Nursing

Nurse's organizations may offer general membership or may target specific roles, such as student nurses or critical care nurses. Professional nurse organizations gain strength through the collaborative exchange of ideas, and members benefit from a foundation built on shared professional experiences. The following professional nurse organizations offer a variety of benefits for any registered nurse looking to enhance their career:

The National Student Nurses Association (NSNA)

This nurse organization offers career development support to students who are preparing for initial nursing licensure. The NSNA offers nursing student resource guides, NCLEX resources, and tools for career planning. This professional nurse organization serves as an excellent resource for students who are seeking networking opportunities and information about potential career pathways.

Sigma Theta Tau International Honor Society of Nursing (Sigma)

This organization has 135,000 members and 700 chapters in institutions of higher learning around the world. Sigma was the first organization in the United States to fund nursing research and continues to offer continuing education opportunities, career advice, and leadership development programs to its members.

The American Nurses Association (ANA)

Founded in 1896, the American Nurses Association (ANA) serves as one of the oldest and largest professional nurse organizations in the country. Subsidiaries of the ANA include the American Academy of Nursing, the American Nurses Foundation, and the American Nurses Credentialing Center, making it one of the most comprehensive nurse organizations available to professionals.

The National League for Nursing (NLN)

The NLN was founded in 1893 and is the oldest of the professional nurse organizations in the United States. The NLN represents nursing education in healthcare organizations and institutions of higher learning. The NLN offers extensive opportunities for networking, continuous education, and professional development.

The American Board of Nursing Specialties (ABNS)

The ABNS promotes specialty nurse certification and represents approximately 750,000 certified nurse's around the world. The ABNS promotes lifelong learning and career development as a means to enhance patient safety and improve healthcare outcomes across a variety of practice settings.

Academy of Medical-Surgical Nurses (AMSN)

With more than 11,500 members, the Academy of Medical-Surgical Nurses (AMSN) represents the largest subspecialty of the nursing profession. The AMSN offers clinical practice resources, career guidance, professional development tools, and publications specifically related to the medical-surgical nursing role.

The Emergency Nurses Association (ENA)

This nurse organization currently has more than 42,000 members who practice in diverse emergency department settings across the world. The ENA offers members access to clinical resources, job opportunities, free continuing education, and global networking.

American Association of Critical Care Nurses (AACN)

With over 100,000 national and international members, the American Association of Critical Care Nurses (AACN) is the world's largest specialty nursing organization. The AACN offers critical care certification resources, continuing education opportunities, and networking events that help to support its core values of accountability, innovation, leadership, and collaboration.

American Academy of Nursing

Members of the American Academy of Nursing are among the most educated in our profession, with 90% holding doctoral degrees and the remaining 10% holding masters degrees. The Academy places a heavy focus on advancing the nursing profession through innovative leadership and the distribution of expert nursing knowledge.

State Nurses Organizations

Nurse professionals at all levels should also join their state nurse's organization. Each state may have unique policies and procedures that govern healthcare in that geographic region. Membership in your state nurse's organization provides easy access to leadership and information that directly impacts your day-to-day practice and professional role.

■ RESEARCH ACTIVITIES IN NURSING

The word research means 'to search again' or 'to examine carefully'. More specifically, research is diligent, systemic inquiry or study to validate and refine existing inquiry or study to validate and refine existing knowledge and develop new knowledge. Diligent, systematic study indicates planning, organization and persistence.

- The ultimate goal of research is the development of a body of knowledge for a discipline or profession, such as nursing.
- Research essential to develop and refine knowledge that can be used to improve clinical practice.
- Nursing practice need to be able to read research reports to identify effective interventions for practice and to implement these interventions to promote positive outcomes for patients and families.
- Nursing search is also need to generate knowledge about nursing education, nursing administration, healthcare services, characteristics of nurses and nursing roles.
- The finding from the studies indirectly influences nursing practice and thus adds to nursing body of knowledge.

Purpose of Research

- It unravels the mysteries of life.
- It aims to analyze interrelations between variables and to derive causal explanations.
- It aids planning and helps in national development.
- It aims at finding solutions to problems.
- It helps in the development of general laws.
- It aims at developing new tools, concepts and theories for better study of unknown phenomena.
- It extends knowledge of human being regarding social life and environment.
- It verifies existing facts and theory and these in turn help in improving our knowledge and ability to handle situations and events.

Need of Research in Nursing

- To molding the attitudes and intellectual competence and technical skill.
- Filling the gaps in the knowledge and practice.
- Fostering a commitment, accountability to client.
- Provide basis for professionalism.
- Provide basis for Professional accountability.
- Identity the role of nurse in changing society.
- Discovering new measures for nursing practice.
- Helping to take prompt decisions by the administration to related problems.

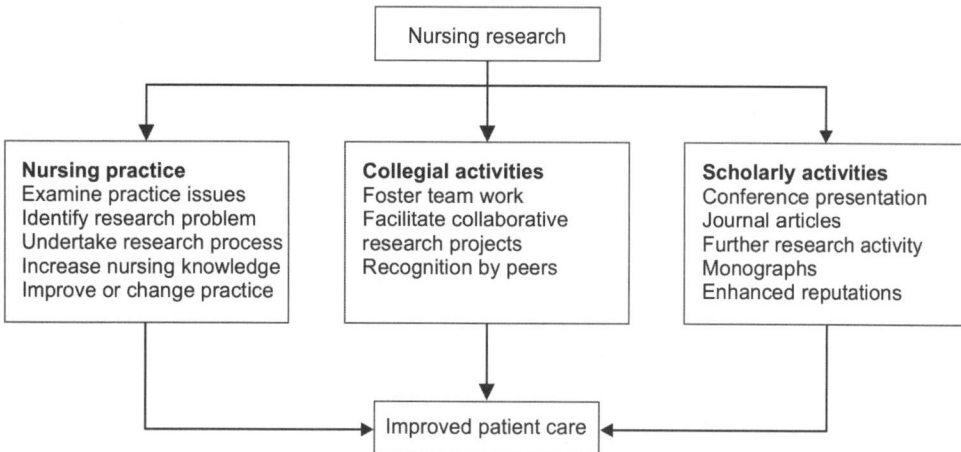

Fig. 25.14: Nursing research areas.

- Helping to improve standards in nursing education.
- Refining existing theories and discovering new theories

Area of Nursing Research (Fig. 25.14)

- **Nursing education:** Research in nursing education may include study of effectiveness of educational programs, strength and weakness of teaching learning process.
- **Nursing administration:** The study includes effectiveness and efficiency of nurse's roles and functions, development of nursing standards, study of planning for nursing manpower, strategies to strengthen nurse's knowledge and performance.
- **Nursing practice:** Research enables nurses to describe the characteristics of a particular nursing situation. It explains the phenomena that must be considered in planning nursing care or to predict the probable outcomes of certain nursing decisions made in relation to client care.
- **Community health nursing:** Several studies are conducted especially relevant to primary healthcare concepts. The spiraling cost of healthcare and the cost containment practices being instituted in healthcare facilities. Nurses are being asked more than ever to document the relevancy and the efficiency of their nursing practice to other, such as consumers of nursing care, administrators of healthcare facilities and government agencies

Characteristics of Nursing Research (Box 25.4)

- Research strives to be objective and logical.
- Research emphasizes the development of generalization, principles or theories.
- Research demands accurate observation and description.
- Research is characterized by patience and unhurried activity.
- Research is directed to solution of problem
- Research is carefully and scientifically recorded and reported.
- Research requires expertise
- Research sometimes requires courage

> **Box 25.4:** Characteristics of nursing research.
>
> - It involves the new and existing data from new sources.
> - It is directed toward the solution of the problem.
> - It emphasizes the development of generalizations, principles, theories that may be helpful in predicting future occurrence.
> - It requires expertise. The researcher must be adequately prepared to undertake such behavior.
> - It is empirical. It is based on direct experience and demands accurate observation and description of what is being studied.
> - It is honest and characterized patient and unhurried activities.
> - It is enable the researcher to achieve valid and comprehensive results.

- Research emphasizes the development of generalization, principles or theories.

Scope of Nursing Research

- To improve the standard of nursing care
- To redefine the existing theories and discovering new theories
- To discover new measures for nursing practice
- To foster a commitment to client
- To provide basis for professional accountability
- To impart professionalism in nursing
- To help in decision making
- To improve standards in nursing education
- To help in documentation
- To bridge the gap between knowledge and practice
- To build the body of knowledge in nursing profession
- To validate improvement in nursing profession
- To make healthcare efficient and cost effective
- To act as a basis for standard setting and quality assurance
- To find solution on immediate practical problems of nursing
- To discover new facts about a known phenomenon
- To discover new message for nursing practice
- To identify the role of the nurse in changing society

Importance of Nursing Research (Box 25.5)

Nursing profession is accountable to society for providing high-quality care patients and families. The healthcare

> **Box 25.5:** Importance of nursing research.
> - To adopt an evidence-based nursing practice (EBP)
> - To improve competent nursing practice
> - To increase body of knowledge
> - To develop new ideas and approaches
> - To improve personal and professional development
> - To improve patient outcomes

provided by nurses must be constantly evaluated and improved based on new information. Nursing's scientific knowledge base is expanding rapidly with the generation of new findings by nurses and other health professional s using a variety of research methods. The knowledge generated through research is essential to provide a scientific basis for description, explanation prediction and control of nursing practice.

Descriptive descried involves identifying the nature and attributes of nursing phenomena and sometimes the relationship among these phenomena (Chinn and Kramer 1995). These studies are often called descriptive or explanatory. This descriptive research is essential ground work for studies that will focus on explanation, prediction and control of nursing phenomena.

Explanation: Relationship among variables is clarified and the reasons why certain events occur are identified. Explanation determining relationships among variables provides a basis for conducting studies for the purpose of predicting and controlling patient outcomes.

Prediction: Through prediction, one can estimate the probability of a specific outcome in a given situation (chin and Kramer 1995). Health promotion research is being conducted to predict the effects of healthy behaviors, such as exercising regularly, eating a balanced diet and not smoking on health status and longevity.

Control: It can be described as the ability to write a prescription to produce the desired results. Control involves imposing condition on the research situation so that biases and confounding factors are minimized based on the research of Meek (1993), nurses could prescribe slow stroke back massage to promote comfort and relaxation in hospice patients.

Objectives of Conducting Nursing Research

- **Improvements in nursing care:** The nursing profession exists to provide a service to society, and this service should be based on accurate knowledge. Scientific research has been determined to be the most reliable means of obtaining knowledge. Clinical nursing research parallels the nursing process. Research finding enable the nurse to describe, explain, predict and control phenomena related to the health of clients.
- **Credibility of the nursing profession nursing:** It has traditionally borrowed knowledge that is distinct from the natural and social sciences, and only in recent years have nurses concentrated on establishing a unique body of knowledge that would allow nursing to be clearly identified as a distinct a unique body of knowledge that would allow nursing to be clearly identified as a distinct profession. The most valid means of developing this knowledge base is scientific research.
- **Accountability for nursing practice:** As nurses have become more independent in making decisions about the care of clients, their independence has brought about a greater need for accountability. Nurses must have sound rationales for their actions, based on knowledge that is gained through scientific research. Nurses have the responsibility of keeping their knowledge base current and one of the best sources of current knowledge is the scientific literature.
- **Documentation of the cost:** effectiveness of nursing care—nursing services can consume a large percentage of a hospital's budget. With prospective payment systems determining the amount of reimbursements that hospitals receive, nursing care services are being closely examined. There are many studied in the literature that demonstrates the cost-effectiveness of nursing care. Ventura et al (1985) conducted a study to examine the cost saving of nursing interventions with patients with peripheral vascular disease. **Figure 25.15** shows short term and long term impact of nursing research. **Box 25.6** describes directions of nursing research.

Research-related Activities in Nursing

- Organizing journal club in a practice setting, which involves regular meeting among nurses to discuss and critique research articles.
- Attending research presentations at professional conferences.

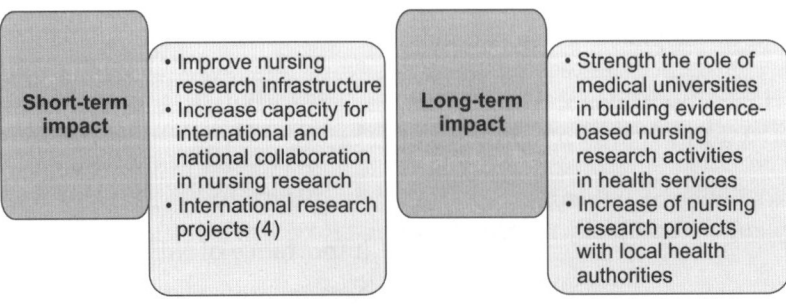

Fig. 25.15: Short-term and long-term impact of nursing research.

Box 25.6: Directions of nursing research.

- Promoting competency for personal care
- Preventing health problems
- Decreasing the negative impact of health problems
- Ensuring that the care needs of particularly vulnerable groups are met through appropriate strategies
- Designing and developing healthcare systems
- Attending research presentations at professional conferences
- Evaluating completed research for its possible use in practice
- Discussing the implications and relevance of research findings with clients
- Giving clients information and advice about participation in studies
- Assisting in the collection of research information (e.g., distributing questionnaires to clients)
- Reviewing a proposed research plan for its applicability in clinical settings
- Assisting with the development of an idea for a clinical research project

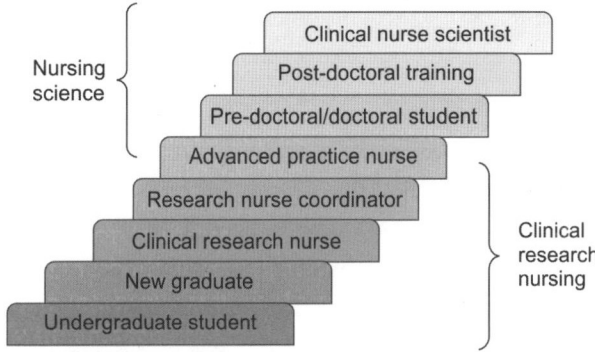

Fig. 25.16: Nursing career path in research at the NIH center.

- Formal evaluation of completed research, for its possible utilization in the practice setting.
- Discussion with clients about the implications and relevance of research findings.
- Providing assistance in collection of research information.
- Review of proposed methods for gathering research information with respect to their feasibility in a clinical setting.
- Contribution in the development of an idea for a research project.
- Participation on an institutional committee whose mission is to review the ethical aspects of proposed research before it is undertaken.
- Incorporation of research findings into nursing practice or nursing education. **Figure 25.16** shows nursing career path in research at the NIH center.

Roles of Nurses in Research

- **Principal investigator:** Nurses can and should serve as principal investigators in scientific investigations. To be a principal investigator, special research preparation is necessary.
- **Members of a research team:** Nurses may act as data collectors or administer the experimental intervention of the study. As nurses increasingly participate in research, it is possible that interest and enthusiasm to conduct their own investigations may grow.
- **Evaluator of research findings:** All nurses should be involved in the evaluation of research findings. As research consumers, nurses have the obligation to become familiar with research findings and determine the usefulness of these findings in the practice area. The evaluation of research is not an easy task.
- **User of research findings:** After evaluating research findings, nurses should use relevant finding in their practice. The primary goal of nursing research, as has been mentioned, is the improved care of clients. However, nurses must be judicious in their use of research findings.
- **Client advocate during studies:** Nurses have the responsibility to act as client advocates when clients are involved in research. Nurses can help answer questions and explain a study to potential participants before the study begins. They also can be available during the study to answer questions or provide support to study participants.
- **Subject in studies:** Nurses also can act as subjects in research. Many nurses are involved in a long-term survey study that is being conducted by researcher at Harvard Medical School, with funds provided by the National Institute of Health.

Nurses use research to provide evidence-based care that promotes quality health outcomes for individuals, families, communities and healthcare systems. Nurses also use research to shape health policy in direct care, within an organization, and at the local, state and federal levels. Nurses conduct research, use research in practice, and teach about research. **Figure 25.17** shows participatory action research goals.

PUBLICATIONS IN NURSING

Writing for publication in nursing is essential to disseminate evidence, share initiatives and innovations with others, provide new information to keep nurses up-to-date, communicate the findings of research studies, and develop the science base of the profession. Writing manuscripts is hard work, but the process can be simplified by understanding how to develop a manuscript and submit it for publication. Writing for publication in nursing was prepared for beginning and experienced authors, for nurses who want to learn how to write for publication, and for graduate students in nursing who need to learn how to write research reports, clinical articles, systematic reviews, and other types of articles.

Need of Good Writing Skills in Nursing

Nurses of all levels use writing to convey information to a wide variety of audiences. Clear written communication is vital for the care of patients as well as for research and staff supervision. Good writing promotes the use of critical thinking and analysis and ensures that different audiences of a nurse's writings will understand what is being said.

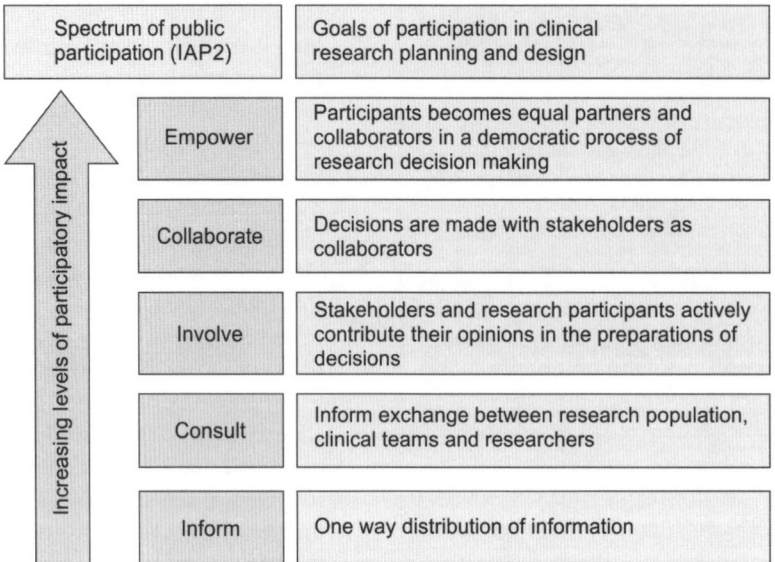

Fig. 25.17: Participatory action research goals.

Writing for peers: Nurses may write case studies, lab reports or research findings, depending on what area of nursing they work in. Having technical writing skills, the ability to research and analyze treatments and processes, for example, is important in sharing nursing information with peers. Other staff nurses can benefit from such studies, and research is further advanced when one nurse's ideas and observations are clearly shared with other nurse researchers. Dissemination of research and case studies that are in written form further new ideas in nursing, helping nurses stay on top of the latest developments in their fields.

Faculty: College nursing faculty find it more and more common to write and publish articles in their discipline. Some undergraduate nursing students are also publishing more. As the Internet becomes more widely available, some journals are going online, providing nurses another area in which to publish. It is vital, therefore, that nurses develop good writing skills that focus on researching, supporting findings and evaluating findings and cases with a critical eye.

Policy: Nurses may work in teams to write policy suggestions for health boards or for politicians. Good writing skills are necessary to explain and persuade audience members who do not have nursing backgrounds. Understanding how to convey information to audience members who are not aware of nursing language and issues is important to effectively advocate for positive change in the healthcare field.

At work: Nurse administrators must be able to communicate effectively in writing with their staff members. Staff meetings require clear and succinct agendas. Reports require clear communication of cases and findings, which are often written for supervisors or board members of healthcare facilities. Email communications with staff also necessitate having good writing skills. Writing manuals and policy or procedure documents also means that nurses must be able to coherently put together a paragraph and logically construct a document. Staff nurses who write on charts and document changes in status must also be able to write clearly, even if it is usually in sentence fragments or using abbreviations. **Box 25.7** shows different types of publications and **Figure 25.18** shows steps in writing in nursing.

Box 25.7: Different types of publications.
- Newsletter
- Professional magazine
- Popular magazine
- Academic (peer-reviewed) journal
- Hybrid journal
- Poster
- Book review
- Book chapter
- Book (single author)
- Book (edited collection)
- Other opportunities—conference presentation, radio broadcast, television, social media

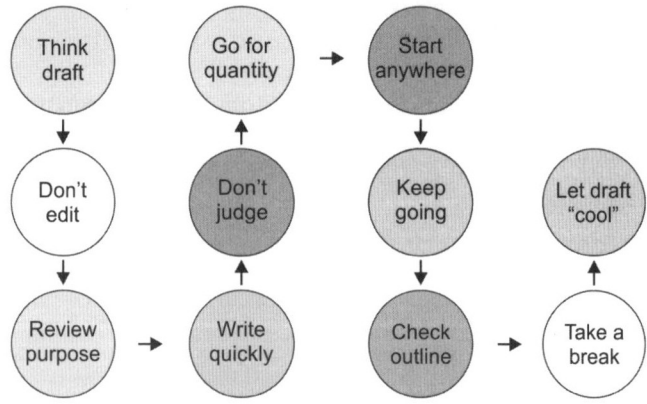

Fig. 25.18: Steps in writing in nursing.

Reason for Writing in Nursing

Writing for publication is an important skill for nurses to develop. By communicating initiatives and innovations in clinical practice, findings of research studies and evidence-based practice projects, and new ideas, nurses direct the future of their practice and advance the development of the profession. As nursing attempts to build its evidence base, it is increasingly important for nurses to write about studies they are doing in their clinical practice: the findings of these studies provide the evidence for practice.

There are five main reasons to write for publication:
1. To share ideas and expertise with other nurses;
2. To disseminate evidence and the findings of nursing research studies;
3. For promotion, tenure, and other personnel decisions;
4. For development of own knowledge and skills; and
5. For personal satisfaction

Share Ideas and Expertise

- Writing for publication provides a way of sharing ideas with other nurses. Through publications, nurses can describe best practices; innovations developed for patients, staff, and students; and new techniques they are using in clinical practice, teaching, management, and administration.
- Publications keep nurses abreast of new developments in nursing. McGaghie and Webster (2009) identified the opportunity to share knowledge with others as an intrinsic motive to write for publication.

Disseminate Evidence and Research Findings

- For nurses involved in research studies and evidence-based practice projects, writing for publication is critical: disseminating research findings and the outcomes of projects to evaluate the effectiveness of nursing interventions are essential to build the knowledge base of nursing, provide new evidence for practice, and develop studies that build on one another.
- Many clinicians are engaged currently in evidence-based practice projects. Some of these projects are to review and synthesize the available evidence to decide on best practices or if a change in practice is warranted

Meet Promotion, Tenure, and Other Job Requirements

- For nursing faculty in colleges and universities, writing for publication is required for promotion, tenure, and other personnel decisions. Not all articles carry the same weight in these decisions.
- Typically, database papers, which report the findings of a research study, published in peer-reviewed journals are highly valued and more important in tenure and promotion decisions than other types of publications, such as non-database articles, chapters, and books.
- McGaghie and Webster (2009) suggested that articles that report original research data (database) and are published in peer-reviewed journals are the "gold standard" for faculty in academic settings.

Expand Personal Knowledge and Skills

- Another reason to write for publication is the learning gained in the process of preparing the manuscript.
- Rarely is the nurse able to write a manuscript without completing a thorough review of the literature.
- This literature review and the thinking that is done in developing the manuscript contribute to the knowledge base and understanding of the author.
- Writing skills are useful in many settings as nurses fulfill both professional and personal roles.
- Writing about a topic facilitates understanding it and oneself. A good writer, i.e., a well-practiced writer, brings a valuable skill to endeavors that range far beyond writing for publication.

Gain Personal Satisfaction

- Writing also gives the nurse a sense of personal satisfaction in sharing expertise with other nurses and contributing to the development of their profession.
- Most journals do not pay authors for their manuscripts; however, writing for publication is personally fulfilling.
- Winslow, Mullaly, and Blankenship (2008) suggested that through publications, nurses share with a wider audience their stories about personal and professional challenges they experience in the work setting on a daily basis and their satisfactions.

Steps in Writing for Publication

Every article written for publication begins with a planning phase; progresses to writing a draft, revising it, and submitting the final copy to the journal; and concludes with its publication. These phases, which provide a framework for the organization of the book, are discussed in more detail in later chapters.

I. **Planning phase:** Prior to writing the manuscript, the author proceeds through a series of steps. These steps are important to assist the author in selecting a topic that is publishable, choosing an appropriate journal with readers who are interested in the topic, and gearing the content and format for the journal. The unpublished document submitted to a journal for review is called the manuscript or paper (American Medical Association, 2007). Once that document is published, it is referred to as an article.

Identify purpose of manuscript: The first step in the planning phase is to identify the topic and purpose of the manuscript. In some cases, the purpose is to present research findings, describe evidence-based practices, and explain how practice changes were made based on a review of the evidence. The intent of other manuscripts may be to present new nursing interventions and approaches to managing patient problems, describe nursing interventions for patients with particular health problems, analyze trends and issues in practice, and present new directions in nursing education or management.

Decide on importance of topic: After deciding on the purpose of the manuscript, the author needs to ask if the ideas to be presented are worth writing about. Will the paper present important information that readers need? The goal in this step in the writing process is to avoid preparing a manuscript that has a limited chance of being accepted for publication. The author can ask to evaluate if the manuscript is worth writing and if the content is important enough to warrant publication. The author should answer these questions before spending any more time on the manuscript.

II. **Writing phase:** The writing phase involves preparing the first and subsequent drafts of the manuscript, completing the final revision, and submitting the manuscript to the journal. The steps in the writing phase include:
1. Develop a formal or an informal outline to guide writing.
2. Write the first draft focusing on presenting the content rather than on grammar, spelling, punctuation, and writing style.
3. Revise the first and later drafts continuing to focus on the content of the manuscript.
4. Then revise the manuscript for grammar, spelling, punctuation, and writing style.
5. Prepare tables, figures, and the references paying close attention to the journal's format for references.
6. Prepare the final version of the manuscript, accompanying materials required by the journal, and the submission or cover letter, and
7. Submit the manuscript to the journal.

III. **Publishing phase:** The final phase in writing for publication occurs after the manuscript is submitted to the journal. The manuscript is critiqued by peer reviewers who have expertise in the topic or methodology and can assess its quality. Peer reviewers provide feedback to authors on needed revisions to strengthen the manuscript and to the editor on the suitability of the manuscript for publication in the journal. It is through this process that the best papers are accepted for publication, ensuring quality of the information and meeting ethical standards. Editors of nursing journals are nurses who have expertise in the content area of the journal. The final decision on acceptance of a manuscript is made by the editor, considering the peer reviews, the editor's own assessment of the quality and suitability of the paper for the journal, and other factors, such as how many similar papers have been published or are in the queue to be published and upcoming themes planned for the journal **(Figs. 25.19 and 25.20)**.

Importance of Writing in Nursing

- Writing for publication is an important skill for nurses to develop. By disseminating new initiatives and innovations in clinical practice, research findings, and other ideas

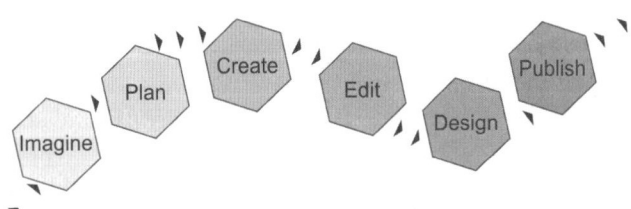

Fig. 25.19: Publication in nursing.

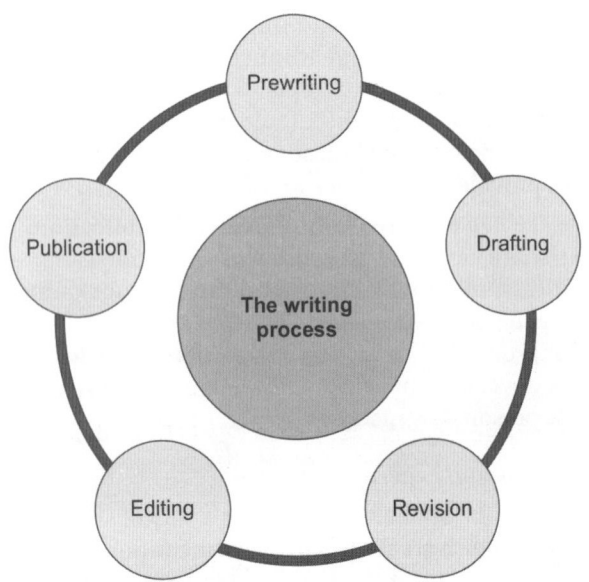

Fig. 25.20: Writing process.

about nursing, nurses direct the future of their practice and advance the development of the profession.
- There are barriers to writing, but the nurse can overcome these by setting due dates for completion of writing projects, meeting these deadlines, and using wisely the available time for writing.
- Every article written for publication begins with a planning phase; progresses to writing a draft, revising it, and submitting the final copy to the journal; and concludes with its publication.
- The manuscript or paper is the unpublished document submitted to a journal for review; once published it is referred to as an article.
- The first step in the planning phase is to identify the topic and purpose of the manuscript.
- After deciding on the purpose of the manuscript, the author needs to assess if the ideas to be presented are worth writing about. Will the paper present important information that readers need? To determine this, the author should do a literature review on the topic and related content areas.

Barriers to Writing (Fig. 25.21)

Writing is time consuming, and authors may be frustrated as to their progress.

In preparing the manuscript, developing a publishable paper requires practice, and the more writing the author does, the easier will be completion of the manuscript. Similar to the development of clinical skills, writing improves with practice. Some of the barriers to writing are a lack of understanding of this process, writer's block, lack of time, and fear of rejection.

Lack of understanding of how to write for publication: Many faculty members have had limited experience in writing for publication and are unsure of the process but need to publish in their academic settings. Similarly, clinicians may be reluctant to assume the role of author because they too are

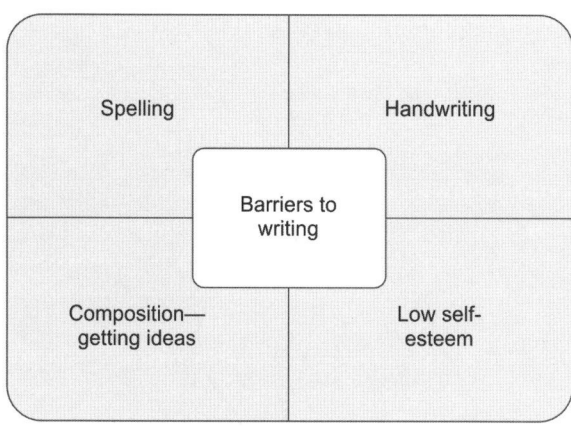

Fig. 25.21: Barriers to writing.

unsure of the process of manuscript development and have never been prepared for this role in their nursing education programs.

Writer's block: Some authors experience writer's block that keeps them from writing. This may occur from anxiety about the project, uncertainty as to how to proceed, and past unsuccessful experiences with writing. It is important for authors to be clear about the topic and intent of their writing project-recording these on paper before beginning, discussing them with colleagues, and "presenting" ideas to others often help to avoid writer's block.

Lack of time: The extensive time for preparing a manuscript is another barrier to writing. Time is needed for preliminary work, such as developing the idea and reviewing the literature, for preparing the draft and rewriting it until suitable for submission, and for subsequent revisions suggested by the editor and reviewers. In a qualitative study of 16 novice researchers, many viewed writing as complex and demanding, particularly when considering their other responsibilities; they identified barriers, such as a lack of time, procrastination, and anxiety, among others. Time for writing is a problem encountered by both novice and experienced authors.

Fear of rejection: One other barrier to writing is fear of rejection. In submitting a manuscript, the author is open to criticism and possible rejection; for some nurses this is a barrier to writing for publication. Having a manuscript rejected is part of the writing process and may not be related to the quality of the writing. The manuscript may be rejected because a similar one has already been accepted, or the information in the manuscript is not new enough for publication in that particular journal. Rejections for reasons, such as these do not mean that the ideas are questionable or poorly presented

CONCLUSION

Continuing professional advancement activities for nurses are planned and organized learning experiences, designed to advance personal and professional development. Activities can include the attendance of workshops or conferences, reading of journal articles and the undertaking of postgraduate nursing course. Professional development may be undertaken in the form of postgraduate courses, vocational education and continuing professional development. Continuing professional advancement is defined as a means by which members of profession maintain their knowledge and skills and develop qualities in their professional lives. The conscious updating of professional knowledge and the improvement of professional competence throughout a person's working life. It is a commitment to begin professional, keeping up to date and continuously seeking to improve. It is key to updating a person's career opportunities.

REVIEW QUESTIONS

Long Essays
1. Define continuing education; explain the need, goals and philosophy.
2. Explain the types of continuing education.
3. Describe career opportunities in nursing.
4. Enumerate the functions of professional bodies.

Short Essays
1. Principles of continuing education.
2. Continuing education in nursing.
3. Principles of continuing education.
4. Scope of continuing education.
5. Benefits of continuing education.
6. Different education levels in nursing.
7. Professional organization membership.
8. International professional organizations in nursing.
9. Research activities in nursing.
10. Publications in nursing.

Short Answers
1. Planning for continuing education.
2. Importance CNE in nursing.
3. Changing technology.
4. Career advancement.
5. Online courses.
6. Critical care nurse.
7. Nurse practitioner.
8. Nurse entrepreneurs.
9. Need of research in nursing.
10. Research-related activities in nursing.
11. Steps in writing for publication.
12. Barriers to writing.

Index

Page numbers followed by *b* refer box, *f* refer to figure, and *t* refer table.

A

Academic audit, principles of 550
Academy of Medical-Surgical Nurses 608
Accident investigation 78
Accountability 106, 260, 499, 610
   creation of 260
Accounting 401
Accreditation
   agencies, types of 579
   concept of 491
   functions of 579
   laws, absence of 316
   objectives of 492
   purpose of 491, 578
Accrediting nursing institutions,
   benefits of 492
Accuracy 306, 423
Achieving organizational objective 88
Activity
   grouping of 88, 89
   plan 330
   principles 501
Actual performance, measurement of 283
Acute care
   hospitals 112
   types of 98*f*
Adaptability 115
Additional revenue stream 431
Ad-hoc committee 387
Administration 8, 9*f*, 413
Administrative
   law 571
   records 423, 519
   statistics 110
Administrator, role of 520
Admission
   discharge and transfer 425, 428
   eligibility for 464, 465, 479, 481, 486
Adult education 184
   scope of 181
Adult learner, characteristics of 180, 181, 181*b*
Adult learning 180*f*, 184*f*
   characteristic of 180*b*
   principles of 182, 183*f*
Adult nurse practitioner 582
Advanced practice nurse 582, 589, 591
Advanced professional development 256
Advertisements 131, 446
Advisory committees 386
Advocacy 41
Affiliation 478
   criteria for 478
Agreement 276
All-round development, principle of 218
Ambulance attendants, police,
   mass media room 81
Ambulatory care nurses 591
American Board of Nursing Specialties 608
American Nurses Association 608
Analysis 413
   paralysis 230
   three levels of 336, 337*f*
Analytical procedures 206, 300
Analytical review 203, 298
Analytical skills 394
Annual leave 165, 540
Annual performance reviews 138
Annual reports 360
Anticipating organizational events 339
Anti-ragging committee 524
Apie charting 425
Appointment letter 448
Appropriate language, principle of 382
Appropriate techniques, principle of 212
Arousal theory, optimum level of 374
Assault 572
Assertive communication
   model 384, 384*f*
   techniques of 385*f*
Assignment 90, 230
   purposes of 155, 230
Assistant professor, job description 496
Assisted living center support 432
Assisting school staff 544
Associate nurse 159
Associate professor, job description 495
Attention, principle of 382
Audio-visual aid 473
   room for 477, 483
Audit 199, 296
   benefits of 203, 298
   characteristics of 200, 297, 406, 517
   committee 204, 205, 299, 387
      duties of 204
      powers of 387
      responsibilities of 204
   cycle 405*f*
      advantages of 208*t*
      disadvantages of 208*t*
      steps of 206, 207*f*
   essential features of 201*f*
   evidence
      procedure for obtaining 205, 299
      reliability of 205 205*b*, 299
   methods of 201
   objectives of 200, 200*f*
   procedure 203*f*, 205*f*
   process 201, 206, 207
      steps in 201
   report examples 407*f*
   risk 203*f*
   techniques 202
   types of 201, 201*f*, 297, 299*f*, 405, 517
Auditing 200, 297, 405, 517
   principles of 202, 202*f*, 297, 406, 517
   six principles of 297*f*
   techniques of 202, 298
Auditorium 476, 482
Authoritative leaders 250
Authority 15, 260
   classical theory of 21*f*
   distribution of 89
   grant of 260
   lack of 262
   lines of 107*b*, 400, 401, 516
   responsibility structure 88
   threat 261
   three bases for 21
Authorization 403
Autocratic coaching 268
Autocratic leadership 245, 245*f*, 246*b*
Autocratic style 237
Auxiliary nurse midwife 154, 471
   roles of 474*b*
AYUSH 58

B

Backward pass 332
Balance 244
   sheet 515
Balancing act 46
Bargaining 367
   types of 370*b*
Basic amenities, lack of 433
Basic managerial functions,
   performance of 8
Basic policies 292
Beds, distribution of 478
Bedside nurses, classes for 179
Behavior
   behearsal 385
   in in-service program, observation of 178
   organizational 336, 336*f*
Behavioral bias 339
Behavioral issues 166
Behavioral parameters 226
Behavioral science 19*t*
   theories on 22
Behavioral theories 243, 271

Benchmarking 313
   concept of 327
   cost of 329
   cycle 329f
   limitations to 329
   principles of 328t
   process 328, 328f
   types of 328, 328f
Beneficence 565
Benefits 119
   discounting future value of 409
   plans 144
Bill, purpose of 144
Bioinformatics 429
Bottom level behaviors 337
Brainstorming 273, 314
Breach sanctions, practice standards for 573
Brochure 356
BSc nursing program, objectives of 480
Budget 75, 396, 396f, 400, 400b, 402, 515
   audit 405, 517
   benefits of 400, 515
   characteristics of 397, 515
   classifications of 398, 515
   committee 401, 516
   essential requisition for 401, 516
   limitations of 400, 401f, 516
   period of 401, 516
   plan, stages of 404
   preparation 399
   principles of 397, 397b
   purpose of 397, 397b, 515
   types of 398, 398f
Budgetary control 285
Budgeting 25, 32, 188, 396
   objectives of 396, 396f, 514
   process, steps in 399
   purposes of 403
   terminology 514
Build self-regulation skills 454
Build work environment 242
Building resilience, components of 453
Bureaucratic leaders 245
Burns
   care of 82
   units 153
Business
   cycle, principle of 392
   diversification of 95
   lending 35
   objectives orderly achievement of 8
   policies 401
   sense 39

C

Camp nurse 591
Canteen 477, 484
   facilities 539
Capital
   composition, determination of 392
   expenditure budget 398, 515
   requirements, estimation of 392
   structure management 395
Cardiac care nurse 591
   role of 592f
Cardiothoracic beds 488
Care
   and services, delineate scope of 318
   continuity of 97
   delays 433
   environment of 112
   giver 354, 552, 580
   philosophy of 499
   standards of 574
   type of 97
Career
   advancement 587
   anchors 459
   development 136, 533
      process 136
   elements of 459
   growth 140
   planning 458, 459
      and career development, features of 459
      benefits of 460
      limitations of 461
      nature of 459
      objectives of 459
      process, steps in 459, 460f
Carrot and stick approach of motivation 375
Cash
   budget 398
   management of 392, 393
Casual callers 131
Casual leave 165, 540
Casualty officers 82
Catastrophes 83
C-charts 314
Celebrate wins 230
Center level healthcare administration 50
Central Council of Health 53
Central Council of Indian System of Medicine 492
Central Government Health Scheme 52, 57
Central Health Education Bureau 52
Centralized in-service training 178
Certification 137, 320, 578
Certified nurse midwife 582, 592
Channel conflict management 274f
Character building, principle of 502
Charismatic leaders 245
Charismatic power 262
Chief medical and health officer 54
Chief nursing officer 146
Child-centered curriculum 501
Christian Medical Association of India 365, 607
Civil law 571
   penalties 573
Classic organization theory 20
Clear vision 242, 251
Client advocate 354, 611
Clinical alert system 414
Clinical expertise 39, 40
Clinical facilities 473, 478, 485
Clinical instructor
   job description 497
   responsibility of 513
Clinical nurse
   leader 593
   managers 40
   performance appraisal, problems of 531f
   specialist 582, 593
Clinical nursing practice, uses of computers in 425b, 428
Clinical posting faculty role in 233, 514
Clinical rotation plan 232, 512, 513f
Coaching 42, 251, 253, 268
   leaders 250
   leadership
      cons of 269
      elements and characteristics of 268
      pros of 269
   mind-set 269
   styles of 268
Code learning events 509
Coercive leaders 250
Coercive power 262
Cognitive interest 182
Cognitive theories 374
Collaboration 268, 360, 499
Collaborative care giver 552
Collective bargaining 365, 367, 367f, 370
   advantages of 366t, 371
   characteristics of 369b
   disadvantages of 366t
   essential prerequisites for 368
   features of 368
   functions of 370, 370b, 370f, 371
   history of 367
   levels of 371
   objectives of 367, 367b
   principles of 368, 369b
   process of 366f, 369, 369f
   pros and cons of 371
   types of 370, 370f
College management committee 485
Commitment 256, 376, 558
Committees 385, 520, 605
   advantages of 388
   common types of 387
   disadvantages of 388
   members of 386f
   organization, purposes of 386
   types of 386, 387
Common ethical dilemmas 566b
Common law 571
Common legal issues 572
Common nursing service
   activities 130
   approaches 130f
Commonwealth nurses federation 363
Communicable diseases, programmes for 58
Communicating guidelines and standards 317
Communication 83, 105, 112, 138, 151, 212, 213, 228, 274, 276, 311, 312, 343, 352, 380, 381f, 394, 403, 419, 420, 463, 464, 518, 534, 552, 570
   advantages of 384

Index

barriers of 383, 383f
disadvantages of 384
elements of 381, 381f
facilitating flow of 215
nature of 380
principle of 211
skills 40, 453, 558
theories of 382
types of 382
Communicative methods 359
Communicator 354, 581
Community 203, 298
   clinical facilities 511
   health center 55
   health nurse 154, 559, 609
      role of 154f
   level healthcare administration 55
   public relations in 358, 359
   records used in 519
   relations 356
   resilience 453
   setting 427b
Company, organizational aspects of 350
Compensation 119, 121, 533
   decisions 533
Compensatory holidays 165, 540
Competency 436
Competition 32, 76, 120
Competitive benchmarking 327
Competitors 33
Complete communication 158
Compliance 203, 298, 413
   issues 166
   test 203, 298
Composite bargaining 370
Comprehensive guidance and counseling, planning for 548
Computer assisted
   charting 425
   surgery 427
Computer
   and nursing, historical perspectives of 428
   in education 428
   in hospital, use of 425, 426, 426b
   in nursing 428f
   skills 416
   techniques, use of 203, 298
   uses of 425b, 426, 428
Concessionary bargaining 370
Concurrent audit 201, 297, 405, 517
Conducting nursing research, objectives of 610
Confidence 240, 242, 376
   development of 215
   establishment of 215
Confidential report 531
Confidentiality 306, 424, 561, 565
Confirmation 203, 205, 298
Conflict 115
   causes of 549
   management 273
      skills 273, 274
      styles 273, 273f
      concept of 273

Confusion 251
Conservative principles 501
Consistency 202, 297, 517
   principle of 382
Constitutes good protocol 294
Constitutional law 571
Consultation 413, 519, 580
Consultative system 24
Consumer Protection Act 575, 575f, 576
Contingency theories 243
Continuing education 164, 175, 177, 535, 536, 585f
   philosophy of 585
   planning for 586
   principles of 586, 586b
   scope of 586
   types of 587, 587f
Continuing nursing education 61, 523
   benefits of 588f
   certification, process for 587f
   purpose of 584
Continuity, principle of 219
Continuous internal assessment 553
Contribution plans 144
Control over
   cost 287
   organization 287
   personnel 287
   wages and salaries 287
Control responsibility, principle of 284
Controlling 15, 30, 32, 281
   climate 44
   function, features of 281
   process of 283, 283f, 381
Convenience 431, 439
Cooperation, principle of 219
Coordinating 25, 30-32, 249
   home, school, and society 543
Coordination 89, 90, 94, 95, 95f, 213, 242, 286, 387, 403, 544
   benefits of 95
   essential elements of 95
   features of 95
   principles of 94
   types of 95
Coping skills 451, 453
Corporate hospitals 98
Corrective actions, limitations of 284
Correlation faculty nurses 593
Cost
   documentation of 610
   effectiveness 37, 127
   efficiency 329
Cost-benefit analysis 407, 407f
   approach 409
   principles of 408, 408b
   purpose of 408
   steps in 408f
   use of 408, 409b
Council mission and vision of 470
Counseling 542, 544
   characteristics of 544
   concept of 544
   levels of 546

   objectives of 544
   principles for 544
   process 546, 546f
   services, scope of 545
   skills 545
   steps of 545, 545f
Counselor 354
   qualities of 546
Coworker negotiations 277
Crafting strategic plan, process for 68
Crashing critical path 325
Creating PERT chart 324
Creative activity 211
Creativity 181, 240
Credential management services 137
Credentialing 137, 320
   purpose of 137
Criminal law 571
Critical care
   beds 488
   nurse 593
Critical incident technique 531
Critical management system 320
Critical path 325, 332
   analysis 313, 331
      model 332f
   diagnosis 160
   estimating 326
   method 332
Critical theory 26
Critical thinking 26, 558
   principles of 25f
Critical-point control, principle of 284
Cumulative record 424, 520
Curriculum 500
   and evaluation committee 521
   change 505
   components of 501
   concept of 500
   design models of 503, 503f
   development
      principles of 501, 502b
      stages of 502f
   evaluation 504
      approaches 505
      functions of 505
   implementation 504
   innovation 505
   modern concept of 501
   planning 500, 501
      levels of 501
   purpose of 500
   types of 503
Customer
   focus 310
   service 529
Cyclic development 506

D

Dampen human initiation 293
Data collection
   and analysis 69
   for research, facilitation of 418
Death and dying, responsibility for 572

Debates 115
Debt repayment, principle of 391
Decentralized in-service education 178
Decibel theory 382
Decision
    support systems 32
    types of 270
Decision-making 44, 72, 269, 282, 505, 518, 546
    advantages of 271
    based on facts 310
    characteristics of 270, 270b
    in management 271f
    little opportunity for 160
    power 236
    process 270f
    slows down 221
    steps in 270
    styles 270
    techniques of 270, 270t
    theories of 271
Dedication 561
Defamation 572
Delegate
    function 211
    tasks
        effectively 229
        guidelines for 261
Delegation 92, 213, 229, 259, 403
    advantages of 94, 261, 261f
    barriers in 261, 261f
    characteristics of 260
    disadvantages of 262
    elements of 260, 260b
    prerequisites for 261
    principles of 93, 93f, 260, 260b
    process 259f
    purpose of 92, 259
    steps in 93
    types of 93, 94f, 260
Delivering staff development program, methods of 536f
Delivery 106, 192
    model 158
Demerits 246, 247
Democratic coaching 268
Democratic leadership 246, 247b, 247f
Democratic style 237
Department of family welfare, functions of 52
Department of medical and public health, functions of 51
Departmental policies and plans, coordination of 521
Deployment 133
    in nursing 133
    management
        cycle 133f
        process 133
Deputy nursing superintendent 559
Dermatology nurse 594
Design training programs 445
Desirable turnover 160

Determining capital
    requirements 393
    structure 393
Develop self-awareness 454
Develop written quality assurance plan 319
Developing employment programs 445
Developing in-service program, steps in 176f
Development, characteristics of 136
Developmental job assignment 253
Dignity of labor, principles of 502
Direct communication, principle of 212
Direct mail 357
    packages 357
Direct objectives, principle of 212
Direct observation 205
Direct patient care 151, 152, 296
Direct supervision
    and observation 285
    principle of 211
Direction 210
    advantages of 214
    characteristics of 211, 211f
    functions of 212
    nature of 211, 211b
    principles of 211f
Directorate general of health service organization of 52f
Disaster 83
    management, phases of 82f
Discharge 168
    information 519
    planning 158
Disciplinary committee 168, 522
Disciplinary practices 167
Discipline 17, 103, 366, 387
    advantages of 233
    approaches of 168b
    errors in 234
    maintenance of 212, 213, 233
    nature of 166
    principles for maintenance of 167
    process 166f
    significance of 167
Discretionary income 514
Disease, prevention of 97
Dismissal compensation 143
Disseminate quality assurance experience 320
Disseminator role 12
Distributive bargaining 370
Distributive negotiations 276
District forum 575
District health system, functions of 54
Disturbance handler role 12
Diversification, principle of 391
Diversity 499
Divisional structure 101
Documentation 206, 300, 419, 574, 577
    principles of 423
    purpose of 419, 420
    records and reports 304
Domestic violence
    nurse 595
    training 588

Donabedian model 316
Downward communication 312
Drinking water 538
Drive reduction theory 373
Drug standards, control of 52
Dry promotion 140
Dummy activity 332
Duty roster 126, 126b
    objectives of 126
    purpose of 126
    principles of 126f
Dynamic models 506
Dynamism 115

E

Echocardiogram 429
Economical factors 34, 502
Economy 32 76, 283
    principle of 382
Education 495, 518
    and development 152, 413
Educational administrator public relations
    aims of 355, 361
    objectives of 355, 361
Educational function 148, 153
Educational institutions 131, 447
    audit of 551
    public relations in 359
Educational qualifications 148, 152
Educational standards 120
Effective administration 90
Effective budget, benefits of 400f
Effective communication 8, 38, 379
    skills 380f
    principles of 382
Effective control system 282f
    elements of 282
Effective coordination 73
Effective decision-making, guidelines for 271
Effective manager
    behaviors of 44b
    qualities of 39, 40f
Effective nurse mentor, qualities of 256
Effective safety management, principles of 322, 322f
Effective team management tips and strategies 228
Efficiency 88, 103, 339
    of controls, principle of 284
Efforts, coordination of 215
Electrocardiogram 429
Electronic health record 427, 429, 438, 439f
    advantages of 439, 440f
    benefits of 420f, 438, 438f
    disadvantages of 440
Electronic medical record 418, 436
    benefits of 437, 437f
    systems 437
Elements 270
Eligibility 488
    criteria 466, 490
E-mail 357
Emergency
    admission 83

Index

and disaster, planning for 80
funds 514
management 81f
medical care, principles of 83b
nurse 595
    association 608
preparedness program 78
response
    organization 81
    planning 81, 81f
    staffing pattern 82
Emotional barriers 384
Emotional intelligence 274, 449, 449f, 450
    benefits of 450
    components of 449
    cons of 451
    domains and competencies 449t
    pros of 450, 451f
    skills 449
    types of 450
Emotional regulation 453
Emotional resilience 453
Emotions
    perceiving 450
    reflective regulation of 450
Empathy 269, 274, 449, 558
Employee
    absenteeism 161
        reasons for 161, 161f
    assistance programs 539
    benefits for 552, 558f
    compensation 138
    conduct and discipline 166f
    counselor 379
    development 533
        level 251
    different phases in career of 460
    disadvantages of rotation of 233
    disciplinary measures 168f
    discipline 165, 166, 166f
    engagement and performance 106
    grievance 169, 169b, 169f
    improves morale of 448
    involvement 310
    management participation 226
    morale 162
    motivation 8, 222, 339
    nature of 339
    objectives 225
    promotion
        benefits of 140
        criteria for 140f
        types of 140
    reduces contribution of 142
    referral scheme 539
    relations 169, 356
    retention 251
        strategies 139f
        techniques 138f
    satisfaction 165f, 222
    skills, knowledge of 262
    state insurance 57
    termination 143f
    training of 448, 448f, 533

transfer method 141f
turnover 160, 160f
    causes of 160
welfare
    schemes 538
    types of 539b
Employers, benefits for 257
Employment 446
    agencies 131, 447
    exchanges 447
    interviews 447
Empowered employee 265f
Empowerment 264, 264f
    concept of 264, 264f
    pros and cons of 266
Energy 244, 376
    benchmarking 329
English laws 579
Enterprise resource planning 32
Entrepreneur role 12
Environmental factors 503
    affecting management 33
Equipment 80, 82, 403
    procurement of 191
Equity 17
Equivalence committee 605
Essential physical skills 496
Establish team mission 229
Estate planning 394
Ethical decision making process 566, 566f
Ethical dilemmas 566
Ethical principles 203, 564, 564f
Ethical responsibility 567
Ethics
    code of 567, 568, 568f
    committee 387
    concept of 564f
Euthanasia 572
Evaluating 90, 155 231
    alternatives 291
    information 44
    internal control system, methods of 298f
Evaluation 60 69, 100
    and research 97
    methods used 178
Evidence based practice 61, 464
Examination
    grading of 479
    regulations for 489
Excellent communication 240
Executive
    committee 387, 605
    function 211
    program 402
    responsibility 402
Existing support manpower 55
Expand personal knowledge and skills 613
Expanded career roles 354
Expectancy theory 374, 374f
Expectation 140
Expense budget 405
Expensive 103
Experience 559
Expert power 262

Exploitive-authoritative 23
Extension, principle of 219
External auditor 203, 299
External benchmarking 327
External factors 33
    affecting staffing 120
External influence 167, 182
External lecturers 478
External recruitment 446
Extrinsic motivation 373
Eye contact 384

F

Face-to-face meetings 357
Facilitates
    change 214
    decentralization 286, 287
    delegation 286
    growth and diversification 88
    reflective learning opportunities 182
Facilitating change 44
Factors affecting
    curriculum development 502
    employee
        morale 379
        retention 138f
    financial management 34
    group dynamics 341, 342f
    human relations 350
    in-service program 174
    interpersonal relationship 343, 343f
    leadership style 244b
    morale 379b
    negotiation 275
    organizational behavior 337f
    performance appraisal 528, 529f
    planning 75
    recruitment 131
    staffing 119, 119t
Factors considered 233, 513
Factors influencing
    adult learning 181
    leadership 244
    nursing service 129
    patient satisfaction 300
    policies 292
Faculty 612
    improvement techniques 162, 539
    members, office for 476, 483
Fair remuneration 17
Fairness 169
False imprisonment 572
Familiarity, degree of 167
Family
    member reports 425
    nurse practitioner 582, 595
    planning 398
    records 520
    welfare 51
Fast tracking 325
Fax 357
Feedback 75, 138, 228, 269
    and recognition, lack of 160

principle of 382
system 283
Female health workers 154
Filing records 520
Financial analysis 399
Financial audit, procedures of 406, 406f
Financial benchmarking 328
Financial control 391, 392
Financial decision 393
  making 391
Financial factors 33
Financial forecasting 399
Financial incentives 439
Financial management 45, 390, 390f, 392
  concept of 390
  function of 392, 392f
  objectives of 391, 391f
  principles of 391, 391b
  process of 391b
  scope of 393, 393f
  types of 395
Financial managers
  role of 394
  skills for 394
Financial motivation 373
Financial planning 391, 393, 394
  analysis and control management 395
  components of 393, 393f
  objectives of 393
  types of 393f
Financial regulations 34
Financial statement 285
  audit 407
    phases of 406f
Financing, ideal principle of 391, 392
Fire extinguisher 477, 483
First aid 78
  appliances 538
First level manager, main role of 9
First-line managers 10
Fixed budget 403
Fixed ceiling budget 398
Fixed expenses 514
Fixed responsibility, lack of 103
Flat organizational design 104f
Flatarchy structure 101
Flexibility, principle of 382
Flexible budget 398, 403, 515
Flexible controls, principle of 284
Flexible method 531
Flexible work schedule, lack of 161
Flexi-time 539
Florence nightingale's environmental theory 27f
Focal objects, method of 273
Focus charting 425
Fogging 385
Follett theory 22
Forced-choice method 530
Force-field analysis 314
Forces influence health system 49
Forecasting 401, 516
Forensic nurse 595
Formal and informal committees 386
Formal counseling 546
Formal curriculum 503
Formal delegation 93, 260
Formal groups 340
Formal organization 101, 101f
  advantages of 101
Formal power 262
Formal training 253
  program 135f
Formulating derivative plans 75
Fostering teamwork 138
Foundation 312
Fracture room 82
Freedom 114, 565
Free-rein leadership style 247, 247f
Friendship groups 340
Fringe benefits 366
Functional benchmarking 327, 329
Functional method 91, 156, 231
  purpose of 91f
Functional nursing 156b
  care delivery model 68f, 91f
Functional organization 103, 103f
Functional planning 66
Functional structure 101, 101f
Fundamental barriers 409
Funds
  investment of 392
  source of 392
Future growth plans 120

G

Gain personal satisfaction 613
Gantt chart 70, 71, 71f, 330, 330f, 331
  advantages of 71
  disadvantages of 71
  history of 330
  key parts of 330
  purpose of 331
Gastroenterology beds 489
Gastroenterology nurse 595
Gathering information 44
General and loose supervision 216
General delegation 260
General faculty committee 521
General hospitals 98
General nursing and midwifery program
  aims of 474
  objectives of 474
  organization of 474
General policies 292
General staff 108
General wards 144, 152
Generic benchmarking 327
Geriatric care nurse manager 40
Geriatric nurse 595
Gestures 384
Global leadership competencies 249
Goal 38
  and ideology 341
  orientation 226
Golden hour 85
Good appraisal system, essentials of 529
Good budget, characteristics of 397
Good hospital information system, lack of 316
Good in-service education, characteristics of 174
Good leader, qualities of 243
Good manager
  functions of 42
  skills of 41b
Good performance appraisal, essentials of 529b
Good planning, essentials of 14, 73
Good rapport 574
Good recording and reporting, characteristics of 422, 518
Good relationship characteristics of 346
Good Samaritan Act 571, 574
Good transfer policy, essentials of 142
Government service conduct rules 579
Graduate nurse 153
Great man theories 242
Green tags 84
Grievance
  causes of 169
  effects of 170
  features of 169
  procedures 366
  redresses 380
Gross death rate 110
Group
  classifications of 340 340b
  development 341f
    stages of 341
  dynamics 339, 339f
    characteristics of 340
    principles of 341, 341f
  efforts, direction, coordination and control of 8
  features of 340
  leader, role of 342
Growth
  and diversification 90
  and progression, lack of 160
  chart and developmental history 421
  objectives 225
Guest room 477, 484
Guidance 7, 218, 542
  aims of 218
  and counseling 542, 547, 548
    functions of 547, 547f
  concept of 542
  elements of 542
  nature of 218
  objectives of 218
  principles of 218, 219b, 542
  purpose of 218, 428, 543
  services 543f
    areas of 218f
  types of 218f, 219
Guidelines establishing new school 472
Guiding subordinates 212, 213

H

Hand signals 510
Handle unforeseen disasters 438

Harassment policy 539
Hardware types 506
Harmony of objectives, principles of 212
Head nurse 150, 158, 590
   in nursing rounds, role of 303
Health 48
   informatics
      and technology 464
      history of 410
   information systems 32
   insurance system 56
   intelligence 52
   promotion of 97
   secretariat 53
   service planning 420
   system 48, 61
      aim of 49
      benchmarking in 329
      challenges in 59
      determinants of 49
      functions of 49
      in India, organization and administration of 50
      infrastructures 222
Healthcare 48, 143
   collaborator in 223f
   computers application in 429
   current trends and issues in 48b
   delivery 112
      system 50, 50f, 56, 57f, 59
   information system 414
   providers
      benefits for 431
      disadvantages for 433
   settings and services 112
   system 48
      goals of 49
      history of 49
      objectives of 49b
   team members 112
   uses for computers in 426
Henry Mintzberg's managerial roles 12t
Hersey and Blanchard's situational leadership theory 250
Hertzberg and Maslow models 375f
Herzberg's two factor theory 26
Hiring flexibility 222
Histograms 314
Holistic development, principle of 218
Holistic nurses 596
Home healthcare nurse 590, 591, 596
Horizontal promotion 140
Hospice nurse 596
Hospital 511
   administration control 107
   administrator responsibilities 107
   beds 109
   budget 396
      principles of 404
   care evaluation statistics 109
   classifications of 97, 97b
   functions of 96, 97
   nurses 589
   objectives of 96
   organization 96
   planning 78
      factors in 79
      guiding principles for 79
   public relations in 356, 356f
   records for 424
   scope of 96
   service statistics 110
   size of 478
   statistics 109
      types of 109, 109b
      uses of 109, 109b
   structure of 96f
   types 96
   utilization
      indices 109
      statistics 109
Hostel block 472, 477, 483
Hostel
   committee 525
   facilities 477, 483
   room 477, 483
Hull's drive-reduction theory 374f
Human genome project 429
Human relations 19t, 38, 348, 348f, 349f, 352b, 353, 354
   characteristics of 348
   concept 4
   concept of 4, 349f
   in health care team 351f
   in nursing 352b
   in team work 352
   philosophy of 348
   principles of 350
   scope of 350, 351f
   skill 216, 350, 351
   theories 21
      principles of 22b
Human resources 45, 264
   approach 338
   management 117, 443t, 447t
   planning 119, 533
      steps in 445f
   use of 261
Human skills 11
Human uniqueness, principle of 218
Humility 251
Hypothesis
   formulation of 272
   testing 273

I

Idealized influence 252
Implementing policy 292
Implementing vision 44
Implicit policies 293
Impression management 263
Improve employee retention, methods of 138
Inaccurate information 440
Incentives 541
Incident reports 306, 425
Incremental budget 398
Independent nurse
   contractor 596
   practitioners 61
Indian Nursing Council 363
   Act 579
   role of 550
Indirect patient care 296
Individual staff records 422
Induction training 535, 536
Industrial nurses 559
Industrial safety 134
Infection
   control nurse 597
   slowing spread of 431
Influence mentoring relationship 257f
Informal curriculum 503
Informal delegation 93, 260
Informal groups 340
Informal organization 102
Informality, principle of 382
Informatics
   knowledge 417
   nurse 417
      specialist 417
   skills 417
Information 33, 76
   education and counseling 552
   listing and prioritizing of 359
   management 220
   power 262
   sharing of 521
   source of 381
   systems 416
Informational roles 12
Informational services 544
Informed consent 573
Innovation planning 506
Inquiry 203, 298
In-service education 164, 172, 174, 175, 179, 179b, 535, 536
   components of 174, 174f
   organization of 175
   principles of 174
   scope of 173
In-service program 173
   concept of 179f
   orientation in 176f
Inspection 77, 205
Inspirational motivation 252
Installing sound communication system 88
Institutional barriers 409
Institutional curriculum 501
Institutional ethics committee 523
Institutional holidays 165, 540
Instructional curriculum 501
Insurance
   and risk management 395
   assessment 394
   coverage 433
Intake and output chart 422f
Integrated system 310
Integrative bargaining 370
Integrative negotiations 277
Integrity 243, 251, 312, 499

Intellectual stimulation 252
Intelligence 242
Intensive care 124
    units 112
Intentional torts 571
Interactions and allergies, faster identification of 438
Interactive telenursing services 434
Interest
    conflict of 566
    lack of 262
Internal assessment 478
Internal auditor 203, 298
Internal benchmarking 327
    advantages of 327
Internal control 202, 298, 406, 517
Internal factors 33, 131
    affecting staffing 119
Internal financing, principle of 391
Internal recruitment 446
Internal relationship 33
International Association of Forensic Nurses 365
International Council of Nurses 605
International health relations and quarantine 52
International relationships 605
Internship period 480
Interpersonal communication, theories of 344
Interpersonal relationship 343f, 570
    nature of 343
    skills 344f
Interprofessional collaboration 222, 222f
    concept of 222
    in healthcare, benefits of 223
    strategies 223
Interviews 178
Intra-organizational bargaining 370
Intrinsic motivation 373
Intuition theory 271
Inventory
    advantages of 196
    classifications of 196t
    control 188, 195, 195f
        functions of 196
        steps in 196
    disadvantages of 196
    management 193, 193f
        principles of 196
    objectives of 195
Investment management 394
Invoice
    approval and payment 193
    verification 190
Isolation
    hospitals 98
    room 82
Issue budget 399

J

James Mooney theory 21
Job
    analysis 119
    description 495
    enrichment 379
    functions 493
    orientation 536
    requirements 495
    responsibilities 493
    role 151
    rotation
        advantages of 233
        benefits of 233t
        drawbacks of 233t
    satisfaction 122, 221
    security 379
    summary 152
Joint committee 387
Junior staff nurse 152

K

Keeping records, purposes of 424
Kerr's model 504
Knowledge and skill 376
    effective communication 376
Kurt Lewin's three-step change model 277, 277f

L

Labor
    and delivery nurse 597
    contractors 447
    division of 16
    laws 120
    staff 82
    turnover
        effects of 161
        reduction of 161
Laboratory 476, 482
    and radiology 519
Lactation consultant 597
Lag time 325
Laissez-faire
    leadership 247f
    style 237
Language barriers 383
Lateral delegation 94, 260
Law, types of 571, 571t
Layoff decisions 533
Lead time 325
Leader 350, 354
    decisions, subject to change 248
    functions of 237
    role 11
Leadership 8, 37t, 39, 105, 212, 213, 236, 236f, 239, 239f, 242, 242f, 244, 244t, 312, 413, 464, 558
    activities 248
    and decision making concept 4
    and management 177
    characteristics of 236, 236f, 240, 241f
    competencies 248f, 249
    development 174, 252, 253f
        general electric model of 254
        methods of 252
        models 253
    elements of 240
    goal-oriented 241
    nature of 239, 240f
    position 216
    principles of 211, 241, 241b
    qualities of 240f, 243f
    roles 129
    style 237, 245, 245f, 254, 380
    techniques 241
    theories of 242, 243f
    training 177
    trait 235f
        theory of 243f
Leading organization 249
Learn coping skills 454
Learning 507
    experiences, selection of 507b
    theories 503
    time, reduction of 134
Leave 164
    facilities 164, 540
Legal
    accountability 419, 420
    documentation 424, 518
    framework 202, 298, 407, 517
    issues in nursing 571, 572
        informatics 418
    nurse consultant 597
    protection 423
    reports 306
    terms 571
Legible chart notes 437
Legitimate power 262
Leisure, training for 502
Less supervision requirements 222
Liability 572
Liaison role 11
Library 476, 482
    committee 521
    cum-study 473
Licensed practical nurse 588, 597
Licensing issues 433
Licensure, renewal of 579
Life-long learning 552
Likert scale, factors measured by 23
Line and staff organization 108
    advantages of 108
    disadvantages of 108
Line committees 386
Line organization 102, 102f
Linear development 506
Liquidity
    and profitability, principle of 391
    control of 515
Listening 383
    and learning 267
Literacy rate 433
Liveliness 115
Long-term care nurse 597
Love and belonging needs 26, 27
Low employee engagement 161
Loyalties, principle of 501
Ludwig von Bertalanffy system theory 24f

M

Macroeconomic factors 34t
Macro-environment factors 34
Mail 357
Major punishment 167
Make sound and timely decisions 241
Malpractice 572, 576
   liability concerns 440
Manage care nurse 597
Management 1, 1b, 2, 5, 7, 7b, 8, 8f, 9t, 29, 32, 35, 244, 244t, 413
   audit 285
   benefits of 226
   by objectives
      advantages of 227f
      elements of 225, 225f
   characteristics of 7, 226, 226b
   concept of 1, 1f, 4
   control system 33, 33f, 287b
   factors of 29
   features of 7f
   functional concept of 4, 4f
   functions 16f, 20, 29, 29f, 31, 130, 211
      classifications of 31, 31f
      types of 31f
   Haimann's concept of 5, 5f
   human activity 8
   imperfections in 284
   information system 285
   leadership in 235, 235f
   levels of 9, 9f, 10f, 63f
   lower level of 10
   middle level of 9
   nature of 6, 6f
   negotiations 277
   policy
      quality of 323
      statement 77
   principles of 14, 16, 16f, 225
   process 14, 15f, 16f
      components of 15b
      elements of 14, 15b, 16f, 29
   scope of 5 6f
   signifies authority 8
   skills 10, 11f, 177, 249f
      domains of 11f
   span of 88
   standards 287f
   support 167
   systems of 23f
   theories 14, 18t, 26, 243
   top level of 9
   training and development, principle of 122
Manager 33, 76, 354
   implications for 263
   responsibilities 136
   role of 44
Managerial appraisal, principles of 121
Managerial communication, principle of 212
Managing budget, skills needed for 399
Manpower
   budget 398

planning 444-446
   steps of 445, 445b
   requirements 122, 123
Maslow's needs theory 26, 26f
Mass production 103
Master nursing, degree of 465
Master rotation plan 232, 511
   principles of 512
   purpose of 512
Material determination 189
Material handling 190
Material management 186, 187, 189
   advantages of 194, 194b
   components of 188f
   goals of 187, 187b
   objective of 188
   planning
      aim of 187, 189
      basic principles of 189
      elements of 189
      purpose of 187, 189
   process 186f, 189, 190f
   role of nurse in 194
   scope of 187 188f
   selective controls in 196
Maternal child health 398
Maternity leave 165, 541
Math skills 395
Matrix
   organizational structure 103f
   structure 101, 103
Matrons rounds 302
Maturity 41
Max Webber theory 21
McClelland's theory 375
Media relations 356
Medical
   and nursing research 97
   assistants 598
   databases 427
   education 52
      and training 97
   encounters 421
   examination 448
   imaging 426
   laboratory 429
   practitioners, perspective of 433
   research 52, 427
   store depots 52
Medicine
   and homeopathy, system of 51
   indigenous system of 58
   system of 97
Medi-claim insurance scheme 539
Membership 362, 365
   group 341
Mental
   activity 70
   health
      and addiction treatment centers 511
      issues 162
Mentor
   activities of 267
   responsibility of 267

role of 256f
skill of 255
Mentoring
   and training management 220
   concept of 266
   program, objectives of 268
   techniques 267
Mentorship
   benefits of 268
   programs 138
   purpose of 266
   usefulness of 256
Mercy killing 572
Message and media 360
   implementation of 360
Metacognition 181
Microeconomic factors 34t
Micro-environment factors 33
Middle level behavior 337
Midwives, benefits for 257
Milestone chart 70, 72
   advantages of 72
Military nurse 559, 598
Mini white boards 510
Minimal care 124
Minimet theory 382
Minimum cost of capital, principle of 392
Minor punishment 167
Misconception 508, 510
Mission 36, 118, 500, 537
   and objectives 33
   and purpose 64
   statements, dimensions of 37
Missionary nurse 598
Modern management theories 24
Modular nursing 92, 157, 158b, 231, 462
Monitor role 12
Monitoring client 580
Morale
   building 377
      strategies 379
   features of 378
Morbidity statistics 110
Morphological analysis 273
Mortuary and chaplain facility 358
Motivate subordinates 237
Motivation 212, 213, 221, 228, 242, 251, 372, 380, 403, 449, 521, 529, 534
   A to Z steps in 376
   and control policies 292
   and productivity 140
   concept of 372f
   elements of 373
   key elements of 372b
   nature of 372
   process of 373, 373f
   raising level of 215
   seven rules of 376
   theories of 373, 374f
   types of 373
Motivational theory, application of 377
MSc nursing program, organization of 487
Multipurpose hall 476, 482

N

National agencies 492, 579
National Health Program 52, 55, 58, 58b
National League for Nursing 608
National Medical Library 53
National Professional Accrediting
    Agency 492, 579
National Service Scheme 522, 524
National Student Nurses Association 607
Negative motivation 373
Negligence 572, 573, 576
    elements of 577
Negotiate towards win-win outcome 276
Negotiation 275, 275f
    principles of 275
    skills 276, 276f
    stages of 275, 275b
    types of 276
Negotiator role 12
Neonatal intensive care nurse 598
Nephrology nurse 598
Nephrourology specialty beds 489
Net cash flows, principle of 391
Net death rate 111
Networks and digital communication 427
Neuroscience nurses 598
Neuro-speciality beds 489
New nursing schools 469
Night duty nurses, room for 477, 484
Nominal group technique 314
Non-financial motivation 373
Nonmaleficence 565
Nonnursing tasks 296
Nonprofessional nursing personnel 129
Non-specialist counseling 546
Nonstatutory schemes 539
Norm-referenced evaluation 505
Nurse
    administrator 583
        role of 321
    advocate 598
    aides 156, 159
    and community 552
    and healthcare system 552
    and profession 552
    anesthetist 582, 598
    attorney 599
    benefits for 257
    classifications of 589
    client relationship, elements of 346
    commits 569
    community relationships 353
    continuing education units for 586
    duties of 580
    educator 582, 599
    entrepreneurs 599
    executives 599
    expanded role of 580
    family relationships 353
    health team relationships 353
    in informatics, duties of 418
    in providing quality care,
        challenges of 320
    informatics specialist, roles of 417
    leader
        motivational qualities of 376
        qualities of 254
    leadership style for 255f
    management rounds 302
    manager 32, 37, 37b, 39, 599
        clinical responsibility of 42, 43f
        common problems of 46
        concept of 39
        dual role of 42b
        functions of 208
        future of 46
        in legal issues, role and
            functions of 572f
        job duties 44
        role of 36, 40f, 41f, 91 194, 208, 342,
            402, 404, 404b 549
        skills needed for 40
        strategical techniques of 45
        supervisory role 36f
        types of 40
        wear 42
    midwifery program, guiding
        philosophy of 499
    patient helping relationship 353
    patient relationship 112
        phases of 346
    practice act 572, 579
    practitioner 582, 590, 599
        regulation for 580
    researcher 583, 599
    responsibility 305, 307, 425
    rights and responsibilities of 579
    role of 195b, 320
    service condition for 471
    supervisor 590
        job duties 149
        job purpose 149
Nursing
    administration 414, 609
        and management 552
    administrator 208
    art of 560
    associates, benefits for 257
    audit 61, 199, 297, 320
        advantages of 204, 299, 299t
        characteristics of 200
        disadvantages of 204, 299, 299t
        goals of 200
        history of 199
        objectives of 200, 297
        process 206f, 298f
        system 204, 299
        uses of 208
    auditor 203, 298
    budget 396
    care 80, 146
        delivery systems and trends 111
        improvements in 610
        records, lack of 316
        responsibilities 154
        services 208
    career 417
        different branches in 590
        opportunities 588, 591
    case managers 40
    clinical practice 413
    colleges, inspections of 493
    computers in 427
    continuing education in 584, 586
    council, function of 363b
    credentialing 137b
    current trends and issues in 61
    curriculum, development of 502
    delegation in 93f
    department
        budgeting for 402
        goals 38
        orientation to 176
    different education levels in 588
    director of 39, 146, 559
    documentation 425
        format 425
    education 414, 503b, 547b, 609
        aims of 462
        committee 605
        duties and responsibilities in
            relation to 150
        educational audit in 550
        goal and objectives of 463
        issues in 61
        programs, types of 463
        standardization of 471
    educational institutions
        accreditation of 491
        establishment of 462
    effective leadership in 254
    ethics 564, 564f, 567b
    examination board, functions of 607
    grand rounds, potential benefits of 303f
    home 98
        nurses 589
    informatics 410f, 411, 411f, 412, 415
        application of 413, 416b
        areas 414
        competencies of 416
        concept of 411, 412f
        functional areas 417b
        history of 411
        inpatient care 415
        model 416
        role of 412f
        sample applications of 414f
        scope of 412, 413f
    information
        management 410
        model 416f
    in-service education 179
    intensity, dimensions of 125
    issues in 61
    knowledge 552
    laboratory 473
    leadership 254f
    management 14, 36, 37, 37b
        audit 297, 405, 517
        goals of 38
        mission statement of 36

disadvantages of 221
styles 220
Participative theories 243
Participatory action research goals 612f
Participatory management 219
　process of 220
Patient assignment
　methods of 90b, 230b
　principles of 154, 231
Patient care 148
　delivery
　　methods of 155
　　system 154
　unit, planning of 79
Patient classification system 123
Patient management 148f
Patient monitoring 427
Patient movement statistics 110
Patient records 419, 419f
Patient satisfaction 300, 431
Patient's bill of right 573
P-charts 314
Pediatric
　beds 489
　endocrinology nurses 601
　nurse 601
　　practitioner 582, 601
Peer review committee 320
Penalties 577
Peplau's theory 344f
Perception 251
　barriers 384
Perform quality assurance 319f
Performance 106, 528
　appraisal 119, 121, 225, 226, 526, 526f,
　　527, 532, 533f
　　advantages of 533
　　benefits of 532, 532f
　　characteristics of 528
　　components of 526f
　　criteria of 530
　　methods 530, 530f
　　objectives of 527
　　purpose of 527
　　steps 527f
　　tool 531
　benchmarking 328
　budget 398
　collecting data on 207
　concept of 295
　evaluation 123, 225
　　principles of 528, 528f
　feedback 532
　in nursing education, evaluation of 553
　reduces cost of 77
　types of 296
Perianesthesia nurse 601
Perinatal nurse 591
Periodic inspection 493
Permanent formal groups 340
Personnel assignment, principles of 155, 230
Personnel management 442, 442f, 447t
　characteristics of 443
　elements of 444

functions of 444
nature of 443
objectives of 443
principles of 442b
roles of 445f
scope of 444, 444b
Personnel manager 444, 448
Pervasive function 211
Philosophy 474, 480, 490, 499
Phone conference call 357
Physical facilities 472, 475, 481, 487
Physiologic needs 26
　oxygen 27
　physical 27
　sexuality 27
　temperature 27
Pie charts 314
Placement cell 522
Plagiarism 566
Planned change
　models 277
　steps in 278
Planned linkage 506
Planning 14, 25, 29, 31, 32, 63, 72, 73f, 90, 202,
　　231, 276, 297, 395, 403, 406, 517
　advantages of 77, 77t
　and implementation 60
　characteristics of 72, 72f
　client care 518
　components of 75
　disadvantages of 77t
　duty roster 127
　　principles of 126
　elements of 67b, 74f
　encourages innovation and creativity 73
　facilitates decision making 73
　hospital
　　and patient care unit 78
　　nursing services 60, 65
　　units, objectives of 79, 79b
　improve morale 73
　nursing
　　rounds 302
　　services 63
　phase 311
　policies 292
　premises, establishment of 74
　principles of 73, 73f
　process 82
　provides direction 73
　purposes of 70
　teaching and learning experiences 507,
　　508f
Plans
　classifications of 76, 76f
　coordination of 83
　execution and revision of 287
　nature of 70, 512
　types of 76
Plaster room 82
Plastic surgery nurse 601
Policies 75, 290, 291, 294, 612
　advantages of 293
　area 291

classifications of 292, 292f
control 287
development and advocacy 413
formulation 163, 168, 291, 540
　process of 291
limitations of 293
making, organization of 409
management 313
purposes of 291, 291f
selection of 291
Political behavior, factors
　contributing to 263
Political factors 34, 292, 502
Political skills 11
Politics, types of 263
Poor interpersonal relationships, factors
　leading to 344
Poor time management, implications of 458
POSDCORB cycle 25f
Positive motivation 373
Power
　and authority 387
　and organizational politics 264f
　and politics 262, 262f
　bases of 262, 262f
　tactics 262
Practical examination 480, 553
Practice, attributes of 561
Preceptorship 256, 257f, 259f
　benefits of 257
　principles of 257
　program 258
Prediction 610
Pre-independence era 49
Preliminary interviews 447
Prenatal nurse 601
Presentations 360
Press
　conference 357
　kit 357
　release 357
Preventative care support 432
Pride approaches 164f, 538f
Primary group 341
Primary health center level 55
Primary healthcare 580
Primary nursing
　basic concepts in 158
　care 92b
　method 92, 158, 159f, 231
Primary objectives 188
Primary purpose 397
Principal investigator 611
Principal job description 493
Principal's office 476, 482
Principle medical officer 54
Privacy, invasion of 577
Private nursing hospitals 98
Privilege, loss of 168
Problem-solving
　skills 272, 272f, 558
　strategies 272
Procedure, limitations of 294
Process knowledge 529

philosophy of 37
roles 39
vision of 37
mentorship in 255, 255f
notes 519
organization chart in 104f
performance 295
personnel
　categories of 146, 146f
　guidance and counseling for 548
practice 562, 570, 609
　accountability for 610
　legal safeguards in 574f
　personnel, classifications of 129
process recording system 423f
profession 557f
　nursing, credibility of 610
　perspectives of 560
programs 463
　aims of 463
　competencies for 464
protocols 295
publication in 611, 614f
records 421
　types of 423f
registration, legal aspects to 573
regulatory mechanisms 578
research 414, 463, 552, 608, 609, 609f, 610b
　activities in 608
　areas of 609
　characteristics of 609, 609b
　conduct of 61
　directions of 611b
　long-term impact of 610f
　scope of 609
　short-term impact of 610f
resource management, director of 32
role of 112
rounds 301, 301f, 303
　advantages of 303, 303b
　disadvantages of 304
　purposes of 302, 302b
　types of 302
scope of 559
sensitive quality indicators 296
service 59, 65b, 128, 559
　administration 38, 60
　department 66b, 129, 360
　essentials of 64f, 128
　healthcare and development of 48
　in public relations 360
　mission statement of 64
　organization of 59
　philosophy 65
　policies, procedures and manuals 65
　scope of planning in 65
software's 428
staff 32, 82, 203, 298
standards, sources of 288
student, responsibility of 513
superintendent 148, 559
supervisor 32 149, 559
teacher faculty 473, 477, 484, 487, 489

team, orientation to 177
unit 79
　goals 39
　orientation to 177
　specific functions of 129
writing in 614
Nutrition laboratory 473

O

Observation 206, 300, 510
Occupational health nurse 590, 600
Office
　committee 387
　nurses 589
　requirements 476, 482
Omissions 423
Oncology
　nurse 600
　specialty beds 489
Ongoing development, principles of 122
Online courses 587
Open competition, principle of 121
Open-ended budget 398
Operating budget 398, 403
Operating facility 357
Operation room 82
Operation theater management 153
Operational benchmarking 329
Operational planning 67, 69, 70, 70f
　improve efficiency of 73
Operative methods 359
Operative procedures 519
Ophthalmic nurse 600
Opportunities 417
Optimal effectiveness, organize for 509
Optimism 244, 451
Optimistic time 325, 326
Oral communication 384
Oral report 305
Oral reprimand 167
Order 17
　processing system 190
　tracking 190
Organization 51, 53-55, 87, 115, 306, 423
　behavior studies 338f
　benefits for 532
　chart
　　advantages of 104
　　principles of 104
　　types of 104
　　uses of 104, 105
　climate
　　approaches 113f
　　areas 114f
　components of 101
　concepts of 107, 108f
　development 99f
　　interventions 99
　　strategies 99f
　goals 225
　goodwill of 339
　growth of 95
　image of 120

objectives of 292
policy threaten employees 263f
skills of 248
strategies of 292
Organizational behavior 334, 334f, 335, 336, 338, 339, 339b
　characteristics of 336, 336b
　levels of 337
　limitations of 339
　model 338, 338f
　nature of 335, 335f
　objectives of 335, 335f
　principles of 337
　scope of 339
Organizational change 169
Organizational charts 104
Organizational climate
　dimensions of 114
　motives 113f
Organizational development 99
　characteristics of 100
　intervention cycle 100f
　steps of 100, 100f
Organizational effectiveness 105, 105f, 106
　benefits of 106
　systems of 105, 105f
Organizational efficiencies 106, 106f
Organizational objectives 136
Organizational philosophy 38
Organizational policies 292
　types of 263f
Organizational skills 395, 529
Organizational structure 100, 292, 379
　types of 101
Organized manager 256
Organizing 14, 25, 29, 31, 32, 87, 87f, 90
　features of 88
　function 89, 90b
　patient care, process of 90, 155, 231
　principles of 88, 88b
　process 89f
　purposes of 87b
Orientation 174,, 535
　objectives of 175
　skill training program 177
Originated policies 292
Orthopedic nurse 600
Otorhinolaryngology nurse 600
Outcome audit 201, 207
Oversee unit-based operations 42

P

Pain management nurse 601
Pantry 477, 483
Parent-teacher association 522
Participation
　concept of 220
　features of 220
　style 237
Participative group 24
Participative management 219f
　advantages of 221
　benefits of 222

Index

Procurement 190
  cycle 191f
  cycle steps 191
  steps in 192f
  strategy 192f
  system, objectives of 191
Production budget 398, 515
Production
  planning 193
  reduces cost of 122
Productivity 251
  approach 338
  bargaining 370
  lack of 230
Profession
  components of 362
  criteria of 560
Professional
  advancement 570, 584
  bodies 467
    benefits of 467
    functions of 604
  conduct 569
    code of 569, 570, 570b
  considerations 557
  counseling 546
  development 561
  etiquette 570
  misconduct 577
  nurse 157
    qualities of 558, 558f
    responsibility of 562, 563f
    role of 562, 562f
    values of 561
  nursing
    core values of 560f
    personnel 129
  organization membership 604
  practice 562
    model 562
  responsibility 557f
    and accountability 570
  staff nurse 159
Professionalism 41, 464, 561f
  characteristics of 559f
  in nursing, concept of 560
Program 75
  aim of 472
  budget 398
  evaluation and review technique 324, 325
    activity 325
    chart 324, 324f
    disadvantages of 326
    event 325
    in nursing, application of 326b
    planning steps 326
    process 326
    subactivity 325
  evaluation in nursing course 552
  objectives of 472
  philosophy of 464, 486
  planning 70
Progressive patient care 158, 231
  elements of 159f

Project, appraisal of 408
Promotes coordination 287
Promotion 360, 366, 533
  and career planning 121
  and transfer 123, 164, 540
  benefits of 140
  policy 119
Proper medium, principle of 382
Proper time, principle of 382
Prospective audit 201
Protecting medical data 433
Protector and client advocate 581
Protocol 294
  application in nursing 295
Prototype evaluation system 130
Psychiatric
  beds 489
  nurse 602
    practitioner 602
  unit 153
Psychoanalytic theory 375
Psychological forces 341
Psychomotor domain 512
Public diplomacy 360
Public health
  nurse 589, 590f, 602
  records for 424
Public hospitals 97
Public relations 354f, 355
  aims of 355
  elements of 355, 355f
  forms of 356
  functions of 355
  in hospital, method of 357
  objectives of 355
  staff, qualities of 359
  tools in 358f
  types of 360
Public sector, benchmarking in 328
Public service announcement 357
Public trust, erosion of 574
Publications, different types of 612b
Publicity 360, 361
Pulmonary care nurse 602
Punishment 167, 168
Purchase order 192
Purchasing, principles of 189, 189f

Q

Quality assurance 61, 314, 314f, 315, 316, 419, 420, 550
  allocate resources for 319
  areas of 319
  assign responsibility for 319
  benefits of 320, 321b
  concept of 315
  cycle 317, 317f
  disadvantages of 321b
  effort, vision for 319
  model 316, 317f
  planning for 317
  principles of 315b
  program 320

  development of 319
  role of nurses in 321
Quality care 206
Quality control 162
  responsibility in 572
Quality health outcome model 317
Quality improvement 134, 464
Quality management 549
Questionable research 574

R

Radiology nurse 602
Rating scale method 530
Rational legal authority 21
Rational thinking 336
Real-time interactive services 431
Recognition management 220
Records 304, 419, 517
  and reports 424, 517, 518, 520
  examination of 202, 298
  keeping
    and reporting, responsibility for 572
    principles of 306
  purpose of 304
  review of 206
  room 476, 483
  types of 305, 422
  writing, principles of 304
Recovery, principle of 391, 392
Recruiting employees, procedure for 294
Recruitment 121, 123, 130, 131, 446
  and selection 119, 131f
  process 132f
  types of 446
Reflection of plans, principle of 284
Registered nurse 573, 588, 590, 602
  functions of 157
  role of 591f
Registration 137
  renewal of 606
Regulatory bodies 466
  principles of 467
  role of 467
Rehabilitation nurse 602
Rehabilitator 581
Reimbursement 419, 420
Rejection, fear of 615
Relationship
  formation, stages of 345
  theories 243
Release management support 133
Relevant skills, lack of 227
Remote chronic disease management 432
Remote post-hospitalization care 432
Remuneration 123, 380
Rensis Likert's theory 22
Reporting 25, 32, 91 155, 231, 402, 424
Reports
  purpose of 305
  types of 305, 305f, 424
  writing stages 306f
Reproductive nurse 603
Research 273, 419, 518

and recommendations 387
committee 523
consumer 354
findings, evaluator of 611
purpose of 608
roles of nurses in 611
team, members of 611
Residential accommodation 477, 484
Resilience 452f
building 451
characteristics 452f
factors of 453
principles of 452, 452f
scale 454
Resolve dilemma 567
Resolve team issue ASAP 229
Resources
allocator role 12
efficient use of 282
lack of 316
management 152
optimum use of 87
utilization of 77
Responsibility 15, 77, 151, 236, 260
assignments of 154, 260
develop sense of 241
Resuscitation room 82
Retirement planning 394
Retrospective audit 201, 297, 405, 517
Revenue 403
and expense budget 398, 515
expenditure 514
Rewards power 262
Rheumatology nurse 603
Right place, principle of 189
Right quality, principle of 189
Right quantity, principle of 189
Right source, principle of 189
Right time, principle of 189
Risk-return trade-off, principle of 391
Root-cause analysis 273
Rotations 232
Rural health service 56

S

Safeguarding nurse 574
Safety 464
and environmental protection policy 323
and security needs
emotional 27
physical 27
assurance 323
issues 162
management 324
phases of 323t
plan, components of 77
principles of 322
system 323
meetings 78
needs 26
policy and objectives 323
promotion 323
risk management 323
rules 78

Sales budget 398, 515
Satisfactory standards, lack of 284
Scalar chain 17
School
administration 428
building 473
nurse 603
records 518
Scientific management 18
theories 19t
Secrecy 202, 297, 517
Security issue 221
Select implementation method 278
Selection procedures, steps of 132
Self-actualization needs 26, 27
Self-awareness 244, 449, 451
Self-care 124, 451
Self-control 286
Self-directed learning 253
Self-esteem 453
needs 27
Self-examination, skills of 248
Self-improvement 181
Self-motivation 269
Self-regulation 449
Sell theory 382
Sense of humor 558
Service
contents of 96
directors 39
excellence 301
settings of 113t
Set up graded learning program 182
Sexual harassment 263
Shared decision-making management 221
Sick
leave 165
room 477, 483
patient care of 97
Sickness 164
Sideways communication 312
Situational leadership 249
advantages of 251
disadvantages of 251
pros and cons of 251t
style 249, 250f
Situational theories 243
Six M's management 14, 14f
Six sigma 317
Skill 229, 383, 436
communication 248
gaps 261
improvement 339
training 174, 177
objectives of 177
Social
change 60
and nursing 112
costs and social benefits, calculation of 409
diversity 502
exchange theory 344
factors 34, 292
insurance 539

order 17
relationships 182
responsibility 499
sciences, branch of 336
skills 449
support 451, 453
system 336
Societal curriculum 501
Software types 506
Sound
control system 286
policy, characteristics of 291
promotion policy 141b
Speaking engagement 357
Specialized hospitals 98, 113
Spokesperson role 12
Sponsorship 137
Staff 357, 403
and students recruitment and selection committee 524
benefit activities 163f
development 534, 534f, 535, 535b, 585b
activities 535
assessment methods 536
functions of 535
goals of 536
objectives of 534
organization 536
process 535, 535f
program 534, 537f
types of 535f
line hierarchy 108f
management system 149f
nurse 208, 559
projecting requirement for 404
records 519
retention 46
scheduling 124
concept of 124
system 125b
selecting method 140f
types of 108
welfare 162, 537, 537f
activities 163, 538, 539
characteristics of 538
committee 524
objectives of 538
purposes of 162, 537
services 163f
Staffing 15, 25, 30-32, 117, 122, 122f
activities 128, 129b
components of 119, 119f
function 120
basis of 120
mission and philosophy of 118
nature of 118b
objectives of 118, 118f
philosophy of 118
principle of 121, 121f
purpose of 121
process 117f, 120, 123b, 123f
steps involved in 122
schedules, types of 125
staff inspection unit, norms of 145
units 144

Index

Standard
 characteristics of 289, 289f, 289b
 classifications of 289, 290
 education, purposes of 289
 purposes of 288
Standing committee 387
State Commission 575
State Health Directorate 54
State Level Healthcare Administration 53
State Ministry of Health and Family Welfare 53
State Nurses Organizations 608
State Nurses Registration Council, functions of 606
State Nursing Council 606
State Nursing Requirement 587
State Registration Council 469
Static budget 403
Statistical budget 404
Statistical information 401
Statutory law 571
Statutory welfare
 schemes 538
 work 539
Stores 190
 management 188
 room 477, 483
Strategic benchmarking 329
Strategic financial management 395
 elements of 395
Strategic planning 66-68, 68f, 70
 concept of 68b
 phases 67f
 process, phases of 68
Stress 455f, 456f, 464
 management 454, 456
 relief 457
 symptoms of 455
Structure audit 201, 208
Structured method 531
Student nurse 153
 Association 364, 364f, 523, 607
 counseling, purposes of 548
Student response systems 510
Student welfare committee 522
Study
 course of 464, 490
 objectives of 464
Subacute care facilities 113
Subordinates, faith in 261
Substance abuse 162
 nurse 603
Substantive test 203, 298
Successful manager, characteristic of 42, 43f
Suggestion schemes 314
Sunset budget 398
Superannuation 143, 144b
 benefit, types of 144, 144f
Supervising nurses 42
Supervision 15, 169, 212-214, 215f, 352
 functions of 215
 methods 217
 objectives of 215

principles of 216, 216b
 techniques of 217, 217f, 286f
Supervisor
 benefits for 532
 fear of 261
 functions of 215
 qualities of 217
Supplementary examination 479
Surgical nurse 603
Surgical procedures, computers for 426
Surplus, disposal of 392
Suspension pending enquiry 168
Synergy 95
System-based practice 464

T

Tally charts 314
Target audiences 356
Task group 340
Tax planning 394
Taylor's scientific management theory 20f
Teaching
 block 475, 482t
 cum-research hospital 98
 learning process 428, 428b
 load 163
 management 221
 rounds 302
 staff, responsibility of 512
 work load 540
Team
 activity 313
 approach 96
 building 228
 leader 157
 management 228
  techniques 229
 managers 229
 nursing 91, 91b, 156, 156b, 156f, 231, 231b
  concept of 157
  functions of 157
Teamwork 528
 advantages of 353
 and collaboration 464
 disadvantages of 353
Technical nurse 156, 159
Technical skills 11
Technology 336
 and production methods, innovations in 351
 update 135, 552
Telehealth 414, 430
 barriers in 433
 major barriers of 433f
 nurses provide nursing care 435
Telemedicine 113, 427, 429, 430f, 432b
 benefits of 430, 431f, 432t
 challenges of 432t, 433
 history of 430f
 principles of 432, 432b
 system, advantages of 432

types of 431
 uses of 430
Telenursing 433, 434f
 application of 435f, 436
 benefits of 435, 435t
 concept of 434
 guidelines for 434
 principles of 434
 role of nurses in 435, 435f
 types of 434
 uses of 435
Telephone reports 425
Terminal cleaning procedure 80
Termination
 letters, types of 143, 143b
 cause of 143b
Theme identification 383
Theory examination 479
Therapeutic nurse behaviors 346
Thinking, flexibility in 181
Time cost 329
Time management 456, 456f, 457, 558
 benefits of 457
 objectives of 456
 skills 457, 457f
 tips 458f
Time matters 408
Time value of money, principle of 391
Timing, flexibility in 402
Top management 65
Total quality management 309, 309f, 310f
 components of 312
 concept of 309
 elements of 311, 311f
 functions of 314
 history of 309
 objectives of 310
 phases of 311, 311f
 principles of 310, 310f
 tools 313, 313f
Toxicology nurse 603
Track attendance 162
Traditional
 authority 21
 methods 231
 theory 271
Trained Nurses Association of India 203, 362, 362b, 470, 471f, 560, 605
Training 78, 133, 134, 229, 448
 and development 119, 121, 123, 136, 136f, 138
 benefits of 448
 methods of 448
 objectives, principle of 122
 process, steps in 135f
 types of 134
Trait theories 243
Transactional theories 243
Transfer 131, 141, 168, 533
 policy, principles of 142
 purposes of 141f
 reports 306
 types of 141f

Transformational leadership 252f
　style 251
　　theory, implications of 252, 252f
Transplant nurse 603
Transport 190, 477, 484
Trauma nurse 603
Triage nurse, characteristics of 85b
Trust and confidence, climate of 261
Trust lack of 262
Tuckman's five stages 341f
Turnover and absenteeism, reduction of 134
Turnover interval calculation of 110, 111f
Two-way budget organization 402
Tyler's model 504

U

Ultrasonography 429
Union Ministry of Health and Family Welfare 51
Unit management 112, 153
Unity of command, principle of 212
Universal application 7
Universal Immunization Program 398
Universal principles 21
University, functions of 468
Urban health services 56
Urban healthcare delivery model 58f
Urology nurse 604

V

Vacation-friendly corporate culture 162
Validate bonus plans 399
Value system 33
Vendor negotiations 277
Ventilation 546
Vertical charts 104
Vision 537
　and mission 537
　statements 64
Vital statistics 420, 518
Voice 384
Voluntary health agencies 58
Voluntary welfare work 539

W

Ward
　clerk 159
　management 147, 148, 153
　　and supervision, duties and responsibilities to 150
　system 149f
　managers shift patterns 127
　reception 358
　records 423
　sister 559
Warden's room 477, 484

Website 357
Wheeler's model 504
White tags 84
Work
　division of 88, 89
　group 350
　hours of 163, 540
　load statistics 109
　plan, execution and control of 38
Worker's participation 379
Working paper preparation 202, 298, 407, 517
Workplace
　burnout 161
　harassment 162
　stress, prevention of 455
　wellness programs 162
Wound care nurse 604
Written communication 384
Written policies 292

Y

Youth red cross unit 524
　activities of 525

Z

Zero based budgets 398